AF698290

EPILEPTIC SEIZURES AND SYNDROMES

with some of their theoretical implications

EPILEPTIC SEIZURES AND SYNDROMES

with some of their theoretical implications

Edited by
Peter Wolf

British Library Cataloguing in Publication Data

Epileptic Seizures and Syndromes
I. Wolf, P.
616.853

Current Problems in Epilepsy: 10
ISSN: 0950-4591
ISBN: 0 86196 430 6

Published by

John Libbey & Company Ltd, 13 Smiths Yard, Summerley Street, London SW18 4HR, England.
Telephone: 0181–947 2777: Fax 0181–947 2664
John Libbey Eurotext Ltd, 127 avenue de la République, 92120 Montrouge, France.
John Libbey - C.I.C. s.r.l., via Lazzaro Spallanzani 11, 00161 Rome, Italy

© 1994 John Libbey & Company Ltd. All rights reserved.
Unauthorised duplication contravenes applicable laws.

Printed in Great Britain by Ashford Colour Press, Gosport, Hampshire, UK.

Introduction

This book reflects debates and results concerning epileptic seizures and syndromes which have developed since the introduction of an international system of classifications in epileptology. The creation of such a system was initiated, in the sixties, mainly for practical reasons: growing international exchange had revealed that divergence of terminology in epilepsy had become important enough to prove a serious obstacle to sensible discussions. In different parts of the world, the same phenomena could be referred to by different names but, likewise, the same terms could have different meanings.

A first version of an International Classification of Epileptic Seizures (ICES) was published in 1970 (Gastaut, 1970). A revised version was proposed and accepted (Commission, 1981), but there is ongoing debate about its merits and defects, and further amendments are under discussion. This debate is reflected in Section I of this volume.

Seizures, even though they are often composed of more than one single sign or symptom, are considered as the symptoms in epilepsy, and their classification was only a preliminary to an International Classification of Epilepsies and Epileptic Syndromes (ICEES). A basic outline of the latter was presented together with the first ICES (Merlis, 1970), but a detailed proposal was first published in 1985 (Commission, 1985), followed by a revision which was accepted by the International League against Epilepsy (ILAE) in 1989 (Commission, 1989).

It soon turned out that a syndrome classification could serve purposes far beyond the provision of a common language. In particular, the publication, during the process of the development of the ICEES, of detailed syndrome descriptions (Roger *et al.*, 1984, updated 1992) drew frequent comments from places with little tradition in epileptology which indicated that these publications had been extremely helpful in developing a modern standard of knowledge as it is indispensable for diagnostics, therapy and research.

The inclusion, in the 1985 ICEES, of a tentative classification according to the anatomical site of an epileptic focus was rightly criticized because it contained more subdivisions than can be distinguished in clinical reality. It also raised suspicions that centres with access to invasive diagnostics were starting to consider themselves superior. But it also increased the awareness of these centres that invasive diagnostics should be considered an intermediate step aimed at collecting information which eventually would make these procedures unnecessary. Finally, it stimulated debate about the concept of the epileptic focus: should it be viewed as a small nest of neurones producing seizure discharge which will spread from there or, rather, as a region with a pathologically altered neuronal interplay resulting in the generation of seizures? Or do both possibilities occur?

A very important result of the ICEES, and perhaps its most unexpected one was its impact on genetic research. The geneticists interested in epilepsy needed this large field to be broken down into more chewable units. The ICEES provided these, and a most fruitful interchange between clinicians and geneticists developed which is repeatedly reflected in this volume, and which has already gone far beyond the narrow limits of classical genetics. It is today reasonable to expect that, when we come to know the genes responsible for epilepsy syndromes more precisely, they will explain structural deviations of ion channels and other elements of the neuronal membrane, of whose functional consequences we will already have a more than rough idea. We can also expect to see the various genes expressed not homogeneously over the brain but with regional accentuations which hopefully we will be able to relate to clinical syndromes. The attentive reader of this book will find food for thought along these lines wherever he/she opens it.

Thus, one of the most exciting features of recent epileptology is an increasing interaction between clinical and basic research, and in many parts of this volume this convergence of interests is palpable. Clinical papers frequently raise questions to which experimental studies suggest at least tentative answers, and in many of the chapters on basic mechanisms the authors are clearly aware of the possible clinical relevance of their research. But critical questions across the clinical–experimental border also become possible, and the scholars of secondary epileptogenesis are confronted, here, with the existence of large provinces in human epilepsy where secondary epileptogenesis has never been observed.

At first glance, there seems to be a great diversity of subjects in this book. A closer look, however, will reveal that the discussions constantly return to a small handful of central themes. One of these are the similarities and differences of the generation and evolution of seizure activity in the different seizure types and syndrome groups. Another is the relation of 'focal' and 'generalized' varieties of epilepsy. The 'generalized' concept, in particular, seems to be in need of a revision where increased attention must be paid to the significance of regional accentuations of the primary bilateral discharges, and their relation to and difference from unilateral regional or focal ictogenesis and epileptogenesis.

It is the intention of this book to stimulate multifaceted considerations of this kind which hopefully will lead the way towards a comprehensive theory of the epilepsies, where both more general pathomechanisms and the more specific ones responsible for the differences between the various types of epilepsy will fall into place to provide the full picture. It is my conviction that we are well on our way to approaching this aim.

Peter Wolf
Bielefeld, August 1994

Acknowledgements: It is a great pleasure for me to thank all the authors who enthusiastically contributed to this book and without any exception gracefully responded to the editor's whims and wishes. The help of my secretary, Mrs Irene Kujath, with the editorial work was again invaluable. It was extremely pleasant to work with a publisher who is as efficient, experienced and understanding as Mr John Libbey.

References

Commission on Classification and Terminology of the ILAE (1981): Proposal for revised clinical and electroencephalographic classification of epileptic seizures. *Epilepsia* **22,** 489–501.

Commission on Classification and Terminology of the ILAE (1985): Proposal for classification of epilepsies and epileptic syndromes. *Epilepsia* **26,** 268–278.

Commission on Classification and Terminology of the ILAE (1989): Proposal for revised classification of epilepsies and epileptic syndromes. *Epilepsia* **30,** 389–399.

Gastaut, H. (1970): Clinical and electroencephalographical classification of epileptic seizures. *Epilepsia* **11,** 102–113.

Merlis, J.K. (1970): Proposal for an international classification of the epilepsies. *Epilepsia* **11,** 114–119.

Roger, J., Dravet, Ch., Bureau, M., Dreifuss, F.E. & Wolf, P. (1984): *Epileptic syndromes in infancy, childhood and adolescence.* London: John Libbey.

Roger, J., Dravet, Ch., Dreifuss, F.E., Perret, A. & Wolf, P. (1992): *Epileptic syndromes in infancy, childhood and adolescence,* 2nd edn. London: John Libbey.

Contents

Section I

Some problems concerning classification and terminology concepts

In the lively discussions of classifications in epilepsy over the past three decades, little attention was paid to terminology. However, behind each term there is at least one concept and sometimes more than one. Some of them have changed over time, and not all are clearly perceived any longer. Thus, an initial chapter about terms appeared timely.

Then, this section is mainly concerned with the seizures, and some of the ongoing controversy about their classification is presented.

The last chapter passes beyond seizures and comes back to concepts. Do the clinical conditions in epilepsy represent a series of different diseases or do they result at random from a complex interplay of heterogeneous pathogenic factors? The Montreal group attempts a comprehensive view of their traditional concept of a 'neurobiological continuum' and the syndromatic approach.

Epileptic Seizures and Syndromes, Edited by Peter Wolf
© 1994 John Libbey & Company Ltd., pp. 3–7

Chapter 1

Epileptic seizures and syndromes: terms and concepts

Peter Wolf

Epilepsie-Zentrum Bethel, Klinik für Anfallskranke, Mara I, Maraweg 21, 33617 Bielefeld, Germany

Introduction

At the beginning of a book on seizures and syndromes, it appears to be useful to give some consideration and discussion to the terminology we currently use and the concepts behind it, as well as some controversial matters related to it.

The very title seizures and syndromes reflects the dual system which we have today in the international epilepsy classification: a classification of seizures, and a classification of epilepsies and epileptic syndromes. There are controversial issues in both, but the more important controversies at present concern the classification of seizures rather than the syndrome classification – probably because the seizure classification is somewhat older and the problems with it have become clearer. Therefore, the focus will be on this part of the classification. However, both parts should always be considered together as they are supposed to make sense as a whole. One question is whether they do. Their origin is not homogeneous. They were worked out by four successive commissions of the International League Against Epilepsy, and between the two commissions responsible for the seizure classification and the two commissions responsible for the syndrome classification there was very little personal overlap. More importantly, they were founded on different backgrounds.

The seizure classification was based on a trial to classify, as objectively as possible, by a consensus of experts, a small number of video-documented seizures. There was some controversy whether electroencephalography (EEG) should or should not be included in the criteria of classification, and finally it *was* included.

A seizure is a well-defined event, and its classification is a question of correct description much more than a problem of conceptualization – although there is an important conceptual angle to which I will come back. The task of a syndrome classification is different. To outline a syndrome is indeed a matter of conceptualization, and of interpretation of descriptive data which may long have been available but not been related to each other. A syndrome is 'a cluster of signs and symptoms customarily occurring together' (Commission, 1989), and the international syndrome classification is again the result of consensus but this time a consensus upon concepts rather than crude facts.

Syndromes

Even the just-mentioned definition of an epileptic syndrome is a convention in which an epileptic seizure is considered as a symptom. Most seizures, however, consist of more than just one symptom and therefore could well be considered as syndromes in themselves.

Syndromes can belong to various levels. A good example is the triad, ptosis, miosis and enophthalmus, known as Horner's syndrome. It is a simple syndrome which indicates a lesion somewhere in the cranial sympathetic pathway and, as such, appears as one component of a number of more complex syndromes according to where in this long and complicated pathway the lesion is located.

This example from a field remote from epilepsy is given here as a reminder of the classical diagnostic procedure in neurology: in a first step we try to define the anatomical site where a lesion would explain all pathological findings of the neurological investigation; in a second step we try to get a look at this anatomical site to find out what the lesion is and what could be done about it.

In the seizure classification, we have not really come as far as this. We have a taxonomic system which invites us to compile and label all individual seizure symptoms and to define their sequence. This is highly useful and was an important step forward, but it remains merely descriptive and thus only provides the prolegomena for an anatomical seizure semiology. Here is a gap between the seizure classification and the syndrome classification which the syndrome classification has only partially filled by its attempts to describe epilepsy syndromes according to the localization of the epileptic focus.

Then, if the very use of the term syndrome in the epilepsy classification requires some comment, some of its most important terminology is even more problematic.

The seizure classification (Commission, 1981) and the classification of epilepsies and epileptic syndromes (Commission, 1989) are connected by the use of a dichotomy between two major classes of seizures and syndromes, one class which is called 'generalized' and the other, 'partial', 'focal' or 'local' or, as far as syndromes are concerned, 'localization-related'. This multiplicity of nomenclature obviously indicates terminological problems, and each of the terms seems to belong to a different stage in the development of the epileptological theory in the last century and a half.

Partial

The oldest of these terms, and the one which has probably changed its significance most is 'partial'. It seems first to have been used by Prichard (1822), who called 'partial epilepsy' those motor seizures which only involved part of the body. It was relatively new that such seizures were accepted as epilepsy at all. They had mostly been termed 'epileptiform', whereas 'epilepsy' was restricted to generalized tonic–clonic seizures. The term 'partial' referred only to the phenotypical aspect of the seizures which were characterized by 'local convulsions'. The term was readily and rapidly accepted by French authors: Charcot (1880), Féré (1896) and de la Tourette (1898) all have it in their clinical textbooks. Binswanger, who wrote the most important German textbook on epilepsy of the turn of the century (1899), also used it amply. In England, it became a preferred term early in this century (Turner, 1907; Wilson, 1935) but it is worth noting that the two British nineteenth-century giants in epileptology, Jackson (1931) and Gowers (1885), used the term 'partial' little if at all.

Local

It may appear as a paradox that this has to do with Jackson's high concern with the very phenomenon for which the term was used. Whereas, formerly, epileptiform or partial seizures were disregarded because they were considered as atypical, the Jacksonian revolution was to focus on these seizures because he understood that they provided much better preconditions than the grand mal seizure to study the elements of epileptogenesis. In this respect, however, the partial aspect of the convulsions did not provide any new insights. For Jackson, the keyword was 'local' because he was able to relate the local convulsions of some muscles to local discharges of the grey matter. Jackson did not create this terminology. As mentioned above, Prichard (1822) talked of 'local convulsions' along with 'partial epilepsy', and Bright, a forerunner of Jackson, had already, in 1831, started to use it analytically as he opposed local to general cerebral excitement.

The impact of Jackson's much more thorough analysis is perhaps most clearly felt in Horsley's 1886 report of his first neurosurgical interventions on patients with local convulsions. It is widely known that his first operated patient had been in the care of Jackson, who was present at the operation. This patient had traumatic epilepsy due to a depressed skull fracture, and Horsley removed a deep cortical scar.

It is much less known that Horsley's second patient was also referred to him by Jackson, and this patient is perhaps even more interesting because the aetiology was not known and there were no overt localizing signs. The patient had Jacksonian seizures which started with a peculiar movement of the left thumb and forefinger. As the same type of movement had been obtained by Horsley in an experiment of cortical stimulation in monkeys, both he and Jackson felt confident of the locus of onset of the patient's seizures, and, when Horsley operated, he found a tuberculoma at exactly the site to which the anatomical interpretation of the seizure semiology had led the way (Horsley, 1886).

All this detail is given here because it illustrates, at a crucial point in the history of epileptology, the high importance of terms and their underlying concepts. The designation of non-generalized-tonic–clonic (GTC) motor seizures as 'partial' had remained merely descriptive and did not stimulate research, whereas the equation of local convulsions with local cerebral discharge opened new horizons for epileptology which remain important to our own day.

Focal

Jackson's term local has, in most connections, been replaced by the term 'focal', the origin of which is not quite clear. The idea of a focus is of course clearly influenced by Jackson but he seems not to have used the term. It seems that it had come into use by the end of the last century, probably in the wake of the first great wave of epilepsy surgery. Fedor Krause, one of the pioneers of epilepsy surgery, in his 1911 monograph amply used *Herdepilepsie* (focal epilepsy) as a term which needed no explanation (Krause, 1911).

The Latin meaning of focus is hearth, signifying a fire within limits but with a potential danger of spreading more widely – a very appropriate image for what happens in epilepsy. The term came increasingly into use in Germany during the first quarter of our century and has been the preferred term in epileptology in the German language since then. It seems that also in epileptology in the English language it is now being used much more frequently, especially in papers concerning epilepsy surgery, where indeed we are always looking for an epileptic focus to take out.

The second revolution in modern epileptology, the one following the introduction of EEG, has very much supported the concept of an epileptic focus because now a functional measurement was available which often demonstrated focal abnormalities even when all other investigations gave normal results. At present it is under discussion whether we should imagine an epileptic focus as localized within narrow limits or, rather, as involving regional neuronal aggregates with complex interactions.

The term partial is of course still in use, even as the preferred term of the International Seizure Classification, where it has undergone a redefinition. In an intermediate stage, it had been defined as seizures *involving* part of one hemisphere but the problem was that seizures had to be integrated into that part of the classification which definitely involved both hemispheres – psychomotor and secondarily generalized motor seizures. Partial seizures are now defined as seizures *originating* in part of one hemisphere (Commission, 1981), which makes the term an almost perfect synonym of focal. Still, the term 'complex partial' is paradoxical because 'complex' requires, according to the definition, impairment of consciousness where the ictal EEG shows frequently bilateral discharge.

This is certainly not consistent with the idea of partial involvement, which is still to some extent present as long as an evolution to generalized convulsions has not occurred.

This terminological situation is somewhat unfortunate because now we have no term for seizures which remain restricted to parts of the brain – one or both hemispheres – and such a term could be useful, for example, for a subdivision of focal seizures into local (isolated auras), partial and secondarily generalized, or for the discussion of regionality in idiopathic epilepsy (see, Chapter 32). It could be that more changes of significance lie ahead for this time-honoured term.

Generalized

The term for the other major part of the classification – generalized – seems at first glance unproblematic as there are no competing synonyms. But there are problems all the same. Generalized seizures are defined as 'those in which the first clinical changes indicate initial involvement of both hemispheres' and where 'the ictal EEG patterns initially are bilateral' (Commission, 1981). In the class of focal seizures, however, there is a subclass of focal seizures evolving to secondarily generalized seizures. This is of course in contradiction with the above definition and echoes a much earlier concept where the term generalized referred to generalized convulsions.

The term comprises still other meanings. Bright (1838) opposed fits depending on a local injury to those of general or constitutional aetiology. The latter concept of a constitutional disorder involving the brain in general is still prevalent when we investigate genetic factors in the aetiology of epilepsies. Today we have become used to calling bilaterally symmetric spikes and waves 'generalized' and to viewing various types of them as indicators of a general genetic predisposition.

It was in fact the detection of such discharge as the ictal pattern of minimal seizure types, such as absences or the short bilateral jerks of juvenile myoclonic epilepsy, that led to their classification as 'generalized' seizures for taxonomical reasons.

The term 'generalized' comprises at least three different concepts on three different levels of consideration: phenotypical, EEG and anatomical or functional. In the International Seizure Classification, the EEG aspect prevails, whereas, on both the phenotypical and the anatomical level, we have the unsatisfactory situation that some minimal seizure types which certainly do not involve the whole brain are considered as generalized because they are ambincipient (starting on both sides) while the much more prominent and probably anatomically more widespread psychomotor seizures are labelled as 'partial'.

But, even on the EEG level, the term generalized is open to criticism because the bilateral discharge may be accentuated on or even restricted to the anterior or, more rarely, other parts of the derivations.

In the syndrome classification, the functional anatomical aspect of the term generalized prevails, and a disorder like the Lennox–Gastaut syndrome is classified as generalized because of its widespread functional disturbance although it may comprise partial seizures. There is, thus, an inconsistency in the significance of terms between the seizure classification and the syndrome classification which has received too little attention and discussion.

Conclusion

Many terms which we use in epileptology – those discussed here as well as some others – have a long history, in the course of which the concepts they are supposed to express have undergone a series of changes. Changes of concepts are a necessary consequence of scientific progress, and our terminology, which is supposed to serve science, must not be considered as static. This should justly be remembered at the outset in a book in which questions of classification, concepts of ictogenesis and the relation of regional to generalized mechanisms in epileptogenesis will be widely discussed.

References

Binswanger, O. (1899): *Die Epilepsie*. Vienna: Hölder.

Bright, R. (1831): *Reports of medical cases,* vol. 2, part II. London: (cited in Temkin, 1945).

Bright, R. (1838): Cases illustrative of the effects produced when the arteries and brain are diseased. *Guy's Hosp. Rep.* **1,** 9–40 (cited in Temkin, 1945).

Charcot, J.-M. (1880): *Leçons sur les maladies du système nerveux,* 4th edn. Paris: Delahaye & Lecrosnier.

Commission on Classification and Terminology of the ILAE (1981): Proposal for revised clinical and electroencephalographic classification of epileptic seizures. *Epilepsia* **22,** 489–501.

Commission on Classification and Terminology of the ILAE (1989): Proposal for revised classification of epilepsies and epileptic syndromes. *Epilepsia* **30,** 389–399.

de la Tourette, G. (1898): *Leçons de clinique thérapeutique sur les maladies du système nerveux.* Paris: Plon.

Féré, Ch. (1896): *Die Epilepsie,* trans. P. Ebers. Leipzig: Engelmann.

Gowers, W.R. (1885): *Epilepsy and other chronic convulsive diseases.* London: Wood.

Horsley, V. (1886): Brain-surgery. *Br. Med. J.* **2,** 670–674.

Jackson, J.H. (1931): *Selected Writings.* London: Hodder & Stoughton.

Krause, F. (1911): *Chirurgie des Gehirns und Rückenmarks nach eigenen Erfahrungen.* Berlin: Urban & Schwarzenberg.

Prichard, J.C. (1822): *A treatise on diseases of the nervous system,* part 1. London: (cited in Temkin, 1945).

Temkin, O. (1945): *The falling sickness.* Baltimore: Johns Hopkins Press.

Turner, W.A. (1907): *Epilepsy – a study of the idiopathic disease.* London: Macmillan.

Wilson, S.A.K. (1935): The epilepsies. In: *Handbook der Neurologie,* Vol. 17, eds. O. Bumke & O. Foerster, pp. 1–87. Berlin: Springer.

Epileptic Seizures and Syndromes, Edited by Peter Wolf
© 1994 John Libbey & Company Ltd., pp. 9–14

Chapter 2

The International Classification of Seizures and Epilepsies: advantages

Fritz E. Dreifuss

Department of Neurology, School of Medicine, University of Virginia Health Sciences Center, Charlottesville, VA 22908, USA

Introduction

The context of this contribution is a discussion comparing the advantages and disadvantages of the International Classification of Epileptic Seizures and the Epilepsies. I would like to preface this by pointing out that the greatest disadvantage of the classification is the need for it. Yet, from the earliest days of epileptology, there have been attempts to classify the observed phenomena into groups. Thus Galen, as early as the second century, classified epilepsies into the idiopathic and the symptomatic with the implication that the former arose in the brain and the latter elsewhere. In turn, epileptic seizures were classified according to their severity by Poupart, Tissot, Delasiauve, Calmeil and Jackson. The rationale for the various classifications has differed but may be summarized as (1) subserving communication, (2) for a better understanding of mechanisms of disease, (3) attempts at creating a uniformity of communication to allow poolability of data among investigators, (4) for comparison of aetiologies across cultures, (5) for purposes of basic research, which has now reached the molecular level in the human genome, and (6) aiding in the choice of the most appropriate antiepileptic drug.

Words are the basic coin of the realm, the common currency, for the transaction of communication and human interaction. Words are the descriptive units which might be described as the individual keys on a keyboard which, when depressed by the sender, cause the homologous key to be activated in the receiver so that the latter sees in his/her mind's eye that which the sender transmits. Without such a mechanism we would be dependent on our own discretionary judgement or merely on chance. I realize that the definition of the words used in a classification does not have mathematical exactness and to some extent depends upon the concept, the limits of which are vague. At the same time the definition, categorization or classification as applied to philosophical rather than mathematical concepts must maintain some flexibility, for, with increase in knowledge, an increase in accuracy of concepts can be further assured. The classification will therefore contribute to the acquisition of knowledge, which in turn will modify the classification in the light of this increased knowledge. In the words of Thomas Jefferson, 'We can tolerate error so long as reason is left free to combat it.' Or, in the words of Immanuel Kant, 'Allow, therefore, your opponent to speak in the name of reason, and combat him only with weapons of reason' (Kant, 1781). Any classification, therefore, must be flexible and take into account the likelihood that continuous change as in a living thing will take place. Otherwise one would engage in the sin of Procrustes, who would stretch or amputate according to preconceived notions rather than adjust to the realities of the observed phenomenon.

Gastaut *et al.* in 1969 proposed a classification for epileptic seizures which was based on observed phenomena as well as electroencephalographic (EEG) data (Gastaut, 1970). This classification led to conceptual advances and these, in turn, coupled with improved quality of observation by virtue of the introduction of time-locked video EEG technology, led to an evolution of the clinical and EEG classification of epileptic seizures. The concatenation of these together with the imperative of uniformity imparted by the international partnership in testing new putative anticonvulsant drugs led to the stimulus for improving the classification, exemplified in the 1981 approved updating (Commission on Classification and Terminology of the ILAE, 1981).

The development of new antiepileptic drugs has provided a further rationale for the classification of epileptic seizures. It has become recognized that there are quite different mechanisms involved in the evolution of different seizure types. The physiology and pathophysiology of generalized convulsive seizures are quite different from thoseof generalized non-convulsive seizures and those of simple partial seizures are different from those of complex partial seizures. Moreover, there is presumably a major distinction between primarily generalized seizures and those which secondarily generalize after a focal onset. The design of the newer antiepileptic drugs (AEDs) is conceived with specific pathophysiological and pharmacophysiological mechanisms in mind. Apart from one or two relatively broad-spectrum AEDs, the majority have a fairly narrow focus of action. For example, some drugs mimic the action of agents on γ-aminobutyric acid ($GABA_A$) receptors and others on $GABA_B$ receptors. Still others are manufactured to occupy glycine receptors while yet others tend to block glutamatergic receptors of the *N*-methyl-D-aspartate (NMDA) variety. Before long, there will be a menu of AEDs to pick from for specific seizure types, which requires as refined a knowledge of the individual seizure type as can be achieved.

The 1981 classification has become the standard means of identifying seizure types over the past 12 years and in that time the Commission on Classification has received many comments and critiques, which in turn have led to proposals for refinement of the 1981 classification. Persistent problems in the use of the classification have included the recognition that a single seizure in its evolution may transcend classification criteria and evolve from one type to another. For example, a simple partial seizure may become a complex partial seizure, and either of them may end as a secondarily generalized tonic–clonic seizure. Similarly, an absence seizure may progress immediately to a generalized tonic–clonic seizure. A further problem frequently encountered is that of defining whether consciousness is or is not impaired and to what degree. This is a matter of importance because the distinction between simple partial seizures and complex partial seizures hinges on this observational point, where analytic logic and sophistry diverge and where intuitiveness remains in the diagnostic process. This leads to such questions as to how one classifies a seizure if the patient appears to remain in contact during the attack and afterwards has amnesia for it. Furthermore, the question can be raised regarding what represents an eye movement *vs.* a mimetic automatism. It is also difficult always to distinguish accurately between inability to speak and impairment of consciousness; the problems of epileptic aphasia, postictal aphasia, ictal and postictal amnesia *vis-à-vis* diminution of consciousness remain problematic points at this time.

Other considerations which are being addressed include the reintroduction as specific seizure types of epileptic spasms associated with hypsarrhythmia and of seizures which are clinically predominantly unilateral but encephalographically generalized in their manifestations.

Table 1. Classification of Epileptic Seizures

I. Partial (focal, local) seizures

Partial seizures are those in which, in general, the first clinical and electroencephalographic changes indicate activation of a system of neurones limited to part of one cerebral hemisphere. A partial seizure is classified primarily on the basis of whether or not consciousness in impaired during the attack. When consciousness is not impaired, the seizure is classified as a simple partial seizure. When consciousness is impaired, the seizure is classified as a complex partial seizure. Impairment of consciousness may be the first clinical sign, or simple partial seizure may evclve into complex partial seizures. In patients with impaired consciousness, aberrations of behaviour (automatisms) may occur. A partial seizures may not terminate, but instead progress to a generalized motor seizure. Impaired consciousness is defined as the inability to respond normally to exogenous stimuli by virtue of altered awareness and/or responsiveness.

There is considerable evidence that simple partial seizures usually have unilateral hemispheric involvement and only rarely have bilateral hemispheric involvement; complex partial seizures, however, frequently have bilateral hemispheric involvement.

Partial seizurcs can be classified into one of the following three fundamental groups:

A. Simple partial seizures

(consciousness not impaired)

1. With motor symptoms
2. With somatosensory or special sensory symptoms
3. With autonomic symptoms
4. With psychic symptoms

B. Complex partial seizures

(with impairment of consciousness)

1. Beginning as simple partial seizures and progressing to impairment of consciousness

a. With no other features
b. With features as in A. 1–4
c. With automatisms

2. With impairment of consciousness at onset

a. With no other features
b. With features as in A. 1–4
c. With automatisms

C. Partial seizures secondarily generalized

II. Generalized seizures (convulsive or non-convulsive)

Generalized seizures are those in which the first clinical changes indicate initial involvement of both hemispheres. Consciousness may be impaired and this impairment may be the initial manifestation. Motor manifestations are bilateral. The ictal electroencephalographic patterns initially are bilateral, and presumably reflect neuronal discharge which is widespread in both hemispheres.

A. 1. Absence seizures
   2. Atypical absence seizures
B. Myoclonic seizures
C. Clonic seizures
D. Tonic seizures
E. Tonic–clonic seizures
F. Atonic seizures

III. Unclassified epileptic seizures

Includes all seizures that cannot be classified because of inadequate or incomplete data and some that defy classification in hitherto described categories. This includes some neonatal seizures, e.g. rhythmic eye movements, chewing and swimming movements.

Adapted from *Commission on Classification and Terminology of the ILAE* (1981)

I mention these efforts in order to reassure the epileptological community on behalf of the Commission on Classification and Terminology of the International League Against Epilepsy that there is not, nor has there ever been, any intent to carve any classification in stone. Rather, the recognition that a classification, leads to increase in knowledge, which in turn mandates periodic updating of the classification has been the ongoing philosophy with which this task has been approached.

Classification of the epilepsies
(Commission on Classification and Terminology of the ILAE, 1989)

An epileptic seizure is a symptom of the condition which is responsible for it. In this way it resembles a pain or a cough and it is the occurrence of this which brings the patient to the physician. Not everybody with a tendency to epilepsy has epileptic seizures. As early as 1770, Tissot pointed out that there are two processes at work in the elicitation of an epileptic seizure, namely an underlying predisposition, which may be the result of inherited traits or acquired structural or metabolic lesion, and a precipitating factor, which elicits the seizure in those whose trait predisposes them to the appropriate provocation of electric-like activity. Such provoking factors may be represented by sleep deprivation, the ingestion of certain drugs such as theophylline, the withdrawal of sedatives including alcohol, stimulation by light, sound and other external factors, hormonal changes, changes in blood sugar, etc. It is the nature of the underlying condition that determines the epilepsy and it is the epilepsy which determines the patient's prognosis. Thus an epilepsy or epileptic syndrome is either idiopathic and the epilepsy a primary epilepsy, or symptomatic and the epilepsy a secondary epilepsy. Idiopathic or primary epilepsy is virtually synonymous with genetic epilepsy. The epilepsies occurring on the basis of structural disease or major identifiable metabolic derangements belong in the category of the symptomatic epilepsies. Cryptogenic epilepsy is considered as a secondary epilepsy but the causation remains hidden. Idiopathic epilepsy often has a family history of a similar ailment, it usually begins early in life and there are as a rule no signs of structural neurological disease or intellectual retardation. The EEG background is usually normal and the condition is frequently self-limited. Symptomatic or cryptogenic epilepsies are less benign with more frequent intellectual or neurological findings. The EEG background is frequently slow and disorganized and the condition, while it may remain static, may on the other hand frequently deteriorate. Response to medication is less good than in the idiopathic epilepsies, and spontaneous remission does not usually occur. It is thus obvious that such questions as the likelihood of recurrence of seizures after a single attack, the likelihood of a person remaining seizure-free after withdrawal of AEDs, whether a person can safely operate a motor vehicle or not and whether offspring are likely to be affected can only be answered in the context of the condition causing the epileptic seizure. This means that a rational treatment plan can be developed only after the classification of the epileptic seizure has been determined as well as the classification of the epileptic syndrome of which the seizure is a symptom. While frequency of seizures and a duration of the seizure disorder may contribute somewhat to the prognosis by far the most important factor on which prognosis, is based is the causation of the epilepsy.

Finally, both partial seizures and generalized seizures may be representative of idiopathic epilepsies and both partial and generalized seizures may be representative of symptomatic epilepsies under different circumstances. Many of the epileptic syndromes will be further discussed in this book.

The advantage of classification should by now be quite evident. Every advance in the design of rational therapy of the person with epilepsy is predicated on the classification of both seizures and epilepsies. While this is generally acknowledged, it is also true that there is still much to be done to perfect the classification process. In the words of Leonardo de Vinci, 'Trifles make perfection but perfection is no trifle'.

Table 2. International Classification of Epilepsies, Epileptic Syndromes and Related Seizure Disorders (ICES)

1. Localization-related (focal, local, partial)	2. Generalized	3. Undetermined epilepsies	4. Special syndromes
Idiopathic (primary) 1.1 • Benign childhood epilepsy with centrotemporal spike • Childhood epilepsy with occipital paroxysms • Primary reading epilepsy	Idiopathic (primary) 2.1 • Benign neonatal familial convulsions • Benign neonatal convulsions • Benign myoclonic epilepsy in infancy • Childhood absence epilepsy (pyknolepsy) • Juvenile absence epilepsy • Juvenile myoclonic epilepsy (impulsive petit mal) • Epilepsies with grand mal seizures (GTCS) on awakening • Other generalized idiopathic epilepsies	3.1 With both generalized and focal seizures • Neonatal seizures • Severe myoclonic epilepsy in infancy • Epilepsy with continuous spike waves during slow–wave sleep • Acquired epileptic aphasia (Landau–Kleffner syndrome) Other undetermined epilepsies 3.2 Without unequivocal generalized or focal features	4.1 Situation-related seizures (*Gelegenheitsanfälle*) • Febrile convulsions • Isolated seizures or isolated status epilepticus • Seizures occurring only when there is an acute or toxic event due to factors such as alcohol, drugs, eclampsia, non-ketotic hyperglycaemia • Reflex epilepsies
Symptomatic (secondary) 1.2 • Temporal lobe epilepsies • Frontal lobe epilepsies • Parietal lobe epilepsies • Occipital lobe epilepsies • Chronic progressive epilepsia partialis continua of childhood			
Cryptogenic 1.3 Defined by: Seizure type (see ICES) Clinical features Aetiology Anatomical localization	Cryptogenic or symptomatic 2.2 • West syndrome (infantile spasms, Blitz–Nick–Salaam Krämpfe) • Lennox–Gastaut syndrome • Epilepsy with myoclonic–astatic seizures • Epilepsy with myoclonic absences		

GTCS = generalized tonic–clonic seizure.
Adapted from *Commission on Classification and Terminology of the ILAE* (1989).

References

Commission on Classification and Terminology of the ILAE (1981): Proposal for revised clinical and electroencephalographic classification of epileptic seizures. *Epilepsia* **22,** 489–501.

Commission on Classification and Terminology of the ILAE (1989): Proposal for revised classification of epilepsies and epileptic syndromes. *Epilepsia* **30,** 389–399.

Gastaut, H. (1970): Clinical and electroencephalographic classification of epileptic seizures. *Epilepsia* **11,** 102–113.

Kant, I. (1781): *Kritik der reinen Vernunft.*, J.F. Hartknoch, Riga.

Tissot, S.A. (1770): *Traité de l'épilepsie. Tome troisième du traité des nerfs et leurs maladies.* Didot le Jeune, Paris.

Epileptic Seizures and Syndromes, Edited by Peter Wolf
© 1994 John Libbey & Company Ltd., pp. 15–20

Chapter 3

The International Classification today: disadvantages

Hans Otto Lüders*, Richard Burgess*, Soheyl Noachtar† and Youssef Comair*

**The Cleveland Clinic Foundation, 9500 Euclid Avenue, Cleveland, OH 44195, USA; †Department of Neurology, Klinikum Grosshaderm, University of Münich, Marchionistrasse 15, 81377 Münich, Germany*

In 1970 the Commission on Classification and Terminology of the International League Against Epilepsy (ILAE) presented a classification of epileptic seizures based on clinical semiology and electroencephalographic criteria (Gastaut, 1970). In 1981 a similar Commission of the ILAE presented a revised version of this classification (Commission, 1981) as an appendix to a preceding manuscript of F.E. Dreifuss. As stressed in the manuscript of F.E. Dreifuss, a standardized, universally accepted classification is an essential tool for appropriate communication among epileptologists around the world. At the same time, it is crucial that no classification system, even if officially accepted by a representative body of internationally famous epileptologists, should be 'cast in stone'. A classification system not only is an effective communication tool but certainly also reflects our current understanding of the entity which we are trying to classify. A better understanding of the entity itself, in this case epileptic seizures, should also lead to new classification systems which may greatly facilitate future scientific work and also enhance the everyday utility of the classification system. In other words, revisions of a classification system not only should be allowed but should definitely be encouraged. It is in this spirit that we would like to criticize the current International Classification of Epileptic Seizures (ICES) and offer some alternative classification system which, we feel, would have significant advantages.

One of the major disadvantages of the ICES is the fact that an epileptic seizure is defined by a combination of clinical symptoms and signs and also the results of ancillary tests. Officially these ancillary tests should only include the electroencephalography (EEG) but the practical reality is quite different, as we explain below. For example, lapses of consciousness associated with some automatisms occurring in a patient with a normal EEG but a focal lesion in one of the mesial temporal lobes would be called 'complex partial seizures' because we would assume that the patient is suffering from focal epilepsy. On the other hand, identical seizures in a patient with a normal EEG but occasional drop attacks and generalized myoclonic seizures would be labelled as 'absence seizures' because we would assume that the patient has a generalized type of epilepsy. In other words, for clinically identical seizures we would be using different terminology depending on what epileptic syndrome we suspect is giving rise to the epileptic seizures. This certainly produces great confusion regarding the difference between epileptic syndromes and epileptic seizures. In the classification system we propose, seizures are classified exclusively by their clinical symptomatology. On the other hand, the epileptic syndrome is defined by all the available clinical information, including seizure types, EEG, neuroimaging, clinical history, etc. In the case illustrated above we would use the label 'psychomotor seizures', which, in our terminology, can be produced by focal or generalized epileptic syndromes. The first example would be a patient with mesial temporal epilepsy and psychomotor seizures, and the second a patient with Lennox–Gastaut syndrome and psychomotor seizures. With this system of seizure classification, we can study the type of epileptic seizures occurring in different epileptic syndromes using a uniform terminology for all seizures that have a similar clinical semiology. For example, in the classification we propose, absence seizures are classified as episodes of loss of consciousness not accompanied by any significant motor movements except some minor automatisms or rhythmical myoclonic jerks like eye blinking. We can now study the incidence of such 'absences' in different epileptic syndromes like pyknolepsy, Lennox–Gastaut syndrome, mesial temporal sclerosis or frontal lobe epilepsy. The special characteristics of the absences in different epileptic syndromes can also be analysed. These studies could tell us the specificity of any given clinical seizure for a certain epileptic syndrome. At the same time, such a classification system permits very clear differentiation between epileptic seizures and epileptic syndromes. As pointed out above, this differentiation is unclear in the present ICES because of the inclusion of ancillary test results when classifying any given epileptic seizure.

Differentiation between seizures of focal or generalized origin is frequently difficult when we can only analyse the seizure semiology and interictal EEG. It is not unusual that such a differentiation is only possible after analysing the whole clinical picture including clinical history, physical examination, EEG and particularly neuroimaging. In other words, only a study of the epileptic syndrome will allow us to define if a seizure was of focal or generalized origin. In more sophisticated epilepsy centres, we usually have all this ancillary available, allowing us to make a fairly accurate distinction between focal and generalized epilepsies. However, when such information has not yet been obtained or is not available, which is frequently the case in less sophisticated epilepsy clinics, we cannot decide if the epileptic syndrome we are dealing with is generalized or focal. Therefore, we are also unable to classify the seizure itself because in the ICES we have to categorize seizures first as generalized or focal. Seizures that cannot be categorized as generalized or partial are labelled as unclassifiable. However, seizure semiology can contain highly valuable information even when it does not allow us to decide if the underlying epileptic syndrome is generalized or focal. For example, there is certainly an important difference between patients who have absence seizures (see definition above), psychomotor seizures (lapses of consciousness associated with prominent, distal automatisms) or clonic seizures, independent of whether the underlying epilepsy syndrome is focal or partial. In the classification we propose, the somatotopic distribution of the seizure symptoms is only an optional modifier that can be used when the seizure semiology gives clear somatotopic information (for example, left-hand clonic seizures or generalized clonic seizures).

Similarly, the ICES requires classifying partial seizures into simple partial seizures and complex partial seizures. As Dreifuss indicated in his chapter it is frequently difficult to define if a patient did or did not lose consciousness during a seizure. Those patients, according to the ICES, would then be just classified as partial seizures even if we have detailed knowledge about the clinical semiology during the seizures. This problem is avoided in the classification we are proposing by paying equal attention to alteration of consciousness and also other essential clinical symptoms like automatisms or other motor manifestations.

Most epileptologists now use the term complex partial seizures as almost a synonym for what was known as psychomotor seizures in the old literature. When dealing with other types of focal seizures, like motor seizures, there is a tendency to deviate from the terminology partial *vs.* complex and to return to the old terminology like 'focal motor seizures' or 'focal tonic seizures', avoiding particularly in those cases the expression complex partial seizures. In these cases, little attention is paid to alterations of consciousness, which are not infrequently seen during focal motor seizures, particularly when the seizure discharge involves more extensive brain regions. Actually, alterations of consciousness occur almost consistently immediately preceding secondary generalization in patients with focal motor seizures. However, epileptologists try to avoid the term 'complex partial seizures' in patients in which the initial symptom is a focal motor seizure (preceding 'simple partial seizure'). This is most probably because conceptually they think of psychomotor seizures when they use the expression 'complex partial seizure'. In other words, in everyday practice the new ICES has not created a new subdivision of seizures, but only replaced a new terminology for old concepts. The problem is that the definition of the new terms does not correspond precisely with the actual seizure type that is being identified.

Another practical problem derived from the dichotomy 'simple *vs.* complex' partial seizures is that essential clinical symptomatology is frequently ignored because of the necessity always to classify seizures according to this dichotomy first. Epileptologists are getting used to talking just about complex and simple partial seizures, ignoring the subclassification because the terminology becomes too complicated when it is included. However, in most cases the essential clinical semiology is contained in this subclassification. This problem can be avoided if alterations of consciousness are only one of the many essential clinical features to which we pay attention. For example, when we are talking about simple partial seizure, we are lumping together all seizures in which the patient is conscious during the seizure. These include all the auras and also motor seizures or psychomotor seizures not associated with loss of consciousness. What then is the value of defining this category? The same is also true when we talk of evolution from a simple partial seizure to a complex partial seizure. The great majority of patients with focal epilepsy have simple partial seizures which evolve into complex partial seizures. As mentioned above, all patients with focal epilepsy will have, just before secondary generalization, a phase of variable duration during which there are alterations of consciousness. In other words, they almost invariably pass through a phase of 'complex partial seizures'. In patients with epilepsy from the perirolandic region this phase tends to be shorter than in patients with temporal lobe epilepsy and is frequently overshadowed by the violent motor movements that occur simultaneously with the convulsions. In patients with temporal lobe epilepsy, the alteration of consciousness is much more obvious because this phase of alteration of consciousness tends to be longer and seizures in these patients are usually associated only with limited movements (like distal automatisms) or even with no significant movements at all. In other words, the alteration of consciousness is frequently the essential sign in these seizures. It is usually very easy to define the most obvious symptomatology which occurs during a seizure (for example, alteration of consciousness associated or not with automatisms in patients with temporal lobe epilepsy or different types of motor phenomena for patients with seizures from the perirolandic region). To determine if the patient did or did not have alterations of consciousness is, however, difficult or even impossible, particularly if other symptoms like violent motor phenomena are in the forefront. In cases in which other symptomatology is most notorious (like, for example, motor seizures), it is also extremely artificial to classify the seizure primarily by the presence or not of alterations of consciousness. For example, a patient has a seizure which starts with clonic movements of the right hand and then the clonic convulsions extend to involve the whole right side of the body together with loss or alteration of consciousness. To speak in this case of a simple partial seizure which evolves into a complex partial seizure really misses the main clinical information we have obtained from observation of this seizure. Applying the ICES in this case only tells us that the patient had a seizure during which initially he/she was conscious and later on had an alteration of consciousness. The essential clinical symptomatology, which contains valuable information for localization of the epileptogenic zone, is not even mentioned unless we include the subclassification, which is very cumbersome. We would have to talk about a 'simple partial seizure with focal motor signs with march,' which evolved into a 'complex partial seizure with focal motor signs with march'. Notice that this more detailed classification still does not contain any somatotopic information. It is certainly not only simpler but also much more informative if we just talk about right-hand clonic seizures and neglect the clinically less relevant feature in this seizure, which is the alteration of consciousness that accompanied the spreading of the seizure discharge.

What is actually the significance of alterations of consciousness during focal seizures? As we mentioned above, in the ICES alteration of consciousness is the essential clinical symptom used to classify focal seizures. In the classification we are proposing, it also represents an important clinical feature, but an equally important place is given to other seizure symptoms that we feel in many seizures represent the essential clinical semiology that should be used to classify and identify the seizure. We know also, as mentioned above, that almost all focal seizures will eventually evolve to loss of consciousness when the epileptiform discharge spreads. In other words, most focal seizures, independent of the location of the epileptogenic zone (in other words, independent of the type of focal epilepsy), will evolve from 'simple partial seizures' to 'complex partial seizures'. Therefore, specifying this evolution, which occurs almost invariably when we analyse the focal seizures more carefully, is clinically meaningless. Nevertheless, the presence or not of consciousness during a seizure while other symptoms are occurring is extremely important in order to specify the epileptic syndrome. For example, patients with mesial temporal sclerosis always have a phase of alteration of consciousness which precedes motor phenomena like clonic twitching of the face or an ictal version. Consciousness in these patients is altered when the epileptiform discharge extends to the primary motor strip. On the other hand, patients with perirolandic epilepsy will almost invariably be completely conscious when the first motor manifestations attributable to the activation of the motor strip occur. In these patients, loss of consciousness always follows the clonic motor twitching characteristic of perirolandic motor seizures. In the classification we are proposing the sequence of events in regard to loss of consciousness, even if not mentioned specifically, can be easily deduced by analysing the evolution of the seizure. For example, seizures which start with a focal motor manifestation are always associated with preserved consciousness (for example, right-hand clonic seizure) and focal seizures in which a psychomotor seizure or an absence seizure evolves into a focal motor seizure will always be associated with loss of consciousness before the focal motor manifestations (examples: abdominal aura → psychomotor seizure → left versive seizure). Notice also that the two seizures which we presented as an example, could be classified as simple partial seizures that evolve into complex partial seizures, indicating how little information is contained in that terminology.

How useful is it actually to classify seizures into 'simple' or 'complex partial seizures'? As mentioned above, both types of seizures occur from an epileptogenic focus localized to any region of the brain. It has, therefore, no localizing value. In addition, when selecting anticonvulsants the classification into simple or complex partial seizures is of essentially no value since all patients with focal epilepsy, independent of whether they have simple or complex partial seizures, will respond equally well to the same type of anticonvulsants. The main value of this classification is that, by distinguishing seizures in which the patient suffers or does not suffer loss of consciousness during the seizures, it gives an index of the impact a seizure could have on the quality of life of the patient. Therefore, when the clinician is particularly interested in the impact of an intervention on the quality of life of the patient, the use of this classification system, or a modification of it which is specially designed to define quality of life, would be most suitable. However, in everyday practice, a classification system which not only highlights the presence or absence of consciousness during a seizure but in addition gives a summarized impression of the essential seizure semiology certainly has great advantages. For example, a patient who had surgery for epilepsy and remained seizure-free except for the presence of frequent 'simple partial seizures' could reflect a patient who still has visual auras, abdominal auras or left clonic motor seizures. Classifying the 'simple partial seizure' according to the classification we are proposing certainly contains a wealth of clinically relevant information.

In a previous publication (Lüders *et. al.*, 1993) other shortcomings of the International Classification are outlined. We will not insist on these shortcomings here, because they could easily be corrected by introducing minor modifications to the current ICES. In this chapter we have addressed what we feel are the most essential disadvantages of the ICES, which most probably can only be addressed by a radical overhaul of the classification itself, requiring a major revision of the philosophical way we look at seizures and weight the importance of different seizure symptoms.

Classifications of seizures in different types, with precise definition of each type, and also universal acceptance of a classification system are essential for effective communication between epileptologists. At the same time, we have to be cognizant of the fact that a seizure classification system can mould our thinking and understanding of epileptic seizures. It sets the framework within which most of the clinical research research related to epileptic seizures will be performed. It is important, therefore, that we continue looking for ways to improve our seizure classification systems to reflect better the continuous advance in our understanding of seizure symptomatology. We feel that the current ICES has been a valuable effort in standardizing the language epileptologists use to communicate among themselves. However, there are still some major shortcomings and criticisms. We feel, therefore, that new proposals to improve the classification should be welcomed. One classification system, which does not suffer from the disadvantages listed above and has been tested intensively in our laboratories will be presented elsewhere (Lüders & Noachtar, in press). A brief summary appears in the Appendix 1. Its principal advantages are: (1) classification of seizures only at the basis of observable semiology; (2) greater precision (a) showing seizure evolution and (b) permitting modifiers where relevant – permitting definition of lateralization and/or somatotopic information; (3) independence of seizure classification from EEG or imaging results, knowledge of whether it is focal or generalized in origin, or an absolute determination of alteration of consciousness; (4) simplicity in writing or speaking; and (5) avoidance of non-standard meanings of terms like 'complex' and 'simple'. We hope that other epileptologists also get a chance to present their views and that these proposals are eventually considered by the ILAE Commission on Classification and Terminology.

Appendix

Seizure classification

1. Aura

a. Somatosensory aura
b. Visual aura
c. Olfactory aura
d. Gustatory aura
e. Auditory aura
f. Psychic aura
g. Autonomic aura
h. Abdominal aura

2. Absence seizure

3. Psychomotor seizure

4. Hypermotor seizure

5. Motor seizure

a. Myoclonic seizure
b. Clonic seizure
c. Tonic seizure
d. Tonic–clonic seizure
e. Atonic seizure
f. Versive seizure

6. Unclassified epileptic seizure

7. Unclassified event

Modifiers

a. To be used preceding the seizure type:
(indicate portion of the body participating in the seizure symptomatology)

1. Generalized
2. Left
3. Right
4. Somatotopic: face, hand, arm, foot, leg

b. Evolution

Arrow (→) linking two seizure types indicates seizure evolution

A detailed description of this seizure classification will be published elsewhere. The following are some examples of how this seizure classification can be used to characterize selected seizures. The corresponding classification according to the ICES is also given.

1. Abdominal aura – psychomotor seizure

ICES: simple partial seizure with autonomic symptomatology evolving into a complex partial seizure.

2. Left visual aura – left-hand clonic seizure – generalized tonic–clonic seizure.

ICES: if the patient loses consciousness during the left-hand clonic seizure: simple partial seizure with visual symptomatology evolving into complex partial seizure and then into a generalized tonic–clonic seizure.

3. Tonic seizure – left face clonic seizure – generalized tonic–clonic seizure.

ICES: if the patient loses consciousness during the left face clonic seizure: Simple partial seizure with postural signs evolving into complex partial seizure and then into a generalized tonic–clonic seizure.

4. Gustatory aura – psychomotor seizure – left versive seizure – generalized tonic–clonic seizure.

ICES: Simple partial seizure with gustatory symptomatology evolving into complex partial seizure and then into a generalized tonic–clonic seizure.

Notice that the last three seizures, although of very different semiology, are classified almost identically in the ICES (except the modifier for the simple partial seizure). The critical differences between these seizures, concealed by the ICES, are what provide the greatest help in localizing and lateralizing the seizure onset and seizure spread accurately.

References

Commission on Classification and Terminology of the ILAE (1981): Proposal for revised clinical and electroencephalographic classification of epileptic seizures. *Epilepsia* **22,** 489–501.

Gastaut, H. (1970): Clinical and electroencephalographic classification of epileptic seizures. *Epilepsia* **11,** 102.

Lüders, H., Burgess, R.C. & Noachtar, S. (1993): An Expansion of the International Classification of Seizures to Provide Localization Information. *Neurology* **43** (9), 1650–1655.

Lüders, H.O. & Noachtar, S. (eds.): *Atlas epileptischer Anfälle und Syndrome*, Ciba-Geigy, in press.

Lüders, H.O. & Noachtar, S. (eds.): *Epileptic Seizures: Pathophysiology and Clinical Semiology.* New York: Churchill Livingstone, in preparation.

Epileptic Seizures and Syndromes, Edited by Peter Wolf
© 1994 John Libbey & Company Ltd., pp. 21–23

Chapter 4

Current problems of the international seizure classification being addressed by the ILAE Commission on Classification and Terminology

Fritz E. Dreifuss

Department of Neurology, School of Medicine, University of Virginia Health Sciences Center, Charlottesville, VA 22908, USA

The Classification of Epileptic Seizures of 1981 and the Classification of Epileptic Syndromes of 1989 were largely accomplished through the aid of simultaneously viewed electroencephalograms (EEG) and clinical information through the technique of closed-circuit television and simultaneous EEG (CCTV-EEG). Though this represented a significant refinement of technique it failed to answer all of the requirements for a definitive classification. Subsequent meetings of the Commission on Classification and Terminology of the International League Against Epilepsy have been occupied in an attempt to resolve some of the remaining issues and these were highlighted by a video-EEG conference held in Bielefeld in March 1993.

The purposes of the Classification of Epileptic Seizures were reviewed. It was recalled that an epileptic seizure is a symptom, a recurrent event occurring intermittently in a person suffering from epilepsy. The epilepsy is the underlying disease responsible for the symptom and may be of idiopathic, symptomatic or cryptogenic aetiology. Once a person has acquired the epileptic propensity this remains as a lifelong predisposition and the individual seizures are events which are probably not unprovoked but triggered by a concatenation of circumstances in persons so predisposed. Such triggering events might include intercurrent illnesses, sleep deprivation, metabolic disturbances, relatively mild trauma, hormonal changes, intoxications, reflexly exciting conditions such as photic stimulation, certain sounds or other afferent stimuli. The individual's seizures are either generalized or localization-related and it is for purposes of their individual description that the classification has been developed.

The purposes of classification include a uniformity of terminology for communication among physicians and coding of hospital records. This becomes especially important when such communication allows the pooling of patient records for purposes of collaborative research, for example, in testing novel antiepileptic drugs in a collaborative manner between various centres. Likewise it is important for communication among basic researchers and in particular in the delineation of syndromes in a manner such that the idiopathic epilepsy can be assigned a place in the human genome. For this purpose extreme care must be taken to assure descriptive uniformity.

It was recognized from the beginning that the classification of epileptic seizures as proposed had certain shortcomings but that continued use would highlight these and lead to a consensus for the improvement of the classification over time. The present Commission on Classification and Terminology has deemed it desirable to review the situation at this point in time in order to build in some refinements to meet the further goals of the classification. The problems had been highlighted by an international meeting in Marseille of paediatric neurologists who were asked to classify all seizures seen during a 1-year period on a world-wide basis. This led to a collection of 4309 seizures, the majority of which were classifiable by both seizure type and responsible syndrome. However, there was a very wide discrepancy between centres, which indicated either that an inordinate number of children were referred to an individual centre by virtue of its expressed interest or that there was a wide discrepancy in understanding between the individual paediatric neurologists and that there was, in fact, an undue conceptual disparity.

In Bielefeld, individual seizures were displayed and difficulties fell into certain major categories. For example, some patients appeared to have automatisms without any impairment of consciousness. The question was raised as to whether these really represented automatisms or involuntary movements of which the patient was aware but which he/she was unable to influence. Another patient was reviewed illustrating postictal amnesia but no impairment of responsiveness during the seizure. At the time, she was able to respond appropriately to questions but after the seizure was over she was amnesic for a large part of the episode. A child was noted with simple partial seizures progressing to complex partial seizures and thereafter to tonic and tonic–clonic symmetrical or asymmetrical seizures, leading to a discussion as to the progression of various epileptic seizures in any one attack. It was evident that one has to occasionally deal with the question as to the nature of the initial symptom, which is then followed by sequencing from one type of seizure to the next, indicating a dynamic process. Another such example was immediate progression from an absence seizure to a generalized tonic–clonic seizure and the inability of the present classification to define this type of primarily generalized seizure progressing to a secondarily generalized tonic–clonic attack. A further question arose by viewing automatisms of mimicry without affective involvement as to whether these represent responses to interoceptive stimuli, as postulated by Penry and Dreifuss (1969), or whether they represent merely epiphenomena. In one seizure, atonic lower-extremity weakness was suggestive of a negative motor phenomenon and the occurrence of such negative phenomena will have to be addressed in revisions of the classification. These have to be distinguished from other causes of loss of movement, including, in one patient whose seizures were viewed, an epileptic paralysis, which in turn had to be distinguished from a post-ictal paralysis and from unilateral neglect due to parietal lobe involvement.

The subject of unilateral seizures in childhood was raised in the context of a patient suffering from alternating unilateral seizures in the face of a consistently generalized EEG discharge.

The question of the elucidation of alteration of consciousness was again discussed, as this is a critical factor in distinguishing between simple partial seizures and complex partial seizures and is occasionally extremely difficult to evaluate *vis-à-vis* such occurrences as epileptic aphasia, postictal aphasia and ictal and postictal amnesia as opposed to a true diminution of consciousness.

Some of these issues raised major conceptual dilemmas and others centred around semantic discussions, as in the case of the syndrome of myoclonic absence whose seizures are, strictly speaking, clonic. This syndrome, furthermore, has to be distinguished from absence with myoclonic components and benign myoclonic attacks of childhood without loss of consciousness.

From these discussions, emanating from well-documented individual cases, an improved updated version of the classification of epileptic seizures is being developed, a process of refinement which is continually ongoing. Continual incorporation of refinements will ultimately enhance an understanding of the processes involved in the spatial evolution of seizure spread.

Reference

Penry, J.K. & Dreifuss, F.E. (1969): Automatisms associated with the absence of petit mal seizures. *Arch. Neurol.* **21,** 142–149.

Epileptic Seizures and Syndromes, Edited by Peter Wolf
© 1994 John Libbey & Company Ltd., pp. 25–37

Chapter 5

The epilepsies: specific syndromes or a neurobiological continuum?

Samuel F. Berkovic*†, David C. Reutens*†, Eva Andermann† and Frederick Andermann†

**Department of Neurology, Austin Hospital, Melbourne, and Department of Medicine (Neurology), The University of Melbourne, Australia; †Montreal Neurological Institute and Hospital, Montreal, Quebec, Canada*

The concept of epilepsies as specific syndromes or diseases can be found in the writings of Hughlings Jackson and other early epileptologists (reviewed by Gastaut & Zifkin, 1985). In 1970 a preliminary attempt to formalize an international classification of epilepsies was published (Merlis, 1970). Subsequently, the more detailed current classification was developed (Commission, 1985; Commission, 1989; Roger *et al.*, 1992). This classification is imperfect, and will doubtless undergo future modification. It does, however, provide a workable scheme for classifying most patients with epilepsy and, as such, it represents a major advance in epileptology.

There has been resistance by some practitioners to accept and use this classification. In some cases this resistance relates to a lack of understanding of the classification, or to an incorrect perception that it is too complex. Others believe that there are more fundamental problems with the classification, when the epilepsies are viewed in terms of their neurobiological basis. Simply put, this latter issue represents a dispute between 'lumpers' and 'splitters'. This is not a new controversy. As pointed out by Reynolds (1988), a century-old version of this problem can be found in the books on epilepsy by Russell Reynolds (a splitter) and Henry Sieveking (a lumper), who were both appointed to the National Hospital for the Paralysed and Epileptic in 1864, ahead of Hughlings Jackson. This review attempts to provide a modern perspective and reconciliation of the polarized positions in this dispute with particular emphasis on recent knowledge from molecular genetic studies.

Lumping and splitting in epileptology

'Splitters' regard epilepsy syndromes as a discrete series of entities that are sharply defined, with little or no overlap. The purpose of splitting is twofold. First, on a practical clinical level, if a specifically defined entity can be clearly identified, the physician can offer precise advice regarding treatment, prognosis and genetic risk. Secondly, at the research level, a clearly identified syndrome may offer the best chance to allow identification of the cause/s of that syndrome, be they genetic or acquired. Currently, much interest focuses on the search for genes in specific epilepsy phenotypes.

An extreme position of the 'lumpers' is that 'all epilepsy is one' (Mackay, 1960). In this view there is a constitutional epileptic predisposition, a concept that goes back to Tissot (1772), upon which other acquired factors are engrafted to cause the spectrum of epileptic phenotypes observed. A more modern and scientific development of this idea is that of a neurobiological continuum of the epilepsies based on the multifactorial hypothesis (Gloor, 1977; Andermann, 1982; Gloor *et al.*, 1982; Berkovic *et al.*, 1987). Lumpers would emphasize that some, and perhaps many, patients do not accurately fit into the syndromes defined by the splitters, and that it is inappropriate and unhelpful to 'squeeze' cases into categories where they do not strictly belong. Scientifically, lumpers can criticize the splitters' classification in that it is artificial and based on 'soft' clinical and electroencephalographic (EEG) criteria, and that it has a debatable neurobiological basis.

A vindication of the splitters' syndromic approach would be the identification of a causative gene from identical phenotypes in different families. So far this approach, has led to inconclusive results for the common epilepsies.

Phenotypes in homogeneous epilepsy genotypes

As one of the main aims of the syndromic classification is to use phenotypes to lead us to genotypes, it is instructive to look at the problem in reverse. That is, in epilepsies where a single genetic defect has been identified, which epilepsy phenotypes are observed, and how much phenotypic variation occurs? Specific genetic defects have been found in only a few epilepsies to date, but these disorders do provide some insight into the phenotype-genotype problem.

Progressive myoclonus epilepsies (PME)

This group of rare epilepsies is currently the best understood at the molecular level. Indeed, disputes about classification and phenotypic relationships of disparate geographic clusters have been resolved by advances in molecular biology (Marseille Consensus Group, 1990; Berkovic *et al.*, 1993).

Unverricht–Lündborg disease, the prototypic PME, is an autosomal recessive disorder linked to chromosome 21q (Lehesjoki *et al.*, 1991; Malafosse *et al.*, 1992b). The specific gene involved is not yet known. The phenotype is relatively homogeneous with a well-defined age of onset although there is some variation in the severity of the myoclonus and in the rate of progression. Heterogeneity in the spectrum of dementia may at least in part be related to the previous inappropriate use of phenytoin in these patients (Eldridge *et al.*, 1983). The similarity of the phenotype amongst different individuals with this disorder, both within families and between families, even in different racial groups, is characteristic of autosomal recessive conditions.

In contrast, myoclonus epilepsy and ragged red fibres (MERRF), which is another distinct form of PME, shows remarkable phenotypic variation between and within families. In most families with MERRF the molecular defect is a single base pair substitution at position 8344 of the mitochondrial genome, resulting in a mutation in tRNA for lysine (Shoffner *et al.*, 1990; Yoneda *et al.*, 1990; Zeviani *et al.*, 1991). In individuals proved to have this mutation, the phenotype can vary from being clinically unaffected, to a late-onset ataxic–myoclonic syndrome, to a severe childhood-onset PME with or without associated dementia and pyramidal and cerebellar signs. At post-mortem, milder cases show a system degeneration whereas severely affected children may have the pathological features of Leigh's disease. Still other cases with this mutation present with myopathy and lipomas without myoclonus epilepsy (Berkovic *et al.*, 1989, 1991; Graf *et al.*, 1993; Hammans *et al.*, 1993; Silvestri *et al.*, 1993). Prior to the recognition of the molecular defect, and in the absence of family data, it would have been unthinkable that such a wide spectrum of phenotypes could be caused by the same mutation. Whilst the phenotypic heterogeneity in cases with the MERRF mutation is extraordinary, probably due to the peculiarities of mitochondrial inheritance, it highlights the difficulties in extrapolating from epilepsy phenotype to genotype.

Epilepsies with autosomal dominant inheritance

Benign familial neonatal convulsions have been linked to chromosome 20q in a number of families,

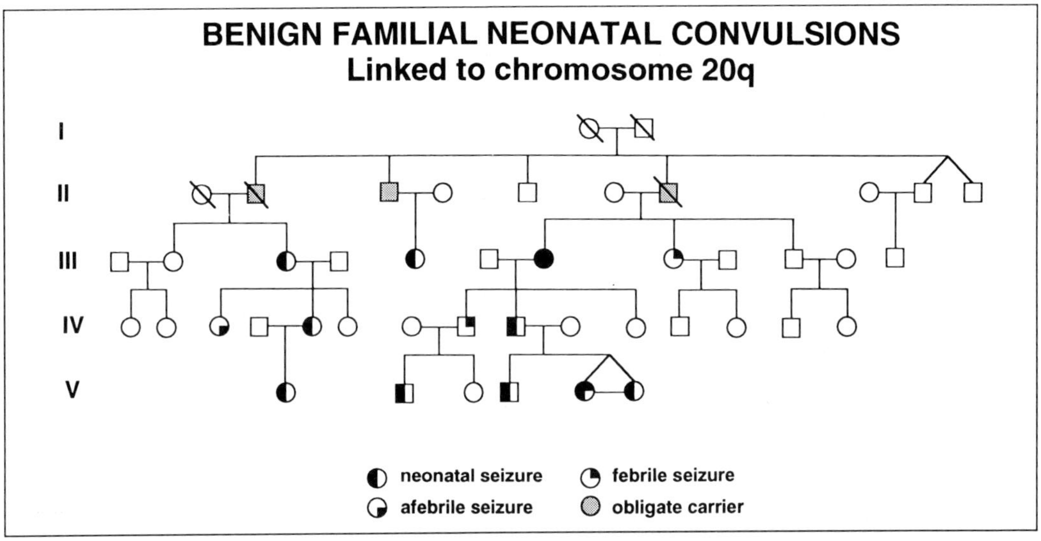

Fig. 1. Phenotypic heterogeneity in a family with benign familial neonatal convulsions linked to chromosome 20 (modified from Berkovic et al., 1993b).

although at least one phenotypically similar family links to another locus on chromosome 8q (Leppert *et al.*, 1989; Ryan *et al.*, 1991; Malafosse *et al.*, 1992a; Berkovic *et al.*, 1994; Lewis *et al.*, 1993; Ronen *et al.*, 1993). This 'simple' autosomal dominant disorder has a number of complexities when the epilepsy phenotypes of affected individuals are examined (Fig. 1). Affected individuals may have neonatal convulsions, febrile seizures and/or later afebrile seizure (Plouin, 1992; Berkovic *et al.*, 1994; Ronen *et al.*, 1993). For example, case IV-3 (Fig. 1) had no neonatal or febrile seizures and at age 15 years had three generalized tonic–clonic seizures over a few months. Seen in isolation, her epilepsy phenotype would be regarded as unrelated to benign familial neonatal convulsions, but the genotype data suggest that her adolescent seizures were probably due to the same gene.

Neurofibromatosis 1 (NF 1) is due to defects in a guanosine triphosphatase-activating protein, which regulates oncogenes (Gutmann & Collins, 1992), causing a highly variable phenotype including peripheral and central nervous system tumours. Although NF 1 is not usually regarded as an 'epilepsy syndrome', seizures occur in some cases, usually due to intracerebral lesions or dysplasia. Figure 2 shows a pair of identical twins with NF 1. One has epilepsy on the basis of a glioma and he underwent cranial irradiation, leading to short stature and other changes in appearance. The striking difference in phenotype between these two genetically identical individuals can be understood in terms of slight variation in expression of the tumour-predisposition gene, causing a variable pattern of intracranial tumours and other lesions, with superimposed acquired factors, including radiotherapy.

What does the example of NF 1 show us regarding the more general genotype–phenotype problem in the epilepsies? Consider if, in a similar, but hypothetical, autosomal dominant disease, the gene product did not result in structurally obvious tumours. Rather, it increased neuronal excitability due to a change in conformation of an ion channel or to altered binding characteristics of a neurotransmitter receptor. Such a structurally invisible abnormality could cause an 'idiopathic' epilepsy. If the variability in expression of the gene in this hypothetical disorder were similar to that in NF 1, the potential variation in epilepsy phenotype would be extremely difficult to understand without detailed molecular knowledge of the gene product.

Perspective on the phenotype–genotype problem

The above examples of phenotypes in epilepsies with known single-gene defects can be summarized

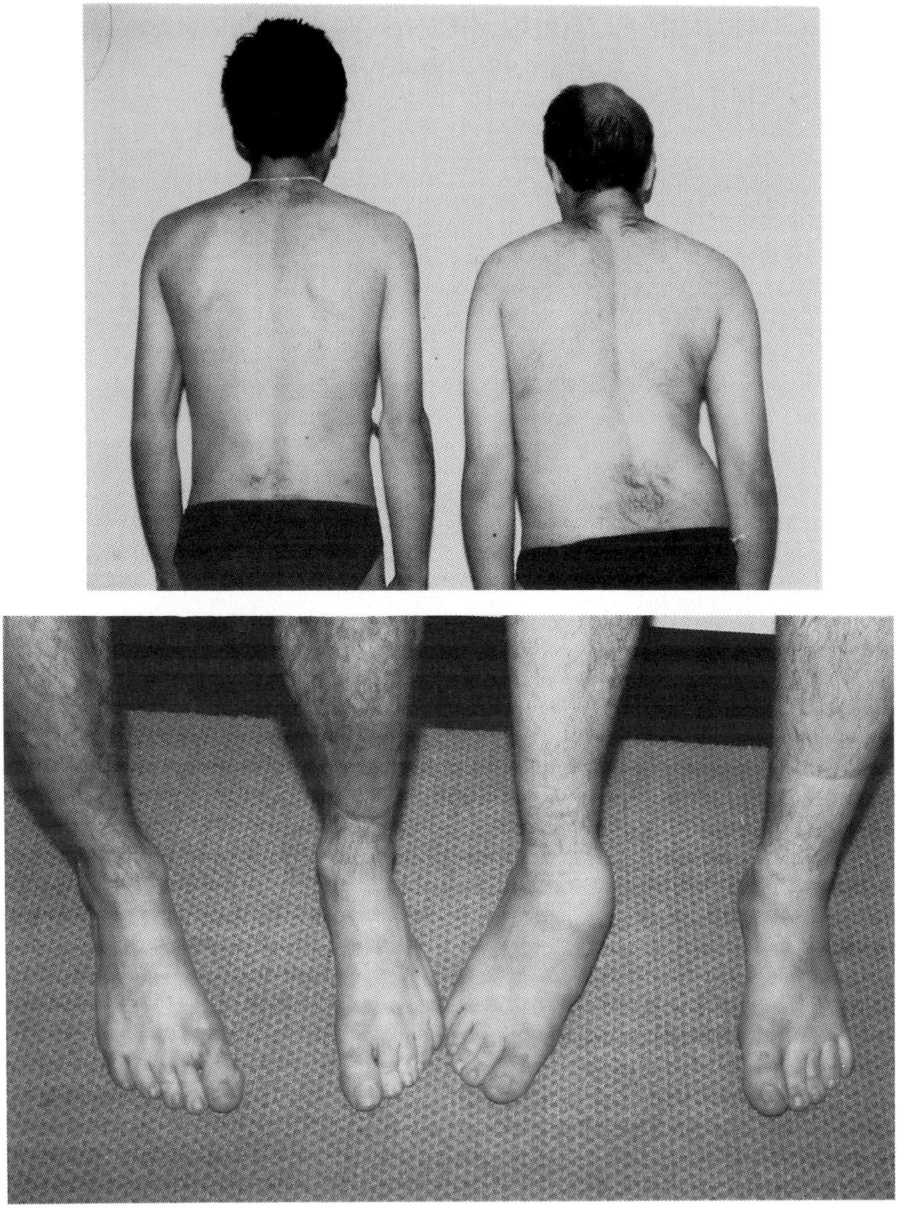

Fig. 2. Identical twins with neurofibromatosis 1.
Fig. 2a (top). The shorter twin, who has a scoliosis, has partial epilepsy associated with a parietal tumour treated with radiotherapy. Fig. 2b (bottom). He also has a plexiform neurofibroma of his right ankle; note the similarity of foot and toe shape.

thus. In general, phenotypic variability is relatively minor in autosomal recessive disorders, very marked in mitochondrial diseases and intermediate in autosomal dominant conditions. Autosomal recessive epilepsies are uncommon, and therefore we can expect considerable variability in most single-gene epilepsies.

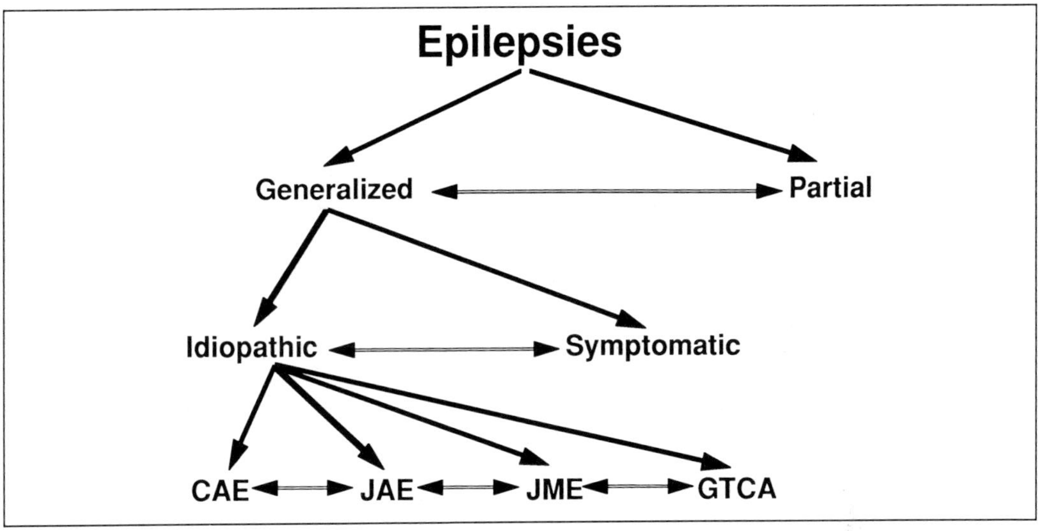

Fig. 3. Simplified classification of the epilepsies emphasizing the generalized epilepsies. Solid arrows indicate subdivisions of higher categories. Double-headed arrows indicate overlap between categories (CAE = childhood absence epilepsy; JAE = juvenile absence epilepsy; JME = juvenile myoclonic epilepsy; GTCA = generalized tonic–clonic seizures on awakening).

Other observations suggest further complexities in the phenotype–genotype problem. First, most common epilepsies are unlikely to be single-gene disorders. Current evidence suggests that they are polygenic or mutifactorial in origin (Andermann, 1982; Blandfort *et al.*, 1987; Doose & Baier, 1989). Second, new unconventional modes of inheritance are increasingly being recognized in neurological diseases. These include triplet repeat expansions and imprinting, which can cause hitherto unexplained variations in clinical phenotypes (Sutherland *et al.*, 1991; Hall, 1992; Ross *et al.*, 1993). With this background of the phenotypes occurring in certain single-gene epilepsies, we now examine the validity of the syndromic classification.

Epilepsy syndromes

Figure 3 is a simplified view of the classification of epilepsy syndromes (Commission, 1989), emphasizing the generalized epilepsies. We will examine the validity of 'splitting' the epilepsies at the three hierarchical levels shown by the horizontal double arrows.

Level 1: generalized and partial epilepsies

The classification recognizes two major groups of epilepsies; the generalized and the partial (localization-related) epilepsy syndrome.* In practice, it is usually possible to accurately categorize the majority of carefully studied patients into one of these two broad groups (Gastaut *et al.*, 1975; Juul-Jensen & Foldspang, 1983; Viani *et al.*, 1988; Eslava-Cobos & Narino, 1989; Loiseau *et al.*, 1991; Manford *et al.*, 1992; see also Berkovic *et al.*, Chapter 20). This has important implications regarding the search for an aetiology of the epilepsy, the choice of antiepileptic medication and other aspects of management.

The classification is based on both clinical and EEG evaluation, but the EEG can sometimes provide

* The group of special epileptic syndromes, including febrile convulsions, isolated seizures etc. are not considered here.

apparently contradictory data. For example, in certain partial epilepsies, generalized spike-and-wave discharges may occur, in addition to focal epileptiform abnormalities. Such partial epilepsies include benign partial epilepsy of childhood with centrotemporal spikes, where generalized spike-and-wave discharges can be found; the significance of this is discussed elsewhere in this volume. Secondly, some patients with chronic temporal lobe epilepsy also have generalized spike-and-wave discharges (Sadler & Blume, 1989). These patients do not usually suffer from seizures generalized from onset and they do well after temporal lobectomy, attesting to the focal nature of their epilepsy. Conversely, certain generalized epilepsies may also have focal epileptiform discharges. The epileptic syndrome associated with hypothalamic hamartomas has generalized seizures and generalized epileptiform discharges (Berkovic *et al.*, 1988). Some patients have seizures apparently arising from one temporal lobe, but the outcome from temporal lobectomy is dismal (Cascino *et al.*, 1993). Similar pseudofocalization may occur in patients with Lennox–Gastaut syndrome. The knowledgeable epileptologist has no difficulty in correctly classifying these cases, despite the apparently confusing EEG data.

It is well known, however, that there are epilepsies that defy the dichotomous division into generalized and partial epilepsies. The classification recognizes these as a subgroup undetermined as to whether they are partial or generalized epilepsies. Some appear to have both partial and generalized seizures, such as certain neonatal and early infantile epilepsies, Landau–Kleffner syndrome and epilepsy with continuous spike-waves during slow-wave sleep (Commission, 1989). There are also patients with diffuse frontal abnormalities where the interpretation of the epilepsy as a generalized or a multifocal problem can be extremely difficult, if not impossible.

Thus, whilst there is some overlap between the generalized and partial epilepsies, for the most part this can be resolved in the individual patients and an appropriate broad classification made.

Level 2: idiopathic and symptomatic generalized epilepsies

The division of generalized epilepsies into idiopathic and symptomatic forms is also a useful dichotomy (Fig. 3). For purposes of clarity, the term cryptogenic generalized epilepsy is avoided here; these cases are grouped together with symptomatic generalized epilepsy.

Idiopathic generalized epilepsies typically have the association of absence, myoclonic seizures and/or tonic–clonic seizures in a child or adolescent with a normal intellect and no neurological signs. The EEG shows generalized epileptiform spike-and-wave discharges at 3 Hz or faster, with normal background activity. These epilepsies are usually easily treatable and spontaneous remission may occur. In contrast, patients with symptomatic generalized epilepsies have atypical absences, tonic seizures and/or atonic seizures as well as tonic–clonic and myoclonic seizures, they often have intellectual disability and they may have focal neurological signs. The EEG shows a pattern of slow spike-and-wave discharges with abnormal background activity. The prognosis for both seizure control and spontaneous remission is much more gloomy.

This dichotomy is useful but it shows much greater blurring of boundaries than that between the generalized and partial epilepsies. One subgroup that lies between the idiopathic and symptomatic generalized epilepsies is epilepsy with myoclonic absences (Tassinari *et al.*, 1992) and another more ill-defined subgroup is so-called 'intermediate petit mal' (Lugaresi *et al.*, 1974). Niedermeyer (1972) examined the extent of overlap in his major treatise on the generalized epilepsies, where he attempted to classify 300 cases of generalized epilepsy. Sixty-one cases had pure idiopathic generalized epilepsy and 125 had symptomatic generalized epilepsy (Lennox–Gastaut syndrome). In addition, there were 72 patients with 'atypical' idiopathic generalized epilepsy, 26 cases regarded as secondary bilateral synchrony and 16 miscellaneous cases. Obviously the proportion of cases in different categories will vary greatly depending of the method of ascertainment.

The greatest difficulty in distinguishing idiopathic from symptomatic generalized epilepsies remains in the confusing area of the myoclonic epilepsies of infancy and early childhood (Jeavons, 1977;

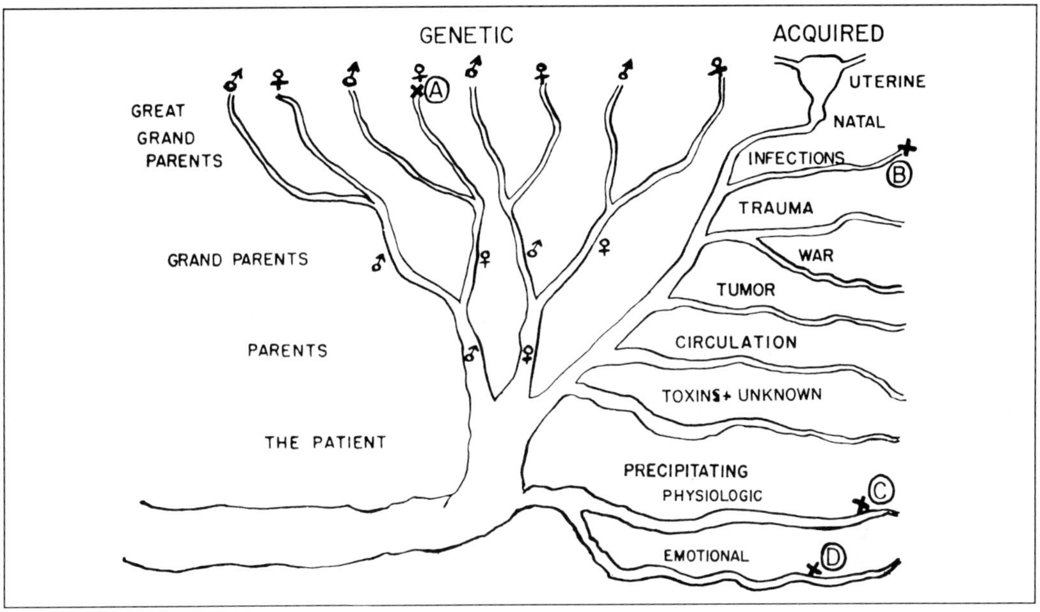

Fig. 4. William Lennox's concept of a 'river of epilepsy' illustrating how many factors may contribute to epilepsy in an individual patient (from Lennox & Lennox, 1960, p. 529).

Lombroso, 1990; Doose, 1992). Even in the area of absence epilepsies, however, where the distinction between typical and atypical absences appears relatively straightforward, critical study reveals evidence of a spectrum of features (Holmes *et al.*, 1987).

The neurobiological approach to the generalized epilepsies

The neurobiological approach allows us to conceptualize epileptic disorders in individual patients that do not fit into a described syndrome. The modern view of this has its roots in the work of William Lennox and was subsequently enunciated by Gloor and ourselves (Lennox & Lennox, 1960; Gloor, 1977; Andermann, 1982; Gloor *et al.*, 1982; Berkovic *et al.*, 1987). Lennox believed that the majority of patients with epilepsy had components of both genetic and acquired factors, which he colourfully described as a 'river of epilepsy' (Fig. 4) and illustrated diagrammatically (Fig. 5). This shows that every individual can have a seizure if exposed to enough convulsant such as metrazol (a purely acquired seizure 'disorder'), whereas a relatively pure genetic disorder would be represented by concordant identical twins with a typical idiopathic generalized epilepsy. In the middle are a large number of cases in whom there is a mixture of common genetic factors with superimposed acquired factors such as head injury, birth trauma, cerebral infection, etc. Perhaps the only major modification that one would make to this general scheme is that the influence of perinatal factors is now known to be far less than generally believed in Lennox's era. Expressed another way, the idiopathic and symptomatic generalized epilepsies lie at the ends of a spectrum; idiopathic generalized epilepsies are due to an inherited spike-wave trait or traits and the symptomatic generalized epilepsies are due to diffuse grey matter pathology (Fig. 6). In certain cases such grey matter pathology can be identified, be it inherited, such as in storage disorders (e.g. Lafora disease, ceroid lipofuscinosis), or acquired (e.g. diffuse anoxic injury), leading to symptomatic generalized epilepsies (Berkovic *et al.*, 1987). More commonly, the precise pathology is unknown although neuroimaging may show non-specific cerebral atrophy. In many cases the diffuse grey matter pathology is thought to be acquired but there

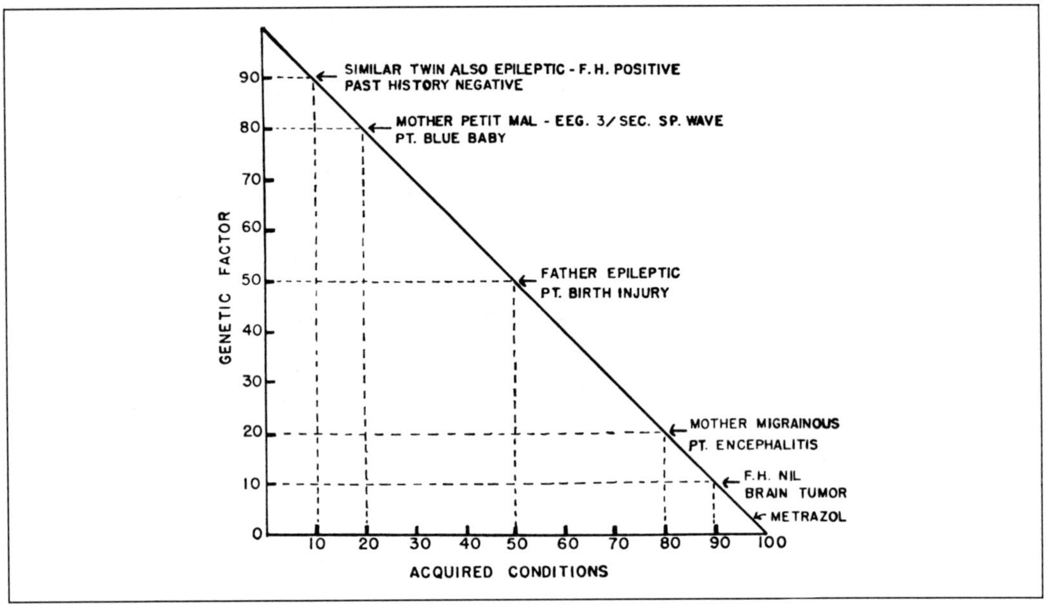

Fig. 5. William Lennox's diagram of the reciprocal contributions of genetic and acquired factors in various individuals with epilepsy (from Lennox & Lennox, 1960, p. 572).

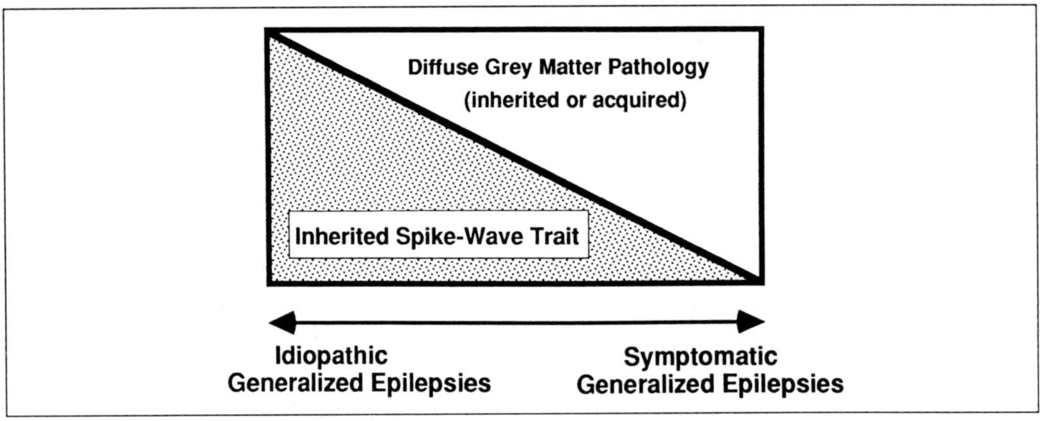

Fig. 6. Spectrum of the idiopathic and symptomatic generalized epilepsies (modified from Berkovic et al., 1987).

is increasing evidence for a more important genetic component in these epilepsies than previously appreciated (Janz *et al.*, 1992; Berkovic *et al.*, Chapter 20).

The complexities of the genetics of generalized epilepsies are beginning to be appreciated from family studies. Most affected relatives of probands with idiopathic generalized epilepsy will also have idiopathic generalized epilepsy, although not necessarily of the same subsyndrome (Janz *et al.*, 1992; Bianchi & the Italian League, 1993). In some families, however, one may see a wide spectrum of generalized epilepsy phenotypes, ranging from benign idiopathic generalized epilepsies to typical symptomatic generalized epilepsy (Scheffer & Berkovic, 1992). Janz *et al.* (1992) found 4.3 per cent of first-degree relatives of probands with symptomatic generalized epilepsies had seizures; 20 per cent of these relatives had symptomatic and 80 per cent had idiopathic generalized epilepsy syndromes.

Clinical application of the neurobiological approach

We must accept that the clinical and EEG features of some patients do not fit specific epilepsy syndrome phenotypes, that the spectrum of idiopathic and symptomatic generalized epilepsies is a real clinical phenomenon and that the multifactorial aetiology with genetic and acquired factors may be a useful model to explain this spectrum. In using the neurobiological approach in a patient in whom a specific epilepsy syndrome cannot be identified, we try to assess their individual epilepsy phenotype. This requires a detailed family history to search for genetic factors; the presence of a strong family history usually indicates a more benign type of generalized epilepsy. A careful history is taken for significant perinatal events and postnatal insults such as head trauma, cerebral infection, prolonged or complicated febrile convulsions, status epilepticus, etc. Care must be taken not to attribute too much significance to minor perinatal abnormalities, such as slight prematurity, cord around the neck, breech birth etc., or trivial postnatal head trauma that previously may have been given inappropriate emphasis. The neurological examination may detect subtle or overt neurological signs. A neuropsychological evaluation is important to detect intellectual impairment, both global and focal, that may reflect acquired brain damage. The EEG will show the characteristics of the spike-and-wave abnormality and of the background activity, which will aid in the assessment of the place in the spectrum of a particular case. Magnetic resonance imaging (MRI) is now essential for accurate classification of such patients. There is increasing realization of the importance of neuronal migration disorders that may present as generalized epilepsies. Moreover, MRI may also be of value in the assessment of the significance of a history of perinatal or postnatal injury.

These data are then amalgamated to formulate an overall profile of the patient's seizure disorder, which reflects both aetiology and prognosis. With an increased weighting of factors suggesting acquired brain disease, the prognosis becomes more guarded. For example, in a family with a number of affected individuals with idiopathic generalized epilepsy, the occurrence of a severe head injury or encephalitis in one affected member would explain why his/her phenotype is more refractory.

Level 3: subsyndromes of idiopathic generalized epilepsies

The international classification recognizes a number of subsyndromes of the idiopathic generalized epilepsies, including childhood absence epilepsy, juvenile absence epilepsy, juvenile myoclonic epilepsy and epilepsy with generalized tonic–clonic convulsions on awakening (Fig. 3). It is known that there is a degree of overlap between them, as acknowledged by Janz, one of the pioneers of this classification (Janz *et al.*, 1992).

Recently we evaluated by a standardized questionnaire a group of 101 patients with idiopathic generalized epilepsy beginning in adolescence (Table 1) in an attempt to determine how robust these categories were (Reutens, 1992). Thirty-seven cases had juvenile absence epilepsy and 21 juvenile myoclonic epilepsy but 28 had both prominent absence and myoclonus and represented a major overlap between these two subsyndromes. The category of generalized tonic–clonic seizures on awakening has been described as a broad syndromic category, encompassing others such as juvenile myoclonic epilepsy (Commission, 1989). Whilst we recognized patients that could fit into this broad group, we did not find this subsyndrome very useful. Of 17 patients with tonic–clonic seizures alone and diagnostic generalized epileptiform discharges on EEG, 10 had seizures predominantly on awakening and seven did not; these seven patients are currently not described within the subsyndromes of the international classification (Reutens, 1992).

What is the meaning of the obvious clinical and EEG overlap of these subsyndromes? Family studies show that there is a close genetic relationship between these subsyndromes. Different subsyndromes often appear in one family, although sometimes the same subsyndrome occurs in siblings or other close relatives (Janz *et al.*, 1992; Bianchi & the Italian League, 1993). Monozygous twins have identical subsyndromes, indicating that there are subtle genetic determinants of specific subsyndromes (Berkovic *et al.*, Chapter 20). The data suggest that these epilepsies are determined by multiple genes, with a probable small role for acquired factors. The frequent occurrence of different subsyndromes in single families suggests that some of the genes determining phenotype are very common. Minor variations in phenotype in similar subsyndromes from the same or different families can thus be explained. Excessive further splitting of these phenotypes on the basis of slight phenotypic differences is unlikely to be meaningful from either the clinical or the neurobiological perspective.

Table 1. Phenotypes in 101 cases of idiopathic generalized epilepsy in adolescence (Reutens, 1992)

Absence ± tonic–clonic (JAE)			37
Myoclonus ± tonic–clonic (JME)			21
Myoclonus ± Absence ± tonic–clonic			26
Tonic–clonic alone			17
	On a wakening	10	
	Not on awakening	7	

JAE = juvenile absence epilepsy; JME = juvenile myoclonic epilepsy.

Conclusion

There is no doubt that the syndromic classification can be valuable for clinical purposes. Knowledge of these syndromes helps in the diagnosis of new cases and allows rapid identification of the correct form of treatment, including drugs and lifestyle management. It must be acknowledged, however, that the syndromes cannot be applied to all patients. We already know that single-gene disorders can cause heterogeneous epilepsy phenotypes by a number of known mechanisms but probably also by numerous unknown mechanisms. It is likely that the common epilepsies are determined by multiple genes plus acquired factors. The view that these syndromes are 'pure' and tightly defined cannot be defended on the basis of current clinical data, and rigid adherence to this view is unlikely to lead to advances in the understanding of the biological basis of the epilepsies.

We can encapsulate the historical and long-running battle between 'lumpers' and 'splitters' in a modern practical context as follows. The clinician must be familiar with the details of the syndromic classification to provide his/her patients with accurate diagnostic, prognostic, genetic and management information. The assessment of each individual with epilepsy should include an attempt at using the syndromic classification. The clinician must, however, be wary of cases that stray from the description of specific syndromes from the clinical, EEG, anatomical, aetiological or therapeutic points of view and be prepared to use a neurobiological approach to understand and manage such patients. On the other hand, the basic scientist should use the hierarchical syndromic approach as a general guide to the epilepsies, but adopt a broad neurobiological perspective in formulating specific questions to be addressed in the laboratory.

Future classifications of the epilepsies could incorporate a multi-armed formulation similar to the Diagnostic and statistical manual of mental disorders, 4th edition (DSM-IV) used in psychiatry. Any additional effort may well be justified by leading to a more accurate and comprehensive description of human epilepsies.

Acknowledgements

Supported by grants from the National Health & Medical Research Council (NH&MRC) of Australia and the Austin Hospital Medical Research Foundation to Dr Berkovic, and by a Ciba-Geigy (Australia) Epilepsy Fellowship and an NH&MRC Postgraduate Fellowship to Dr Reutens.

References

Andermann, E. (1982): Multifactorial inheritance of generalized and focal epilepsy. In: *Genetic basis of the epilepsies*, eds. V.E. Anderson, W.A. Hauser, J.K. Penry & C.F. Sing, pp. 129–145. New York: Raven Press.

Berkovic, S.F., Andermann, F., Andermann, E. & Gloor, P. (1987): Concepts of absence epilepsies: discrete syndromes or biological continuum? *Neurology* **37,** 993–1000.

Berkovic, S.F., Andermann, F., Melanson, D., Ethier, R., Feindel, W. & Gloor, P. (1988): Hypothalamic hamartomas and associated evolution of the characteristic epileptic syndrome and diagnostic value of magnetic resonance imaging. *Ann. Neurol.* **23,** 429–439.

Berkovic, S.F., Carpenter, S., Evans, A., Karpati, G., Shoubridge, E.A., Andermann, F., Meyer, E., Tyler, J.L., Diksic, M., Arnold, D., Wolfe, L.S., Andermann, E. & Hakim, A.M. (1989): Myoclonus epilepsy and ragged-red fibers (MERRF) 1. A clinical, pathological, biochemical, magnetic resonance spectroscopic and positron emission tomographic study. *Brain* **112,** 1231–1260.

Berkovic, S.F., Shoubridge, E.A., Andermann, F., Andermann, E., Carpenter, S. & Karpati, G. (1991): Clinical spectrum of mitochondrial DNA mutation at base pair 8344. *Lancet* **338,** 457.

Berkovic, S.F., Cochius, J., Andermann, E. & Andermann, F. (1993): Progressive myoclonus epilepsies: clinical and genetic aspects. *Epilepsia* **34** (Suppl. 3), S19–S30.

Berkovic, S.F., Kennerson, M.L., Howell, R.A., Scheffer, I.E., Hwang, P.A. & Nicholson, G.A. (1994): Phenotypic expression of benign familial neonatal convulsions linked to chromosome 20. *Arch. Neurol.* (in press).

Bianchi, A. & the Italian League Against Epilepsy (1993): The concordance of clinical forms of epilepsy in families with several affected members. *Epilepsia* **34,** 819–816.

Blandfort, M., Tsuboi, T. & Vogel, F. (1987): Genetic counseling in the epilepsies. *Hum. Genet.* **76,** 303–331.

Cascino, G.D., Andermann, F., Berkovic, S.F., Kuzniecky, R.I., Sharbrough, F.W., Keene, D.L., Bladin, P.F., Kelly, P.J., Oliver, A. & Feindel, W. (1993): Gelastic seizures and hypothalamic hamartomas: evaluation of patients undergoing chronic intracranial EEG monitoring and outcome of surgical treatment. *Neurology* **43,** 747–750.

Commission on Classification and Terminology of the International League Against Epilepsy (1985): Proposal for classification of epilepsies and epileptic syndromes. *Epilepsia* **26,** 268–278.

Commission on Classification and Terminology of the International League Against Epilepsy (1989): Proposal for revised classification of epilepsies and epileptic syndromes. *Epilepsia* **30,** 389–399.

Doose, H. (1992): Myoclonic astatic epilepsy of early childhood. In: *Epileptic syndromes in infancy, childhood and adolescence*, eds. J. Roger, M. Bureau, Ch. Dravet, F.E. Dreifuss, A. Perret & P. Wolf, pp. 103–114. London: John Libbey.

Doose, H. & Baier, W. (1989): Genetic aspects of childhood epilepsy. *Clev. Clin. J. Med.* **56** (suppl.), S105–S11O.

Eldridge, R., Iivanainen, M., Stern, R., Koerber, T. & Wilder, B.J. (1983): 'Baltic' myoclonus epilepsy: hereditary disorder of childhood made worse by phenytoin. *Lancet* **ii,** 838–842.

Eslava-Cobos, J. & Narino, D. (1989): Experience with the Interational League Against Epilepsy proposals for classification of epileptic seizures and the epilepsies and epileptic syndromes in a pediatric outpatient clinic. *Epilepsia* **30,** 112–115.

Gastaut, H. & Zifkin, B.G. (1985): Classification of the epilepsies. *J. Clin. Neurophysiol.* **2,** 313–326.

Gastaut, H., Gastaut, J., Goncalves, E., Silva, G. & Fernandes Sanchez, G. (1975): Relative frequency of different types of epilepsy: a study employing the classification of the International League Against Epilepsy. *Epilepsia* **16,** 457–461.

Gloor, P. (1977): The EEG and differential diagnosis of epilepsy. In: *Current concepts in clinical neurophysiology*, eds. H. van Duijn, D.N.J. Donker & A.C. van Huffelen, pp. 9–21. The Hague: Trio.

Gloor, P., Metrakos, J., Metrakos, K., Andermann, E. & Van Gelder, N. (1982): Neurophysiological, genetic and biochemical nature of the epileptic diathesis. *Electroencephalogr. Clin. Neurophysiol.* (Suppl. 35), 45–56.

Graf, W.D., Sumi, S.M., Copass, M.K., Ojemann, L.M., Longstreth, W.T. Jr, Shanske, S., Lombes, A. & DiMauro, S. (1993): Phenotypic heterogeneity in families with the myoclonic epilepsy and ragged-red fiber disease point mutation in mitochondrial DNA. *Ann. Neurol.* **33,** 640–645.

Gutmann, D.H. & Collins, F.S. (1992): Recent progress towards understanding the molecular biology of von Recklinghausen neurofibromatosis. *Ann. Neurol.* **31,** 555–561.

Hall, J.G. (1992): Genomic imprinting and its clinical implications. *N. Engl. J. Med.* **326,** 827–829.

Hammans, S.R., Sweeney, M.G., Brockington, M., Lennox, G.G., Lawton, N.F., Kennedy, C.R., Morgan-Hughes, J.A. & Harding, A.E. (1993): The mitochondrial DNA transfer RNA^{Lys} $A \rightarrow G^{(8344)}$ mutation and the syndrome of myoclonic epilepsy with ragged-red fibers (MERRF). *Brain* **116,** 617–632.

Holmes, G.L., McKeever, M. & Adamson, M. (1987): Absence seizures in children: clinical and electroencephalographic features. *Ann. Neurol.* **21,** 268–273.

Janz, D., Beck-Mannagetta, G. & Sander, T. (1992): Do idiopathic generalized epilepsies share a common susceptibility gene? *Neurology* **42** (Suppl. 5), 48–55.

Jeavons, P.M. (1977): Nosological problems of myoclonic epilepsies in childhood and adolescence. *Dev. Med. Child Neurol.* **19,** 3–8.

Juul-Jensen, P. & Foldspang, A. (1983): Natural history of epileptic seizures. *Epilepsia* **24,** 297–312.

Lehesjoki, A.E., Koskiniemi, M., Sistonen, P., Miao, J., Hästbacka, J., Norio, R. & de la Chapelle, A. (1991): Localization of a gene for progressive myoclonus epilepsy to chromosome 21q22. *Proc. Nat. Acad. Sci. USA* **88,** 3696–3699.

Lennox, W.G. & Lennox, M.A. (1960): *Epilepsy and related disorders.* Boston: Little Brown.

Leppert, M., Anderson, V.E., Quattlebaum, T., Stauffer, D., O'Connell, P., Nakamura, Y., Lalouel, J.-M. & White, R. (1989): Benign familial neonatal convulsions linked to genetic markers on chromosome 20. *Nature* **337,** 647–648.

Lewis, T.B., Leach, R.J., Ward, K., O'Connell, P. & Ryan, S.G. (1993): Genetic heterogeneity in benign familial neonatal convulsions: identification of a new locus on chromosome 8 q. *Am. J. Hum. Genet* **53,** 670–676.

Loiseau, P., Duche, B. & Loiseau, J. (1991): Classification of epilepsies and epileptic syndromes in two different samples of patients. *Epilepsia* **32,** 303–309.

Lombroso, C.T. (1990): Early myoclonic encephalopathy, early infantile epileptic encephalopathy, and benign and severe infantile myoclonic epilepsies: a critical review and personal contributions. *J. Clin. Neurophysiol.* **7,** 380–408.

Lugaresi, E., Pazzaglia, P., Roger, J. & Tassinari, C.A. (1974): Evolution and prognosis of petit mal. In: *Epilepsy: proceedings of the Hans Berger centenary symposium,* eds. P. Harris & C. Mawdsley, pp. 151–153. Edinburgh: Churchill Livingstone.

Mackay, R.P. (1960): All epilepsy is one. *Arch. Neurol.* **2,** 237–246.

Malafosse, A., Lehesjoki, A.E., Genton, P., Labauge, P., Durand, G., Tassinari, C.A., Dravet, Ch., Michelucci & de la Chapelle, A. (1992a): Identical genetic locus for Baltic and Mediterranean myoclonus. *Lancet* **339,** 1080–1081.

Malafosse, A., Leboyer, M., Dulac, O., Navelet, Y., Plouin, P., Beck, C., Laklou, H., Mouchnino, G., Grandscene, P., Vallee, L., Guilloud-Bataille, M., Samolyk, D., Baldy-Moulinier, M., Feingold, J. & Mallet, J. (1992b): Confirmation of linkage of benign familial neonatal convulsions to D20S19 and D20S20. *Hum. Genet.* **89,** 54–58.

Manford, M., Hart, Y.M., Sander, J.W.A.S. & Shorvon, S.D. (1992): National General Practice Study of Epilepsy: the syndromic classification of the Interational League Against Epilepsy applied to epilepsy in a general population. *Arch. Neurol.* **49,** 801–808.

Marseille Consensus Group (1990): Classification of progressive myoclonus epilepsies and related disorders. *Ann. Neurol.* **28,** 113–116.

Merlis, J.K. (1970): Proposal for an international classification of the epilepsies. *Epilepsia* **11,** 114–119.

Niedermeyer, E. (1972): *The generalized epilepsies.* Springfield, Illinois: Charles C. Thomas.

Plouin, P. (1992): Benign idiopathic neonatal convulsions (familial and non-familial). In: *Epileptic syndromes in infancy, childhood and adolescence,* 2nd edn, eds. J. Roger, M. Bureau, C. Dravet, F.E. Dreifuss, A. Perret & P. Wolf, pp. 3–11. London: John Libbey.

Reutens, D.C. (1992): Aspects of the nosology and pathophysiology of the idiopathic generalised epilepsies of adolescence. University of Melbourne: PhD thesis.

Reutens, D.C. (1993): Idiopathic generalised epilepsy of adolescence: relationship between the syndromes. *Brain* (in press).

Reynolds, E.H. (1988): Hughlings Jackson: a Yorkshireman's contribution to epilepsy. *Arch. Neurol.* **45,** 675–678.

Roger, J., Bureau M., Dravet C., Dreifuss, F.E., Perret, A. & Wolf, P. (1992): *Epileptic syndromes in infancy, childhood and adolescence,* 2nd edition, London: John Libbey.

Ronen, G.M., Rosales, T.O., Connolly, Y., Anderson, V.E. & Leppert, M. (1993): Seizure characteristics in chromosome 20 benign familial neonatal convulsions. *Neurology* **43,** 1355–1360.

Ross, C.A., McInnis, M.G., Margolis, R.L. & Li, S.H. (1993): Genes with triplet repeats: candidate mediators of neuropsychiatric disorders. *TINS* **16,** 254–260.

Ryan, S.G., Wiznitzer, M., Hollman, C., Torres, C.M., Szekeresova, M. & Schneider, S. (1991): Benign familial neonatal convulsions: evidence for clinical and genetic heterogeneity. *Ann. Neurol.* **29,** 469–473.

Sadler, R.M. & Blume, W.T. (1989): Significance of bisynchronous spike-waves in patients with temporal lobe spikes. *Epilepsia* **30,** 143–146.

Scheffer, I.E. & Berkovic, S.F. (1992): Phenotypic heterogeneity in an exceptional multiplex family with generalized epilepsy. *Epilepsia* **33** (Suppl. 3), 74.

Shoffner, J.M., Lott, M.T., Lezza, A.M.S., Seibel, P., Ballinger, S.W. & Wallace, D.C. (1990): Myoclonic epilepsy and ragged-red fiber disease (MERRF) is associated with a mitochondrial DNA $tRNA^{Lys}$mutation. Cell **61,** 931–937.

Silvestri, G., Ciafaloni, E., Santorelli, F.M., Shanske, S., Servidei, S., Graf, W.d., Sumi, M. & DiMauro, S. (1993): Clinical features associated with the A→G transition at nucleotide 8344 of mtDNA ('MERRF mutation'). *Neurology* **43,** 1200–1206.

Sutherland, G.R., Haan, E.A., Kremer, E., Lynch, M., Pritchard, M., Yu, S. & Richards, R.I. (1991): Hereditary unstable DNA: a new explanation for some genetic questions? *Lancet* **338,** 289–292.

Tassinari, C.A., Bureau, M. & Thomas, P. (1992): Epilepsy with myoclonic absences. In: *Epileptic syndromes in infancy, childhood and adolescence,* 2nd edn, eds. J. Roger, M. Bureau, C. Dravet, F.E. Dreifuss, A. Perret & P. Wolf, pp. 151–160. London: John Libbey.

Tissot, S.A. (1772): *Traité de l'épilepsie.* p. 419. Paris.

Viani, F., Beghi, E., Atza, G. & Gulotta, M.P. (1988): Classifications of epileptic syndromes: advantages and limitations for evaluation of childhood epileptic syndromes in clinical practice. *Epilepsia* **29,** 440–445.

Yoneda, M., Tanno, Y., Horai, S., Ozawa, T., Miyatake, T., Tsuji, S. (1990): A common mitochondrial DNA mutation in the $tRNA^{Lys}$ of patients with myoclonic epilepsy and ragged-red fibers. *Biochem. Int.* **21,** 789–796.

Zeviani, M., Amati, P., Bresolin, N., Antozzi, C., Piccolo, G., Toscano, A. & DiDonato, S. (1991): Rapid detection of the A→G (8344) mutation of mtDNA in Italian families with myoclonus-epilepsy and ragged red fibers (MERRF). *Am. J. Hum. Genet.* **48,** 203–211.

Section II

From seizures to syndromes

Seizures may be precipitated by specific stimuli, simple as well as complex. How correct is it to call these 'reflex' seizures? What can they teach us about the part played by normal neuronal activity in the basic mechanisms of seizure generation? To what extent are they fortuitous individual additions to the clinical picture, traits common to patient groups extending across the syndromes (e.g. photosensitivity), or the pivotal feature of syndromes which otherwise would not exist (e.g. reading epilepsy)?

In the discussions on complex reflex epilepsies (reading, praxis, eating) two different theoretical concepts arise which at first glance only are similar: a concept of functional complexity of the tasks leading to seizure precipitation (Wolf, Chapter 9; Inoue *et al.*, Chapter 11); and a 'critical mass' concept where epileptic neurones of a 'group two' are temporarily recruited to produce a seizure (Zifkin *et al.*, Chapter 13). Whereas the former concept is qualitative and highly specific, the latter is quantitative and rather non-specific. Zifkin *et al.* seem to suggest that their hypothesis should be applied universally to all complex modalities of seizure precipitation. Alternatively, some of these modalities could follow the one and others the other model. In fact, the authors of the first-mentioned chapters have good reason to treat their subjects as syndromes, whereas the authors of seizure precipitation by eating have good arguments that this does not constitute a syndrome.

Specific seizure precipitation may occur in both focal and generalized epilepsies but may raise the question of how generalized 'generalized' epilepsies really are. In relation to the problem of the epileptic focus, analysis of focal 'reflex' epilepsies seems to indicate that their specificity is a matter of well-established functional interplay rather than spatial delimitation.

Absences are another case: at first glance they may seem to be one of the least ambiguous, most straightforward seizure types. Are not all absence epilepsies really one, previously called petit mal? Most authors in this section, however, do not believe that, and new subvarieties – regarding both semiology and syndromatology – are discussed. To the views presented here, the even more radical one of Lüders *et al.* (Chapter 3) may be added that absences should be diagnosed without reference being made to the EEG, and the term should not be kept restricted to generalized epilepsies.

Epileptic Seizures and Syndromes, Edited by Peter Wolf
© 1994 John Libbey & Company Ltd., pp. 41–48

Chapter 6

Photosensitive epilepsy as an age-related genetic disorder

Dorothée G.A. Kasteleijn-Nolst Trenité*, Walter van Emde Boas* and Colin D. Binnie†

**IDepartment of Clinical Neurophysiology, Instituut voor Epilepsiebestrijding, Achterweg 5, 2103 SW Heemstede, The Netherlands; †The Maudsley Hospital, Denmark Hill, London SE5 8AZ, UK*

Summary

Photosensitivity can be regarded as a separate syndrome. About 5 per cent of epileptic Caucasian patients are photosensitive, i.e. show generalized epileptiform discharges in their electroencephalogram during intermittent photic stimulation (IPS), outlasting the stimulus train. The peak prevalence is between 10 and 25 years of age, with a female-to-male ratio of 1.5.

Sixty-three per cent of the photosensitive patients have a history of visually induced seizures, such as provoked by television, sunlight and artificial lighting. Although 60 per cent of these patients belong to the idiopathic generalized epilepsy group, they do not exclusively belong to this category.

Follow-up of 64 patients for an average of 7 years reveals no consistent relationship between intake of antiepileptic drugs (AEDs) and occurrence of classical photoparoxysmal responses to IPS. Evaluation of patients without AEDs (in order to investigate the natural history) shows a gradual decrease after puberty, with a more clear reduction at the age of 25. This striking age dependency of the phenotypical expression of the response to IPS strongly suggests expression of a genetic trait.

Introduction

Visual stimuli can induce seizures in about 5 per cent of epileptic patients. Although some authors have suggested the use of the term sensory-evoked or stimulus-sensitive epilepsy (Aicardi, 1986), most clinical investigators nevertheless use the term reflex epilepsy, in which attacks can be triggered by external stimuli, when referring to this special form of epilepsy.

Photosensitive epilepsy, the most common form of sensory-evoked epilepsy, was first described in detail by Gowers in 1885 (Gowers, 1964). His patient had seizures when looking into bright sunlight. After the invention of the electroencephalograph (EEG) by Berger in 1929, various methods were tried out to influence normal brain rhythms. Walker *et al.* described the phenomenon of photic driving in 1944. Subsequently, Walter *et al.* discovered in 1946 that flickering light could evoke epileptiform discharges in some subjects. Furthermore, absence seizures could be triggered by intermittent light stimulation. It has since then become general practice to use photic stimulation as one of the activating

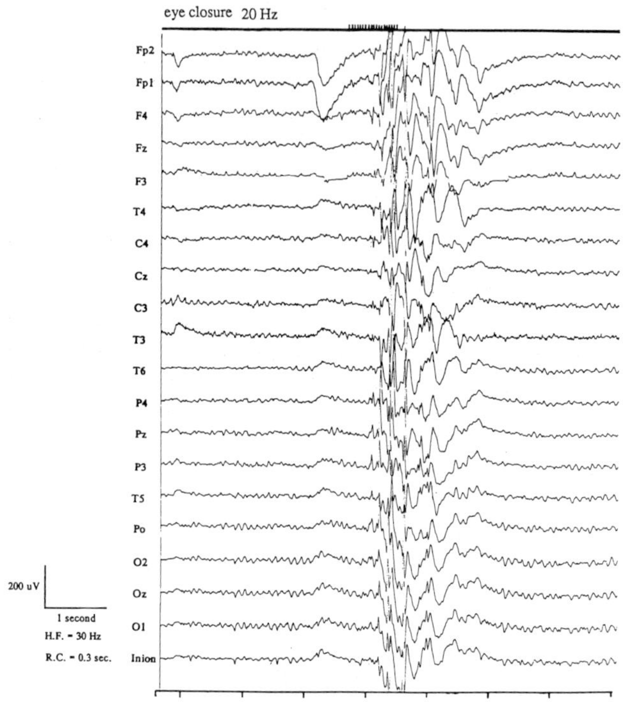

Fig. 1. An example of a classical photoparoxysmal response (CPPR) to intermittent photic stimulation (IPS) with 20 Hz performed during eye closure.

methods in routine EEG recordings in the investigation of patients with suspected epilepsy. Many different EEG reactions can be evoked by intermittent photic stimulation (IPS), ranging from photic driving with harmonics and subharmonics, occipital spiking and generalized spikes at the stimulus frequency up to pathological responses such as generalized polyspike-wave discharges. This last-mentioned response is known as the Bickford criterion and is strongly related to a history of epilepsy, especially when associated with myoclonic jerks. The positive association with clinical epilepsy is more than 90 per cent if the generalized discharges outlast the stimulus train (Reilly & Peters, 1973; see Fig. 1 for an example).

In order to establish the relation between the occurrence of this 'classical photoparoxysmal response' to IPS in the EEG laboratory and the occurrence of visually induced seizures in daily life, we performed in the 1980s a prospective prevalence study in patients attending the EEG clinic of a tertiary referral epilepsy centre. Special emphasis was given to seizure history and electrophysiological findings.

Of the 100 extensively investigated photosensitive patients, 64 were followed-up for an average of 7 years. Using the standardized IPS method repeatedly at different ages, their photosensitivity could be measured quantitatively and qualitatively, i.e. range and type of response (see Kasteleijn-Nolst Trenité, 1989). Antiepileptic drugs (AEDs) are, however, known to influence the response IPS to both acutely (Binnie *et al.*, 1985) and chronically (Jeavons *et al.*, 1986). Whether or not pharmacodynamic or pharmacokinetic tolerance to the drugs occurs still has to be established. Therefore, we selected the IPS results of photosensitive patients not taking AEDs in order to establish the natural history of photosensitivity.

Methods

Between 1980 and 1983 all patients found to be photosensitive on routine clinical EEG investigation were eligible for admission to the study. During that period a total of 2342 patients were referred for EEG examination. On initial screening 138 patients (5.6 per cent) appeared to be photosensitive, whereas 40 (1.8 per cent) showed a reaction to IPS that did not meet our criteria of a classical photoparoxysmal response. Eventually, after a second extended EEG examination, 100 patients who were consistently photosensitive were studied. Because of the predominance of the female sex and the 10- to 25-year age-group in photosensitive patients, they were compared with age- and sex-matched controls in our prospective study. Furthermore, this control group was matched on the variable in- and out-patient, the majority being out-patients.

A standardized procedure in performing IPS has been developed in our laboratory. This makes it possible to determine lower and upper limits of flash frequencies to which the individual patient is sensitive (the photosensitivity range, as it is called by Jeavons & Harding, (1975)). This seems to be a reliable, reproducible measure of epileptogenicity in photosensitive patients. This photosensitivity range was subsequently determined during control EEG recordings in 64 of the previously selected 100 patients, as well as in 84 patients referred to our laboratory in the mid- and late 1980s. This was done for several clinical reasons, such as evaluation of the effect of medication on the visual sensitivity or prediction of relapse of seizures after (partial) AED withdrawal. Furthermore, it gave information on age-dependent diminution or abolition of the photosensitivity range. In order to determine the natural history of photosensitivity, only those data on IPS had been used when the patient was without any AEDs for at least 2 months.

Results and discussion

Prevalence study

In Fig. 2 the sex and age distribution of the photosensitive patients in relation to the distribution in the whole EEG population is given. The prevalence of about 5 per cent with a preponderance of females among Caucasians with epilepsy is a general finding. Wolf and Goosses (1986) found a prevalence of 9.9 per cent in about 1000 epileptic patients. They, however, used a less restricted definition of a photoparoxysmal response. The peak prevalence between the age of 10 and 25 years old was also established by Jeavons and Harding (1975) and Wolf and Goosses (1986). The female-to-male ratio of 1.5 proved in our series to be independent of age. Although many authors

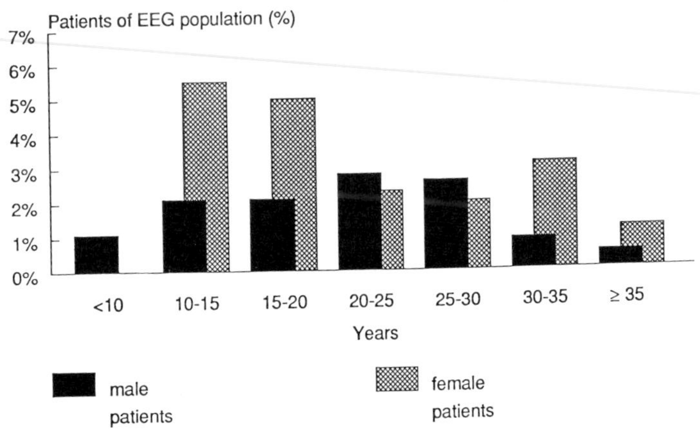

Fig. 2. Percentage photosensitive patients of EEG population in different age-groups.

suggested fluctuating hormonal influence in photosensitivity because of the greater prevalence in women, especially at puberty, our results of unaltered female-to-male ratios at different ages make it more likely that genetic influences play a major role in these sex differences. Furthermore, female photosensitive patients do not show consistent changes when examined on different days of their menstrual cycle.

A total of 94 of the photosensitive patients had a history of epilepsy, including five patients with additional psychogenic seizures, whereas a history of true epilepsy was only found in 84 of the 100 control subjects. Thus, indeed, the finding of a classical photoparoxysmal response is indicative for a history of epilepsy. No significant difference was found in age of onset of seizures between photosensitive patients and controls. The photosensitive group had a mean age of onset of 8.8 years, with a range of 6 months to 48 years. Jeavons and Harding (1975) found a higher mean age of onset (13.7 years), which cannot be explained other than by the selected population in their study.

In agreement with the study of Jeavons and Harding (1975), a high prevalence of myoclonic and absence seizures was found. Photosensitive patients more often have a history of either absences or myoclonic seizures, whereas the control patients more often have partial seizures (see Tables 1 and 2). As is commonly accepted, photosensitive patients do indeed have predominantly generalized seizures, usually in combination with absence seizures, myoclonus or both.

Table 1. Seizure type distribution in percentages per patient in 94 photosensitive patients and 84 non-photosensitive controls

	Photosensitive patients	Control patients
One type only	29%	37%
Tonic–clonic	16	17
Absence	7	3
Myoclonus	2	–
Partial	4	8
Psychogenic	–	9
More than one type	71%	63%
± tonic–clonic ± absence ± myoclonus	38	8
± tonic clonic ± partial	20	45
Other	13	10

A total of 63 per cent of the 94 photosensitive patients had a history of visually and sometimes self-induced seizures, while no relationship was found between an individual seizure type and a history of visually evoked or self-induced seizures. The spontaneously occurring seizures could, however, also be visually precipitated, while patients are often not aware of possible provocative stimuli such as escalators, venetian blinds etc. The television set was most often reported as visual stimulus (35 patients), followed by sunlight (31 patients) and artificial lighting (21 patients).

Beside the occurrence of generalized epileptiform discharges evoked by IPS, photosensitive patients more often presented a poorly organized posterior-dominant rhythm than the controls, although a higher mean frequency of alpha rhythm was found. No other differences were found with regard to occurrence of spontaneous focal or generalized epileptiform activity. Although most patients are sensitive in the range of 10–30 flashes/s, individual differences can be found. Patients with a greater photosensitivity range are more likely to experience response to visual stimuli in daily life.

Table 2. Seizure type and relation to circumstances of occurrence in 94 photosensitive patients with a history of seizures

	Total number of points	Spontaneous seizure only	Visual evoked seizure only	Both
Primary generalized				
Tonic–clonic	43	25	7	11
Absence	34	20	6	3
Myoclonus	31	18	5	4
Tonic	2	1	1	–
Secondary generalized				
Tonic–clonic	34	21	2	11
Atonic/akinetic	5	3	1	–
Unilateral	5	2	1	2
Simple partial	7	6	–	1
Complex partial	26	13	3	10
Unclassifiable	4	3	1	–
Psychogenic	5	5	–	–

Note: more than one seizure type in 69 out of 94 patients.

A total of 40 per cent of photosensitive patients did not have an idiopathic generalized epilepsy. If our patients should therefore be classified according to the revised epilepsy classification as proposed in 1989, they would be subdivided. Although this new classification recognizes the existence of epilepsies with seizures precipitated by specific modes of activation, photosensitivity, as such, is not in this classification (Commission on Classification and Terminology of the International League Against Epilepsy, 1989)).

Table 3. IPS results at latest EEG examination in relation to use of antiepileptic drugs (AEDs) in 64 photosensitive patients

AED/IPS	Positive	Negative	Total
Yes	29	16	45*
No	13	6	19
Total	42	22	64

* 40 out of these 45 patients used valproic acid medication (15 polytherapy).

Follow-up

A total of 64 of these patients were followed up during an average of 7.3 years, with a range of 1–13 years. The average age of latest IPS examination was 25.6 years (range 9 to 71 years), while 43 patients were at least 21 years of age. Thus the majority of the unselected patient group were followed for many years. Of these 64 patients (24 male/40 female), a total of 22 (30 per cent) did not show a classical photoparoxysmal response to IPS (see Table 3). Most of the IPS-negative patients were on medication. Remarkably, however, there was no significant relation between use of AEDs and whether or not the patient was still photosensitive (see Table 3). A total of 40 out of the 65 (63 per cent) patients took valproic acid, a drug which is known to be very effective in treatment of photosensitive patients. On initial investigation, 44 of the 100 (44 per cent) photosensitive patients took valproic acid. A possible explanation is the occurrence of tolerance – either pharmacokinetic tolerance, due to liver enzyme autoinduction and subsequent lowering of the drug plasma levels, or pharmacodynamic tolerance, i.e. loss of sensitivity of the target organ for the drug itself. Although some patients seem to develop pharmacodynamic (functional) tolerance, a standardized prospective study in initially naïve photosensitive patients is necessary to answer this adequately. Jeavons *et al.* (1986) followed up 86 patients with a mean age on final assessment of 22.5 ± 4.6 years, with a follow-up length varying from 2–23 years. A total of 64 of their 86 patients (74 per cent) took valproic

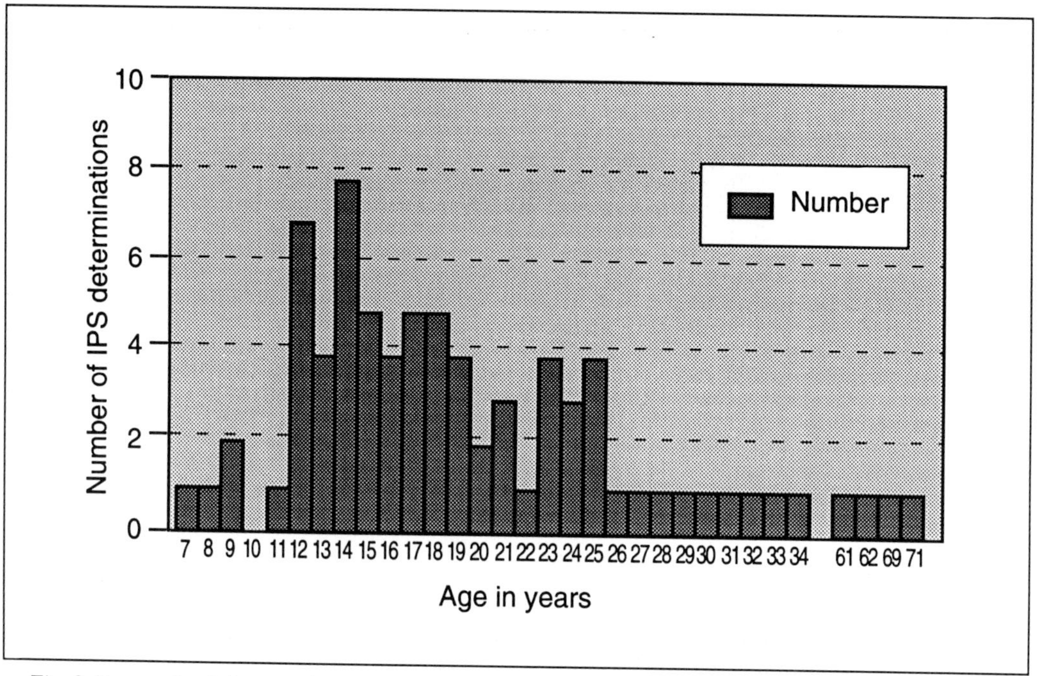

Fig. 3. Prognosis of photosensitivity in 26 patients without AEDs. Number of JPS determinations vs. age.

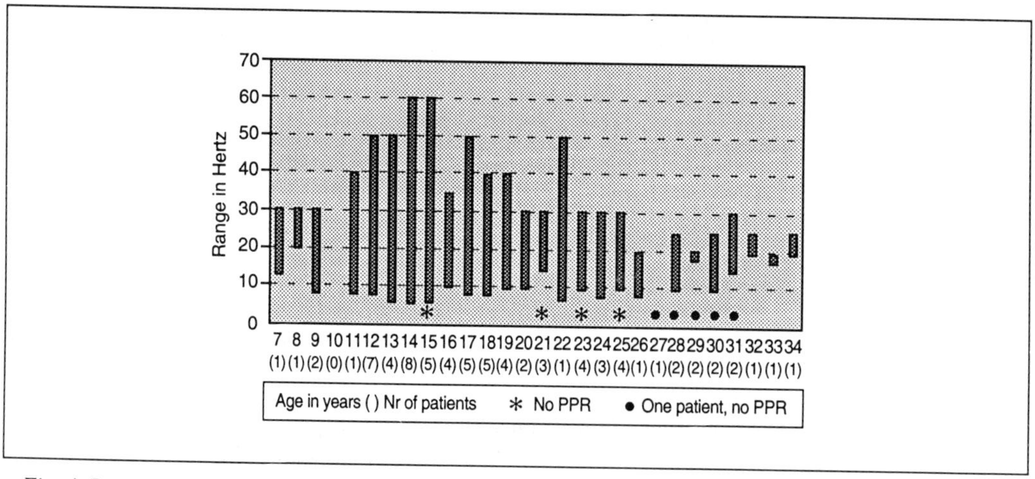

Fig. 4. Prognosis of photosensitivity in 26 patients without AEDs. Maximal photosensitivity range, derived from ranges determined at that age.

acid in mono- or polytherapy. Moreover, their patients were more likely to be photosensitive with valproic acid medication than without. Jeavons *et al.* (1986) used relatively high dosages of valproic acid, up to 2.5 g; development of pharmacodynamic tolerance seems therefore more likely, provided there was an intermediate stage where they did better.

Because of the confounding factor of AEDs, for the present study we selected those patients who were investigated at different ages without AEDs. In order to have a sufficient number of patients,

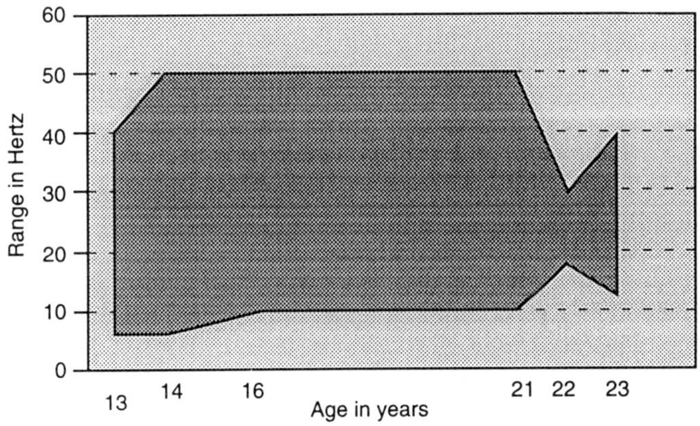

Fig. 5. Follow-up of photosensitivity ranges in a patient without AED treatment.

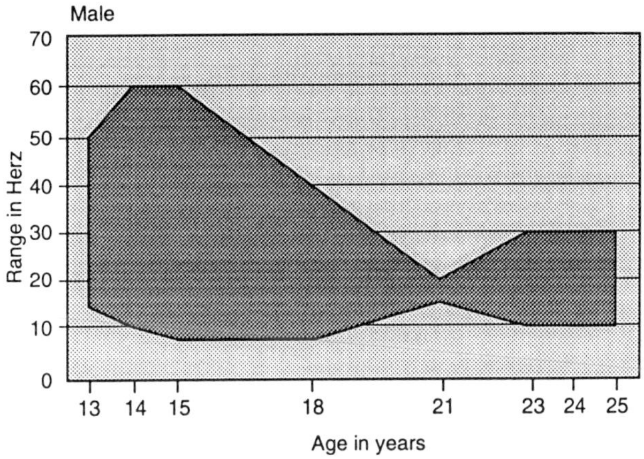

Fig. 6. Follow-up of photosensitivity ranges in patient without AED treatment.

we also included photosensitive patients known since 1983, thus enlarging our cohort to 148 patients. Twenty-six of these patients (18 per cent) without AEDs were selected; all of them (male 7, female 19) were investigated at least twice. In Fig. 3 the number of IPS determinations *vs.* age is given in these 26 patients. The distribution seems to be the same as the prevalence distribution of photosensitive epileptic patients (Fig. 2), which is not surprising. In Fig. 4 maximal upper and lower limits are given in relation to age. In accordance with the findings of Jeavons *et al.* (1986), the lower limit seems to be more or less stable when patients grow older. The upper limit first increases and decreases only gradually after puberty. At the age of 25 a more clear reduction in photosensitivity range is seen. Thereafter, again a slight increase seems to occur, although the number of patients is very low. The results described above are in agreement with the age-dependent penetrance of the photoparoxysmal response in relatives of photosensitive patients, as investigated by Waltz *et al.* (1992). This striking age dependency of the phenotypical expression of the response to IPS strongly suggests expression of a genetically determined trait. Even in two individual patients this effect on photosensitivity range was found (see Figs. 5 and 6). Two other patients without AEDs proved to be 60 years or more. Whether or not these patients belong to a specific subgroup of all photosensitive patients is yet unknown. Although the trait to respond to IPS in the laboratory with epileptiform discharges may depend on single genes, many additional genes and environmental factors will eventually determine the various clinical characteristics of these patients: whether visually induced seizures or spontaneous seizures occur, type of seizures, etc. Some overlap exists between photosensitivity and the epilepsy syndromes juvenile myoclonic epilepsy (JME) and certain progressive myoclonus epilepsies (Unverricht–Lundborg, Baltic type, ceroid lipofuscinosis). These syndromes, all characterized by myoclonic jerks, have been localized on chromosomes 6, 16, 20 and 21 (Berkovic *et al.*, 1993). It seems therefore worthwhile to perform genetic linkage studies in photosensitive patients with and without a history of myoclonic jerks. Whether the fact that the majority of photosensitive patients, as well as all patients with JME, belong to the idiopathic generalized epilepsy group is of importance in the search for common genes still has to be established.

Conclusion

Photosensitive patients, i.e. patients who show photoparoxysmal responses to IPS, can be identified not only by this specific EEG pattern but also by a number of clinical characteristics. It can be argued therefore that photosensitive epilepsy should constitute a separate entity in the classification of epilepsies and epileptic syndromes. Furthermore, age- and sex-dependent expression of this syndrome indicates a common genetic background; the EEG response on IPS can be used as a genetic marker.

Acknowledgements

The study was supported by a grant from the Commissie Landelijk Epilepsieonderzoek (CLEO). We thank our colleagues, in particular J.A.P. van Parys, O.G. Mulder, M. Engelsman and H. Stroink, who referred patients for investigation, and the EEG technicians, with special thanks to E. Dekker. We also thank G.J.F. Brekelmans for help in making the figures and A. Tierlier-Long for preparing the text.

References

Aicardi, J. (1986): Stimulus-sensitive epilepsies. In: *Epilepsy in children*, pp. 260–268. New York: Raven Press.

Berkovic, S.F., Cochius, J., Andermann, E. & Andermann, F. (1993): Progressive myoclonus epilepsies: clinical and genetic aspects. *Epilepsia* **34** (suppl. 3), S19–S30.

Commission on Classification and Terminology of the International League Against Epilepsy (1989): Proposal for revised classification of epilepsies and epileptic syndromes. *Epilepsia* **30,** 389–399.

Gowers, W.R. (1964): *Epilepsy and other chronic convulsive diseases: their causes, symptoms and treatment.* Reprint of the work first published by William Wood, New York, 1885. American Academy of Neurology, reprint series, Vol. I. New York: Dover.

Jeavons, P.M. & Harding, G.F.A. (1975): *Photosensitive epilepsy.* London: Heinemann.

Jeavons, P.M., Bishop, A. & Harding, G.F.A. (1986): The prognosis of photosensitivity. *Epilepsia* **27,** 569–575.

Kasteleijn-Nolst Trenité, D.W.G. (1989): Photosensitivity in epilepsy: electrophysiological and clinical correlates. *Acta Neurol. Scand.* **80** (suppl. 25*)*, 121–125.

Reilly, E.L. & Peters, J.F. (1973): Relationship of some varieties of electroencephalographic photosensitivity to clinical convulsive disorders. *Neurology* **23,** 1050–1057.

Walker, A.E., Woolf, J.I., Halstead, W.C. & Case, T.J. (1944): Photic driving. *Arch. Neurol. Psychiat.* **52,** 117–125.

Walter, V.J., Dovey, V.J. & Shipton, H. (1946): Analysis of the electrical response of the human cortex to photic stimulation. *Nature* **158,** 540.

Waltz, S., Christen, H.-J. & Doose, H. (1992): The different patterns of the photoparoxysmal response – a genetic study. *Electroencephalogr. Clin. Neurophysiol.* **83,** 138–145.

Wolf, P. & Goosses, R. (1986): Relation of photosensitivity to epileptic seizures. *J. Neurol. Neurosurg. Psychiat.* **49,** 1386–1391.

Epileptic Seizures and Syndromes, Edited by Peter Wolf
© 1994 John Libbey & Company Ltd., pp. 49–54

Chapter 7

Human and simian photosensitivity

Colin D. Binnie

The Maudsley Hospital, Denmark Hill, London SE5 8AZ, UK

Introduction

A general problem of clinical and basic research in epilepsy is the unpredictable occurrence of the relevant clinical and electrographic manifestations, both ictal and interictal. For this reason particular interest centres on those experimental models which produce seizures when required, and on the human reflex epilepsies which allow subclinical, or minor ictal, events to be elicited repeatedly and on demand. It may seem, therefore, particularly fortunate that two apparently analogous models exist in animals and humans, the photosensitive baboon, *Papio papio*, and human photosensitive epilepsy.

The photosensitive baboon

Killam *et al.* in 1966 found in four out of 10 baboons a response to intermittent photic stimulation (IPS), characterized by myoclonus of the eyelids and face, sometimes spreading to involve the entire body, and accompanied by paroxysmal activity commencing in the occipital regions but rapidly becoming generalized. The seizures and discharges were not self-sustaining and ceased abruptly when IPS was terminated. In subsequent research, both naturally photosensitive baboons have been studied, and also those rendered sensitive by administration of allyl-glycine; these two models are closely similar.

Aetiological factors

Formal genetic studies have not been performed; however, apes captured in the forested area of Casamance in Senegal are more often photosensitive than those from the desert regions. It is interesting to speculate what adaptive advantage enhanced sensitivity to light stimulation might confer on the arboreal apes from the jungle (Stevens, 1977). Photosensitivity is not present in the infant but appears at 6 months of age and is most prevalent at 9 months to 4 years. Females are more often affected. No neuropathological abnormalities are reported (Riche *et al.*, 1971).

Clinical phenomenology

The optimal IPS frequency for inducing photosensitive phenomena is some 25 Hz. The clinical effects are not all or none in nature but show a progressive increase of severity, depending on the susceptibility of the individual animal and the duration of stimulation. Four grades of response are distinguished

(Meldrum *et al.*, 1970): (1) ocular myoclonus; (2) ocular myoclonus spreading to involve facial and cranial muscles; (3) massive generalized myoclonus affecting the entire body; (4) self-sustaining myoclonic seizures persisting after termination of IPS and sometimes evolving to tonic–clonic convulsions.

Electroencephalogram (EEG) phenomenology

The optimal flash frequency is 25/s and the graded response develops gradually, at a rate depending on the degree of sensitivity of the particular animal, during sustained stimulation over some tens of seconds. In apparent contradiction of the original account of Killam *et al.* (1966) the spike-and-wave discharges are usually described as having a frontorolandic onset. Later, as clinical manifestations become more marked, discharges may invade other regions and may be recorded from subcortical structures (Fischer-Williams *et al.*, 1968). Similar discharges may occur on eye closure and in sleep.

Pathophysiology

In paralysed animals, single unit recordings from frontorolandic cortex demonstrate high frequency bursts of action potentials synchronous with EEG spikes and intervals of reduced activity corresponding to the slow waves (Ménini *et al.*, 1980). Such activity is not found in other regions, in particular the visual cortex, where burst firing is phase-locked to the flashes but not to the frontal spike-and-wave activity. Similarly, spike-and-wave discharges are not found in other cortical or subcortical structures before their onset in the frontal region (Fischer-Williams *et al.*, 1968). The discharges appear first in layer III of area 4, appear to be of dendritic origin and are elicited by corticocortical efferents (Silva-Barrat *et al.*, 1988). Following a conditioning train of flashes, single stimuli elicit abnormal 'paroxysmal visual evoked potentials' (PVEPs) resembling spike-and-wave discharges (Ménini *et al.*, 1980; Silva-Comte *et al.*, 1982). PVEPs are maximal in the precentral region, are of lower amplitude and greater latency in adjacent areas, and are not found in the visual cortex (Silva-Barrat & Ménini, 1984). However, the striate cortex is apparently involved, if only as part of the afferent pathway, as bilateral or unilateral occipital cortical ablations eliminate photosensitivity (Lanoir & Dimov, 1971; Wada *et al.*, 1973).

Bilateral synchrony, but not the generation of the discharges, is disrupted after section of the corpus callosum (Naquet *et al.*, 1972). Hemifield stimulation (achieved by monocular stimulation after laser coagulation of the temporal part of the retina) produces bilateral discharges in the otherwise intact ape, but only contralateral after callosotomy (Fukuda *et al.*, 1989).

Pharmacology

Papio papio has been used extensively as a model for pharmacological studies. Benzodiazepines and gabaergic agents appear most effective (Meldrum *et al.*, 1975; Meldrum & Horton, 1978), whereas phenytoin and carbamazepine are inactive except at toxic levels (Meldrum *et al.*, 1978). Conversely, antagonists of benzodiazepines and γ-aminobutyric acid (GABA) enhance photosensitivity (Meldrum *et al.*, 1979; Meldrum & Braestrup, 1984; Stutzmann *et al.*, 1984). Chronic infusion of GABA into both motor and occipital regions suppresses photosensitivity, whereas infusions in the premotor and prefrontal areas did not have this effect (Brailowski *et al.*, 1989). Curiously, sodium valproate, which is highly effective in human photosensitive epilepsy and is presumed to be gabaergic, shows relatively little activity in *Papio papio* (Meldrum, 1977). Dopamine agonists, however, do suppress photosensitivity as they do in humans (Meldrum *et al.*, 1978).

Summary of photosensitivity in the baboon

In summary, the naturally occurring photosensitivity of some baboons is genetically determined and involves a gradual recruitment of discharges in the frontorolandic cortex in response to corticocortical afferents which are transmitted via the primary visual area. The underlying mechanisms are probably gabaergic.

Human photosensitivity

The first unequivocal account of photosensitive epilepsy in humans is probably that by Radovici *et al.* (1932) of a patient with visually self-induced seizures. Photosensitivity has come to be generally recognized since the introduction of photic stimulation into routine EEG practice (Cobb, 1947). IPS elicits a range of effects, from typical photic following, through various more or less atypical responses to frank epileptic seizures. Various anomalous responses are genetically determined (Doose & Gerken, 1973) and some are positively associated with epilepsy. The strongest clinical association is with generalized spike-wave activity, or occasionally multiple spikes, described by Bickford *et al.* (1952) as a 'photoconvulsive response', or PCR, particularly if it is self-sustaining and continues for 100 ms or longer after the stimulus train ceases (Reilly & Peters, 1973). In the present text the term 'photosensitive' is applied only to subjects with a prolonged PCR.

Among patients undergoing clinical EEG examination 47 per cent of those with occipital spikes and 95 per cent of those with a prolonged PCR have epilepsy. On close examination and questioning it appears that in over 70 per cent of instances the PCR is itself accompanied by clinical ictal events (Kasteleijn-Nolst Trenité *et al.*, 1987). In many photosensitive patients epileptiform discharges can also be elicited by viewing linear patterns: 30 per cent of IPS-sensitive patients show sensitivity to static patterns and 70 per cent do so if the patterns oscillate in the direction orthogonal to the line orientation (Wilkins *et al.*, 1980). The occurrence of pattern sensitivity in the absence of sensitivity to IPS has not been convincingly established.

Aetiology

The association of photosensitivity with epilepsy is determined by multifactorial inheritance. Forty per cent of siblings of photosensitive patients with epilepsy are themselves photosensitive (Doose & Gerken, 1973). In a tertiary referral centre for epilepsy, the prevalence of photosensitivity was 21 per cent in idiopathic generalized epilepsy, 5.1 per cent in symptomatic or cryptogenic generalized epilepsy and only 2.8 per cent among patients with partial epilepsy (Binnie *et al.,* 1989). Five and a half per cent of patients were photosensitive, of whom 43 per cent had idiopathic epilepsy. There are, however, particularly strong associations with specific epilepsy syndromes (Gooses, 1984). As in the baboon, photosensitivity is more common in females and presents in childhood and adolescence.

Clinical phenomenology

Forty per cent of photosensitive patients with epilepsy have no spontaneous seizures (the syndrome of 'pure photosensitive epilepsy'). Only 20 per cent have never experienced a seizure induced by visual stimuli. Most patients report multiple seizure types, tonic–clonic, absence and myoclonic seizures being the most common (Kastelijn-Nolst Trenité, 1989). As in the baboon, myoclonus appears often to start in or be confined to the eyelids. During photic stimulation in the laboratory, IPS is limited to avoid seizure induction; nevertheless, 44 per cent of patients exhibit myoclonus and 75 per cent exhibit some form of clinical ictal manifestations (Kastelijn-Nolst Trenité *et al.*, 1987).

EEG phenomenology

The PCR consists of generalized spikes or multiple spikes and slow waves, which are self-sustaining and are not phase-locked to the stimulus. Recruitment is more rapid than in the baboon; usually discharges commence within 2 s of starting IPS and may appear generalized from onset. However, sometimes discharges can be seen starting posteriorly, with a breakup of the regular photic following response and the development of irregular spikes, which then generalize. In 41 per cent of subjects there are consistent asymmetries in onset of the discharges (Binnie *et al.*, 1981). The stimulus frequency is a critical determinant of the occurrence of a PCR; subjects are sensitive to a restricted range of flash rates, 15–18/s being most likely to be epileptogenic.

Pathophysiology

Few experimental data are available concerning the mechanisms of human sensitivity to IPS. However, pattern provides a stimulus more suitable for physiological studies. The liability of a pattern to elicit discharges depends on its physical characteristics, and a substantial body of knowledge concerning mechanisms of pattern vision allows very specific physiological interpretation of the findings.

Epileptogenesis and onset of frank epileptiform discharges take place in the visual cortex. This may be inferred from three lines of evidence (which are reported by Wilkins *et al.*, 1980, unless otherwise stated):

1. Stimulus characteristics which determine the occurrence of discharges are similar to those which determine the activity of striate and prestriate cortical neurones. Epileptogenicity (as assessed by the probability of a discharge occurring under standardized conditions) is increased by:

(a) Length of line contours within the pattern; stripes are more effective than chequer-boards.
(b) Binocular fusion; under conditions of binocular rivalry pattern sensitivity is much reduced.

2. Suitable stimuli elicit discharges confined to the posterior regions:

(a) Hemifield stimulation elicits focal epileptiform discharges over the contralateral posterior quadrant.
(b) Discharge onset to both pattern and IPS may remain confined to the posterior regions for some seconds before generalizing; this is demonstrable with stimuli which are marginally supraliminal (with respect to pattern size of IPS frequency) and after suppression of generalization by sodium valproate.
(c) Subliminal IPS at 8 Hz may elicit abnormal steady-state visual evoked potentials (VEPs) over the visual area, 'occipital spikes' (Herrick, 1978). These persist after generalized discharges have been abolished by sodium valproate.

3. Discharges arise when the pattern projects to a critical area of visual cortex, within either hemisphere:

(a) Peripheral and central stimuli (e.g. annuli and discs) have equivalent effects after correction for the cortical magnification factor.
(b) Spatial summation occurs within each visual field independently.
(c) Threshold pattern area may show marked interhemispheric differences. IPS-induced discharges commence over the hemisphere with the lower pattern threshold.
(d) Sodium valproate in doses which do not totally abolish photosensitivity selectively suppresses generalized discharges and reduces the probability of posterior discharges, but does not change threshold pattern size (Darby *et al.*, 1985).

Pharmacology

Acute administration of a wide range of antiepileptic drugs, both established and experimental, suppressed photosensitivity at clinically relevant plasma concentrations (Binnie *et al.*, 1986). With chronic administration benzodiazepines, sodium valproate and succinimides are most effective. As in *P. papio*, apomorphine also has a suppressant effect.

Summary of photosensitivity in humans

Photosensitivity in humans is familial and strongly associated with idiopathic generalized epilepsy, but occurs sporadically in patients with symptomatic epilepsies and no known family history. Robust evidence from pattern-sensitive subjects, but supported also by findings in patients sensitive only to IPS, indicates that the trigger mechanism involves binocularly innervated cells in the striate or prestriate cortex with 'complex' properties. Epileptogenesis depends on the intensity of activation and on stimulation of a critical area of cortex. Spatial summation occurs within but not between hemispheres. Despite the association of photosensitivity with idiopathic generalized epilepsy and the finding of more widespread cortical hyperexcitability as evidenced by abnormal somatosensory evoked potentials (SEPs) (Broughton *et al.*, 1969), in this model stimulation of a specific sensory system can elicit epileptic phenomena which are localization-related. Generalized discharges arise by secondary epileptogenesis and are suppressed by GABA antagonists.

Conclusion

From a neurobiological standpoint human and simian photosensitivity may appear similar, as reflecting a common deficiency of gabaergic inhibitory neurotransmission (Meldrum & Wilkins, 1984). It may be considered, however, that, as they share this feature with some symptomatic, including partial, epilepsies, the similarity is non-specific. As clinical syndromes they appear very different. The photosensitivity of the baboon serves as a model of generalized corticoreticular epilepsy, hyperexcitable cortex responding abnormally to normal afferent activity in diffuse, non-specific systems. Human photosensitivity, in contrast, may be considered a form of reflex partial epilepsy arising in the visual cortex, with a marked tendency to secondary generalization.

References

Bickford, R.G., Sem-Jacobsen, C.W., White, P.T. & Daly, D. (1952): Some observations on the mechanism of photic and photometrazol activation. *Electroencephalogr. Clin. Neurophysiol.* **4,** 275–282.

Binnie, C.D., Darly, C.E., Kasteleijn-Nolste Trenité, D.G.A. & Wilkins, A.J. (1989): Photosensitive epilepsy: clinical features. In: *Colloquium on Reflex Epilepsy,* eds. A. Beaumanoir, H. Gastaut & R. Naquet, pp. 163–170. Geneva: Edition Medicine et Hygiene.

Binnie, C.D., Kasteleijn-Nolst Trenité, D.G.A. & De Korte, R. (1986): Photosensitivity as a model for acute antiepileptic drug studies. *Electroencephalogr. Clin. Neurophysiol.* **63,** 35–41.

Binnie, C.D., Wilkins, A.J. & de Corte, R.A. (1981): Interhemispheric differences in photosensitive epilepsy: II. Intermittent photic stimulation. *Electroencephalogr. Clin. Neurophysiol.* **52,** 469–472.

Brailowski, S., Silva-Barrat, S., Ménini, C., Riche, D. & Naquet, R. (1989): Effects of localized, chronic GABA infusions into different cortical areas of the photosensitive baboon, *Papio papio. Electroencephalogr. Clin. Neurophysiol.* **72,** 147–156.

Broughton, R., Meier-Ewart, K.-H. & Ebe, M. (1969): Evoked visual, somato-sensory and retinal potentials in photosensitive epilepsy. *Electroencephalogr. Clin. Neurophysiol.* **27,** 375–386.

Darby, C.E., Park, D.M., Smith, A.T. & Wilkins, A.J. (1985): Electroencephalographic characteristics of epileptic pattern sensitivity and their relation to the nature of pattern stimulation and the effect of sodium valproate. *Electroencephalogr. Clin. Neurophysiol.* **63,** 517–525.

Doose, H. & Gerken, H. (1973): On the genetics of EEG-anomalies in childhood. IV. Photoconvulsive reaction. *Neuropaediatrie* **4,** 162–171.

Fischer-Williams, M., Ponset, M., Riche, D. & Naquet, R. (1968): Light induced epilepsy in the baboon *Papio papio*: cortical and depth recordings. *Electroencephalogr. Clin. Neurophysiol.* **25,** 557–569.

Fukuda, H., Valin, A., Ménini, C., Boscher, C., de-la-Sayette, V., Riche, D., Kunimoto, M., Wada, J.A. & Naquet, R. (1989): Effect of macular and peripheral retina coagulation on photosensitive epilepsy in the forebrain bisected baboon *Papio papio. Epilepsia* **30,** 623–630.

Gooses, R. (1984): Die Beziehung der Fotosensibilität zu den verschiedenen epileptischen Syndromen. Thesis: Berlin.

Herrick, C.E. (1978): An investigation into the stimulus characteristics of photosensitive epilepsy with regard to therapeutic procedures. University of Aston: PhD thesis

Kasteleijn-Nolst Trenité, D.G.A. (1989): Photosensitivity in epilepsy: electrophysiological and clinical correlates. *Acta Neurol. Scand.* (Suppl. 125), 80.

Kasteleijn-Nolst Trenité, D.G.A., Binnie, C.D. & Meinardi, H. (1987): Photosensitive patients: symptoms and signs during intermittent photic stimulation and their relation to seizures in daily life. *J. Neurol. Neurosurg. Psychiatry* **50,** 1546–1549.

Killam, K.F., Killam, E.K. & Naquet, R. (1966): Mise en évidence chez certains singes d'un syndrome myoclonique. *C.R. Acad. Sci. Sér. D (Paris)* **262,** 1010–1012.

Lanoir, J. & Dimov, S. (1971): Effets des foyers corticaux chroniques frontaux, temporaux et rolandiques chez le *Papio papio* photosensible. In: *Pathogenesis of epilepsy*, ed. Usunoff, pp. 319–326. Sofia: Bulgarian Academy of Sciences.

Meldrum, B.S. (1977): L'épilepsie photosensible du *Papio papio*: un modèle animal pour l'évaluation de drogues anticonvulsivantes. *C.R. Ren. Ann. Ligue Franc. Epilepsie* 64–90.

Meldrum, B.S. & Braestrup, C. (1984): GABA and the anticonvulsivant action of benzodiazepines and related drugs. In: *Actions and interactions of GABA and benzodiazepines*, ed. N.G. Bowery, pp. 133–153. New York: Raven Press.

Meldrum, B.S. & Horton, R.W. (1978): Blockage of epileptic responses in the photosensitive baboon, *Papio papio*, by two irreversible inhibitors of GABA-transaminase, gamma-acetylinic GABA (4-amino-hex-5-ynoic acid) and gamma-vinyl GABA (4-amino-hex-5-ynoic acid). *Psychopharmacology* **60,** 277–280.

Meldrum, B.S. & Wilkins, A.J. (1984): Photosensitive epilepsy in man and the baboon: integration of pharmacological and psychophysical evidence. In: *Electrophysiology of epilepsy*, eds. P. Schwartzlcroin & H.V. Wheal, pp. 51–77. London: Academic Press.

Meldrum, B.S., Balzamo, E., Gadea, M. & Naquet, R. (1970): Photic and drug induced epilepsy in the baboon (*Papio papio*): the effect of isoniazid, thiosemicarbazide, pyridoxine and aminooxyacetic acid. *Electroencephalogr. Clin. Neurophysiol.* **29,** 333–347.

Meldrum, B.S., Anlezark, G., Balzamo, E., Horton, R. & Trimble, M. (1975): In: *Advances in neurology*, eds. B.S. Meldrum & C.D. Marsden, pp. 117–128. New York: Raven Press.

Meldrum, B.S., Brailowski, S. & Naquet, R. (1978): Approche pharmacologique de l'épilepsie photosensible du *Papio papio. Actualités Pharmacol.* **8,** 81–99.

Meldrum, B.S., Ménini, C., Naquet, R., Laurant, H. & Stutzmann, J.M. (1979): Proconvulsant, anticonvulsant and other actions of the D and L stereo-isomers of allylglycine in the photosensitive baboon *Papio papio. Electroencephalogr. Clin. Neurophysiol.* **47,** 383–395.

Ménini, C., Stutzmann, J.M., Laurent, H. & Naquet, R. (1980): Paroxysmal visual evoked potentials (PVEPs) in *Papio papio*: I. Morphological and topographical characteristics, comparison with paroxysmal discharges. *Electroencephalogr. Clin. Neurophysiol.* **50,** 356–364.

Naquet, R., Ménini, C. & Catier, J. (1972): Photically induced epilepsy in *Papio papio*: the initiation of discharges and the role of frontal cortex and of the corpus callosum. In: *Synchronization of the EEG in the epilepsies*, eds. M.A.B. Brazier & H. Petsche, pp. 347–367. Vienna: Springer Verlag.

Radovici, A., Misirliou, V. & Gluckman, M. (1932): Epilepsie réflexe provoquée par excitations des rayons solaires. *Rev. Neurol.* (Paris) **1,** 1305–1308.

Reilly, E.L. & Peters, J.F. (1973): Relationship of some varieties of electroencephalographic photosensitivity to clinical convulsive disorders. *Neurology* **13,** 1050–1057.

Riche, D., Gambarelli-Dubois, D. & Naquet, R. (1971): Repeated seizures and cerebral lesions in photosensitive baboons (*Papio papio*): a preliminary report. In: *Brain hypoxia*, eds. J.B. Brierley & B.S. Meldrum, pp. 297–301. London: Spastics International Medical Publications.

Silva-Barrat, C. & Ménini, C. (1984): The influence of light stimulation on potentials evoked by single flashes in photosensitive and non-photosensitive *Papio papio. Electroencephalogr. Clin. Neurophysiol.* **57,** 448–461.

Silva-Barrat, C., Brailowski, S., Levesque, G. & Ménini, C. (1988): Epileptic discharge induced by intermittent light stimulation in photosensitive baboons: a current source density study. *Epilepsy Res.* **2,** 1–8.

Silva-Barrat, C., Velluti, J. & Ménini, C. (1982): Characteristics and origin of frontal paroxysmal responses induced by light stimulation in the *Papio papio* under allylglycine. *Electroencephalogr. Clin. Neurophysiol.* **53,** 479–490.

Stevens, J.R. (1977): The EEG spike: signal of information transmission. *Ann. Neurol.* **1,** 309–314.

Stutzmann, J.M., Cepeda, C. & Naquet, R. (1984): Action of suriclone in naturally and allylglycine-induced photosensitive baboon *Papio papio. Exp. Neurol.* **86,** 379–386.

Wada, J.A., Catier, J., Charmasson, G., Ménini, C. & Naquet, R. (1973): Further examination of neural mechanisms underlying photosensitivity in the epileptic Senegalese baboon *Papio papio. Electroencephalogr. Clin. Neurophysiol.* **34,** 786.

Wilkins, A.J., Darby, C.E. & Binnie, C.D. (1980): Visually induced seizures. *Prog. Neurobiol.* **15,** 85–117.

Epileptic Seizures and Syndromes, Edited by Peter Wolf
© 1994 John Libbey & Company Ltd., pp. 55–66

Chapter 8

Fixation-off-sensitive epilepsies: clinical and EEG characteristics

Chrysostomos P. Panayiotopoulos*
with comments and contributions from Colin D. Binnie† and Takeo Takahashi‡

**Department of Clinical Neurophysiology and Epilepsy, St Thomas's Hospital, London SE1 7EH, England; †The Maudsley Hospital, Denmark Hill, London SE5 8AZ, England; ‡Division of Neuropsychiatry, Sendai City Hospital, 3–1, Shimizukoji, Sendai 980, Japan*

Introduction and definitions

Fixation-off sensitivity (FOS) denotes the form or forms of epilepsy and electroencephalographic (EEG) abnormalities which are elicited by elimination of central vision and fixation (Panayiotopoulos, 1977, 1978, 1979, 1980, 1981, 1987a, b, 1989a, b, c, 1993b).

In routine EEG, performed in an illuminated room and conditions allowing preservation of fixation and central vision, FOS may be suspected if the EEG abnormalities appear and persist as long as the eyes remain closed and disappear when the eyes are opened, i.e. they show a similar reactivity to that of the α-rhythm (Figs. 1–4).

FOS is related to 'eyes-closed' not 'eye-closure' EEG abnormalities (Fig. 1).

The significance of differentiating the 'eyes-closed'-from 'eye-closure'-related EEG abnormalities

It is crucial to differentiate (Fig. 1) between 'eyes-closed'- (seen mainly in FOS) and 'eye-closure'- (seen mainly in photosensitive epilepsies and eyelid myoclonia with absences) related abnormalities.

'Eyes-closed' is the state which lasts and persists as long as the eyes remain closed (Fig. 1) while 'eye-closure' is the transient state which immediately follows closing of the eyes, lasting less than 3s (Fig. 1) and does not persist in the remaining period of eyes-closed.

'Eye-closure'-related EEG abnormalities are often seen in photosensitive, not FOS, patients and consist of brief generalized discharges occurring within 1–3 s after closing of the eyes (Fig. 1). Eye-closure-related abnormalities occur only if the recording room is illuminated; they do not occur in total darkness (see review and other opinions in Panayiotopoulos, 1974; Fabian & Wolf, 1987). However, there are reports describing eye-closure abnormalities in darkness and also emphasizing

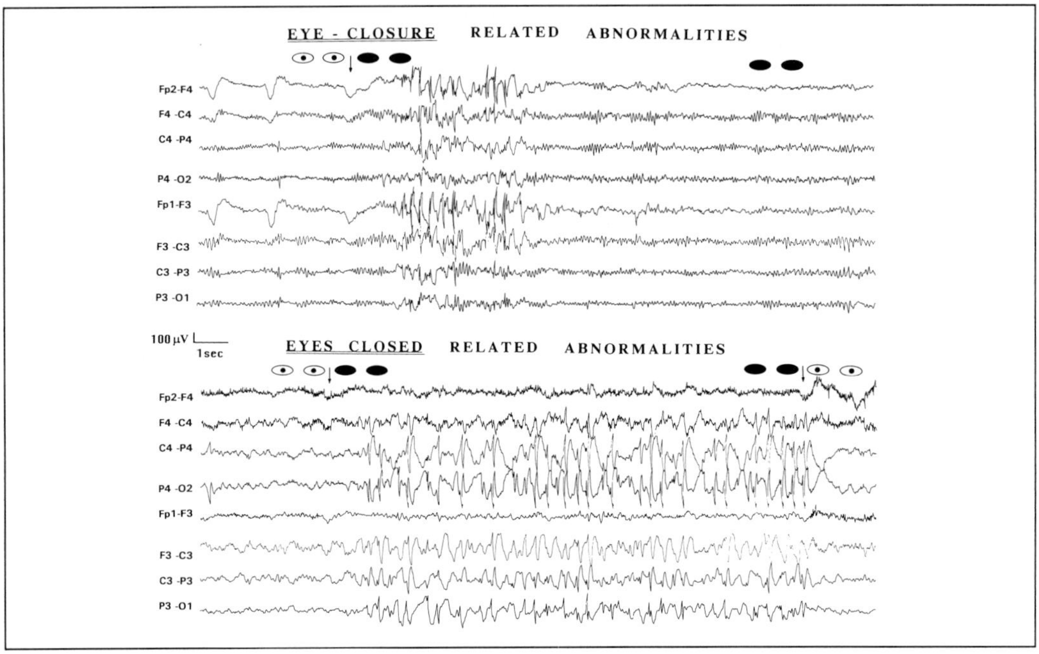

Fig.1. Eye-closure (upper) abnormalities are induced within a few seconds after closing of the eyes, are short and do not persist in the remaining period that the eyes are closed. Eye-closure-induced abnormalities are eliminated in darkness and occur mainly in photosensitive patients. Eye-closed-related (lower) abnormalities last as long as the eyes remain closed and disappear when the eyes are opened. They are often, not in all patients, associated with FOS. Arrows indicate when the eyes are opened (symbols with open eyes) or closed (symbols with closed eyes).

the siginificance of proprioceptive impulses from closing the eyelids or movements of the eyes (Green, 1968; Lewis, 1972; Vignaendra *et al.*, 1976; Fabian & Wolf, 1987). This may indicate different mechanisms of precipitation but it is also likely that some of these patients have not been tested in total darkness.

Total darkness means elimination of all possible light sources like small light indicators of the EEG and other equipment or light coming from door or window openings; if total darkness is not achieved, central vision and fixation may not be eliminated during the testing and the results may be jeopardized. Switching off the lights in the EEG recording room is not adequate and this may be the reason for the conflicting results in the relevant literature (see Panayiotopoulos, 1974, 1987b). Furthermore, 'eye-closure' and 'eyes-closed' should be distinguished during both intermittent photic stimulation (IPS)and the recording and interpretation of the resting EEG (Jeavons, 1966; Panayiotopoulos, 1972, 1974).

Eye-closure abnormalities in photosensitive patients were attributed to the 'off-light' effect of closing the eyelids (Panayiotopoulos, 1972, 1974). However, I cannot support this view any more because I, like Fabian and Wolf (1987), have seen eye-closure-related abnormalities in photosensitive patients, particularly eyelid myoclonia with absences, who have 'lost' their sensitivity to IPS (either because of antiepileptic drugs or because of an age-related improvement or remission) while the eye-closure-related abnormalities persist. See for other views in Gobbi *et al.* (1989).

Eyes-closed-related EEG abnormalities of FOS epilepsies are due to the elimination of central vision and fixation by the closed eyelids because:

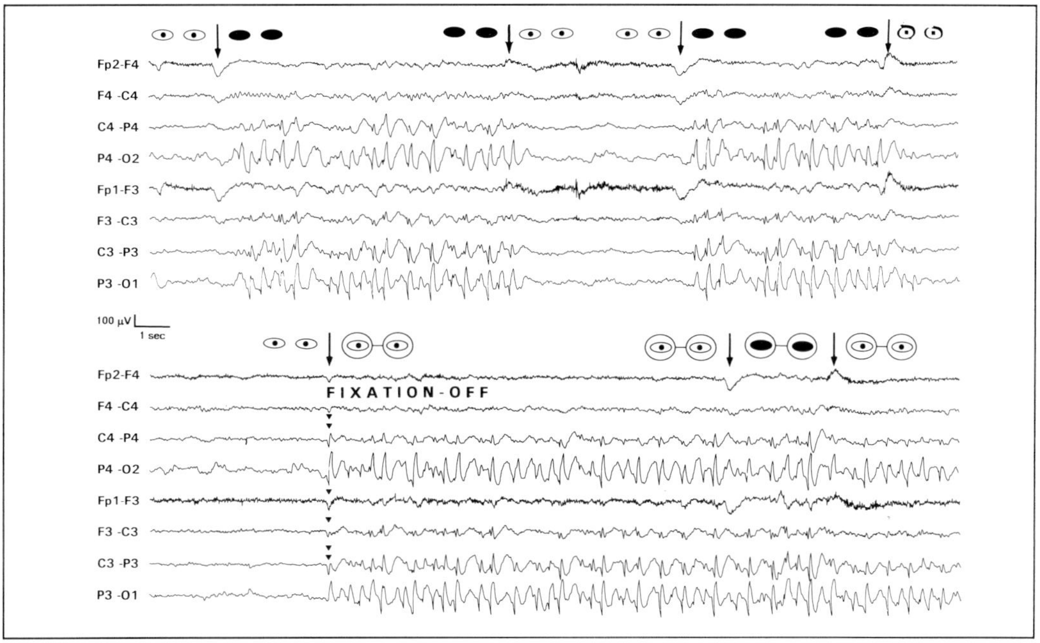

Fig. 2. Video-EEG recording. Fixation-off sensitivity in an 11-year-old boy with benign childhood epilepsy and occipital paroxysms (case 7 in Panayiotopoulos, 1993b). High-amplitude sharp- and slow-wave occipital paroxysms are induced by binocular fixation-off. The results are identical whether fixation-off is achieved with closed eyelids or complete darkness or +10 spherical lenses in the presence of light or underwater goggles covered with semitransparent tape. Monocular fixation-off is not effective in eliciting occipital paroxysms irrespective of means by which central vision and fixation are eliminated; similarly occipital paroxysms are inhibited with binocular or monocular fixation. Occipital paroxysms are not inhibited by eyes-open in conditions of elimination of central vision and fixation, thus excluding the contribution of proprioceptive impulses from the eyelids or oculomotor muscles in the activation of the EEG abnormalities (see also Fig. 4). Imaginary fixation (asking the patient to 'look' at his/her thumb) in conditions of elimination of central vision does not alter (does not inhibit) the occipital paroxysms. Arrows indicate when the eyes are open (symbols of open eyes) or closed (symbols of closed eyes). Eyes with glasses indicate that the patient has been deprived of central vision and fixation.

(a) The EEG paroxysms can also be elicited when eyes are opened in complete darkness or with unpatterned vision either through +10 spherical lenses or through underwater goggles covered with semitransparent paper, i.e. when fixation and central vision are eliminated (Figs. 2–4).

(b) the EEG paroxysms disappear on binocular or monocular fixation (Figs. 1–4).

Imaginary fixation (by asking the patient to 'look, fixate' his/her thumb) in conditions when fixation and central vision are eliminated does not alter the occipital paroxysms (Fig. 2).

Proprioceptive impulses from ocular and eyelid muscles are not implicated because the EEG paroxysms are not altered when eye closing and eye opening are performed in conditions where fixation and central vision are eliminated (Fig. 2). They are inhibited by central vision and fixation (Fig. 2).

The clinical manifestations of patients having eyes-closed and eye-closure EEG abnormalities appear to be different (Gobbi *et al.*, 1989); in this important paper all of their patients were tested for photosensitivity, most of them had sleep EEG studies but none were tested for FOS; a difference was found between the two groups regarding the latency of the onset of the discharges in light and darkness

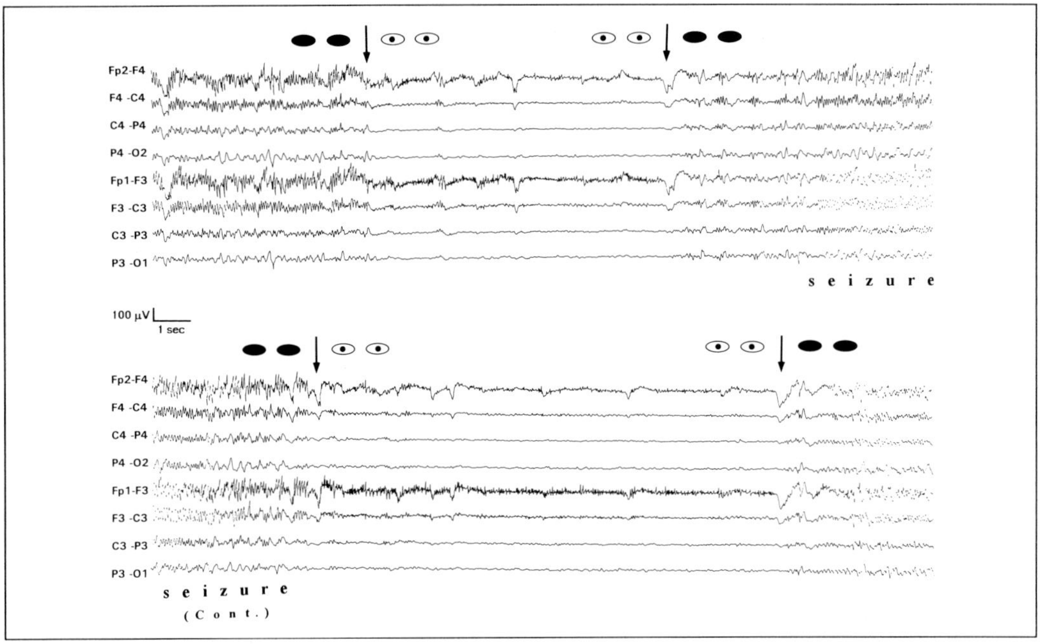

Fig. 3. Video-EEG recording of a patient reported as 'fixation-off-sensitive epilepsy with eyelid myoclonia and absences' (Panayiotopoulos, 1987b). I re-evaluated the same patient with video-EEG recording in 1992 and confirmed the previously published results and observations regarding fixation-off sensitivity, in this rare form of idiopathic generalized epilepsy. However, the seizures of this patient are markedly different from those of photosensitive patients with eyelid myoclonia with absences (Appleton et al., 1993). They consist of fast eyelid clonic movements associated with marked tonic spasm of the eyelids and the eyes, which are deviated upwards and laterally. The seizures occurred only when eyes were closed or on elimination of central vision and fixation. The patient has a long clinical and EEG follow-up which consistently demonstrated eyes-closed related EEG rhythms which were induced by elimination of central vision and fixation . She never showed any evidence of photosensitivity. Symbols are the same as in Figs. 1 and 2.

(total darkness or darkened room?). We may learn more about these patients and the underlying mechanisms if testing of FOS is introduced in the routine EEG examinations of these patients.

Electroencephalographic aspects of fixation-off sensitivity

The EEG abnormalities consist of:

(a) occipital paroxysms, i.e. high-amplitude, long runs of repetitive occipital spike-wave or sharp and slow-wave complexes, morphologically similar to the centrotemporal spikes, which are often bilateral and are eyes-closed-related (Fig. 1) or
(b) generalized discharges of spike or multiple and slow waves which are eyes-closed-related, or
(c) generalized slow theta and delta activity intermixed with spikes or multiple spikes which continuously occur as long as the eyes remain closed but disappear on eyes being opened.

Other types of EEG abnormalities may be found if FOS testing is introduced in the EEG departments, as is the practice with IPS and photosensitive epilepsy.

The prevalence of FOS-related EEG abnormalities appears, in my experience, to be as frequent as that of photoconvulsive responses in children younger than 12 years of age (Panayiotopoulos, 1988).

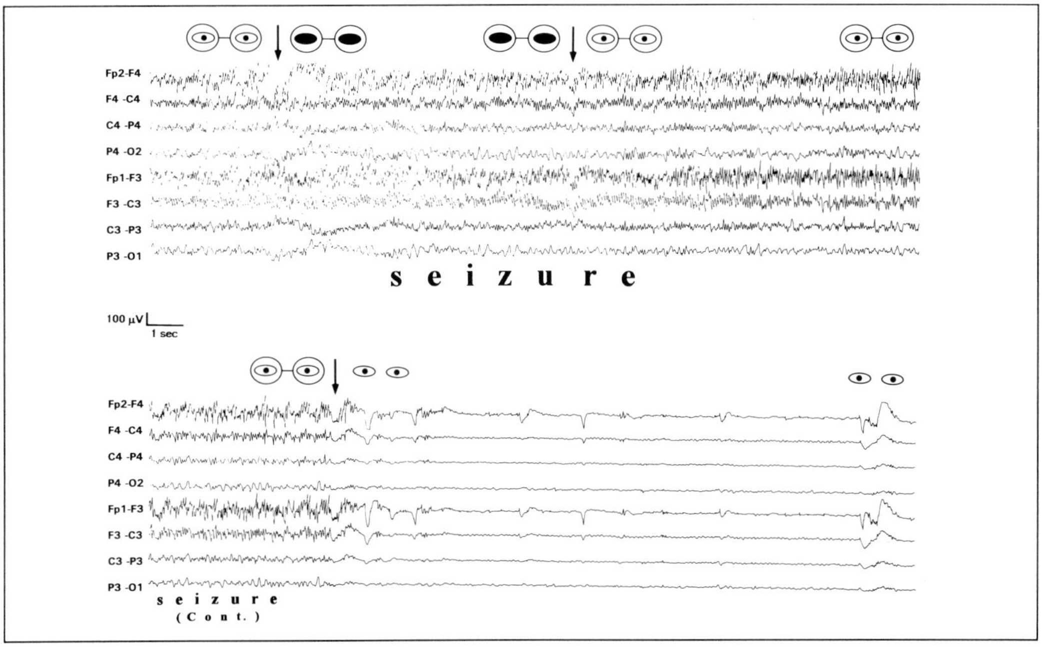

Fig.4. Video-EEG recording of the same patient as in Fig. 3 during fixation-off (eyes with glasses). Complete inhibition by fixation-on (eyes without glasses). Symbols are the same as in Figs. 1 and 2.

Clinical syndromes of fixation-off sensitivity

Benign childhood epilepsy with occipital paroxysms (BCEOP)

FOS is probably more frequently associated with benign childhood epilepsy with occipital paroxysms (BCEOP) than with any other epileptic condition (Panayiotopoulos, 1980, 1981, 1989a, b, 1993 a, b; Panayiotopoulos & Siafacus, 1980).

BCEOP has been extensively reviewed recently (Panayiotopoulos, 1993a, b; Roger & Bureau, 1992).

Generalized epilepsies with tonic and clonic manifestations from the eyes and eyelids

I have previously published a case with absences and generalized tonic–clonic seizures who had eyes-closed-, not eye-closure-related clinical and EEG manifestations (Panayiotopoulos, 1987b). Clinically, her eyelids showed fast, small-range clonic movements associated with tonic spasm of the eyelids and eyes which were deviated upwards and laterally; they occasionally spread to involve the neck muscles. These attacks were always related to eyes closed and the patient was not photosensitive. I called this 'eyelid myoclonia with absences', a name which should probably be reserved only for the syndrome described by Jeavons (1977), where all patients are photosensitive and show eye-closure, not eyes-closed, abnormalities (Appleton *et al.*, 1993; Binnie & Jeavons, 1992; see comments by C.D. Binnie below). Eyelid myoclonia with absences should not be always equated with self-induction; none of our 11 adult patients with this syndrome had any evidence of self-induced seizures (see also comments by C.D. Binnie below)

The neurophysiological manifestations of patients with eyelid-related epileptic seizures may be more interesting and more complex than initially thought because some may show photosensitivity, others have FOS, and others exhibit features common to photosensitivity and FOS (Panayiotopoulos *et al.*, unpublished).

FOS has been confirmed by other authors (Lugaresi *et al.,* 1984; Beaumanoir *et al.,* 1989). Cirignota *et al.* (1987) described a case of BCEOP in whom occipital paroxysms were not induced immediately but with a long delay of 20 s to 4 min after eyes closed, darkness or vision through semitransparent glasses. Beaumanoir *et al.*, (1989) have shown an inhibitory effect on functional occipital spikes by 'visual perception'.

In addition, FOS may operate in other epleptic (not necessarily of the spike-and- wave type only) or non-epileptic (α-rhythm, slow posterior waves) conditions with EEG manifestations recorded in association with 'eyes closed'.

Scotosensitive or fixation-off sensitive epilepsy?

Scotosensitive epilepsy was rarely reported in the literature before the recent papers on BCEOP (Pazzaglia *et al.*, 1970). BCEOP was recently described as scotosensitive epilepsy, a term which is inappropriate for BCEOP because darkness is not a prerequisite for the cortical 'epileptogenic' excitation of the occipital paroxysms (see above, Figs. 2–4). Darkness, like the closed eyelids, induces the occipital abnormalities because of elimination of central vision and fixation (Figs. 2 and 4). Occipital paroxysms can be induced with eyes opened and in the presence of light if central vision and fixation are eliminated (Figs. 2–4). Do true cases of scotosensitive epilepsy exist? That is are there cases where the excitatory role of darkness is not secondary to FOS? I have not found a convincing case so far, although in some patients with FOS a grading response may be seen, i.e. darkness may be more effective than +10 spherical lenses. A case which I described in 1979 as scotosensitive epilepsy was probably another example of FOS (Panayiotopoulos, 1979).

In conclusion, darkness is not a prerequisite for eliciting the EEG paroxysms; thus the term scotosensitive epilepsy is not appropriate. Genuine cases of scotosensitivity may exist but their documentation would require exclusion of FOS.

Confirmation of fixation-off sensitivity

First, it is essential to confirm that the EEG abnormalities observed in routine EEG recording are eyes-closed related. The patient is asked to open and close his/her eyes every 5 s six times consecutively; ensure fixation in the eyes-opened state by instructing the patient to look at a fixed point (the tip of a pencil would do).

Second, test for FOS by instructing the patient to perform the same sequence of eyes-opened and eyes-closed as above (six sequential trials of 5 s eyes-opened and eyes-closed) in conditions where central vision and fixation are eliminated. There are many ways to achieve this; a practical method is to ask the patient to wear a pair of underwater goggles which are fitted with +10 spherical lenses or semitransparent tape.

Elimination of central vision and fixation through total darkness is difficult to achieve in routine EEG departments because of the light indicators of EEG and other machines as well as light coming through door and window openings; it should be remembered that FOS EEG abnormalities introduced in total darkness are dramatically inhibited when the patient fixates on a small red spot of light (Panayiotopoulos, 1981, 1989a, c). It is our practice to test the effect of darkness with the patient wearing another pair of underwater goggles in which light has been totally blanked out with an opaque (non-transparent) tape.

Photosensitive *vs.* FOS epilepsy

Photosensitive epilepsy appears to have opposite mechanisms of excitation and inhibition to that of FOS:

a. The resting EEG of photosensitive patients frequently shows eye-closure (not eyes-closed) EEG abnormalities, which are inhibited by total darkness and probably by elimination of central vision and fixation (Jeavons, 1966; Panayiotopoulos, 1972, 1974).

b. Photosensitivity is mainly mediated through central vision and fixation (Jeavons *et al.*, 1971a, b, 1972; see also more recent views in Binnie, Chapter 7; Wilkins *et al.,* 1980; Takahashi, 1989). Photoconvulsive responses are induced only if the patient 'looks'at the centre of the stroboscope. 'Sometimes a shift of gaze from the centre of the lamp to the edge (12° or 15°) will inhibit responses, including photic driving' (Jeavons *et al.*, 1971b).

c. Occipital spikes induced by photic stimulation are elicited when IPS is combined with patterns (Panayiotopoulos *et al.*, 1970a, b, Panayiotopoulos, 1972). The occipital spike appeared to emerge from the negative component of a triphasic W-shaped P100 visual evoked response (VER) and made us support the view that an increased sensitivity of the occipital cortex is implicated in the pathophysiology of photosensitive epilepsy. This well-documented view of a regional (I use the word regional as opposed to partial or focal) occipital lobe sensitivity has been well established (Wilkins *et al.*, 1980).

Despite the above marked differences between photosenitivity and FOS, there are examples of patients in whom both the 'photosensitive' and the 'FOS' mechanisms are jointly apparent, particularly in patients with eyelid-related ictal clinical manifestations. Video-game induced seizures should not always be equated with photosensitivity (70 per cent of the patients). FOS may be operative in some of them (Ferrie *et al.*, 1994).

Conclusions and proposals

The phenomena I have described in this review are extremely interesting from a clinical and neurophysiological point of view. There are more issues which are unknown than clarified. In 1991 we probably know for FOS and other related conditions as much as we knew for photosensitivity in 1946 when Gray Walter induced a photoconvulsive response on a patient while experimenting with his stroboscobe. Gastaut and his team in Marseille promoted IPS in the study of patients with epileptic seizures, photosensitivity has been studied extensively in man and animals all over the world (see Chapter 7) and no routine EEG is performed without application of IPS. FOS, is as interesting as photosensitivity. FOS which is mainly related to occipital lobes (occipital paroxysms) but also appears with more generalized EEG manifestations, may be easily studied in routine EEG (it is less time-consuming and the required equipment is less expensive than a stroboscope), and may be associated with many epileptic conditions. Moreover, the possible inhibitory effect of elimination of central vision and fixation on the α-rhythm makes the study of FOS more attractive.

The invited comments and opinions of Dr Colin Binnie and Dr Takeo Takahashi, leading experts in the field of photosensitive epilepsy, would certainly promote further research and understanding of FOS.

Comments by Colin D. Binnie

A problem highlighted by Dr Panayiotopoulos is the distinction between eyelid myoclonia with absences and self-induction by eye-closure. Both are found in highly photosensitive subjects and are characterized by generalized spike-wave activity, possibly of posterior onset, on eye-closure in an illuminated environment but not in darkness. The first point at issue must be whether of not these are in fact distinct syndromes.

That some patients use their photosensitivity to induce seizures and/or discharges is not in doubt.

However, the early accounts concern patients, usually mentally handicapped, who induced their attacks by flicker, waving the outspread fingers of one hand in front of the eyes whilst gazing at the sun (Andermann *et al.*, 1962). Green in 1966 described self-induction by eye closure and more recent studies by the writer and his collaborators suggest this to be a more common method and used by some 30 per cent of photosensitive subjects (Binnie *et al.*, 1980; Darby *et al.*, 1980; Kasteleijn-Nolst Trenité, 1989). Some features of this phenomenon (described in these reports) are listed below (after Binnie & Jeavons (1992). Those most important for the recognition of self-induction by eye-closure are asterisked and those which are considered to support the claim that it is not identical to myoclonia with absences are shown in bold type.

1. *The eye movement precedes the epileptiform discharge.

2. ***The eye and lid movement, as assessed by electrooculography, video recording or a mechanical transducer, is different from that accompanying normal eye-closure, either spontaneous or to command.** The main upward rotation of the eye is of greater magnitude and more sustained than the normal Bell's phenomenon, and there is often a superimposed lid flutter at about 6 Hz.

3. ***The manoeuvre undergoes rapid extinction when the patient is placed in darkness**, and fails to induce discharges.

4. ***The behaviour is increased by stress.**

5. Patients display guilt when the matter is discussed.

6. ***About 60 per cent of patients admit to self-induction**, variously describing it as compulsive or pleasurable.

7. ***A pleasant sensation is often reported,** sometimes with a sexual component occasionally leading to orgasm. Only a minority of patients express a wish to be relieved of their habit.

8. ***There may be a history of self-induction by hand-waving,** and some patients use both manoeuvres together, initiating the discharge by eye movement and prolonging it by hand-waving.

9. **There is a greater prevalence of mental handicap in self-inducing patients than among other photosensitive subjects,** although the majority are of normal intelligence.

10. **There is a greater prevalence of current and past psychiatric disorder in self-inducing patients than among other photosensitive subjects.**

11. ***Self-inducing patients are more often therapy-resistant than is usual in photosensitive epilepsy.**

12. The behaviour may be abolished by dopaminergic drugs, despite the fact that these probably increase photosensitivity.

13. **Some patients induce not only 'subclinical' discharges and absences or myoclonic attacks but also tonic–clonic seizures.**

The information necessary to resolve the differential diagnosis in favour of self-induction may be readily available if the patient indulges in obvious hand-waving (present in only about 10 per cent of our subjects) or indeed admits (as eventually do some 60 per cent) to self-induction. Mental handicap, psychiatric problems and therapy resistance should all heighten the suspicion of self-induction. Positive features for establishing with certainty that the observed behaviour is involuntary and that the patient does not self-induce may be more difficult to find. However, although self-induction can be very frequent, occurring sometimes as often as once a minute, it is elective, and is produced only by a particular type of eye movement. A patient who produces discharges on virtually every eye-closure, including those carried out to command, is unlikely to be self-inducing. There remains a need for careful phenomenological studies of the behavioural, oculographic and EEG features of these two syndromes, so that they can be distinguished by direct observation.

Another intriguing issue raised by Dr Panayiotopoulos is the apparent paradox that epileptic activity can be induced both by high levels of physiological activation of visual cortical neurones involved in pattern vision and also by withdrawal of such stimulation. This can possibly be resolved, albeit *post hoc*, as follows. Epileptogenesis in general involves excessive and/or hypersynchronous neuronal activity. Both are involved in conventional photosensitive epilepsy (Binnie *et al.*, 1980; Wilkins *et al.*, 1980), and stimulation of neuronal activity (whether or not the stimulus is inherently synchronizing) presumably underlies those more specific reflex epilepsies in which cognitive or other activity involving a specific brain region or system induces seizures. However, activation of a specific region can have an antiepileptic action, as demonstrated by some patients who discover manoeuvres for aborting their partial seizures, usually by moving or rubbing the part of the body in which the initial symptoms occur. Here, stimulation presumably has a desynchronizing effect. Isolated, interconnected neuronal populations have a tendency to spontaneous oscillatory burst firing, particularly when deprived of afferent input. Functional deafferentation is presumably the mechanism underlying the increase of epileptiform activity and seizure liability often seen during sleep, and the activating effects on epileptogenic foci of intravenous barbiturates, including some which under other circumstances are anticonvulsant.

The paradox of photic and FOS activation may not be easily explained, but is at least consistent with other aspects of the phenomenology of epilepsy. Stimulation of hyperexcitable cortex can be epileptogenic, particularly if it also synchronizes neuronal activity, as is the case with IPS. However, withdrawal of desynchronizing afferents can also have an epileptogenic effect in cortex which already has a liability to hypersynchronous discharge.

Comments by Takeo Takahashi

Regarding EEG aspects of FOS provocation of paroxysms by the fixation-off method appears to have a similar underlying mechanism to that of the Ganzfeld (homogeneous visual field) effect, as has already been reported (Gumnit *et al.*, 1965; Takahashi, 1976).

As a simple method for yielding a Ganzfeld stimulation, we used the following technique (Takahashi, 1976). A thick white paper, 18 × 26 cm in size, was placed 20 cm before the eyes of a subject, who looked at a fixation point in the centre for 10 s. This paper was then quickly replaced by a thin white paper; the subject kept his/her eyes open for 30 s. The luminosity of both papers was kept at 40 nt. The latter condition was regarded as a Ganzfeld stimulation. Using this pair of visual stimuli, EEG changes in response to looking at a fixation point and a Ganzfeld effect were investigated in a total of 77 subjects. They consisted of five adults, 66 epileptics and six patients with neuropsychiatric disorders. Of these 77 subjects, 16 showed normal and 61 abnormal EEGs while awake.

The EEG changes could be divided into the following two groups: (1) desynchronization by gazing at a fixation point and synchronization by Ganzfeld stimulation and (2) no significant changes by either stimuli. The first group included α activity (16 cases), posterior slow activity (12 cases), diffuse slow activity (three cases), generalized paroxysms (23 cases) and focal paroxysms over the posterior regions (10 cases). The second group included only focal paroxysms over the anterior regions (13 cases).

In a total of 46 epileptics who showed paroxysms of the anterior (13 patients), posterior (10 patients) and generalized (23 patients) regions, EEG activation by red flicker and flickering geometric pattern stimuli by the use of a visual stimulator (Tsukahara & Takahashi, 1973) were performed. Provocation of similar paroxysms was found in one (7.6 per cent), three (30 per cent) and 20 (86.9 per cent) patients respectively. Namely, a provocative rate of photoparoxysmal responses was the highest in epileptics in whom Ganzfeld stimulation produced generalized paroxysms, followed by posterior and anterior ones. The higher rate of the posterior paroxysms over the anterior one may indicate a closer link to the function of the occipital lobe in the genesis of FOS epilepsy. This is conceivably true in patients with FOS epilepsy.

On the other hand, we have demonstrated that patients with photosensitive epilepsy are particularly sensitive to red flicker and/or flickering geometric patterns stimuli when a decreased luminance, such as 10 nt, is used as a stimulating light source (Takahashi, 1989).

Therefore, a question may arise whether the patients with FOS are particularly sensitive to such stimuli or not. It has also been shown that epileptics sensitive to Ganzfeld stimulation are often sensitive to opening and closing their eyes and eye deviation in a dark room (Takahashi, 1976). Accordingly, in addition to the fixation-off method, EEG activation by the aforementioned visual stimuli and eye movements may help to further clarify the nature of FOS epilepsy.

Additionally, in order to state clearly that the paroxysms in FOS epilepsy are elicited by elimination of central vision in particular, non-effectiveness by any peripheral stimulation during the testing of FOS may necessarily be validated. Testing the colour effect and keeping the luminance constant, such at 5 nt, may provide valuable information because of the valid efficacy of red flicker stimulation in eliciting photoparoxysmal responses.

References

Andermann, K., Oaks, G., Berman, S., Cooke, P.M., Dickson, J., Gastaut, H., Kennedy., A., Margerison, J.H., Pond, D.A. & Tizard, J.P. (1962): Self-induced epilepsy. *Arch. Neurol.* **6,** 49–79.

Appleton, R., Panayiotopoulos, C.P., Acomb, A.B. & Beirne, M. (1993): Eyelid myoclonia with absences: an epilepsy syndrome. *J. Neurol. Neurosurg. Psychiatry* **56,** 1312–1316.

Beaumanoir, A., Capizzi, G., Nahori, A. & Yousfi, Y. (1989): Scotogenic seizures. In: *Reflex seizures and reflex epilepsies*, eds. A. Beaumanoir, H. Gastaut & R. Naquet, pp. 219–223. Geneva: Médecine and Hygiène.

Binnie, C.D. & Jeavons, P.M. (1992): Photosensitive epilepsies. In: *Epileptic syndromes of infancy, childhood and adolescence*, 2nd edn., eds. J. Roger, M. Bureau, C. Dravet, F.E. Dreifuss, A. Perret & P. Wolf, pp. 299–305. London: John Libbey.

Binnie, C.D., Darby, C.E, de Corte, R.A. & Wilkins, A.J. (1980): Self induction of epileptic seizures by eye closure: incidence and recognition. *J. Neurol. Neurosurg. Psychiatry* **43,** 386–389.

Cirignotta, F., Lugaresi, E. & Montagna, P. (1987): Occipital EEG activity induced by darkness: the critical role of central vision. In: *Migraine and epilepsy,* eds. F. Andermann & J. Lugaresi, pp. 139–143. New York: Raven Press.

Commission on Classification and Terminology of the International League Against Epilepsy (1989): Proposal for classification of epilepsies and epileptic syndromes. *Epilepsia* **30,** 389–399.

Darby, C.E., De Corte, R.A., Binnie, C.D. & Wilkins, A.J. (1980): The self-induction of epileptic seizures by eye-closure. *Epilepsia* **21,** 31–41.

Fabian, A. & Wolf, P. (1987): Epileptic dischargesd after eye-closure: relation to photosensitivity. In: *Advances in Epileptology,* eds. P. Wolf *et al.,* pp. 259–264. New York: Raven Press.

Ferrie, C.D., De Marco, P., Grunewald, R.A., Giannakodimos, S. & Panayiotopoulos, C.P. (1994): Video-game induced seizures. *J. Neurol. Neurosurg. Psychiatr.* in press.

Green, J.B. (1968): Seizures on closing the eyes: EEg studies. *Neurology* **18,** 391–396.

Gobbi, G., Bruno, L., Mainetti, A., Parmegianni, A., Tullini, A., Salvi, F., Tassinari, C.A., Santanelli, P., Bureau, M., Dravet, C.H. & Roger, J. (1989): Eye-closure seizures. In: *Reflex seizures and reflex epilepsies*, eds. A. Beaumanoir, H. Gastaut & R. Naquet, pp. 181–191. Geneva: Médècine et Hygiene.

Green, J.B. (1966): Self-induced seizures: clinical and electroencephalographic studies. *Arch. Neurol.* **15,** 579–586.

Gumnit, R.J., Niedermeyer, E. & Spreen, O. (1965): Seizure activity uniquely inhibited by patterned vision. *Arch. Neurol.* **13,** 363–368.

Jeavons, P.M. (1977): Nosological problems of myoclonic epilepsies in childhood and adolescence. *Dev. Med. Child. Neurol.* **19,** 3–8.

Jeavons, P.M. (1966): Summary of papers on abnormalities during photic stimulation. *Proc. electrophysiol. Technol. Ass.* **13,** 153–157.

Jeavons, P.M., Harding, G.F.A. & Panayiotopoulos, C.P. (1971a): Photosensitive epilepsy and driving. *Lancet* **i,** 1125.

Jeavons, P.M., Harding, G.F.A., Panayiotopoulos, C.P. (1971b): The effect of lateral gaze and lateral illumunation on photoconvulsive responses to intermittent photic stimulation. *Electroencephalogr. Clin. Neurophysiol.* **32,** 445.

Jeavons, P.M., Harding, G.F.A. & Panayiotopoulos, C.P. & Drasdo, N. (1972): The effect of geometric patterns combined with intermittent photic stimulation in photosensitive epilepsy. *Electroencephalogr. Clin. Neurophysiol.* **33,** 221–224.

Kasteleijn-Norst Trenité, D.G.A. (1989): Photosensitivity in epilepsy: electrophysiological and clinical correlates. *Acta Neurol. Scand.* (Suppl. 125), pp. 80.

Lewis, J.E. (1972): Eye closure as a motor trigger for seizures. *Neurology* **22,** 1145–1150.

Lugaresi, E., Cirignotta, F. & Montagna, P. (1984): Occipital lobe epilepsy with scotosensitive seizures. *Epilepsia* **25,** 115–120.

Panayiotopoulos, C.P. (1972): A study of photosensitive epilepsy with particular reference to occipital spikes induced by intermittent photic stimulation. PhD Thesis, University of Aston in Birmingham.

Panayiotopoulos, C.P. (1974): Effectiveness of photic stimulation on various eye states in photosensitive epilepsy. *J. Neurol. Sci.* **23,** 165–173.

Panayiotopoulos, C.P. (1977): 'Eye closure' and 'eyes closed' EEG abnormalities: discrimination and effectiveness of light and dark. *Electroencephalogr. Clin. Neurophysiol.* **43,** 523.

Panayiotopoulos, C.P. (1978): Occipital epilepsy. *Mat. Med. Greca* **30,** 557–564.

Panayiotopoulos, C.P. (1979): Conversion of photosensitive to scotosensitive epilepsy. *Neurology* **30,** 1550–1555.

Panayiotopoulos, C.P. (1980): Basilar migraine? Seizures and severe epileptiform EEG abnormalities. *Neurology* **30,** 1122–1125.

Panayiotopoulos, C.P. (1981): Inhibitory effect of central vision on occipital lobe seizures. *Neurology* **31,** 1331–1333.

Panayiotopoulos, C.P. (1987a): Difficulties in differentiating migraine and epilepsy based on clinical and electroencephalographic findings. In: *Migraine and epilepsy*, eds. F. Andermann & J. Lugaresi, pp. 31–46. New York: Raven Press.

Panayiotopoulos, C.P. (1987b): Fixation-off sensitive epilepsy in eye-lid myoclonia with absence seizures. *Ann. Neurol.* **22,** 87–89.

Panayiotopoulos, C.P. (1988): Vomiting as an ictal manifestation of epileptic seizures and syndromes. *J. Neurol. Neurosurg. Psychiatry* **51,** 1448–1451.

Panayiotopoulos, C.P. (1989a): Benign nocturnal childhood occipital epilepsy: a new syndrome with nocturnal seizures, tonic deviation of the eyes, and vomiting. *J. Child. Neurol.* **4,** 43–48.

Panayiotopoulos, C.P. (1989b): Benign childhood epilepsy with occipital paroxysms: a 15 year prospective study. *Ann. Neurol.* **26,** 51–56.

Panayiotopoulos, C.P. (1989c): Fixation-off-sensitive epilepsies. In: *Reflex seizures and reflex epilepsies*, eds. A. Beaumanoir, H. Gastaut & R. Naquet, pp. 203–217. Geneva: Médecine et Hygiène.

Panayiotopoulos, C.P. (1993a): Benign childhood partial epilepsies: benign childhood seizure susceptibility syndromes. *J. Neurol. Neurosurg. Psychiatry* **56,** 2–5.

Panayiotopoulos, C.P. (1993b): Benign childhood epilepsy with occipital paroxysms In: Occipital seizures and epilepsies in children, eds. F. Andermann, A. Beaumanoir, L. Mira, J. Roger & C.A. Tassinari, pp. 151–196. London: John Libbey.

Panayiotopoulos, C.P. & Siafacas, A. (1980): Triggering factors in occipital lobe epilepsy. *Acta Neurol. Scand.* Suppl. 79, 112.

Panayiotopoulos, C.P., Jeavons, P.M. & Harding, G.F.A. (1970a): Relation of occipital spikes evoked by intermittent photic stimulation to visual evoked responses in photosensitive epilepsy. *Nature* **228,** 566–567.

Panayioutopoulos, C.P., Jeavons, P.M. & Harding, G.F.A. (1970b): Occipital spikes and their relation to visual evoked responses in epilepsy with particular reference to photosensitive epilepsy. *Electroencephalogr. Clin. Neurophysiol.* **32,** 179–190.

Pazzaglia, P., Sabattini, L. & Lugaresi, E. (1970): Crisi occipitali precipitate dal buio. *Riv. Neurol.* **40,** 184–192.

Roger, J., Bureau, M. (1992): Benign epilepsy of childhood with occipiral paroxysms: up-date. In: *Epileptic syndromes in infancy, childhood and adolescence,* eds. J. Roger, M. Bureau, Ch. Dravet, F.E. Dreifuss, A. Perret & P. Wolf, pp. 205–217. London:John LIbbey.

Takahashi, T. (1976): Influence on EEGs of gazing at a fixation point and of Ganzfeld. *Brain. Nerve* **28,** 95–103.

Takahashi, T. (1989): Techniques of intermittent photic stimulation and paroxysmal responses. *Am. J. EEG Technol.* **29,** 205–208.

Tsukahhara, Y. & Takahashi, T. (1972): Visual stimulator for EEG activation. *Electroencephalogr. Clin. Neurophysiol.* **35,** 333–335.

Vignaendra, V., Thiam, G., Loh, G.L & Lim S.T.C (1976):Epileptic discharges triggered by blinking and eye closure. *Electroencephalogr. Clin. Neurophysiol.* **40,** 491–498.

Wilkins, A.J., Binnie, C.D. & Darby, C.E. (1980): Visually-induced seizures. *Prog. Neurobiol.* **15,** 85–117.

Epileptic Seizures and Syndromes, Edited by Peter Wolf
© 1994 John Libbey & Company Ltd., pp. 67–73

Chapter 9

Reading epilepsy

Peter Wolf

Epilepsie-Zentrum Bethel, Klinik für Anfallskranke, Mara I, Maraweg 21, 33617 Bielefeld, Germany

Introduction

The precipitation of epileptic seizures by specific stimuli was at first considered as an interesting feature which was present in some cases for reasons which were difficult to assess, but which could be worth studying for the understanding of some basic mechanisms of epilepsy (Bickford & Klauss, 1969). The handy term 'reflex epilepsy' for such cases has been criticized for two reasons: first, because many of the precipitating stimuli cannot be explained by reflex mechanisms in the proper sense; and second, because precipitation of seizures was observed in many types of epilepsy, but did not characterize these epilepsies because other patients with the same epileptic syndromes did not have provoked seizures.

A typical example for this is photosensitivity, which is observed frequently in all variants of generalized idiopathic epilepsy (Wolf & Goosses, 1986) but only in minorities of these patients, and sometimes it may be found in patients with epilepsies not belonging to the idiopathic generalized class (see Kasteleijn-Nolst Trenité *et al.*, Chapter 6; Binnie, Chapter 7). Reading epilepsy became the first and is still the only example where a specific mode of seizure precipitation was recognized as the presenting and therefore name-giving feature of a well-delimited epilepsy syndrome which is classified as one of the age-related idiopathic epilepsies which are in some way related to an anatomical location or region.

Syndrome classification

The characteristics of the syndrome, as they emerged from the meta-analysis of 111 cases (Wolf, 1992), are listed in Table 1.

The hereditary predisposition is most frequently specific. Of 20 first-degree family members with sufficient information on the type of epilepsy, 11 also had reading epilepsy. But there seems also to exist some genetic relation to idiopathic generalized epilepsies, as three affected first-degree relatives had some type of idiopathic generalized epilepsy. Two had febrile convulsions.

Concerning the age of onset, especially the lower boundary seems to be quite definite. There were only three patients with an onset before their twelfth birthday whereas five started at an age over 25.

The semiology of the partial motor seizures is remarkably uniform. They develop in clear consciousness, after a certain amount of reading, in the musculature which is involved in reading and talking:

tongue, throat, jaw, lips and face. Such symptoms have been reported in all cases but four. They have been described as stiffness, numbness, tightness, clicking sensation, stammering, etc., and the movements observed were myoclonic, or, more rarely, tonic. These symptoms and signs are usually bilateral, but in some cases they were asymmetric or unilateral.

Table 1. Clinical characteristics of reading epilepsy

Hereditary predisposition in 40–45%
Exogenous causes absent
Age of onset 12–25 years (mean: 17.7 years)
Sex ratio males/females: 1.8
Seizures: simple partial: orofacial motor, visual, dyslexic; secondary generalized tonic–clonic
Precipitation by reading (100%), talking (27%), writing (11%), reading figures (4–7%), reading Braille or music (rare)
Unprovoked seizures: absent in 95%, very rare in 5% of patients
Therapy: behavioural; valproic acid, clonazepam
Benign course in all longitudinal observations

A minority of patients described some kind of visual or ocular manifestation in addition to the motor seizures, and in a few cases this is the presenting symptom or the only partial seizure type. These manifestations are not uniform but can be differentiated into paroxysmal alexia or dyslexia, visual hallucinations (both simple and complex), and probably oculomotor.

Generalized tonic–clonic (GTC) seizures are usually rare. Most patients with the syndrome have experienced less than five grand mal seizures in total – probably because the preceding partial seizures helped them to prevent generalization. In some reported cases, secondary generalization had never occurred, but these were mostly discovered as affected relatives of patients with reading epilepsy, and their condition had not previously been identified as epileptic.

Modes of precipitation

Seizure precipitation by reading is of course mandatory for the diagnosis. One-quarter of the patients get motor seizures also when talking, and usually the conversation has to be vivid or vigorously argumentative. In most cases where writing was provocative, the motor seizure manifestations involved the writing arm, which would jerk or stiffen. Likewise, in three individuals where the reading of music was provocative, the arms would be jerking when they played an instrument. There seems to be a transition to seizure precipitation by other complex cognitive tasks, such as board or card games or calculation where simular motor involvements seem to occur (see Inoue *et al.*, Chapter 11). Such games have been provocative in three out of the 111 patients with reading epilepsy.

The mechanisms by which the seizures are precipitated have long been highly controversial, as was discussed in detail elsewhere (Wolf, 1992). Today it is clear that much of the controversy was due to individual variability, and the oniy feature of the precipitating mechanism which is common to all patients is the formal act of transforming linguistic material displayed in some graphic system into phonetic speech (audible or internal), which need not be semantically understood. The more difficult this formal task (unusual scripts, nonsense texts, known and unknown foreign languages), the more it becomes provocative. Reading aloud is more provocative than silent reading, and turbulences which disturb a smooth performance are often crucial. These may be caused by graphic, phonetic or semantic difficulties and anomalies.

Spontaneous seizures occur rarely and were reported by only five patients. They are consistent with the diagnosis if all other typical features are present.

Therapy and prognosis

Quite a few patients with reading epilepsy decide not to take antiepileptic drugs but to prevent secondary generalization by reacting to the partial seizure and stopping to read. This is possible whenever there is no rapid progress to a convulsive seizure. In some patients, there is rapid progress and this possibility does not exist. A few completely give up reading, which is, however, an important drawback in literate societies. Thus, many patients ask for antiepileptic drug treatment. The only antiepileptic drugs which have been reported as highly effective in this syndrome are valproic acid and clonazepam. In view of the problems with benzodiazepine treatment, valproic acid in monotherapy would today be considered by most authors as the drug of first choice. The prognosis of reading epilepsy is good because, even if untreated, the seizures usually remain strictly bound to precipitation by reading or whatever related additional stimulus may be active. Of the 111 cases reported, 29 had a history of 10 years or more, and in none of them was a tendency observed to develop spontaneous seizures.

In a volume where the controversial issue of secondary epileptogenesis is discussed at some length, it may be worth mentioning that in this as in all other idiopathic localization-related epilepsy syndromes, secondary epileptogenesis has never been observed.

Electroencephalography (EEG)

Reading epilepsy is not a variant of photosensitivity. The seizures are not provoked by intermittent light stimuli, and only 9 per cent of the patients were photosensitive at EEG investigation. This is, however, a much higher rate than in symptomatic focal epilepsies, and points again to a nosological and genetic relation to the generalized idiopathic epilepsies. Likewise, a certain proportion of the patients (11 per cent) have bilateral spike waves in their interictal EEG (Table 2), which otherwise remains mostly unrevealing.

Table 2. EEG findings in reading epilepsy

Routine EEG:	Negative	84	(80%)
	Bilateral SW	11	(11%)
	Paroxysmal temporal	5	(5%)
	Unclear	4	(4%)
Photic stimulation:	Negative	59	(91%)
	Epileptiform	6	(9%)
Other findings:	Generalized SW in sleep or 24 h EEG, $n = 2$		
Reading provocation:	Paroxysmal	73	(77%)
	Negative	15	(16%)
	Questionable	7	

In the ictal EEG (Table 3) the typical discharge is a single or a very short volley of steep or sharp wave(s), spike(s) or spike-and-wave complex(es). In many instances, these findings were reported as 'generalized' or, rather, bilateral, with inconsistent regional accentuation. This notion, however, is somewhat problematic because, of the illustrated reports, several tracings show clear asymmetries, which were not always pointed out by the authors. Table 3 combines the information of the reports with that of the illustrations. Still, as not all case reports include EEG illustrations, the one-third of symmetric bilateral findings could be too high a figure. The most common type of discharge was bilateral with unilateral accentuation, whereas unilateral or focal discharge was more rarely seen. Lateralization to the language-dominant hemisphere was more common (78 per cent) than to the non-dominant side (10 per cent) or shifting lateralization (12 per cent). The regions involved in unilateral or bilateral localized discharges were preferentially temporoparietal (with occasional extension to central or occipital (80 per cent) whereas frontal discharges (sometimes extending to central or anterior temporal leads) were found in only 20 per cent.

Table 3. Reading epilepsy, paroxysmal findings with reading provocation

Bilateral, symmetric	23	(32 per cent)
Bilateral, lateralized	28	(38 per cent)
Unilateral and focal	22	(30 per cent)
Lateralization		
Left	39	
Right	5	(1 left-hander)
Shifting	6	(1 left-hander)
Regional distribution		
Frontal (+ central, temp. ant.)	11	
Parietotemp. (+ central, occip.)	44	

The EEG findings are thus much less uniform and much less specific than in other idiopathic localization-related epilepsies.

Pathophysiology

The above-mentioned relative variability of EEG findings may have to do with the fact that the anatomy of reading is functional rather than topographic, and involves multiple subsystems of both cerebral hemispheres, and not only the angular region of the dominant hemisphere as could have been suspected from the alexias caused by lesions at that site (Hoff *et al.*, 1954).

Positron emission tomography (PET) studies of silent reading, reading aloud and semantic processing have demonstrated the *bilateral* activation of not only the striate cortex but also the visual association cortex during semantic reading (Posner *et al.*, 1988).

Semantic surprises which activate the N 400 component of the event related brain potential (Bentin, 1989) belong to the anomalies which may be provocative in reading epilepsy, such as in an example reported by Forster (1977, case 6), which comes close to the semantic priming experiment in the study of N 400 (Kutas *et al.*, 1988). N 400 is topographically widespread, with prominence in the temporal and parietal regions and right predominance. Reading is today considered to be a bihemispheric co-operative performance (Taylor, 1988), where the phonological representation is more on the left and the semantic representation more on the right side. Involvement of the phonological track is indispensable for the mechanism of reading epilepsy but semantics may become involved through the constant interhemispheric exchange in the reading process. Primarily semantic reading as it occurs in logographic script systems such as Chinese, would be expected to be less provocative, and it has indeed been noted (Y. Inoue, personal communication) that reading epilepsy is perhaps unexpectedly rare in Japan, where the script is a combination of logograms and phonograms.

Thus, the modern concepts of the neurophysiology of reading are very much in accord with the ictal EEG findings in reading epilepsy.

Open questions

As a consequence of this outline of the clinical and some theoretical aspects of reading epilepsy, three questions emerge in the argumentative context of this volume.

The nosological place of the syndrome

The hallmark is partial seizures involving parts of the nervous system which are active during reading: the orolaryngeofacial musculature subserving speech, the visual and oculomotor systems, the muscles of the arm in the cases where writing, playing music from a score or reading Braille is provocative. These may, with further provocation, proceed to a secondary GTC seizure, the least specific of all seizure types but often the event which concludes the diagnosis.

Partial seizures indicate a relation to an anatomical localization. In focal symptomatic epilepsies, the localization is circumscribed; in multifocal cases more than one circumscribed epileptogenic locus can be identified. In the prototype of idiopathic localization-related epilepsies, benign centrotemporal epilepsy of childhood, seizure discharge may flare up bilaterally in various locations within topographic boundaries, the lower parts of the perirolandic regions of both hemispheres. This may be considered as a bilateral functional instability of this region. The disorder is transient and genetically predetermined. It is still not known if the transient character is caused by an age-dependent transient activity of the responsible gene or by an interaction of a genetic disorder with non-specific factors of regional brain maturation. The first explanation, however, is more likely, considering the strictness of the age dependence. Similar to reading epilepsy, this syndrome has EEG relations to idiopathic generalized epilepsy (Beaumanoir *et al.*, 1974; Dalla Bernardina *et al.*, 1992), and possibly also genetic relations to the same, but these have both been less clearly established than in reading epilepsy.

The difference from perirolandic idiopathic epilepsy is that, in reading epilepsy, the anatomical relation is functional rather than topographic, notwithstanding bilateral involvement, with a bias to the language-dominant hemisphere. Although one region, the left orofacial segment of the motor strip, is involved in both types of idiopathic localization-related epilepsy, transitions between the two syndromes have never been described, which is in interesting contrast to idiopathic generalized epilepsy, where transitions and overlap between syndromes are frequent (Janz *et al.*, 1992).

Why is the phenotype of this genetic syndrome regional rather than generalized?

This is a question to be asked with respect to all localization-related idiopathic epilepsies, and is addressed in Chapter 32 of this volume. There is some reason to believe that in idiopathic epilepsies the inheritance is polygenic. The idiopathic localized epilepsies share some traits with idiopathic generalized epilepsy such as bilateral spike-wave discharge, or, in reading epilepsy, photosensitivity, and there may be some genetic overlap in families. These disorders could have a gene in common, along with others which separate them. In the localization-related syndromes, the distinctive genes seem to be limited in action, and the message from reading epilepsy is that the limitation need not necessarily be spatial but may be functional. It could depend on disturbances of subsets of transmitter interactions which are used for highly complex cerebral performances such as reading. Something similar may be discovered in seizure precipitation by praxis (see Inoue *et al.*, Chapter 11).

What makes the brain produce seizures in reading epilepsy?

Certainly not any circumscribed morphological changes. This, with the nosological relation to generalized idiopathic epilepsy, suggests that the basic mechanisms of ictogenesis may be similar to those which generate the typical seizures of idiopathic generalized epilepsies, absences and bilateral myoclonus, rather than to those responsible for local lesional ictogenesis. The notion that turbulances, overload and multiple feedback in the systems involved in reading are crucial for the precipitation of seizures indicates that maximal interactive neuronal performance is at least a facilitating factor in this condition.

Reading epilepsy as a 'reflex' epilepsy

The pathological functional system which appears to be responsible for reading epilepsy has some interesting properties. It has usually to be 'warmed up' before it fires (Wolf, 1992). It can be modulated by non-specific factors such as fatigue, stress, emotions, fasting, lack of sleep, and alcohol intake (Wolf, 1992). When some discharge has been provoked in the usual way, the system may become 'sensitized' (Geschwind & Sherwin, 1967; Brooks & Jirauch, 1971) and start to respond to less specific input such as talking. It has 'plastic' abilities which may integrate new pathways. Thus, one patient of Forster and Daly (1973) learned to read Braille in order to avoid seizures but then had them provoked by reading Braille.

Therefore, a puzzling situation arises. The pathophysiology of reading epilepsy involves multiple sensorimotor, cognitive and integrative processes which are so complex that they seem to be far remote from reflex theories. However, the pathological system is able to respond, at its periphery, in simple veritably reflex-like ways: the 'proprioceptive bombardment' from the speech musculature results in 'reflex firing through the same motor segment' (Bickford *et al.*, 1956). A similar relation has been suggested for eye movements and oculomotor seizures (Wolf, 1992). Another such relation clearly exists when the active hands start jerking in a patient who writes or plays from a musical score (Stevens, 1957; Forster & Daly, 1973).

There is only one other 'reflex' epileptic condition where a similarly close relation of stimulus and response has been noted, eyelid myocloni in eye-closure sensitivity (Guirao Bringas *et al.*, 1987). This, again, is a rather marginal feature in a pathological system which produces absences. In other types of 'reflex' epilepsy, such as photosensitivity, pattern sensitivity or musicogenic epilepsy, the relations of stimulus and response are clearly of a different kind.

Theories concerning 'reflex' epilepsies will have to account for these complex and variable conditions.

References

Beaumanoir, A., Ballis, T., Varfis, G. & Ansari, K. (1974): Benign epilepsy of childhood with rolandic spikes. *Epilepsia* **15,** 301–315.

Bentin, S. (1989): Electrophysiological studies of visual word perception, lexical organization, and semantic processing: a tutorial review. *Lang. Speech* **32,** 205–220.

Bickford, R.G. & Klass, D.W. (1969): Sensory precipitation and reflex mechanisms. In: *Basic mechanisms of the epilepsies*, eds. H.H. Jasper, A.A. Ward & A. Pope, pp. 543–564. London: Churchill.

Bickford, R.G., Whelan, J.L., Klass, D.W. & Corbin, K.B. (1956): Reading epilepsy: clinical and electroencephalographic studies of a new syndrome. *Trans. Am. Neurol. Assoc.* **81,** 100–102.

Brooks, J.E. & Jirauch, P.M. (1971): Primary reading epilepsy: a misnomer. *Arch. Neurol.* **25,** 97–104.

Dalla Bernardina, B., Sgrò, V., Fontana, E., Colamaria, V. & La Selva, E. (1992): Idiopathic partial epilepsies in children. In: *Epileptic syndromes in infancy, childhood and adolescence*, 2nd edn, eds. J. Roger, M. Bureau, Ch. Dravet, F.E. Dreifuss, A. Perret & P. Wolf, pp. 173–188. London: John Libbey.

Forster, F.M. (1977): *Reflex epilepsy, behavioural therapy and conditional reflexes.* Springfield: Thomas.

Forster, F.M. & Daly, R.F. (1973): Reading epilepsy in identical twins. *Trans. Am. Neurol. Assoc.* **98,** 186–188.

Geschwind, N. & Sherwin, I. (1967): Language-induced epilepsy. *Arch. Neurol.* **16,** 25–31.

Guirao Bringas, I.P., Behl, I. & Wolf, P. (1987): Epileptic discharge after eye closure: relation to epileptic syndromes. In: *Advances in epileptology*, Vol. 16, eds. P. Wolf, M. Dam, D. Janz & F.E. Dreifuss, pp. 255–258. New York: Raven Press.

Hoff, H., Gloning, I. & Gloning, K. (1954): Über Alexie. *Wien. Zschr. Nervenheilk.* **10,** 149–162.

Janz, D., Beck-Mannagetta, G. & Sander, T. (1992): Do idiopathic generalized epilepsies share a common susceptibility gene? *Neurology* **42** (suppl. 5), 48–55.

Kutas, M., Van Petten, C. & Besson, M. (1988): Event-related potential asymmetries during the reading of sentences. *Electroencephalogr. Clin. Neurophysiol.* **69,** 218–233.

Posner, M.I., Petersen, S.E., Fox, P.T. & Raichle, M.E. (1988): Localization of cognitive operations in the human brain. *Science* **240,** 1627–1631.

Stevens, H. (1957): Reading epilepsy. *N. Engl. J. Med.* **257,** 165–170.

Taylor, M.M. (1988): The bilateral cooperative model of reading. In: *The alphabet and the brain*, eds. D. De Kerckhove & Ch. J. Lumsden, pp. 322–361. Berlin, Heidelberg: Springer.

Wolf, P. (1992): Reading epilepsy. In: *Epileptic syndromes in infancy, childhood and adolescence*, 2nd edn, eds. J. Roger, M. Bureau, Ch. Dravet, F.E. Dreifuss, A. Perret & P. Wolf, pp. 281–298. London: John Libbey.

Wolf, P. & Goosses, R. (1986): Relation of photosensitivity to epileptic syndromes. *J. Neurol. Neurosurg. Psychiatry* **49,** 1386–1391.

Epileptic Seizures and Syndromes, Edited by Peter Wolf
© 1994 John Libbey & Company Ltd., pp. 75–80

Chapter 10

Three new cases of reading epilepsy

Antonio Martins da Silva,*‡ Ana Paula Correia† and Margarida Santiago§

**Serviço de Neurofisiologia and †Serviço de Neurologia, Hospital de Santo Antonio; ‡Unidade de Fisiologia Humana, Instituto Ciências Biomédicas 'Abel Salazar', Universidade do Porto, 4000 Porto, Portugal; §Clinica Neurologica, Hospital da Universidade de Coimbra, 3000 Coimbra, Portugal*

Summary

Three epileptic patients (two males and one female) had seizures precipitated by reading and generalized tonic–clonic seizures starting in adolescence or early adulthood (15, 17 and 21 years). In one patient the first seizures were not induced by reading and he had scarce generalized tonic–clonic seizures and paroxysmal activity also induced by board games and mental calculation. This patient had left temporal lobe atrophy on CT scan, and was the only one with a family history of epilepsy. The other ones had normal physical and CT scan examination at the time of the diagnosis.

During EEG and video recordings, the frequency of discharges and/or myoclonic jerks was increased by progressive reading difficulties (reading of texts in foreign language and of longer and complex sentences) or by reading aloud. The EEG discharges (spike-wave; polyspike-wave) were more frequent, had longer duration, and progressed to generalized myoclonus if the tests were prolonged. All patients had scarce interictal EEG recording abnormalities: generalized or left temporal and temporoparietal paroxysmal activity.

Two important aspects arise from these cases: the relevance of both the lexical and phonological components of reading and the possible role of a structural lesion as a generator of seizures or epileptiform discharges precipitated by or secondary to reading.

Introduction

As in many other reflex epilepsies, primary reading epilepsy seems to be a homogeneous clinical entity. It is benign in its clinical course and expression, more frequent in adolescents or young adults, and idiopathic localization-related, with specific precipitating mechanisms (Wolf, 1989). Although the first reports were published almost 40 years ago (Bickford *et al.*, 1956; Chavany *et al.*, 1956) and in spite of the large number of cases investigated, speculations and controversies about the role of a number of presumed factors involved still remains open to discussion. Among others, suggested factors comprise hyperexcitation of a determined cortical area by sensory stimuli such as proprioceptive impulses from speech and eye muscles (Bickford *et al.*, 1956; Alajouanine *et al.*, 1959); the role of attention or of emotional involvement in the reading material (Bingel, 1957; Critchley *et al.*, 1960); possible lesions on optic pathways predisposing or being a pathogenic factor (Bingel, 1957); the influence of the disturbed transcoding process of reading words into specific acoustic–speech motor entities (Wolf, 1978); and cognitive factors such as interpretation of difficult texts and foreign languages (Mesri & Pagano, 1987) and difficulties of comprehension (Kartsounis, 1988). In some of these studies a genetic preponderance of epilepsy was mentioned (Daly & Forster, 1975). Multifactorial triggering mechanisms have been evoked to explain this type of epilepsy and have been recognized by some authors as one of the reasons why these patients were treated by different kinds of antiepileptic drugs (Zagury *et al.*, 1989).

Recent advances in the investigation of reading epilepsy are more concerned with the influence of reading sequences on seizure generation. In normal situations, highly complex functions are activated at the same time as the eyes are reading the text. The eye movements when reading texts anticipate the words or are just ahead of them. These systems interact smoothly and constantly and can be disturbed by foreign languages or complex or nonsense texts that cause misreading. This may induce reprocessing of the sequences and act as turbulence on the reading systems (Wolf, 1992), increasing excitatory mechanisms of seizures or discharges in the cases of 'primary reading epilepsy'.

The clinical, electroencephalographic (EEG) and imaging data of three cases in which reading is the eliciting factor of seizures are reported. The authors discuss the role of the sensitization of the cortical networks by the repetitive stimuli of reading, and the role of structural lesions as determinant factors in the generation of seizures or discharges.

Report of cases

The three patients studied have common clinical and EEG features which are summarized in Tables 1 and 2. The tables include details of patients' characteristics and of the EEG at rest and during reading tests. Taking into account the time duration of the EEG recording, in each patient the number of discharges at rest EEG was plotted against the number of discharges obtained during reading tests. Chi-square statistics was applied. In all patients the number of discharges occurring during reading sessions was significantly higher ($P < 0.001$) than at rest.

Table 1. Patients' characteristics

		Not reading sz			Reading sz					
Pt	Sex	Age	Sz type	Pp	Age	Sz type	Heredity	Clin. ex	CT	Tt
1	F	21	1 GTC	Sl. Depr.	26	SPM > My > 2 GTC	No	N	N	PB PHT
2	M	15 24	5 GTC 1 SPM	? Speaking	36	SPM > My	Uncle	N	LT pole atrophy	PHT
3	M	–			17	SPM > My > GTC	No	N	N	CBZ

Pt = patient; Sz = seizure; Pp = precipitating factor; Clin. ex. = clinical examination; CT = computerized tomography scan; Tt = treatment; GTC = generalized tonic–clonic seizures; SPM = single partial motor seizures; My = myoclonic seizures; Sl. depr. = sleep deprivation; LT = left temporal; PB = phenobarbital; PHT = phenytoin; CBZ = carbamazepine.

Case 1

A 36-year-old female nurse, right-handed, started seizures at age 21 years. She had a generalized tonic–clonic (GTC) seizure on awakening after a sleep-deprived night. She was free of seizures during 3 years, under phenobarbital. Treatment was discontinued. Two years later (at 26) she began to experience episodes of jaw jerking after a certain amount of reading. Two of the episodes were followed by GTC seizures. Prolonged reading and emotional and/or physical stress such as sleep deprivation increased the frequency of attacks. Family history was negative. Past medical history and clinical examinations were unremarkable. Computerized tomography (CT) scan was normal.

EEG recorded at rest or during intermittent photic stimulation (IPS) and hyperventilation (HV) was normal. During reading, paroxysmal generalized EEG abnormalities were recorded. The patient was submitted to a time-indexed monitoring session with continuous EEG and video recording including resting EEG, naps, HV, IPS and neuropsychological testing. The neuropsychological test battery was similar for all the three cases, and included spatiotemporal orientation; memory tests; drawing; calculation, writing and dictation; board games; and talking and reading (native and foreign languages, silent or aloud). In each test session we calculated the recording time (during tests or at rest), the duration of the reading tests, the discharge rates (number of discharges per minute) and the latency, i.e. the time between the beginning of the tests session and the time of the first discharge. In this patient, during the EEG/video monitoring session, we recorded at rest two generalized bursts of spikes and waves (GSW). When the patient was reading Portuguese and French texts (silent or aloud) generalized bursts of spikes and waves were recorded. Discharges were more frequent, had longer duration and shorter latency when the test was repeated, or when the patient was reading a foreign language (namely when reading aloud). Jaw myoclonic jerks were noticed, inducing reading errors. Writing calculation induced three GSW without clinical involvement (see Table 2). Treatment with phenytoin failed to suppress reading seizures.

Table 2. Paroxysmal activity

Pt	Rest EEG/ duration	PS/ HV	Sleep	Duration in minutes	Reading Test Test	Disch/min	Lat.	Mental calcul board games	Writing calcul.
1	2 GSW (60′)	0	0	26	PT Al	1	50" – 8"	0	3 SW
					PT S	2	18" – 14"		
					F Al	4	4"		
					F S	2	8"		
2	2 SW LT (36′)	0	0	25	PT S	1	70"	+ (?)	0
					PT Al	1	60"		
					PT S	9	10"		
3	Rare SW LT (270′)	0	+ (focal)	56	PT S	5	20"	0	3 SW
					PT Al	6	10"		
					E S	7	7"		
					E Al	6	5"		
					SP S	10	8"		
					SP Al	16	5"		

PS = photosensitivity; HV = hyperventilation; Duration in minutes = total recording time; Disch/min = number of discharges per minute; Lat. = latency: time between onset of the tests and the beginning of the discharges; Calcul. = calculation; SW = spike and wave; G = generalized; LT = left temporal; languages (S = silent; Al = aloud): PT = Portuguese; F = French, E = English, SP = Spanish.

Case 2

A 41-year-old male casino croupier, right-handed, started spontaneous generalized seizures at 15 years. Four years later he suffered, on the same day, three spontaneous GTC seizures. By the age of 24, while talking or reading aloud, he stared and had tongue and jaw myoclonic jerks which prevent him from speaking. After a short rest he again had normal speech. From the age of 36 he experienced occasional jaw jerking, tiredness and drowsiness while reading. Past medical history and neurological examination were normal but there was an uncle with GTC seizures. CT scan showed a left temporal lobe atrophy with larger left ventricle and enlargement of the sylvian fissure (Fig. 1). Rest EEG showed left temporal sharp and slow waves with bilateral involvement. Board games and mental calculation induced scarce left temporal or GSW of short duration without clinical involvement. Reading Portuguese in silence and especially aloud induced left temporal and generalized spike-and-wave bursts with eyelid myoclonus. The patient felt tired and drowsy while reading and had to stop. The discharges occurred faster if the tests were repeated. Phenytoin treatment was unsuccessful.

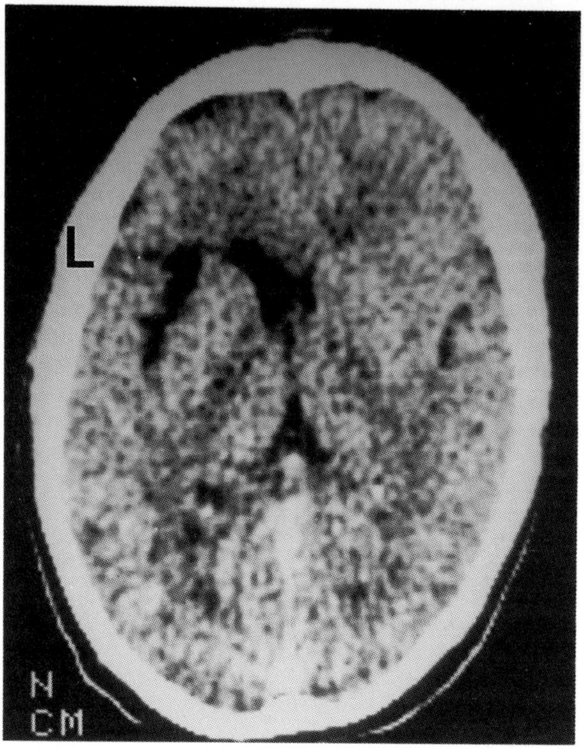

Fig. 1. Case 2. CT scan showing left (L) temporal lobe atrophy and enlargement of the sylvian fissure.

Case 3

A 28-year-old man, right-handed, started seizures at 17 years. While reading he experienced episodes of confusion and myoclonic jaw jerks, followed by GTC seizures. His medical history and clinical examination were unremarkable. No history of epilepsy in the family was found. Rest EEG showed rare sharp waves in the left parietotemporal region. IPS and HV did not induce abnormalities. Writing calculations, with difficult multiplication and division, induced three GSW. Reading in silence or aloud in Portuguese and foreign languages induced left temporal and generalized discharges (Fig. 2). The discharge rate increased strongly and the latency became shorter when the time between tests was shortened and when longer texts with foreign languages were used. The EEG recording showed GSW and frequently the patient had myoclonic jerks of the head and trunk. Under carbamazepine he continued to suffer occasional myoclonic jerks while reading.

Discussion

The three patients showed evidence of reading epilepsy and may contribute to the discussion of some of its aspects. The first aspect to discuss is what kind of reading epilepsy could be considered. Some authors suggested that reading seizures could be of secondary origin, caused by IPS induced by the scanning eye movements involved in reading (Alajouanine *et al.*, 1959; Mayersdorf & Marshal, 1970). However, if primary reading epilepsy is considered a syndrome, a secondary form would be considered a symptom. In general, disturbances caused by lesions of the sentence-implementation structures or of the mediation structures of the brain systems for language (Damasio & Damasio, 1992) could elicit epileptiform discharges or seizures when reading is processed. In such circumstances, reading-induced seizures have been considered as secondary or as symptoms of these

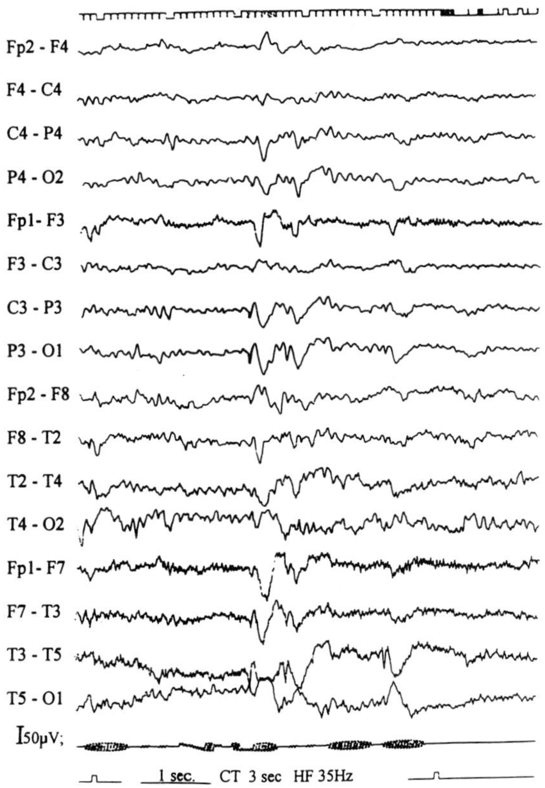

Fig. 2. Case 3. EEG recording during reading aloud native language texts.

disturbances which may frequently be associated with a constellation of other neurological deficits. Some authors claim that in such cases the patients had two types of seizures: spontaneous or induced by reading. To some extent this type of patient could be represented by case 2.

Two out of the cases reported (cases 1 and 3) also had few epileptiform discharges during complicated and sequential calculations. Case 2 also had seizures induced by talking. In general, these patients presented the usual picture of reading epilepsy (Wolf, 1992). They had few or no spontaneous GTC seizures, starting in adolescence, followed by seizures induced by reading, especially when reading difficulties increased (longer texts, foreign languages) or when reading aloud. Semantic ambiguities increased the inducing effect. In cases 1 and 3 the lexical component of reading seemed to contribute as well as the phonological component. Both patients had more discharges and shorter latency with foreign languages or reading aloud, especially when the stimuli became more frequent. This could be the result of sensitization of neuronal networks involved in reading. The phonological component seems to be more important in case 2. In this patient, a structural lesion was found in the left temporal lobe and in the sylvian fissure corresponding to areas involved in the phonological components of the language process that can be stimulated by the sensory stimuli generated by talking or reading aloud. This stimulation can induce instability of the neighbouring areas and can interfere with local networks and elicit discharges or seizures.

As a feature in favour of sensitization of the systems operating in reading as a causative factor, all patients had more frequent, longer and earlier discharges or seizures if the tests were repeated or if the test intervals were decreased, similar to that reported by Christie *et al.* (1988). It seems that the tests act as repetitive firing on determined areas (in the cases of structural lesions) or on the overall networks involved in reading processes. To some extent, this may be compared to the provocative effect of the animal kindling model of epilepsy. These findings could explain some of the typical clinical features of reading epilepsy.

The patients know the type of stimuli evoking the seizures, the duration of reading without causing disturbances and how to prevent them. This can explain why, in spite of frequently unsuccessful pharmacotherapy, generalized seizures are rare.

References

Alajouanine, T.H., Nehlil, J. & Gabersek, V. (1959): A propos d'un cas d'épilepsie déclenchée par la lecture. *Rev. Neurol.* **101,** 463–467.

Bickford, R.G., Whelan, J.L., Klass, D.W. & Corbin, K.B. (1956): Reading epilepsy: clinical and electroencephalographic studies of a new syndrome. *Trans. Am. Neurol. Assoc.* **81,** 100–102.

Bingel, A. (1957): Reading epilepsy. *Neurology* **7,** 752–756.

Chavany, J.A., Fischgold, H., Messimy, R. & Arfel-Capdevielle, G. (1956): Étude clinique et EEG d'un cas d'épilepsie provoquée électivement par la lecture. *Rev. Neurol.* **95,** 381–387.

Christie, S., Guberman, A., Tansley, B.W. & Couture, M. (1988): Primary reading epilepsy: investigation of critical seizure-provoking stimuli. *Epilepsia* **29 (3),** 288–293.

Critchley, M., Cobb, W. & Sears, T.A. (1960): On reading epilepsy. *Epilepsia* **1,** 403–417.

Daly, R.F. & Forster, F.M. (1975): Inheritance of reading epilepsy. *Neurology* **25,** 1051–1054.

Damasio, A.R. & Damasio, H. (1992): Brain and language. *Sc. Am.* **267 (3),** 63–71.

Kartsounis, L.D. (1988): Comprehension as the effective trigger in a case of primary reading epilepsy. *J. Neurol. Neurosurg. Psychiatry* **51,** 128–130.

Mayersdorf, A. & Marshall, C. (1970): Pattern activation in reading epilepsy: a case report. *Epilepsia* **11,** 423–426.

Mesri, J.C. & Pagano, M.A. (1987): Reading Epilepsy. *Epilepsia* **28,** 301–304.

Wolf, P. (1978): Reading epilepsy: evidence for a cognitive factor in seizure precipitation. In: *Advances in epileptology*, eds. H. Meinardi & A.J. Rowan, pp. 85–90. Amsterdam, Lisse: Swets & Zeitlinger.

Wolf, P. (1989): Reflex epilepsies and syndrome classification: an argument for considering primary reading epilepsy as an idiopathic localisation-related epilepsy. In: *Reflex seizures and reflex epilepsies*, eds. A. Beaumanoir, H. Gastaut & R. Naquet, pp. 283–286. Geneva: Médecine et Hygiène.

Wolf, P. (1992) Reading epilepsy. In: *Epileptic syndromes in infancy, childhood and adolescence*, 2nd edn, eds. J. Roger, M. Bureau, Ch. Dravet, F.E. Dreifuss, A. Perret & P. Wolf, pp. 281–298. London: John Libbey.

Zagury, S., Daniele, O. & Salas-Puig, J. (1989): Primary reading epilepsy. In: *Reflex seizures and reflex epilepsies*, eds. A. Beaumanoir, H. Gastaut & R. Naquet, pp. 275–282. Geneva Médecine et Hygiène.

Epileptic Seizures and Syndromes, Edited by Peter Wolf
© 1994 John Libbey & Company Ltd., pp. 81–91

Chapter 11

Epilepsy with praxis-induced seizures

Yushi Inoue, Masakazu Seino, Hidemoto Kubota, Kimiaki Yamakaku, Masaki Tanaka and Kazuichi Yagi

National Epilepsy Center, Shizuoka Higashi Hospital, Urushiyama 886, Shizuoka 420, Japan

Summary

Clinical characteristics of epilepsy with induced seizures we examined can be summarized as followed:

(1) Seizure onset occurs around puberty, with male preponderance. Clinical seizure types are absence seizures with or without clonic components, massive myoclonic jerks or generalized convulsions. The seizures may be asymmetrical and can be localized in a part of the body concurrently moved or intended to be moved. Partial motor seizures are exceptional. The EEG shows a burst of bisynchronous spike-and-wave or polyspike-and-wave discharges with or without focal accentuation predominating in the centroparietal regions. Photoconvulsive response is rare. Almost all patients experience non-precipitated spontaneous seizures. The vast majority of the cases are diagnosed as juvenile myoclonic epilepsy.

(2) The precipitating factors include ideation or execution of complicated movements, including sequential spatial processing, such as playing games, construction, calculation, complicated finger manipulation, drawing and writing. Concentration of attention and stress associated with these activities may contribute to precipitation.

This particular type of reflex epilepsy may be called praxis-induced epilepsy.

Introduction

Various higher brain functions may contribute to the precipitation of epileptic seizures. This study is limited to precipitation by non-verbal higher brain activities relating to spatial processing and ideation or execution of movements, including handwriting. Various terminologies have been used to describe epileptic seizures or epilepsy induced by these activities: epilepsia arithmetices (Ingvar & Nyman, 1962); seizures induced by thinking (Wilkins *et al.*, 1982), or thinking epilepsy; game-playing epilepsy (Siegel *et al.*, 1992), or chess and card epilepsy (Ch'en *et al.*, 1965); drawing-induced seizures (Brenner & Seelinger, 1979); graphogenic epilepsy (Asbury & Prensky, 1963), or writing epilepsy (Sharbrough *et al.*, 1977). Language-induced epilepsy (Geschwind & Sherwin, 1967) includes seizures induced by reading. However, the clinical and electroencephalographic (EEG) features of the induced epileptic seizures seem to be equivocal. In some patients, the EEG and clinical seizure characteristics remind us of juvenile myoclonic epilepsy (JME).

In this study, we compared the clinical and EEG features of induced seizures that we observed with those reported in the literature, and scrutinized the relationship between clinical features of patients having induced seizures and those of JME patients. The study shows that the basic processes underlying the various precipitating factors are relatively common, and may be described by the term 'praxis'.

Patients and methods

The patients consisted of two groups that were partly overlapping. The first group consisted of 32 patients who had a history of seizures induced by non-verbal higher brain activities. In 21 of the 32 patients, various neuropsychological examinations were performed under video-EEG monitoring to elucidate the clinical and EEG features of the induced seizures and the modalities of their precipitation. These findings were compared with those of 79 cases of induced seizures associated with higher brain function reported in the literature.

The second group consisted of 132 patients who were diagnosed as having JME for the past 2 years, according to criteria proposed by the Commission on Classification and Terminology of the International League Against Epilepsy (1989). These JME patients served as control subjects in terms of EEG features and other clinical characteristics.

Results

Patients with induced seizures

In 13 of the 21 patients who had a history of induced seizures, certain neuropsychological tasks induced paroxysmal EEG discharges, with accompanying clinical manifestations in 12 patients. The clinical profiles of three such cases are presented below. Ten of the 12 patients, including case 3, were reported previously (Inoue *et al.*, 1987, 1992).

Case 1

A 32-year-old right-handed woman had five febrile convulsions between 3 and 4 years of age. Family history of seizure disorders was negative. Neurological examination results were normal. Since the age of 14, she had had myoclonic jerks several times a day and two generalized tonic–clonic seizures (GTCs). Myoclonic jerks of both arms were prone to occur when she used a word processor. The myoclonic jerks also occurred, though rarely, in the perioral area when she was talking in a stressful situation. She realized then an error of pronunciation. EEG background activities were normal, and there was no photoconvulsive response. During the neuropsychological examination, generalized polyspike-and-wave complexes were induced frequently (Fig. 1). Word processing was the most effective precipitator of her seizures (Table 1).

Table 1. Induced epileptic EEG discharges by type of task (case 1)

Task	Test time (min)	Induced sp-w-c (s)	Sp-w-c index (sp-w-c/test time)
Word processor	17.1	120	6.76
Block design	22.0	142	6.45
Playing puzzle	9.5	60	6.32
Calculating (mental)	5.0	23	4.60
Calculating (writing)	5.0	16	3.20
Writing (kanji)	8.5	24	2.82
Writing (kana)	3.0	4	1.33
Reading	3.2	6	1.85
Resting	29.8	19	0.64

Sp-w-c = (poly)spike-and-wave complexes.

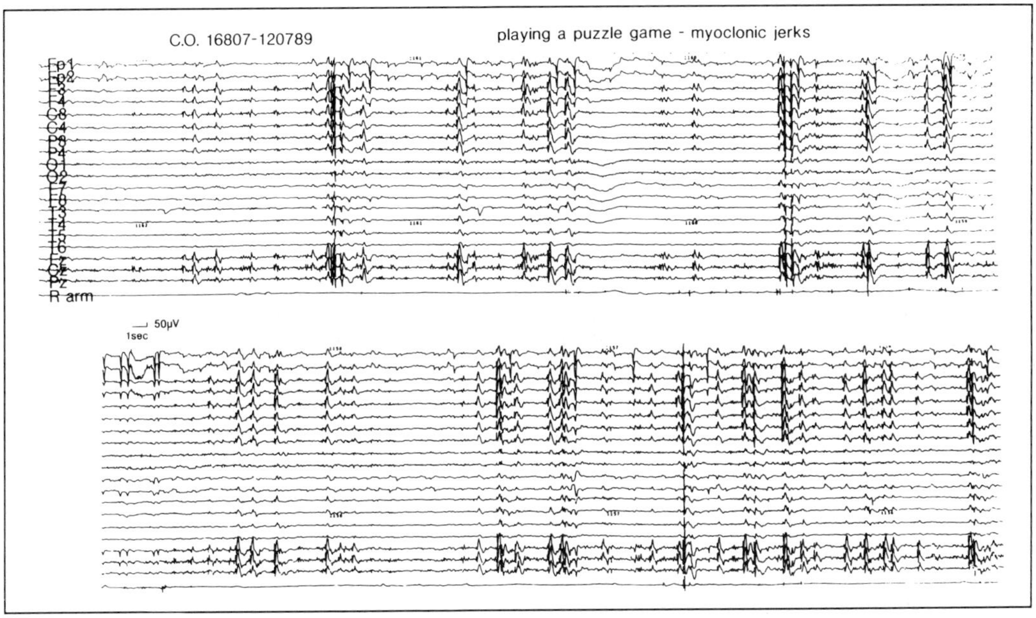

Fig. 1. Frequent bisynchronous and symmetrical polyspike-and-wave discharges accompanying myoclonic jerks induced by playing a puzzle game (case 1).

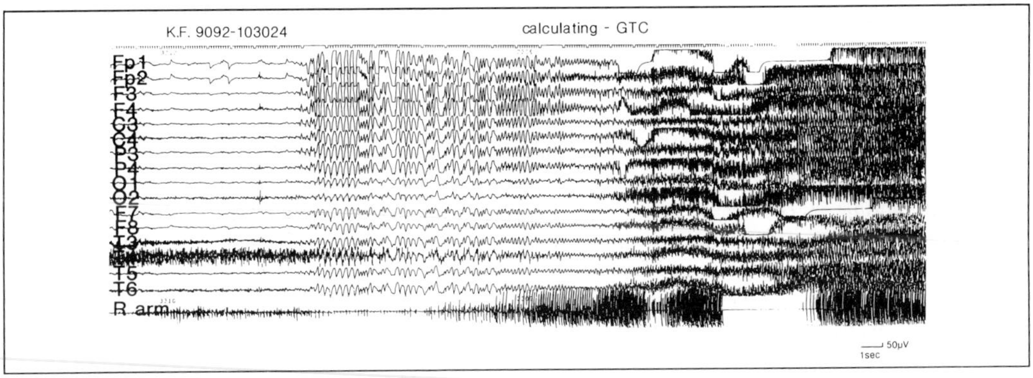

Fig. 2. Ictal EEG abnormalities precipitated by calculation using soroban (case 2). Myoclonic jerks of the right hand followed by tonic extension of right arm and retraction of the mouth to the right evolved to a generalized convulsion.

Case 2

A 28-year-old right-handed man was affected by meningitis at the age of 2 years. Family history of seizure disorders was negative. Neurological examination results were normal. Since the age of 9 years, he had had myoclonic jerks of both arms and eyelids, rarely involving the legs, but occasionally associated with falling. The jerks occurred several times a month, progressing occasionally to GTCs. The seizures were prone to induction by writing or calculating, especially by using a soroban (Japanese abacus). Interictal EEGs were normal, and no photoconvulsive responses were observed. During neuropsychological examination (Table 2), myoclonic movements of the right hand were induced, especially during soroban practice. The movements occasionally resulted in tonic extension of the right arm and retraction of the mouth to the right followed by a generalized convulsion. Ictal EEGs were bisynchronous and symmetrical from the onset (Fig. 2), and ictal single photon emission computed tomography (SPECT) executed during a major convulsive seizure indicated an asymmetrical hyperperfusional area that included the left putamen.

Table 2. Induced epileptic EEG discharges by type of task (case 2)

Task	Test time (min)	Induced sp-w-c (s)	Sp-w-c index (sp-w-c/test time)
Calculating (soroban)	32	25	0.78
Calculating (mental)	13	3	0.23
Writing	30	12	0.4
Copying Rey's figure	2	1	0.5
Copying letters	6	2	0.33
Playing puzzle	8	1	0.13

Sp-w-c = (poly)spike-and-wave complexes.

Case 3

A 22-year-old right-handed man had, since the age of 10 years, had absence seizures with clonic components several times a day, and occasionally had myoclonic jerks eventually evolving to GTCs. Neurologically he was normal, and his IQ was 74. His grandfather suffered from epilepsy. No photoconvulsive response was observed. Seizure-precipitating factors consisted of writing, calculating, playing games, constructing spatial tasks and complicated finger manipulations. Myoclonic movements accompanying rhythmic elevation of the arm occurred predominantly in the arm he was using or intended to use. The ictal EEG showed bursts of bisynchronous spike-and-wave discharges predominating in the centroparietal region (Fig. 3). The ictal EEG of an induced major convulsive seizure was also bisynchronous from the outset. The seizures were medically refractory. Epilepsy with myoclonic absences may well be an appropriate diagnosis (C.A. Tassinari, personal communication).

The clinical and EEG features of the induced seizures in the 13 patients (nine males, four females) are summarized in Table 3. The mean age of seizure onset was 12.2 ± 3.82 years (range, 6–21 years). The seizure manifestations were generalized both clinically and electrographically. The myoclonic jerks were, not rarely, asymmetrical or localized in the part of the body concurrently moved or

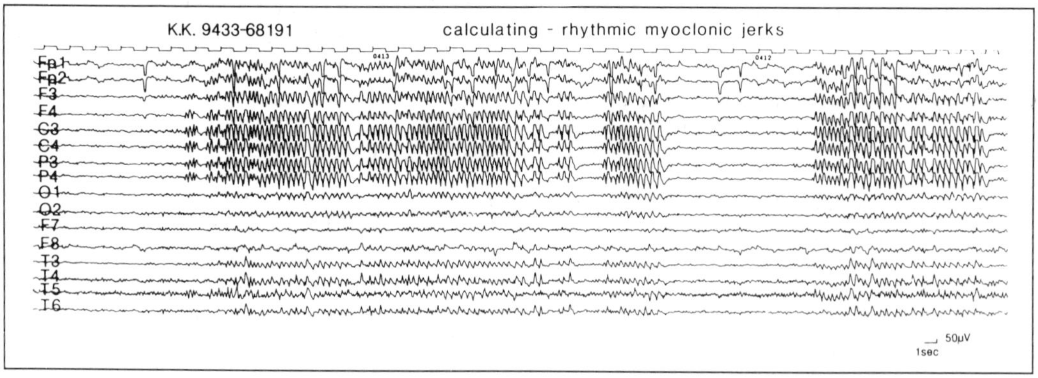

Fig. 3. Bursts of bisynchronous spike-and-wave or wave discharges predominating in the centroparietal region induced by calculation using soroban (case 3). Myoclonic movements accompanying elevation of the arms were observed predominantly in the arm the patient was using or intended to use.

intended to be moved. The seizure-precipitating factors consisted of various higher brain activities associated with spatial processing and/or ideation or execution of complicated movements. Complicated tasks, rather than simple ones, were prone to elicit clinical seizures, EEG discharges or both. Writing complexly composed sentences was also an effective precipitator. Rarely, reading or speaking, which was tested after non-verbal tasks, induced seizures. Concentration of attention or stress may contribute to the precipitation of seizures.

Table 3. *Clinical features, ictal EEG findings and precipitating factors in induced seizures*

Induced clinical seizures (12 patients)	
Absences with or without clonic components	5
Myoclonic jerks	8
Major convulsive seizures	3
Induced EEG paroxysms (13 patients)	
Bisynchronous (poly)spikes-and-waves	12
Focal (poly)spikes-and-waves	1
Precipitating factors	
Calculating	10
Drawing	5
Spatial constructing	11
Writing	9
Playing chess	8
Playing cards	9
Complicated manipulation	8
Reading	1
Speaking	1

Relation to JME

The clinical seizure characteristics and ictal EEG findings described above resembled those of JME. On the basis of the clinical characteristics, including seizure semiology and ictal EEG, 21 of the 32 patients who had a history of reflex seizures were diagnosed as having JME. The diagnoses of the other 11 patients were juvenile absence epilepsy (three cases), idiopathic generalized epilepsy (four cases), and undetermined epilepsy (four cases).

Reflex seizures were predominant and habitual in 19 (14.4 per cent) of the comparison cohort of 132 JME patients, and incidental or rare in 24 of them (18.2 per cent). In the predominant group, the number of males exceeded that of females. Age at epilepsy onset and family and personal history of seizures did not differ from those of JME patients who did not have reflex seizures (Table 4). With regard to seizure types, all patients in the predominant group had experienced GTCs in the past. The routine interictal EEGs of all patients in the predominant group showed bisynchronous spike-and-wave or polyspike-and-wave discharges, but no photoconvulsive responses.

Medical refractoriness was investigated for 3 years (Table 5). While 69 per cent of JME patients without reflex seizures were free from seizures for the 3-year period, only 31 per cent of those in the predominant group were free from seizures. Two patients were particularly medically refractory. Almost all patients in the predominant group could recognize the likelihood of occurring seizures and tried to avoid the precipitating stimuli in their daily lives. Valproate, clonazepam and zonisamide were the most effective drugs.

Comparison with reported cases

The clinical and EEG characteristics of 79 reported cases of induced seizures (references: 1–13,

Table 4. Frequency of induced seizures in JME patients

	Reflex seizure		
	None ($n = 89$)	Incidental ($n = 24$)	Predominant ($n = 19$)
Demographic features			
Female/male	46/43	15/9	4/15
Age at onset (years)	13.9 ± 3.28 (7–29)	13.0 ± 3.17 (8–21)	14.1 ± 2.71 (10–21)
Epilepsy in family	19 (21.3%)	2 (8.0%)	3 (15.8%)
Personal history			
Febrile seizures	23 (25.8%)	8 (32%)	7 (36.8%)
Birth asphyxia	1	2	2
Minor head injury	3	0	1
Meningitis	0	0	1
Seizure types			
Myoclonic jerks only	8	2	0
Myoclonic + absences	1	0	0
Myoclonic + GTCs	73	16	13
Myoclonic + absences + GTCs	7	6	6
Interictal EEG findings			
Gen. spikes-and-waves (GSW)	67	22	16
GSW + focal spikes	12	1	2
Focal spikes only	2	1	0
Normal	8	0	1
Photoconvulsive response	14 (15.7%)	5 (20.8%)	0

Table 5. Drug response in JME patients during a 3-year period

	Reflex seizures		
	None ($n = 71$)	Incidental ($n = 17$)	Predominant ($n = 16$)
Seizure-free (> 3 years)	49 (69%)	5 (29.4%)	5 (31.2%)
Occasional seizures	22 (31%)	12 (70.6%)	9 (56.3%)
No improvement	0	0	2 (12.5%)

15–50, 52–56) were closely similar to those shown in our cases (Table 6). The age at initial seizure onset was around puberty, and there was male preponderance. In regard to the patients' nationality, the incidence of non-verbal-induced epilepsy was obviously high in Japan. Focal paroxysmal discharges on the EEG were exceptional, and the incidence of photosensitivity was obviously low.

Precipitating factors included various non-verbal higher brain activities, as also indicated in our cases. Some patients whose seizures were induced not only by non-verbal performances but also by reading, speaking or both were reported as having language-induced epilepsy.

Table 6. Seventy-nine cases of induced seizures reported in the literature

Age at onset ($n = 77$)	15.7 ± 6.70 (6–46) years
Female/male ($n = 79$)	29/50
Epilepsy in family ($n = 70$)	20 (28.6%)
Personal history ($n = 74$)	
Childhood convulsions	9
Other causative disorders	13
Nationality	
Japanese	33
Other	46
Paroxysms on EEG ($n = 78$)	
Bisynchronous (poly) spikes-and-waves	69
Focal accentuation	12
Additional focal spikes	3
Other generalized discharges	4
Focal spikes	3
Normal	2
Photosensitivity ($n = 50$)	7 (14%)
Precipitating factors	
Calculating	51
Drawing	19
Spatial constructing	23
Writing	30
Playing chess	22
Playing cards	29
Complicated manipulation	20
Reading	13
Speaking	1

Discussion

Most patients with induced seizures have two or more precipitating factors in various combinations. An attempt of cluster analysis to elucidate which precipitating factors are likely to be combined (Inoue *et al.*, 1992; Fig. 4) indicated that reading and speaking may play similar roles as precipitators, but rarely combine with non-verbal performances. Writing tended to combine with the nonverbal performances in place of reading or speaking. Non verbal performances such as calculation, drawing, construction, playing games and complicated finger movements were likely to combine.These results suggest that the processes underlying activation of reflex seizures may be relatively identical, although the range of stimuli was apparently broad. Forster (1977) reported that the three factors of complex decision-making, sequential decision-making and stress may play a deterministic role in seizure evocation, although their threshold effects might vary. Cirignotta *et al.* (1980) stressed the importance of foreseeing the consequence of decision and introduced the term strategic thinking. Goossens *et al.* (1990) suggested that various stimuli leading to activation of reflex seizures seemed related to and involved in mathematical or spatial thinking, which is referable to parietal lobe function. Daniele *et al.* (1989) further noticed that the stimuli involved not only decision-making but also praxic abilities. Likewise, our observations indicated that the seizures were precipitated when the patients were obliged to contemplate complicated spatial tasks in a sequential fashion, to make decisions and to practically respond by using a part of their body under the stress of circumstances. In other words, transcoding processes of thinking into voluntary or intentional acts seem to be affected in this particular type of reflex epilepsy. These processes may be called praxic ability. Therefore, the term 'praxis-induced seizures' may be applied in this type of reflex epilepsy.

Although the stimuli are apparently referable to certain regional brain areas, the activated EEG and,

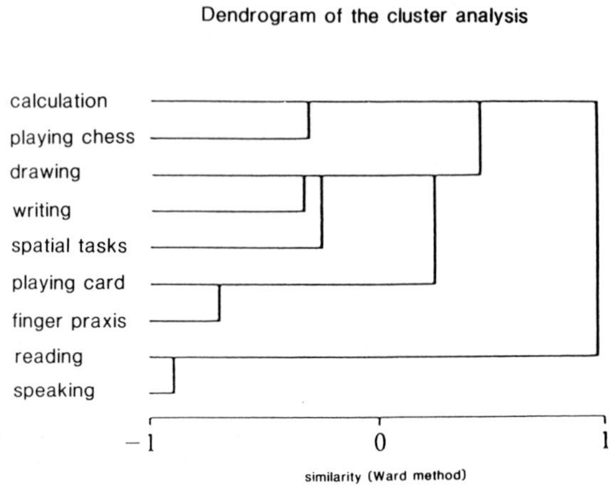

Fig. 4. Cluster analysis of the precipitating factors performed in 93 patients with praxis-induced epilepsy and language-induced epilepsy.

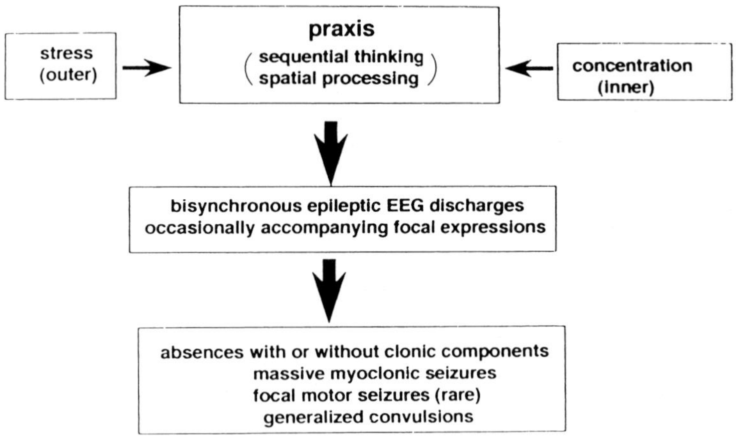

Fig. 5. Schematic representation of precipitating processes and EEG and clinical expressions in praxis-induced epilepsy.

to some extent, clinical seizure patterns are of a generalized nature. All patients with induced seizures in our series had generalized seizures, and no patients were distinctly recognized as having focal (localization-related) epilepsy. Focal epilepsy was also an exceptional diagnosis among the cases reported in the literature. Goossens *et al.* (1990) postulated that parietal cortical dysfunction eventually activated generalized epileptogenic mechanisms analogous to the occipital cortical activation leading to generalized epileptic abnormalities in patients with photosensitive epilepsy. The fact that the induced seizures can be asymmetrical and localized in a part of the body concurrently moved or intended to be moved indicates an expression of focal or regional accentuation of generalized epileptic bombardments.

The vast majority of the patients were under the umbrella of idiopathic generalized epilepsy, particularly JME. The relation of this kind of reflex epilepsy to JME was confirmed by the fact that one-seventh of our patients with JME experienced induced seizures as habitual attacks. However,

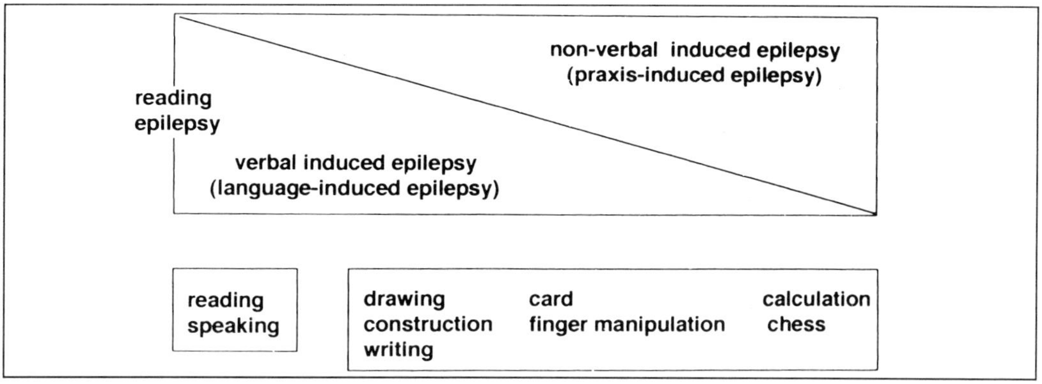

Fig. 6. Schematic representation of the spectral continuum between reading epilepsy, language-induced epilepsy and praxis-induced epilepsy, and the modalities of precipitation.

certain characteristics, such as male preponderance and a lower incidence of photoconvulsive response in the patients with induced seizures than those without induced seizures, suggest a dispositional difference even in the realm of JME.

Figure 5 illustrates a possible reflex mechanism involving stress and concentration. Physiological variables such as lack of sleep may, of course, also play a role in seizure precipitation.

Forster (1977) noticed that reading epilepsy and decision-making epilepsy are closely related. As case 1 in this study indicated, praxis-induced epilepsy may occasionally have seizures induced by reading and, conversely, reading epilepsy may have seizures induced by other higher brain activities (see Wolf, this volume). Those cases in which seizures are induced by reading, speaking and writing are denoted as language-induced epilepsy. It may be reasonable to postulate a spectral continuum between these three types of epilepsy induced by higher brain activities. The relationship of these is schematically represented in Fig. 6.

As already mentioned, the incidence of praxis-induced epilepsy is high in Japan. This fact may not only be a reflection of interest among Japanese epileptologists in this particular type of reflex seizure, but also represent a transcultural difference in terms of practising higher brain function associated with seizure precipitation, when we consider the fact that reading epilepsy is found to be low in Japan (Wolf, 1992).

Therapeutically, it is important to identify which factors do precipitate seizures and which do not, because the patients can learn or be advised to avoid precipitating circumstances, even when the seizures are medically refractory.

Acknowledgement

We are grateful to Prof. Dr P. Wolf of Bethel, who encouraged us to pursue this work.

References

Andermann, F., Goossens, L. & Andermann, E. (1989): Clinical features and diagnosis of epilepsy induced by thinking. In: *Reflex seizures and reflex epilepsies*, eds. A. Beaumanoir, H. Gastaut & R. Naquet, pp. 317–322. Geneva: Médecine & Hygiène.

Anderson, N.E. & Wallis, W.E. (1986): Activation of epileptiform activity by mental arithmetic. *Arch. Neurol.* **43,** 624–626.

Aoki, Y. & Ogasawara, N. (1975): Petit mal absence precipitated by calculation. *Psychiatry* (Japan) **17,** 135–142.

Asbury, A.K. & Prensky, A.L. (1963): Graphogenic epilepsy. *Trans. Am. Neurol. Assoc.* **88,** 193–194.

Bennet, D.R., Mavor, H. & Jarcho, L.W. (1971): Language induced epilepsy: report of a case. *Electroencephalogr. Clin. Neurophysiol.* **30,** 159.

Bingel, A. (1957): Reading epilepsy. *Neurology* **7,** 752–756.

Brenner, R.P. & Seelinger, D.F. (1979): Drawing-induced seizures. *Arch. Neurol.* **36,** 515–516.

Brooks, J.E. & Jirauch, P.M. (1971): Primary reading epilepsy: a misnomer. *Arch. Neurol.* **25,** 97–104.

Bruns-Malzahn, B., Wolf, P. & Janz, D. (1978): Seizure precipitation by decision making. *Epilepsia* **19,** 110.

Ch'en, H., Ch'in, C. & Ch'u, C. (1965): Chess epilepsy and card epilepsy. *Chin. Med. J.* **84,** 470–474.

Ch'ien, L.T. & Little, S.C. (1971): Reading epilepsy. *Ala. J. Med. Sci.* **8,** 227–231.

Cirignotta, F., Cicogna, P. & Lugaresi, E. (1980): Epileptic seizures during card games and draughts. *Epilepsia* **21,** 137–140.

Cirignotta, F., Zucconi, M., Mondini, S. & Lugaresi, E. (1986): Writing epilepsy. *Clin. Electroencephalogr.* **17,** 21–23.

Commission on Classification and Terminology of the International League Against Epilepsy (1989): Proposal for revised classification of epilepsies and epileptic syndromes. *Epilepsia* **30,** 389–399.

Daniele, O., Raieli, V., Mattaliano, A. & Natale, E. (1989): Seizures precipitated by unusual epileptogenic tasks. In: *Reflex seizures and reflex epilepsies*, eds. A. Beaumanoir, H. Gastaut & R. Naquet, pp. 333–336. Geneva: Médecine & Hygiène.

Egawa, I., Yamamoto, J., Yamamoto, S. & Shimizu, A. (1989): Two cases of reflex epilepsy evoked by decision making. *Clin. Electroencephalogr.* (Japan) **31,** 138–143.

Espadaler Medina, J.M., Espadaler Gamissans, J.M. & Seoane, J.L. (1992): Reflex epilepsy. *Clin. Neurol. Neurosurg.* **94,** 70–72.

Forster, F.M. (1977): *Reflex epilepsy, behavioral therapy and conditional reflexes,* pp. 94–134. Springfield: Thomas.

Geschwind, N. & Sherwin, I. (1967): Language-induced epilepsy. *Arch. Neurol.* **16,** 25–31.

Goossens, L., Andermann, F., Andermann, E. & Remillard, G.M. (1990): Reflex seizures induced by calculation, card or board games, and spatial tasks: a review of 25 patients and delineation of the epileptic syndromes. *Neurology* **40,** 1171–1176.

Hasegawa, T., Matsuoka, H., Takahashi, T. & Okuma, T. (1981): Myoclonic seizures induced by writing, calculation with figures and constructive acts – with special reference to neuropsychological EEG activation. *Psychiatry Neurol. Japan.* **83,** 199–210.

Ingvar, D.H. & Nyman, G.E. (1962): Epilepsia arithmetices. *Neurology* **12,** 282–287.

Inoue, Y., Yagi, K., Muramatsu, R., Morikawa, T., Tottori, T. & Seino, M. (1987): Three cases of reflex epilepsy evoked by non-linguistic higher cerebral activities. *J. Japan. Epilepsy Soc.* **5,** 106–114.

Inoue, Y., Suzuki, S., Watanabe, Y., Yagi, K. & Seino, M. (1992): Non-lesional reflex epilepsy evoked by non-verbal higher cerebral activities. *J. Japan Epilepsy Soc.* **10,** 1–9.

Kalina, P., Pristasova, E. & Papayova, M. (1984): Reflex epilepsy evoked by specific psychic activity, a case report. *Acta Neurol. Belg.* **84,** 204–208.

Martin da Silva, A., Pinto, R. & Coutinho, P. (1989): Thinking epilepsy: cognitive processes and cortical structures involved. In: *Reflex seizures and reflex epilepsies*, eds. A. Beaumanoir, H. Gastaut & R. Naquet, pp. 323–331. Geneva: Médecine & Hygiène.

Maruko, K., Ishige, K., Takahashi, Y. & Sato, Y. (1975a): On reading epilepsy: case reports and review of the literature. *Clin. Electroencephalogr. (Japan)* **17,** 106–114.

Maruko, K., Ono, T., Ishige, K., Takaya, Y. & Yashima, Y. (1975b): A case of Mah-jong induced epilepsy. *Psychiatry* (Japan) **17,** 709–715.

Masaoka, S., Sugita, Y., Nanno, H., Yamamoto, J., Hishikawa, Y., Kaneko, Z. & Kemeda, H. (1975): Reading epilepsy: epileptic seizures induced by mental activity. *Clin. Electroencephalogr.* (Japan) **17,** 595–605.

Matsuoka, H., Hasegawa, T., Takahashi, T. & Okuma, T. (1981): Myoclonic seizures induced by decision making and psychic tension – with special reference to the findings obtained by neuropsychological EEG activation. *Psychiatr. Neurol. Japan* **83,** 211–221.

Matsuoka, H. (1989): A clinical and electroencephalographic study of juvenile myoclonic epilepsy: its pathophysiological considerations based on the findings obtained from neuropsychological EEG activation. *Psychiatr. Neurol. Japan* **91,** 318–346.

Murphy, M.J. & Yamada, T. (1981): Clonazepam therapy in reading epilepsy. *Neurology* **31,** 233.

Mutani, R., Ganga, A. & Agnetti, V. (1980): Epilessia riflessa decisionale: descrizione di un caso. *Schweiz Arch. Neurol. Neurochir. Psychiatr.* **127,** 61–67.

Ohtaka, T. & Miyasaka, M. (1977): A case of language-induced epilepsy precipitated mainly by writing. *Psychiatry Neurol. Japan* **79,** 587–601.

Okazaki, K., Kato, N., Toshida, S., Fukuyama, Y., Kazamatsuri, H. (1981): Reflex epilepsy evoked by fine movements of upper limbs and accompanying stressful situation: report of two cases. *Psychiatry* (Japan) **23,** 1241–1249.

Oller F.-V. L. (1989): Absences provoked by mental activity. In: *Reflex seizures and reflex epilepsies*, eds. A. Beaumanoir, H. Gastaut & R. Naquet, pp. 341–345. Geneva: Médecine & Hygiène.

Rosciszewska, D. & Motta, E. (1989): Reflex decision-making epilepsy. In: *Reflex seizures and reflex epilepsies*, eds. A. Beaumanoir, H. Gastaut & R. Naquet, pp. 337–340. Geneva: Médecine & Hygiène.

Saenz-Lope, E., Herranz-Tanarro, F.J. & Masdeu, J.C. (1985): Primary reading epilepsy. *Epilepsia* **26,** 649–656.

Saito, A. & Anzai, S. (1975): A case of epilepsia arithmetices. *Psychiatry* (Japan) **17,** 127–134.

Senanayake, N. (1987a): Epileptic seizures evoked by card games, draughts and similar games. *Epilepsia* **28,** 356–361.

Senanayake, N. (1987b): Epileptic seizures evoked by the Rubik's cube. *J. Neurol. Neurosurg. Psychiatry* **50,** 1553–1559.

Senanayake, N. (1989): Epilepsia arithmetices revisited. *Epilepsy Res.* **3,** 167–173.

Sharbrough, F.W., Westmoreland, B.F. & Campa, H.K. (1977): Writing epilepsy. *Electroencephalogr. Clin. Neurophysiol.* **43,** 506.

Siegel, M., Kurzrok, N., Barr, W.B. & Rowan, A.J. (1992): Game-playing epilepsy. *Epilepsia* **33,** 93–97.

Stoupel, N. (1968): On the reflex epilepsy: epilepsy caused by reading. *Electroencephalogr. Clin. Neurophysiol.* **25,** 416–417.

Striano, S., Orsini, A. & Vitolo, S. (1983): Epilepsia arithmetices: clinical and EEG study of a case and characteristics of precipitating factors. *Acta Neurol.* (Napoli) **38,** 14–19.

Takahashi, T. (1979): A case of graphogenic epilepsy induced by writing associated with psychic tension. *Brain Nerve* **31,** 159–165.

Wiebers, D.O., Westmoreland, B.F. & Klass, D.W. (1979): EEG activation and mathematical calculation. *Neurology* **29,** 1499–1503.

Wilkins, A., Zifkin, B., Andermann, F. & McGovern, E. (1982): Seizures induced by thinking. *Ann. Neurol.* **11,** 608–612.

Wolf, P. (1978): Reading epilepsy – evidence for a cognitive factor in seizure precipitation. In: *Advances in epileptology*, eds. H. Meinardi & A.J. Rowan, pp. 85–90. Amsterdam: Swets and Zeitlinger.

Wolf, P. (1992): Reading epilepsy. In: *Epileptic syndromes in infancy childhood and adolescence*, eds. J. Roger, M. Bureau, Ch. Dravet, F.E. Dreifuss, A. Perret & P. Wolf, pp. 281–298. London: John Libbey.

Yamamoto, J., Egawa, I., Shimizu, A. (1987): Two cases of reflex epilepsy induced by calculation using a 'soroban' (Japanese traditional abacus). *Clin. Electroencephalogr.* (Japan) **29,** 25–30.

Yamamoto, J., Egawa, I., Yamamoto, S. & Shimizu, A. (1991): Reflex epilepsy induced by calculation using a 'soroban', a japanese traditional calculator. *Epilepsia* **32,** 39–43.

Yamamoto, S., Egawa, I., Yamamoto, J., Kawasaki, T., Yamashita, K., Shiraisha, J & Shimizu, A. (1990a): A case of reflex epilepsy induced by higher mental activities, mainly by arithmetices. *J. Japan. Epil. Soc.* **8,** 22–28.

Yamamoto, S., Yamamoto, J., Egawa, I., Kawasaki, T., Yamashita, K., Shiraisha, J & Shimizu, A. (1990b): Two cases of reflex epilepsy induced mainly by writing. *Clin. Electroencephalogr.* (Japan) **32,** 764–767.

Yamamoto, S., Yamamoto, J., Kawasaki, T., Shiraishi, J & Shimizu, A. (1992): A pathophysiological consideration of reflex epilepsy induced by higher mental activity. *Ann. Rep. Japan. Epilepsy Res. Found.* **4,** 204–214.

Epileptic Seizures and Syndromes, Edited by Peter Wolf
© 1994 John Libbey & Company Ltd., pp. 93–98

Chapter 12

Two cases of reflex epilepsy with response to games of chance, calculations and spatial decisions

Javier Salas-Puig, Valentín Mateos, Apolinar G.-D. Castroverde*, Enrique Vera† and Carlos H. Lahoz

*Neurological Department and †Neuropsychological Department, Hospital General de Asturias, 33006 Oviedo, Spain; *Neurological Department, Hospital Cabueñes, Gijon, Spain*

Summary

We report two patients with reflex epilepsy triggered by complex cognitive stimuli. such as mathematical calculations, taking decisions or playing board games. Paroxysmal EEG discharges were observed during exposure to the precipitating agents.

The clinical and neurophysiological characteristics of this type of reflex epilepsy, and its similarities with idiopathic generalized epilepsies of adolescence, especially with Janz's juvenile myoclonic epilepsy, are discussed. We emphasize the need to recognize the reflex character of the seizures since the elimination of the causative agent may be very important in achieving a satisfactory clinical control.

Introduction

Ingvar and Nyman (1962) coined the term 'epilepsia arithmetices' to refer to a type of reflex epilepsy (RE) in which the precipitating factor was the execution of arithmetical operations. Since then, scarcely 30 cases have been described with seizures induced by calculation (Wiebers *et al.*, 1979; Wilkins *et al.*, 1982) and similar intellectual activities such as thought (Wilkins *et al.*, 1982; Gil-Néciga *et al.*, 1986; Martin da Silva *et al.*, 1989; Oller, 1989), drawing (Brenner & Seelinger, 1979), manipulative praxic activities (Senanayake, 1987b; Daniele *et al.*, 1989), taking decisions (Forster *et al.*, 1975; Rosciszewska & Motta, 1989) and board games (Cirignotta *et al.*, 1980; Senanayake, 1987a; Siegel *et al.*, 1992).

We present the clinical and neurophysiological characteristics in two patients with RE responding to complex stimuli, and analyse the relationship with idiopathic generalized epilepsies (IGE) of adolescence, especially with Janz's juvenile myoclonic epilepsy (JME).

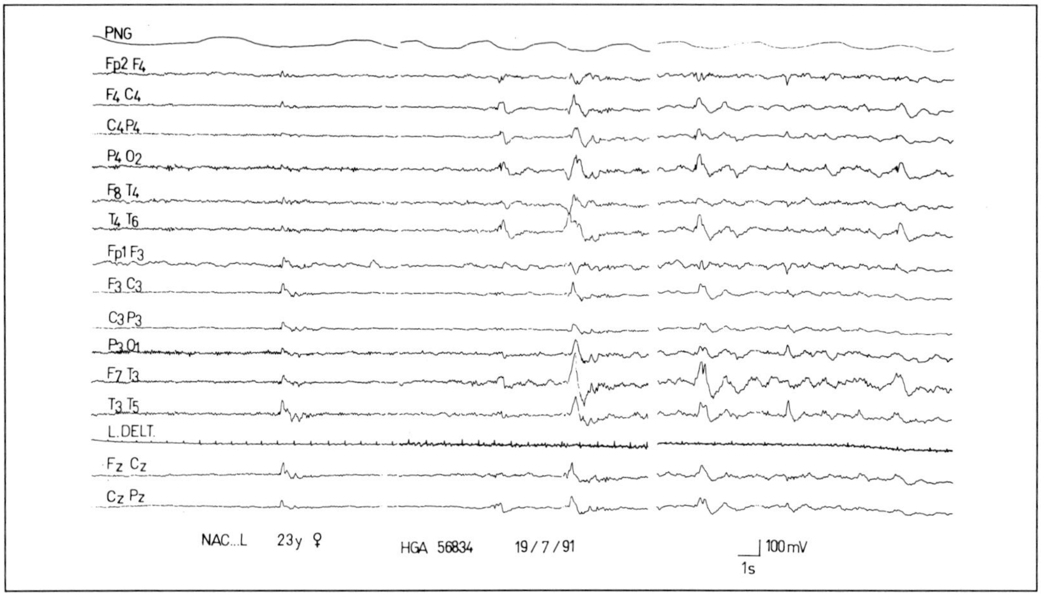

Fig. 1. EEG recorded during waking and sleeping stages showing a normal background activity and paroxysms of generalized SW–PSW as well as isolated spikes in the right parietotemporal area and, to a lesser extend, in the homonymous left area.

Clinical observations

Case 1

A 24-year-old woman with an unremarkable personal history. Two epileptic cousins. Since the age of 10, she has shown seizures of various types: (a) generalized tonic–clonic, in the daytime, once or twice a month, generally triggered by board games; (b) myoclonic, short, affecting the upper limbs, with no change of consciousness, favoured by calculations and games of chance; and (c) absences triggered by the same activities. Furthermore, she had generalized seizures with no apparent precipitating factor, both during the day and when asleep. She had been treated with multiple antiepileptic drugs (phenobarbital (PB), phenytoin (PHT), carbamazepine (CBZ), valproic acid (VPA)) in different combinations, with a poor clinical control. Electroencephalograph (EEG) recordings showed, both when awake and asleep, a normal background activity and paroxysms of generalized spike waves (SW) and polyspike waves PSW), as well as isolated spikes in the right parietotemporal area and, independently and in lesser amount, in the left homonymous area (Fig. 1). During games of chance, bursts of generalized SW at 3 Hz, lasting 1–2 s, were observed; these were not accompanied by any external signs, although the patient did refer to the existence of brief lapses with interrupted consciousness (Fig. 2). The neurological examination and neuroimaging studies computerized tomography (CT) and magnetic resonance (MR) were normal. The IQ was 85 and the neuropsychological studies did not show any focal dysfunctions. Treatment was started with VPA (2000 mg/day), clobazam (CLB) (10 mg/day) and CBZ 600 mg/day), and a good clinical control of the seizures has been achieved in the last 12 months. The patient was also told to avoid games of chance.

Case 2

A 34-year-old man with an unremarkable personal or family history. Since the age of 11, he had suffered generalized tonic–clonic seizures and brief absences which were triggered off when he played cards. He had never had myoclonias. He was kept asymptomatic under treatment with VPA

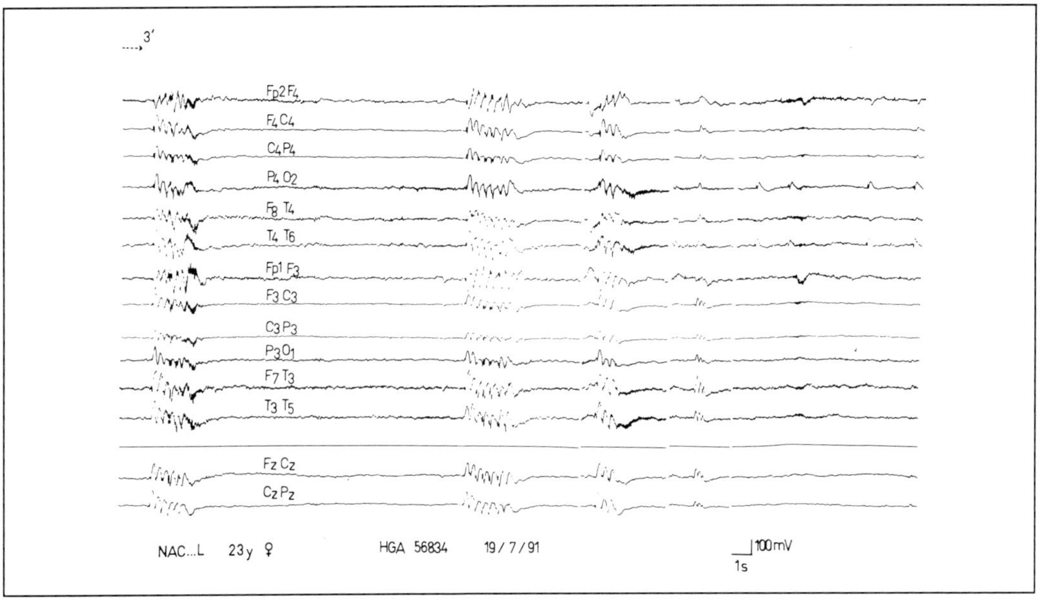

Fig. 2. EEG recorded whilst the patient was practising games of chance, in which we noted erratic, generalized burst of SW at 3 Hz, lasting 1–2 s, during which the patient reported brief lapses of consciousness.

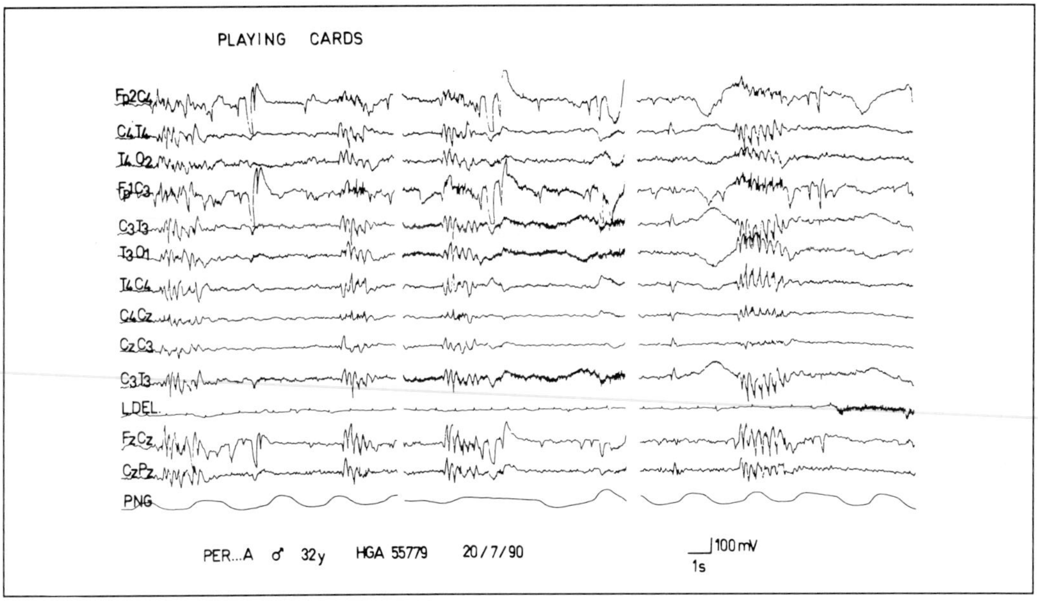

Fig. 3. EEG recorded during card games in which we noted a number of bursts of generalized and degraded SW–PSW.

(1500 mg/day) until he was 20. Subsequently, he started once more to have generalized seizures and absences when he focused on taking decisions, generally when they involved spatial components. The conventional EEG recordings had been normal, as well as the neurological examination. An EEG-polygraphic sleep recording presented paroxysms of generalized SW and PSW (3–4 Hz), which were isolated or in bursts lasting 2 s. During card games, we noted a number of bursts of fast generalized and degraded SW and PSW, lasting up to 4 s, without any clinical or polygraphic findings, although the patient did report experiencing microabsences (Fig. 3). There were no changes when drawing, reading or speaking, ocular following or manipulating the Rubik's cube, or after mental calculations. Paroxysmal abnormalities appeared, however, during written calculations, especially complex multiplications and divisions. Discharges with the same characteristics also appeared when the patient was asked to put different-sized cubes into the appropriate order. The intermittent photic stimulation was negative. The IQ was 124 and no neuropsychological disturbances were observed. Erratic administration of VPA was accompanied by persistence of the seizures, be they absences or generalized tonic–clonic. He is now following the treatment properly (VPA 1500 mg/day) and has proved asymptomatic for the last 10 months. The EEG is normal despite activations (card games and Wechsler Adult's Intelligence Scale (WAIS) cube test).

Discussion

The two cases illustrate the essential findings, both clinical and neurophysiological, of RE with seizures induced by complex stimuli, which may be called 'epilepsy of thought and spatial decision' (Salas-Puig *et al.*, 1992) – whereas Inoue *et al.* in Chapter 11 suggest the term 'praxisinduced'. It is characterized by the presence of seizures triggered by specific activities which combine, to a greater or lesser extent, praxic, visual/spatial, decision-making and emotional components. It is not uncommon for several of these mechanisms to act on the same patient, or for the seizures to appear in an apparently spontaneous manner (Goosens *et al.*, 1990).

In a review of the literature, Goosens *et al.* (1990) verified the following characteristics: male predominance, lack of pathological history, start of the seizures in adolescence, normal neurological and neuroimaging findings, and a family history of epilepsy in 25 per cent. The seizures can be generalized tonic–clonic (95 per cent of cases), myoclonic (75 per cent) or absences (50 per cent), frequently combined in the same patient (80 per cent). EEG anomalies consist of bursts of generalized SW or PSW on a normal background activated during exposure to the specific precipitating factor.

Thus, this group of RE shares many of the characteristics, both clinical (occurrence in adolescence, family history, normal neurological examination, a combination of generalized tonic–clonic, myoclonic and absence seizures) and neurophysiological (normal background activity, generalized paroxysms of SW and PSW), of IGE and, more specifically, of JME (Goosens *et al.*, 1990). With respect to the latter, it may also be noted that some patients report myoclonic seizures triggered by concentrating on carrying out manual tasks. Matsuoka *et al.* (1988) studied the effect, in patients with JME, of mental and manipulative activities performed in a situation of psychic stress, and paroxysmal discharges were noted in 21 of the 25 patients studied. Yamamoto *et al.* (1991) reported an activation in 52.5 per cent of a series of 40 patients with JME. However, it is most common in JME for the spontaneous myoclonic seizures to appear on waking up (Janz & Christian, 1957), whilst in RE through spatial decision there seems to be no circadian rhythm. JME has a high index of positive responses with a favouring effect of photic stimulation and eye closure (Wolf & Goosses, 1986). It has been reported that in RE through spatial decision 25–30 per cent of the patients have a photoparoxysmal response (Goosens *et al.*, 1990), but the figures of Inoue *et al.* (see Chapter 11) are lower. Focal EEG changes have occasionally been described in patients with RE when taking decisions, generally with reference to the non-dominant hemisphere (Ingvar & Nyman, 1962; Goosens *et al.*, 1990). Asymmetric paroxysmal anomalies may also appear in up to 33 per cent of JME patients, which may be a source of diagnostic error in these patients (Obeid & Panayiotopoulos, 1986; Grünewald *et al.*, 1992). In our case 1, focal anomalies occurred in different EEG recordings referring to the right parietal area, although the absence seizures were characterized by generalized SW. Considering the relationship between the trigger mechanism (essentially decisions with spatial components) and the functions attributed to the parietal lobe, it has been suggested that a parietal dysfunction could be at the origin of the epileptogenic discharge (Daniele *et al.*, 1989; Goosens *et al.*, 1990) similar to the occipital cortical activation in patients with generalized epilepsy and photosensitivity (Goosens *et al.*, 1990). Other authors have postulated emotional factors (Ingvar & Nyman, 1962) or the visual pattern (Senanayake, 1987a) as the probable responsible mechanisms. The need for decisions, apart from being complex, to be accomplished in a sequential order (strategic thinking) has also been underlined (Cirignotta *et al.*, 1980; Daniele *et al.*, 1989; Goosens *et al.*, 1990). In the cases described, as in other complex RE such as reading epilepsy (Vercelletto *et al.*, 1985), prolonged stimulus exposure is necessary before the paroxysmal anomalies and seizures appear. In RE with simple stimuli, such as photogenic epilepsies, the seizures appear, on the contrary, after a few seconds (Jeavons & Harding, 1975).

In our patients strategic thought appears to be the common item, influencing other factors like spatial decision in case 2. Both patients had a normal or above-average intelligence and no global or located dysfunctions were observed during neuropsychological testing (WAIS, Hooper visual organization test, Rey-Osterrieth complex figure, Trail-making test, symbol digit modality test, go–no-go test), and there were no personality changes in the Cattell 16 PF test.

The pharmacological treatment recommended for this type of RE consists of drugs like VPA and the benzodiazepines, most often in association, which generally gives good results, although the long-term prognosis is difficult to establish (Goosens *et al.*, 1990). Of our patients, the combination of VPA, CBZ and CLB was required in case 1, and in case 2 VPA in monotherapy was sufficient. Just as in JME, and probably also in reading epilepsy, relapses seem to be common after discontinuation of the medication, as in case 2.

Apart from the pharmacological treatment, the elimination, prevention or reduction of specific triggering stimuli should be attempted (Niedermeyer, 1990). This task must begin when the medical history is taken and the existence of factors which precipitate the seizures is inquired into, especially in patients with IGE (Goosens *et al.*, 1990).

References

Brenner, R.P. & Seelinger, D.F. (1979): Drawing-induced seizures. *Arch. Neurol.* **36,** 515–516.

Cirignotta, F., Cicogna, P. & Lugaresi, E. (1980): Epileptic seizures during card games and draughts. *Epilepsia* **21,** 137–140.

Daniele, O., Raieli, V., Mattaliano, A. & Natalè, E. (1989): Seizures precipitated by unusual epileptogenic tasks. In: *Reflex seizures and reflex epilepsies*, eds. A. Beaumanoir, H. Gastaut & R. Naquet, pp. 333–336. Geneva: Médecine & Hygiène.

Forster, F.M., Richards, J.F., Panitch, H.S., Huisman, R.E. & Paulsen, R.E. (1975): Reflex epilepsy evoked by decision making. *Arch. Neurol.* **32,** 54–56.

Gil-Néciga, E., Boza, F., Bautista Lorite, J. & Villalobos, F. (1986): Epilepsia refleja inducida por el pensamiento. *Neurologia* **1,** 260–262.

Goosens, L.A.Z., Andermann, F., Andermann, E. & Remillard, G.M. (1990): Reflex seizures induced by calculation, card or board games, and spatial tasks: a review of 25 patients and delineation of the epileptic syndrome. *Neurology* **40,** 1171–1176.

Grünewald, R.A., Chroni, E. & Panayiotopoulos, C.P. (1992): Delayed diagnosis of juvenile myoclonic epilepsy. *J. Neurol. Neurosurg. Psychiatry* **55,** 497–499.

Ingvar, D.H. & Nyman, G.E. (1962): Epilepsia arithmetices: a new psychologic trigger mechanism in a case of epilepsy. *Neurology* **12,** 282–287.

Janz, D. & Christian, W. (1957): Impulsive-petit mal. *Dtsch. Z. Nervenheilk.* **176,** 346–386.

Jeavons, P.M. & Harding, G.F.A. (1975): *Photosensitive epilepsy: a review of the literature and a study of 460 patients.* pp. 1–121. London: William Heinemann.

Martin da Silva, A., Pinto, R. & Coutinho, P. (1989): Thinking epilepsy: cognitive processes and cortical structures involved. In: *Reflex seizures and reflex epilepsies*, eds. A. Beaumanoir, H. Gastaut & R. Naquet, pp. 323–331. Geneva: Médecine & Hygiène.

Matsuoka, H., Takahashi, T. & Sato, M. (1988): The clinical and electroencephalographic studies of juvenile myoclonic epilepsy. *Japan. J. Psychol. Neurol.* **42,** 556–557.

Niedermeyer E. (1990): Triggering mechanisms of epileptic seizures. In: *The epilepsies: diagnosis and management,* ed. E. Niedermeyer, pp. 187–192. Baltimore, Munich: Urban Schwarzenberg.

Obeid, T. & Panayiotopoulos, C.P. (1986): Juvenile myoclonic epilepsy: a study in Saudi Arabia. *Epilepsia* **29,** 280–282.

Oller L. (1989): Absences provoked by mental activity. In: *Reflex seizures and reflex epilepsies,* eds. A. Beaumanoir, H. Gastaut & R. Naquet, pp. 341–345. Geneva: Médècine & Hygiène.

Rosciszewska, D. & Motta, E. (1989) Reflex decision-making epilepsy: report of a case. In: *Reflex seizures and reflex epilepsies,* eds. A. Beaumanoir, H. Gastaut & R. Naquet, pp. 337–340. Geneva: Médècine and Hygiène.

Salas-Puig, J., Mateos, V. & Colosía, V.P. (1992): Epilepsias reflejas. In: *Actualizacion de las Epilepsias,* vol.2, eds. J.L. Herranz & J.A. Armijo, pp. 57–81. Barcelona: Ediciones Consulta.

Senanayake, N. (1987a): Epileptic seizures evoked by card games, draughts and similar games. *Epilepsia* **28,** 356–361.

Senanayake, N. (1987b): Epileptic seizures evoked by Rubik's cube. *J. Neurol. Neurosurg. Psychiatry* **50,** 1553–1554.

Siegel, M., Kurzrok, N., Barr, W.B. & Rowan, A.J. (1992): Game-playing epilepsy. *Epilepsia* **33** (1), 93–97.

Vercelletto, P., Cler, J.M. & Friol, M. (1985): Epilepsie primairede la lecture: onze cas. *Rev. Neurol.* (Paris) **141,** 379–385.

Wiebers, D.O., Westmoreland, B.F. & Klass, D.W. (1979): EEG activation and mathematical calculation. *Neurology* **29,** 1499–1503.

Wilkins, A.J., Zifkin, B., Andermann, F. & McGovern, E. (1982): Seizures induced by thinking. *Ann. Neurol.* **11,** 608–612.

Wolf, P. & Goosses, R. (1986): Relation of photosensitivity to epileptic syndromes. *J. Neurol. Neurosurg. Psychiatry* **49,** 1385–1391.

Yamamoto, S., Yamamoto, J., Shimizu, A., Kawasaki, T., Yoshida, J. & Shirvaishi, J. (1991): 1231 IMP Simple-photon emission computed tomography in juvenile myoclonic epilepsy. *Epilepsia* **32** (suppl. 1), 8.

Epileptic Seizures and Syndromes, Edited by Peter Wolf
© 1994 John Libbey & Company Ltd., pp. 99–105

Chapter 13

Epilepsy with seizures induced by eating

Benjamin G. Zifkin, Frederick Andermann* and Guy-M. Rémillard

*Epilepsy Clinic, Montréal Neurological Hospital, *Montréal Neurological Institute and Hospital, 3801 rue University, Montréal, Québec, Canada H3A 2BF*

Definition and classification

Eating seizures are those which reliably occur in close relation to eating. The very sight or smell of food may be an effective seizure trigger in some patients. Many eating seizures are identical to those of complex reflex epilepsies of temporal lobe origin, characterized by relatively elaborate triggering stimuli whose specific pattern is the determining factor in seizure evocation. Such seizures are precipitated by integration of higher cortical function and may be evoked by anticipation of the stimulus. Latency from stimulus onset to the clinical or electroencephalographic event is typically longer than in the seizures of simple reflex epilepsies such as photosensitive epilepsy. A second type of seizure induced by eating appears to be of suprasylvian origin, triggered at least in part by proprioceptive or somatosensory afferents, and resembles those described with simple reflex epilepsies. These properties, enunciated in the 1985 proposal for classification of epilepsies (Commission on Classification, 1985), were first systematically described in the pioneering work of Forster (1972). Although described as eating epilepsy, seizures triggered by eating often occur in patients who also have spontaneous seizures and are not considered to constitute a separate epileptic syndrome. Some cases may be described as 'epilepsies characterized by specific modes of seizure precipitation' (Commission on Classification, 1989).

Eating seizures have been reported in childhood, youth and adult life. Most cases of eating seizures are reported in patients with symptomatic localization-related epilepsies. Patients with frequent reflex attacks, particularly those with suprasylvian onset, may avoid eating, and weight loss and nutritional deficiency can result. Patients considered to have idiopathic generalized epilepsies are exceptional and not as well documented. Eating seizures are rare. A prevalence of approximately 1 per 1000–2000 epileptic patients has been reported (Vizioli, 1962; Nagaraja & Chand, 1984). The unusually high figures reported for Sri Lanka (Senanayake, 1990) may be related to ascertainment methods. The phenomenon may be more common: patients may not be aware of the association between their seizures and eating, and discovery of a case often depends on detailed and at times repeated questioning of the patients and those around them.

Clinical manifestations

Seizures induced by eating are usually simple or complex partial attacks which may be followed by a generalized convulsion. Cases in which seizures have been shown to be generalized from the start are less frequent (see Fiol *et al.*, 1986; Koul *et al.*, 1989). While each patient may report specific trigger characteristics, there are a few obvious common points among them. Some report seizures at the sight or smell of food while others may have them only when beginning to eat or shortly thereafter. The types of food trigger may also differ. Some early reports (Boudouresques & Gastaut, 1954; Symonds, 1959) noted reflex seizures at or near the end of a meal, but later studies suggest that most such attacks occur at or near the beginning of eating, whether in the setting of a full meal or not (Koul *et al.*, 1989). Ahuja *et al.* (1980) reviewed the importance of factors such as smell, visualization of food, the effect of mastication and a familiar environment and noted that nine of their 10 patients had reflex seizures only when eating at home.

Eating seizures occur with symptomatic localization-related epilepsies and patients may be divided into those with temporolimbic seizure onset and those with apparent extralimbic, perirolandic suprasylvian onset. The latter may have ictal and interictal clinical findings usually associated with lesions of this region, such as simple partial seizures, and fixed hemiparesis or intellectual deficit. These are usually related to a static encephalopathy. Other lesions, such as the deep forebrain glioma reported by Robertson and Fariello (1979), are rare.

Rémillard *et al.* (1989) proposed two clinical syndromes of eating seizures, differentiating temporolimbic from extralimbic seizure onset. They suggested that patients with temporolimbic seizures activated by eating have fewer spontaneous attacks and are more likely to have such attacks from the onset of their epilepsy than are those with extralimbic suprasylvian seizure onset, who have less constant activation by eating, more obvious extratemporal structural lesions, and possible activation by specific thalamocortical afferents. It is our impression that patients with extralimbic onset of eating seizures are particularly sensitive to either somatosensory or proprioceptive stimuli during eating. A representative case of each type is described (adapted from Rémillard *et al.*, 1989).

Temporolimbic onset

A 32-year-old man had a 10-year history of complex partial seizures with an initial *déjà vu* phenomenon. He had two to eight attacks per month, mostly during breakfast, at times with other meals, and rarely without eating. Interictal EEGs showed active epileptiform activity over the right anterior and inferomesial temporal regions. A seizure was recorded while he was eating a boiled egg at breakfast. The localization of onset was not precise, but very early in the seizure, ictal activity predominated over the right anterior and inferomesial temporal regions. He has been seizure-free for several years following right temporal resection, including the amygdala and anterior hippocampus.

Extratemporal onset

A 46-year-old woman with left hemiparesis and hemianopia had seizures from the neonatal period. The reflex epileptic response to eating started at age 22 years. She estimated preoperatively that about 75 per cent of attacks were related to eating. These consisted of numbness of the left arm and side of the face, followed by raising the left arm and turning of the head to the left. She had stopped eating toast and crackers because she felt that the crackling induced seizures and found that hot food could induce a startle reaction and precipitate an attack. Spontaneous seizures were recorded with poorly localized right frontocentroparietal epileptiform activity. Right frontal resection and temporoparieto-occipital lobectomy were performed. The pre- and postcentral gyri were spared because of some useful finger movement, but residual spikes were recorded from these regions in the postexcision electrocorticogram. At 10-year follow-up, there was about 90 per cent reduction in all attacks: about 25 per cent of the residual seizures were still precipitated by eating.

Pathogenesis

Some shared characteristics of reflex seizures with different triggers suggest that recruitment of a 'critical mass' of epileptogenic cortex in response to the epileptogenic stimulus can result in epileptiform EEG activity or a clinical seizure. This recruitment can be understood as relatively direct in some, but in other cases may involve the participation and interaction of several cortical areas or of cortex and subcortical structures activated by the external trigger. Studies in pattern-sensitive subjects suggest that generalized seizures can occur if normal excitation of visual cortex involves a 'critical mass' of cortical area with synchronization and subsequent spread of excitation from the occipital lobe trigger (Binnie *et al.*, 1985). Wilkins *et al.* (1982) documented the increased likelihood of thinking-induced paroxysmal EEG activity with increasing task difficulty. They suggested that increasing difficulty of parietal lobe and possibly frontal lobe epileptogenic stimuli led to increasing regional recruitment to reach a critical mass of epileptogenic cortex with activation of generalized epileptiform activity, analogous to the activation of such generalized activity by the occipital cortical stimuli of pattern-sensitive epilepsy. Studies of reading epilepsy also suggest that increased task difficulty, complexity or duration increase the chance of EEG or clinical activation (Christie *et al.*, 1988). Based on an experimental model of a chronic epileptic focus (Wyler & Ward, 1980) Wieser (1989) has proposed a pathophysiological explanation of these observations, suggesting that epileptogenic stimuli produce temporary recruitment of group 2 epileptic neurones into the effective quantity of epileptic cortex to reach a critical mass. Ritaccio *et al.* (1992) suggest that reading epilepsy is a form of cortical reflex myoclonus (Obeso *et al.*, 1985) with an unstable motor response to afferent volleys to a hyperexcitable Brodmann's area 6. The basis for cortical hyperexcitability may be dysregulation of extracellular Ca^{2+} concentration (Pumain *et al.*, 1985) or imbalances of excitatory and inhibitory amino acids similar to those reported in feline generalized penicillin epilepsy and human epilepsy (Gloor *et al.*, 1982; Lloyd *et al.*, 1986; van Gelder, 1987). The concept of a critical mass of cortex recruited to produce a clinical reflex seizure may also be applied to eating seizures, both those seen with partial seizures and those rare attacks apparently generalized from the start. While this approach is speculative, there seem to be no strong arguments against it and much in its favour.

Both classical and more recent anatomical and neurophysiological studies show that afferent impulses related to eating are represented in cortical regions involved in the onset or progression of eating seizures. Fibres subserving taste project from the pons to the nucleus ventralis posteromedialis (VPM) of the thalamus, and thence to the cerebral cortex. Penfield and Jasper (1954) described the cortical representation of taste in man 'where the upper Sylvian bank joins the insula' and more recent texts describe one cortical representation of taste within or near the primary somaesthetic tongue area in the opercular part of the postcentral gyrus. The limbic system is also involved in the sensation of taste, with projections from the pons to the lateral hypothalamus and the central nucleus of the amygdala. In monkeys, there is a fine-tuning of neuronal responses to taste stimuli that becomes progressively sharper through the brainstem, thalamus and primary and secondary taste cortices in the frontal operculum and insula, and orbitofrontal cortex (Rolls, 1989). Some neurones in these regions are also sensitive to non-taste stimuli related to eating, such as mouth and tongue movements and even approach or anticipation of a taste stimulus (Smith-Swintosky *et al.*, 1991). The parietal lobe second somatosensory area, located in the upper bank of the sylvian fissure near the insula, is also of particular interest because each one contains both ipsilateral and contralateral representations of the face, mouth and throat.

We have noted that two clinical syndromes of eating seizures emerged from a review of intensively monitored patients with activation by eating, many treated surgically for intractable seizures. In those with temporolimbic seizure onset, reflex activation was usually present from the start of their seizures, most seizures occurred during eating, without spontaneous cessation or reduction of reflex activation, and reflex seizures could occur at any time during a meal. Subjects with extratemporal, perirolandic suprasylvian seizure onset often had large lesions and corresponding neurological deficits. They developed reflex activation by eating during the course of their epilepsy, sensitivity to eating could wax and wane or even cease spontaneously, and reflex attacks were more commonly unrelated to a full meal and usually occurred at or near the beginning of taking food into the mouth. The type, consistency and temperature of food as well as drink were more important in these subjects.

Many reported patients have eating seizures only with obvious combinations of stimuli (Aguglia & Tinuper, 1983; Fiol *et al.*, 1986). Proprioceptive or similar stimuli seem necessary to trigger attacks in many patients, and may be sufficient on their own.

The important role of proprioceptive afferent stimuli has been shown convincingly by Reder and Wright (1982) in a patient whose eating seizures disappeared after accidental amputation of the fingers. Further circumstantial evidence for parietal lobe involvement in the pathogenesis of eating seizures is provided by the occurrence of seizures with drinking in a subject with right parieto-occipital cortical dysplasia (Verdu & Ruiz-Falco, 1991). It is of interest that simple mouth and tongue movements do not usually trigger seizures and that patients do not usually have attacks with recitation or singing. One of our patients with previous surgery in the left central face area, however, reported seizures with talking on the phone or chewing gum as well as with eating. He became seizure-free after additional removal of the postcentral face area. Another patient with bilateral perirolandic macrogyria had seizures with hot or cold drinks or on eating juicy fruit, and reported brief attacks when kissing her boyfriend, also suggesting the importance of more complex behaviour in many effective triggering stimuli.

Considering these observations, it appears that the occurrence of eating seizures may also be related to the excitation of a critical mass of epileptogenic cortex by a variety of afferent stimuli. When this abnormal cortex is located in regions responding to proprioceptive and other sensory afferents (especially lingual, buccal or pharyngeal) activated by the extensive sensory input generated by a complex and often relatively prolonged behaviour such as eating, patients may be more sensitive to the physical manipulation of food, texture, temperature and chewing. This would correspond to those patients with extralimbic seizure onset. This mechanism may be similar to that described for other proprioceptive-induced seizures (Chauvel & Lamarche, 1975; Brick *et al.*, 1989). A similar mechanism, but in this instance with afferents recruiting hyperexcitable temporolimbic structures, may also operate in subjects with temporolimbic seizure onset, who may be more sensitive to gustatory, olfactory, affective or emotional stimuli, or to stimuli arising from more distal parts of the gut.

Fiol *et al.* (1986) have also suggested that interaction between limbic and extralimbic cortices operates in many cases, and contributions of brainstem and hypothalamus have been suggested by Gastaut and Poirier (1964), Scollo-Lavizzari and Hess (1967) and Robertson and Fariello (1979). Arousal stimuli are reported to prevent some reflex induction by eating, also suggesting brainstem or thalamic participation in modulating effectiveness of the seizure trigger (Ganga *et al.*, 1988).

Diagnostic investigation

Patients with eating seizures require investigation similar to others with epilepsy. History-taking must be particularly painstaking when reflex seizures are suspected. In pursuing more detailed investigation, one fundamental question must be 'What is epileptogenic about the triggering stimulus'? The answers can be important for studying both epileptogenesis and cognition. It is always of interest to determine whether all of a subject's seizures appear to be reflex-induced, and as precise a history as possible should be obtained of the details of presumed seizure triggers. With eating seizures, particular attention should be given to the timing of attacks during the day and with respect to the act of eating, whether attacks occur with snacks or only with full meals, any possible food characteristics that may be important such as temperature, texture or bulk, and any associated emotional factors. It is also important to note whether any oral activities not specifically involved with eating may trigger attacks, such as kissing, chewing gum or brushing the teeth.

As almost all reported cases occur with partial seizures, extensive imaging studies are indicated and magnetic resonance imaging should be performed. New functional methods such as echo-planar imaging may make it possible to study cortical activation during eating more directly. There has as yet been no systematic study of eating seizures with positron emission tomography.

The EEG remains the cornerstone of laboratory investigation in reflex epilepsy. Complex reflex epilepsies introduce special problems because it is often difficult to separate the effective stimulus into components for study, and because the latency from stimulus to EEG effect can be longer than in simple reflex epilepsies and complicate the demonstration of a cause-and-effect relation between possibly epileptogenic components of the stimulus and the recorded EEG changes (Wilkins *et al.*, 1982; Zifkin, 1989). Testing should begin with routine EEG recording including hyperventilation, photic stimulation and a sleep tracing. While recording the effects of the reported trigger may be useful in screening, it is common practice to break down the trigger into components that can be presented individually during EEG and video monitoring. In eating seizures, these would include components such as the isolated sight or smell of food, handling food, other proprioceptive tasks not related to eating, chewing without swallowing (e.g. chewing gum), or the effects of various temperatures and food textures. Non-epileptogenic tasks should be identified and should ideally remain non-epileptogenic throughout evaluation, excluding a conditioned epileptiform response. Non-epileptogenic stimuli should also be used repeatedly at different levels of difficulty to control for the effects of attention, effort and relaxation; and to occupy time to prevent contamination of the recording by long-latency induced epileptiform activity. As in many other forms of reflex seizures, a stimulus may not always be effective. This may depend on levels of antiepileptic drugs and other factors. The presence of a refractory period after a precipitated or spontaneous attack must also be considered and is particularly obvious in some patients with suprasylvian onset of seizures. Inability to demonstrate the reflex activation at any given time does not in itself represent sufficient evidence against the diagnosis. Statistical considerations for such EEG monitoring have been reviewed by Wilkins *et al.* (1982) and by Fiol *et al.* (1986). Cases which do not respond adequately to medical treatment should undergo intensive monitoring with the usual video-EEG techniques.

Treatment

Treatment of eating seizures involves stimulus avoidance or modification, antiepileptic drugs and resective surgery. Unless some special circumstance or food characteristic can be identified as a specific trigger, stimulus avoidance is impractical. Indeed, the tendency to avoid eating during periods of frequent seizures suggests that an aggressive approach to management is often warranted. Stimulus modification may be very helpful. It is our impression that patients with eating epilepsy and extralimbic seizure onset are more sensitive to either somatosensory or proprioceptive stimuli during eating and are more likely to report that seizure induction can be prevented by altering the sensory characteristics of their food. Some will drink through a straw rather than from a cup, avoid biting into a whole fruit by cutting it into small pieces, or avoid extremes of food temperature such as hot soup or ice cream. Stimulus modification can reduce seizure frequency in what can otherwise be an intractable or socially disabling condition. Most subjects, however, also have spontaneous seizures, usually of local or regional onset. Drugs effective for partial seizures are necessary, and carbamazepine is currently the treatment of choice. While clobazam can be a useful adjunct, and new drugs such as vigabatrin, lamotrigine, felbamate and gabapentin may prove helpful, medically intractable patients should be recognized early and assessed for possible surgical treatment.

References

Aguglia, U. & Tinuper, P. (1983): Eating seizures. *Eur. Neurol.* **22,** 227–231.

Ahuja, G.K., Mohandas, S. & Narayanaswamy, A.S. (1980): Eating epilepsy. *Epilepsia* **21,** 85–89.

Binnie, C.D., Findlay, J. & Wilkins, A.J. (1985): Mechanisms of epileptogenesis in photosensitive epilepsy implied by the effect of moving patterns. *Electroencephalogr. Clin. Neurophysiol.* **61,** 1–6

Boudouresques, J. & Gastaut, H. (1954): Le mécanisme réflexe de certaines épilepsies temporales. *Rev. Neurol.* **90,** 157–158.

Brick, J.F., Gutrecht, J.A. & Ringel, R.A. (1989): Reflex epilepsy and nonketotic hyperglycemia in the elderly: a specific neuroendocrine syndrome. *Neurology* **39,** 394–399.

Chauvel, P. & Lamarche, M. (1975): Analyse d'une 'épilepsie du mouvement' chez un singe porteur d'un foyer rolandique. *Neurochirurgie* **21,** 121–137.

Christie, S., Guberman, A., Tansley, B.W. & Couture, M. (1988): Primary reading epilepsy: investigation of critical seizure-provoking stimuli. *Epilepsia* **29,** 288–293.

Commission on Classification and Terminology of the ILAE (1985): Proposal for classification of epilepsies and epileptic syndromes. *Epilepsia* **26,** 268–278.

Commission on Classification and Terminology of the ILAE (1989): Proposal for revised classification of epilepsies and epileptic syndromes. *Epilepsia* **30,** 389–399.

Fiol, M.E., Leppik, I.E. & Pretzel, K. (1986): Eating epilepsy: EEG and clinical study. *Epilepsia* **27,** 441–445.

Forster, F.M. (1972): The classification and conditioning treatment of the reflex epilepsies. *Int. J. Neurol.* **9,** 73–86.

Ganga, A., Sechi, G.P., Porcella, V., Traccis, S., Rosati, G. & Agnetti, V. (1988): Eating seizures and distraction-arousal functions. *Eur. Neurol.* **28,** 167–170.

Gastaut, H. & Poirier, F. (1964): Experimental or 'reflex' induction of seizures: report of a case of abdominal (enteric) epilepsy. *Epilepsia* **5,** 256–270.

Gloor, P., Metrakos, J., Metrakos, K. & Van Gelder, N. (1982): Neurophysiological, genetic, and biochemical nature of the epileptic diathesis. In: *Henri Gastaut and the Marseille school's contribution to the neurosciences*, ed. R. Broughton, pp. 45–56. Amsterdam: Elsevier.

Koul, R., Koul, S. & Razdan, S. (1989): Eating epilepsy. *Acta Neurol. Scand.* **80,** 78–80.

Lloyd, K.G., Scatton, B., Voltz, C., Brière, P., Valin, A. & Naquet, R. (1986): Cerebrospinal fluid amino acid and monoamine metabolite levels of *Papio papio*: correlation with photosensitivity. *Brain Res.* **363,** 390–394.

Nagaraja, D. & Chand, R.P. (1984) Eating epilepsy. *Clin. Neurol. Neurosurg.* **86,** 95–99.

Obeso, J.A., Rothwell, J.C. & Marsden, C.D. (1985): The spectrum of cortical myoclonus. *Brain* **108,** 193–224.

Penfield, W. & Jasper, H.H. (1954): *Epilepsy and the functional anatomy of the human brain.* Boston: Little, Brown.

Pumain, R., Menini, C., Heinemann, U., Louvel, J. & Silva-Barrat, C. (1985): Chemical synaptic transmission is not necessary for epileptic seizures to persist in the baboon *Papio papio*. *Exp. Neurol.* **89,** 250–258.

Reder, A.T. & Wright, F.S. (1982): Epilepsy evoked by eating: the role of peripheral input. *Neurology* **32,** 1065–1069.

Rémillard, G.M., Andermann, F., Zifkin, B.G., Olivier, A. & Rasmussen, T. (1989): Eating epilepsy: a study of ten surgically treated patients suggests the presence of two separate syndromes. In: *Reflex seizures and reflex epilepsies*, eds. A. Beaumanoir, H. Gastaut & R. Naquet, pp. 289–300. Geneva: Éditions Médecine et Hygiène.

Ritaccio, A.L., Hickling, E.J. & Ramani, V. (1992): The role of dominant premotor cortex and grapheme to phoneme transformation in reading epilepsy: a neuroanatomic, neurophysiologic, and neuropsychological study. *Arch. Neurol.* **49,** 933–939.

Robertson, W.C. & Fariello, R.G. (1979): Eating epilepsy with a deep forebrain glioma. *Ann. Neurol.* **6,** 271–273.

Rolls, E.T. (1989) Information processing in the taste system of primates. *J. Exp. Biol.* **146,** 141–164.

Scollo-Lavizzari, G. & Hess, R. (1967): Sensory precipitation of epileptic seizures: report on two unusual cases. *Epilepsia* **8,** 157–161.

Senanayake, N. (1990): Eating epilepsy – a reappraisal. *Epilepsy Res.* **5,** 74–79.

Smith-Swintosky, V.L., Plata-Salaman, C.R. & Scott, T.R. (1991): Gustatory neural coding in the monkey cortex: stimulus quality. *J. Neurophysiol.* **66,** 1156–1165.

Symonds, C. (1959): Excitation and inhibition in epilepsy. *Brain* **82,** 134–146.

van Gelder, N.M. (1987): Contributions of basic neurochemistry towards a novel concept of epilepsy. *Neurochem. Res.* **12,** 111–119.

Verdu, A. & Ruiz-Falco, M.L. (1991): Eating seizures associated with focal cortical dysplasia. *Brain Dev.* **13,** 352–354.

Vizioli, R. (1962): The problem of human reflex epilepsy and the possible role of masked epileptic factors. *Epilepsia* **3,** 293–302.

Wieser, H.G. (1989): Seizure-inducing and preventing mechanisms. In: *Reflex seizures and reflex epilepsies*, eds. A. Beaumanoir, H. Gastaut & R. Naquet, pp. 49–55. Geneva: Éditions Médecine et Hygiène.

Wilkins, A.J., Zifkin, B., Andermann, F. & McGovern, E. (1982): Seizures induced by thinking. *Ann. Neurol.* **11,** 608–612.

Wyler, A.R. & Ward, A.A., Jr (1980): Epileptic neurons. In: *Epilepsy: a window to brain mechanisms*, eds. J.S. Lockard & A.A. Ward, Jr, pp. 51–68. New York: Raven Press.

Zifkin, B.G. (1989): Some considerations in the intensive EEG investigation of reflex epilepsy. In: *Reflex seizures and reflex epilepsies,* eds. A. Beaumoir, H. Gastaut & R. Naquet, pp. 457–462. Geneva: Éditions Médicine et Hygiène.

Epileptic Seizures and Syndromes, Edited by Peter Wolf
© 1994 John Libbey & Company Ltd., pp. 107–114

Chapter 14

Olfactory activation in epilepsy

Vladimír Komárek

Department of Child Neurology, Charles University, 2nd Medical School, 150 18 Prague 5 Motol, Czech Republic

Introduction

At the first symposium on reflex epilepsy (RE) in Prague, 1960, Kamil Henner (1963) reserved the term RE for those rare cases in which seizures were explicitly elicited by specific types of stimulation. Gastaut (1989) proposed a less restrictive definition, according to which all or most seizures are unmistakably provoked by natural or artificial stimulations of one or several receptors. Visual stimuli have been identified as RE elicitors more frequently than other forms of stimuli; conversely, olfactory stimuli have not yet been reported in this connection till now.

However, Henner's collaborator Servít (1977) observed epileptic changes in human EEG due to nasal air flow and identified them as specific responses to mechanical or chemical stimulation of olfactory epithelium that had been known to cause burst activity in the olfactory bulb (Adrian, 1950). This activity increases during inhalation and stops if nasal air flow has been interrupted (Domino & Ueki, 1960).

Repetitive and/or forced introduction of air into the nostrils is more effective than inhalation of odours during eupneic breathing (Gault & Coustan, 1965).

Provocation of phasic acceleration in neuronal firing in the olfactory bulb leads to the following consequences:

(1) Afteractivation in the pyriform cortex through the lateral olfactory tract, and in the corticomedial part of the amygdala; bursts spreading towards the septum, area subcalosa (through stria olfactoria medialis), and towards trigonum olfactorium (through stria olfactoria intermedia).
(2) Transition to theta waves and destabilization of limbic structures (Stewart, 1993).
(3) Arousal response in electroencephalogram (EEG) mediated by the projection of olfactory impulses into the mesencephalic reticular formation (through the medial forebrain bundle) (Motokizawa & Furuya, 1973).

Servít was the first to mention the possibility that such reflex olfactory responses could play some role in the appearance of early EEG changes during hyperventilation (HV) (Servít, 1977; Servít *et al.*, 1981). HV had been known as an activation procedure since Berger's time. The main effect of this procedure is based upon metabolic changes, due to decrease in the CO_2 level with vasoconstrictive cerebral hypoxaemia (Blinn & Noell, 1949; Gotoh *et al.*, 1965; Sherwin, 1984). In the experimental study of Gotoh *et al.* (1965), 80 s appeared to be the shortest period of latency in this hypocapnic effect. Servít assumed, therefore, that fast EEG responses can only be caused by other than hypocapnic mechanisms; for their closer investigation he suggested a method of differentiated HV (DHV). The DHV-test consists of 4 min of deep nasal breathing, separated from 4 min of oral breathing by a break of 5 min.

Very recently Stefan (1992) recommended 4 min of oral hyperventilation followed by 1 min of nasal HV.

In clinical studies, Servít (1977) confirmed differential effects of nasal and oral forms of HV upon EEG. In our first common study with Servít and co-workers (unpublished data), we learned that the DHV test was uncomfortable for children; therefore, we tried to elaborate a more convenient method.

The aim of the present studies was to evaluate the effectiveness of the new method and to assess the clinical relevance of olfactory stimulation.

Methods

Three studies are summarized in this presentation:

(1) In the first study, we used power spectral analysis of EEG to measure the effects of nasal and oral forms of HV as consecutively applied in random order in 20 5–15-year-old healthy children. In comparison with Konishi's method (1987a, b) we used the lower respiration rate (20/min). Effects on alpha and theta power-bands were analysed within 20 s sections of EEG during every 2 min of the DHV test. We then introduced a new method of combined HV (the CHV test) which consisted of 2 min of intensive nasal breathing with closed mouth, followed by 2 min of oral HV. This method was applied in 380 children and the results (positive responses in 201 children) were then compared with results provided by the former method of non-differentiated HV (NDHV) in 259 children (positive responses in 100 children).

(2) In the second study, our new CHV test was applied in 638 children within 2 years: data obtained during each of those 2 years were analysed separately and compared with one another in order to test the stability of applied procedures.

The total sample of 638 children was divided into two groups: children with epileptic seizures (n = 397) and children with other, non-epileptic brain disorders (n = 241) . The purpose of this analysis was to find out how reliably epilepsy was characterized by specific changes in EEG.

(3) The third study evaluated our attempt to improve the diagnostic classification of epilepsies and epileptic syndromes with the help of neurophysiological methods including the CHV test and long-term EEG monitoring. From a sample of 431 children referred to our Department of Child Neurology for a detailed neurological examination, we selected 154 children with symptomatology of complex partial seizures and different forms of non-convulsive attacks. Children with evidence of organic brain disorders were excluded. After a careful analysis of the patient's history and detailed clinical examination, we applied our new CHV-test together with long-term monitoring. The Siemens Elema 21, Bioscript 2100, eight-channel Medilog 9000 Oxford system and/or Biomedical Monitering System Incorporated (BMSI) video-EEG system were used for EEG recordings during the CHV test and for intensive monitoring.

Results

In the first study, the oral form of HV appeared to influence the EEG spectrum more strongly than the nasal form, and this effect was particularly evident during the fourth minute of HV (see Table 1). On the whole, the new CHV method elicited epileptic abnormalities in EEG more frequently (in 22.6 per cent) than the former NDHV method (in 2.2 per cent); that difference was significant (χ^2 [3]= 99.1; $P < 0.01$) – see Table 2.

In the second study, the comparison between findings from the first year of application and from the second year indicated a relative stability in applied procedures (no significant differences between the same forms of responses (see Fig. 1)) and thus justified an aggregation of data for further analyses.

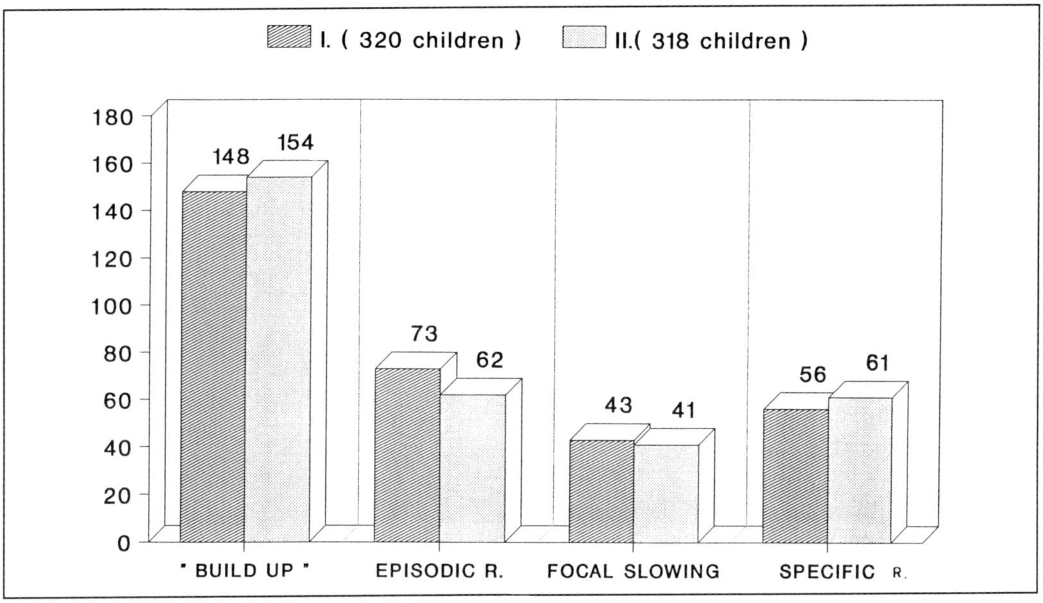

Fig. 1. EEG changes in responses to CHV test in the first (I) and second (II) year of study. Build-up, episodic and specific responses: see Table 2, focal slowing: unilateral or focal delta waves, χ^2 [3] =1.27, P <0.05.

An analysis of the diagnostic validity of EEG changes during the CHV test was carried out in this part of the study, in which findings in children with evident epilepsy were compared with non-epileptic neurological disorders (see Table 3). Our data showed that epilepsy-specific abnormalities appeared with a higher frequency (26.2 per cent) in epileptic disorders than in non-epileptic disorders (0.4 per cent), and the difference was significant ($P < 0.01$).

Table 1. Changes in per cent power averages during hyperventilation (HV)

	Resting EEG	Nasal HV	Nasal HV	Oral HV	Oral HV
	4′	2′	4′	2′	4′
Alpha %	32	28[a]	26	22[b]	17[b]
Theta %	17	19	20	26[b]	28[b]

Values of power spectral analysis of background activity in the bilateral centroparietal area in 20 healthy children.
[a]Statistically significant difference compared with resting ($P < 0.05$).
[b]Significant difference compared with resting and with nasal HV ($P < 0.01$).

Table 2. EEG changes in response to hyperventilation

	NDHV (n = 138)	NDHV (n = 138)	CHV (n = 201)	CHV (n = 201)
Responses	n	%	n	%
Build-up	100	72.5	134	66.6
Episodic*	35	25.3	20	10.0
Specific	3	2.2	47	23.4†

NDHV: 3–4 min of non-differentiated hyperventilation (mostly oral); CHV: 2 min of nasal HV followed by 2 min of oral HV. Build-up: slowing of background activity (Konishi, 1987a).
*Episodes of υ or δ waves
†Significant difference compared with epileptiform responses during NDHV test ($P < 0.01$).

Table 3. Results of CHV test in 638 children

	Group 1	Group 1	Group 2	Group 2
	n	%	*n*	%
Build-up	167	42.1	135	56.0
Episodic	84	21.1	51	21.2
Focal slowing	30	7.6	54	22.4
Specific	116	29.6	1	0.4
Total	397		241	

Group 1 : children with epilepsy 5–15 years old
Group 2 : controls, non-epileptic children 5–15 years old; χ^2 [3] = 99.1, $P < 0.01$.

During nasal HV, early activation of epileptic focal abnormalities (during the first 30 or 60 s) concerned anterior temporal and prefrontal areas of olfactory projection. Middle activation (at the end of the first minute and during the second minute) led to asymmetric, generalized irregular spikes and waves with a unilateral maximum in frontal areas. Lack of fundamental changes in the background EEG activity during this time allowed the conclusion that metabolic and vascular factors were not yet involved. EEG abnormalities characterizing pyknoleptic absences appeared during the third and fourth minutes (late response).

Figure 2 illustrates graphic appearances of EEG abnormalities in children with different types of absences.

The third study made it evident that the aforementioned methodological improvements increased the reliability of diagnostic tools. Original clinical diagnoses – based on symptom assessment and routine EEG – were substantially corrected in 49 children. Pseudoseizures were detected in 10 of them, benign epilepsy with Rolandic spikes (BERS) in 15 and frontal absences in 24. Diagnoses were improved in

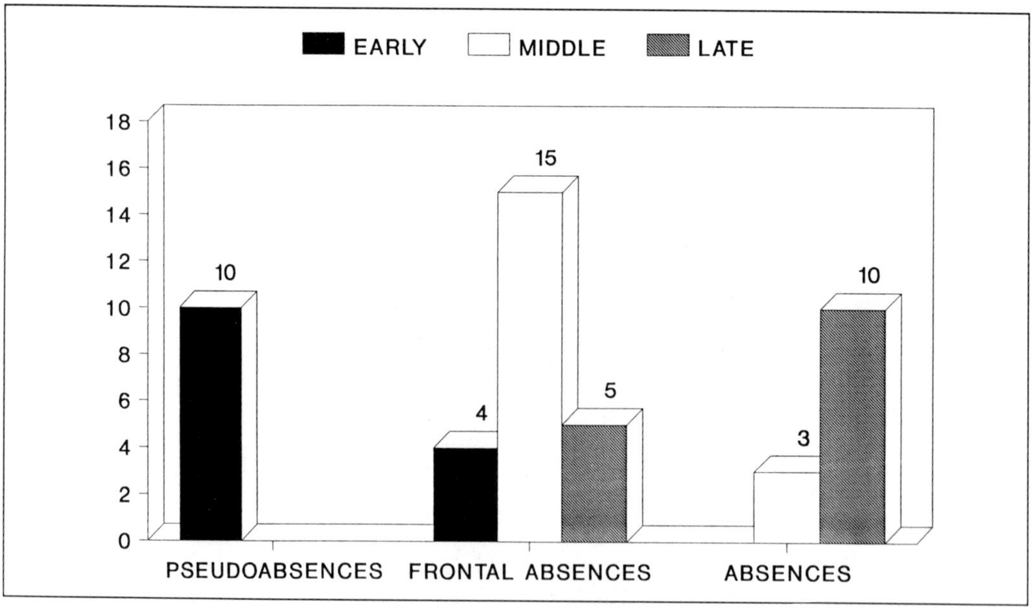

Fig. 2. Appearance of three main types of EEG responses to CHV in children with absences. Early response: during the first minute of nasal HV (NHV), middle: during the second minute of NHV, late: during the third and fourth minutes of oral HV (OHV).

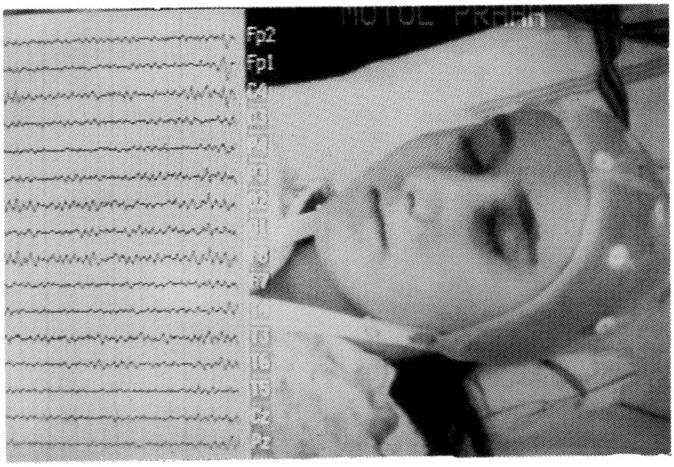

Fig. 3a. Frontal absence seizure in a 15-year-old girl elicited only during nasal hyperventilation (65 s latency). Ictal EEG showing discharges of irregular sharp wave activity with left frontal onset. No changes of background activity.

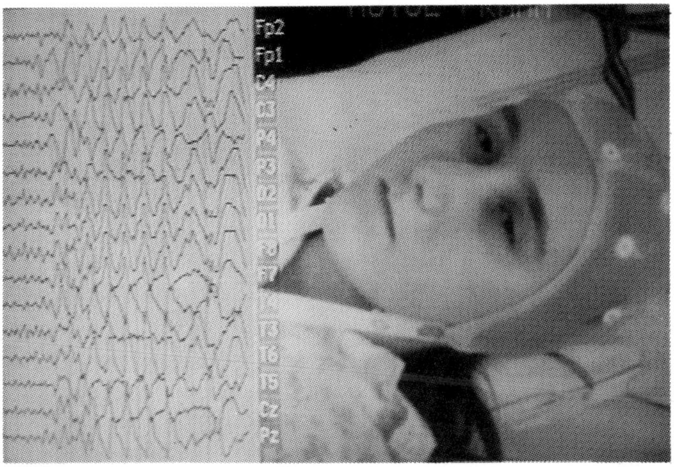

Fig. 3b. Brief episode of staring (opened eyes with 'blank face'), no answer to simple questions.

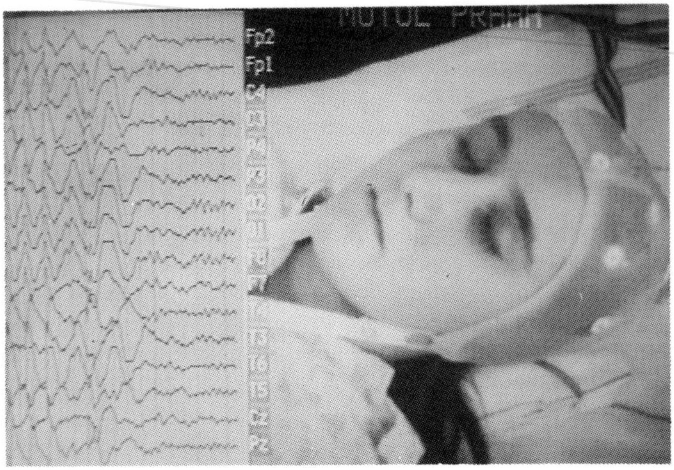

Fig. 3c. The end of seizure, no EEG changes during the next 2 min of oral hyperventilation. The seizure lasted 5 s.

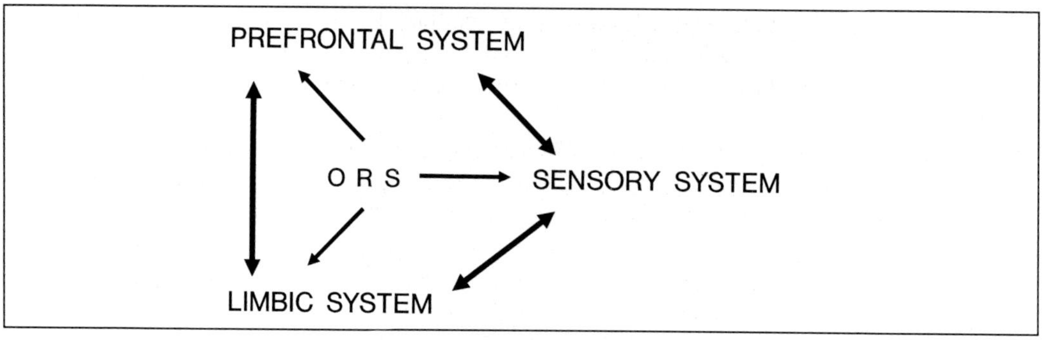

Fig. 4. The role of the olfactory system; with the permission of F. Koukolik (unpublished data).

the additional 27 children with the so-called Glaser syndrome – complex partial seizures occurring after a silent period in children with prolonged generalized seizures in early childhood ('scenario II' – Glaser, 1987).

Occasionally intensive nasal breathing elicited clinical seizures (frontal absences) – see Fig. 3a, b, c.

Discussion

The fact that olfactory stimulation during nasal HV can activate specific symptoms in EEG as well as clinical seizures deserves attention from the point of view of pathogenic mechanisms of these phenomena (Lehovsky & Komárek, 1989). According to Servít (1976), nasal insufflation of air activates penicillin's foci in the anterior thalamus and in the frontal lobe in amphibians. Freeman (1986) supposed that forebrain structures are destabilized under the influence of olfactory stimulation and thus abnormal activity in the limbic system leads to behavioural disturbances and absence-like seizures.

The possible role of the olfactory system (ORS) in the fragile balance among brain systems is shown in Fig. 4. Stewart (1993) demonstrated that the hippocampal interneurones are actively inhibited during transititons into theta rhythm. Consequently, experimental animals (rats) may be particularly susceptible for seizures at the time of transitions.

Thus, we can speculate that a forced inhalation or sniffing may activate processes mentioned by Freeman or Stewart, and that, in healthy subjects, these processes are responsible for awakening or orientation, and also participate in learning (Freeman & Grajski, 1987). However, in epileptic patients, these processes may lead to activation of epileptiform abnormalities in EEG or to clinical 'pseudoabsences' or absences.

Another interesting aspect is the type of stimuli that result from intensive nasal breathing. Both specific chemical stimuli (odorants), and other physical stimuli, such as the force or the temperature of the air stream, come into consideration.

Livermore (1992) discriminated three fundamental categories of stimulation: purely olfactory (such as vanillin or acetaldehyde), purely trigeminal (such as ammonium or sulphur dioxide) and dichorhinic (such as menthol or eucalyptol). Investigating chemosensory events-related potentials (CSER), Hummel and Kobal (1992) demonstrated that – unlike information processing in the somatosensory system – processing of olfactory sensations does not involve structures contralateral to the stimulated nostril. The authors considered the orbitofrontal cortex as the area in which evoked olfactory potentials may be generated. However, they did not find a linear correlation between stimulus concentration and response qualities when olfactory and trigeminal systems were activated simultaneously.

Neurophysiological evidence on the mechanisms of differential effects of various olfactory stimulations helps to understand our own clinical experience with the differentiated and combined forms of HV. In particular, we can now better interpret and diagnose non-convulsive seizures, so-called absences.

The CHV test helps distinguish three types of attacks taking the form of absence:

(1) Typical age-dependent absences, including only a generalized 'reticulothalamocortical' (RTC) component, with a 'late response' to CHV (regular spike wave 3/s with maximum in central area).

(2) Pseudoabsences (motionless staring) occurring as initial phase of complex partial seizures, including only a focal 'limbic' component, and with an 'early response' to CHV (sharp waves/spikes in temporal/frontal areas or flattening in surface EEG).

(3) Frontal absences as 'middle response' to CHV, characterized with asymmetrical, generalized irregular spike waves of a focal origin, including both a focal 'cortical' and generalized RTC components.

Although we have occasionally observed clinically manifest seizures during the CHV test, we can neither exclude nor confirm the possibility that some forms of olfactory stimulations may elicit epileptic seizures independently of activation methods. It is possible that further research on the effects of olfactory stimulation upon limbic functions in humans elucidate further aspects relevant not only for epileptology, but also for research on human brain functions involved in behavioural regulation in general.

References

Adrian, E.D (1950): The electrical activity of the mammalian olfactory bulb. *Electroencephalogr. Clin. Neurophysiol.* **2,** 377–388.

Blinn, K.A. & Noell, W.K. (1949): Continuous measurement of alveolar CO_2 tension during the hyperventilation test in routine electroencephalography. *Electroencephalogr. Clin. Neurophysiol.* **1,** 333–342.

Domino, E.F. & Ueki, S. (1960): An analysis of the electrical phenomenon in some rhinencephalic structures of the dog and monkey. *Electroencephalogr. Clin. Neurophysiol.* **12,** 635–648.

Freeman, W.J. (1986): Petit mal seizure spikes in olfactory bulb and cortex caused by runaway inhibition after exhaustion of excitation. *Brain Res. Rev.* **11,** 259–284.

Freeman, W.J. & Grajski, K.A. (1987): Relation of olfactory EEG to behavior: factor analysis. *Behav. Neurosci.* **101,** 766–777.

Gastaut, H. (1989): Synopsis and conclusions of the international colloquium on reflex seizures and epilepsies. In: *Reflex seizures and reflex epilepsies*, eds. A. Beaumanoir, H. Gastaut & R. Naquet, pp. 497–507. Geneva: Médecine & Hygiène.

Gault, F.P. & Coustan, D.R. (1965): Nasal air flow and rhinencephalic activity. *Electroencephalogr. Clin. Neurophysiol.* **31,** 617–624.

Glaser, G.H. (1987): Natural history of temporal lobe epilepsy. In: *Surgical treatment of the epilepsies,* ed. J. Enger, pp. 19–30. New York: Raven Press.

Gotoh, F., Meyer, J. & Takagi, Y. (1965): Cerebral effects of hyperventilation in man. *Arch. Neurol. Psychiatr.y* **12,** 410–423.

Henner, K. (1963): Reflex epileptic mechanisms. In: *Reflex mechanisms in the genesis of epilepsy*, ed. Z. Servít, pp. 28-42. Amsterdam: Elsevier.

Hummel, T. & Kobal, G. (1992): Differences in human evoked potentials related to olfactory or trigeminal chemosensory activation. *Electroencephalogr. Clin. Neurophysiol.* **84,** 84–89.

Livermore, A., Hummel, T. & Kobal, G. (1992): Chemosensory event-related potentials in the investigation of interactions between the olfactory and the somatosensory (trigeminal) systems. *Electroencephalogr. Clin. Neurophysiol.* **83,** 201–210.

Konishi, T. (1987a): The standardization of hyperventilation on EEG recording in childhood I. The quantity of hyperventilation activation. *Brain Dev.* **9,** 16–20.

Konishi, T. (1987b): The standardization of hyperventilation on EEG recording in childhood II. The quantitative analysis of build-up. *Brain Dev.* **9,** 21–25.

Lehovsky, M. & Komárek, V. (1989): Olfactorhinencephalic system activation in epilepsy. In: *Reflex seizures and reflex epilepsies,* eds. A. Beaumanoir, H. Gastaut & R. Naquet pp. 261–263. Geneva: Médecine & Hygiène.

Motokizawa, F. & Furuya, N. (1973): Neural pathway associated with the EEG arousal response by olfactory stimulation, *Electroencephalogr. Clin. Neurophysiol.* **35,** 83–91.

Servít, Z. (1977): Ätiopathogenetische Diagnostik und Therapie der Epilepsie. *Z. EEG EMG* **8,** 113–125.

Servit, Z. Strejckova, A. (1976):Influence of nasal respiration upon normal EEG and epileptic electroencephalographic activities in frog and turtle. *Physiol. B.* **25,** 109–114.

Servít, Z., Krištof, M. & Kolínová, M. (1981): Activating effect of nasal and oral hyperventilation on epileptic electrographic phenomena: reflex mechanisms of nasal origin. *Epilepsia* **22,** 321–329.

Sherwin, M. (1984): Hyperventilation: mode of action and application in electroencephalography. *A. J. Electroencephalogr.* 24, 201–211.

Stefan, H. (1992): *Epilepsien, Diagnose und Behandlung,* 2nd edn, p. 72. Weinheim: VCH.

Stewart, M. (1993): Disinhibition of hippocampal pyramidal cells during the transition into theta rhythm. Exp. Brain. Res. 93, 1–5.

Epileptic Seizures and Syndromes, Edited by Peter Wolf
© 1994 John Libbey & Company Ltd., pp. 115–126

Chapter 15

Childhood absence epilepsy (pyknolepsy) and juvenile absence epilepsy: one or two syndromes?

Dieter Janz, Gertrude Beck-Mannagetta, Barbara Spröder, Jürgen Spröder and Stefan Waltz*

Abteilung für Neurologie, Klinikum Rudolf Virchow, Freie Universität, Augustenburger Platz 1, D-13353, Berlin;
**Abteilung für Neuropädiatrie, Kinderklinik der Universität Kiel, Schwanenweg 20 D-24105, Kiel, Germany*

Introduction

Scarcely any statement in the International Classification of Epilepsies and Epileptic Syndromes has caused more hesitation and doubts than the subclassification of the absence epilepsies in a childhood absence epilepsy and a juvenile absence epilepsy. Before the International Classification was established in 1985, this distinction was used only in German publications. In 1965 Doose *et al.* described a late infantile and a juvenile form, while Janz reported an epilepsy with pyknoleptic absences and an epilepsy with nonpyknoleptic absences in 1969. Therefore it is only just that the first author has been asked to comment on the utility and correctness of this distinction in the light of the new syndrome classification.

In 1955, Janz reported in a study on 'the clinical position of pyknolepsy' that the form with 'pure' (i.e. simple) absences usually develops between the ninth and fourteenth years, which is somewhat later than the other types of absences in pyknolepsy (Janz, 1955). In a study on 'Impulsiv-Petit mal' published in 1957, Janz and Christian mentioned that epilepsies with simple absences constitute a clinical and electroencephalographic (EEG) disease entity situated nosologically between the retropulsive petit mal and impulsive petit mal forms. Doose *et al.* (1965) studied 149 children with absences in the course of their illness and attempted to determine whether or not all cases with 'spike-wave absences' represented a uniform syndrome. In addition to the late infantile form occurring between the ages of 4 and 8 years, termed pyknolepsy, they identified a group of patients with early onset, which they called infantile absence epilepsy, as well as a further group with late onset at or immediately before puberty, which they termed juvenile absence epilepsy. Infantile absence epilepsy is more common in boys, while pyknolepsy occurs more often in girls. There is no gender difference among patients with juvenile absence epilepsy. The absences are less frequent than in pyknolepsy and occur either in clusters (the 'cycloleptic' form) or sporadically (the 'spanioleptic' form).

In a comparison of 505 cases of pyknoleptic absences and 197 patients with non-pyknoleptic absences

Janz (1969) confirmed these differences in age of onset, frequency of seizures, the sex distribution and differences in the frequency of spike wave patterns noted by Doose *et al.* in 1965.

This raises the question whether both forms are nothing but age-dependent variants of a biological entity or essentially distinct disease states. Analysis of their genetic characteristics might provide the answer to this question.

The present study

Therefore, we recently undertook a clinical, EEG and genetic investigation of all cases of absence epilepsy treated in our hospital from 1973 to the present (Purucker & Spröder, 1992). After exclusion of all cases in which absences occurred in connection with other syndromes such as juvenile myoclonic epilepsy and the Lennox–Gastaut syndrome, 306 cases remained from a total 3245 patients with non-febrile epileptic seizures. Two hundred and thirty-four cases – 113 with pyknoleptic and 121 with non-pyknoleptic absences – were treated in Berlin during the period 1973–1988. Seventy-two additional patients – 40 with pyknoleptic absences and 32 with non-pyknoleptic absences – treated in Heidelberg before this period were contacted by letter.

The initial question concerns criteria for discrimination between the two forms of absence epilepsy. One might choose age of onset or the frequency of the absences. Doose *et al.* (1965) were the first to note that the age of onset demonstrates two peaks, a finding later confirmed by Oller-Daurella & Sanchez (1981) and Weber (1967). A trough at age 10 convinced Doose *et al.* (1965) that a late infantile absence epilepsy, usually with a pyknoleptic course, was distinct from a juvenile type, usually with a cycloleptic or spanioleptic mode of recurrence. This trough is evident in graphs demonstrating the age of onset in 197 cases from our early study (Janz, 1969: p. 126), from a recent epidemiological study of 134 cases published by Olsson (1988) and in the series of 210 patients (with known age of onset of absences) of the present study (Fig. 1). Therefore, the two peaks in the age of onset might provide a criterion for discrimination between absence epilepsies with onset before and after the age of 10 years (Fig. 2). The semantic distinction between childhood absence epilepsy and juvenile absence epilepsy implies use of the age of onset as the criterion for differentiation.

However, the fact that absences recur more frequently with early age of onset and less frequently with later age of onset suggests that the frequency of absences might also be a useful criterion for

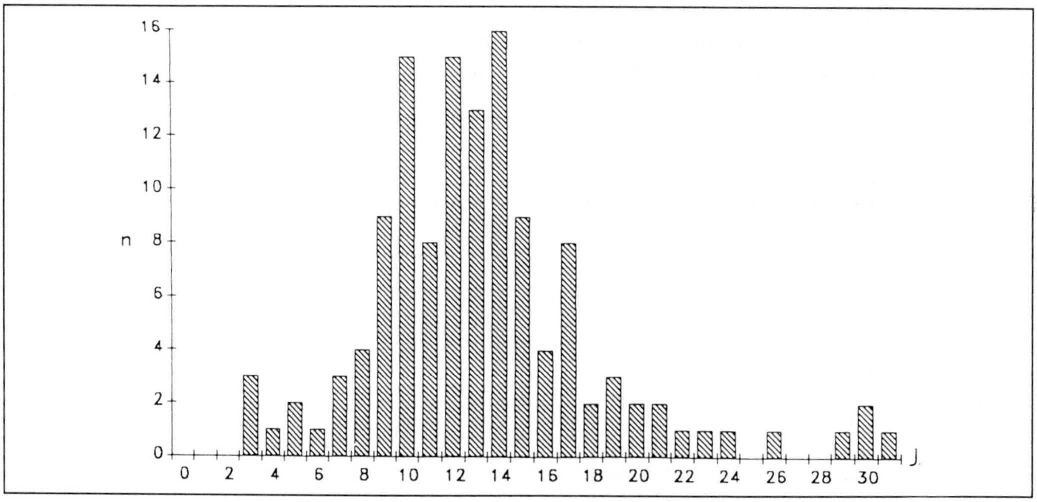

Fig. 1. Age-specific distribution of the onset of absences in 210 cases of epilepsy with absences (except Lennox–Gastaut syndrome and juvenile myoclonic epilepsy).

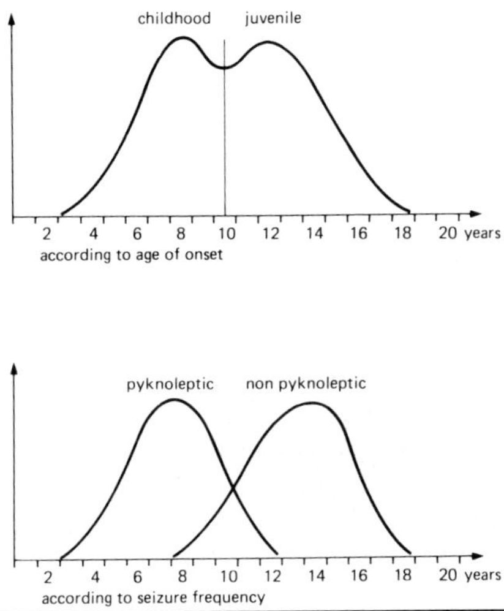

Fig. 2. Syndrome definition of absence epilepsy either by age of onset or by seizure frequency.

discrimination. Therefore, one might distinguish between epilepsies with pyknoleptic absences and those with non-pyknoleptic absences (Fig. 2). We elected to use seizure frequency as the criterion and chose daily recurrence as the measure of pyknoleptic seizures and a lower frequency – which means less than one seizure per day – as a characteristic of non-pyknoleptic absences. It is no more difficult to elicit the frequency of absences during the first months of illness than it is to determine the age of onset.

Age of onset

Distinction between the absence epilepsies according to the age of onset of absences reveals that pyknoleptic absences first occur between the third and fifteenth years of life with the peak between the fifth and ninth years and the average age of onset at 7.5 years. The onset of epilepsies with non-pyknoleptic absences demonstrates a broader range, with the age of onset from 4 to 30 years, a peak between the tenth and sixteenth years and a mean age of onset at 13.3 years (Table 1). This represents a difference in average age of onset of 5.8 years (Fig. 3).

Table 1. Absence epilepsies: comparison of various factors

Epilepsy	With pyknoleptic absences *n*	With non-pyknoleptic absences *n*
Number	153	153
Birth trauma	6	–
Age at investigation	36.9 years	36.3 years
Duration of disease	22.3 years	28.2 years
Age of onset (epilepsy)	7.3 years	12.7 years
Age of onset (absences)	7.5 years	13.3 years
Age of onset (grand mal)	13.5 years	15.6 years
Absence status	35	42
Grand mal status	7	6

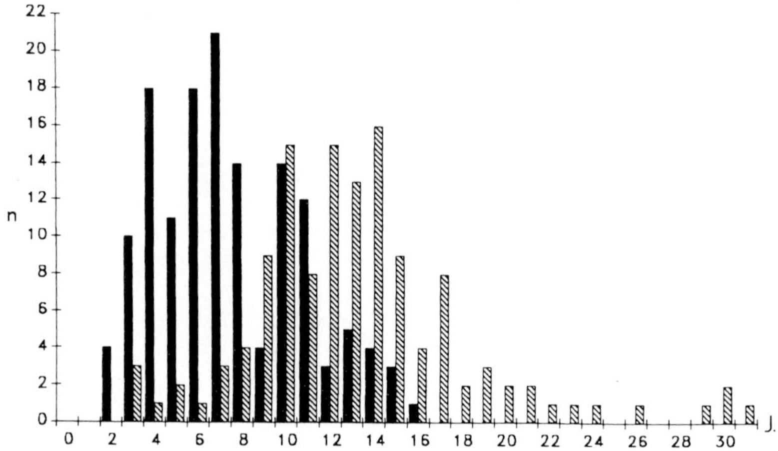

Fig. 3. Age-specific distribution of the onset of absences in 142 cases with pyknoleptic and in 128 cases of non-pyknoleptic absences.

Sex distribution

Both types of absence epilepsy are slightly more common among females (Table 2). According to the literature pyknolepsies are significantly more common in girls than in boys. Sixty to 76 per cent of all affected children are females (Doose *et al.*, 1965; Loiseau, 1992). In juvenile absence epilepsy, Doose *et al.* (1965) and Janz (1969) found a less pronounced preponderance of females, although Wolf and Inoue (1984) reported the opposite.

According to our study, the preponderance of females in both forms of epilepsy is limited to early age of onset (between the ages of 5 and 10 in cases of pyknolepsy and between 7 and 14 in juvenile absence epilepsies), while males predominate among patients with later onset.

Table 2. Absences epilepsies: sex ratio

	With pyknoleptic absences		With non-pyknoleptic absences	
Epilepsy	*n*	%	*n*	%
Male	67	44	69	45
Female	86	56	84	55
Total	153	100	153	100

Exogenous aetiological factors

Only six of 153 patients (3.9 per cent) with pyknoleptic absences had prenatal, perinatal or postnatal complications as possible relevant aetiological factors. None of the 153 patients with non-pyknoleptic absences had a relevant aetiological factor in the history (Table 1).

A review of the literature shows that exogenic factors as possible causes were elicited in 4 to 8 per cent of patients with pyknolepsy (Lugaresi & Volterra, 1963; Weber, 1967; Janz, 1969) and in 3.5 per cent of patients with non-pyknoleptic absences (Janz, 1969).

Symptomatology of absences

The type of absences in patients with non-pyknoleptic absences is limited to simple absences in a significant percentage of cases, while patients with pyknoleptic absences show a significantly higher proportion of complex absences (Table 3). Complex absences in patients with non-pyknoleptic absences are often characterized by eyelid myoclonus, while complex absences in patients with pyknoleptic absences more often show 'retropulsive' movements (upward gaze and/or retro-movements of the head and/or trunk). Automatisms are equally common in both forms of absence epilepsy (Table 4). Differentiation between the patterns of absences is supported by video-EEG recordings.

Table 3. Absence epilepsies: type of absences

	With pyknoleptic absences		With non-pyknoleptic absences	
Epilepsy	*n*	%	*n*	%
Simple	54	35	100	66
Complex	65	43	38	25
Both	34	22	14	9
Total	153	100	153	100

Table 4. Absence epilepsies: subtype of complex absences

	With pyknoleptic absences		With non-pyknoleptic absences	
Epilepsy	*n*	%	*n*	%
Myoclonic	47	39	31	57
Retropulsive	47	39	12	22
Versive	6	5	4	7
Propulsive	8	7	–	–
Automatisms	12	10	7	13
Total	120	100	54	100

Panayiotopoulos *et al.* (1989) demonstrated that disorders of consciousness manifested by interruption of speech and hyperventilation are more readily interrupted by external stimuli in juvenile absences than in absences in childhood absence epilepsy. Simple absences were more common in cases of juvenile absence epilepsy, and these patients almost never demonstrated upward gaze during their absences. However, the authors did not find differences between the two patient groups in the duration of absences, as other investigators have supposed (Janz, 1969; Doose, 1991).

Type of seizure at the onset of disease

Pyknoleptic absence epilepsy usually begins with absences. In rare cases one or more grand mal seizures may precede frequent absences (Table 5). The onset of epilepsy with non-pyknoleptic absences is often identified by the appearance of the first grand mal seizures. An initial presentation with grand mal seizures rather than with absences has been reported in patients with non-pyknoleptic absences (Janz, 1969; Wolf & Inoue, 1984). However, these figures certainly do not represent reality in these patients. The average duration of illness is 22 and 28 years (Table 1). Since mild non-pyknoleptic absences may easily escape notice by the patient and the doctor, one might suspect that these seizures might also have been overlooked or forgotten when they occurred as the initial manifestation.

Table 5. Absence epilepsies: initial seizure type

	With pyknoleptic absences		With non-pyknoleptic absences	
Epilepsy	*n*	%	*n*	%
Absences	117	82	45	36
Grand mal	6	4	20	16
Myoclonic jerks	–	–	2	2
Absences and grand mal in the same year	19	13	58	46
Total	142	100	126	100

Clinical course

Nineteen cases (12.4 per cent) of pyknoleptic and six patients (3.9 per cent) with non-pyknoleptic absences remained free of grand mal seizures during periods averaging 10.2 and 9.5 years, respectively. Grand mal seizures begin on average at the age of 13.5 years in patients with pyknolepsy and at 15.6 years in cases of non-pyknoleptic absence epilepsy. All patients with 'pure' absence epilepsies were older than the average age at which grand mal seizures occur, but they were still at the younger end of the age spectrum in our series, averaging 27.4 and 28.2 years, respectively, in comparison with mean ages of 36.9 and 36.3 years in the whole group (Table 1).

If one takes the number of grand mal seizures as a criterion of the severity of disease, 28 per cent of patients from both groups with grand mal seizures might be considered as suffering from relatively mild disease, because they had fewer than seven grand mal seizures. Of the remaining patients with grand mal seizures related to the sleep–wake rhythm, most suffered from grand mal on awakening (Table 6).

Table 6. Absence epilepsies: type of grand mal

	With pyknoleptic absences		With non-pyknoleptic absences	
Epilepsy	*n*	%	*n*	%
Awakening	92	96	93	91
Sleep	1	1	3	3
Random	3	3	6	6
Total	96	100	102	100
Not classifiable yet because fewer than seven seizures	38	28	40	28
Total	134		142	

Combinations with other types of seizures have been observed, but the only significant difference between non-pyknoleptic and pyknoleptic absences concerned myoclonic jerks of the impulsive petit mal type, which were observed in 19.6 per cent of patients with non-pyknoleptic absences as compared with 3.3 per cent in combination with pyknoleptic absences (Table 7). Febrile convulsions in early childhood occur with equal frequency in both types of absence epilepsies, although the incidence in our series was lower than the 15–20 per cent reported by other authors (Penry *et al.*, 1975; Rocca *et al.*, 1987).

Table 7. Absence epilepsies: type of preceding, accompanying or following seizures

	With pyknoleptic absences, n = 53		With non pyknoleptic absences, n = 153	
Epilepsy	n	%	n	%
Grand mal	134	88	142	93
Myoclonic jerks	5	3	30	20
Astatic seizures	2	1	2	1
Focal seizures	2	1	3	2
Febrile convulsions	15	10	11	7

Cases with absence status were observed more often in our patients than in other series in the literature (Table 1), where an incidence of 10–16 per cent has been reported (Livingston *et al.*, 1965; Dieterich *et al.*, 1985). Paediatricians have reported them rarely, and Aicardi (1986) described them as extremely rare in childhood absence epilepsy. This implies that absence status in pyknolepsy develops with increasing age.

EEG

Differences in EEG findings between the two forms of absence epilepsy have been described rather impressionistically up to the present (Doose *et al.*, 1965; Janz, 1969; Christian, 1982). During interictal periods in juvenile absences, somewhat faster (3.5–4/s) and more irregular spike-wave patterns have been observed than the monomorphic 3/s spike-wave complexes usually found in pyknolepsy. However, the ictal patterns observed were apparently somewhat longer than those found in childhood absence epilepsy, although this finding was based on a comparison of only three and six cases (Panayiotopoulos *et al.*, 1989). Photosensitivity was found significantly less often in epilepsy with non-pyknoleptic absences than in pyknoleptic absence epilepsy when patients with additional myoclonic seizures were excluded (Wolf & Goosses, 1986).

A systematic comparison was undertaken recently by Waltz (1993). He analysed EEG findings from 88 patients with pyknoleptic and 92 patients with non-pyknoleptic absences. There were no significant differences in the basal rhythm, which was normal in 83 and 84 per cent, respectively, the incidence of focal findings – inconstant in most cases (18 *vs.* 28 per cent), occipital delta waves (5 *vs.* 2 per cent) and activation or provocation of specific potentials by hyperventilation (75 *vs.* 72.5 per cent). In contrast to the findings published by Wolf & Goosses (1986), Waltz found no difference in photosensitivity between the two forms (19.5 *vs.* 21 per cent). There was no difference when absence epilepsies combined with myoclonic jerks – which are more photosensitive (29 per cent) – were eliminated from the evaluation (19 *vs.* 18 per cent). It is noteworthy that patients with non-pyknoleptic absences demonstrated greater eyelid closure sensitivity than patients with pyknoleptic absences (15.2 *vs.* 5.7 per cent). This difference was at the limit of statistical significance.

Regarding the various frequency-related spike-wave patterns, Waltz confirmed earlier impressions reported in the literature (Fig. 4). The only statistically significant difference was the fact that patterns with the classical frequency between 2.5 and 3.5/s were more common in pyknoleptic absence epilepsies than in non-pyknoleptic absences. Correspondingly, spike-wave patterns with higher frequencies were more common in the latter group. Slow spike-wave patterns were equally rare with both forms of epilepsy. A systematic analysis failed to confirm the impression that polyspike-wave and irregular spike-wave patterns are more common in non-pyknoleptic absences (Doose *et al.*, 1965).

In patients with a combination of absences and myoclonic jerks such as occur in juvenile myoclonic epilepsy, there is an increase in the incidence of fast spike-wave and polyspike-wave complexes with corresponding decreases in the other two groups, as one might expect (Waltz, 1993).

Waltz found a clear distinction between pyknoleptic and non-pyknoleptic absences in the sex distribution of photosensitivity. The latter was equally common among males and females with pyknoleptic absences, while there was a significantly higher incidence of photosensitivity among

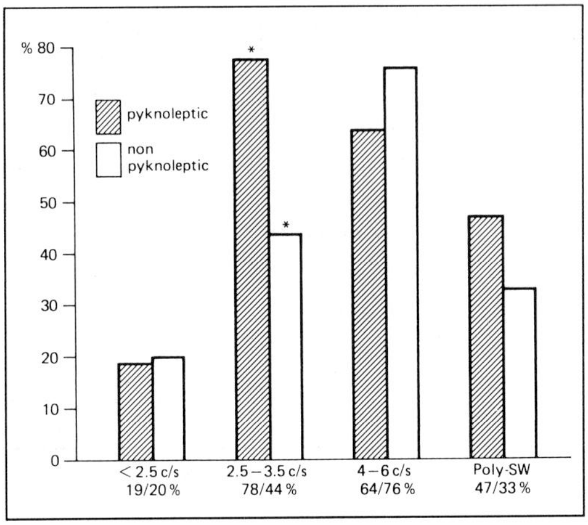

Fig. 4. Spike-wave pattern in absence epilepsies (Waltz, 1993).

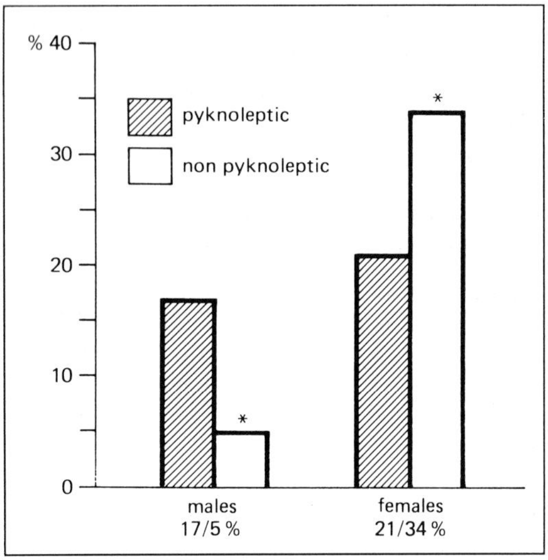

Fig. 5. Photosensitivity and gender in absence epilepsies (Waltz, 1993).

females with non-pyknoleptic absences. The graph shows these relations after elimination of cases with a combination of myoclonic jerks and absences (Fig. 5). Wolf and Goosses (1986) reported that almost half of all females with juvenile myoclonic epilepsy are photosensitive. There was also a significant difference in sensitivity to eyelid closure between males and females with both types of absence epilepsy. This is not surprising, since one may assume that photosensitivity and sensitivity to eyelid closure are related (Wolf *et al.*, 1986).

Since it is unlikely that the age of onset and the age at examination, both of which might influence the incidence of photosensitivity and sensitivity to eyelid closure, are different in males and females, these findings suggest genuine biological differences between the two forms of absence epilepsy. Photosensitivity is a genetically determined characteristic. Since the two forms of absence epilepsy differ in their significance between the sexes, it may well be that the different clinical presentations of absence epilepsy are the expression of differences in their genetic disposition.

Genetic disposition

The incidence of non-febrile epileptic seizures among close relatives of patients with pyknoleptic and non-pyknoleptic absences is 5.3 and 4.5 per cent, respectively. Male relatives were affected almost twice as often as females in both groups (Table 8).

The only comparable investigation in families of patients with pyknolepsy (Weber, 1967) reported the opposite result. In juvenile myoclonic epilepsy female relatives are more often affected than males (Tsuboi & Christian, 1973; Janz *et al.*, 1989).

In epilepsy with pyknoleptic absences, relatives of male patients are affected less often than the relatives of female patients (3.5 per cent *vs.* 6.3 per cent), a finding which has also been reported in juvenile myoclonic epilepsy (Tsuboi & Christian, 1973; Janz *et al.*, 1989). The proportions are almost equal in non-pyknoleptic absences (4.7 *vs.* 4.4 per cent).

Type of familial epilepsies

In addition to determining the familial incidence of afebrile seizures, we compared the types of epilepsies and epileptic syndromes between affected members of families with absence epilepsies in index cases. There were only generalized epilepsies among close (first-degree) relatives of the patients. The relatively high proportion of absence epilepsies in both groups (Table 9) suggests that absence epilepsies are more common in families of patients with absence epilepsy than would be expected from a normal distribution (Janz *et al.*, 1989). The fact that both types of absence syndrome occur in relatives of patients with both forms seems to argue against a homologous inheritance. That juvenile myoclonic epilepsy is not rare among relatives of patients with absence epilepsies supports the hypothesis that absence epilepsies and juvenile myoclonic epilepsy share a close genetic relationship (Janz *et al.*, 1992).

Table 8. Absence epilepsies: incidence of non-febrile epileptic seizures in first degree relatives

	With pyknoleptic absences			With non-pyknoleptic absences		
Epilepsy	*N*	*n*	%	*N*	*n*	%
Father	69	5	7	82	5	6
Mother	69	3	4	82	2	2
Parents	**138**	**8**	**6**	**164**	**7**	**4**
Brother	67	3	6	68	5	7
Sister	58	2	6	57	3	5
Siblings	**125**	**5**	**4**	**125**	**8**	**6**
Son	32	3	9	35	1	3
Daughter	27	1	4	25	–	–
Children	**59**	**4**	**7**	**175**	**11**	**6**
First degree male relatives	167	11	7	185	11	6
First degree female relatives	155	6	4	168	5	3
First degree relatives	**322**	**17**	**5**	**353**	**16**	**5**

Table 9. Absence epilepsies: epileptic syndromes in first degree relatives

	With pyknoleptic absences		With non-pyknoleptic absences	
Epilepsy	*n*	%	*n*	%
Generalized epilepsies	16	100	13	100
Pyknoleptic absences	2	13	2	15
Non -pyknoleptic absences	3	19	1	8
Not classifiable absences	1	6	–	–
Juvenile myoclonic epilepsy	5	31	1	8
Pure grand mal	5	31	8	62
West/Lennox–Gastaut	1	6	1	8

While preparing molecular genetic studies, we collected the family trees of 21 families in which the index subject and at least one relative had absence epilepsy. A comparison of the subsyndromes of absence epilepsy within the families produced the following results. In one family it was not possible to classify the type of familial absence epilepsy. Different absence syndromes were observed only within four of the 20 remaining families. In nine families there were two and in three families there were three close relatives affected with pyknoleptic absence epilepsy. Seven other families comprised individuals with juvenile absence epilepsy alone. This result confirms the findings published by

Berkovic *et al.*, 1990), who investigated identical twins with absence epilepsies and found the same type of disorder in pairs of twins in every case. Five of the twin pairs in their series suffered from childhood absence epilepsy, while the remaining two pairs had juvenile absence epilepsy. Therefore, they concluded 'that the fidelity of subsyndromes in monozygous pairs indicates that the syndromes are genetically distinct'.

Conclusion

Berkovic, the Andermanns and Gloor published a highly regarded article in 1987 in which they proposed a concept of absence epilepsy. In the subtitle of their article they asked whether the observed differences were sufficient to discriminate between discrete syndromes or whether the differences were points on a biological continuum. Even though it is certain that the findings which we have presented do not permit discrimination between the two absence epilepsies as 'fundamentally different conditions', one should consider the similarities and dissimilarities among epileptic syndromes before assuming that this is but a manifestation of an undifferentiated broad neurobiological continuum. Biological phenomena, including disease – which is a biological phenomenon – are not easily classified either as simple dichotomous alternatives or as elements of a continuous spectrum.

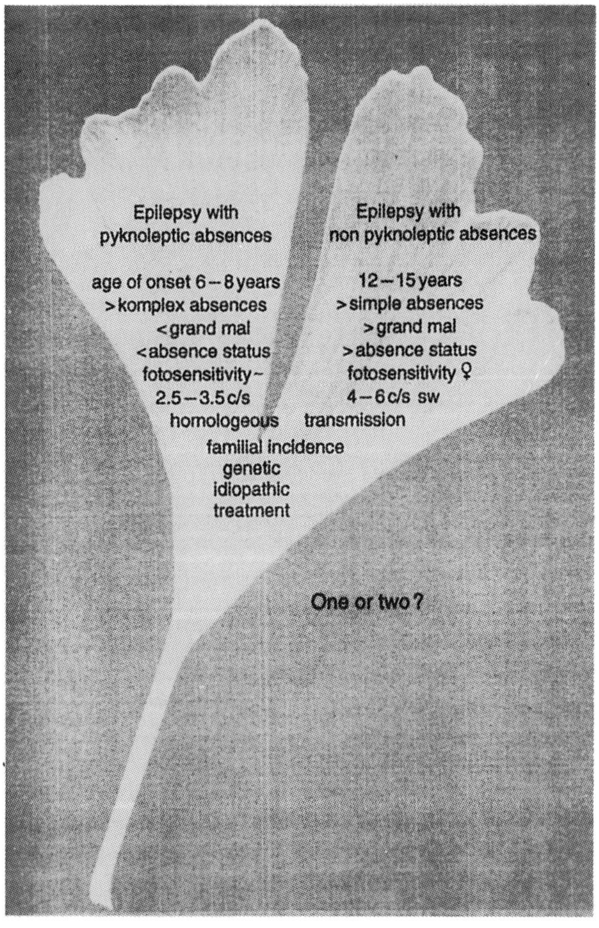

Fig. 6. Ginkgo biloba leaf as a symbol for the answer to the title question.

It is also possible to describe different degrees of relationships. The two forms of absence epilepsy are members of the group of idiopathic generalized epilepsies which also includes juvenile myoclonic epilepsy and epilepsy with grand mal on awakening. Within this group there are closer relationships in symptomatology, genetic components and treatment than are found within other forms of generalized epilepsies which may also present as idiopathic forms. The latter differ especially in terms of clinical presentation and therapeutic approach. Within this complex of idiopathic generalized epilepsies it is possible to recognize close sibling relationships between the two absence epilepsies of a type that suggests biological and even poetic analogies.

Goethe was inspired by the leaf of the ancient *Ginkgo biloba* – the most ancient extant tree in the earth's history – to write a poem in which he posed a question which we share:

> By itself in twain divided,
> Does it have the life of One?
> Is it two, who have decided
> As a unit to be known?

Unfortunately we cannot share his answer:

> Answering these, with little trouble
> On the very sense I hit;
> For I am that One and Double;
> In my songs thou feelest it.

A song may not suffice but a picture might suggest the close relationship between these two syndromes, similar to the leaf of the *Ginkgo biloba* tree (Fig. 6), which represents a division within a unity.

References

Aircardi, J. (1986): *Epilepsy in children.* New York: Raven Press.

Berkovic, S.F., Andermann, F., Andermann, E. & Gloor, P. (1987): Concepts of absence epilepsies: discrete syndromes or biological continuum? *Neurology* **37,** 993–1000.

Berkovic, S.F., Howell, R.A., Hopper, J.I., Hay, D.A. & Anderman, E. (1990): A twin study of the epilepsies (abstr.). *Epilepsia.* **31,** 813.

Christian, W. (1982): *Klinische Elektroenzephalographie: Lehrbuch und Atlas,* 3rd edn. Stuttgart: Thieme.

Dieterich, E., Baier, W.K., Doose, H. & Tuxhorn J. (1985): Longterm follow-up of childhood epilepsy with absences. I: Epilepsy with absences at onset. *Neuropediatrics* **16,** 149–154.

Doose, H. (1991): Verlauf und Prognose von Absence-Epilepsien. In: *Epilepsien des Kindesalters.,* eds. G. Jacobi & K. Meier-Ewert, pp. 55–66. Stuttgart, Jena, New York: Gustav Fischer.

Doose, H., Völzke, E. & Scheffner, D. (1965): Verlaufsformen kindlicher Epilepsien mit spike wave-Absencen. *Arch. Psychiatr. Nervenkr.* **207,** 394–415.

Janz, D. (1955): Die klinische Stellung der Pyknolepsie. *Dtsch. Med. Wschr.* **80,** 1392–1394.

Janz, D. (1969): *Die Epilepsien.: Spezielle Pathologie und Therapie.* Stuttgart: Thieme.

Janz, D. & Christian, W. (1957): Impulsiv-Petit mal. *Dtsch. Z. Nervenheilk..* **176,** 346–386.

Janz, D., Beck-Mannagetta, G. & Sander, T. (1992): Do idiopathic generalized epilepsies share a common susceptibility gene? *Neurology* **42** (suppl. 5), 48–55.

Janz, D., Durner, M., Beck-Mannagetta, G. & Pantazis, G. (1989): Family studies on the genetics of juvenile myoclonic epilepsy. In: *Genetics of the Epilepsies,* eds. G. Beck-Mannagetta, V.E. Anderson, H. Doose & D. Janz, pp. 43–52. Berlin: Springer.

Livingston, S., Torres, I., Pauli, L.L. & Ridder, R.V. (1965): Petit mal epilepsy: results of prolonged follow-up study of 117 patients. *J. Amer. Assoc.* **194,** 113–118.

Loiseau, P. (1992): Childhood absence epilepsy. In: *Epileptic syndromes in infancy, childhood and adolescence,* 2nd edn., eds. J. Roger, M. Bureau, Ch. Dravet, F.E. Dreifuss, A. Perret & P. Wolf, pp. 135–160. London: John Libbey.

Lugaresi, E. & Volterra, V. (1963): Considerazioni cliniche et EEG sull'assenza Piccolo Male. *Clin. Paediatr. (Bologna)* **45,** 3–18.

Oller-Daurella, L. & Sanchez, M.E. (1981): Evolucion de las ausencias tipicas. *Rev. Neurol. (Barcelona)* **9,** 81–102.

Olsson, I. (1988): Epidemiology of absence epilepsy. 1: Concept and incidence. *Acta Paediatr. Scand.* **77,** 860–866.

Panayiotopoulos, C.P., Obeid, T. & Waheed, G. (1989): Differentiation of typical absence seizures in epileptic syndromes: a video EEG study of 224 seizures in 20 patients. *Brain* **112,** 1039–1056.

Penry, J.K., Porter, R.J. & Dreifuss, F.E. (1975): Simultaneous recording of absence seizures with video tape and electroencephalography: a study of 374 seizures in 48 patients. *Brain* **98,** 427–440.

Purucker, B. & Spröder, J. (1992): Epilepsie mit pyknoleptischen Absencen und juvenile Absence-Epilepsie: Eine vergleichende klinische und genetische Untersuchung. Inaugural dissertation. Berlin: Freie Universität.

Rocca, W.A., Sharbrough, F.W., Hauser, W.A., Annegers, J.F. & Schoenberg, B.S. (1987): Risk factors for absence seizure: a population-based case-control study in Rochester, Minnesota. *Neurology* **37,** 1309–1314.

Tsuboi, T. & Christian, W. (1973): On the genetics of the primary generalized epilepsy with sporadic myoclonias of impulsive petit mal type. *Humangenetik* **19,** 155–182.

Waltz, St. (1993): Elektroenzephalographische Befunde bei der Epilepsie mit pyknoleptischen Absencen und der juvenilen Absencen-Epilepsie. Inaugral dissertation, Berlin: Freie Universität.

Weber, H.P. (1967): Genetische Untersuchungen bei Pyknolepsie. Inaugural dissertation, Heidelberg Universität.

Wolf, P., Behl, I., Fabian, A. & Guirao Bringas, P. (1986): Provokation epileptisches Potentiale und Anfälle durch Lidxchluss: Untervariante der Iotosensibilität oder eigenständiges Phänomen? Rundbrief der deutschen liga gegen. *Epilepsie* 5–9.

Wolf, P. & Goosses, R. (1986): Relation of photosensitivity to epileptic syndromes. *J. Neurol. Neurosurg. Psychiatr.* **49,** 1386–1391.

Wolf, P. & Inoue, Y. (1984): Therapeutic response of absence seizures in patients of an epilepsy clinic for adolescence and adults. *J. Neurol.* **231,** 225–229.

Epileptic Seizures and Syndromes, Edited by Peter Wolf
© 1994 John Libbey & Company Ltd., pp. 127–131

Chapter 16

Absences are non-specific symptoms of many epilepsies

Frederick Andermann

Montreal Neurological Institute and Hospital, 3801, rue University, Montréal, Québec, Canada, H3A 2B4

Prior to the development of electroencephalography (EEG) there was still discussion as to whether isolated absence attacks, e.g. ones not associated with other, more obvious seizure patterns, were in fact epileptic in nature (Friedmann, 1906). The problems appeared resolved when the characteristic discharge was demonstrated in the EEG and electroclinical correlations were first established (Gibbs *et al.,* 1935, 1943).

In the early 1960s, at the time when the first US centres of excellence for the study of epilepsy were conceived, Robb, Masland, Penry, Dreifuss, Schmidt and others thought that absence attacks, irrespective of whether they were manifestations of generalized or focal epilepsy, would be an ideal seizure pattern for study. Such studies would permit validation of multicentre observations and serve as a prototype of future investigations of what were considered to be more complicated seizure patterns. However it soon became apparent that such a phenomenological study, completely ignoring the electroclinical correlation and the anatomical basis, was unpractical. Most patients entered in these studies had absences as a manifestation of idiopathic generalized epilepsy. This led to the pioneering studies of Dreifuss and Penry (Penry, 1973; Penry *et al.*, 1975), which addressed the degree of impairment of awareness and responsiveness as a function of the duration and pattern of the spike-and-wave discharges.

At that time also the concept of typical and atypical 3 Hz spike-and-wave was still discussed (Lennox, 1945; Lennox & Davis, 1950). Typical or classical spike-and-wave was considered more characteristic of primary generalized epilepsy. Normal intelligence, normal background EEG activity and normal neurological examination were prerequisites of this form. Atypical spike-and-wave was not thought to be as heavily weighted in favour of the primary, more intensely genetic form of the disease. Atypical or more irregular spike-and-wave had a lesser correlation with good intelligence, normal EEG background and neurological examination. It soon became apparent that such a sharp distinction was artificial, and that the configuration of discharges as well as the background activity and the person's level of functioning changed over time and that one was dealing with a continuum of EEG patterns which were subject to change in relation to age and presumably also as a function of medications, seizure control, trauma, anoxia, etc.

In early descriptions William Lennox referred to the petit mal triad – absence, myoclonus and drop attacks (Lennox & Lennox, 1960). It later became clear that drop attacks were usually associated with

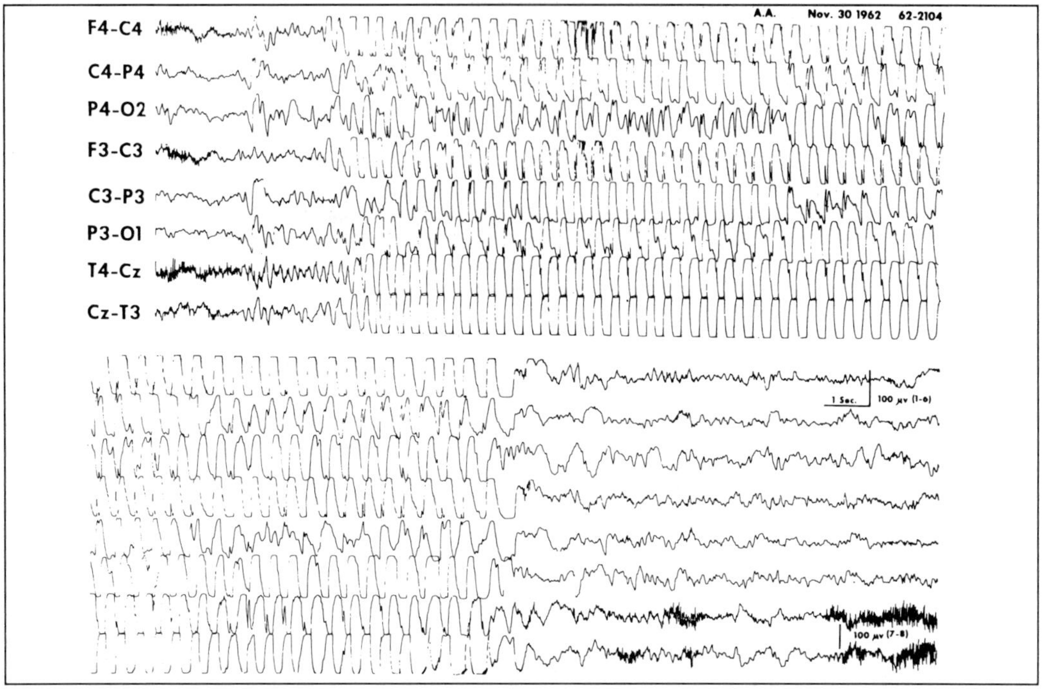

Fig. 1. A spontaneous burst of bilaterally synchronous symmetrical spike-and-wave lasting 25 s, accompanied by a clinical absence attack in a child with histologically proven Batten's disease.

slow spike-and-wave and Lennox began to refer to the slow, 1½–2½ Hz discharges as atypical. The concept of secondary (or symptomatic) generalized epilepsy then evolved, with the Lennox–Gastaut syndrome as one of the prototypes of this form of epilepsy. Atypical absence was one of the associated seizure patterns, atypical because of its association with slow spike-and-wave and because of the often indistinct onset and cessation of absence attacks. The responsiveness or lack of response to treatment of atypical absences has never been easy to assess, probably because of the severity of the epilepsy and because of the abundant or ongoing epileptogenic discharges which made evaluation difficult.

The pathophysiology of absence associated with primary (idiopathic) generalized epilepsy was the subject of much debate. Abnormality in thalamocortical relationships and frontal cortical abnormalities were the main anatomical substrates invoked. Otherwise normal brain structure and function were considered essential features of pyknoleptic absence. Soon, however, exceptions to this rule appeared. These cases, though anecdotal, were important far beyond their number, since they conclusively demonstrated that diffuse neuronal disorders could cause absences which were at first indistinguishable from the idiopathic genetic variety.

Examples of such absences occurring early in the course of the illness were described in juvenile cerebromacular degeneration Batten's disease, (Andermann, 1967) (Figs. 1 and 2), Lafora's disease (Roger *et al.*, 1983) and in subacute sclerosing panencephalitis (Broughton *et al.*, 1973).

Atypical absences are well known, on the other hand, to be symptomatic of a wide variety of anatomical syndromes which lead to secondary generalized epilepsy. An example of this is a young girl whose absence attacks were unresponsive to antiepileptic medication and who functioned just

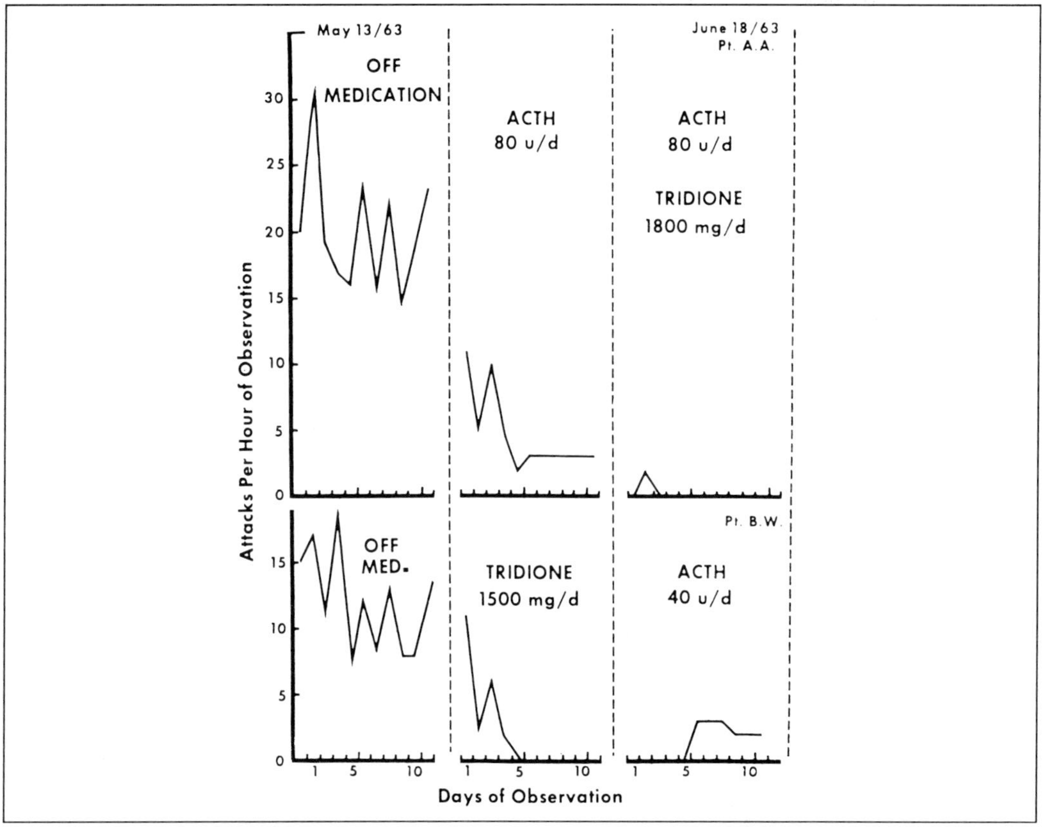

Fig. 2. Frequency and response to medication for absence in a child with Batten's disease (top panels) compared with a child with the idiopathic form (lower panels).

below the borderline range of intelligence. Her spike-and-wave discharges, though irregular, were fairly well organized and the failure of medication was difficult to understand. She was therefore admitted for further investigation: at that time we explained to the mother that it was difficult to imagine what such investigation could contribute to our management of her problem. Her magnetic resonance image (MRI) showed the typical picture of generalized band heterotopia or the double cortex syndrome (Fig. 3). This led to a clearer understanding of the cause of her epilepsy and of her developmental delay but unfortunately did not change the treatment of her absence attacks.

Simple absence may also be manifestations of temporolimbic epilepsy. Only the timing, the frequency and at times the presence of aura or the fatigue that follows allow one to distinguish this type of absence from the generalized form, particularly when information about other aspects of history and investigation are not yet available. Absences, usually brief and more frequent, occur as manifestations of frontal lobe epilepsy. Even lesions remote from mesial temporal lobe structures may manifest with absences and with epileptogenic abnormalities involving anterior and inferomesial temporal structures (Fig. 4). Presumably the mechanism of development of attacks in these patients is one of secondary epileptogenesis.

Thus a wide range of aetiologically and anatomically diverse processes may lead to the appearance of epileptic absence attacks. It is therefore not meaningful to refer to absence attacks as a diagnosis

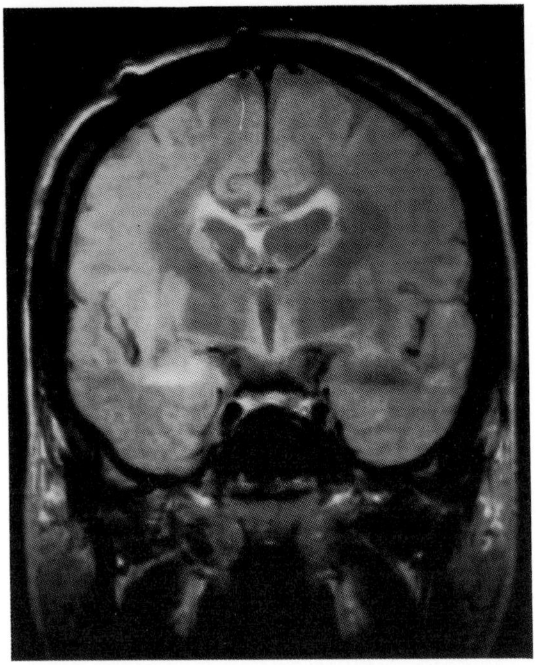

Fig. 3. Band heterotopia or the double cortex syndrome (MRI): an unsuspected finding in a child with medically refractory absence attacks.

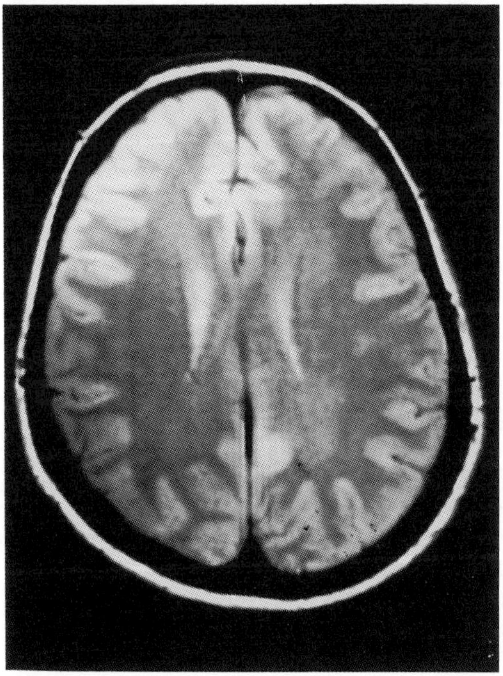

Fig. 4. Posterior cingulate lesion in a patient with anterior and inferomesial epileptogenic temporal abnormalities and simple absence attacks: an example of secondary epileptogenesis.

without qualifying the type and aetiology of the epilepsy since our understanding and treatment of the attacks certainly depend on these factors.

What remains unexplained at the core of the problem is the mechanism of interference with awareness and responsiveness, while other functions like tone and stance are either partially or totally preserved. The attraction of the centrencephalic hypothesis is easy to understand but the neuronal networks subserving the functions lost or impaired during absence are still not identified. It is important to keep in mind not only that the attacks subsumed under the term absence are diverse aetiologically and anatomically, but also that they vary in intensity, ability of the subject to respond and react and, in particular, that they vary in their natural history and in their response to antiepileptic medication.

References

Andermann, F. (1967): Absence attacks and diffuse neuronal disease. *Neurology* **17,** 205–212.

Broughton, R., Nelson, R., Gloor, P. & Andermann, F. (1973): Petit mal epilepsy evolving to subacute sclerosing panencephalitis. In: *Evolution and prognosis of epilepsies*, eds. E. Lugaresi, P. Pazzaglia & C.A. Tassinari, pp. 63–72. Bologna: Aulo Gaggi.

Friedmann, M. (1906): Über die nichtepileptischen Absencen oder kurzen narkoleptischen Anfälle. *Dtsch. Z. Nervenheilk.* **30,** 462–492.

Gibbs, F.A., Davis, H. & Lennox, W.G. (1935): The EEG in epilepsy and in conditions of impaired consciousness. *Arch. Neurol. Psychiatr.* **34,** 1134–1148.

Gibbs, F.A., Gibbs, E.L. & Lennox, W.G. (1943): Electroencephalographic classification of epileptic patients and control subjects. *Arch. Neurol. Psychiatr.* **50,** 111–128.

Lennox, W.G. (1945): The petit mal epilepsies. *JAMA* **129,** 1069–1073.

Lennox, W.G. & Davis, J.P. (1950): Clinical correlates of the fast and slow spike-wave electroencephalogram. *Pediatrics* **5,** 626–644.

Lennox, W.G. & Lennox, M.A. (1960): *Epilepsy and related disorders*, Vol. 1. Boston: Little Brown and Co.

Penry, J.K. (1973): Behavioural correlates of generalized spike-wave discharge in the electroencephalogram. In: *Epilepsy, its phenomena in man*, UCLA Forum in Medical Sciences, No. 17, pp. 171–178. New York: Academic Press.

Penry, J.K., Porter, R.J. & Dreifuss, F.E. (1975): Simultaneous recording of absence seizures with video tape and electroencephalography: a study of 374 seizures in 48 patients. *Brain* **98,** 427–440.

Roger, J., Pellissier, J.F., Bureau, M., Dravet, C., Revol, M. & Tinuper, R. (1983): Le diagnostic précoce de la maladie de Lafora: importance des manifestations paroxystiques visuelles et intérêt de la biopsie cutanée. *Rev. Neurol.* **139,** 115–124.

Epileptic Seizures and Syndromes, Edited by Peter Wolf
© 1994 John Libbey & Company Ltd., pp. 133–135

Chapter 17

Discussion: absence epilepsy of early childhood

Hermann Doose

Norddeutsches Epilepsie-Zentrum, Epilepsie-Forschungsstelle, 24223 Raisdorf, Germany

The International Classification distinguishes three types of absence epilepsy: childhood absence epilepsy (CAE), with absences as the presenting symptom (Loiseau, 1992), juvenile absence epilepsy (Janz & Christian, 1957; Doose *et al.*, 1965; Wolf, 1992), with and without generalized tonic–clonic seizures (GTCS), and epilepsy with myoclonic absences (Tassinari *et al.*, 1992). Early childhood absence epilepsy, often with GTCS at onset, has not yet been included in the International Classification.

In 1965 we gave a first description of this epilepsy (Doose *et al.*, 1965), based on a series of 47 children with spike-wave (SW) absences and an onset during the first 5 years of life. We demonstrated some peculiarities which allow a delineation from CAE. By a retrospective study, comprising only cases aged more than 18 years, Dieterich *et al.* (1985a, b) showed that the course as well as the psychomental and social prognosis of children with this type of epilepsy, especially if starting with GTCS, is less favourable than that of patients with CAE. Finally, we performed a family study in 140 cases to analyse the genetic background (Doose, 1994).

From these studies the main characteristics of this type of early childhood epilepsy can be summarized as follows.

Age at onset

Due to selection criteria, the age at onset (absences or GTCS) is between 0 and 4 years.

Gender

In cases with initial GTCS there is a significant preponderance of boys (58/32), whereas in cases with absences at onset boys and girls are equally often affected (26/24; Doose, 1994).

Seizure symptomatology

According to case ascertainment, every case shows absences with generalized SW. Mostly, the occurrence of absences is not pyknoleptic but spanioleptic. GTCS as presenting seizure type could be observed in about two-thirds of the cases, in boys more often than in girls. The age at onset is different in cases with and without GTCS. In GTCS cases the distribution shows a maximum in the first 3 years of age, whereas in the non-GTCS group the distribution increases continuously up to age 5 years. In about 40 per cent of the cases additional myoclonic and/or myoclonic astatic seizures occur, in boys as often as in girls, but more often in cases with GTCS as compared to those without.

Psychomental and social development

Signs of primary psychomental retardation are more frequent than in CAE. In cases of prolonged status, mental deterioration can occur (Doose & Völzke, 1979.) The long-term social prognosis is more often unfavourable than in cases with CAE.

Electroencephalography (EEG)

The seizure pattern with generalized SW is often more irregular than in CAE; especially in cases with myoclonias, polyspikes may occur. The end of the paroxysm may not be abrupt but can fade with slower SW. The background activity is mostly dominated by 4–7/s rhythms. Focal abnormalities may sometimes occur but not as a consistent phenomenon.

Genetics

The clinical and EEG family data of 140 cases support the assumption of genetic heterogeneity (Doose, 1994). Cases with GTCS and those with absences at onset turn out to be different in many respects. In the first group the incidence of seizures in the parental generation is twice as high as in the second group. Early-onset GTCS prevail in the affected relatives, whereas in the relatives of cases with absence onset absences are found more frequently. These results are in accordance with the data of a former family study of 399 cases with generalized minor seizures (Doose & Baier, 1987), which leads to the conclusion that the liability to early-onset convulsive seizures (so-called A-liability: Doose & Baier, 1987) is genetically different from the disposition to later-onset absence epilepsy (B-liability).

EEG investigations of the relatives revealed an increased incidence of generalized SW and photosensitivity in both groups indicating common genetic factors. However, in parents of the group with absences at onset, EEG pathology is significantly more frequent than in those of the GTCS group. Thus, the EEG findings contrast with the clinical finding of a higher seizure risk in parents of the GTCS group. Possibly, the A-liability which is decisive in the pathogenesis of the GTCS type has no correlate in the adult EEG, i.e. in parents.

Table 1. Spectrum of idiopathic generalized epilepsies in childhood and adolescence

Epilepsy with generalized tonic–clonic seizures and alternating hemigrand mal
Severe myoclonic epilepsy
Benign myoclonic epilepsy
Myoclonic astatic epilepsy
Early childhood absence epilepsy
Childhood absence epilepsy
Epilepsy with myoclonic absences
Juvenile absence epilepsy
Juvenile myoclonic epilepsy
Juvenile epilepsy with GTCS

Early childhood epilepsy with absences seems to be a heterogeneous subgroup within the idiopathic generalized epilepsies. There is a distinct overlap with early childhood epilepsy with GTCS and myoclonic astatic epilepsy (Doose *et al.*, 1965) on the one side and with CAE on the other. Thus, it should not be regarded as a special syndrome. It seems more reasonable to consider this type of epilepsy with its different kinds of clinical manifestation as another peak of a broad spectrum (Table 1). This spectrum reaches from early childhood idiopathic epilepsy with GTCS to juvenile epilepsy with GTCS. As shown by family EEG studies (elevated incidences of SW and photosensitivity), early childhood and juvenile epilepsies have some genetic factors in common. The distinctive genetic factors, possibly among others, are the A- and B-liability (Doose & Baier, 1987).

References

Dieterich, E., Baier, W.K., Doose, H., Fichsel, H. & Tuxhorn, I. (1985a): Longterm follow-up of chilhood epilepsy with absences. I. Epilepsy with absences at onset. *Neuropediatrics* **16,** 149–154.

Dieterich, E., Baier, W.K., Doose, H. & Fichsel, H. (1985b): Longterm follow-up of childhood epilepsy with absences. II. Epilepsy with initial grand mal. *Neuropediatrics* **16,** 155–158.

Doose, H. (1994): Absence epilepsy of early childhood – genetic aspects. *Eur. J. Pediatr.* **153,** 372–377.

Doose, H. & Baier, W.K. (1987): Genetic factors in epilepsies with primarily generalized minor seizures. *Neuropediatrics* **18** (Suppl. I), 1–64.

Doose, H. & Völzke, E. (1979): Petit mal-status in early childhood and dementia. *Neuropädiatrie* **10,** 10–14.

Doose, H., Völzke, E. & Scheffner, D. (1965): Verlaufsformen kindlicher Epilepsien mit spike wave-Absencen. *Arch. Psychiatr. Nervenkr.* **207,** 394–415.

Janz, D. & Christian, W. (1957): Impulsiv-Petit mal. *Dtsch. Z. Nervenheilk.* **176,** 346–386.

Loiseau, P. (1992): Childhood absence epilepsy. In: *Epileptic syndromes in infancy, childhood and adolescence*, eds. J. Roger, M. Bureau, Ch. Dravet, F.E. Dreifuss, A. Perret & P. Wolf, pp. 135–150. London: John Libbey.

Tassinari, C.A., Bureau, M. & Thames, P. (1992): Epilepsy with myoclonic absences. In: *Epileptic syndromes in infancy, childhood and adolescence*, eds. J. Roger, M. Bureau, Ch. Dravet, F.E. Dreifuss, A. Perret & P. Wolf, pp. 151–160. London: John Libbey.

Wolf, P. (1992): Juvenile absence epilepsy. In: *Epileptic syndromes in infancy, childhood and adolescence*, eds. J. Roger, M. Bureau, Ch. Dravet, F.E. Dreifuss, A. Perret and P. Wolf, pp. 307–312. London: John Libbey.

Epileptic Seizures and Syndromes, Edited by Peter Wolf
© 1994 John Libbey & Company Ltd., pp. 137–141

Chapter 18

Epilepsy with myoclonic absences: a reappraisal

Carlo Alberto Tassinari and Roberto Michelucci

Department of Neurology, University of Bologna, Bellaria Hospital, Via Altura 3, 40139 Bologna, Italy

Summary

The clinical and neurophysiological features of epilepsy with myoclonic absences are described based on 36 cases from the Centre Saint-Paul of Marseille and 13 new cases observed in Bologna in the last 10 years. Follow-up study of these patients suggests that myoclonic absences are refractory to treatment in about half of the cases whereas they may promptly disappear in the remaining half. The response to treatment seems to depend on a variety of factors, such as the type and frequency of associated seizures and the correct medical therapy (valproic acid and ethosuximide at high doses). Mental impairment is usually observed in patients with refractory myoclonic absences, whereas it is absent in patients with rapid remission of the seizures.

Introduction

Myoclonic absences (MA) represent a specific seizure type, whose diagnosis rests on two major criteria, i.e. direct clinical observation and ictal polygraphic recording. *Clinical observation* discloses that MA are absence seizures accompanied by rhythmic and bilateral myoclonic jerks of severe intensity. *Polygraphic recording* (electroencephalogram (EEG) + electromyogram (EMG) of deltoid muscles) shows a rhythmic spike-and-wave (SW) discharge at 3 c/s, bilateral, synchronous and symmetrical (as observed in childhood absence epilepsy) associated with an EMG discharge of myoclonias at 3 c/s and an increasing tonic contraction.

Since the early description of MA (Tassinari *et al.*, 1969; Lugaresi *et al.*,1973; Tassinari & Bureau, 1985), it has been felt that an epileptic syndrome characterized by the presence of MA as the only or predominant seizure type could be identified and separated from other forms of generalized epilepsy, such as childhood absence epilepsy. Indeed, MA were shown to be often associated with some degree of mental retardation and a clear-cut resistance to medical treatment, so that the prognosis was less favourable than in idiopathic generalized epilepsy. Eventually, epilepsy with MA was classified as a separate syndrome in the group of cryptogenic or symptomatic generalized epilepsies (Commission, 1989).

Over the years, we have repeatedly described the essential features of the syndrome, mainly based on the analysis of 36 cases from the Centre Saint-Paul of Marseille (Tassinari & Bureau, 1985; Tassinari *et al.*, 1992). Now we add 13 new cases observed in Bologna in the last decade and, on the basis of the overall clinical material, we outline the clinical, neurophysiological and evolutive features of epilepsy with MA.

Clinical data

General

MA are a rare seizure type, accounting for 0.5–1 per cent of the epilepsies observed in a selected population of epileptics of the Centre Saint Paul. There is a male preponderance (69 per cent), at variance with the female preponderance in childhood absence epilepsy. Aetiological factors are absent, except for a genetic susceptibility, as demonstrated by a positive family history of epilepsies in about 20 per cent of cases. The mean age of onset of MA is 7 years, with a range from 11 months to 12.2 years.

Myoclonic absences

MA are characterized by:

– *Impairment of consciousness*, which is quite variable in intensity, ranging from a mild disruption of contact to a complete loss of consciousness. Sometimes the patients are aware of the jerks and may recall the words pronounced by the examiner during the seizures.

– *Motor manifestations*, which consist of bilateral myoclonic jerks, often associated with a discrete tonic contraction. The myoclonias mainly involve the muscles of shoulders, arms and legs. When facial myoclonias occur, they are more evident around the chin and the mouth, whereas eyelid twitching is typically absent or rare. Due to concomitant tonic contraction, the jerking of the arms is accompanied by a progressive elevation of the upper extremities, giving rise to a quite constant and recognizable pattern. When the patient is standing, falling is uncommon. Head and body deviation can be a feature present in some patients.

– *Autonomic manifestations*, which consist of an arrest of respiration and, sometimes, loss of urine.

MA last for 10–60 s and recur at a high frequency (many seizures per day). They are often precipitated by hyperventilation or awakening. MA may also be observed during the early stages of sleep. Episodes of MA status are distinctly rare.

Seizures other than MA

In about one-third of cases, MA represent the only seizure type. In the remaining patients, other seizures occur either before the onset of MA or in association with MA. They consist of rare generalized tonic–clonic seizures, simple absences or falling seizures.

Neurological and neuropsychological examination

Neurological examination is normal in all cases. Mental retardation is present in about 45 per cent of cases before the onset of MA. During the course of MA, mental retardation occurs in a further 25 per cent of cases, so that a total of 70 per cent of patients present mental impairment at some time of their evolution. These data constitute a very significant difference as compared with mental status observed in childhood absence epilepsy.

Neurophysiological data

Interictal EEG

The interictal EEG shows a normal background activity in all cases, with generalized SW (in one-third of cases) or, more rarely, focal or multifocal SW.

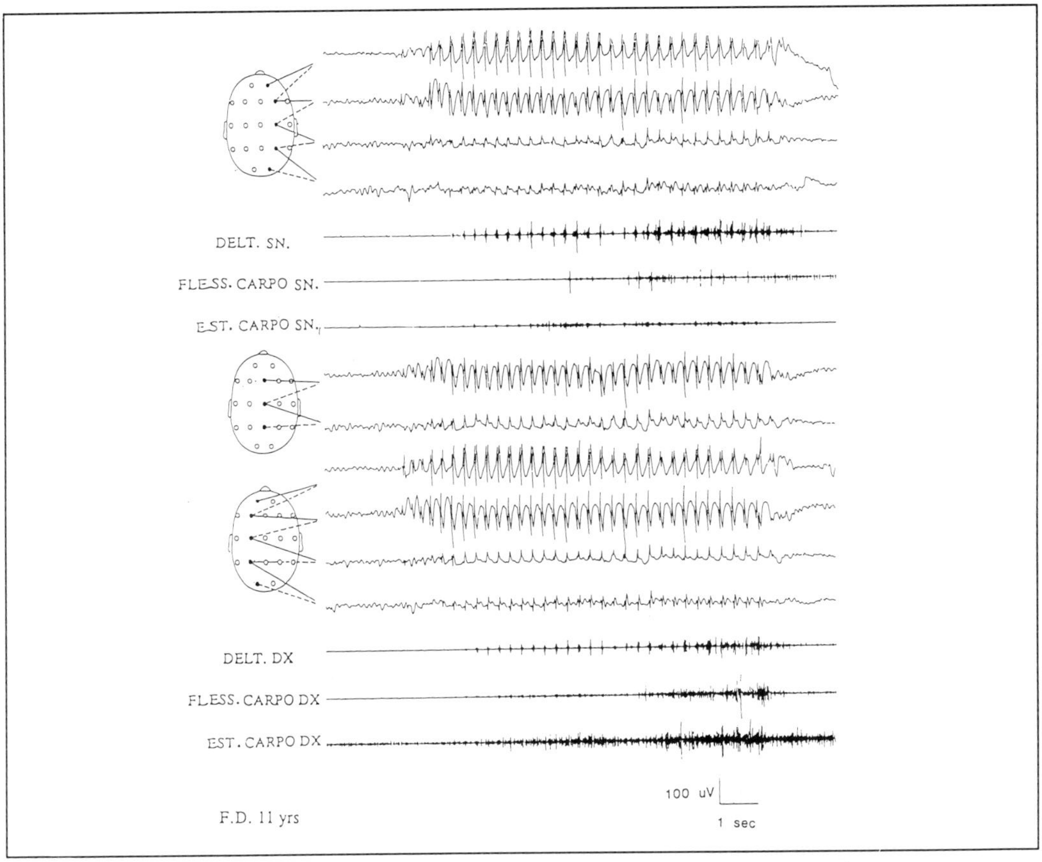

Fig. 1. Spontaneous MA. Rhythmic SW discharge at 3 c/s. Rhythmic myoclonias begin 1 s after the onset of EEG paroxysmal discharges and are progressively associated with a tonic contraction.

Ictal EEG

The ictal EEG consists of rhythmic SW discharge at 3 c/s, bilateral, synchronous and symmetrical, as observed in childhood absences (Fig. 1). The onset and the end of SW are abrupt. Polygraphic (EMG) recording discloses the appearance of bilateral myoclonias, at the same frequency as the SW, which begin about 1 s after the onset of EEG paroxysmal discharges and are followed by a tonic contraction, maximal in the shoulder and deltoid muscles (Fig. 1). Tassinari *et al.* (1969, 1971) provided a detailed analysis of the relationships between the EEG SW and motor events by means of high-speed oscilloscopic recording. They found that there is a strict and constant relation between the spike of the SW discharge and the myoclonia, as the spike, morphologically related to a positive transient (Weir, 1965) of high amplitude, is followed on the EMG by a myoclonia with a latency of 15–40 ms for the more proximal muscles and of 50–70 ms for the more distal muscles. This myoclonia is again followed by a brief silent period (60–120 ms) which interrupts the tonic contraction.

Sleep EEG

Sleep organization is constantly normal and physiological patterns are symmetrically present. During sleep, the evolution of the SW discharges is fundamentally similar to that observed in childhood absence epilepsy (Tassinari *et al.*, 1974).

MA may occur during stage I of sleep, where they are followed by awakening. During stage II, SW discharges of brief or long duration are also observed, and are sometimes associated with bursts of myoclonias.

Evolution

At the time of the last observation, MA were still present in one-half of the cases followed up for a mean period of 10.7 years, whereas they had disappeared in the remaining patients, after a mean period of 5.5 years from the onset. The two groups of patients differed for the frequency and type of associated seizures: patients with 'refractory' MA had a high incidence (85 per cent) of associated seizures, mainly of grand mal and atonic type. On the contrary, patients with remitting MA had a lower incidence (50 per cent) of associated seizures, and these were mainly of absence type.

Another factor which seemed to influence the evolution was medical therapy. This point was particularly evident from the analysis of our last 13 cases observed in Bologna in recent years. Of these patients, six had a rapid remission of MA after receiving a primary combination of valproic acid (VPA) and ethosuximide (ETS) at high doses (with serum plasma levels ranging from 80–130 μg/ml for VPA and 60–110 μg/ml for ETS). The remaining seven cases, who had a long history of refractory MA, had been treated with lower doses of the above drugs, in combination, or with different medical therapies. Interestingly, the six cases who promptly stopped having MA during VPA/ETS therapy experienced, for a brief period (lasting for 1–3 months), sudden and isolated diffuse jerks with an EEG correlate of generalized polyspike-and-wave discharge, as in juvenile myoclonic epilepsy.

The long duration of MA is likely to be an important factor for the appearance of mental retardation. Indeed, in our last 13 patients, severe mental impairment occurred in four of the seven cases with refractory MA, whereas it remained absent in the six cases with rapid remission of MA.

A particular evolution of epilepsy was described in five of the 36 cases observed in the Centre Saint-Paul of Marseille. In these patients, the disappearance of MA was followed by the onset of other seizure types, namely absences with atypical SW discharges, clinical and subclinical tonic seizures, giving rise to a clinical picture similar to the Lennox–Gastaut syndrome (Tassinari *et al.*, 1992).

Treatment

Evolutive data seem to suggest that correct medical therapy for MA consists of the associated use of VPA and ETS at high doses, with constant determination of serum plasma levels.

In individual cases, a good seizure control was achieved by using a combination of phenobarbital, VPA and benzodiazepines. Lamotrigine has been recently reported to be effective in suppressing MA in 'refractory' cases (Manonmani & Wallace, 1994).

Diagnosis

The diagnosis of MA rests mainly on the polygraphic demonstration of SW discharges at 3 c/s accompanied by rhythmic myoclonias. Therefore, polygraphic recording is mandatory when the clinical suspicion of MA is raised. Since the anamnestic data may sometimes be misleading (asymmetrical MA may be misdiagnosed as partial motor seizures, MA with mild myoclonias may be misdiagnosed as typical petit mal absences, etc.), we suggest that polygraphic recording should also be performed in patients with 'drug-resistant' absence seizures and in cases with refractory 'myoclonic' or 'partial motor' seizures.

Conclusions

MA represent a specific seizure type, whose recognition rests on direct clinical observation and polygraphic recording of the seizures. The diagnosis of MA is *per se* sufficient for the identification of a syndrome, namely *epilepsy with myoclonic absences*, which is included in the International

Classification of the Epilepsies and Epileptic Syndromes (Commission, 1989) among generalized epilepsies of cryptogenic or symptomatic nature.

The reasons which have allowed the identification of a specific syndrome, distinct from the other forms of generalized epilepsy, include the very remarkable electroclinical aspect of MA, male preponderance, and a less favourable prognosis than in childhood absence epilepsy, due to the resistance to therapy, mental retardation and possible evolution toward other types of epilepsy, such as Lennox–Gastaut syndrome.

Therefore epilepsy with MA seems to be an intermediate type of epilepsy between idiopathic and symptomatic generalized epilepsies.

Future research will be aimed to better define the follow-up of MA once correct medical treatment is instituted, with special emphasis on the evolution of the epilepsy and neuropsychological assessment.

Acknowledgements

We thank Prof. G. Avanzini and Dr S. Franceschetti from the Neurological Institute C. Besta of Milan for providing a case of MA. The financial support mof Telethon (grant no. 109) is gratefully acknowledged.

References

Commission on Classification and Terminology of the International League Against Epilepsy (1989): Proposal for revised classification of epilepsies and epileptic syndromes. *Epilepsia* **30,** 389–399.

Lugaresi, E., Pazzaglia, P., Franck, L., Roger, J., Bureau-Paillas, M., Ambrosetto, G. & Tassinari, C.A. (1973): Evolution and prognosis of primary generalized epilepsies of the petit mal absence type. In: *Evolution and prognosis of epilepsy*, eds. E. Lugaresi, P. Pazzaglia & C.A. Tassinari, pp. 2–22. Bologna: Aulo Gaggi.

Manonmani, V. & Wallace, S.J. (1994): Epilepsy with myoclonic absences. *Arch. Dis. Child* **70,** 288–290.

Tassinari, C.A. & Bureau, M. (1985): Epilepsy with myoclonic absences. In: *Epileptic syndromes in infancy, childhood and adolescence*, eds. J. Roger, C. Dravet, M. Bureau, F.E. Dreifuss & P. Wolf, pp. 123–131. London: John Libbey.

Tassinari, C.A., Lyagoubi, S., Santos, V., Gambarelli, F., Roger, J., Dravet, C. & Gastaut, H. (1969): Etude des décharges de pointes ondes chez l'homme. II. Les aspects cliniques et electroencephalographiques des absences myocloniques. *Rev. Neurol.* **121,** 379–383.

Tassinari, C.A., Lyagoubi, S., Gambarelli, F., Roger, J. & Gastaut, H. (1971): Relationships between EEG discharge and neuromuscular phenomena. *Electroencephalogr. Clin. Neurophysiol.* **31,** 176.

Tassinari, C.A., Bureau-Paillas, M., Dalla Bernardina, B., Mancia, D., Capizzi, G., Valladier, C. & Roger, J. (1974): Generalized epilepsies and seizures during sleep: a polygraphic study. In: *Brain and sleep*, eds. H.M. Van Praag & H. Meinardi, pp. 154–166. Amsterdam: De Erven Bhon.

Tassinari, C.A., Bureau, M. & Thomas, P. (1992): Epilepsy with myoclonic absences. In: *Epileptic syndromes in infancy, childhood and adolescence*, 2nd edn, eds. J. Roger, M. Bureau, C. Dravet, F.E. Dreifuss, A. Perret & P. Wolf, pp. 151–160. London: John Libbey.

Weir, B. (1965): The morphology of the spike-wave complex. *Electroencephalogr. Clin. Neurophysiol.* **19,** 284–290.

Epileptic Seizures and Syndromes, Edited by Peter Wolf
© 1994 John Libbey & Company Ltd., pp. 143–153

Chapter 19

Perioral myoclonia with absences: a new syndrome

Chrysostomos P. Panayiotopoulos, Colin D. Ferrie, Stelios E. Giannakodimos and Richard O. Robinson*

Department of Clinical Neurophysiology and Epilepsy, St Thomas's Hospital, London SE1 7EH, UK, and
**Department of Child Neurology, Guy's Hospital, London SE1 9RT, UK*

Summary

Six patients are presented with idiopathic generalized epilepsy. They display unique clinical and EEG features and it is suggested these may constitute a new syndrome of absence epilepsy. We propose the term perioral myoclonia with absences as the most suitable name for the syndrome. The syndrome is characterized by typical absence seizures which are accompanied by rhythmic myoclonus of the perioral muscles and more rarely the muscles of mastication. These have their onset from childhood to early adolescence, are of variable frequency and are associated with differing degrees of impairment of consciousness. All patients also suffer generalized tonic–clonic seizures (GTCS), which may be frequent or rare and often have their onset before that of the absences. GTCS may be preceded by absences and absence status is relatively common. The ictal EEG shows generalized, relatively short, irregular spike- and more often polyspike-and-wave discharges at around 3–4 Hz, sometimes with fragmentations. There is no photosensitivity. Response to drugs is often poor and there is no age-related tendency for spontaneous remission.

Introduction

The International League Against Epilepsy (ILAE) classification of epileptic seizures (Commission, 1981) recognized six types of absences plus a class of 'atypical' absences. In the ILAE classification of epilepsies and epileptic syndromes (Commission, 1989), three syndromes of idiopathic generalized epilepsy with 'typical' absence seizures (TAS) were included: childhood absence epilepsy (CAE), juvenile absence epilepsy (JAE) and juvenile myoclonic epilepsy (JME). Differences in the semiology and electroencephalography (EEG) of the characteristic absences of these three syndromes have been studied by Panayiotopoulos *et al.* (1989a). These refer mainly to the degree of impairment of consciousness, the duration of the ictal discharge, the delay in eye opening from the start of the ictus and qualitative differences in the EEG discharges. Epilepsy with myoclonic absences was included as an additional absence syndrome within the class of generalized symptomatic or cryptogenic epilepsies (Commission, 1989).

In this paper we wish to draw attention to a further type of TAS and discuss its place in the syndrome classification. We describe six patients who do not fit within the existing syndromes of absence epilepsy and who have perioral myoclonus as a consistent symptom of their absences. Analysis suggests the clustering of other clinical and EEG manifestations in a non-fortuitous manner supporting their designation as a new epilepsy syndrome.

Methods

As a consequence of our particular interest in idiopathic generalized epilepsies, patients presenting with absences are extensively investigated, including interviews with witnesses and scrutinization of old records and routine EEG and in many cases video-EEG recordings (34-channel Telefactor). Impairment of consciousness is assessed during spike-wave discharges by asking the patients to count out loud during hyperventilation (Panayiotopoulos *et al.*, 1993). Additionally, in the patients presented here all ictal EEG discharges available were evaluated for the duration, frequency of opening, initial and terminal phases, regularity and morphology of their complexes and, where video recordings were available, impairment of consciousness and the nature and timing of clinical events were assessed. Details of the methods used have been previously reported (Panayiotopoulos *et al.*, 1989a). The six patients are described in detail below and in Table 1.

Table 1. Clinical data for the five patients

	Patient 1	Patient 2	Patient 3	Patient 4	Patient 5	Patient 6
Age now (years)	11	29	22	22	37	18
Onset of TAS (years)	3	11	7	13	2	11
POM during TAS	Yes	Yes	Yes	Yes	Yes	Yes*
Onset of GTCS (years)	3	11	7	22	2	11
Other seizures	Nil	Nil	Nil	Nil	Nil	Yes†
Frequency of TAS	Frequent	Frequent	Frequent	Infrequent	Unknown	1–2/week
Frequency of GTCS	1/month	0–12/year	0–3/year	1/life	3/life	3–6/year
IOC during TAS	Severe	Moderate	Moderate	Moderate	Mild	Moderate
TAS now stopped	No	No	No	No	No	No
Last GTCS (years)	7	22	21	22	36	18
Family history	Yes	No	Yes	Yes	No	No
CT scan	Not done	Normal	Abnormal‡	Not done	Normal	Normal
Intellectual status	Normal	Normal	Normal	Normal	Normal	Normal
TAS leading to GTCS	Not apparent	Yes	Yes	No	Yes	Yes
Absence status	No	Yes	Possible	No	Yes	Possible

POM = perioral myoclonus; IOC = impairment of consciousness; CT = computerized tomography.
*with jaw myoclonus; †infrequent myoclonic limb jerks; ‡slight asymmetry of the temporal horns.

Case 1

This patient had an unremarkable history until the age of 3 years when she had the onset of GTCS occurring mainly on awakening and at a frequency of around 1/month. Initial therapy with sodium valproate was substituted for carbamazepine because of abnormal hepatic enzyme results. A few months later TAS began. These were characterized by profound impairment of consciousness. Marked perioral movements described as 'lip smacking' were consistently observed. Ethosuximide was added and control was achieved such that therapy was stopped after 2 years. Seizures, however, relapsed at 6 years of age and have since proved refractory to sodium valproate alone and in combination with ethosuximide and clobazam.

This patient has a strong family history of epilepsy. She is one of four sisters: one died of aspiration following a fit at 14 months of age. Another, now a young adult, had absences as a child. These have now subsided but she is still suffering occasional GTCS.

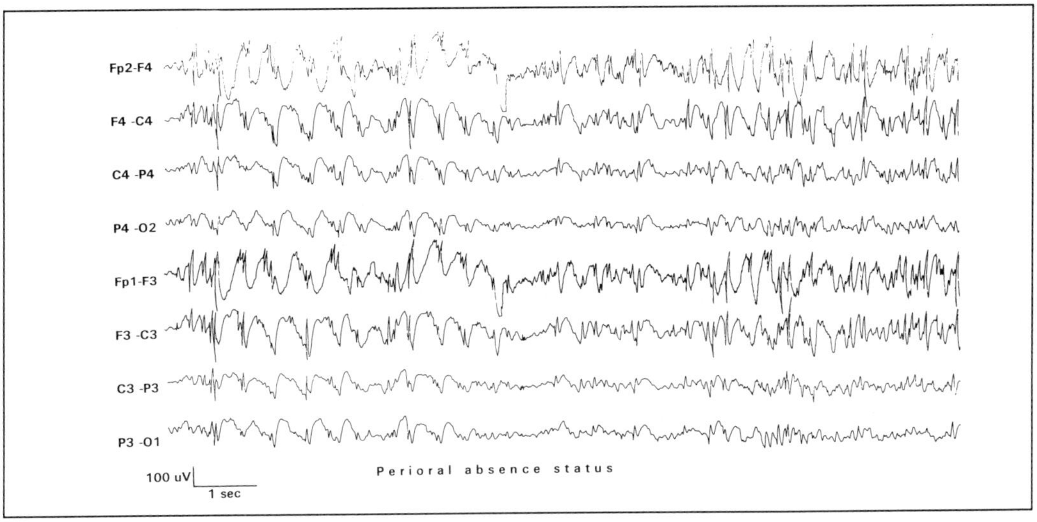

Fig. 1. EEG of patient 2 during absence status. Continuous perioral movements were noticed by the technician.

Case 2

This female patient had an uneventful childhood apart from a simple febrile convulsion with measles at 4 years of age. She presented at 11 years of age following two GTCS. Her mother noted that before the second attack she had become 'quiet' and that there was facial 'twitching'. A third GTCS was preceded by her 'wandering around the school in a dazed condition'. Absences were not initially recognized but in retrospect she reports having experienced them frequently throughout her teenage years and described them as 'vacancies' 'sticking on words', 'feeling dreamy' and 'can't understand what others say'.

Partial motor epilepsy with secondary generalization was diagnosed and a number of drug combinations were tried during her childhood and adolescence. Absences did not respond to any of them but both the combination of phenytoin with nitrazepam and carbamazepine alone controlled the GTCS for some years. At 22 years of age she was admitted to our hospital after a GTCS. During the admission she had two episodes of absence status during which continuous perioral 'twitching' was noticed. One was recorded on EEG (Fig. 1) and ended in a GTCS.

All seizures ceased with the introduction of sodium valproate but recently absences have recurred and control has necessitated the combination of valproate with clonazepam.

Case 3

This patient was born at 36 weeks' gestation but suffered no significant complications related to this. She presented at 7 years of age following two GTCS. No mention was made of absences. During an EEG frequent generalized spike-and-wave discharges were noticed but were not accompanied by clinically discernible changes. Within 2 months of presentation, however, 'vacancies' had become noticeable to her mother and, on EEG, spike-and-wave discharges were accompanied by impairment of consciousness as assessed by her failure to respond to stimuli given during the discharges.

The patient was initially commenced on phenytoin and ethosuximide was added when the absences were diagnosed. Control was felt to be satisfactory but around the age of 10 years her school performance was deteriorating and it became apparent that she was suffering frequent daily absences in which impairment of consciousness appears to have been moderate. Substitution of phenytoin for carbamazepine was of no benefit but the introduction of sodium valproate at 11 years of age was followed by a number of years of good control. Seizures (both absences and GTCS) occurred on attempts to withdraw valproate. By the age of 19 years carbamazepine had been successfully discontinued.

Since her early twenties her condition has deteriorated, particularly with an increase in GTCS to approximately one every 2–3 months. She also experiences absences, which, however, are less frequent than previously. During them her fiancé has consistently noticed 'twitching' around her mouth. On some occasions he describes this as continuing and then progressing to a GTCS. High dosage of valproate required to achieve control has not been well tolerated, necessitating the combination of sodium valproate, ethosuximide and phenobarbitone to relatively good effect. This patient has a maternal aunt with epilepsy but no details are available.

Case 4

Absences began in this patient at around the age of 13 years. They were mild and therefore went unreported. At 22 years she presented following a GTCS, and the history of TAS was revealed. These were described as 'like a light switching off and on' and sometimes caused her to stop in mid-sentence. They were reported as lasting only a few seconds and witnesses describe a characteristic 'quivering' around her mouth during the absences. Following the GTCS and the retrospective diagnosis of TAS with perioral myoclonus, sodium valproate was commenced.

The patient's sister (now 16 years old) also suffers TAS, with perioral twitching and occasional GTCS, but we have not been able to examine her.

Case 5

This patient's absences probably had their onset around the age of 2 years. However, he has been unaware of them except during episodes of absence status, which have often progressed to a GTCS. This probably happened for the first time at 2 years of age during an upper respiratory tract infection. His parents noticed he appeared 'vacant' and after an undetermined period of time he suffered a GTCS more marked on the right side.

At the ages of 11 and 12 years he had two episodes in which he felt strange and was aware of twitching involving his face and possibly his left hand. These lasted many hours and subsided spontaneously. At the age of 14 years, during a flu-like illness, the patient awoke and for 30 min felt 'dizzy' and was aware of his lips twitching. This resolved but later the same day recurred and progressed to a GTCS. Following this he was treated with phenobarbitone until the age of 19 years. At the age of 36 years, after sleep deprivation and moderate alcohol consumption, the patient awoke and was again aware of his lips twitching. This was so intense that it prevented him from drinking water but was not associated with any noticeable impairment of consciousness. The episode continued for 12 h and finally ended in a short GTCS.

After this last event, a video-EEG revealed multiple TAS accompanied by minor mistakes on counting and consistent perioral myoclonus. These had not previously been noted by the patient or witnesses but since their recognition he has been aware of brief episodes of twitching around his mouth. Sodium valproate was commenced.

Case 6

This patient had an unremarkable history until the age of 11 years. One morning she awoke and was aware of some jerking of her hands and then 'passed out'. This was not, however, witnessed and she did not come to medical attention until the age of 13 years when she experienced three GTCS within a few weeks. A history of infrequent TAS was also obtained. These were described as 'she loses concentration and misses what others say'. They are accompanied by prominent jerking around the

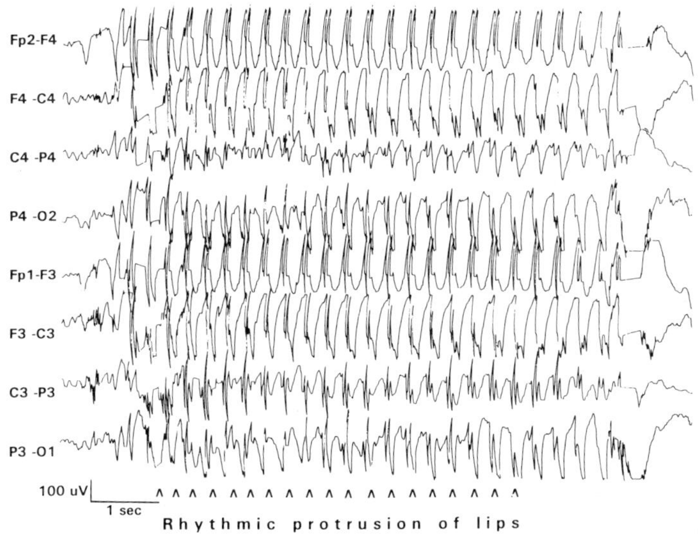

Fig. 2. Ictal video-EEG from patient 1 which is annotated to show the timing of perioral myoclonus. This discharge was associated with profound impairment of consciousness.

mouth and of the jaw. The absences are generally short but occasionally last longer and characteristically GTCS are preceded by a prolonged absence, during which the perioral/jaw myoclonus may spread to involve her upper limbs. Jerks of her upper limbs independent of any discernible absences have also occurred, particularly in the morning, but these have been infrequent.

Incomplete control of seizures was achieved with sodium valproate but, because of adverse effects and because the jaw jerks were diagnosed as partial motor seizures, other drug combinations with phenytoin, carbamazepine and lamotrigine have been tried, with little success. Currently sodium valproate combined with clonazepam is being assessed.

EEG and video-EEG recordings

All but patient 4 had one or more video-EEG recordings. Patients 2 and 3 had no ictal events during the recordings. In the remaining three, clinical absences accompanied by EEG discharges occurred (Figs. 2, 3 and 4). Analysis of these are presented in Table 2.

The major findings are the relative shortness of the discharges, the irregularities of the discharges in terms of the number of spikes per spike-wave complex, the fluctuations in spike amplitude, the inconstant relationship of spike to slow wave and the occurrence of fragmentations. Additionally, although there appears to be a slowing from start to finish in the discharge frequency, this is not consistent.

Perioral myoclonia was seen in virtually all TAS recorded on video-EEG. It consists of rhythmic contractions of the orbicularis oris muscle, causing protrusion of the lips, contractions of the depressor anguli oris, causing twitching of the corners of the mouth, or rarely more widespread involvement, including the muscles of mastication, causing jaw jerking. It begins within the first second of the discharge (often coinciding with the first polyspike-wave complex) and lasts for most of its duration. There is a close relationship of each myoclonic jerk to the polyspike component and the frequency of the myoclonia thus varies with that of the discharge.

Table 2. Analysis of the video-EEG-documented electroclinical discharges from patients 1, 5, and 6

	Patient 1	Patient 5	Patient 6
No of discharges	3	18	13
Total duration (s)*	8.7 ± 0.8 (8.0 – 9.5)	2.5 ± 1.1 (1.5 – 6.0)	2.4 ± 0.9 (1.5 – 4.5)
OP (1 s)*	3.7 ± 0.3 (3.5 – 4.0)	3.3 ± 0.3 (2.6 – 4.0)	3.5 ± 0.2 (3.0 – 3.8)
IP (3 s)*	3.4 ± 0.1 (3.3 – 3.5)	2.4 ± 0.2 (2.0 – 3.0)	2.7 ± 0.3 (2.2 – 3.1)
TP (3 s)*	3.1 ± 0.2 (2.9 – 3.3)	2.4 ± 0.2 (2.2 –2.5)	2.2 (1 discharge)
Fragmentations	Uncommon	Common	Common
Max no. of polyspikes	4 (Mean = 3.7)	6 (Mean = 5.1)	6 (Mean = 4.5)
S-amplitude fluctuation	Uncommon	Common	Common
S–SW relation	Inconstant	Inconstant	Inconstant
POM delay (s)*	1.0	0.3 ± 0.3 (0.0 – 1.0)	No delay
POM duration (s)*	6.8 ± 0.3 (6.5 – 7.0)	1.40 ± 0.9 (0.5 – 4.5)	1.5 ± 0.8 (0.5 – 3.0)
Impairment of consciousness	Severe	Moderate	Mild

OP, IP, TP = frequencies of opening, initial and terminal phases respectively.
* = mean ± SD (max – min), S = spike, SW = slow wave, POM = perioral myoclonus.

Standard EEG recordings were available for all patients except case 5. No consistent background abnormalities were seen in any patient, although some individual records contained excessive slow activity. Focal abnormalities consisting either of single spikes and spike–slow wave complexes or of

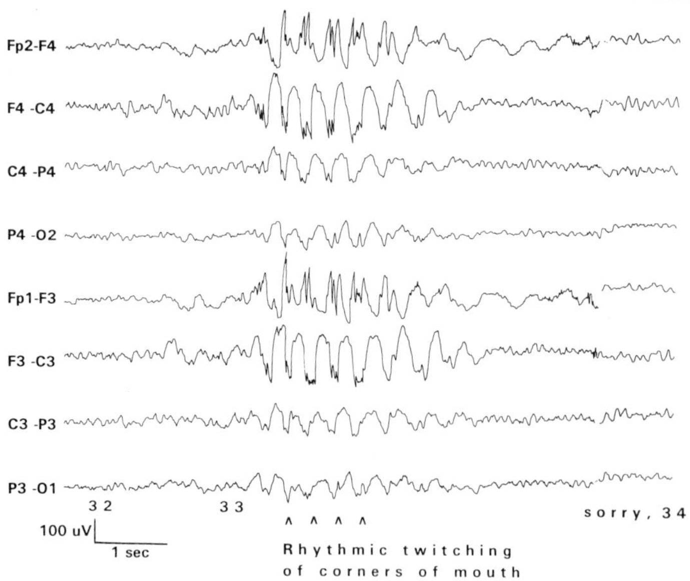

Fig. 3. Ictal video-EEG from patient 5. The timing of perioral myoclonus is shown. Impairment of consciousness was mild but, as shown, counting was delayed.

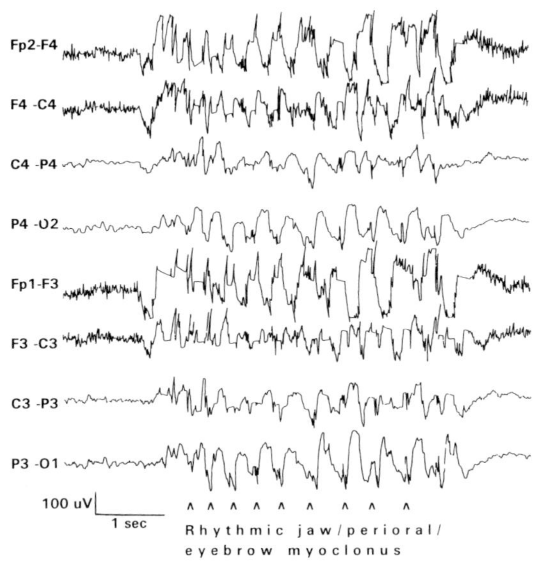

Fig. 4. Ictal video-EEG from patient 6 which is annotated to show the timing of perioral myoclonus.

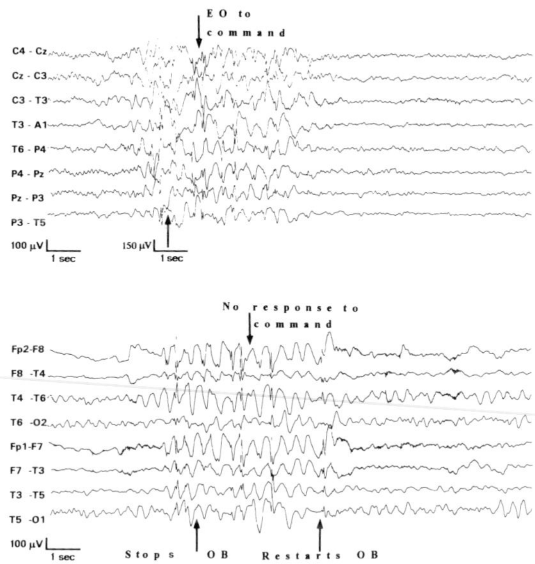

Fig. 5. EEG discharges recorded from patient 3 at 7 (top) and 7.5 (bottom) years of age. The discharges are annotated to show clinical events. Note the intradischarge irregularities (see text). EO = eye opening; OB = overbreathing.

focal theta waves were common and were seen at some time in all patients except patient 1. However, they tended to be inconstant in their side emphasis and between records.

Nine records were available from patient 3. Electrical events during ictal discharges were analysed

Table 3. Analysis of the EEG ictal discharges from patient 3 from ages 7 to 19 years

Age (years)	Discharges (no.)	Duration (s)*	OP (s)*	IP (s)*	TP (s)*	Fragmentations	Poly-Ss (max)	S-amplitude fluctuation	S-SW relation
7	7	4.14 ± 1.4 (2.5 – 6.0)	2.9 ± 0.2 (2.5 – 3.1)	2.5 ± 0.2 (2.2 – 2.7)	2.3 ± 0.1 (2.2 – 2.3)	Common	5	Common	Inconstant
7.5	4	6.3 ± 3.2 (4.5 – 11.0)	3.4 ± 0.2 (3.2 – 3.5)	2.6 ± 0.2 (2.4 – 2.8)	2.9 ± 0.3 (2.6 – 3.2)	Common	4	Common	Inconstant
8	Nil	Nil	Nil	Nil	Nil	Nil	Nil	Nil	Nil
9	1	3.0	3.5	2.5	(–)	Common	Nil	Uncommon	Inconstant
10	3	6.5 ± 3.3 (3.0 – 9.5)	3.1 ± 0.1 (3.0 – 3.2)	2.6 ± 0.1 (2.5 – 2.6)	2.4 ± 0.1 (2.3 – 2.4)	Nil	4	Common	Constant
12	1	5.5	3.3	2.6	1.8	Uncommon	5	Common	Inconstant
14	7	6.3 ± 1.8 (4.0 – 8.5)	3.6 ± 0.1 (3.5 – 3.8)	2.9 ± 0.1 (2.8 – 3.0)	2.7 ± 0.2 (2.5 – 2.9)	Common	6	Common	Inconstant
15	2	6.5 ± 1.4 (5.5 – 7.5)	3.2 ± 0.2 (3.0 – 3.3)	3.0 ± 0.1 (2.9 – 3.0)	2.8 ± 0.1 (2.7 – 2.8)	Common	4	Common	Inconstant
19	1	2.0	4.0	3.0	(–)	Common	4	Common	Inconstant

OP, IP, TP = frequencies of opening, initial and terminal phases respectively.
* = mean ± SD (max – min), S = spike, SW = slow wave, POM = perioral myoclonus.

in a similar way to those occurring during video-EEG (Table 3) and show that the irregularities of the EEG discharges persist through childhood and into adult life. However, individual recordings may have more regular discharges, as in Figs. 5 and 6, illustrating the danger of over-interpreting single EEG events.

Discussion

All patients in this series would be difficult or impossible to classify within existing epilepsy syndromes. Patients 1, 2 and 3 resemble CAE in the frequency of their absences and their age of onset. Additionally, in patient 1 the impairment of consciousness was severe. However, in all three the onset of GTCS was before that of clinical absences and in patients 2 and 3 the impairment of consciousness was milder than that usually seen in CAE. In patient 5 the timing of onset of absences is difficult to judge but it is likely that he suffered absences throughout childhood and from the evidence of video-EEG they may have had a pyknolepsy-type frequency. However, they were so mild as to have gone virtually unnoticed and the initial presentation was with a GTCS and absence status. In patients 4 and 6 the age of onset of seizures and their frequency would be compatible with JAE. However, the severity of the jaw/perioral myoclonus in patient 6 was too severe for this diagnosis to be accepted and she has been far more resistant to therapy than is usual in JAE. In patient 4 absences were accompanied by mild impairment of consciousness than is usual in JAE.

Analysis of EEG and video-EEG data gives further support to our contention that these patients merit separate classification. The mean ictal discharge duration is short (3.05, range 2.7–8.9) and the discharges are very irregular, as discussed previously. In both respects the discharges more resemble those seen in JME than in CAE or JAE (Panayiotopoulos *et al.*, 1989a, b, 1992, 1994). The clinical hallmark of the patients is the ictal rhythmic perioral myoclonia, whose features have been described earlier. Failure to recognize its significance may lead to misdiagnosis of a focal motor seizure.

Myoclonus may be seen during TAS in a number of different epileptic syndromes. Aicardi (1986)

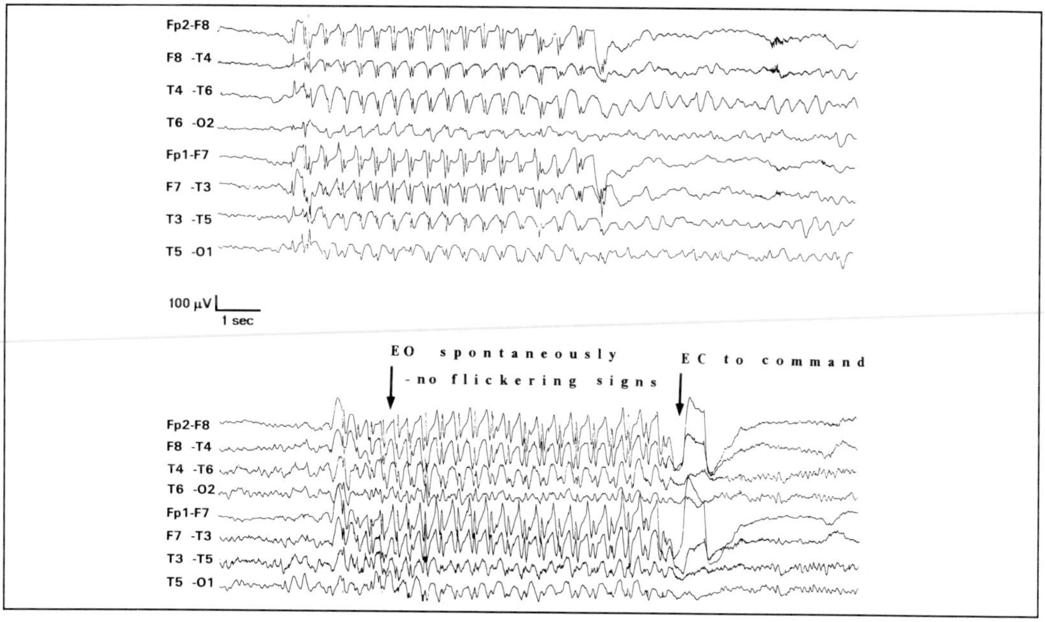

Fig. 6. EEG discharges recorded from patient 3 at 14 (top) and 15 (bottom) years of age. The sensitivity scale refers to the bottom trace and is double that of the top. The upper discharge is more regular (see text). EO = eyes open; EC = eyes closed; '– no flickering signs' = technician's annotation.

considers that in CAE and JAE phasic muscle contractions during absences are limited to the eyelids and occasionally the deltoids. Loiseau (1992) recognizes that in some cases of CAE clonic components may involve the chin and lips, but this has not been assessed prognostically. In our patients perioral myoclonus was prominent, being reported by witnesses in all cases and some patients being aware of it. In eyelid myoclonia with absences myoclonia of the eyelids is a defining feature of the syndrome and perioral myoclonia is not described (Jeavons, 1977; Appleton *et al.*, 1993). In epilepsy with myoclonic absences (Tassinari *et al.*, 1992) myoclonia mainly involves the shoulders, arms and legs. Less frequently, facial myoclonia occurs, particularly around the mouth and chin. However, in contrast to our patients, intellectual impairment is common, ictal discharges resemble those of CAE and more males than females are affected (Tassinari *et al.*, 1992). It is possible that idiopathic, but not symptomatic or cryptogenic, cases of epilepsy with myoclonic absences belong to the new syndrome we describe.

At present, epidemiological data are scant. After seeing the first two cases (Panayiotopoulos *et al.*, 1992) it took a further year to collect the other four. During this time we saw around 40 children and adults with typical absences. Of these, six had eyelid myoclonia with absences, suggesting the two syndromes may have a similar prevalence, i.e. 8 per cent of all patients with TAS. As in CAE, but not JAE and JME, there is a strong female predominance (five out of six patients). The frequency of a family history of epilepsies (three out of six) is similar to that which might be expected in idiopathic generalized epilepsies.

Definition

We suggest the name 'perioral myoclonia with absences' for a syndrome of idiopathic generalized epilepsy with TAS characterized by rhythmic myoclonia of the perioral and, rarely, jaw muscles accompanying the ictus. Onset of absences is from childhood to early adolescence. Frequency and associated impairment of consciousness are variable. GTCS are seen in all patients and often have their onset prior to that of the absences. They may be frequent or rare and are often preceded by showers of absences or absence status. Absence status is more common than in other typical absence syndromes. The ictal EEG shows generalized, relatively short, irregular discharges with spike, more often polyspike and slow wave complexes at around 3–4 Hz. Inter- and intradischarge frequency variations and fragmentations occur. Photosensitivity is not seen. Response to therapy isoften poor and the condition may be lifelong. Family history is often positive for epilepsies.

More recently we have seen two additional adult patients with perioral myoclonia with absences also had absence status and GTCS. In adddition, other clinicians have notified us of at least another six patients who had the same characteristics as the patients described in this report. The misdiagnosis of perioral myoclonia as partial seizures, the occurrence of absence status and GTCS, the lack of remission and the resistance to treatment are striking features. Some of the patients may initially respond to medication by relapses may be common. In others, the absences may be so mild in adult life that the patient may erroneoulsy be considered cured until an absence status followed by a GTCS occurs.

Prevalence of perioral myolclonia with absences in adults older than 20 years of age is 1.8 per cent of all epilepsies, 5.9 per cent of idiopathic generalised epilepsies and 9.3 per cent of epileptic syndromes with absences. The prevalence of perorial myoclonia with absences may be lower; we have seen only one child amongst 50 with video-EEG recorded typical absences.

References

Aicardi, J. (1994): Epilepsies with typical absence seizures. In: *Epilepsy in children*, 2nd edn. ed J. Aicardi, pp. 94–117. New York: Raven Press.

Appleton, R.E., Panayiotopoulos, C.P., Acomb, A. & Beirne, M. (1993): Eyelid myoclonia with typical absences: an epilepsy syndrome. *J. Neurol. Neurosurg. Psychiatr.* **56,** 1312–1316.

Commission on Classification and Terminology of the International League Against Epilepsy (1981): Proposal for revised clinical and electroencephalographic classification of epileptic seizures. *Epilepsia* **22,** 489–501.

Commission on Classification and Terminology of the International League Against Epilepsy (1989): Proposal for revised classification of epilepsies and epileptic syndromes. *Epilepsia* **30,** 389–399.

Jeavons, P.M. (1977): Nosological problems of myoclonic epilepsies in childhood and adolescence. *Dev. Med. Child Neurol.* **19,** 3–8.

Loiseau, P. (1992): Childhood absence epilepsy. In: *Epileptic syndromes in infancy, childhood and adolescence,* 2nd edn, eds. J. Roger, M. Bureau, Ch. Dravet, F.E. Dreifuss, A. Perret & P. Wolf, pp. 135–150. London: John Libbey.

Panayiotopoulos, C.P., Obeid, T. & Waheed, G. (1989a): Differentiation of typical absence seizures in epileptic syndromes: a video EEG study of 224 seizures in 20 patients. *Brain* **112,** 1039–1056.

Panayiotopoulos, C.P., Obeid, T. & Waheed, G. (1989b): Absences in juvenile myoclonic epilepsy: a clinical and video-electroencephalographic study. *Ann. Neurol.* **25,** 391–397.

Panayiotopoulos, C.P., Chroni, E., Daskalopoulos, C., Baker, A., Rowlinson, S. & Walsh, P. (1992): Typical absence seizures in adults: clinical, EEG, video EEG findings and diagnostic/syndromic considerations. *J. Neurol. Neurosurg. Psychiatr.* **55,** 1002–1008.

Panayiotopoulos, C.P., Baker, A., Grunewald, R., Rowlinson, S. & Walsh, P. (1993): Breath counting during 3 Hz generalized spike and wave discharges. *J. Electrophysiol. Technol.* **19,** 15–23.

Panayiotopoulos, C.P., Obeid, T. & Tahan, A.R. (1994): Juvenile myoclonic epilepsy: a 5 year prospective study. *Epilepsia* **35,** 285–296.

Panayiotopoulos, C.P., Ferrie, C.D., Giannakodimos, S. & Robinson, R.O. (1994): Perioral myoclonia with absences. In: *Typical absences and related epileptic syndromes,* eds, J.S. Duncan, C.P. Panayiotopoulos. London: Churchill Livingstone (in press).

Tassinari, C.A., Bureau, M. & Thomas, P. (1992): Epilepsy with myoclonic absences. In: *Epileptic syndromes in infancy, childhood and adolescence,* 2nd edn, eds. J. Roger, M. Bureau, Ch. Dravet, F.E. Dreifuss, A. Perret & P. Wolf, pp. 151–160. London: John Libbey.

Section III

Idiopathic epilepsy syndromes

Traditionally, epilepsies are first divided into generalized and focal. In this book, a different approach is taken which considers all idiopathic epilepsies, both generalized and localization-related, together as distinct from symptomatic epilepsies, and attempts to look into their similarities and differences. Idiopathic epilepsies, i.e. epileptic disorders *sui generis*, not caused or occasioned by some other disease or insult to the brain, are today mostly viewed as genetically determined. Although the exclusiveness of this view will be challenged later in this book (see Introduction to Section V), this section therefore starts with some genetic aspects including a first attempt to bridge the gap between clinical and basic (receptor) approaches (Chapter 23).

A feedback takes place: geneticists have been induced by clinicians to investigate juvenile myoclonic epilepsy because this was a well-described syndrome with an obvious genetic background. They now come back asking the clinicians to take a closer look because linkage studies have indicated that this may not be one uniform syndrome.

Chapter 31 describes the discovery of a new idiopathic epilepsy syndrome which was made by the traditional method of studying twins, combined with a differentiated evaluation of the clinical phenotype.

The term 'localization-related' has been introduced because in the idiopathic epilepsies belonging in this category there is no circumscribed focus, and the seizures may even originate in corresponding regions of either hemisphere. When all idiopathic epilepsies are viewed together, regional accentuations of the 'generalized' varieties again attract attention (see Introduction to Section II). The possible consequences are discussed at large in the concluding chapter of this section.

Epileptic Seizures and Syndromes, Edited by Peter Wolf
© 1994 John Libbey & Company Ltd., pp. 157–164

Chapter 20

Epilepsies in twins

Samuel F. Berkovic*, R. Anne Howell*, David A. Hay † and John L. Hopper‡

**Department of Neurology, Austin Hospital, Heidelberg, Melbourne, Victoria 3084, Australia, and Department of Medicine (Neurology), The University of Melbourne; †Department of Psychology, LaTrobe University, Bundoora, Victoria 3083, Australia; ‡The Australian NHMRC Twin Registry, The University of Melbourne, Parkville, Victoria 3052, Australia*

Summary

Twins provide a unique model to disentangle the genetic and acquired components of epilepsies and to study the complex genetic interrelationships of inherited epilepsy syndromes. It is essential to understand these relationships to identify appropriate families for molecular genetic study. Here we present an analysis of 245 twin pairs where one or both have seizures. Twins were ascertained from community-based registries (70 per cent) and by referral (30 per cent), and were personally examined and classified according to the international classification of epilepsy syndromes. Twins were not found to have a higher risk of seizures than their non-twin siblings and 91 per cent of those affected could be classified according to the international classification. Among the monozygotic twin pairs, there was a high concordance for idiopathic generalized epilepsies (65 per cent) and symptomatic/cryptogenic generalized epilepsies (71 per cent) with lower concordance for the localization-related epilepsies (20 per cent). Analysis of the subsyndromes amongst monozygous and dizygous twins with idiopathic generalized epilepsies suggest that these epilepsies are determined by more than one gene.

Inheritance of epilepsy

Hippocrates (*circa* 400 BC) first observed that epilepsy could be inherited. Since that seminal observation, however, the relative contribution of genetic and acquired factors to the causation of epilepsies has remained a controversial and unresolved issue (Metrakos & Metrakos, 1974; Newmark & Penry, 1979; Anderson *et al.*, 1982; Andermann, 1985; Blandfort *et al.*, 1987; Treiman & Treiman, 1993).

Much of the confusion in the literature regarding the genetics of the epilepsies is due to inadequacies in diagnosis. In some early studies, 'epilepsy' was regarded as a relatively homogeneous entity, and, in later work, epileptic seizures were studied. It cannot be emphasized too strongly that epileptic seizures are symptoms and not disease entities. Study of the genetics of symptoms is of limited value and cannot lead to proper clarification of the inheritance of diseases. Moreover, studies predating the current International League Against Epilepsy (ILAE) classification of epileptic seizures (Commission, 1981) used old terminology, which has been shown to be potentially misleading by contemporary video-electroencephalographic (EEG) monitoring studies. For example, some studies of the genetics of 'petit mal' probably contained a mixture of absence seizures and complex partial seizures, seizure types that have totally different mechanisms and are seen in quite separate epileptic syndromes.

The systematized classification of epileptic syndromes developed by the ILAE (Commission, 1989) represents a major advance in understanding the epilepsies. Although difficulties remain in applying the ILAE classification to all patients with epilepsy (Berkovic *et al.*, 1987; see also Berkovic *et al.*, Chapter 5), it now provides a basis to begin the proper genetic analysis of specific epilepsies. However, with the exception of a number of rare epilepsies that are inherited in a classic Mendelian fashion, the inheritance patterns of most epileptic syndromes are complex (Andermann, 1982; Blandfort *et al.*, 1987).

Twins provide a useful natural model for examining the genetics of complex diseases. Interpretation of genetic data obtained from twin studies is considerably simplified compared with that of ordinary family studies. There have been a number of previous twin studies of epilepsy based largely on selected twin samples (Table 1). All have shown a higher concordance for monozygotic twins compared with dizygotic pairs, strongly suggesting a major inherited component contributing to 'epilepsy'. The variability in concordance rates in these studies probably reflects the different methods of ascertainment of twins.

Table 1. Concordance rates in previous studies of twins with epilepsy

		Concordances (%)	
	Twin pairs	Monozygous	Dizygous
Rosanoff *et al.*, 1934	107	61	24
Conrad, 1935	157	67	3
Lennox & Lennox, 1960	225	62	15
Inouye, 1960	40	54	7
Braconi, 1962	51	80	32
Harvald & Hauge, 1965	127	37	10

These studies predated the ILAE classifications of seizures and epilepsies and thus it is difficult to interpret them in terms of the current understanding of the epilepsies. Two more recent epidemiological studies of twins have confirmed the higher concordance in monozygous twins but these studies used self-reported questionnaire data and thus the diagnoses were imprecise (Corey *et al.*, 1991; Sillanpää *et al.*, 1991).

We have used the large community-based twin registries at LaTrobe University, Australia and the National Health and Medical Research Council (NHMRC) based at the University of Melbourne to examine the inheritance of specific epilepsies (Berkovic *et al.*, 1990, 1991a, b, 1993). Twins were screened by a questionnaire to determine the possible occurrence of seizures.

In contrast to previous studies of twins ascertained from twin registries, those with possible seizures were then examined personally to attempt to classify their epileptic seizure type(s) and their epileptic syndrome according to the ILAE classifications. We have addressed a number of questions using these data.

Are epilepsies more common in twins?

Twin pregnancies have an increased incidence of antenatal and perinatal complications, congenital malformations and perinatal deaths (Campbell & MacGillivray, 1988). Epilepsy is often attributed to abnormal perinatal events. Therefore, it has been widely assumed that epilepsy has an increased incidence in twins. If epilepsies were disproportionately represented in twins, it would be difficult to generalize the genetic conclusions to non-twin subjects with epilepsy.

We examined this question by determining the cumulative incidence of epilepsies and febrile convulsions in the LaTrobe twin cohort and their non-twin siblings (Berkovic *et al.*, 1993). A previously validated seizure questionnaire was mailed to all 627 families with multiple births on the LaTrobe register. Non-responders were sent a second questionnaire and recalcitrant non-responders were followed up by telephone. Responses were obtained from 549 families (88 per cent); the remaining 78 (12 per cent) were no longer at the address given and were untraceable by telephone. All positive responders were personally examined.

A total of 63 positive responses were obtained, where one or both twins had suffered seizures or possible seizures. All were evaluated and classified as affected (37 pairs) or false positives (26 pairs). The false positive pairs comprised syncope (12), hyperventilation (7) and miscellaneous (7). Of the 37 true positive pairs, both twins were affected in five, making a total of 42 affected individual twins (3.8 per cent, Table 2). The age-specific cumulative incidence rate rose rapidly from 1.5 per cent at 1 year to 3.4 per cent (5 years), reflecting the 30 cases of febrile seizures. Thereafter, the rise was more gradual from 3.6 per cent (6 years) to 4.2 per cent (10 years).

The 549 responders from the LaTrobe register had 29 affected siblings (3.9 per cent, Table 2). The non-twin siblings were older than the twins (mean age 9.4 ± 4.8 for twins, 12.4 ± 7.0 for siblings, $P < 0.0001$). Based on the age-specific cumulative incidence in twins, the expected number of affected siblings was 30.5 (4.1 per cent), being only slightly greater than the observed number of 29. This estimate was well within the 95 per cent confidence interval of the twins estimate (2.6–5.0 per cent).

Table 2. Seizures in twins and non-twin siblings (La Trobe twin study)

	Twin individuals (n = 1110)		Non-twin individuals (n = 751)	
Afebrile seizures	18	1.6%	11	1.5%
Febrile seizures	30	2.7%	19	2.5%
All seizures*	42	3.8% (2.6, 5.0)†	29	3.9% (2.3, 5.4)†

*Six twins and one singleton had both afebrile and febrile seizures; † 95% confidence intervals.

The types of epilepsy syndrome diagnoses for affected twins and non-twin siblings were similar, and comprised mainly neonatal seizures and idiopathic generalized and idiopathic localization-related epilepsies in addition to febrile convulsions. The epilepsies observed in the 18 twins with afebrile seizures were benign and self-limited in 12 cases, controlled on treatment in four, whereas only two were poorly controlled (Berkovic *et al.*, 1993).

These data strongly suggest, contrary to previous belief, that twin birth is not a major risk factor for epilepsy or febrile convulsions. Moreover, this implies that the data obtained from the twin subjects can be extrapolated to the population as a whole.

How practical is the ILAE classification of epilepsies?

Proper classification is a prerequisite to meaningful genetic analysis. The ILAE classification of epileptic syndromes (Commission, 1989; Roger *et al.*, 1992) was developed largely on the basis of carefully studied patients in hospital clinics. It is therefore important to determine if it can be used for patients ascertained from the wider community. The twin registries provide a very good test of this, because the twins are unusually compliant in responding to questionnaires, resulting in higher ascertainment rates than those achieved by many other methods. To date we have studied 359 pairs who reported that one or both twin individuals had seizures. These 359 pairs comprised 74 pairs referred from other neurologists or twin clubs, 63 from the LaTrobe Registry and 222 from the NHMRC Twin Registry.

Of the 359 pairs studied to date, 163 have epilepsy, 82 have febrile convulsions alone and 114 pairs were false positives. The false positives largely comprise cases of syncope, convulsive syncope, breath-holding attacks, etc. The 245 true positive pairs ascertained from epidemiological sources (LaTrobe and NHMRC Registries) and by referral were classified following a clinical history and examination, routine EEG, and after obtaining old clinical records and EEG reports, etc. (Table 3).

Table 3. Diagnoses in 245 twins with epilepsy

	Referred twins*	Registry twins†	Total
Generalized epilepsies			
Idiopathic	19	22	41
Symptomatic/cryptogenic	11	2	13
Generalized/unclassified	5	0	5
Partial epilepsies (localization-related)			
Idiopathic	1	8	9
Symptomatic/cryptogenic	26	26	52
Other epileptic syndromes			
Neonatal seizures	0	10	10
Febrile convulsions	5	77	82
Miscellaneous	2	9	11
Unclassified	5	17	22
Total	74	171	245

*Twins ascertained by referral from neurologists or twin clubs; †twins ascertained from community-based registries (La Trobe, NHMRC).

These data show that 223/245 pairs studied to date (91 per cent) could be classified into subdivisions of the epilepsies. Similar success in classification was achieved with twins ascertained from community-based registries (90 per cent), compared with referred twins (93 per cent). There were, however, some important differences in the patterns of epileptic syndromes depending on the mode of ascertainment. As expected, the community-based twin registry group largely comprised cases with benign epileptic syndromes such as febrile convulsions, idiopathic generalized and idiopathic localization-related epilepsies. In contrast, the referred group had many more cases of symptomatic generalized and localized epilepsies, which are often resistant to therapy.

What are the concordance rates in different epilepsy subgroups?

The twin pairs where a broad syndromic diagnosis was made were then analysed according to concordance in monozygous and dizygous pairs (Table 4). Zygosity was determined by a clinical questionnaire, by clinical examination and by a panel of red cell antigens and human leucocyte antigens (HLA). Proper analysis of these data requires further consideration of the specific epilepsy syndromes.

Table 4. Concordance rates for specific epilepsies

	Twin pairs	Concordance			
		Monozygous		Dizygous	
Generalized epilepsies					
Idiopathic	41	65%	(13/20)	24%	(5/21)
Symptomatic/cryptogenic	13	71%	(5/7)	0%	(0/6)
Localization-related epilepsies					
Idiopathic	9	20%	(1/5)	0%	(0/4)
Symptomatic/cryptogenic	52	21%	(4/19)	0%	(0/33)
Febrile convulsions	82	39%	(11/28))	7%	(4/54)

Idiopathic generalized epilepsies

These epilepsies are known to have a major inherited component (Lennox & Lennox, 1960; Metrakos & Metrakos, 1961; Matthes & Weber, 1968; Doose *et al.*, 1973; Tsuboi & Christian, 1973; Degen *et al.*, 1990). The nature of this inherited component and the genetic relationships between the subsyndromes of idiopathic generalized epilepsy (childhood absence epilepsy, juvenile myoclonic epilepsy, etc.) are, however, unclear (Berkovic *et al.*, 1987; Greenberg *et al.*, 1992; Janz *et al.*, 1992).

The high concordance in our monozygous twins (Table 4) confirms the major genetic component in these epilepsies. Of the 41 pairs studied to date, 20 were monozygous and 13 of these were clinically concordant for seizures. The other seven monozygous pairs were discordant, but in three of these pairs the clinically unaffected twin had unequivocal generalized epileptiform abnormalities on EEG. Thus the concordance rate was 65 per cent (13/20) for clinical epilepsy, but rose to 80% (16/20) if EEG abnormalities were taken into account. These data are similar to those reported by Lennox & Lennox (1960) for twins with 'petit mal'. A striking observation in our twins was that in all 13 concordant pairs the specific syndrome of generalized epilepsy was the same in both twins, namely childhood absence epilepsy (eight pairs), juvenile absence epilepsy (one pair), juvenile myoclonic epilepsy (two pairs) and others (two pairs).

Only five of the 21 dizygous pairs were concordant for seizures, and the twins had different subsyndromes in four of these pairs. For example, in one pair the proband developed mild benign myoclonic epilepsy of infancy and, at age 4 years, when his seizures had spontaneously resolved, his co-twin developed mild childhood absence epilepsy. In two of the 16 clinically discordant dizygous pairs, the unaffected twin had unequivocal generalized epileptiform abnormalities on EEG.

These data lead to some important conclusions. First, the high rate of concordance for specific epileptic syndromes in monozygous pairs strongly supports the primacy of genetic factors in the idiopathic generalized epilepsies. Second, the fidelity of subsyndromes in monozygous pairs indicates that the subsyndromes have some genetic differences. Third, the low rate of concordance in dizygous pairs and in non-twin relatives (data not shown) and lack of fidelity of subsyndromes make simple dominant or recessive inheritance extremely unlikely. Perhaps the most likely explanation for these data is that a complex or complexes of multiple genes underlie the idiopathic generalized epilepsies, as first suggested by Andermann (1982). This has great importance for planning molecular genetic approaches to these epilepsies, as strategies based on single-gene hypotheses may yield misleading data.

Symptomatic and cryptogenic generalized epilepsies

This category contains cases that are more difficult to classify, including the Lennox–Gastaut syndrome and other myoclonic epilepsies of early childhood. Patients usually have mental retardation and refractory seizures, and acquired factors have been thought to be paramount. Doose has described an inherited subgroup amongst these patients (Doose *et al.*, 1970; Doose & Baier, 1987), but his views have been the subject of major controversy.

We have studied 13 pairs to date, and five of the seven monozygous pairs were concordant. Two concordant pairs have known genetic disorders: one with late-infantile neuronal ceroid lipofuscinosis and the other pair with West syndrome due to tuberose sclerosis. The other three concordant pairs have symptomatic generalized epilepsies with myoclonic seizures and drop attacks. None of the six dizygous pairs are concordant, but one has an affected sibling. Although our numbers are small, these data suggest that genetic factors are far more important than previously thought, and support the concept of Doose's subgroup.

Idiopathic localization-related epilepsies

In this group our data are more difficult to reconcile with previous family studies. We have examined seven pairs (four monozygous, three dizygous) with benign childhood epilepsy with centrotemporal spikes. This is a common, well-defined, self-limited epileptic syndrome with good evidence for a genetic basis (Bray & Wiser, 1964; Heijbel *et al.*, 1975). None of our pairs were concordant for seizures or EEG abnormalities, although concordant monozygous pairs have been described previously (Kajitani *et al.*, 1980). Our anomalous results may be in part explained by the fact that three of the monozygous twins were studied late in the second decade, when this benign syndrome has remitted.

One monozygous pair was concordant for primary reading epilepsy. Although presently classified as an idiopathic partial epilepsy (Commission, 1989), there is evidence that this unusual syndrome is a form of idiopathic generalized epilepsy (Wolf, 1992), a view that we favour.

Symptomatic focal epilepsies

This category has the least nosological precision. It includes all cases of focal epilepsy, except those fulfilling criteria for specific idiopathic partial epilepsies. Cases studied most intensively are those with medically refractory seizures, and acquired factors are clearly most important for those patients (Andermann, 1982, 1985). Little is known about the more benign cases. Amongst the 19 monozygous pairs, four were concordant. All four pairs had mild, easily controlled, temporal lobe epilepsy of adult onset. One of these pairs had two other similarly affected relatives. These data strongly suggest that there is a hitherto unsuspected familial form of temporal lobe epilepsy with a benign course beginning in adult life. We believe that these cases should be reclassified as a new form of idiopathic partial epilepsy (see Chapter 31).

Conclusions

These observations show the power of the twin method when applied to a complex group of disorders such as the epilepsies. The method may yield important clues to aetiology, in even small numbers of cases, and may help identify new genetic syndromes that would be difficult to recognize by conventional genetic studies. It is hoped that the genetic patterns will become even clearer as larger numbers of twins are studied and that this will lay the basis for molecular genetic studies.

Acknowledgements

Supported by the NHMRC of Australia, the Australian NHMRC Twin Registry, the Austin Hospital Medical Research Foundation, and the Epilepsy Foundation of Victoria. We thank the staff of the NHMRC Twin Registry, the LaTrobe twin study, the EEG laboratory of the Austin Hospital, and the Departments of Neurology of the Royal Perth Hospital, Westmead Hospital, Royal Hobart Hospital and Launceston Hospital. We are also grateful to the Red Cross Blood Bank (Melbourne) for HLA typing, to Dr John Mitchell for red cell typing, and to innumerable neurologists, paediatricians and other medical practitioners who provided information on twins treated by them.

References

Andermann, E. (1982): Multifactorial inheritance of generalized and focal epilepsy. In: *Genetic basis of the epilepsies*, eds. V.E. Anderson, W.A. Hauser, J.K. Penry & C.F. Sing, pp. 129–145. New York, Raven Press.

Andermann, E. (1985): Genetic aspects of the epilepsies. In: *Genetic aspects of human behaviour*, eds. T. Sakai & T. Tsuboi, pp. 129–145. Tokyo: Igaku-Shoin.

Anderson, V.E., Hauser, W.A., Penry, J.K. & Sing, C.F. (eds.) (1982): *Genetic basis of the epilepsies*. New York: Raven Press.

Berkovic, S.F., Andermann, F., Andermann, E. & Gloor, P. (1987): Concepts of absence epilepsies: discrete syndromes or biological continuum? *Neurology* **37**, 993–1000.

Berkovic, S.F., Howell, R.A., Hopper, J.L., Hay, D.A. & Andermann, E. (1990): A twin study of the epilepsies. *Epilepsia* **31,** 813 (abstract).

Berkovic, S.F., Howell, R.A., Hopper, J.L. & Hay, D.A. (1991a): Generalized epilepsies: genetics as revealed by twins. *Neurology* **41** (suppl 1), 127 (abstract).

Berkovic, S.F., Howell, R.A., Hay, D.A. & Hopper, J.L. (1991b): Epilepsy in twins. In: *Epilepsy update*, eds. F.J.E. Vajda, S.F. Berkovic & G.A. Donnan, pp. 32–38. Melbourne: The University of Melbourne.

Berkovic, S.F., Howell, R.A., Hay, D.A. & Hopper, J.L. (1993): Twin birth is not a risk factor for seizures. *Neurology* 43, 2515–2519.

Blandfort, M., Tsuboi, T. & Vogel, F. (1987): Genetic counseling in the epilepsies. *Hum. Genet.* **76,** 303–331.

Braconi, L. (1962): La ricera gemellologica nell'epilepssia. *Acta Genet. Med. Gemellol.* (Roma) **11,** 138–157.

Bray, F.P. & Wiser, W.C. (1964): Evidence for a genetic etiology of temporal central abnormalities in focal epilepsy. *N. Engl. J. Med.* **271,** 926–933.

Campbell, D.M. & MacGillivray, I. (1988): Outcomes of twin pregnancies. In: *Twinning and twins*, eds. I. MacGillivray, D.M. Campbell & B. Thompson, pp. 179–202. New York: John Wiley.

Commission on Classification and Terminology of the International League Against Epilepsy (1981): Proposal for revised clinical and electroencephalographic classification of epileptic seizures. *Epilepsia* **22,** 489–501.

Commission on Classification and Terminology of the International League Against Epilepsy (1989): Proposal for revised classification of epilepsies and epileptic syndromes. *Epilepsia* **30,** 389–399.

Conrad, K (1935): Erbanlage und Epilepsie: Untersuchungen an einer Serie von 253 Zwillingspaaren. *Z. Ges Neurol. Psychiatr.* **153,** 271–326.

Corey, L.A., Berg, K., Pellock, J.M., Sollas, M.H., Nance, W.E. & DeLorenzo, R.J. (1991): The occurrence of epilepsy and febrile seizures in Virginian and Norwegian twins. *Neurology* **41,** 1433–1436.

Degen, R., Degen, H.E. & Roth, C. (1990): Some genetic aspects of idiopathic and symptomatic absence seizures: waking and sleep EEGs in siblings. *Epilepsia* **31,** 784–794.

Doose, H. & Baier, W.K. (1987): Epilepsy with primarily generalized myoclonic-astatic seizures: a genetically determined disease. *Eur. J. Pediatr.* **146,** 550–554.

Doose, H., Gerken, H., Leonhardt, R., Volzke, E. & Volz, C. (1970): Centrencephalic myoclonic-astatic petit mal. *Neuropädiatrie* **2,** 59–78.

Doose, H., Gerken, H., Horstmann, T. & Volzke, E. (1973): Genetic factors in spike-wave absences. *Epilepsia* **14,** 57–75.

Greenberg, D.A., Durner, M. & Delgado-Escueto, A.V. (1992): Evidence for multiple gene loci in the expression of the common generalized epilepsies. *Neurology* **42** (suppl. 5), 56–62.

Harvald, B. & Hague, M. (1965): Hereditary factors elucidated by twin studies. In: *Genetics and the epidemiology of chronic diseases*, eds. J.V. Neel, M.W. Shaw & W.J. Schull, pp. 61–96. Washington: USDHEW, PHS.

Heijbel, J., Blom, S. & Rasmuson, M. (1975): Benign epilepsy of children with centrotemporal EEG foci: a genetic study. *Epilepsia* **16,** 285–293.

Inouye, E. (1960): Observations on forty twin index cases with chronic epilepsy and their co-twins. *J. Nerv. Ment. Dis.* **130,** 401–416.

Janz, D., Beck-Mannagetta, G. & Sander, T. (1992): Do idiopathic generalized epilepsies share a common suseptibility gene. *Neurology* **42** (suppl. 5), 48–55.

Kajitani, T., Nakamura, M., Ueoka, K. & Kobuchi, S. (1980): Three pairs of monozygotic twins with rolandic discharges. In: *Advances in epileptology X*, eds. J.A. Wada & J.K. Penry, pp. 171–175. New York: Raven Press.

Lennox, W.G. & Lennox, M.A. (1960): *Epilepsy and related disorders,* pp. 548–574. Boston: Little Brown.

Matthes, A. & Weber, H. (1968): Klinische und elektroenzephalographische Familienuntersuchungen bei Pyknolepsien. *Dtsch. Med. Wschr.* **93,** 429–435.

Metrakos, K. & Metrakos, J.D. (1961): Genetics of convulsive disorders. II. Genetic and electroencephalographic studies in centrencephalic epilepsy. *Neurology* **11,** 474–483.

Metrakos, K. & Metrakos, J.D. (1974): Genetics of epilepsy. In: *Handbook of clinical neurology*, Vol. 15, eds. P.J. Vinken & G.W. Bruyn, pp. 429–439. Amsterdam: North Holland.

Newmark,, M.E. & Penry, J.K. (1979): *Genetics of epilepsy: a review,* 122 pp. New York: Raven Press.

Roger, J., Bureau, M., Dravet, C., Dreifuss, F.E., Perret, A. & Wolf, P. (1992): *Epileptic syndromes in infancy, childhood and adolescence*, 2nd edn, 418 pp. London: John Libbey.

Rosanoff, A.J., Handy, L.M. & Rosanoff, I.A. (1934): Etiology of epilepsy with special reference to its occurrence in twins. *Arch. Neurol. Psychiatr.* **31,** 1165–1193.

Sillanpää, M., Koskenvuo, M., Romanov, K. & Kaprio, J. (1991): Genetic factors in epileptic seizures: evidence from a large twin population. *Acta Neurol. Scand.* **84,** 523–526.

Treiman, L.J. & Treiman, D.M. (1993): Genetic aspects of epilepsy. In: *The treatment of epilepsy: principles and practice,* ed. E. Wyllie, pp. 145–156. Philadelphia: Lea and Febiger.

Tsuboi, T. & Christian, W. (1973): On the genetics of primary generalized epilepsy with sporadic myoclonias of impulsive petit mal type. *Humangenetik* **19,** 155–184.

Wolf, P. (1992): Reading epilepsy. In: *Epileptic syndromes in infancy, childhood and adolescence,* 2nd edn, eds. J. Roger, M. Bureau, C. Dravet, F.E. Dreifuss, A. Perret & P. Wolf, pp. 281–298. London: John Libbey.

Epileptic Seizures and Syndromes, Edited by Peter Wolf
© 1994 John Libbey & Company Ltd., pp. 165–168

Chapter 21

Genetic aspects of epilepsies with myoclonic-astatic seizures

Gertrude Beck-Mannagetta, Claudia Dehe-Steffens, Bettina Schmitz and Dieter Janz

Abteilung für Neurologie, Klinikum Rudolf Virchow, Augustenburger Platz 1, D-13353 Berlin, Germany

Introduction

The documented medical history of what we call today myoclonic-astatic seizures starts with Jackson's observation from 1886 of a 7-year-old boy who had started to fall by the age of 2½ (Jackson, 1931). Jackson used the term 'falls' and by this described the consequence of what pathophysiologically is still not entirely clear.

The phenomenon stayed but terms have changed since, for instance: static seizures (Hunt, 1922), akinetic seizures (Lennox, 1945), petit mal variant epilepsies (Gibbs & Gibbs, 1952), myoclonic amyotonic petit mal (Gastaut, 1961), akinetic petit mal (Doose, 1964), Lennox syndrome (Gastaut *et al.,* 1966), myoclonic astatic petit mal (Kruse, 1968) centrencephalic myoclonic petit mal (Doose *et al.*, 1970). What was a description of a seizure type initially has become part of syndromes comprising other seizure types too.

The International Classification of Epilepsies and Epileptic Syndromes (ICEES) (Commission, 1989) lists under category 2.2 (cryptogenic or symptomatic generalized epilepsies) the Lennox–Gastaut syndrome and epilepsy with myoclonic-astatic seizures. With regard to clinical signs and symptoms these syndromes are clearly generalized but the Lennox–Gastaut syndrome may comprise focal seizures and especially a multifocal electroencephalogram (EEG). With respect to aetiology there is a controversy as to whether some of the affected should be listed under the idiopathic generalized syndromes. The attempt to distinguish 'benign' and 'severe' syndromes is mainly motivated by the need of paediatricians to offer prognostic criteria to parents.

Systematic clinical genetic studies dedicated to the cryptogenic or symptomatic generalized syndromes are rare, molecular genetic studies are lacking completely so far. Figures referring to the rate of what is called 'hereditary' (= positive family history) range between 2.5 per cent and 48 per cent in the various studies (Chevri & Aicardi, 1972; Boniver *et al.,* 1987). These differences are due to incomparable ascertainment procedures: febrile convulsions and single seizures may be included without specification, the degree of relationship in affected family members is often not defined, the age structure of relatives is unknown, and in general the total number of relatives in the different degrees is missing.

Method

The present study is part of the Berlin Pedigree Study and based on pooled data from the Neurological and the Neuropaediatric Department of the Klinikum Rudolf Virchow (Free University, Berlin) and the Paediatric Department of the Rittberg Krankenhaus, Berlin. Probands with a confirmed diagnosis of an epilepsy of early childhood with myoclonic-astatic seizures who attended one of the three departments between 1973 and 1988 were included.

Case records were retrospectively analysed with respect to clinical data. Information on the state of affectedness in the families was obtained by structured interviews of probands and their relatives.

Results

The study group comprised 159 probands (95 male, 64 female). The aetiology was considered to be cryptogenic or idiopathic in 106 cases, symptomatic in 53 cases. A symptomatic aetiology was stated according to unequivocal historical data and/or findings of structural imaging techniques. Most frequent were perinatal events (n = 31), followed by prenatal (n = 13) and postnatal (n = 8) complications. In one case the aetiology could not be specified. The mean age of onset was 4.1 years with a peak of age distribution around 2 years and a second less prominent peak in puberty.

Complete pedigrees could be obtained from 102 patients. A first-degree relative was affected by febrile or afebrile seizures or both in 16 probands (15.7 per cent), a first- or second-degree relative in 19 probands (18.6 per cent), and a first-, second- or third-degree relative in 30 probands (29.4 per cent). The total number of first-degree relatives was 363. Among these, 11 (3 per cent) suffered from afebrile seizures, and nine (2.5 per cent) from febrile convulsions. Looking at afebrile seizures, there were three of 204 parents (1.5 per cent) affected, seven of 152 siblings (4.6 per cent) and one of seven children (14.3 per cent). With respect to febrile convulsions, parents were affected in 2.5 per cent, siblings in 2.6 per cent and there was no affected offspring. The type of epileptic syndromes seen in first-degree relatives were distributed as follows: infantile spasms, $n = 1$; epilepsies with myoclonic-astatic seizures, $n = 1$; epilepsies with absence seizures, $n = 4$; juvenile myoclonic epilepsy (JME), $n = 1$; pure grand mal epilepsies, $n = 4$.

*Table 1. Clinical features in hereditary and non-hereditary forms of epilepsies with myoclonic-astatic seizures**

	Hereditary $n = 16$	Non-hereditary $n = 72$
Females/males	0.45	0.67
Age of onset	5.2 years	5.6 years
Symptomatic aetiology	13%	44%†
Tonic seizures	51%	44%
Focal seizures	0%	3%
Status epilepticus	38%	38%
Febrile convulsions	19%	13%
BNS seizures	6%	11%

*Hereditary refers to probands with affected first-degree relatives. Non-hereditary refers toprobands without affected relatives. Probands with affected second- or third-degree relatives are excluded from this analysis. †$P < 0.05$, chi-square test. BNS = Blitz-Nick-Salaam.

Table 2. Prevalence of seizures in first-degree relatives of 102 probands related to aetiology

	Idiopathic		Symptomatic	
Afebrile seizures	10/232	4.3%	1/131	0.8%*
Febrile convulsions	8/232	3.4%	1/131	0.8%

*$P < 0.05$, chi-square test.

Comparing clinical data in the patients with hereditary epilepsies (those who had first-degree relatives with afebrile seizures or febrile convulsions) *vs.* non-hereditary epilepsies, there were no differences with respect to age of onset, the occurrence of tonic seizures, focal seizures or febrile convulsions, a history of status epilepticus and preceding infantile spasms (Table 1). Thirty-two out of the 72 non-hereditary cases (44 per cent) had been diagnosed as symptomatic in contrast to only two out of 16 hereditary probands (13 per cent) (Table 1). Exploring the relationship between aetiology and heredity related to the total number of first-degree relatives, this difference could be confirmed (Table 2). Ten out of 65 patients with an idiopathic aetiology had first-degree relatives with afebrile seizures (15.3 per cent), in contrast to only one out 37 'symptomatic patients' (2.7 per cent).

Discussion

The rate of hereditary cases among our patients with myoclonic-astatic seizures was 15.7 per cent. Comparing this figure to the frequency of hereditary cases among patients with other generalized epilepsies, it appears that genetic mechanisms are less important for the manifestation of myoclonic–astatic seizures. However, our patient material comprises of both idiopathic cases separately, the rate of heredity rises up to 21.5 per cent, a figure much closer to juvenile myoclonic epilepsies and epilepsies with absence seizures (Beck-Mannagetta & Janz, 1991). This finding suggests that the idiopathic form of epilepsies with myoclonic–astatic seizures represents a variant of generalized epileptic syndromes with age-dependent onset. Looking at the spectrum of epileptic syndromes seen in relatives, it is remarkable that epilepsies with seizures dominate, exceeding the frequency which would be expected by chance distribution. This obsevation fits well with previous findings from family studies of probands with juvenile myoclonic epilepsies (Janz *et al.* 1989) and gives further evidence for the close relationship between the idiopathic form of the epilepsies with myoclonic–astatic seizures and the other idiopathic generalized epileptic syndromes. In one case there was a first degree family member suffering from myoclonic–astatic seizures; in another family a diagnosis of infantile spasms was made, a syndrome which frequently evolves into an epilepsy with myoclonic–astatic seizures. The numbers are too small to draw any definite conclusions. However, these two cases are interesting because they suggest that although there is a predisposition to the whole range of generalized epilepsies, the type of epilepsy is biased towards a syndrome-specific expression.

There was a significant link between idiopathic aetiology and heredity on the one hand, underlining the crucial role of aetiology for classification of epileptic syndromes. Apart from aetiology, there were no clinical features which differentiated between hereditary and non-hereditary cases. This is a remarkable finding, since there have been several attempts to identify subentities on the basis of specific symptom patterns, resulting in the acknowledgement of two separate syndromes in the recent International Classification Syndrome and the epilepsy with myoclonic–astatic siezures. Our data co not support such subdivisions. From a biological point of view it appears to be more reasonable to simply distinguish idiopathic (cryptogenic) and symptomatic variants of the syndromes with the leading symptom of astatic seizures, a proceeding already establisshed for the diagnosis of infantile spasms.

References

Beck-Mannagetta, G. & Janz, D. (1991): Syndrome-related genetics in generalized epilepsies. In: *Genetic strategies in epilepsy research* (*Epilepsy Res.* Suppl. 4), eds. V.E. Anderson, W.A. Hauser, J.E. Leppik, J.L. Noebels & S.S. Rich. Amsterdam: Elsevier.

Boniver, C., Dravet, C., Bureau, M. & Roger, J. (1987): Idiopathic Lennox–Gastaut syndrome. In: *Advances in Epileptology,* Vol. 16, eds. P. Wolf, M. Dam, D. Janz & F.E. Dreifuss. pp. 195–200. New York: Raven Press.

Chevri, J.J. & Aicardi, J. (1972): Childhood epileptic encephalopathy with slow spike-waves: as statistical study of 80 cases. *Epilepsia* **13,** 259–271.

Commission on Classification and Terminology (1989): Proposal for revised clinical and electroencephalographic classification of epilepsies and epileptic syndromes. *Epilepsia* **30,** 389–395.

Doose, H. (1964): Das akinetische petit mal. *Arch. Psychiatr. Neurol.* 205, 638–654.

Doose, H., Gerken, H., Horstmann, T., Völzke, E. & Völz, C. (1970): Centrencephalic myoclonic-astatic petit mal.: clinical and genetic investigations. *Neuropädiatrie* **2,** 59–78.

Gastaut, H., Roger, J., Soularyol, R., Tassinari, C.A., Regis, H. & Dravet, C. (1966): Childhood epileptic encephalopathy with diffuse slow spike-waves (otherwise known as 'petit mal variant') or Lennox–Gastaut syndrome. *Epilepsia* **7,** 139–179.

Gastaut, H. & Regis, H.(1961): On the subject of Lennox's 'akinetic' petit mal: in memory of W.G. Lennox, *Epilepsia* **2,** 298–305.

Gibbs, F.A. & Gibbs, E.L. (1952): *Atlas of electroencephalography*. Cambridge, Mass.: Addison Wesley Press

Hunt, J.R (1922): On the occurrence of static seizures in epilepsy. *J. Nerv. Ment. Dis.* **56,** 351.

Jackson, H. (1931): On a case of fits resembling those artificially produced in guinea-pigs. *Med. Soc. Proc.* 10 (1886b) 78. In: *Selected writings of John Hughlings Jackson*, ed. J. Taylor, Vol. 1, p. 362. London: Hodder & Stoughton.

Janz, D., Durner, M., Beck-Mannagetta, G. & Pantazis, G. (1989): Family studies on the genetics of juvenile myoclonic epilepsy (epilepsy with impulsive petit mal). In: *Genetics of the epilepsies,* eds. G. Beck-Mannagetta, V.E. Anderson, H. Doose & D. Janz, pp. 44–52. Berlin, Heidelberg, New York: Springer.

Kruse, R. (1968): Das myoklonisch–astatische petit mal. Berlin, Heidelberg, New York: Springer.

Lennox, W.G. (1945): The petit mal epilepsies: their treatment with tridione. JAMA **129,** 1068–1073.

Epileptic Seizures and Syndromes, Edited by Peter Wolf
© 1994 John Libbey & Company Ltd., pp. 169–173

Chapter 22

Genetics of juvenile myoclonic epilepsy

Martina Durner

Eberhard-Karls Universität, Klinikum Schnarrenberg, Abteilung Neurologie, Hoppe-Seyler Str. 3, 7400 Tübingen, Germany

Summary

JME is an epilepsy form which is almost exclusively genetically determined. The mode of inheritance is complex and probably more than one gene is needed for the expression of the disease. A two locus model of inheritance fits the observed data from segregation analysis, twin studies and perspective studies. With a likelihood of $10^{7.4}$: 1 there is strong evidence that a dominantly inherited gene is found on chromosome 6. But there are also indications that JME is genetically heterogeneous and clinical differentiation criteria should be found to distinguish the different genetic forms.

Introduction

It has been known for a long time that genetic factors play a role in epilepsy. Recent developments in genetic techniques have given us tools to enhance our understanding of the genetic basis of epilepsy and hence the underlying causes of the disease, with the ultimate goal of finding better treatment for these patients.

In this chapter the following questions will be addressed:

1. Why did we choose juvenile myoclonic epilepsy (JME) out of the diversity of epileptic syndromes for genetic studies?
2. What indication do we have for a genetic basis of JME and how strong is it?
3. What is the possible mode of inheritance of JME?
4. How close are we in finding a gene for JME?

Why JME?

One of the most feared confounding factors in genetic studies is that of heterogeneity. Heterogeneity refers to clinically similar or even indistinguishable diseases that have different aetiologies (which can be different genes or environmental factors). Obviously a heterogeneous data set makes the detection of a gene for one of the diseases very difficult. To minimize the possibility of heterogeneity an epileptic syndrome was chosen which by virtue of its clinical characteristics can be clearly differentiated from other forms of epilepsies.

JME seemed to fulfil all these criteria. JME is characterized by short jerks of the shoulders and arms and is the only form of idiopathic generalized epilepsy (IGE) which is experienced without loss of consciousness. The jerks occur mostly in the morning after awakening and are precipitated by lack of sleep and/or consumption of alcohol. These clear-cut symptoms made JME a better candidate for genetic studies than, for example, absence epilepsy. There are already clinical debates as to whether all absences are the same or whether they should be subdivided into childhood absences and juvenile absences, pyknoleptic *vs.* non-pyknoleptic absences (Janz, this volume), early childhood absences (Doose, this volume), myoclonic absences and absences with oral myoclonias, etc. (Tassinari & Michelucci, this volume; Panayiotopoulos *et al.*, this volume).

Another prerequisite was that the epilepsy chosen for genetic studies had to show a strong genetic component. About 30 per cent of patients with JME have a positive family history, a percentage as high as in all the other forms of idiopathic (and therefore believed to be more genetic) generalized epilepsies with age-dependent onset, but clearly higher than in symptomatic forms of epilepsy or focal epilepsy (Janz *et al.*, 1989).

Furthermore we wanted to study an epilepsy form with no known exogenous factors contributing to the aetiology of the disease. Janz (1969) called JME 'the prototype of essential epilepsy or the only form of epilepsy where the symptomatology alone excludes a symptomatic epilepsy' because he was not able to find any causal factors in his patients with JME nor were later investigators.

Indication for heritability of JME

Seventeen to fifty per cent of patients with JME have a genetic predisposition for epilepsy (Janz *et al.*, 1989). This proportion is similar to that found in other forms of IGE (idiopathic infantile spasms, 25 per cent (Doose, 1964), myoclonic astatic petit mal, 29 per cent (Kruse, 1968), childhood absences, 32 per cent (Matthes & Weber, 1968)), of which JME is part.

Tsuboi and Christian (1973) found 3.3 per cent of parents, 4.4 per cent of siblings and 5.1 per cent of children with epilepsy in families of JME patients. About the same proportions were found by Janz *et al.* (1989).

Since the family electroencephalographic (EEG) study in centrencephalic epilepsy by Metrakos & Metrakos (1961), it has been believed that epileptic activity in the EEG of otherwise healthy individuals can be a subclinical marker for epilepsy. When abnormal EEG findings in family members of JME patients are added to those who have epilepsy, the percentage of affected parents is 5.2 per cent, siblings 6.7 per cent and children 13.8 per cent.

Twin studies in IGE show an almost 100 per cent concordance rate in monozygotic twins compared with about 15 per cent in dizygotic twins (Conrad, 1935; Gedda & Tatarelli, 1971; Bercovic *et al.*, 1990). The ratio of the almost complete concordance in monozygotic twins versus the low dizygotic twin rate is an indication for an almost exclusive genetic aetiology of IGE.

Mode of transmission

Several modes of inheritance have been proposed for different epilepsies. From family studies and from everyday clinical experience it is clear that IGE, and JME specifically, does not follow a simple autosomal dominant or recessive mode of inheritance. The mode of inheritance must be more complex and the observed data cannot be explained by one fully penetrant gene. It was therefore thought that a single gene with reduced penetrance might better fit the data. Reduced penetrance is a phenomenon in which a person has the disease gene but does not express the clinical symptoms of the disease. The reduced penetrance was believed to depend upon environmental factors. The results of twin studies contradict this hypothesis. If, for example, the penetrance of a disease would be reduced by 30 per cent, one would expect that only 70 per cent of monozygotic twins are concordant for the disease.

The observed concordance rate of almost 100 per cent in IGE indicates that the disease is fully penetrant and that environmental factors play no role.

Tsuboi and Christian (1973) were the first to propose a polygenic mode of inheritance for JME. A polygenic mode of inheritance is defined by the inheritance of several genes, each contributing to the expression of the phenotype by a small and additive effect. Hodge *et al.* (1989) tested a polygenic model in two different data sets and found it unfavourable but could not reject this model. A model requiring two interacting loci was also tested. Greenberg *et al.* (1988a) performed a formal segregation analysis in 21 families of JME patients. They were able to exclude a simple recessive mode of inheritance and a two-locus model where both the genes are dominantly inherited. They could not reject models of a two-gene inheritance with one gene dominantly and the other recessively or both recessively inherited.

Further support of a two-locus model comes from twin studies and from prospective studies of children where one parent has epilepsy. Under a two-locus – dominant and recessive – model of inheritance, the expected concordance rate in monozygotic twins is 100 per cent, whereas in dizygotic twins the concordance rate is 12.5 per cent, which is close to the observed rate of 15 per cent in IGE. Follow-up studies of children of epileptic parents have the advantage that they have less ascertainment bias, a crucial point which confounds many segregation analyses. Beck-Mannagetta *et al.* (1989) found that about 9–13 per cent of children of an epileptic parent with IGE also have epilepsy and/or spike-wave discharges in the EEG. Under the assumption of simple dominant inheritance 50 per cent of the children would be expected to be affected and under a recessive mode of inheritance around 4 per cent, because only when the unaffected parent is a carrier is there a chance of a child being affected. Under a two-locus model the expected rate of affected children is 15 per cent when one gene is dominantly and the other recessively transmitted and 10 per cent when both genes are recessive (Greenberg *et al.*, 1992). Therefore the observed epilepsy and/or spike-wave rate in children of epileptic parent of 9–13 per cent would fit a two-locus model.

Linkage analysis in JME

One of the frequently used methods to find a gene is linkage analysis. The basic principle for this method is that two genes on the same chromosome are usually inherited together and therefore are called linked, as long as they are not separated through crossing over during meiosis. The further apart they are from each other, the more likely it is that a crossing over between them occurs. In linkage analysis one looks for the co-segregation (common inheritance) of the disease gene and a marker gene whose chromosomal localization is known. The likelihood of the observed constellation under linkage is compared with the likelihood under no linkage. The ratio of these two likelihoods is called the lod score. A lod score of 3 or $10^3 : 1$ in favour of linkage is generally considered significant evidence for linkage, whereas a lod score of –2 means there is no linkage between the marker and the disease.

Greenberg *et al.* (1988b) tested 31 markers randomly scattered over the genome for linkage in families ascertained through JME patients. They considered family members with idiopathic generalized epilepsy and/or spike wave in the EEG as affected. Only the marker Bf/human leucocyte antigen (HLA) provided them positive evidence for linkage. The updated highest maximum lod score was 4.2 under a dominant mode of inheritance and 90 per cent penetrance (Greenberg *et al.*, 1993). This linkage was confirmed by an independent study group (Durner *et al.*, 1991), who found a lod score of 4.1, also assuming a dominant mode of inheritance and 90 per cent penetrance and classifying family members with JME, epilepsy with absences or generalized tonic–clonic seizures (GTCS) or generalized epileptic activity in the EEG as affected. When family members who only had abnormal EEGs but no epilepsy were called normal for the analysis, the lod score was 3.9 at 70 per cent penetrance. The combined lod score of these two studies is 7.4, indicating 25 million : 1 in favour of linkage.

Since these studies were published, more families have been collected by several other groups. Their results are not as clear, even though they still provide positive evidence for linkage with HLA. Whitehouse *et al.* (1993) reported a small positive lod score of 1.4 in mostly multiplex families of JME patients at a higher recombination rate than reported by Greenberg *et al.* (1993) or Durner *et al.* (1991). Therefore these results may invite a hypothesis of heterogeneity in JME. The New York group found a lod score of 1.7 in their JME families under a dominant mode of inheritance but at 50 per cent penetrance. This penetrance value probably reflects better the 'true' or expected penetrance because both the above-mentioned studies are biased towards multiplex families (i.e. families with more than one affected family member). Some of these families in New York show negative lod scores, also indicating that there might be genetic heterogeneity within JME. However, the dataset is too small to make statistical inferences about heterogeneity. Therefore the linkage data from Greenberg *et al.* (1993) and Durner *et al.* (1991) and the New York study group were pooled to perform a heterogeneity test. The admixture test (Hodge *et al.*, 1983) was chosen to test for heterogeneity. But even then we were unable to demonstrate heterogeneity. This failure to *prove* heterogeneity does not mean that heterogeneity is *excluded.* For this many more families are needed (Cavalli-Sforza & King, 1986; Martinez & Goldin, 1989).

Heterogeneity in neurological genetic diseases is no longer an uncommonly observed phenomenon. For example, in Charcot–Marie–Tooth disease, a hereditary motor and sensory neuropathy, linkage was first established to the Duffy blood group on chromosome 1 by several groups (Bird *et al.*, 1982; Guiloff *et al.*, 1982). Soon thereafter, families with clear absence of linkage were found, thus demonstrating heterogeneity. In those families unlinked to Duffy, linkage was then found with chromosome 17 markers (Vance *et al.*, 1989). Another example is benign familial neonatal seizures, a rare epilepsy form which ranks first on the age scale among age-related forms of IGE. Even in this distinct syndrome with a simple autosomal dominant inheritance, there is evidence that some families are linked to chromosome 20 (Leppert *et al.*, 1989) and some are unlinked (Ryan *et al.*, 1991). Recently, linkage to the same markers on chromosome 20 was found with low-voltage EEG (Steinlein *et al.*, 1992), but only in about 30 per cent of the families. It would not be surprising to find that in a complex disease group like epilepsy even subsets (syndromes) are genetically heterogeneous.

The goal for future studies is to find possible clinical features which might help us to differentiate different forms of JME. It is of utmost importance to be more stringent in the selection criteria to ensure a more homogeneous patient group and to avoid possible misdiagnosis.

References

Beck-Mannagetta, G., Janz, D., Hoffmeister, U., Behl, I. & Scholz, G. (1989): Morbid risk for seizures and epilepsy in offspring of patients with epilepsy. In: *Genetics of the epilepsies*, eds. G. Beck-Mannagetta, V.E. Anderson, H. Doose & D. Janz, pp. 119–126. Berlin: Springer Verlag.

Bercovic, F.S., Howell, R.A., Hopper, J.L., Hay, D.A. & Andermann, E. (1990): A twin study of the epilepsies. *Epilepsia* **31,** 813.

Bird, T.S., Ott, J. & Giblett, E.R. (1982): Evidence for linkage of Charcot–Marie–Tooth neuropathy to the Duffy locus on chromosome 1. *Am. J. Hum. Genet.* **34,** 388–394.

Cavalli-Sforza, L.L. & King, M.C. (1986): Detecting linkage for genetically heterogeneous diseases and detecting heterogeneity with linkage data. *Am. J. Hum. Genet.* **38,** 599–616.

Conrad, K. (1935): Erbanlage und Epilepsie: Untersuchungen an einer Serie von 253 Zwillingspaaren. *Z. Ges. Neurol. Psychiatr.* **153,** 271–291.

Doose, H. (1964): Zur Nosologie der Blitz-Nick-Salaamkraempfe. *Arch. Psychiatr. Nervenkr.* **206**, 28–48.

Durner, M., Sander, T., Greenberg, D.A., Johnson, K., Beck- Mannagetta, G. & Janz, D. (1991): Localization of idiopathic generalized epilepsy on chromosome 6p in families of juvenile myoclonic epilepsy patients. *Neurology* **41,** 1651–1655.

Gedda, L. & Tatarelli, R. (1971): Essential isochronic epilepsy in MZ twin pairs. *Acta Genet. Med. Germellol.* **20,** 380–383.

Giuloff, R.J., Thomas, P.K., Contreras, M., Armitage, S., Schwarz, G. & Sedgwick, E.M. (1982): Evidence for linkage of type 1 hereditary motor and sensory neuropathy to the Duffy locus on chromosome 1. *Ann. Hum. Genet.* **46,** 25–27

Greenberg, D.A., Delgado-Escueta, A.V., Maldonado, H.M. & Widelitz, H. (1988a): Segregation analysis of juvenile myoclonic epilepsy. *Genet. Epidemiol.* **5,** 81–94.

Greenberg, D.A., Delgado-Escueta, A.V., Widelitz, H., Sparkes, R.S., Treiman, L., Maldonado, H.M., Park, M.S. & Terasake, P.I. (1988b): Juvenile myoclonic epilepsy (JME) may be linked to the Bf and HLA loci on human chromosome 6. *Am. J. Med. Genet.* **31,** 185–192.

Greenberg, D.A. & Delgado-Escueta, A.V. (1993): The chromosome 6p epilepsy locus: exploring mode of inheritance and heterogeneity through linkage analysis. *Epilepsia* **34 (Suppl),** S12–S18.

Greenberg, D.A., Durner, M. & Delgado-Escueta, A.V. (1992): Evidence for multiple gene loci in the expression of the common generalized epilepsies. *Neurology* **42** (Suppl.), 56–62.

Hodge, S.E., Anderson, C.E., Neiswanger, K., Sparkes, R.S. & Rimoin, D.L. (1983): The search for heterogeneity in insulin dependent diabetes mellitus (IDDM): linkage studies, two-locus models, and genetic heterogeneity. *Am. J. Hum. Genet.* **35,** 1139–1155.

Hodge, S.E., Greenberg, D.A., Durner, M., Delgado-Escueta, A.V. & Janz, D. (1989): Is juvenile myoclonic epilepsy polygenic? In: *Genetics of the epilepsies*, eds. G. Beck-Mannagetta, V.E. Anderson, H. Doose & D. Janz, pp. 62–67. Berlin: Springer Verlag.

Janz, D. (1969): *Die Epilepsien*. Berlin: Springer Verlag.

Janz, D., Durner, M., Beck-Mannagetta, G. & Pantazis, G. (1989): Family studies on the genetics of juvenile myoclonic epilepsy (epilepsy with impulsive petit mal). In: *Genetics of the epilepsies*, eds. G. Beck-Mannagetta, V.E. Anderson, H. Doose & D. Janz, pp. 43–52. Berlin: Springer Verlag.

Kruse, R. (1968): *Das myoclonisch-astatische Petit mal.* Berlin: Springer Verlag.

Leppert, M., Anderson, V.E., Quattlebaum, T., Stauffer, D., O'Connell, P., Nakamura, Y., Lalouel, J.M. & White, R. (1989): Benign familial neonatal convulsions linked to genetic markers on chromosome 20. *Nature* **337,** 647–648.

Martinez, M.M. & Goldin, L.R. (1989): The detection of linkage and heterogeneity in nuclear families for complex disorders: one versus two marker loci. *Am. J. Hum. Genet.* **44,** 552–559.

Matthes, A. & Weber, H. (1968): Klinische und elektroencephalographische Familienuntersuchungen bei Pyknolepsien. *Dtsch. Med. Wschr.* **93,** 429–435.

Metrakos, K. & Metrakos, J.D. (1961): Genetics of convulsive disorders. II. Genetics and electroencephalographic studies in centrencephalic epilepsy. *Neurolgy* **11,** 414–483.

Ryan, S.G., Wiznitzer, M., Hollman, C., Torres, M.C., Szekeresova, M. & Schneider, S. (1991): Benign familial neonatal convulsions: evidence for clinical and genetic heterogeneity. *Ann. Neurol.* **29,** 469–473.

Steinlein, O., Anokhin, A., Yping, M., Schalt, E. & Vogel, F. (1992): Localisation of a gene for the human low-voltage EEG on 20q and genetic heterogeneity. *Genomics* **12,** 69–73.

Tsuboi, T. & Christian, W. (1973): Genetics of primary generalized epilepsy with sporadic myoclonias of impulsive petit mal type. *Humangenetik* **19,** 155–182.

Vance, J.M., Nicholson, G.A., Yamaoka, L.H., Stajich, J., Stewart, C.S., Speer, M.C., Hung, W.Y., Roses, A.D., Barker, D. & Pericak-Vance, M.K. (1989): Linkage of Charcot–Marie–Tooth neuropathy type 1a to chromosome 17. *Exp. Neurol.* **104,** 186–189.

Whitehouse, W.P., Rees, M., Curtis, D., Sunquist, A., Parker, K., Chung, E., Baralle, D. & Gardiner, R.M. (1993): Linkage analysis of idiopathic generalized epilepsy (IGE) and marker loci on chromosome 6p in families of patients with juvenile myoclonic epilepsy: no evidence for an epilepsy locus in the HLA region. *Am. J. Hum. Genet.* **53,** 652–662.

Epileptic Seizures and Syndromes, Edited by Peter Wolf
© 1994 John Libbey & Company Ltd., pp. 175–181

Chapter 23

Genetically determined changes of glutamate receptors: implications for epilepsy

Georg Köhr

ZMBH, Universität Heidelberg, Im Neuenheimer Feld 282, 69120 Heidelberg, Germany

Summary

Ionotropic glutamate receptors in the central nervous system comprise a gene family of more than 16 members. The molecular and functional diversity is increased by post-transcriptional modifications (alternative splicing and RNA editing). Structure–function studies in defined, recombinantly expressed glutamate receptors have elucidated important functional determinants (e.g. calcium permeability of AMPA receptors) which may play an important role in epileptogenesis. In particular, disturbed regulatory mechanisms underlying expression or modification of individual glutamate receptor subunits may be involved in epilepsy. The emerging success of linkage analysis in correlating aspects of familial epilepsies with glutamate receptor genes offers hope to identify epilepsy genes in the future.

Introduction

Genetic approaches have provided important insights concerning neurogenetic diseases. Genes responsible for some neurological and neuropsychiatric disorders have been localized and characterized (e.g. Huntington's disease). In contrast, genes involved in familial epilepsies or seizure generation are as yet unidentified. Linkage analysis and the subsequent identification of candidate genes may help to locate genes responsible for epilepsies (Rise *et al.*, 1991). Excitatory and inhibitory transmitters, both being involved in seizure initiation and their propagation, are potential candidates. Glutamate is the principal excitatory neurotransmitter in the central nervous system. Glutamate activates two different types of cation-selective channels, the non-*N*-methyl-D-aspartate (NMDA) (α-amino-3-hydroxy-5-methyl-4-isoxazole propionate (AMPA), kainate) and the NMDA receptors. These receptors mediate synaptic transmission and neuronal plasticity and also contribute to epileptiform activity and neurotoxicity in a number of experimental and pathological conditions (Dingledine *et al.*, 1990).

Recently, closely related glutamate receptor subunits, all belonging to the same gene family, have been analysed by molecular cloning (for review see Gasic & Hollmann, 1992; Nakanishi, 1992; Sommer & Seeburg, 1992). The glutamate receptor superfamily can be divided into subfamilies because of high amino acid sequence identities and because of common pharmacological properties.

The AMPA receptor family comprises the subunits GluR-A to GluR-D (also called GluR-1 to GluR-4), the high-affinity kainate receptor family the subunits GluR-5 to GluR-7, KA-1 and KA-2 and the NMDA receptor family the subunits NMDAR1 (NR1) and NMDAR2A to NMDAR2D (NR2A–NR2D). Additional subunits have been found (Lomeli *et al.*, 1993). All subunits are approximately 1000 amino acids in length and are predicted to contain four transmembrane regions (TM1 to TM4). After selectively assembling into functional receptor channels, the receptor subunits can be studied, using heterologous expression systems. In the brain, read-out of individual receptor subunit genes is probably controlled by development and pathophysiological events. Depending on the subunit combination, receptor channels with different properties emerge. Additional functional variability can be generated post-transcriptionally (alternative splicing and mRNA editing) or posttranslationally (e.g. phosphorylation; for review see Raymond *et al.*, 1993), resulting in micro-heterogeneity of individual subunits.

This chapter does not want to compete with glutamate receptor overviews referenced above, but rather should stimulate physicians to become acquainted with recent basic research in glutamate receptors. Therefore, this chapter briefly describes alternative splicing and mRNA editing and focuses on possible functional consequences in pathophysiological situations. The last paragraph speculates how glutamate-directed gene expression might participate in epilepsy.

Results and discussion

Alternative splicing

The expression of a single gene can be regulated to produce different forms of a protein by alternative splicing of a single primary RNA transcript. This post-transcriptional regulation exists in some families of ligand-gated ion channels. In general, proteins of comparable function are produced. Within the glutamate receptor superfamily, splice variants impart different (Sommer *et al.*, 1990; Sugihara *et al.*, 1992) or not yet identified (Bettler *et al.*, 1990; Gallo *et al.*, 1992; Sommer *et al.*, 1992) pharmacological and kinetic properties. Functionally different splice products were first found for the AMPA receptor genes (Sommer *et al.*, 1990). In each receptor (GluR-A to GluR-D) a small segment (38 of about 1000) of the amino acid sequence preceding the predicted fourth transmembrane region exists in two versions having different amino acid sequences (Fig. 1). The alternative products (termed Flip and Flop) show different pharmacological and kinetic profiles on agonist-evoked currents. Glutamate-activated currents show an initial fast desensitizing component followed by a steady-state component. Both components are significantly larger in cells expressing the Flip version (Sommer *et al.*, 1990).

In situ hybridization experiments using GluR-Flip or GluR-Flop probes showed distinct expression patterns of alternatively spliced mRNAs in the rat brain, particularly in the hippocampus. The Flip forms are abundantly expressed in CA1 and CA3 pyramidal cells, whereas the Flop forms are virtually lacking in the latter. In the dentate gyrus of the hippocampus a higher expression of Flop relative to Flip forms exists. The cell-specific expression of Flip and Flop correlates with glutamate- or

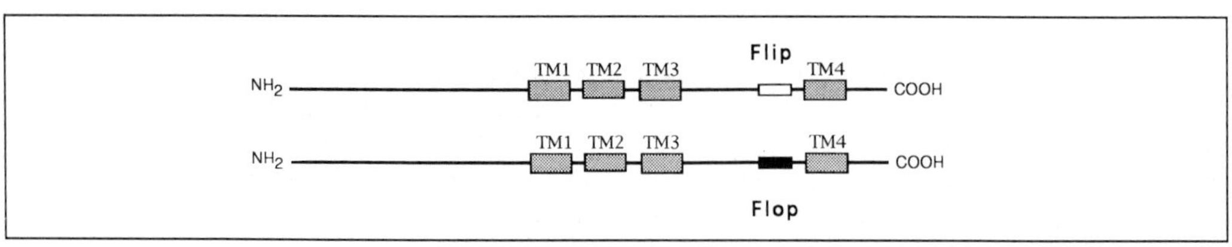

Fig. 1 Relative position of alternatively spliced exons (Flip and Flop) in the coding region of the GluR-A to GluR-D transcripts. The locations of four putative transmembrane regions (TM1-TM4) are indicated. For details see Sommer et al. (1990).

AMPA-activated peak and steady-state currents in rat hippocampal neurones (Jonas & Sakmann, 1992).

If different splice products of one receptor gene coexist in the same cell, their individual expression may vary with neuronal activity. Indeed, the expression of Flip and Flop is controlled by development (Monyer *et al.*, 1991). During postnatal life (postnatal days 1, 8 and 14 (P1, P8 and P14)) the expression of the Flip forms remains largely constant. In contrast, the Flop forms are expressed at low levels prior to P8, reaching adult levels by P14. Thus, the dominance of the Flip module during early development and the delayed addition of the Flop seem crucial for development.

Another condition which clearly involves neuronal activity that might influence alternative splicing is epilepsy. Kindling, an animal model of epilepsy, is induced by repeated application of initially subconvulsive electrical stimulations, which eventually results in long-lasting, generalized tonic–clonic seizures (Goddard *et al.*, 1969). Kamphuis and his colleagues (1992) studied the expression pattern of the GluR-A and GluR-B splice variants in brains of control and kindled rats. Control rats showed a higher expression of Flop relative to Flip mRNAs in dentate gyrus granule cells. In kindled granule cells the expression level of the Flip variant was *bilaterally* enhanced 24 h after the last seizure. However, the increased Flip expression pattern returned to control levels 28 days after the last seizure. Therefore, an increased glutamate receptor sensitivity, due to the presence of the Flip forms, might have contributed to the establishment of the kindling phenomenon.

In order to detect subunit- and splice-form specific differences in AMPA receptor gene expression involved in human epilepsy, expression of the GluR-A to GluR-D genes and their splice forms should be studied in the human brain. Especially studies comparing AMPA receptor expression in human epileptic brains and brains from patients with no neurological disease should be useful. A first study in the human hippocampus using GluR-A and GluR-B probes did not confirm the cell-specific expression of Flip and Flop seen in the rat hippocampus (McLaughlin *et al.*, 1993). Future experiments including GluR-C and GluR-D probes may clarify this discrepancy.

In addition, a potential involvement of the glutamate receptor gene family in inherited human central nervous system (CNS) disorders (including epilepsy) can also be studied by correlating the chromosomal localization of human receptor genes with loci of human diseases. Several glutamate receptor genes and a number of mutant genes underlying different familial epilepsies have already been mapped. GluR-A to GluR-D genes have been mapped to human chromosome 5q32–33, 4q32–33, Xq 25–26 and 11q22–23, respectively (e.g. McNamara *et al.*, 1992), GluR-5 to chromosome 21q21.1–22.1 (Eubanks *et al.*, 1993) and NR1 to chromosome 9q34.3 (Karp *et al.*, 1993). Benign neonatal convulsions (20q), juvenile myoclonic epilepsy (6q), progressive myoclonic epilepsy (21q22.3) and tuberous sclerosis (11q23 in some families, 9q34 in others) were also chromosomally localized (McNamara, 1992). Therefore, GluR-D and NR1 are candidate genes for tuberous sclerosis. To show definitive linkage GluR-D or NR1 genes should be localized and cloned from patients with tuberous sclerosis. Introducing the cloned genes into transgenic animals in order to examine disease expression may confirm their pathological functions.

RNA editing

Studies in native brain membranes suggested a high calcium permeability of NMDA receptor channels and a low calcium permeability of non-NMDA (AMPA, kainate) receptor channels. However, ion flow measurements through recombinant AMPA receptor channels detected differences in their divalent permeability (Verdoorn *et al.*, 1991; Hollmann *et al.*, 1991). Expression of GluR-A, C and D subunits to form homo-oligomeric (homomeric) receptors or co-expression of them to form heteromeric receptors (in the absence of GluR-B) results in receptor channels which show doubly rectifying current voltage (IV) relationships and which are permeable to calcium. In contrast, homomeric GluR-B channels and heteromeric receptor channels containing the GluR-B subunit show simple outward rectiflcation and reduced calcium permeability. These experiments suggested that the

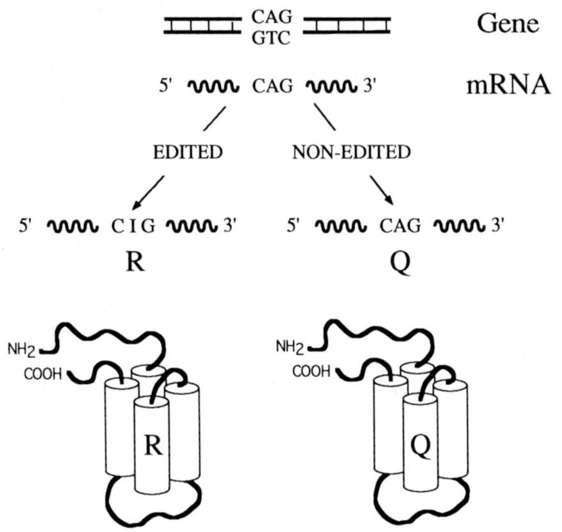

Fig. 2. It is proposed that mRNA editing of an adenosine to inosine gives rise to an arginine (R) instead of a glutamine (Q) in the TM2-coding region of glutamate receptor transcripts. For details see Sommer et al. (1991).

GluR-B subunit, when assembled with other subunits into heteromeric channels, determines ion conductance properties of receptor channel mosaics.

Molecular analysis revealed a single amino acid difference within the putative channel-forming region (TM2) controlling ion flow through AMPA receptor channels (Sommer *et al.*, 1991). GluR-B carries a positively charged arginine (R) where the other three subunits carry the neutral glutamine (Q). This site is referred to as the Q/R site (Fig. 2). The mechanism by which the arginine in GluR-B is generated is called RNA editing, an enzyme-directed, post-transcriptional modification of RNA transcripts. The gene for the GluR-B subunit specifies a glutamine residue as does the gene for the GluR-A, C and D subunits. In the mRNA transcript of GluR-B, however, there is a single nucleotide exchange, giving rise to an R instead of a Q in the TM2 region of the receptor protein. RNA editing in GluR-B is highly selective (as the GluR-A, C and D subunits are not targeted) and highly efficient since virtually no glutamine-containing GluR-B subunit is found in the adult brain.

Therefore, it was predicted that cells with calcium-permeable AMPA receptor channels lack the GluR-B subunit or incorporate the unedited form of GluR-B. Indeed, cerebellar Bergmann glial cells lacking expression of the GluR-B gene (Sommer *et al.*, 1990) contain calcium-permeable AMPA receptor channels (Burnashev *et al.*, 1992; Müller *et al.*, 1992). In contrast, hippocampal CA1 and CA3 pyramidal neurones expressing GluR-B show a very low calcium permeability (Jonas & Sakmann, 1992).

Regulation of GluR-B gene expression might serve to set the level of calcium influx through glutamate-activated receptor channels. Sustained calcium influx resulting in increased cytoplasmic free calcium concentration is thought to play an important role in glutamate-mediated neuronal plasticity (Meldrum & Garthwaite, 1990). To determine the function of GluR-B gene expression in epilepsy, its expression pattern should be studied in epileptic brains. In another pathological state, global ischaemia, relative GluR-B gene expression was reported to be reduced (Pellegrini-Giampietro *et al.*, 1992) but other studies indicate reduced mRNAs of all four AMPA receptors in rat hippocampal CA1 neurones (H. Monyer & T. Wieloch, pers. comm.). Further *in situ* hybridization studies of other brain areas vulnerable to ischaemia may solve this controversy.

RNA editing also occurs in the TM2 segment of GluR-5 and GluR-6 but is less efficient than in GluR-B. Recently, two additional amino acid residues located in TM1 of GluR-6 were reported to be targeted by RNA editing, with functional consequences for glutamate-activated calcium permeability (Köhler *et al.*, 1993). Since edited, hemiedited and unedited TM1 forms coexist with either edited or unedited TM2 forms, eight GluR variants occur at different frequencies, displaying a considerable range of calcium permeabilities.

Glutamate receptor-directed gene expression

In the brain, the maintenance of long-lasting plasticity changes may depend upon protein synthesis involving specific gene expression. The notion that changes in gene expression underlie some of the long-lasting structural and functional alterations observed in epilepsy gains support from several findings. Neurotransmitter-binding sites are known to increase in the epileptic brain (Yeh *et al.*, 1989). Second, the development of kindling-induced epilepsy is impaired if protein synthesis is blocked (Jonec *et al.*, 1979). Third, seizures and a kindled stimulus induce immediate early gene (IEG) expression (Labiner *et al.*, 1993; for review see Morgan & Curran, 1991). Fourth, kindling-induced epilepsy selectively changes expression of a membrane-associated protein (Perlin *et al.*, 1993). Most IEGs (like c-*fos* or c-*jun*; but see Qian *et al.*, 1993) encode transcription factors that bind to DNA at sites known to stimulate or inhibit the transcription of target genes. However, a transiently actived IEG expression cannot account for all persistent structural, functional and behavioural changes associated with neuronal excitability.

Recently, non-NMDA and NMDA receptor stimulation has been shown to activate c-*fos* gene transcription by distinct calcium signalling pathways (Bading *et al.*, 1993; Lerea & McNamara, 1993). Whether this differential signal processing can regulate gene expression of distinct targets is not known. But kindling-induced epilepsy, which critically depends on NMDA receptor activation, induces changes in gene expression that might be involved in the maintenance of kindling (Perlin *et al.*, 1993; Qian *et al.*, 1993). Therefore, genes like NMDA receptor genes, which are involved in activity-dependent synaptic plasticity, are potential candidates in a glutamate-activated and IEG-mediated pathway of effector gene expression. As NMDA receptor expression (H. Monyer, J. Laurie & P.H. Seeburg, unpublished) and NMDA receptor function (Carmignoto & Vicini, 1992; Hestrin, 1992) are regulated during development, they may also be modulated in some forms of long-lasting changes in neuronal excitability. Once kindling-induced epilepsy is generated, the NMDA component of synaptic transmission is enhanced in the hippocampal dentate gyrus of kindled rats (Mody & Heinemann, 1987) and epileptic patients (Urban *et al.*, 1990). The enhanced synaptic excitability in the kindled brain might be due to the prolonged openings of the NMDA receptor channels (Köhr *et al.*, 1993). A switch in NMDA receptor subunit expression or modifications in functionally important domains of the NMDA receptor subunits (e.g. phosphorylation) might be responsible for structural and functional changes in the synaptic efficacy during development as well as following excessive neuronal activity associated with the progression of epileptogenesis.

Acknowledgements

I wish to thank my colleagues, particularly Peter H. Seeburg, Martin Köhler and Rolf Sprengel, for helpful suggestions and comments. Supported by a Bundesministerium für Forschung und Technologie (BMFT) (Helmholtz) Fellowship.

References

Bading, H., Ginty, D.D & Greenberg, M.E. (1993): Regulation of gene expression in hippocampal neurons by distinct calcium signaling pathways. *Science* **260,** 181–186.

Bettler, B., Boulter, J., Hermans-Borgmeyer, I., O'Shea-Greenfield, Deneris, E.S., Moll, C., Borgmeyer, U., Hollmann, M. & Heinemann, S. (1990): Cloning of a novel glutamate receptor subunit, GluR5: expression in the nervous system during development. *Neuron.* **5,** 583–595.

Burnashev, N., Khodorova, A., Jonas, P. Helm, P.J., Wisden, W., Monyer, H., Seeburg, P.H. & Sakmann, B. (1992): Calcium-permeable AMPA-kainate receptors in fusiform cerebellar glial cells. *Science* **256,** 1566–1570.

Carmignoto, G. & Vicini, S. (1992): Activity-dependent decrease in NMDA receptor responses during development of the visual cortex. *Science* **258,** 1007–1011.

Dingledine, R, McBain, C.J. & McNamara, J.O. (1990): Excitatory amino acid receptors in epilepsy. *Trends Pharmacol. Sci.* **11,** 334–338.

Eubanks, J.H., Puranam, R.S., Kleckner, N.W., Bettler, B., Heinemann, S.F. & McNamara, J.O. (1993): The gene encoding the glutamate receptor subunit GluR5 is located on human chromosome 21q21.1-22.1 in the vicinity of the gene for familial amyotrophic lateral sclerosis. *Proc. Natl. Acad. Sci. USA* **90,** 178–182.

Gallo, V., Upson, L.M., Hayes, W.P., Vyklicky, L., Jr, Winters, C.A. & Buonanno, A. (1992): molecular cloning and developmental analysis of a new glutamate receptor subunit isoform in cerebellum. *J. Neurosci.* **12,** 1010–1023.

Gasic, G.P. & Hollmann, M. (1992): Molecular neurobiology of glutamate receptors. *Annu. Rev. Physiol.* **54,** 507–536.

Goddard, G.V., McIntyre, D.C. & Leech, C.K. (1969): A permanent change in brain function resulting from daily electrical stimulation. *Exp. Neurol.* **25,** 295–330.

Hestrin, S. (1992): Developmental regulation of NMDA receptor-mediated synaptic currents at a central synapse. *Nature* **357,** 686–689.

Hollmann, M., Hartley, M. & Heinemann, S. (1991): Ca^{2+} permeability of KA-AMPA-gated glutamate receptor channels depends on subunit composition. *Science* **252,** 851–853.

Jonas, P. & Sakmann, B. (1992): Glutamate receptor channels in isolated patches from CAl and CA3 pyramidal cells of rat hippocampal slices. *J. Physiol.* **455,** 143–171.

Jonec, V., Masuoka, D. & Wasterlain, C.G. (1979): Effect of inhibitors of protein synthesis on the development of kindled seizures in rats. *Exp. Neurol.* **66,** 524–532.

Kamphuis, W., Monyer, H., de Rijk, T.C. & Lopes da Silva, F.H. (1992): Hippocampal kindling increases the expression of glutamate receptor-A Flip and -B Flip mRNA in dentate granule cells. *Neurosci. Lett.* **148,** 51–54.

Karp, S.J., Masu, M., Eki, T., Ozawa, K. & Nakanishi, S. (1993): Molecular cloning and chromosomal localization of the key subunit of the human *N*-methyl-D-aspartate receptor. *J. Biol. Chem.* **268,** 3728–3733.

Köhler, M., Burnashev, N., Sakmann, B. & Seeburg, P.H. (1993): Determination of Ca^{2+} permeability in both TM1 and TM2 of high affinity kainate receptor channels: diversity by RNA editing. *Neuron* **10,** 491–500.

Köhr, G., De Koninck, Y. & Mody, I. (1993): Properties of NMDA channels in acutely isolated epileptic (kindled) neurons. *J. Neurosci.* **13,** 3612–3627.

Labiner, D.M., Butler, LS., Cao, Z., Hosford, D.A., Shin, C. & McNamara, J.A. (1993): Induction of c-*fos* mRNA by kindled seizures: complex relationship with neuronal burst firing. *J. Neurosci.* **13,** 744–751.

Lerea, L.S. & McNamara, J.O. (1993): Ionotropic glutamate receptor subtypes activate c-*fos* transcription by distinct calcium-requiring intracellular signaling pathways. *Neuron* **10,** 31–41.

Lomeli, H., Sprengel, R., Laurie, D.J., Köhr, G., Herb, A., Seeburg, P.H. & Wisden, W. (1993): The rat delta-1 and delta-2 subunits extend the excitatory amino acid receptor family. *FEBS Lett.* **315,** 318–322.

McLaughlin, D.P., Cheetham, M.E. & Kerwin, R.W. (1993): Expression of alternatively-spliced glutamate receptors in human hippocampus. *Eur. J. Pharmacol.* **244,** 89–92.

McNamara, J.O. (1992): The neurobiological basis of epilepsy. *Trends Neurosci.* **15,** 357–359.

McNamara, J.O., Eubanks, J.H., McPherson, J.D., Wasmuth, J.J., Evans, G.A. & Heinemann, S.F. (1992): Chromosomal localization of human glutamate receptor genes. *J. Neurosci.* **12,** 2555–2562.

Meldrum, B. & Garthwaite, J. (1990): Excitatory amino acid neurotoxicity and neurodegenerative disease. *Trends Pharmacol. Sci.* **11,** 379–387.

Mody, I. & Heinemann U. (1987): NMDA receptors of dentate gyrus granule cells participate in synaptic transmission following kindling. *Nature* **326,** 701–704.

Monyer, H., Seeburg, P.H. & Wisden, W. (1991): Glutamate-operated channels: developmentally early and mature forms arise by alternative splicing. *Neuron* **6,** 799–810.

Morgan, J.I. & Curran, T. (1991): Proto-oncogene transcription factors and epilepsy. *Trends Pharmacol. Sci.* **12,** 343–349.

Müller, T., Möller, T., Berger, T., Schnitzer, J. & Kettenmann, H. (1992): Calcium entry through kainate receptors and resulting potassium-channel blockade in Bergmann glial cells. *Science* **256,** 1563–1566.

Nakanishi, S. (1992): Molecular diversity of glutamate receptors and implications for brain function. *Science* **258,** 597–603.

Pellegrini-Giampietro, D.E., Zukin, R.S., Bennett, M.V.L., Cho, S. & Pulsinelli, W.A. (1992): Switch in glutamate receptor subunit gene expression in CA1 subfleld of hippocampus following global ischemia in rats. *Proc. Natl. Acad. Sci. USA* **89,** 10499–10503.

Perlin, J.B., Gerwin, C.M., Panchision, D.M., Vick, R.S., Jakoi, E.R. & DeLorenzo, R.J., (1993): Kindling produces long-lasting and selective changes in gene expression of hippocampal neurons. *Proc. Nat. Acad. Sci. USA* **90,** 1741–1745.

Qian, Z., Gilbert, M.E., Colicos, M.A., Kandel, E.R. & Kuhl, D. (1993): Tissue-plasminogen activator is induced as an immediate-early gene during seizure, kindling and long-term potentiation. *Nature* **361,** 453–457.

Raymond, L.A., Blackstone, C.D. & Huganir, R.L. (1993): Phosphorylation of amino acid neurotransmitter receptors in synaptic plasticity. *TiNS* **16,** 147–153.

Rise, M.L, Frankel, W.N., Coffin, J.M. & Seyfried, T.N. (1991): Genes for epilepsy mapped in the mouse. *Science* **253,** 669–673.

Sommer, B. & Seeburg, P.H. (1992): Glutamate receptor channels: novel properties and new clones. *TiPS* **13,** 291–296.

Sommer, B., Keinänen, K., Verdoorn, T.A., Wisden, W., Burnashev, N., Köhler, M., Takagi, T., Sakmann, B. & Seeburg, P.H. (1990): Flip and Flop: a cell-specific functional switch in glutamate-operated channels of the CNS. *Science* **249,** 1580–1585.

Sommer, B., Köhler, M., Sprengel, R. & Seeburg, P.H. (1991): RNA editing in brain controls a determinant of ion flow in glutamate-gated channels. *Cell* **67,** 11–19.

Sommer, B., Burnashev, N., Verdoorn, T.A., Keinanen, K., Sakmann, B. & Seeburg, P.H. (1992): A glutamate receptor channel with high affinity for domoate and kainate. *EMBO J.* **11,** 1651–1656.

Sugihara, H., Moriyoshi, K., Ishii, T., Masu, M. & Nakanishi, N. (1992): Structures and properties of seven isoforms of the NMDA receptor generated by alternative splicing. *Biochem. Biophys. Res. Comm.* **185,** 826–832.

Urban, L, Aitken, P.G., Friedman, A. & Somjen, G.G. (1990): An NMDA-mediated component of excitatory synaptic input to dentate gyrus granule cells in 'epileptic' human hippocampus studied *in vitro. Brain Res.* **515,** 319–322.

Verdoorn, T.A., Burnashev, N., Monyer, H., Seeburg, P.H. & Sakmann, B. (1991): Structural determinants of ion flow through recombinant glutamate receptor channels. *Science* **252,** 1715–1718.

Yeh, G.C., Bonhaus, D.W., Nadler, J.V. & McNamara J.O. (1989): *N*-Methyl-D-aspartate receptor plasticity in kindling: quantitative and qualitative alterations in the *N*-Methyl-D-aspartate receptor-channel complex. *Proc. Nat. Acad. Sci. USA* **86,** 8157–8160.

Epileptic Seizures and Syndromes, Edited by Peter Wolf
© 1994 John Libbey & Company Ltd., pp. 183–192

Chapter 24

Mapping epilepsy genes: a bridge between clinical and molecular studies

Victor Elving Anderson* and Stephen S. Rich†

**Epilepsy Clinical Research Program, Genetics and Epidemiology, 400 Church Street S.E., Minneapolis, MN 55455–0341, USA; †Box 206 UMHC, Institute of Human Genetics, University of Minnesota, Minneapolis, MN 55455, USA*

Summary

Gene mapping has been reported for three epilepsy syndromes, juvenile myoclonic epilepsy, benign familial neonatal convulsions and progressive myoclonus epilepsy of the Unverricht–Lundborg type. These differ in frequency, mode of inheritance, age at onset and other parameters, and illustrate the range of difficulties and prospective value in such studies. Although gene mapping is heavily dependent on molecular methodologies, clinicians will have a continuing significant role.

The ability to map disease genes by molecular methods is a relatively recent development. It was only some 20 years ago that the recombinant DNA era started, with the discovery of enzymes that are able to cut and to join DNA segments. Fifteen years ago it was recognized that restriction fragment length polymorphisms (RFLPs) could be used to map a disease gene to a specific place on the chromosomes. The first use of this methodology to map a disease gene (for Duchenne muscular dystrophy) was reported in 1982, with the sequencing and cloning of the gene itself (dystrophin) in 1985.

With reference to epilepsy research, Ray White outlined the potential value of gene mapping at a conference in Minneapolis in 1980 (White & Skolnick, 1982). Since that time, three epilepsy loci (to be discussed later) have been identified: juvenile myoclonic epilepsy (JME) (1987), benign familial neonatal convulsions (BFNC) (1989) and one form of progressive myoclonus epilepsy (PME) (1991). The growing use of molecular genetic strategies in epilepsy research, however, does not mean that the role of clinicians is being replaced. It is the purpose of this paper to outline the new areas of collaboration that are emerging.

The purposes of gene mapping

Gene mapping will contribute to our understanding of epilepsy in several ways: (1) The identification of specific chromosome loci confirms the hypothesis that genetic mutations are involved in the aetiology of certain epilepsies. (2) The diagnosis and recognition of subtypes of the epilepsy syndromes may be clarified. (3) Detection of early stages of the disease, and even susceptibility prior to the advent of any clinical signs, may be improved. (4) The ability to determine which family members have a genetic susceptibility to seizures will strengthen studies designed to analyse the contribution of environmental factors to seizure risk. (5) When a gene has been cloned and sequenced, comparison of the sequence with other known genes will permit tentative hypotheses about the nature and function of the gene product. Further molecular, cellular and clinical studies can then determine the pathogenetic mechanisms which lead from altered gene expression to the manifestation of seizures. (6) Finally, more rational modes of therapy can be developed.

There are at least 160 Mendelian, or single-locus, traits that increase the risk of seizures (Anderson & Hauser, 1993), and the genes for some of these (such as tuberous sclerosis and neurofibromatosis) have been mapped recently. It is also clear that seizures occur as part of mitochondrial syndromes resulting from mutations in mitochondrial or nuclear genes (DiMauro *et al.*, 1991). Another class of conditions leading to seizures is detectable at the cytogenetic level, such as Angelman syndrome (Fryburg *et al.*, 1991). Further attention in this paper, however, will be directed to those conditions in which seizures are the main presenting sign.

Gene mapping strategies

The basic goal of gene mapping is to find the specific chromosomal location (locus) of a gene that is involved in the pathogenesis of a specific epilepsy syndrome. This will make it possible to make many copies of that gene (by cloning) and sequence it (determine the DNA code).

The principal method is to test families with DNA markers that have already been mapped to specific loci. In the case of multigenerational families showing an autosomal dominant trait, for example, one looks for a marker that follows the trait down through the pedigree. The earlier studies used RFLPs, DNA segments that show population variation in length (White & Skolnick, 1982) when cleaved by enzymes (restriction endonucleases). Currently, short tandem repeat polymorphisms (STRPs) are commonly used; these include variable numbers of tandem repeats (VNTRs) and dinucleotide (two-base) repeats (Leppert *et al.*, 1991). Recent evidence implying that unstable repeated trinucleotide units may represent a common feature of several disorders that have neurological or behavioural features (Huntington's disease, myotonic dystrophy, spinocerebellar ataxia, and fragile-X syndrome) suggests that a genome-scanning approach (using a battery of polymorphic markers) may be feasible. Seldom does one have sufficient understanding of the pathogenesis of the epilepsies to restrict initial tests to one or a few candidate genes.

Two statistical measures are used in the data analysis. The *recombination frequency* (θ) estimates the distance between the disease locus and a given marker locus, with an upper limit of 0.50, which is equivalent to no linkage. The *lod score* is the $\log_{10}$ of the ratio between two probabilities: the chance of finding a given family if the disease and the marker are linked with a specified θ, divided by the chance if the markers are unlinked. Usually linkage is accepted at a lod score of +3 (odds of 1000 : 1 in favour of linkage) and rejected at a lod score of –2 (odds of 10 : 1 against linkage). Thus, for a given data set, linkage closer than $\theta = 0.10$ may be rejected, but more distant linkage may remain a possibility. If the limits for a gene search have been narrowed to $\theta = 0.01$, the physical distance is still about one million bases in the DNA molecule.

If linkage to a marker is identified, the current linkage map is reviewed to find potential *candidate* genes that can be included in further search. The candidates listed in Table 1 reflect a small sample of the rapidly expanding information about genes expressed in the brain. The list of 321 reference loci in the human, mouse, cattle and cat compiled by O'Brien *et al.* (1993) provides an excellent resource for reviewing animal studies to identify loci that may be relevant for human epilepsy. At this point in the research additional strategies are used to narrow the range and find the gene itself (Evans, 1991). A short cut is possible, however, if an affected individual is found to have a chromosomal break in the gene responsible for the disease. Such an event was a significant aid in identifying the gene which causes neurofibromatosis type 1 (Leppert *et al.*, 1991).

Table 1. Some neuronal candidate genes

MIM no.[1]	Gene product	Symbol	Chromosome[2]
Sodium channel, neuronal polypeptide			
182389	Type I α	NAC 1	21
182390	Type II α-1	NAC 2	2q23
	Type II α-2		2q23–q24
183291	Type III α	NAC3	?
Potassium voltage-gated channel			
176261	ISK-related[3]	KCNE1	21
176260	Shaker-related 1	KCNA1	12p13
176262	Shaker-related 2	KCNA2	12
176263	Shaker-related 3	KCNA3	1p13.3
176266	Shaker-related 4	KCNA4	11p14
176267	Shaker-related 5	KCNA5	12p13
176268	Shaker-related 7	KCNA7	19
	Shaw-related 1	KCNC1	11p15
	Shaw-related 2	KCNC2	12
176264	Shaw-related 3	KCNC3	19
176265	Shaw-related 4	KCNC4	1p21
GABA-A receptor polypeptide[4]			
137160	α-1	GABRA1	5q34
137140	α-2	GABRA2	4p13
305660	α-3	GABRA3	Xq28
	α-5	GABRA5	15q11
137190	β-1	GABRB1	4p13
137192	β-3	GABRB3	15q11.2[5]
137163	δ	GABRD	1p
	γ-1	GABRG1	4p14-q21.1
	γ-2	GABRG2	5q31.1
	ρ-1	GABRR1	6q14-q21
	ρ-2	GABRR2	?

[1]From Mendelian Inheritance in Man (MIM) (McKusick, 1992). First digit 1 = autosomal dominant, 2 = autosomal recessive; [2]p = short arm, q = long arm; followed by location, with band 11 closest to centromere; [3] X-linked recessive; [4] γ-aminobutyric acid receptor polypeptides; [5]in same region as Angelman syndrome.
[3] A new protein that induces a slow K^+ current (designated I_K).

The problems encountered in linkage studies and the potential implications of the identification and sequencing of the genes involved can now be discussed with reference to the three syndromes which are recognized primarily by the presence of seizures and for which linkage has been reported (Table 2).

Juvenile myoclonic epilepsy

JME is the first epilepsy syndrome for which linkage has been reported. The clinical features have been well described by Janz (1989). Photosensitivity is observed in about 30 per cent of the cases and a polyspike-and-wave electroencephalogram (EEG) in 39 per cent. The major finding, the myoclonic jerks, are not always recognized, however, and thus JME tends to be underdiagnosed and misdiagnosed. The estimated frequency of 1 per 2000 in the general population (Table 2) is an approximation based on a 1 per cent population risk for epilepsy by age 20 (Hauser *et al.*, 1993) and an estimate that JME constitutes 5 per cent of the epilepsies by that age.

Table 2. Clinical and genetic features of three epilepsy sydromes

Feature	Juvenile myoclonic epilepsy	Beningn familial neonatal convulsions	Progressive myoclonic epilepsy (Unverricht–Lundborg)
Population frequency	1 in 2000	1 in 100,000	1 in 20,000
Inheritance	Unknown	Autosomal dominant	Autosomal recessive
Penetrance	Unknown	85%	100%
Usual onset	12–18 years	First week	6–15 years
Epilepsy risk in siblings	8%	40–45%	25%
First linkage report	1987	1989	1991
MIM number[1]	254770	121200	254800
Locus	EJM1	EBN	EPM1
Chromosome location[2]	6p21.3	20q13.2–13.3	21p22.3
Linkage heterogeneity	Likely	Yes	None as yet

[1] From Mendelian inheritance in Man (MIM) (McKusick, 1992). First digit 1 = autosomal dominant, 2 = autosomal recessive; [2] p = short arm, q = long arm, followed by location with band 11 closest to centromere.

The risk for unprovoked seizures in siblings of JME cases is about 8 per cent, but only about one-third of the affected siblings have JME, with the others showing absence or generalized tonic–clonic seizures or both. With this low a sibling risk, it is not surprising that the mode of inheritance for underlying genes remains undetermined, with dominant, recessive and two-locus patterns remaining as options. Currently linkage studies are under way in four centres, with some differences in findings and interpretations that need to be reconciled.

(1) The initial positive results came from Los Angeles (Greenberg *et al.*, 1987), with evidence for linkage between JME and serological markers on chromosome 6p (human leucocyte antigen (HLA) and properdin factor Bf). Careful attention has been given to the diagnosis of JME in the probands and EEG studies in unaffected relatives. Linkage analyses have been performed with and without including EEG findings as an indicator of the JME gene. The analysis of 24 families informative for HLA/Bf types (with those having abnormal EEGs considered as affected) produced the highest lod score (4.2) at a recombination fraction of 0.01 under the assumption of dominant inheritance with a penetrance of 0.7 (Greenberg & Delgado-Escueta, 1993). In more recent studies DNA markers in the HLA region have been used, and analysis of the first 12 completed families gave results that are significantly negative for linkage (Delgado-Escueta *et al.*, 1993). Further review of these data, however, shows that only half of the 12 families are informative both for DNA markers and for HLA/Bf, so that the comparison between the HLA/Bf typing and DNA markers is not based on identical family samples. The negative DNA results, however, must mean that the epilepsy in at least some of the DNA-tested families is not mapped to these markers on 6p.

(2) A second series, in Berlin, was based on multiplex families (with two or more affected) and has used DNA markers from the outset. EEG findings in otherwise unaffected relatives have not been considered as evidence for affected status. Linkage analyses have consistently yielded significant evidence for linkage of JME to DNA markers in the HLA region (Durner *et al.*, 1991).

(3) A third series, in England, consists of 25 nuclear families of whom about half were referred from various neurologists in England and the others from a single source in Sweden. EEG data are not considered as a component of the phenotype. The results appear to exclude close linkage to the HLA area, but are weakly positive with more distant markers (Whitehouse *et al.*, 1993).

(4) The final small series, from New York City, yielded modest evidence for linkage between JME and DNA markers in the HLA region. Families with adolescent-onset generalized tonic–clonic

seizures (but not JME), on the other hand, were negative for linkage (D.A. Greenberg, personal communication).

These inconsistent findings emphasize the need for agreement on definition of the phenotype, with some lesser concern for differences in the way that samples of families are collected. There is an even more basic question as to which features of the complex phenotype may be most closely related to gene action. The myoclonic jerks may not be the most fundamental manifestation, and the significance of photosensitivity is not clear. Greenberg and Delgado-Escueta (1993) have also suggested the possibility that the finding of absence seizures in some probands and relatives (but not others) may indicate genetic heterogeneity. There is, however, general agreement that any underlying genetic basis is not for JME alone, but involves a more general susceptibility toward adolescent-onset generalized epilepsy. The four research teams are now in the process of comparing phenotype definitions and case ascertainment. It can be expected that further discussion, together with some new family data (using an agreed-upon common set of markers) and additional data analysis, will help to resolve the major questions.

Benign familial neonatal convulsions

The term 'benign familial neonatal convulsions' (BFNC) was introduced 25 years ago (Bjerre & Corelius, 1968) to describe a condition with onset of seizures usually in the first week of life and often ending spontaneously by 6 months of age, with other causes of neonatal seizures excluded, and with an autosomal dominant pattern of inheritance. The responsible gene was mapped to the long arm of chromosome 20 (Leppert *et al.*, 1989) through DNA analysis of a family published by Quattlebaum (1979). Including the work by Malafosse *et al.* (1992a) and others, about 15 families with BFNC have now been mapped to 20q, with the largest being a Newfoundland family with 69 affected (Ronen *et al.*, 1993).

The developmental history is of considerable interest. In half of the cases in these families the convulsions start on the third day of life, with a total of 80 per cent in the first week. The seizures stop by 4 months in 35 per cent and by 1 year in 70 per cent. Recurrent seizures are seen later in life (after 5 years) in 15 per cent, but these are generally not severe.

The seizure manifestations are mixed, including tonic extension or clonic movements of the limbs, automatisms, ocular signs and autonomic effects. The seizures can be generalized or focal, on one side or the other (even in one individual). The tentative conclusion seems to be that the main effect of the mutant gene is on age at onset.

The interictal EEGs are normal or show only minor non-specific abnormalities, while the ictal EEGs establish the epileptic nature of the seizures. Three studies of ictal EEGs report similar findings – a general diffuse sudden suppression of amplitude, followed by symmetric rhythmic slow waves, interrupted by high-voltage multiple spike and sharp waves (Hirsch *et al.*, 1993; Ronen *et al.*, 1993; Plouin, see Chapter 25). Hirsch *et al.* (1993) interpret the EEG data to suggest that the seizures in BFNC are 'a form of generalized tonic–clonic seizure whose expressio may be asymmetrical probably because of the immaturity of the corpus callosum or other structures ensuring seizure synchronization.

There is, however, evidence for heterogeneity at two levels. Ryan *et al.* (1991) reported two families with neonatal onset, only the second of which mapped to chromosome 20. More recent evidence shows that the locus for the first family is on chromosome 8 (Lewis *et al.*, 1993). Family 1 is different in that no affected members had seizures after the age of 2 months, none had audiogenic or febrile seizures, and there were no asymptomatic obligate carriers (features that were seen in family 2).

Five infants with later onset (4–6 months) and their families were reported by Vigevano *et al.* (1992). These have now been shown by Malafosse (1994) not to be the result of mutations on chromosome 20q. Thus at present we can conclude that most families with neonatal onset map to chromosome 20, but one or more map to 8; on the other hand, families with infantile onset do not map to 20.

Progressive myoclonus epilepsy of the Unverricht-Lundborg type (PME-UL)

The PMEs are a group of genetic disorders characterized by myoclonic seizures, tonic–clonic seizures and progressive neurological decline (Berkovic *et al.*, 1993). One of the commonest types is myoclonus epilepsy and ragged red fibres (MERRF), which is transmitted through the maternal line and results from a mutation in mitochondrial DNA. Juvenile neuronal ceroid lipofuscinosis (NCL) has been mapped to chromosome 16 (Gardiner *et al.*, 1990) and infantile NCL to chromosome 1 (Jarvela *et al.*, 1991).

Of particular interest here is Unverricht-Lundborg disease (PME-UL). The inheritance pattern is autosomal recessive with a penetrance of 100 per cent, so that the risk to the sibling of a proband is 25 per cent (a classic Mendelian ratio). The frequency in Finland is 1 in 20,000 births, with carriers (heterozygotes) at the rate of 1 in 70 births. Two years ago the gene locus was mapped to band q22.3, nearly at the end of the long arm of chromosome 21 (Lehesjoki *et al.*, 1991). In that initial study the maximum multipoint lod score was 10.08, quite enough to establish a firm chromosome location.

Further studies to date provide strong evidence that PME-UL is genetically homogeneous, showing linkage to chromosome 21 in French-Canadian, Japanese and Iranian families (Cochius *et al.*, 1992), and in families of Algerian and Italian extraction (Malafosse *et al.*, 1992b). Thus the previous distinction between Baltic and Mediterranean types of PME does not reflect distinct genetic loci. Furthermore, families with Lafora's disease do not show linkage to chromosome 21 markers, supporting the view that Lafora's disease is genetically distinct (Lehesjoki *et al.*, 1992). The terminology is growing more cumbersome because of the number of types of progressive myoclonic epilepsy. The designation of the gene locus as EPM1 is a start toward simplification.

Discussion

A comparison of the present status of gene mapping for these three epilepsy syndromes provides an excellent background for reflecting on the implications of genetics for epilepsy research in the near future, with special emphasis on the important role that clinicians can and must fill.

Selecting the trait

Clinicians are on the front line in recognizing the combinations of findings and a set of patients that can form the basis of new genetic studies. As Greenberg (1992) has suggested, this may require choosing a specific subform of epilepsy and collecting data on subclinical markers. One important issue is whether to choose a rare or a common trait. Rare conditions are likely to have a simpler genetic base, but informative families are harder to find. Common syndromes are more important in clinical practice, but they may be genetically intractable. It is our opinion that we need both, but a new insight is more important than the frequency of the trait *per se*. Within a few years we should have a better idea as to the relative impact of genetic studies in JME, BFNC and PME-UL.

Defining the phenotype

Usually it is best to select probands according to strict (and relatively narrow) criteria. Furthermore, a consensus must be reached early, so that the different research groups can use the same criteria. Gene mapping is never possible within a single laboratory setting, since a gene mapping report is not considered final until the results have been replicated elsewhere; but any replication requires consistency in criteria. This problem must be resolved, for example, before the several studies of JME can be compared rigorously and the data later pooled for analysis. In the case of relatives the issue is the definition of affected status. In BFNC, for example, many of the data are in the form of reports by mothers or other care-givers. Hence we adopted a threefold designation: clearly affected, not affected (on the informed report of the mother or other relative) and unknown (no convulsions known, but information weak). For all three syndromes, detailed information about other clinical findings will become essential in later stages of the investigation.

Selecting the families

Should one use a few large, dense pedigrees or many small nuclear families? In a comparison of JME and BFNC, Greenberg (1992) has claimed that 'the "specialized" disease seen in large families has not yet shed any light on the common disease, whereas working directly with the common form has contributed to our understanding of the genetics of epilepsy'. This comment, unfortunately, confounds the choice of trait with the selection of families. In our opinion, all three of the traits reviewed above will contribute to our understanding of the genetics of epilepsy, but for each we must use strategic reasoning to select families from those available to us. Breakthroughs in gene mapping may build on surprising combinations of basic molecular techniques, well-organized prospective studies of families and a spark of insight (not to mention luck). In this context we wish to emphasize the long-term careful data collection by clinicians, which requires time and patience.

Recognizing genetic heterogeneity

Godfrey (1993) has pointed out that 'The concept of heterogeneity is one that influences both clinical and molecular genetics. In fact, heterogeneity, with its cousins, pleiotropy and variability, provides the framework for both the understanding of and confusion in medical genetics.' He illustrated this theme with the disorders of connective tissue, but the issues apply equally well to epilepsy.

Heterogeneity can be assessed at several levels: (a) the features of the clinical phenotype; (b) the pattern of inheritance; (c) the primary gene action (a developmental process, an enzyme, receptor, ion channel; or other gene product) or (d) the genetic code itself (Anderson, 1989). In the present context we ask for each of the three syndromes if more than one locus is involved (any one of which can play a major role in the development of epilepsy) or if there is a more complex pattern of inheritance.

JME is widely accepted as a clinical entity, but it does not appear to be a genetic entity. From the presently available evidence it is likely that a locus on 6p is part of the story, but this is not well enough defined to permit a direct search for the gene. There is most likely to be another locus as well, and the possibility of a more complex genetic system is difficult to resolve. (Note in Table 2 that the 6p locus has been designated EJM1.) For BFNC two loci (20q and 8q) have been identified, but we do not yet know if there are distinguishing clinical signs. In later onset cases (benign familial infantile convulsions, or BFIC) the gene locus on chromosome 20q is not involved. PME-UL is the only one of the three syndromes that thus far shows locus homogeneity. Even here, however, the possibility of different mutations within the gene remains, since linkage homogeneity doesn't rule out molecular heterogeneity.

The other two terms introduced by Godfrey (1993) are also relevant for epilepsy. *Pleiotropy* refers to the multiple phenotypic effects that can result from a mutation at a single locus, such as the EEG pattern abnormalities in relatives of JME probands (if we assume that the abnormalities reflect the action of a JME gene). *Variability* indicates the individual differences in phenotype, either intrafamilial or interfamilial, that can result from the same genotype. Variability is usually more apparent in autosomal dominant disorders (as compared with recessive), probably because the affected persons are heterozygotes with one normal and one mutant gene at the main locus. These dimensions of variation must be recognized in gene mapping studies.

Godfrey's (1993) final comments show the continuing interdependence between clinicians and molecular scientists: 'So with what are we left? Do we begin to classify disorders on the basis of molecular lesions or on the basis of clinical criteria? Neither alone seems satisfactory any more. Therefore, we will use both, singly and in combination, but heterogeneity will continue to pose dilemmas in our practices and laboratories.'

Early detection of susceptibility

One of the applications of gene mapping is the use of DNA markers to detect the susceptibility of an individual to a genetic problem, either prenatally or preclinically. This is not now possible for JME. It is theoretically possible for BFNC but uninteresting, because the seizures are not serious enough to warrant such attention. In fact, for neither of these conditions is it obvious that gene mapping has significantly changed any aspect of clinical practice.

The situation is potentially quite different for PME-UL. Once an affected (homozygous) patient and both (heterozygote) parents have been evaluated with DNA markers, it would be possible through the use of amniocentesis to predict with high (but not 100 per cent) accuracy the likelihood that a fetus will develop the disorder. Further studies will be required to determine the level of acccuracy. Once the gene has been isolated and cloned, however, much of the uncertainty will be removed. At this point a new set of ethical problems will be encountered. Is this condition serious enough to justify such a procedure? How will this information be presented to parents?

Similar questions will arise after the birth of a child at risk, but before any signs develop. At what age might testing be considered? How should the results be interpreted to parents? It is not too early to consider such questions, and epileptologists might wish to discuss these issues with medical geneticists and genetic counsellors who have had experience with similar problems.

Pathogenesis and treatment

When the gene and its primary product have been identified for any of these three syndromes, a new level of collaboration between clinicians and molecular biologists will become possible. In order to explore hypotheses concerning pathogenesis at the level of gene regulation and cell biology, patients with a range of specific clinical manifestations will be needed.

Finally, some new modes of therapy may be identified that are directed toward primary steps in gene action, but treatments at a more symptomatic level can be expected to remain appropriate. Direct intervention at the genetic level, such as gene insertion therapy, cannot be considered seriously for any epilepsy syndrome until three criteria have been met: (a) it should be reserved for conditions in which no other adequate or better therapies are available; (b) it must be effective; and (c) it must be safe.

Acknowledgement

Supported in part by NIH grant 5 P50 NS-16308 from the National Institute of Neurological Disorders and Stroke.

References

Anderson, V.E. (1989): Genetic heterogeneity in Alzheimer's disease. In: *Familial Alzheimer's disease: molecular genetics and clinical perspectives*, eds. G.D. Miner, R.W. Richter, J.P. Blass, J.L. Valentine & L.A. Winters-Miner, pp. 57–83. New York: Marcel Dekker.

Anderson, V.E. & Hauser, W.A. (1993): Genetics. In: *A textbook of epilepsy*, 4th ed., eds. J. Laidlaw, A. Richens & D. Chadwick, pp. 47–75. Edinburgh: Churchill Livingstone.

Berkovic, S.F., Cochius, J., Andermann, E. & Andermann, F. (1993): Progressive myoclonus epilepsies: clinical and genetic aspects. *Epilepsia* **34** (Suppl. 3), S19–S30.

Bjerre, I. & Corelius, E. (1968): Benign familial neonatal convulsions. *Acta Paediatr. Scand.* 571, 557–561.

Cochius, J.I., Figlewicz, D.A., Kälviäinen, R., Nousiainen, U., Farrell, K., Patry, G., Söderfeldt, B., Frydman, M., Lerman, P., Andermann, F., Andermann, E. & Rouleau, G.A. (1993): Unverricht–Lundborg disease:absence of nonallelic genetic heterogeniety. *Ann. Neurol.* **34,** 739–741.

Delgado-Escueta, A., Liu, A., Serratosa, J.M., Weissbecker, K., Medina, M.T., Gee, M., Treiman, L.J. & Sparkes, R.S. (1993): JME: evidence for heterogeneity. Presented at an international workshop on idiopathic generalized epilepsies, Le Bischenberg, Alsace, France, April 1993.

DiMauro, D., Ricci, E., Hirano, M. & De Vivo, D.C. (1991): Epilepsy in mitochondrial encephalomyopathies. In: *Genetic strategies in epilepsy research*, eds. V.E. Anderson, W.A. Hauser, I.E. Leppik, J.L. Noebels & S.S. Rich, pp. 173–180. Amsterdam: Elsevier.

Durner, M., Sander, T., Greenberg, D.A., Johnson, K., Beck-Mannagetta, G. & Janz, D. (1991): Localization of idiopathic generalized epilepsy on chromosome 6p in families of juvenile myoclonic epilepsy patients. *Neurology* **41,** 1651–1655.

Evans, G.A. (1991): Recent advances in genetics. In: *Genetic strategies in epilepsy research*, eds. V.E. Anderson, W.A. Hauser, I.E. Leppik, J.L. Noebels & S.S. Rich, pp. 189–198. Amsterdam: Elsevier.

Fryburg, J.S., Breg, W.R. & Lindgren, V. (1991): Diagnosis of Angelman syndrome in infants. *Am. J. Med. Genet.* **38,** 58–64.

Gardiner, M., Sandford, A., Deadman M., Poulton, J., Cookson, W., Reeders, S., Jokiaho, I., Pelton, L., Erberg, H. & Julier, C. (1990): Batten disease (Spielmeyer–Vogt disease, juvenile onset neuronal ceroid lipofuscinosis) gene (CLN3) maps to human chromosome 16. *Genomics* **8,** 387–390.

Godfrey, M. (1993): Molecular heterogeneity: a clinical dilemma. Clinical heterogeneity: a molecular dilemma. *Am. J. Hum. Genet.* **53,** 22–25.

Greenberg, D.A. (1992): There is more than one way to collect data for linkage analysis: what a study of epilepsy can tell us about linkage strategy for psychiatric disease. *Arch. Gen. Psychiatry* **49,** 745–750.

Greenberg, D.A. & Delgado-Escueta, A.V. (1993): The chromosome 6p epilepsy locus: exploring mode of inheritance and heterogeneity through linkage analysis. *Epilepsia* **34** (Suppl. 3), S12–S18.

Greenberg, D.A., Delgado-Escueta, A.V., Widelitz, H., Sparkes, R. S., Treimman, L., Maldonado, H.M., Terasaki, P.Z. & Park, M.S. (1987): A locus involved in the expression of juvenile myoclonic epilepsy and of an associated EEG trait may be linked to HLA and Bf. *Cytogenet. Cell Genet* **46,** 623.

Hauser, W.A., Annegers, J.F. & Kurland, L.T. (1993): Incidence of epilepsy and unprovoked seizures in Rochester, Minnesota: 1935–1984. *Epilepsia* **34,** 453–468.

Hirsch, E., Velez, A., Sellal, F., Maton, B., Grinspan, A., Malafosse, A. & Marescaux, C. (1993): Electroclinical signs of benign neonatal familial convulsions. *Ann. Neurol.* **34,** 835–841.

Janz, D. (1989): Juvenile myoclonic epilepsy: epilepsy with impulsive petit mal. *Cleveland Clin. J. Med.* **56** (Suppl. 1), S23–S33.

Jarvela, I., Schleutker, J., Haataja, L., Santavuori, P., Puhaaka, L., Maminen, T., Palotie, A., Sandkuijl, L.A., Renlund, M., White, R., Aula, P. & Peltonen, L. (1991): Infantile neuronal ceroid lipofuscinosis (CLN1) maps to the short arm of chromosome 1. *Genomics* **9,** 170–173.

Lehesjoki, A.-E., Koskiniemi, M., Sistonen, P., Miao, J., Hästbacka, J., Norio, R. & de la Chapelle, A. (1991): Localization of a gene for progressive myoclonus epilepsy to chromosome 21q22. *Proc. Nat. Acad. Sci. USA* **88,** 3696–3699.

Lehesjoki, A.-E., Koskiniemi, M., Pandolfo, M., Antonelli, A., Kyllerman, M., Wahlström, J., Nergårdh, A., Burmeister, M., Sistonen, P., Norio, R. & de la Chapelle, A. (1992): Linkage studies in progressive myoclonus epilepsy: Unverricht–Lundborg and Lafora's disease. *Neurology* **42,** 1545–1550.

Leppert, M., Anderson, V.E., Quattlebaum, T., Stauffer, D., O'Donnell, P., Nakamura, Y., Lalouel, J.-M. & White, R. (1989): Benign familial neonatal convulsions linked to genetic markers on chromosome 20. *Nature* **337,** 647–648.

Leppert, M., Anderson, V.E. & White, R. (1991): The discovery of epilepsy genes by genetic linkage. In: *Genetic strategies in epilepsy research*, eds. V.E. Anderson, W.A. Hauser, I.E. Leppik, J.L. Noebels & S.S. Rich, pp. 181–188. Amsterdam: Elsevier.

Leppert, M., McMahon, W.M., Quattlebaum, T.G., Bjerre, I., Zonana, J., Shevell, M.I., Andermann, E., Rosales, T.O., Ronen, G.M., Connolly, M. & Anderson, V.E. (1993):Searching for human epilepsy genes: a progress report. *Brain Pathology* **3,** 357–369.

Lewis, T.B., Leach, R.J., Ward, K., O'Connell, P. & Ryan, S.G. (1993): Genetic heterogeneity in benign familial neonatal convulsions: identification of a new locus on chromosome 8q. *Am. J. Hum. Genet.* **53,** 670–675.

McKusick, V.A. (1992): *Mendelian inheritance in man: catalogs of autosomal dominant, autosomal recessive, and X-linked phenotypes*, 10th edn. Baltimore: Johns Hopkins University Press.

Malafosse A. (1993): Data presented at an international conference on idiopathic generalized epilepsies, Le Bischenberg, Alsace, France, April 1993.

Malafosse, A., Leboyer, M., Dulac, O., Navelet, Y., Plouin, P., Beck, C., Laklou, H., Mouchnino, G., Grandscene, P., Vallee, L., Builloud-Bataille, M., Samolyk, D., Baldy-Moulinier, M., Feingold, J. & Mallet, J. (1992a): Confirmation of linkage of benign familial neonatal convulsions to D20S19 and D20S20. *Hum. Genet.* **89,** 54–58.

Malafosse, A., Lehesjoki, A.E., Genton, P., Labauge, P., Durand, G., Tassinari, C.A., Dravet, C., Michelucci, R. & de la Chapelle, A. (1992b): Identical genetic locus for Baltic and Mediterranean myoclonus. *Lancet* **339,** 1080–1081.

Malafosse, A., Beck, C., Bellet, H., Di Capua, M. Dulac, O., Echenne, B., Fusco, L., Lucchini, P., Ricci, S., Sebastianelli, R., Feingold, J., Baldy-Moulinier. & Vigevano, F. (1994): Benign infantile convulsions is not an allelic form of the benign familial neonatal convulsions gene. *Ann. Neurol.* **35,** 479–482.

O'Brien S.J., Womack. J.E., Lyons, L.A., Moore, K.J., Jenkins, N.A. & Copeland, N.G. (1993): Anchored reference loci for comparative genome mapping in mammals. *Nature Genet.* **3,** 103–112.

Quattlebaum, T.G. (1979): Benign familial convulsions in the neonatal period and early infancy. *J. Pediatr.* **95,** 257–259.

Ronen, G.M., Rosales, T.O., Connolly, M., Anderson, V.E. & Leppert, M. (1993): Seizure characteristics in chromosome 20 benign familial neonatal convulsions. *Neurology* **43,** 1355–1360.

Ryan, S.G., Wiznitzer, M., Hollman, C., Torres, M.C., Szekeresova, M. & Schneider, S. (1991): Benign familial neonatal convulsions: evidence for clinical and genetic heterogeneity. *Ann. Neurol.* **29,** 469–473.

Vigevano, F., Fusco, L., DiCapua, M., Ricci, S., Sebastianelli, R. & Lucchini, P. (1992): Benign infantile familial convulsions. *Eur. J. Pediatr.* **117,** 1–5.

White, R. & Skolnick, M. (1982): DNA sequence polymorphism and the genetics of epilepsy. In: *Genetic basis of the epilepsies*, eds. V.E. Anderson, W.A. Hauser, J.K. Penry & C.F. Sing, pp. 311–316. New York: Raven Press.

Whitehouse, W.P., Rees, M., Curtis, D., Sundqvist, A., Parker, K., Chung, E., Baralle, D. & Gardiner, R.M. (1993): Linkage analysis of idiopathic generalised epilepsy and marker loci on chromosome 6p in families with juvenile myoclonic epilepsy: no evidence for an epilepsy locus in the HLA region. *Am. J. Hum. Gen.* **53,** 652–662

Epileptic Seizures and Syndromes, Edited by Peter Wolf
© 1994 John Libbey & Company Ltd., pp. 193–201

Chapter 25

Benign idiopathic neonatal convulsions (familial and non-familial): open questions about these syndromes

Perrine Plouin

INSERM U 29, Hôpital Saint Vincent-de-Paul, 82 avenue Denfert-Rochereau, 75014 Paris, France

Benign neonatal convulsions (NNC) are those showing a favourable neurological outcome, i.e. a normal psychomotor development without secondary epilepsy. This seemingly plain definition may raise practical difficulties in the individual patient. Whereas psychomotor development can be easily assessed in infancy and childhood, the absence of subsequent epilepsy makes benign NNC a retrospective diagnosis and raises the following question: how long should an affected child be followed up to confirm safely that his/her NNC was benign (Matsumoto *et al.*, 1983)? In addition, it may be difficult to document or exclude a causative link between NNC and the eventual occurrence of subsequent convulsions.

We shall focus on the clinical features and the electroencephalographic (EEG) findings in NNC of unknown aetiology and favourable outcome. Two subtypes may be characterized according to the absence or presence of a familial history of NNC: benign idiopathic neonatal convulsions (BINC) or so-called fifth-day fits (Dehan *et al.*, 1977) and benign familial neonatal convulsions (BFNC) (Rett & Teubel, 1964). Following a symposium held in Marseille in 1983 on epileptic syndromes in infancy, childhood and adolescence, the Commission on Classification and Terminology of the International League Against Epilepsy decided to include these subtypes in the classification of epilepsies and epileptic syndromes (1989). They belong to the second section (generalized epilepsies and syndromes), and are classified among idiopathic generalized epilepsies (age-related).

Benign idiopathic neonatal convulsions

We compiled the studies dealing with NNC or neonatal status epilepticus published between 1959 and 1982 (Plouin, 1992) in order to identify those which could be defined as BINC. Among these studies, we paid special attention to the description by Dehan *et al.* (1977) of NNC with unknown aetiology occurring around the fifth day of life. Although it was estimated by Gastaut (1981) that the clinical and EEG characteristics of these NNC were not specific enough to constitute an independent syndrome, the criteria proposed by Dehan *et al.* (1977) may be considered a useful key for the analysis of the published reports of NNC.

We therefore selected reported cases of neonates born after 39 weeks of gestation, having had an APGAR score of 9 or more at the fifth minute of life, in whom a status epilepticus had begun around the 104th hour (day 5) after a symptom-free interval between birth and the beginning of convulsions, lasting for about 20 h, with clonic or apnoeic seizures, 'théta pointu alternant' pattern on the interictal EEG (75 per cent of the first study of Dehan *et al.*, 1977), all other examinations being negative, and subsequently showing a favourable outcome.

The 15 published studies exhibit a great disparity regarding material and methods. Most do not report EEG findings; some take into account convulsions occurring in the first 10 days of life only, while others include convulsions occurring at any time during the first month. These studies were undertaken between 1959 and 1979, and the advances in the diagnosis and treatment of NNC were substantial in those 20 years. Thus, similar cases of NNC might have been considered idiopathic in the 1960s, and linked to some identified aetiology in the late 1970s. Among the 2042 cases reported in these 15 studies, a majority of NNC of unknown aetiology had a good outcome (120 out of 195 documented cases, mean and range: 62 per cent, 28–93 per cent), and cases with unknown aetiology and favourable outcome account for 6.6 per cent of NNC (with a range of 0–28 per cent).

Considering these 120 cases with no aetiology and benign outcome, we tried to focus on two important criteria of Dehan *et al.* (1977): the date of onset of convulsions and the interictal pattern of the EEG. The date of onset was known in only 37 neonates, 33 of whom had begun to have convulsions between the third and sixth day of life. Interictal EEG were described in 39 cases: they were normal in 15 cases, exhibited focal or multifocal abnormalities in 13, and a 'théta pointu alternant' pattern in 11. No traces connected with a poor prognosis were reported (Monod *et al.*, 1972; Plouin *et al.*, 1977). This suggests that cases of BINC had been reported in the literature before their formal description by Dehan *et al.* in 1977. Their prevalence can be evaluated as about 7 per cent of that of NNC, this percentage decreasing to 2 per cent when taking into account only the cases in which the date of occurrence of seizures and the interictal EEG patterns are reported.

Since the first report of Dehan *et al.* (1977), several workers from France (André *et al.*, 1978, 1990; Dreyfus-Brisac *et al.*, 1981; Navelet *et al.*, 1981; Plouin *et al.*, 1981), Australia (Pryor *et al.*, 1981; North *et al.*, 1989) and more recently Germany (Herrmann *et al.*, 1993) have reported BINC. Table 1 summarizes the 299 published cases.

Table 1. Benign idiopathic neonatal convulsions

Authors	Collection period	Number of cases
Dehan *et al.* (1977)	1973–76	20
André *et al.* (1978)	1972–76	4
Pryor *et al.* (1981)	1973–77	90
Dreyfus-Brisac *et al.* (1981)	1974–79	11
Plouin *et al.* (1981)	1966–80	39
Navelet *et al.* (1981)	1976–80	18
North *et al.* (1989)	1972–85	94
André *et al.* (1990)	1980–81	2
Herrmann *et al.* (1993)	1989–91	21
Total ($n = 9$)	1966–1991	299

Estimates of the prevalence of BINC vary from 4 to 38 per cent of NNC, this large scatter probably reflecting differences in patients' referral and recruitment: intensive care units (ICUs), maternity clinics, departments of neonatology or paediatric neurology. A rate of 38 per cent probably overestimates the true prevalence of BINC, whereas the 4 per cent figure is in good agreement with the 2 –7 per cent range cited above.

The sex distribution denotes a majority of boys (62 per cent). In all cases the convulsions occurred between day (D) 1 and D7, including 90 per cent between D4 and D6 and 97 per cent between D3 and D7.

When described, the convulsions were always of the clonic type, mostly partial or apnoeic or both, but never tonic. North *et al.* (1989) reported apnoeic seizures in 31 per cent of their cases. Clonic seizures were often lateralized, starting on one side then affecting the other, and rarely of a generalized type. They lasted from 1 to 3 min. They were frequently repeated, leading to a status epilepticus. The mean duration of status epilepticus was about 20 h, but could be shorter (2 h) or longer (up to 3 days).

The neurological state of the infants is usually normal at the onset of convulsions. Then infants become drowsy and hypotonic, the various antiepileptic drugs given to stop the convulsions being partly responsible for this evolution. Drowsiness and hypotonia may last for several days after the end of the status epilepticus. Then the infants recover a normal neurological state.

Interictal EEG patterns were described in 101 of the 299 published cases. The interictal EEG was normal in 10 infants, was discontinuous in six and showed 'focal or multifocal abnormalities' in 25. The 'théta pointu alternant' pattern was present in the remaining 60 infants. This pattern was first described by Dehan *et al.* (1977) as a dominant theta activity, alternating or discontinuous, unreactive, with sharp waves and frequent interhemispheric asynchrony. The 'théta pointu alternant' pattern may be present in cases of status epilepticus of different aetiologies (hypocalcaemia, neonatal meningitis, subarachnoidal haemorrhage) and cannot be considered as specific of BINC (Navelet *et al.*, 1981; P. Plouin, unpublished data). Nevertheless, it is associated with a favourable neurological prognosis.

Seizures have been recorded in most of the 101 cases. They last from 1 to 3 min and have no remarkable features: mostly rhythmic spikes or rhythmic slow waves. They can be localized in any area but are more frequently present in the rolandic areas. They can be strictly unilateral, immediately generalized or first localized and then generalized. Electroclinical seizures or subclinical discharges (so-called electrical seizures) can be recorded; clinical seizures without EEG modifications have also been reported.

Many antiepileptic drugs have been used for these BINC, often in association, without a consistent effect on the duration of seizures. Most often the convulsions stopped without treatment, but occasionally the end seemed to be related to administration of diazepam or phenytoin. Now Dehan *et al.* (1982) proposes not to treat these infants if alternative diagnoses have been eliminated.

The differential diagnosis is of major importance. BINC remain a diagnosis of exclusion and any other aetiology must be sought, such as metabolic disturbances, neonatal meningitis, viral infections or malformations of the central nervous system.

One aetiological hypothesis was proposed by Goldberg and Sheehy (1983), who, after a 3-year prospective study, found that there was an acute zinc deficiency in the cerebrospinal fluid (CSF) of infants suffering from BINC when compared with a group of infants in whom a cause of convulsions had been identified, and with another group of infants without convulsions but with other health problems. Up to now this hypothesis has not been confirmed. Moreover, in Australia and in France, very complete metabolic, toxic and viral enquiries have been carried out, without any significant result.

More recently, Herrmann *et al.* (1993) reported 21 cases of BINC referred between 1989 and 1991 among 1917 hospitalized neonates during the same period. They tested the faeces of 19 BINC babies as well as 30 healthy controls (age 4–6 days) and 202 sick neonates without convulsions for rotavirus infection. They found rotavirus in the faeces of 18 of the 19 BINC babies (95 per cent) whereas only 40 per cent of the healthy control had positive findings ($P < 0.001$) and 48 per cent of the sick neonates without convulsions ($P < 0.001$). The authors suggest a causal relationship between BINC and rotavirus infections, although rotavirus was not present in the CSF of six rotavirus-positive babies with BINC. They conclude that the pathogenic mechanisms remain unclear.

Finally, the long-term favourable outcome must be confirmed by more numerous and more extensive studies. The 90 cases reported by Pryor *et al.* (1981) have not been followed-up beyond the neonatal period. The 92 cases reported by French authors were followed from 6 months to 6 years: in five cases a transitory psychomotor retardation was noted until the age of 1 year, one child had a simple febrile convulsion and another one had a convulsion without fever at the age of 3 (Dehan *et al.*, 1982).

Among the 94 cases reported by North *et al.* (1989), 33 (38 per cent) have been followed up to an age between 6 months and 2 years. In half of these 33 infants, the authors found abnormalities. Although there is no control group, the percentage of abnormalities seems excessive in this study. One can also think that children with medical problems were more exposed to frequent consultations than children without any problem. Anyway these authors conclude that their own results do not allow them to assess the benignity of this syndrome.

Finally, North *et al.* (1989) insist on the fact that no case of BINC has been observed in their department since 1982. Moreover, the incidence of NNC, which was very high during the 1970s, has decreased since the beginning of the 1980s. The same facts have been noted by other maternity hospitals in Australia, leading to the hypothesis of an epidemic phenomenon of BINC, the aetiology remaining indeterminate. In 1990, M. Dehan, Y. Navelet and A.M. D'Allest performed a retrospective study among neonatology and ICU paediatric departments as well as maternity hospitals concerning the number of cases of BINC referred to them each year between 1979 and 1989. The results were presented at the first Réunion d'Actualités en Epileptologie (in Geneva, 1991). The authors concluded that sporadic cases exist among all departments (0.5–1.5 cases/year/department), with an important peak in 1981 (comparable to the one of 1975 leading to the first report of BINC). The epidemic occurrence of BINC has also been reported by Herrmann *et al.* (1993), with 21 cases referred between 1989 and 1991. The fact that they found a rotavirus infection associated in 95 per cent of their cases reinforces the hypothesis of an epidemic phenomenon but does not explain the relationship with the convulsions.

This syndrome must be isolated with regard to all clinical and paraclinical elements which compose it. Its recognition allows one to forecast a favourable neurological outcome. However the 'théta pointu alternant' EEG pattern is present in only 60 per cent of cases and is not specific. Further reports will perhaps lead to a better understanding of this syndrome and clarify the outcome with a longer follow-up of the babies.

Benign familial neonatal convulsions

Three hundred and thirty-four cases of BFNC have been reported in the literature since the first paper by Rett & Teubel (1964). These neonates belong to 38 families. The number of generations affected varies from 1 to 5 (Table 2). It is not possible to define the prevalence of these BFNC as they are not compared with other NNC in any study.

In 80 per cent of cases, seizures start on the second and third days of life. But some infants begin to convulse later, during the first month of life or even up to the third month of life. Ronen *et al.* (1993) report in their large family that two of the individuals in whom the first seizures occurred at 1 month of age were premature.

In documented cases birth was always at full term (except for three cases of Ronen *et al.*, 1993) with normal birthweight and an APGAR score above 7 at the first minute of life. None of these neonates was in an ICU. There was always a free interval between birth and occurrence of convulsions. The sex ratio shows an equal distribution between boys and girls.

In most cases biological and radiological work-up had been performed and failed to disclose any aetiology except for a single case with transitory hypomagnesaemia.

When described, seizures were of the clonic type, sometimes with apnoeic spells. Tonic seizures were reported in two cases. Clonic or tonic seizures were short (lasting from 1 to 3 min), frequently repeated over 7 days, whereas isolated seizures could occur in some cases during the following weeks. We had the opportunity to record seizures in one case (family 1 in the paper by Malafosse *et al.*, 1992): seizures were stereotyped, starting with a diffuse hypertonia with a short apnoea, followed by clonic movements of the limbs. Seizures had already been described in previous reports(Giacoia, 1982; Crispen & Kelly, 1985; Shevell *et al.*, 1986; Camfield *et al.*, 1991), but there was no evidence for a homogeneous presentation. More recently, Ronen *et al.* (1995) have listed all the clinical components of the 70 seizures they could analyse in their large family. They concluded that most of the times seizures started with tonic, autonomic or oculofacial features, being of a mixed type. No myoclonic seizure has been reported, and no spasm either.

Table 2. Beningn familial neonatal convulsions

Author (date of publication)	No. of cases (per family)	No. of generations (per family)
Rett & Teubel (1964)	8	3
Bjerre & Corelius (1968)	14	5
Steejohnsen (1968)	8	?
Rose & Lombrosco (1970)	3	3
Goutières (1977)	8	3
	2	1
Carton (1978)	9	4
Quattelbaum (1979)	15*	4
Pettit & Fenichel (1980)	5	3
Tibbles (1980)	2	2
	6	2
	3	2
Pavone *et al.* (1982)	7	2
Giacoia (1982)	7	4
Plouin (1984)	2	2
	2	1
Kaplan & Lacey (1983)	12	4
Palencia & Berjon (1985)	4	2
Shevell *et al.* (1986)	5	3
	4	3
Nieto Barrera *et al.* (1986)	14	3
Calero Garcia *et al.* (1988)	17	4
Cunniff *et al.* (1988)	8	2
Giroud *et al.* (1989)	2	2
	2	2
	2	1
Malafosse *et al.* (1990)	6*	3
	4*	3
	4*	2
Webb & Bobele (1990)	9	5
Camfield *et al.* (1991)	5	2
Ryan *et al.* (1991)	14*	3
	15	3
Schiffmann *et al.* (1991)	4	1
Wakai *et al.* (1991)	5	2
Aso & Watanabe (1992)	3	2
Malafosse *et al.* (1992)	9*	4
	3*	2
	9*	4
Mami *et al.* (1993)	4	2
Ronen *et al.* (1993)	69*	5

Total 1964–1993: 334 cases, 38 families.
*Families with BFNC mapped in chromosome 20 (linkage analysis of Quattelbaum's family has been done by Leppert *et al.*, 1989).

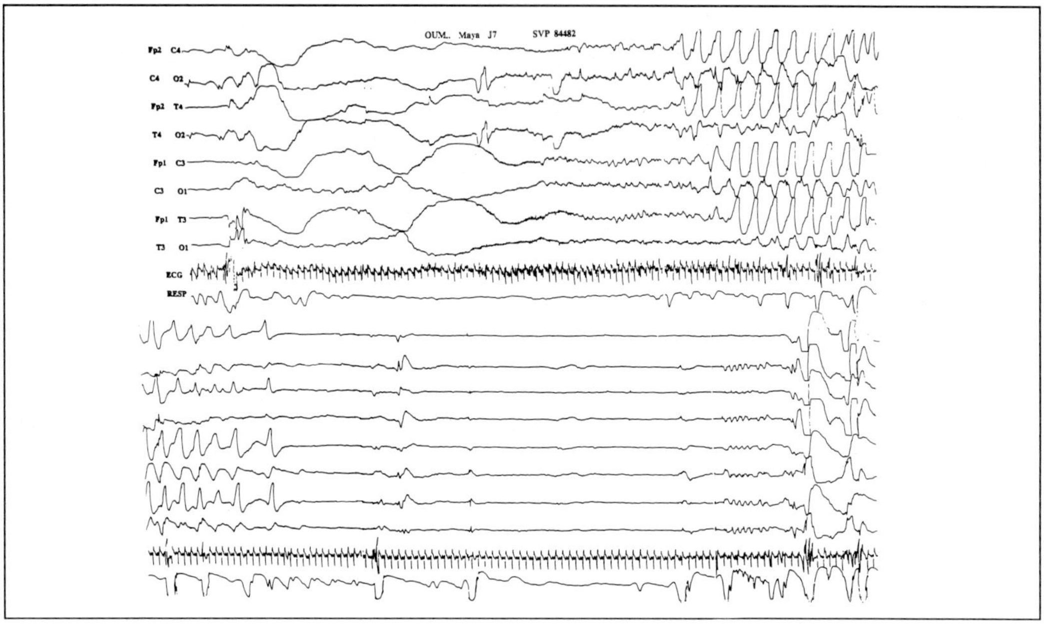

Fig. 1. BFNC: seizure recorded in a 7-day-old neonate; diffuse flattening of the tracing, followed by theta rhythms and by high-amplitude one 1 Hz generalized delta waves for 30 s. Marked generalized depression of the tracing at the end of the seizure. Note the central apnoea at the beginning of the seizure.

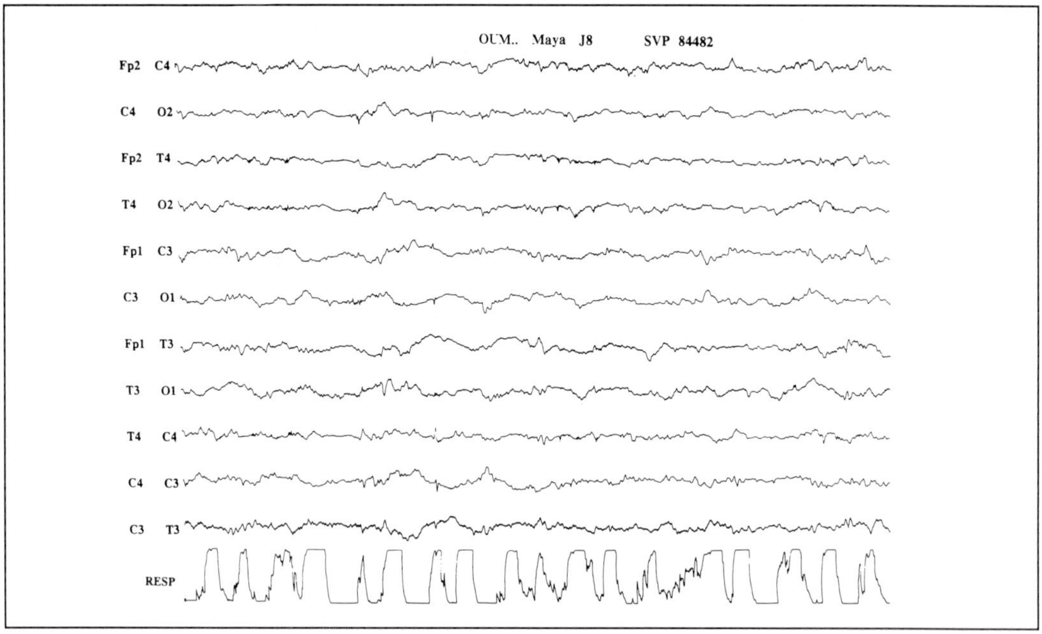

Fig. 2. Same neonate, aged 8 days. No more seizure. Continuous background activity during active sleep. No abnormal EEG pattern.

When described, interictal EEG was either normal, discontinuous or including focal or multifocal abnormalities or with 'théta pointu alternant' pattern. Patterns suggesting poor prognosis, such as a paroxysmal or inactive EEG, were never reported. In previous reports some seizures were recorded but the EEG were not published or were incomplete. In the case we recorded (Figs. 1 and 2), the ictal pattern is very similar to the one published by Ronen *et al.* (1993), and to the cases of Hirsch *et al.* (1993). All these individuals had BFNC mapped in chromosome 20.

The clinical and EEG presentations of these seizures suggest that they are of a generalized type. Aso and Watanabe (1992) discussed this point because they recorded a unilateral seizure in a 3-month-old infant who had BFNC. From this observation, one cannot draw conclusions about the characteristics of the seizures at the neonatal period.

Infants with such BFNC had a favourable psychomotor developmental outcome. In some cases (11 per cent), however, epileptic seizures subsequently occurred in infancy, in childhood and in adulthood. When present, seizures were described as isolated, rare and easily controlled by medication some of these seizures were provoked. No case of severe epilepsy was reported. In addition 5 per cent of the children presented one or more simple febrile convulsions at the usual age. Consequently, overall rates of secondary epilepsy and febrile convulsions were 11 and 5 per cent respectively, the rate for febrile convulsions being comparable to that of the general population (see also Berkovic *et al.*, Chapter 5).

Studies of pedigrees with several affected generations and a sufficient number of siblings show a 1/1 sex ratio and a probability around 1/2, confirming a dominant autosomal transmission. In 1989, Leppert *et al.* studied a family of four generations including 48 individuals, 19 of them having the characteristics of BFNC. They localized the gene to the long arm of chromosome 20, possibly to 20q13.2.A similar study concerning three families was published in 1990 by Malafosse *et al.*. They used the same polymorphic DNA marker loci (RMR6 and CMM6) as Leppert *et al.* (1989) to determine the restriction fragment length polymorphism. Their results suggested the same localization to 20q13.2 of the gene linked to BFNC. They could not draw conclusions from their own data only, but, when adding their lod scores to those reported by Leppert *et al.* (1989), Malafosse *et al.* (1990) were able to establish a reliable linkage and suggest the single-gene origin of BFNC. More recently, Ryan *et al.* (1990) studied two new families with BFNC; in the first one, with only cases of BFNC, they found that both markers (RMR6 and CMM6) were informative; in the second one, with a different evolution of secondary epilepsy, only marker CMM6 was informative. They concluded that the syndrome of BFNC was genetically heterogeneous. Schiffmann *et al.* (1991) reported an autosomal recessive form of BFNC in a consanguineous sibship leading to the same conclusion. In another study, Sander *et al.* (1990), demonstrated that there is an exclusion of linkage in susceptibility locus for BFNC with idiopathic generalized epilepsies in juvenile myoclonic epilepsy families. These data must be confirmed by testing additional families, and the next step should be the identification of the gene or genes.

BFNC are different from BINC on several counts: BFNC are a familial disease with an autosomal mode of inheritance linked to genetic markers localized to the long arm of chromosome 20, at least for the majority of cases; conversely, a family history is very rare in BINC (0.2 per cent). Seizures start earlier in BFNC (D2, D3) and persist longer than in BINC (starting on D4–D5, and lasting no more than 20 h). Occurrence of secondary epilepsy is more frequent in BFNC (11 per cent) compared to 0.5 per cent in BINC. Minor neurological impairment would seem to be more frequent among cases of BINC.

Even if some questions remain open about these two syndromes, they must be identified and recognized but considered as different. Both of them allow the forecast of a favourable neurological outcome from the neonatal period.

References

André, M., Vert, P. & Bouchez, T. (1978): A propos des convulsions du cinquième jour. *Arch. Fr. Pédiatr.* **35,** 922–923.

André, M., Matisse, N. & Vert, P. (1990): Prognosis of neonatal seizures. In: *Neonatal seizures*, eds. C.G. Wasterlain & P. Vert, pp. 61–67. New York: Raven Press.

Aso, K. & Watanabe, K. (1992): Benign familial neonatal convulsions: generalized epilepsy? *Pediatr. Neurol.* **8,** 226–228.

Bjerre, I. & Corelius, E. (1968): Benign neonatal familial convulsions. *Acta Paediatr. Scand.* **57,** 557–561.

Calero Garcia, J.L., Nieto Barrera, M., Moruno Tirado, A. & Gozalvez Bueno, I. (1988): Convulsiones neonatales familiares benignas: aportacion de una nueva familia. *Rev. Esp. Epilepsia* **4,** 32–35.

Camfield, P.R., Dooley, J., Gordon, K. & Orlik, P. (1991): Benign familial neonatal convulsions are epileptic. *J. Child. Neurol.* **6,** 340–342.

Carton, D. (1978): Benign neonatal familial convulsions. *Neuropädiatrie* **9,** 167–171.

Commission on Classification and Terminology of the International League Against Epilepsy (1989): Proposal for revised classification of epilepsies and epileptic syndromes. *Epilepsia* **30,** 389–399.

Crispen, C. & Kelly, T. (1985): Benign familial neonatal convulsions. *Iowa Med.* **75,** 397–401.

Cunniff, C., Wieldlin, N. & Lyons Jones, K. (1988): Autosomal dominant benign neonatal seizures. *Am. J. Med. Genet.* **30,** 963–966.

Dehan, M., Quilleron, D., Navelet, Y., D'Allest, A.M., Vial, M., Retbi, J.M., Lelong-Tisier, M.C. & Gabilan, J.C. (1977): Les convulsions du cinquième jour de vie: un nouveau syndrome? *Arch. Fr. Péiatr.* **34,** 730–742.

Dehan, M., Navelet, Y., D'Allest, A.M., Vial, M., Ropert, J.C., Boulley, A.M. & Gabilan, J.C. (1982): Quelques précisions sur le syndrome des convulsions du cinquième jour de vie. *Arch. Fr. Pédiatr.* **39,** 405–407.

Dreyfus-Brisac, C., Peschanski, N., Radvanyi, M. F., Cukier-Hemeury, F. & Monod, N. (1981): Convulsions du nouveau-né: aspects clinique, électroencéphalographique, étiopathogénique et pronostique. *Rev. EEG Neurophysiol.* **11,** 367–378.

Gastaut, H. (1981): Individualisation des épilepsies dites bénignes ou fonctionnelles aux différents âges de la vie: appréciation des variations correspondantes de la prédisposition épileptiques à ces âges. *Rev. EEG Neurophysiol.* **11,** 346–366.

Giacoia, G.P. (1982): Benign familial neonatal convulsions. *Southern Med. J.* **75,** 629–630.

Giroud, M., Soichot, P., Nivelon-Chevalier, A., Gouyon, J.B., Nivelon, J.L. & Dumas, R. (1989): Les convulsions néo-natales familiales: leurs aspects électrocliniques et génétiques. *Neurophysiol. Clin.* **19,** 47–54.

Goldberg, H.J. & Sheehy, E.M. (1983): Fifth day fits: an acute zinc deficiency syndrome? *Archs. Dis. Child.* **57,** 633–635.

Goutières, F. (1977): Convulsions néonatales familiales bénignes. In: *Congrès de la société de neurologie infantile*, pp 281–286. Marseille: Diffusion générale de librairie.

Herrmann, B., Lawrenz-Wolf, B., Seewald, C., Selb & B., Wehinger, H. (1993): 5-Tages-Krämpfe des Neugeborenen bei Rotavirusinfektionen. *Monatsschr. Kinderheilkd.* **141,** 120–123.

Hirsch, E., Velez, A., Sellal, F., Maton, B., Grinspan, A., Malafosse, A. & Marescaux, C. (1993): Electroclinical signs of benign neonatal familial convulsions. *Ann. Neurol.* **34,** 835–841.

Kaplan, R.E. & Lacey, D.J. (1983): Benign familial neonatal–infantile seizures. *Am. J. Med. Genet.* **16,** 595–599.

Leppert, M., Anderson, V.E., Quattlebaum, T., Stauffer, D., O'Connell, P., Nakamura, Y., Lalouel, J.M. & Whitr, R. (1989): Benign familial neonatal convulsions linked to genetic markers on chromosome 20. *Nature* **337,** 647–648.

Malafosse, A., Leboyer, M., Dulac, O., Plouin, P., Navelet, Y., Feingold, J. & Mallet, J. (1990): Convulsions néonatales familiales bénignes: un modèle d'étude des bases moléculaires des facteurs génétiques des épilepsies. *Epilepsies* **2,** 64–71.

Malafosse, A., Leboyer, M., Dulac, O., Navelet, Y., Plouin, P., Beck, C., Laklou, H., Mouchnino, G., Grandscene, P., Vallee, L., Guilloud-Bataille, M., Samolyk, D., Baldy-Moulinier, M., Feingold, J. & Mallet, J. (1992): Confirmation of linkage of benign familial neonatal convulsions to D20S19 and D20S20. *Hum. Genet.* **89,** 54–58.

Mami, C., Tortorella, R., Manganaro, R. & Gemelli, M. (1993): Les convulsions néonatales familiales bénignes. *Arch. Fr. Pédiatr.* **50,** 31–33.

Matsumoto, A., Watanabe, K., Sugiura, M., Negoro, T., Takaesu, E. & Iwase, K. (1983). Longterm prognosis of convulsive disorders in the first year of life: mental and physical development and seizures persistance. *Epilepsia* **24,** 321–329.

Monod, N., Pajot, N. & Guidasci, S. (1972): The neonatal EEG: statistical studies and prognostic value in full-term and pre-term babies. *Electroencephalogr. Clin. Neurophysiol.* **32,** 529–544.

Navelet, Y., D'Allest, A.M., Dehan, M. & Gabilan, J.C. (1981): A propos du syndrome des convulsions néonatales du cinquième jour. *Rev. EEG Neurophysiol.* **11,** 390–396.

Nieto Barrera, M., Borrego, S. & Aguilar Quero, F. (1986): Convulsiones neonatales familiares benignas y crisis asociadas. *Rev. Esp. Epilepsia* **2,** 66–70.

North, K.N., Storey, G.N.B. & Handerson-Smart, D.J. (1989): Fifth day fits in the newborn. *Aust. Paediatr. J.* **25,** 284–287.

Palencia, R. & Berjon, M.C. (1985): Convulsiones neonatales familiares benignas, crises febriles y epilepsia: su coincidencia en una familia. *An. Esp. Pediatr.* **23,** 65–67.

Pavone, L., Mazzone, D., La Rosa, M., Livolti, S. & Mollica, F. (1982): Le convulsioni familiari benigne: studio di una famiglia. *Pediatr. Oggi* **11,** 375–378.

Plouin, P. (1992): Benign idiopathic neonatal convulsions (familial and non-familial). In: *Epileptic syndromes in infancy, childhood and adolescence*, eds. J. Roger, M. Bureau, Ch. Dravet, F.E. Dreifuss, A. Perret & P. Wolf, pp. 3–11. London: John Libbey.

Pettit, R.E. & Fenichel, G.M. (1980): Benign familial neonatal seizures. *Archs. Neurol.* **37,** 47–48.

Plouin, P., Moussali, F., Lerique, A., Mises, J., Lavoisy, P. & Navelet, Y. (1977): Evolution clinique après un tracé néonatal considéré comme grave. *Rev. EEG Neurophysiol.* **7,** 410–415.

Plouin, P., Sternberg, B., Bour, F. & Lerique, A. (1981): Etats de mal néonataux d'étiologie indéterminée. *Rev. EEG Neurophysiol.* **11,** 385–389.

Pryor, D.S., Don, N. & Macourt, D.C. (1981): Fifth day fits: a syndrome of neonatal convulsions. *Arch. Dis. Child.* **56,** 753–758.

Quattelbaum, T.G. (1979): Benign familial convulsions in the neonatal period and early infancy. *J. Pediatr.* **95,** 257–259.

Rett, A. & Teubel, R. (1964): Neugeborenen Krampfe im Rahmen einer epileptisch belasten Familie. *Wien. Klin. Wschr.* **76,** 609–613.

Ronen, G.M., Rosales, T.O., Connolly, M. Ed., Anderson, V.E. & Leppert, M. (1993): Seizure characteristics in chromosome 20 benign familial neonatal convulsions. *Neurology* **43,** 1355–1360.

Rose, A.L. & Lombroso, C.T. (1970): Neonatal seizure states: a study of clinical pathology and EEG features in 137 full-term babies with a long term follow-up. *Pediatrics* **45,** 405–425.

Ryan, S.G., Wiznitzer, M., Hollman, C., Torres, C., Szekeresova, M. & Schneider, S. (1991): Benign familial neonatal convulsions: evidence for clinical and genetic heterogeneity. *Ann. Neurol.* **29,** 469–473.

Sander, T., Johnson, K. & Janz, D. (1990): Exclusion of linkage between the susceptibility locus for benign familial neonatal convulsions with idiopathic generalized epilepsies in juvenile myoclonic epilepsy. *Epilepsia* **31,** 818.

Schiffmann, R., Shapira, Y. & Ryan, G. (1991): An autosomal recessive form of benign familial neonatal seizures. *Clin. Genet.* **40,** 467–470.

Shevell, M.I., Sinclair, D.B. & Metrakos, K. (1986): Benign familial neonatal seizures: clinical and electroencephalographic characteristics. *Pediatr. Neurol.* **2,** 272–275.

Tibbles, J.A.R. (1980): Dominant benign neonatal seizures. *Dev. Med. Child Neurol.* **22,** 664–667.

Wakai, S., Tachi, N., Chiba, S., Ishikawa, Y., Okabe, M., Minami, R. & Kibayashi, M. (1991): Benign familial neonatal convulsions: clinical features of the propositus and comparison with the previously reported cases. *Acta Paediatr. Japan.* **33,** 77–82.

Webb, R. & Bobele, G. (1990): 'Benign' familial neonatal convulsions. *J. Child. Neurol.* **5,** 295–298.

Epileptic Seizures and Syndromes, Edited by Peter Wolf
© 1994 John Libbey & Company Ltd., pp. 203–211

Chapter 26

Benign myoclonic epilepsy in infancy and idiopathic West syndrome

Charlotte Dravet

Centre Saint Paul, 300 boulevard de Sainte Marguerite, 13009 Marseille, France

Summary

Benign myoclonic epilepsy and West syndrome are briefly described with emphasis on the semiology of seizures, their respective mode and age of onset, the EEG and the psychomotor features, and the response to drug therapy. In the author's opinion, there is no overlap between these well-described epileptic syndromes. Their differences and their respective nosological place are discussed.

Introduction

The West syndrome (WS) seems to be a well-known syndrome and the literature contains so many studies concerning it that it is actually impossible to summarize them. On the contrary, benign myoclonic epilepsy (BME) was described comparatively recently (Dravet & Bureau, 1981), and is not yet recognized by everybody. Some people do not clearly see the difference between the benign and the severe forms of myoclonic epilepsy in infancy (Lombroso, 1990).

It appears that the difference between BME and an idiopathic WS should also be discussed if we accept that WS may be idiopathic. The present International Classification (Commission, 1989) distinguishes only the symptomatic and the cryptogenic forms of WS, but it seems reasonable to accept the existence of an idiopathic type of WS, as discussed by Jeavons and Livet (1992), according to the data of Dulac *et al.* (1986, 1993). In that case idiopathic WS and BME would be the two types of generalized epilepsies with a favourable outcome appearing in the first year of life. In the author's opinion their similarities stop here.

The West syndrome

The definition of WS and its main characteristics are well known: infantile spasms, arrest of psychomotor development, hypsarrhythmia in the electroencephalogram (EEG). Of these, one element may be missing. This triad occurs before the age of 1 year, with a peak between 4 and 7 months. Usually the prognosis is very poor.

Several studies have analysed the *semiology of the spasms* by polygraphic and video recording, first by Gastaut *et al.* (1964), and then by Frost *et al.* (1978), Plouin *et al.* (1987), Glaze *et al.* (1988) and Fusco and Vigevano (1993). The spasm consists of a sudden contraction, usually bilateral and symmetrical, of the muscles of the neck, trunk and limbs. An abrupt contraction lasting less than 2 s is usually followed by a less intense but more sustained contraction lasting 2 to 10 s. But it can be limited to the initial jerk followed by a relaxation of the muscles (like a flash of lightning or a flick knife). The type of the spasm depends on the affected muscles: there are flexor, extensor or most often mixed spasms. They can be asymmetrical, or even unilateral in some of the symptomatic cases, as in hemimegalencephaly. Sometimes they are limited to either a nod of the head, a slight shrug of the shoulders or a stare.

One of their essential characteristics is their frequent occurrence in series: several dozen spasms occur at 5–30 s intervals. Their intensity can either increase or diminish during the course of the cluster. This repetition is an important diagnostic clue. It is observed electively at the end of sleep, upon awakening and during drowsiness just before sleeping. The spasms are less frequent during slow sleep and never occur during rapid-eye-movement (REM) sleep (Plouin *et al.*, 1987). Usually there is a behavioural change during the cluster of spasms: the infant may either cry or smile, sometimes appearing to be aware that something strange is happening and seeming to expect the next spasm. At the end of the series, the infant either comes back to his/her usual behaviour or falls asleep.

Classically, the spasms are accompanied by different EEG patterns: initial high-amplitude sharp and slow waves, often with superimposed diffuse fast rhythms or followed by a period of flattening. This decremental pattern, as well as the rapid rhythms, can occur as an isolated finding. The most recent work of Fusco and Vigevano (1993) has shown that the only true EEG pattern of spasm was the slow wave, with or without associated rapid rhythms, named 'spindle-like' activity by these authors. Figure 1 illustrates one series of spasms of this type. Clinical and EEG characteristics seem thus to indicate that a spasm is a type of seizure which belongs neither to the myoclonias nor to the tonic seizures, and which deserves to have its own place in the classification of seizures, as in the 1970 classification (Gastaut, 1970), whereas it is not mentioned in the 1981 classification (Commission, 1981). However, we must remark that some spasms do not have any visible EEG correlate, particularly at the onset and at the end of a cluster, when the clinical aspect is limited to a small change in the eyes or an extremely slight axial contraction. Hypsarrhythmia can disappear or continue between the repeated spasms. When it disappears, it may be replaced by progressively increasing slow waves, and the cluster of spasms could be considered as a single epileptic seizure (Dulac *et al.*, 1986). However, this aspect is not always easy to distinguish on the recordings because of numerous artefacts.

Hypsarrhythmia has been described by Gibbs and Gibbs (1952). Slow waves of large amplitude are mixed with spikes and sharp waves whose amplitude and topography vary in an asynchronous manner between the two hemispheres. Background activity is not discernible. In slow sleep there is a fragmentation of the hypsarrhythmia, with bursts of polyspike waves which are more diffuse and synchronous, and spindles are visible. This hypsarrhythmic aspect disappears during REM sleep (Fig. 2). All studies of the WS have underlined that hypsarrhythmia was not always present with its typical features in the traces, even in the active phase of the syndrome, being replaced by 'modified hypsarrhythmia' or focal and multifocal, sometimes asymmetrical, abnormalities. Lacy and Penry (1976) indicate that only about 60 per cent of patients described by different authors had a true or modified hypsarrhythmia. In their recent study Watanabe *et al.* (1993) confirm the variability of the interictal patterns in WS.

A delay in psychomotor development or a regression are associated with the spasms in 95 per cent of the cases (Jeavons & Livet, 1992). There is loss of social smiling, of interest in objects, of voluntary prehension and often of ocular pursuit. Infants become irritable, unsatisfied, crying without apparent reason when awake; they do not sleep quietly. The muscular tone decreases, leading to a postural regression.

Classical antiepileptic drugs are usually not effective, even if some patients may have a good response

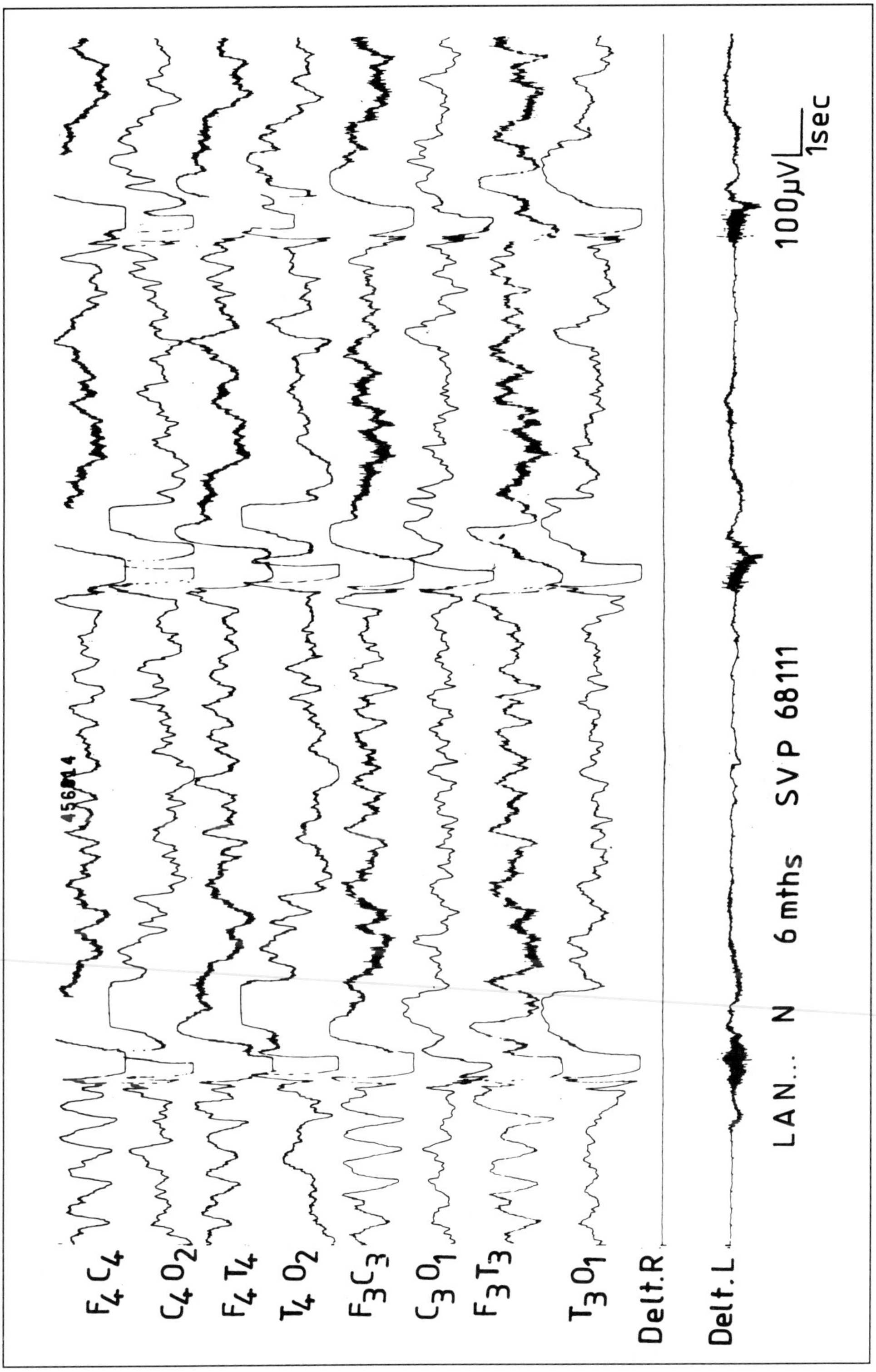

Fig. 1. Infantile spasms: a series of spasms characterized by a brief tonic contraction of the right and left deltoids, accompanied by a diffuse high-amplitude slow wave in the EEG. (With the kind permission of O. Dulac and P. Plouin.)

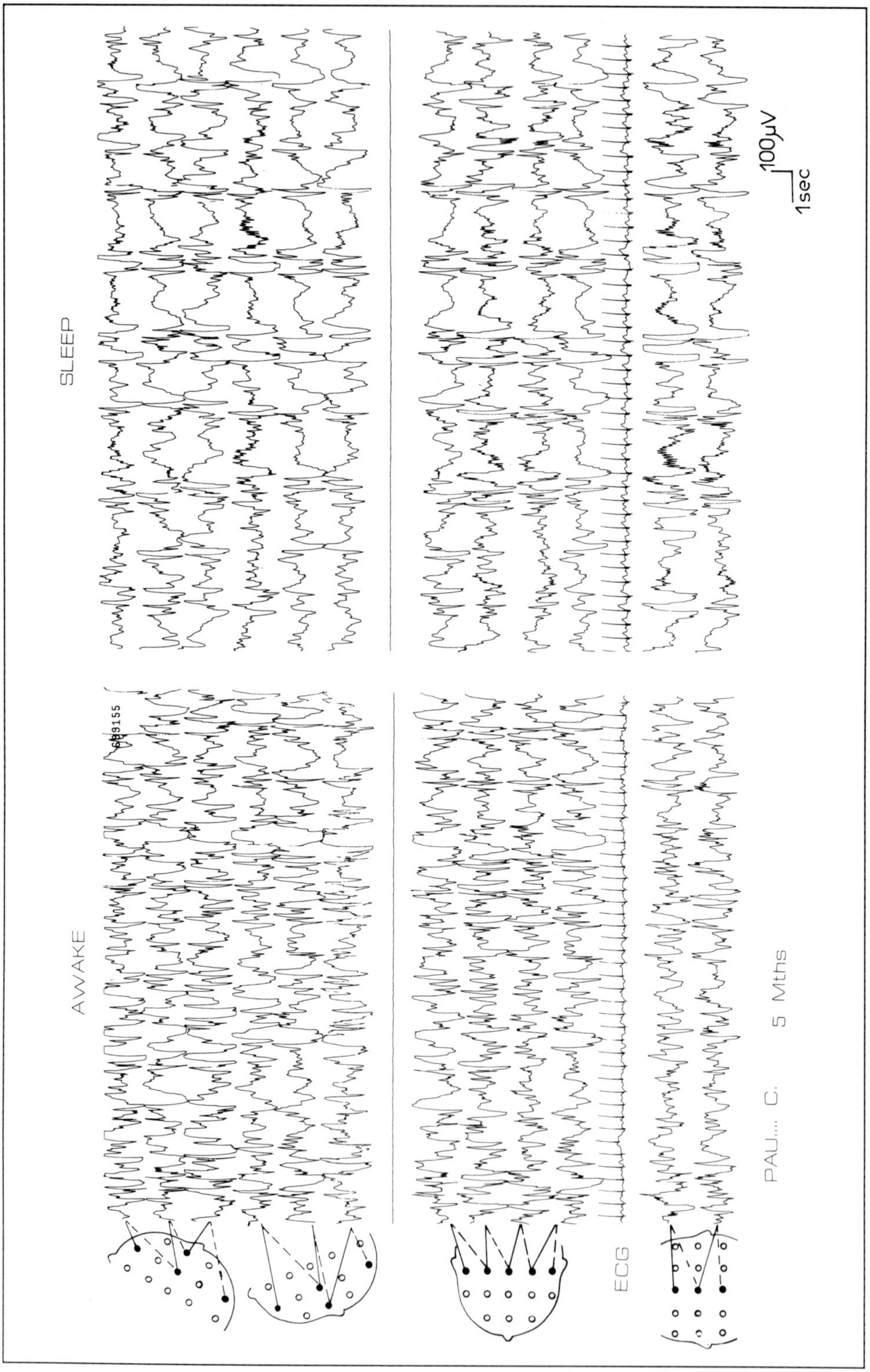

Fig. 2. Infantile spasms: an example of typical hypsarrhythmia. Left: awake recording, showing slow waves of high voltage intermixed with diffuse or asynchronous spikes on both hemispheres. Right: sleep recording, showing fragmentation of the hypsarrhythmia and the presence of spindles.

to high doses of valproate (Bachman, 1982). Treatment by corticosteroids has been found to control the spasms better, but the long term results are not satisfactory (Glaze *et al.*, 1988).

Two forms of WS are recognized: the symptomatic form, with a known aetiology or the previous existence of signs of organic brain damage; and the cryptogenic form, in which no aetiology and no signs of brain damage are found.

What about the idiopathic type? Since the first studies on the outcome of WS, it is known that it can disappear rapidly, even spontaneously in some patients where there is no clear aetiology and who remain normal after the end of the spasms (Jeavons *et al.*, 1973). But it was the merit of O. Dulac and co-workers to have underlined the possible existence of a type of WS with specific characteristics which could be considered as idiopathic and not as cryptogenic (Dulac *et al.*, 1986, 1993). Besides normal development, clinical examination and neuroimaging as in the cryptogenic type, these patients always present symmetric spasms, occurring independently during a series, not associated with other types of seizure, a true hypsarrhythmia in the EEGs, without localized spikes after intravenous diazepam, and a rapid good response when treated. From the psychomotor point of view, they do not lose ocular pursuit during the acute phase of the disease. Of course, the EEG features do not fulfil the criteria of the other types of idiopathic generalized epilepsies (presence of generalized spikes and waves and normal background). It would be necessary to prove that another type of EEG change can be associated with a genetic predisposition in the first months of life, which is the most debatable point of this discussion. This hypothesis remains to be supported by further genetic studies. However, in the series reported by Vigevano *et al.* (1993), there is a group of 17 patients with a favourable outcome and a normal neurological and psychological development, who had a family history of other forms of idiopathic epilepsy or febrile convulsions, or who developed an EEG genetic trait (photo-convulsive response, spike-wave discharges, rolandic spikes) during the follow-up. Up to now almost all the patients with idiopathic WS, in the two groups (Dulac *et al.*, 1993; Vigevano *et al.*, 1993), have been treated by corticosteroids.

Table 1 shows the differential diagnostic of WS, considering every element of the triad. Here we are concerned only with the other type of idiopathic generalized epilepsy occurring at the same age, i.e. BME.

Table 1. Differential diagnosis of West syndrome

Spasms or	Pure myoclonic seizures Myoclonic atonic seizures Tonic seizures Abnormal movements
Hypsarrhythmia or	Generalized spike waves Modified hypsarrhythmia Focal abnormalities Normal EEG (awake and asleep)
Psychomotor development:	Delayed Arrest Regression Normal

Benign myoclonic epilepsy

As described in 1981, it is characterized by the occurrence of generalized myoclonias, before the age of 3 years, in normal infants, without other symptoms, the EEG showing rapid generalized spike waves, the response to drug treatment being good and the psychomotor development remaining normal.

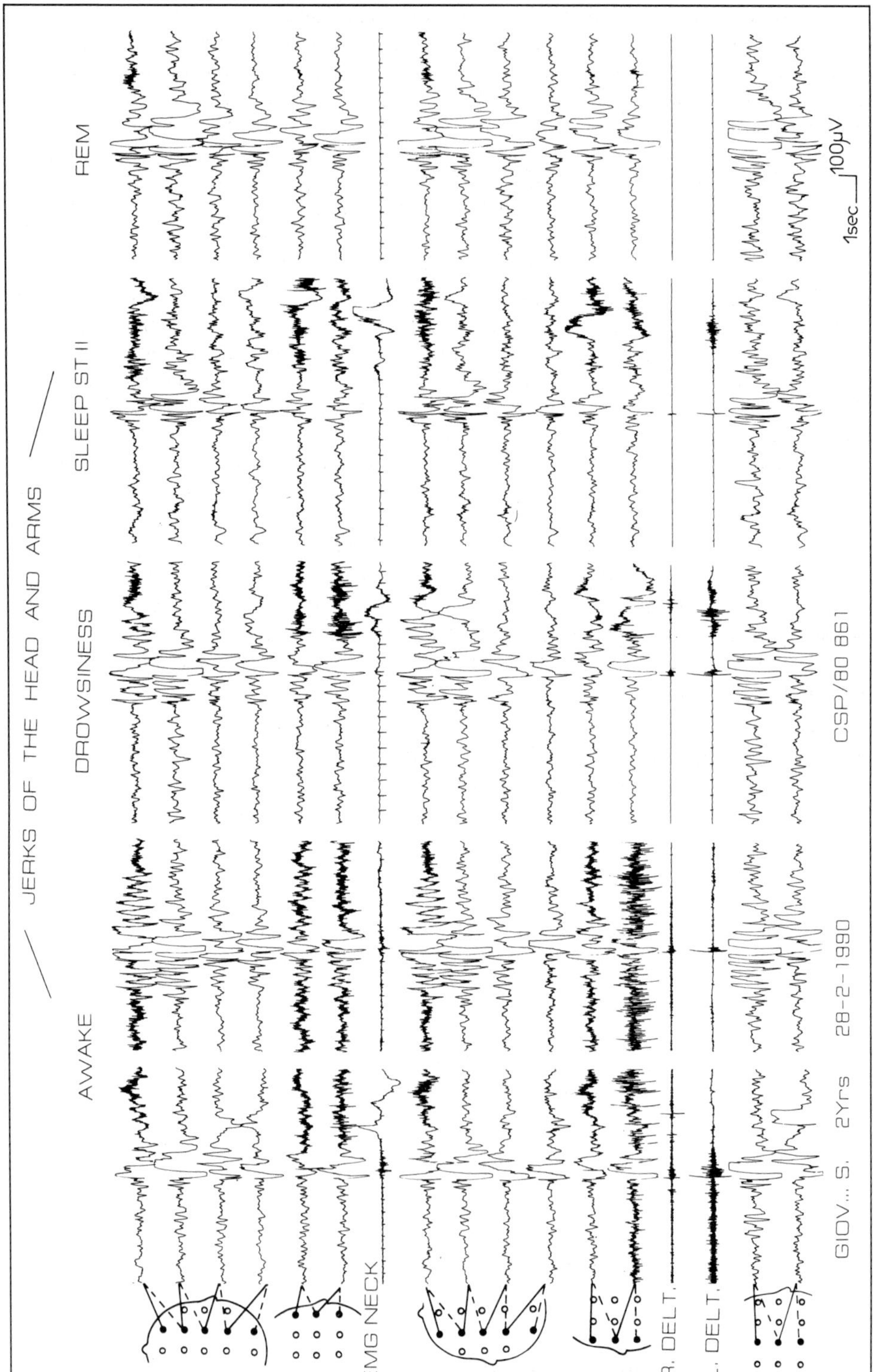

Fig. 3. Benign myoclonic epilepsy of infancy. Several myoclonic jerks are recorded before any treatment, while awake, when drowsy and during sleep stage II. They are associated with generalized spike waves, sometimes preceded by spike waves localized in the anterior areas. Subclinical discharges of the same type are present during REM. R. DELT: right deltoid muscle; L. DELT.: left deltoid muscle.

The *myoclonias* predominate in the head and upper limbs, causing a sudden head drop onto the trunk, and an upward–outward movement of the upper limbs with flexion of the lower limbs. They may also provoke a rolling of the eyeballs. The intensity of the seizures varies greatly from one child to another, and sometimes from one attack to another in the same child. The most severe forms cause the child to fall suddenly and to throw involuntarily any objects he/she may be holding. The mildest forms provoke only brief forward movements of the head or even a simple closing of the eyes. As a rule the myoclonic attacks (MA) are very brief (1–3 s) and there is no apparent loss of consciousness. Sometimes they occur in groups of three or four but they are not repeated in series and they can occur at any time of the day, during drowsiness or activities, without any known triggering factor. They do not influence the behaviour of the infant unless the jerks are strong, leading to crying.

On *EEG recordings* (Fig. 3), polygraphy demonstrates that the MA are always accompanied by a discharge of generalized spike waves or polyspike waves at 3 c/s and by a brief jerk in the recorded muscles. In some patients myoclonias appear to be favoured by intermittent photic stimulation (IPS). They usually, but not always, disappear during slow-wave sleep. The background is normal for the age. Some slow waves may be found over the central areas. During the waking state interictal spike waves are rare, most of the discharges having a clinical expression. IPS does not provoke spike waves without concomitant myoclonia. The organization of sleep is normal. The discharges tend to become less frequent during slow-wave sleep. Exceptionally they can be observed during REM sleep (Fig. 3).

The affected infants are normal at the onset, *psychomotor development continues regularly* and no behavioural change is observed so that parents and paediatricians tend not to worry. These MA can be either preceded or followed by one or two simple febrile convulsions. Neuroimaging investigations are normal. A family history of epilepsy or febrile convulsions is present in 31 per cent of cases. The drug of choice is valproate, which has controlled the seizures in all our patients and in most of the patients of Todt and Müller (1992).

At present there are about 37 cases reported in the literature, including our 12 patients.

There is controversy concerning the long-term outcome and the benignity of this condition. However, few studies describe a long-term follow-up of the patients. According to our own data and to those of Todt and Müller (1992), shown in Tables 2 and 3, the prognosis is usually good.

Table 2. Seizure outcome in BME.

	Dravet *et al.*, 1992 12 patients	Todt & Müller, 1992 14 patients
Seizure-free	9	11
without treatment	5	–
with treatment	4	–
Persistence of seizures	0	3
Lost to follow-up	3	–

Table 3. Psychological outcome in BME.

	Dravet *et al.*, 1992 12 patients	Todt & Müller, 1992 14 patients
Normal	5	11
Slight retardation	3	3
Mild retardation	3	–
Severe retardation	1 (Down's syndrome)	–

Conclusion

Infantile spasms in idiopathic WS and MA in BME are different in their clinical expression, their mode of occurrence, their ictal and interictal EEG and polygraphic expression and their response to drugs. Also the age of onset, clinical history of the affected infant, psychomotor development, behaviour and long-term outcome are different. There is no doubt that we are dealing with two different epileptic syndromes.

BME is probably the earliest form of the generalized idiopathic epilepsies. Its onset is not limited to the first year of life but may take place until age 3 years. The diagnosis is relatively easy through an accurate anamnesis and an EEG recording of the attacks. A good prognosis can be affirmed if all the criteria are met. It must be treated by valproate. If not, the myoclonias persist, there is no other type of seizure, the EEG does not change but the psychomotor development becomes delayed.

If idiopathic WS exists, it never starts after age 1 year, it is characterized by a peculiar type of seizure, accompanied by at least a behavioural change, often by transient psychomotor arrest, and by a specific and very abnormal EEG. The diagnosis of the idiopathic nature of WS and the prognosis are not as easy as in BME and need numerous investigations. On the other hand we do not know whether or not initial treatment by valproate only could give a good result as in BME. At present, the adequate treatment still seems to be steroid therapy.

References

Bachman, D.S. (1982): Use of valproic acid in treatment of infantile spasms. *Arch. Neurol.* **39,** 49–52.

Commission on Classification and Terminology of the International League Against Epilepsy (1981): Proposal for revised clinical and electroencephalographic classification of epileptic seizures. *Epilepsia* **22,** 489–501.

Commission on Classification and Terminology of the International League Against Epilepsy (1989): Proposal for revised classification of epilepsies and epileptic syndromes. *Epilepsia* **30,** 389–399.

Dravet, C. & Bureau, M. (1981): L'épilepsie myoclonique bénigne du nourrisson. *Rev. EEG Neurophysiol.* **11,** 438–444.

Dravet, Ch., Bureau, M. & Genton, P. (1992): Benign myoclonic epilepsy of infancy: the electroclinical symptomatology and differential diagnosis from the other types of generalized epilepsy in infancy. In: Benign localized and generalized epilepsies of early childhood. Epilepsy Res. (suppl. 6) eds, R. Degeu & F.E. Dreifuss, pp. 131–135. Amsterdam: Elsevier.

Dulac, O., Plouin, P., Jambaqué, I. & Motte, J. (1986): Spasmes infantiles épileptiques bénins. *Rev. EEG Neurophysiol. Clin.* **16,** 371–382.

Dulac, O., Plouin, P. & Jamabaque, I. (1993): Predicting favorable outcome in idiopathic West syndrome. *Epilepsia,* **34** (4), 747–756.

Frost, J.D., Hrachovy, R.A., Kellaway, P. & Zion, T. (1978): Quantitative analysis and characterization of infantile spasms. *Epilepsia* **19,** 273–282.

Fusco, L. & Vigevano, F. (1993): Ictal clinical electroencephalographical findings of spasms in West syndrome. *Epilepsia* **34** (4), 671–678.

Gastaut, H. (1970): Clinical and electroencephalographical classification of epileptic seizures. *Epilepsia* **11,** 102–113.

Gastaut, H., Roger, J., Soulayrol, R. & Pinsard, N. (1964): *Encéphalopathie myoclonique infantile avec hypsarythmie (syndrome de West).* Paris: Masson.

Gibbs, F.A. & Gibbs, E.L. (1952): *Atlas of electroencephalography: Epilepsy,* Vol. II. Cambridge, Mass.: Addison-Wesley.

Glaze, D.J., Hrachovy, R.A., Frost, J.D., Kellaway, P. & Zion, T. (1988): Prospective study of outcome of infants with infantile spasms treated during controlled studies of ACTH and prednisone. *J. Pediatr.* **112,** 389–396.

Jeavons, P.M. & Livet, M.O. (1992): West syndrome: infantile spasms. In: *Epileptic syndromes in infancy, childhood and adolescence*, 2nd edn, eds. J. Roger, M. Bureau, Ch. Dravet, F.E. Dreifuss, A. Perret & P. Wolf, pp. 53–65. London: John Libbey.

Jeavons, P.M., Bower, B.D. & Dimitrakoudi, M. (1973): Long-term prognosis of 150 cases of West syndrome. *Epilepsia* **14,** 153–164.

Lacy, J.R. & Penry, J.K. (1976): *Infantile spasms*. New York: Raven Press.

Lombroso, C.T. (1990): Early myoclonic encephalopathy, early infantile epileptic encephalopathy, and benign and severe infantile myoclonic epilepsies: a critical review and personal contributions. *J. Clin. Neurophysiol.* **7** (3), 380–408.

Plouin, P., Jalin, C., Dulac, O. & Chiron, C. (1987): Enregistrement ambulatoire de l'EEG pendant 24 h dans les spasmes infantiles épileptiques. *Rev. EEG Neurophysiol.* **11,** 419–424.

Todt, H. & Müller, D. (1992): The therapy of benign myoclonic epilepsy in infants. In: *The benign localized and generalized epilepsies in early childhood (Epilepsy Res.)*, eds. R. Degen & F.E. Dreifuss, pp. 137–139. Amsterdam: Elsevier.

Vigevano, F., Fusco, L., Cusmai, R., Claps, D., Ricci, S. & Milani, L. (1993): The idiopathic form of West syndrome. *Epilepsia* **34** (4), 743–746.

Watanabe, K., Negoro, T., Aso, K. & Matsumoto, A. (1993): Reappraisal of interictal electroencephalograms in infantile spasms. *Epilepsia* **34** (4), 679–685.

Epileptic Seizures and Syndromes, Edited by Peter Wolf
© 1994 John Libbey & Company Ltd., pp. 213–220

Chapter 27

Pitfalls in the diagnosis of grand mal on awakening

Dieter Janz

Abteilung für Neurologie, Klinikum Rudolf Virchow, Freie Universität Berlin, Augustenberger Plate 1, D-13353 Berlin, Germany

Introduction

A study published last year reported the distribution of epileptic syndromes as defined by the International Classification in patients from 275 general practitioners in England. During a period of 3 years 814 patients with epileptic seizures were identified, but there was not a single case of epilepsy with generalized tonic–clonic seizures (GTCS) on awakening (Manford *et al.*, 1992). However, in the chapter on epilepsy with grand mal on awakening in the revised edition of the 'guide bleu' of epileptic syndromes, published in the same year, Wolf (1992c) reported that the prevalence of epilepsy on awakening among hospitalized patients with grand mal ranges from 22 to 37 per cent. This discrepancy is surprising even if one considers Delgado-Escueta's claim (Delgado-Escueta *et al.*, 1990) that 'pure' epilepsy on awakening is much less common if a history of absences or myoclonic jerks is sought carefully. It is noteworthy that this syndrome has been described primarily by German (Janz, 1953; Beyer & Jovanovic, 1966) and French (Le Camus, 1951; David, 1955; Loiseau, 1964) authors but has been generally neglected by English-speaking authors, with the exception of Niedermeyer (1984). Is there a reason for this?

Has no one encountered a case like the following in the United States or England, or would the patient be evaluated and classified differently?

A 25-year-old student reported that he had suffered his first seizure on Ash Wednesday morning 5 years previously. He had stayed up late at a *mardi gras* party with his girlfriend and had got up early the next morning to go to university. The seizure occurred as he sat down to breakfast. The next seizure occurred 1½ years later under similar circumstances. He had attended a party the previous evening, gone to bed late and got up early. The seizure occurred about 1½ h after he arose. He has taken phenytoin (diphenylhydantoin) 200 mg daily since then. The third seizure occurred 1 year later after he had taken an overnight train from southern Germany to Berlin and had spent the day in town. He was going to rest in the apartment of a friend when the seizure took place. Despite phenytoin (diphenylhydantoin) 300 mg daily he suffered a fourth seizure approximately 3 months later when he was on his way to the station to take a train back to Berlin after the Christmas holidays. The previous evening he had stayed up late with his family and had slept poorly; he had hoped to catch up on his sleep in the train. Subsequent seizures occurred 6 months later – again early in the morning shortly after arising. He had intended to hitchhike home from Berlin and had got up early after sleeping badly because he had been anxious that he might oversleep. He was admitted to hospital, where he slept all morning and suffered his second seizure shortly after the midday meal. He was given phenytoin 300 mg daily but suffered another seizure while watching television in the evening after a hard day.

Several EEGs failed to document epileptiform discharge, and there were no signs of photosensitivity. The patient did not remember involuntary movements in the morning, and neither he nor his family and friends had noticed absences.

This case history contains all the basic characteristics of the syndrome under discussion. Five of seven seizures occurred shortly after awakening, though they may occur in the afternoon or the evening, usually in association with lack of sleep. The intervals between seizures become progressively shorter, and the seizures themselves are usually GTCS.

Even though the diagnosis may seem simple, even evident at the onset of the disorder, there are some potential traps that one must be aware of in order to make the diagnosis.

Morning or awakening?

The association between the seizure and awakening is important. Seizures always occur after awakening and are not associated with arising; therefore, the term 'rising fitters' (Griffiths & Fox, 1938) is not appropriate. Nor are they associated with a particular time of day, so the term 'matutinal epilepsy' is not appropriate either. They may occur while the patient is awake but still in bed or some time after arising. Since the pathomechanism is closely associated with the process of awakening, the question of the time of day at which these seizures occur is entirely inappropriate. A number of occupations, especially those with shift work, and changes in daily habits – quite common at weekends or during vacations – are associated with changes in the hour of awakening. Questions concerning the hour at which seizures occur may be misleading in patients with this type of epilepsy, since their seizures generally occur in exceptional circumstances – when they have gone to bed very late after a long night and awaken at an unusual hour during the day, or when they get up especially early after a short night's sleep – in order to go on a trip, for instance. It is important to realize this in order to pose the appropriate questions. Generally, patients with epilepsy on awakening tend to conceal the circumstances of the seizures. This is comprehensible, since it reveals a conflict which all these patients suffer – a conflict between knowledge and desire. The patients know the special circumstances associated with their seizures and know that they are avoidable. However, the patients do not wish to limit themselves or sacrifice any element of their lifestyle and they desire to live like 'normals'. A diagnosis of epilepsy on awakening presupposes a certain degree of knowledge which leads to the appropriate questions. The necessary prerequisite is interest and comprehension on the part of the physician, and taking the history carefully constitutes the beginning of treatment in these patients.

Variants in the clinical course

While a critical situation 'on awakening' is important in almost all cases, some patients describe an additional situation which disposes to seizures. This is the period at the end of the workday, which we have termed 'about eve'. The primary characteristic of this situation is relaxation after previous effort; this was the case in our patient at his third and at his last seizure, both of which occurred in situations of relaxation during leisure time. These circumstances of leisure are not coupled to a certain time of day and may occur at any time, although it is usual and customary that they occur toward evening after work. Some patients demonstrate clinical courses that one might term 'free time' or 'leisure time' epilepsy, since the seizures occur almost exclusively in situations of relaxation. Patients with epilepsy on awakening usually suffer seizures about eve as well, while those with epilepsy during leisure time usually suffer seizures on awakening also.

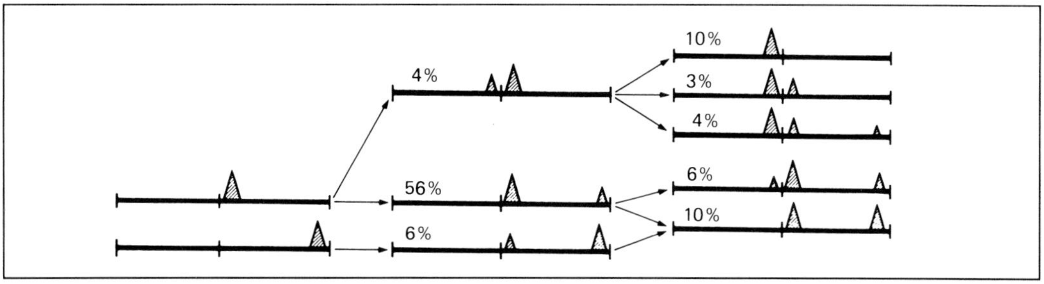

Fig. 1. Variation in the clinical course of 98 patients with grand mal epilepsy on awakening. The horizontal line represents the circadian rhythm of one day, on the left side the sleeping period, on the right side the waking period. The pyramids indicate the circadian predilection of the seizures. The height of the pyramids denotes the relative frequency of the seizures (Janz, 1962).

The temporal distribution of these variants is illustrated in Fig. 1, which shows the seizure peaks in the form of pyramids on a timeline, while the incidence of the variants is expressed in numbers. The illustration shows that epilepsy on awakening is sometimes accompanied by seizures during sleep, which may even predominate during the later clinical course.

These possible variants in the clinical course of this type of epilepsy raise the question whether longitudinal or cross-sectional observation should be used as diagnostic criteria for epilepsy on awakening. When the actual seizure distribution is used, a number of cases originally beginning as epilepsy on awakening will be classified as sleep epilepsy or random epilepsy. Longitudinal observation always carries the uncertain risk of retrospective classification. However, we prefer longitudinal observation for the classification of the cases in our series.

Two additional questions arise in considering variants of this disorder. How many seizures are required and how closely should the seizures be associated with characteristic situations in order to permit a diagnosis of epilepsy with grand mal on awakening? A diagnosis of epilepsy requires repeated seizures, as does identification of a consistent association of the seizures with a certain situation. Therefore, we require at least six grand mal seizures before making a diagnosis of grand mal epilepsy on awakening, during sleep or at random. In cases with fewer than six seizures we refer to isolated grand mal seizures or oligoepilepsy. We define epilepsy on awakening in patients who have suffered grand mal seizures exclusively or predominantly after awakening or at leisure. 'Predominantly' is defined as > 90 per cent of the time in the International Classification. However, we tend to use the general meaning of 'predominantly', which means more than half of the time.

Two or more seizures may occur in a single day, representing a series or a status. In these cases, as in sleep epilepsy, the first seizure is relevant for definition of the syndrome. Fortunately, grand mal series and grand mal status are rare in epilepsy on awakening.

Seizure syndromes

Grand mal epilepsy on awakening may occur with other epileptic seizures, usually with absences or myoclonic jerks or both, but only rarely with simple focal or complex focal seizures (Table 1). There is no apparent cause of grand mal epilepsy on awakening in most cases – in 90 per cent of our patients (Janz, 1969). An analysis of data published in 1969 shows that among all patients with epilepsy in a neurological department, excluding those with isolated seizures and oligoepilepsies, 27 per cent had grand mal on awakening, with 17 per cent in combination with other seizures and 10 per cent as pure grand mal on awakening. Three-quarters of the patients with combined seizures were associated with age-related minor generalized seizures of childhood and adolescence (Table 1).

Table 1. Diagnosis of grand mal on awakening (GMA) in epilepsy patients of a university hospital for neurology (Janz, 1969)

	Hospital in- and out-patients; n = 4816*			
Sample	n	%	n	%
GMA in combination	812	17		
with CAE, JAE, JME			616	13
with other seizures			196	4
GMA pure	508	10		
GMA total	1320	27		

*Without isolated and oligo- (up to 6) grand mal seizures.
CAE = childhood absence epilepsy; JAE = juvenile absence epilepsy; JME = juvenile myoclonic epilepsy.

Delgado-Escueta *et al.* (1990) claimed that epilepsies with 'pure' grand mal seizures (i.e. without initial absences or myoclonic jerks) are rare if verification of the seizures is available on videotape. There is no systematic investigation of this claim. However, clinical data from an exact history and observation indicate that pure grand mal on awakening constitutes less than half of cases, as data from the University of Heidelberg (Janz, 1969; Table 1) and of Schmitz and Wolf (1989) from the Free University of Berlin (Table 2) reveal. It is noteworthy that epilepsy with grand mal on awakening was diagnosed only half as frequently in Loiseau's private practice and was not found a single time during 1 year in his hospital (Loiseau *et al.*, 1991), although one can assume on the basis of his publications that he was well acquainted with this diagnosis (Loiseau, 1964).

Table 2. Syndromes of idiopathic generalized epilepsy: diagnosis in general practice, neurological private practice, neurological hospital

	General practice* n = 592		Hospital** n = 263†		Private practice** n = 570†		Hospital*** n = 699	
Sample	n	%	n	%	n	%	n	%
GMA	–	–	–		12	2.1	32	4.6
CAE }			14	5.3	60	10.5	52	7.5
}	13	2.2						
JAE }			7	2.7	17	3.0	56	8.5
JME	9	1.5	12	5.3	31	5.4	64	9.2

*Manford *et al.* (1992); **Loiseau *et al.* (1991); ***Schmitz & Wolf (1989). †For comparison without the cases under 2.3 and 4 of the International Classification. GMA = epilepsy with grand mal on awakening, CAE = childhood absence epilepsy, JAE = juvenile absence epilepsy, JME = juvenile myoclonic epilepsy.

The present investigation

We recently performed a clinical study of pure grand mal epilepsy on awakening – i.e. grand mal on awakening unassociated with other seizures (Janz & Purucker, 1993). We were primarily interested in genetic aspects of this disorder, especially the incidence and type of familial seizure disorders. In a review of all in-patients and out-patients of the Berlin University Klinikum Charlottenburg from 1973 to 1988 we identified 88 cases with at least six major seizures without focal onset and without other types of seizures. The ratio of males to females was 1.8 to 1 (Fig. 2).

Age of onset ranged from 7 to 45 years and was concentrated in the period of adolescence. Eighty-two per cent of patients suffered their first seizure between 12 and 24 years, 7 per cent before the age of 12 and 11 per cent after the age of 24 years. The average age of onset of epilepsy with grand mal on awakening was 17.1 years. Figure 3 demonstrates that this is the latest peak age of onset among the syndromes of idiopathic generalized epilepsy of childhood and adolescence. The age of onset is the

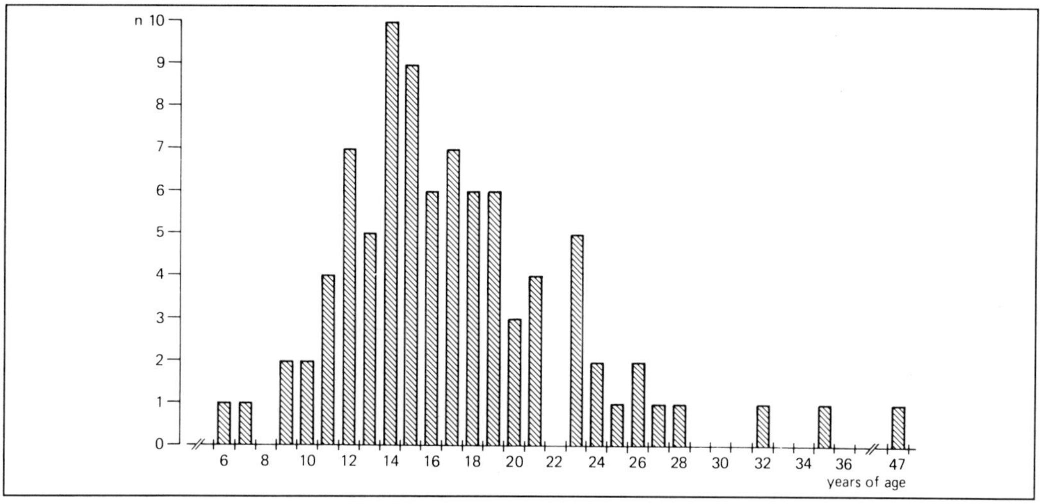

Fig. 2. Age of onset in 88 cases of primary grand mal on awakening.

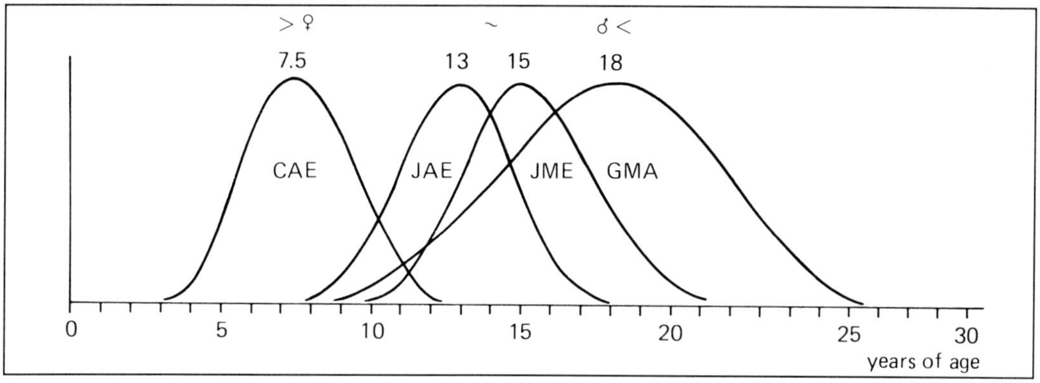

Fig. 3. Schematic manifestation spans and peaks, and sex ratio in childhood absence epilepsy (CAE), juvenile absence epilepsy (JAE), juvenile myoclonic epilspsy (JME) and epilepsy with grand mal on awakening (GMA).

strongest single criterion of a biological difference among the four subsyndromes of idiopathic generalized epilepsy (IGE), which tend to overlap in many ways and which may differ very subtly in some respects (Janz *et al.*, 1992; Beck-Mannagetta & Janz, 1991; Wolf, 1992a, b, c).

The incidence of manifest epileptic disease in close family members of patients with pure grand mal on awakening is virtually the same as that in close family members of patients with IGE associated with minor seizures, i.e. 3.8 per cent. The type of familial disease also suggests a close relationship between pure (genuine) epilepsy on awakening and other forms of IGE (Janz & Purucker, 1993).

Almost all patients (80 per cent) reported that their seizures occurred in association with external influences. The most common factor was lack of sleep (63 per cent), caused by going to bed late, restlessness or early rising, often combined with unaccustomed or excessive alcohol consumption (24 per cent). 'Stress' was reported as a cause by some patients. This referred to a wide variety of circumstances, such as acute conflict within the family, occupational problems, examination situations and problems at school. This raises the question whether the common denominator of these stress situations might also be a disturbance of sleep. Definition of a discrete form of epilepsy termed 'stress convulsions' (Friis, 1991) without reference to the importance of 'stress' in precipitating seizures in epilepsy on awakening (Janz, 1953; David, 1955; Helmchen, 1958; Loiseau, 1964; Beyer & Jovanovic, 1966) is rather unconvincing. Only four of 32 females reported an association between seizures and the menstrual cycle. Three patients reported repeated seizures after febrile episodes and one patient noted an association with the full moon.

The endogenous–exogenous pathogenic circle

One source of confusion in dealing with epilepsy on awakening is the apparently contradictory finding that this type of epilepsy is usually idiopathic and evidently hereditary in some cases, while the seizures are precipitated by external provoking factors, at least at the onset of disease if not during the entire clinical course. It seems paradoxical that this is an endogenous disease which becomes manifest under the influence of external provoking factors. The patient's own behaviour has a major influence on the clinical course. We have encountered patients with a single seizure in association with unaccustomed lack of sleep, who learned the appropriate lesson from their experience and changed their habits, with the result that they did not suffer additional seizures. Among the examples of these spontaneous cures are patients who changed their occupational activities, which were associated with lack of sleep. However, every specialist in epilepsy has encountered patients who refuse to recognize the association between their life style and their seizures and persist in placing themselves in situations which precipitate seizures.

This experience shows that the patient and his/her personality and surroundings are intimately involved in the dynamics of epilepsy. Grand mal epilepsy on awakening is a paradigm of these implications. This comprises a spectrum of patients, ranging from those who draw appropriate conclusions,learn from their experiences and contribute to their own cure to those who develop progredient epilepsy as a result of frivolity or fear of consequences. Reflection on this spectrum is useful in developing a concept of the processes causing epilepsy.

The endogenous component should not be neglected, but it should be emphasized that this is less a matter of fate than a potential factor. The fact that individuals with hypersynchronous EEG potentials may remain free of epilepsy illustrates this point.

Sleep is the common ground of the internal and external influences on this disorder. The clinical impression that the sleep patterns of patients with epilepsy on awakening tend to produce a chronic sleep deficit (Christian, 1960; Janz, 1974) is supported by the results of polygraph sleep studies, which demonstrated that the sleep of these patients is particularly unstable and subject to external influences (Wolf *et al.*, 1984). Clinical experience and EEG data permit the conclusion that these patients suffer from a constitutional inability to compensate for external influences on sleep (Wolf, 1992b). When the compensatory reserves of these patients are exhausted by external circumstances, seizures may result in the phase of awakening.

Additional factors which may appear to be exogenous in nature – a tendency to go to bed too late, to drink alcohol and to exert oneself at unconventional hours – may contain an endogenous component, which might be construed as suggestibility, a tendency to be easily misled or even as a weakness of character which could be described in psychological terms. The psychological aspect should not become a pitfall in the diagnosis of these disorders. This is possible when seizures occurring after extreme situations are described as non-epileptic seizures or 'stress convulsions' or when the clinician believes that simple admonition will suffice to prevent further seizures. The tendency to repetition of similar situations and the inability to withstand temptation should be addressed when establishing the prognosis and defining the treatment together with these patients.

The intervals between seizures get shorter with time, while the precipitating situations become less dramatic, especially when seizures occur during sleep as well (see also Fig. 1). It is possible to claim that the relationship between exogenous disturbances and endogenous disposition changes in the sense that, over time, smaller irritations are sufficient to trigger seizures. The pathophysiology of this phenomenon, described by Gowers as 'seizures beget seizures', is currently the subject of a considerable experimental effort on the topic of 'epileptogenesis'. However, the social consequences and the psychological effects on the patient when seizures occur at decreasing intervals in association with slight external causes should also be investigated more thoroughly. My experience suggests that this process of habituation to the seizures is associated with increasing resignation on the part of the patient, who makes fewer efforts to order his/her life and finishes by despising him/herself. There is no pathophysiological mechanism explaining deterioration of this kind nor can it be prevented by medication or admonition, and I am convinced that this type of patient career can be prevented only when apparently exogenous factors, such as irregular behaviour and sleep disorders, are understood also as components of internal processes. This would permit more adequate recognition of a weakness, which would then be amenable to integration into a therapeutic concept. In this sense, a diagnosis of epilepsy on awakening implies the concept of a pathogenetic mechanism as well as a more comprehensive treatment programme.

References

Beck-Mannagetta, G. & Janz, D. (1991): Syndrome-related genetics in generalized epilepsy. In: *Genetic strategies in epilepsy research*, eds. V.E. Anderson, W.A. Hauser, I.E. Leppik, J.L. Noebels & S.S. Rich, pp. 105–112. Amsterdam: Elsevier.

Beyer, L. & Jovanovic, U.J. (1966): Elektroencephalographische und klinische Korrelate bei Aufwachepileptikern mit besonderer Berücksichtigung der therapeutischen Probleme. *Nervenarzt* **37,** 333–336.

Christian, W. (1960): Bioelektrische Charakteristik tagesperiodisch gebundener Verlaufsformen epileptischer Erkrankungen. *J. Neurol.* **181,** 413–444.

David, J. (1955): L'épilepsie du réveil. Thesis, Lyon.

Delgado-Escueta, A.J., Greenberg, D., Weissbecker, K., Liu, A., Treiman, L., Sparkes, R., Park, M.S Barbetti, A. & Terasaki, P.J. (1990): Gene mapping in the idiopathic generalized epilepsies: juvenile myoclonic epilepsy, childhood absence epilepsy, epilepsy with grand mal seizures, and early childhood myoclonic epilepsy. *Epilepsia* **31** (Suppl. 3), S19–S29.

Friis, M.L. (1991): Stress convulsions. In: *Comprehensive epileptology*, eds. M. Dam & L. Gram, pp. 247–250. New York: Raven Press.

Griffiths, G.N. & Fox, J.T. (1938): Rhythm in epilepsy. *Lancet* **234,** 409–416.

Helmchen, H. (1958): Beitrag zur konstitutionellen Differenzierung im Bereich genuiner Epilepsien. *J. Neurol.* **178,** 541–582.

Janz, D. (1953): 'Aufwach'-epilepsien (als Ausdruck einer den 'Nacht'-oder 'Schlaf'-Epilepsien gegenüberzustellenden Verlaufsform epileptischer Erkrankungen). *Arch. Z. Neurol.* **191,** 73–98.

Janz, D. (1962): The grand mal epilepsies and the sleeping–waking cycle. *Epilepsia* **3,** 69–109.

Janz, D. (1969): *Die Epilepsien: spezielle Pathologie und Therapie.* Stuttgart: Thieme.

Janz, D. (1974): Epilepsy and the sleeping–waking cycle. In: *The epilepsies* (Handbooks of Clinical Neurology, Vol. 15), eds. O. Magnus & A.M. Lorentz de Haas, pp. 457–490. Amsterdam: North-Holland.

Janz, D. & Purucker, H. (1993): Aufwach-Epilepsie: eine klinische und genetische Untersuchung. Manuscript.

Janz, D., Beck-Mannagetta, G. & Sander, T. (1992): Do idiopathic generalized epilepsies share a common susceptibility gene? *Neurology* **42** (Suppl. 5), 48–55.

Le Camus L. (1951): L'épilepsie du réveil. Thesis: Paris.

Loiseau, P. (1964): Crises épileptiques survenant au réveil et épilepsie du reveil. *Sud Méd. Chirurg.* **99,** 11492–11502.

Loiseau, P., Duchét, B. & Loiseau, J. (1991): Classification of epilepsies and epileptic syndromes in two different samples of patients. *Epilepsia* **32,** 303–309.

Manford, M., Hart, Y.M., Sander, J.W.A.S. & Shorvon, S.D. (1992): The national general practice study of epilepsy: the syndromic classification of the International League Against Epilepsy applied to epilepsy in a general population. *Arch. Neurol.* **49,** 801–808.

Niedermeyer, E. (1984): Awakening epilepsy (Aufwach-Epilepsie) revisited 30 years later. In: *Epilepsy, sleep and sleep deprivation*, eds. R. Degen & E. Niedermeyer, pp. 85–96. Amsterdam: Elsevier.

Schmitz, B. & Wolf, P. (1989): Epilepsies and epileptic syndromes in a neurological seizure clinic. In: *Genetics of the epilepsies*, eds. G. Beck-Mannagetta, V.E. Anderson, H. Doose & D. Janz, pp. 19–22. Berlin, Heidelberg, New York: Springer.

Wolf, P. (1992a): Juvenile absence epilepsy. In: *Epileptic syndromes in infancy, childhood and adolescence,* 2nd edn, eds. J. Roger, M. Bureau, Ch. Dravet, F.E. Dreifuss, A. Perret & P. Wolf, pp. 307–312. London: John Libbey.

Wolf, P. (1992b): Juvenile myoclonic epilepsy. In: *Epileptic syndromes in infancy, childhood and adolescence,* 2nd edn, eds. J. Roger, M. Bureau, Ch. Dravet, F.E. Dreifuss, A. Perret & P. Wolf, pp. 313–327. London: John Libbey.

Wolf, P. (1992c) Epilepsy with grand mal on awakening. In: *Epileptic syndromes in infancy, childhood and adolescence,* 2nd edn, eds. J. Roger, M. Bureau, Ch. Dravet, F.E. Dreifuss, A. Perret & P. Wolf, pp. 329–341. London: John Libbey.

Wolf, P., Röder-Wanner, U.U. & Brede, M. (1984): Influence of therapeutic phenobarbital and phenytoin medikation on the polygraphic sleep of patients with epilepsy. *Epilepsia* **25,** 467–475.

Epileptic Seizures and Syndromes, Edited by Peter Wolf
© 1994 John Libbey & Company Ltd., pp. 221–230

Chapter 28

Juvenile myoclonic epilepsy: an underdiagnosed syndrome

Chrysostomos P. Panayiotopoulos

Department of Clinical Neurophysiology and Epilepsy, St. Thomas's Hospital, London SE1 7EH, UK

Introduction

Despite well-defined clinical and electroencephalographic (EEG) features, high prevalence and its importance in genetics, prognosis and treatment, juvenile myoclonic epilepsy (JME) remains underdiagnosed, not only by general physicians but also by experienced neurologists (Delgado-Escueta & Enrile-Bascal, 1984; Janz, 1985, 1989; Obeid & Panayiotopoulos, 1988; Panayiotopoulos *et al.*, 1991, 1992, 1994; Grunewald *et al.*, 1992).

More than 90 per cent of patients with JME are not correctly diagnosed. The factors contributing to this and the consequences for seizure control and the quality of life of these patients have been previously detailed (Panayiotopoulos *et al.*, 1991; Grunewald *et al.*, 1992). Recent detailed reviews on JME (Wolf, 1992; Grunewald & Panayiotopoulos, 1993) and two large studies (Canevini *et al.*, 1993; Panayiotopoulos *et al.*, 1994) can be found elsewhere.

Definition

JME is an idiopathic generalized epileptic disorder which is hereditary. Prevalence is 5–11 per cent amongst adult and adolescent patients with epilepsies and both sexes are equally affected. JME is characterized by myoclonic jerks on awakening, generalized tonic–clonic seizures (GTCS), and absences in more than one-third of the patients. The seizures have an age-related onset, with absences appearing first in either childhood or adolescence, followed by myoclonic jerks and GTCS in the middle teens; all seizures are probably lifelong although absences may become less severe with age, jerks and GTCS probably improving after the fourth decade of life.

Seizure-precipitating factors, such as sleep deprivation and fatigue, alcohol, photosensitivity and mental and psychological arousal, are prominent.

The EEG in untreated patients is usually abnormal, with generalized discharges of an irregular mixture of 3–6 Hz spike/polyspike and slow wave, with intradischarge fragmentations, unstable intradischarge frequency and no constant relations of spikes/multiple spikes with the slow wave of the complexes. One-third show photoconvulsive responses and one-third may also have focal EEG abnormalities.

Inclusion criteria for JME

(a) Unequivocal clinical evidence of generalized seizures with myoclonic jerks on awakening.
(b) No evidence of neurological or intellectual deficit although JME occurs in patients with these deficits caused by other factors unrelated to JME. How JME and other brain insults interact and the clinical product of this interaction are not known.
(c) Abnormal EEG in untreated patients with generalized spike and/or multiple spike-slow wave discharges. Focal or background abnormalities should be accepted if other clinical and EEG criteria are strictly justified. Normal EEGs in treated patients are common.
(d) Normal brain imaging where performed.

Exclusion criteria

(a) Clinical or EEG evidence of myoclonic jerks secondary to brain hypoxia, metabolic diseases or other structural brain abnormalities.
(b) Myoclonic jerks of other epileptic syndromes clinically or genetically defined (e.g. Baltic-Mediterranean myoclonus) or other epileptic syndromes such as eyelid myoclonia with absences, pure forms of photosensitive epilepsy, self-induced epilepsy.
(c) Other generalized seizures without firm documentation of myoclonic jerks.
(d) EEG abnormalities but no clinical evidence of any type of seizures. Healthy members of JME families with unequivocal generalized spike/polyspike and slow wave discharges should probably be included for the purposes of genetic studies.

The rate of misdiagnosis of JME remains high

We have studied the factors of error in the diagnosis of JME in 70 patients with JME in Riyadh (Panayiotopoulos *et al.*, 1991) and 15 patients in London (Grunewald *et al.*, 1992) and concluded that:

(a) JME was unrecognized or misdiagnosed for many years in more than 90 per cent of the patients.
(b) Diagnoses were usually vague and non-syndromic; 'epilepsy', 'grand mal', 'temporal lobe epilepsy'. Pseudoseizures and alcohol-induced fits were often suspected.
(c) Myoclonic jerks and absences were not evaluated either because the patient was not specifically questioned or because relevant questions were not understood by the patients.
(d) Focal epilepsy was diagnosed because absences were mistaken as complex partial seizures, unilaterally reported jerks as partial motor seizures; this erroneous diagnosis was often bolstered by focal EEG abnormalities (Aliberti *et al.*, 1994; Panayiotopoulos *et al.*, 1994).
(e) Drug treatment was unsatisfactory; carbamazepine was prescribed more often than sodium valproate. Medication was reduced or withdrawn in patients who did not have GTCS, despite continuing myoclonic jerks and absences. Sodium valproate was stopped or substituted for carbamazepine in female patients anticipating pregnancy; phenobarbitone was substituted with newer drugs like carbamazepine.
(f) Control of seizures was poor; on substitution of appropriate medication striking improvement was achieved.
(g) Avoidable morbidity in addition to the psychological and social effects and embarrassment of poor seizure control included injury to self or child (death also was recorded), status epilepticus (convulsive and non-convulsive), loss of or prohibition to obtain driving licence, depression, learning and behavioural problems, loss of or inability to obtain employment.

The factors responsible for the delayed diagnosis of JME are often multiple; the most important is that the physicians are not attracted to the syndromic classification of epilepsies. Our traditional teaching is to differentiate 'fits' from 'faints and funny turns'; the next step is to exclude an underlying structural lesion in patients with genuine epileptic seizures. Subsequently, the patient's condition is labelled as 'epilepsy' and treatment is initiated after a second seizure; drugs are withdrawn after 2–3 years' freedom from seizures, management is empirical and no prognosis is conveyed. Avoidable morbidity is the result (Editorial, 1992).

A didactic case diagnosed before the description of JME

The following case (Grunewald & Panayiotopoulos, 1993) was correctly diagnosed in 1949, and is probably the first case of JME accurately described clinically with EEG, 8 years before the classical report of JME by Janz and Christian (1957).

Mr D, a successful businessman born in 1927, was referred to me in 1992 by his general physician to 'review his grand mal epilepsy . . . Attempts in the past to slowly reduce phenobarbitone and replace it with carbamazepine have resulted in an increase in fits, and therefore patient's compliance.'

An excellent description of the patient's seizures (myoclonic jerks on awakening, diurnal absences and GTCS) is reproduced from a district hospital medical notes for didactic and historic purposes:

1949. 'Illness started five years ago. He began by waking up at night about 2 a.m. and shaking violently – tonic spasms – followed by almost uncontrollable clonic movements until falling, but not loss of consciousness, only twice has he been incontinent of urine, once bitten his tongue.

He does not know if he wakes himself at night by shaking or if he wakes to pass water and becomes shaky and falls on getting up.

These fits come on also in the morning on getting up, and recently have recurred several times a week, only on working days except on one occasion; he has not infrequently bruised his head on falling; he often falls whilst walking or drops his tin jug of shaving water, but is able to shave. He takes 1 h 15 min from getting out from bed to leaving the house after breakfast.

The one occasion when the falling fits occurred on a Sunday was when he was cycling early to church and fell from his cycle, he felt embarrassed and went to church.

He never has falling fits by day, but he has transient losses of consciousness strongly resembling petit mal.

Phenobarbitone and various other sedations (what?) tried by local doctor were not effective.'

September, 1949. 'Seen yesterday evening, half an hour later found in fit near bus stop. Readmitted. Had a major fit during the first night.'

March, 1949. 'The EEG shows frequent high-voltage epileptic discharges throughout, of the type associated with myoclonic epilepsy.

These discharges are inhibited when the eyes are opened. There is no focus of abnormality, and the discharges are seen in both hemispheres without asymmetry.' (C.C. Evans. Physician in charge)

Subsequent EEGs, between 1980 and 1992, showed diffuse and non-specific abnormalities, some of which were described as focal.

He was seen by many physicians and by at least three experienced neurologists on many occasions. The myoclonic jerks and absences were not appreciated and the diagnosis was 'epilepsy', 'grand mal', 'seizures'; the differential diagnosis was between idiopathic, temporal lobe and post-traumatic epilepsy. The following is an extract from a neurologist's report:

1982–1987. 'In addition to the major attacks which have varied in frequency from one to two a month to one every two years or so, he has also had periods during which he feels anxious and has a sense of foreboding . . . and sometimes he has myoclonic jerks with them . . . the period of foreboding may lead to a major convulsion . . .

His medication was adjusted a few months ago to phenytoin alone. Despite this he has continued to have frequent fits . . . Intoxication with phenytoin 500 mg daily . . . I would have thought that carbamazepine would be the drug of choice . . . hopefully that will prove more beneficial than phenytoin . . . reassured . . .'

1992. Discharge summary from a teaching hospital in London: 'This 65 years old gentleman has had epilepsy since the age of 17 following head trauma. It is grand mal in nature and is controlled by phenytoin 100 mg tds and phenobarbitone 60 mg tds. He was admitted having had a fit after which he did not fully regain consciousness and continued twitching for several hours. On examination he was slightly drowsy and post-ictal with persistent twitching . . . '.

Clinical symptoms

Myoclonic jerks

The myoclonic jerks of JME generally appear when the patient reaches the mid teens, usually preceding the appearance of GTCS by a few months. Less than 10 per cent of patients with mild forms of JME never develop GTCS, probably as the result of early diagnosis and treatment.

Myoclonic jerks characteristically occur after awakening, particularly after sleep deprivation and excessive alcohol consumption. The question arises whether patients who do not demonstrate this circadian pattern belong to JME; they may belong to other syndromes, some of which may still be unrecognized.

Nocturnal myoclonic epilepsy could be such a syndrome related to JME within the idiopathic generalized epilepsies. I have seen three young female patients who, in their middle teens, developed myoclonic jerks only during slow-wave sleep (as shown by all night video-EEG recordings which demonstrated brief multiple spike discharges). The myoclonic jerks infrequently wake the patient up and proceed to a GTCS. The myoclonic jerks had the characteristics of those seen in JME. The patients were mentally and physically normal. A first cousin of one of these patients had JME with myoclonic jerks on awakening.

The myoclonic jerks of JME are shock-like, irregular and arrhythmic, clonic movements of proximal and distal muscles, mainly of the upper extremities, bilaterally. They are of variable amplitude and force. They are sufficiently violent to cause falls in more than half of the patients. In others, mild jerks were described in the fingers, making the patient clumsy or prone to drop things unexpectedly. None of our patients had facial or eyelid myoclonus. One-fifth of the patients described their jerks as unilateral, mainly in the dominant hand, probably because jerks of the fingers of the dominant hand become more apparent, i.e. dropping things, becoming clumsy.

There is no impairment of consciousness during the jerks but patients with pronounced myoclonic jerks and myoclonic status occasionally complained of lack of awareness. This may be due either to the distress caused by the continuous jerks or absences interspersed with jerks. Myoclonic jerks are independent of absences and do not occur during the absence. A series of myoclonic jerks often heralds a GTCS.

Diagnosing myoclonic jerks

It is often necessary physically to demonstrate mild myoclonic jerks of the fingers and hands, and to enquire about morning clumsiness and tremors. Questions like 'do you spill your morning tea?' 'do you drop things in the morning?', with simultaneous demonstration of how myoclonic jerks produce this effect, may be answered positively by patients who denied myoclonic jerks on direct questioning. If the patient reports normal hypnagogic jactitations, then it is reassuring that the concept of myoclonic jerks has been understood. Diagnostic yield may be improved by emphasizing the close relation of jerks to fatigue, alcohol and sleep deprivation. Some patients assume that jerks are a self-inflicted normal phenomenon related to abuse or excess of alcohol and lack of sleep. 'I thought everyone had it if you overdo it, like a hangover' is a frequent comment on enquiring the reasons for not reporting jerks.

Older patients who have been treated for many years for 'epilepsy' are particularly difficult to diagnose; obtaining old medical and EEG reports may be rewarding (see example of the didactic case presented in this report).

Typical absences in JME

The clinical and EEG manifestations of typical absences in JME have been detailed in four previous reports (Panayiotopoulos *et al.*, 1989a, b, 1992, 1994). They are markedly different from those of other epileptic syndromes, e.g. childhood absence epilepsy (CAE), juvenile absence epilepsy (JAE), myoclonic absence epilepsy, eyelid myoclonia with absences, perioral myoclonia with absences.

The absences in JME are simple absences (in accordance with the International League Against Epilepsy (ILAE) definition), i.e. brief impairment of consciousness (which is mild in JME and severe in CAE), with 3 Hz spike and slow-wave discharges. The characteristic JME patient does not jerk or have automatisms or other motor clinical manifestations like eyelid or perioral myoclonia, during the absence. Furthermore, and unlike CAE or JAE, impairment of consciousness is mild (subjectively perceived by the adult patients as 'momentary lack of concentration', 'like in a distance', 'tiny, little blackouts') and the EEG discharge is characteristically different from that of CAE and JAE, as we have previously demonstrated (Panayiotopoulos *et al.*, 1989a, b, 1992). The EEG discharge of JME is frequently short and fragmented, the spike and slow wave complexes show intradischarge frequency variations with multiple spike components (Ws) and other characteristics which are different from those of CAE and JAE (Panayiotopoulos *et al.*, 1989a, b, 1994).

Studies claiming overlapping of CAE or JAE with JME, CAE evolving to JME and the theory of a biological continuum of absences should not be accepted without great reservations, because no attempt is made to classify the absence syndromes as 'clusters of symptoms and signs which occur in a non-fortuitous manner' (see Commission, 1989). Instead, absences are studied in a unitary fashion and patients are classified as having or not having absences with 3 Hz spike and slow wave. This is an oversimplification which discourages diagnostic precision.

In our studies typical absences were found in 22 (33.3 per cent) of 66 patients with JME with a mean age (± SD) at onset of 10.5 ± 3.4 (range 5–16) years (Panayiotopoulos *et al.*, 1994). In eight of the 22 patients with absences, onset was before the age of 10 years (early-onset absences; median 6). Absences predated myoclonic jerks by 3.4 ± 2.5 years (range 0–9 years). Myoclonic jerks took longer to appear in the eight patients with early onset (4.9 ± 2.6 years) than in the 14 patients with late onset (2.6 ± 2.0 years) of absences. Absences were never antedated by myoclonic jerks or GTCS (Fig. 1). Typical absences predated myoclonic jerks and GTCS in all but two patients, who had simultaneous onset of absences and myoclonic jerks at age 16 years. The clinical severity of absences appeared to be age-related.

Early-onset absences (see above)

Absences were for most of these eight patients superficially similar to those of CAE; the patient would stop, become inactive and unresponsive and stare. There were no postictal symptoms or recollection of ictal events. Automatisms were described in two children. Absences were frequent, diagnosed and treated as pyknolepsy in four patients. All improved on appropriate medication (ethosuximide or sodium valproate). Video-EEG studies and detailed observations of these early-onset absences in childhood are lacking; they would be most important for comparisons with CAE because of age-matching.

Late-onset absences

Fourteen (21.1 per cent) patients had onset after the age of 10 years but in only three of them were absences so severe as to cause ictal interruption of mental and physical activity. There were no automatisms or postictal confusion. The frequency of absences varied from rare (which was more common) to one to 10 per day. Three other patients complained of instantaneous loss of contact and concentration with no objective change and only minimal interference in the activity of daily life. In the remaining eight patients absences consisted of brief impairment of concentration only, without impairment of cognition or daily activity.

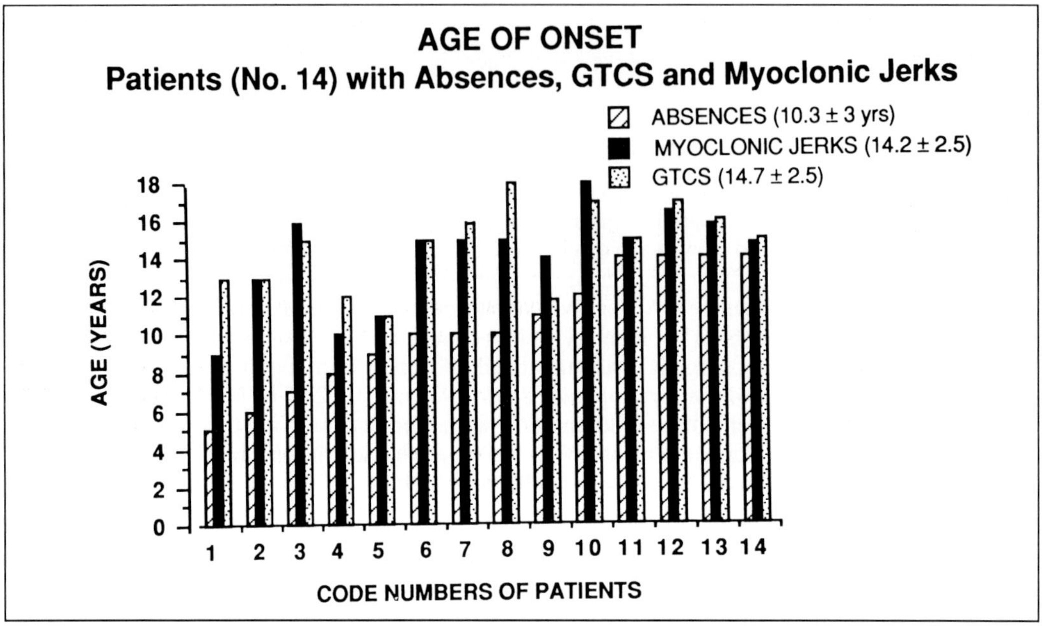

Fig. 1. Age at onset of absences, myoclonic jerks and GTCS in 14 patients with all three types of seizures. Typically, absences start long before the onset of jerks and GTCS.

Asymptomatic absences

Nine (13.7 per cent) patients (seven male and two female) did not admit to absences despite generalized spike–slow wave discharges lasting more than 3 s.

Diagnosing absences in JME

Absences are difficult to reveal and diagnose in JME. In our studies, absence seizures had frequently been unrecognized for years or misdiagnosed as complex partial seizures (Panayiotopoulos *et al.*, 1991, 1992; Grunewald *et al.*, 1992). Clinically, the absences are perceived by the patients as transient sensations of 'momentary lack of concentration', 'flashes of blackouts', 'going to a distance', 'lack of awareness' which may be misinterpreted as normal sensations, as drug-induced in patients, who are often overmedicated, or as complex partial seizures. Derealization and fear may infrequently be experienced (Panayiotopoulos *et al.*, 1992).

Clinicians have been trained to identify absences in their classical form in children, but frequently are not familiar with absences in adults where the level of awareness is not conspicuously impaired. Then, episodes of impairment of consciousness in adults are most likely to be diagnosed as complex partial seizures. Furthermore, absences may escape clinical detection even during conventional EEG. Current practice in EEG is to test the ability of a patient to recall a phrase or number administered during a generalized spike-wave discharge. This is often inadequate. We have frequently seen patients with spike-wave discharges in whom clinical manifestations (such as slowing down of breath-counting, repetition and mistakes, stuttering) became apparent only after careful video-EEG viewing. For practical purposes, we proposed that patients with spike-wave paroxysms should be asked to count their breaths during hyperventilation (Panayiotopoulos *et al.*, 1993); this may show slowing, discontinuity, errors, repetition and other signs of impairment of consciousness and speech which otherwise would escape recognition with the current practice established in EEG departments. This method is sensitive (involves concentration, memory, recollection of learned experience, expressive speech and other cognitive functions), practical (easy for the patient to perform and easy for the observer to evaluate) and is clinically relevant (reflects impairment of daily-life performance).

Generalized tonic–clonic seizures

These are usually preceded by clusters of myoclonic jerks (clonic–tonic–clonic generalized seizures). In other patients, particularly when the jerks occur in the morning after sleep deprivation and fatigue, myoclonic jerks interspersed with absences, or absences alone, may herald a GTCS. In patients on clonazepam alone, GTCS may be violent and not preceded by myoclonic jerks. GTCS occur mainly on awakening but also at any other time of the day and night.

Patients with single or rare GTCS may have frequent absences and myoclonic jerks. It is not unusual for a patient referred or diagnosed as having had one seizure, 'the first seizure', to have suffered numerous other seizures (myoclonic jerks, absences) many years prior to his first GTCS. In many patients, medication is withdrawn because they have been 'free of seizures' for many years, although they continue having many jerks and absences long after their 'last GTCS'. As this often results in a relapse of GTCS, the implication of these errors for driving licence, evaluation of studies referring to the 'first' or 'last' seizure and mainly the well-being of patients is of paramount importance.

Electroencephalographic findings

The EEG is nearly always abnormal in untreated patients or in patients with inappropriate antiepileptic medication. A normal EEG in a patient suspected of having JME should generate an EEG on awakening. Our practice is to ask the patient to wake up at 5 a.m. and have the EEG at 1 p.m. We

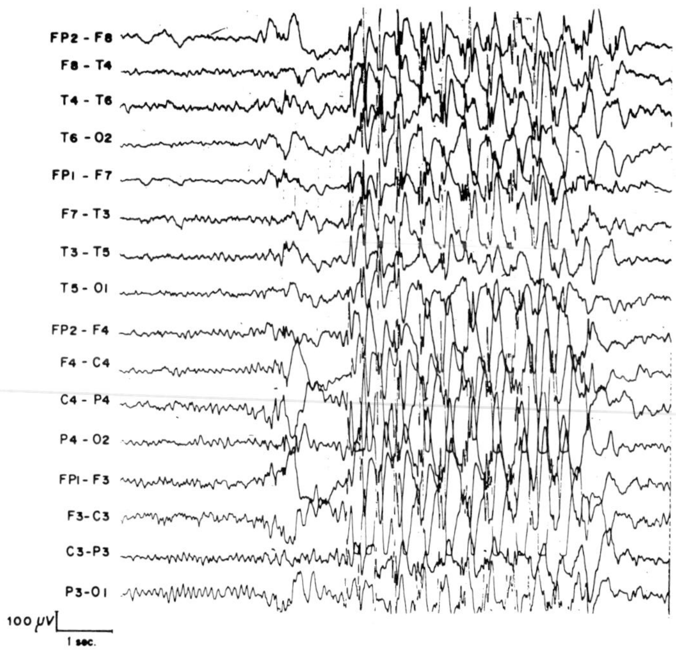

Fig. 2. EEG of a 14-year-old patient with JME. There were no apparent clinical manifestations during the discharge. Note fragmentation of the discharges, multiple spike complexes (Ws), intradischarge irregularities in rhythm and spike/multiple spike–slow wave relations, i.e. features which are unlikely to occur in childhood and juvenile absence epilepsy.

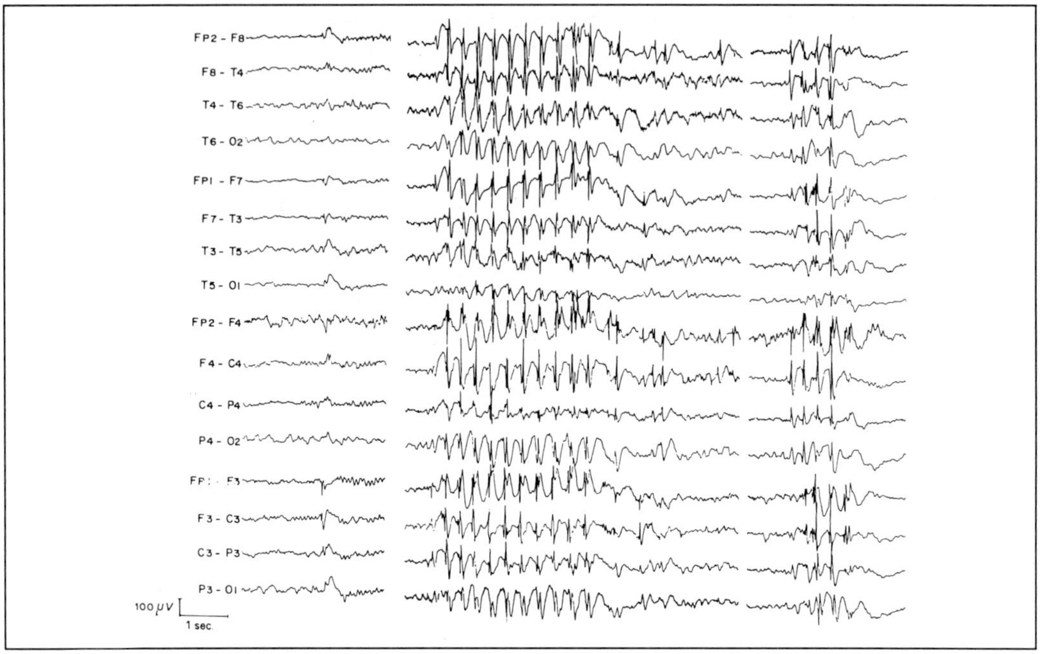

Fig. 3. EEG of a 22-year-old patient. There were no apparent clinical manifestations. Note fragmentation of the discharges, multiple spike complexes (Ws), asymmetries and frequent focal abnormalities independently right and left. (From Panayiotopoulos et al., 1993b. With permission from Epilepsia).

prefer this partial instead of all-night sleep deprivation, because of the fear of inducing GTCS. The ideal is an all-night sleep and 1 h awakening EEG.

In our experience (Panayiotopoulos *et al.*, 1994) paroxysmal abnormalities were recorded in 52 out of 66 patients; 34 (51. 5 per cent) had spike/multiple spike–slow wave discharges and 18 had brief generalized bursts of sharp θ activity with occasionally interspersed small spikes.

Morphology and characteristics of the discharges

The discharges consisted of single, double, treble or multiple spikes, usually preceding or superimposed on slow waves. Multiple spikes consisted of up to eight spikes with a characteristic 'worm-like' or compressed capital W appearance ('Ws'). The number and amplitude of spikes showed considerable inter- and intradischarge variation. The intradischarge frequency of the spike/multiple spike–slow wave complexes varied from 2 to 10 Hz, mainly 3–5 Hz. Frequency was often higher in the first second following onset (opening phase), with no smooth decrease in frequency from the initial to the terminal phase of the discharge. Fragmentations of the discharges were common and characteristic. These were transient interruptions of individual discharges either by brief discontinuation of the spike/multiple spike complexes or abrupt changes in the dominant frequency of the discharges (Panayiotopoulos *et al.*, 1989a, b). 'Ws' and fragmentation of discharges were observed in all patients but varied quantitatively between patients and discharges (Fig. 2). Fragmentations were more frequent in older whilst 'Ws' were more abundant in younger patients.

Duration of the discharges ranged from 1–20 s (mean ± SD = 6.8 ± 4.8 s) with frequent Ws and discharge fragmentations.

Focal abnormalities were recorded in 20 (30.3 per cent) patients. Ten had focal single spikes and spike–slow wave complexes. The other 10 patients showed focal slow waves consisting of sharp, medium- to high-amplitude θ or δ waves; they were independently right or left in nine and had unilateral preponderance in six. Focal paroxysmal abnormalities were recorded in seven patients. These were short transients of localized slow, sharp waves and/or spikes. Focal spikes were either independent or associated with the generalized paroxysms (preceding, following or interspersed). The same patient could have spikes in multiple locations in the same or a previous EEG (Fig. 3). These focal abnormalities had often been interpreted previously as evidence of partial seizures with secondary generalization (Aliberti *et al.*, 1993).

Photoconvulsive responses (PCR) were evoked in 18 (27.3 per cent) patients; three had all type of seizures, 13 myoclonic jerks and GTCS, one myoclonic jerks and absences and one absences alone.

Background abnormalities consisting of a moderate excess of θ activity and/or some slowing of the α rhythm were recorded in 28 (42.4 per cent) patients.

Eyes-closed-related abnormalities were observed in eight, eye-closure-related abnormalities in two and no effect was found in four of 14 patients studied.

Hyperventilation accentuated the abnormalities in all patients.

Treatment

In our studies on the misdiagnosis of JME, therapeutic decisions were influenced by the diagnostic problems (Panayiotopoulos *et al.*, 1991, 1993b; Grunewald *et al.*, 1992). Sodium valproate, which is the drug of choice in idiopathic generalized epilepsies, was prescribed less often than carbamazepine, which is not appropriate treatment for absences or myoclonic jerks. The effect of carbamazepine in GTCS of idiopathic generalized epilepsies has not been clarified; two of our patients with JME needed carbamazepine as an add-on treatment for the control of GTCS. Clonazepam was rarely used despite its controlling myoclonic jerks.

Our patients showed considerable improvement in frequency of all seizure types (absences, myoclonic jerks and GTCS) on sodium valproate alone or combined with small doses of clonazepam. From the new antiepileptic drugs, Lamotrigine appears to be promising particularly when combined with valproate-controlled studies are urgently needed.

Unfortunately, studies on the effectiveness of old and new anti-epileptic drugs are not syndrome-related. JME, a lifelong disorder, with absences, myoclonic jerks and GTCS, would be ideal for this type of study in patients who are not controlled with the above medication or suffer unacceptable side- effects. We have still to learn a lot about the most effective and most realistic treatment of JME.

References

Aliberti, B., Grunewald, R. & Panayiotopoulos, C.P. (1993): Focal electroencephalographic abnormalities in juvenile myoclonic epilepsy. *Epilepsia* **35** (2), 297–301.

Canevini, M., Mai, R. Di Marco, C., Bertin, C. Minotti, L., Pontrelli, V., Saltareli, A. & Canger, R. (1992): Juvenile myoclonic epilepsy of Janz: clinical observations in 60 patients. *Seizure* **1**.

Commission on Classification and Terminology of the International League Against Epilepsy (1989): Proposal for classification of epilepsies and epileptic syndromes. *Epilepsia* **30,** 389–399.

Delgado-Escueta, A.V. & Enrile-Bascal, F. (1984): Juvenile myoclonic epilepsy of Janz. *Neurology* **34,** 285–294.

Editorial (1992): Diagnosing juvenile myoclonic epilepsy. *Lancet* **340,** 759–760.

Grunewald, R. & Panayiotopoulos, C.P. (1993): Juvenile myoclonic epilepsy: a review. *Arch. Neurol.* **50,** 594–598.

Grunewald, R., Chroni, E. & Panayiotopoulos, C.P. (1992): Delayed diagnosis of juvenile myoclonic epilepsy. *J. Neurol. Neurosurg. Psychiatr.* **55,** 497–499.

Janz, D. (1985): Epilepsy with impulsive petit mal (juvenile myoclonic epilepsy). *Acta Neurolog. Scand.* **72,** 339–359.

Janz, D. (1989): Juvenile myoclonic epilepsy: epilepsy with impulsive petit mal. *Cleveland Clin. J. Med.* **56** (Suppl., part I), S23–S33.

Janz, D. & Christian, W. (1957): Impulsive petit-mal. *Dtsch. Z. Nervenheilk.* **176,** 346–386.

Obeid, T. & Panayiotopoulos, C.P. (1988): Juvenile myoclonic epilepsy: a study in Saudi Arabia. *Epilepsia* **29,** 280–282..

Panayiotopoulos, C.P., Obeid, T. & Waheed, G. (1989a): Absences in juvenile myoclonic epilepsy: a clinical and video-electroencephalographic study. *Ann. Neurol.* **25,** 391–397.

Panayiotopoulos, C.P., Obeid, T. & Waheed, G. (1989b): Differentiation of typical absence seizures in epileptic syndromes: a video EEG study of 224 seizures in 20 patients. *Brain* **112,** 1039–1056.

Panayiotopoulos, C.P., Tahan, R. & Obeid, T. (1991): Juvenile myoclonic epilepsy: factors of error involved in the diagnosis and treatment. *Epilepsia* **32,** 672–676.

Panayiotopoulos, C.P., Chroni, E., Dascalopoulos, C., Baker, A, Rowlinson, S. & Welsh, P. (1992): Typical absences in adults: a clinical, EEG, video-EEG study and syndromic/diagnostic considerations. *J. Neurol. Neurosurg. Psychiatr* **55,** 1002–1008.

Panayiotopoulos, C.P., Baker, A., Grunewald, R., Rowlinson, S. & Welsh, P. (1993a): Breath counting during 3 Hz generalised spike and wave discharges. *J. Electrophysiol. Technol.* **19,** 15–23.

Panayiotopoulos, C.P., Obeid, T. & Tahan, A.R. (1994b): Juvenile myoclonic epilepsy: a 5-years prospective study. *Epilepsia* **35** (2), 285–296.

Wolf, P. (1992): Juvenile myoclonic epilepsy. In: *Epileptic syndromes in infancy, childhood and adolescence,* 2nd edn., eds. J. Roger, M. Bureau, C. Dravet, F.E. Dreifus, A. Perret & P. Wolf, pp. 313–327. London: John Libbey.

Epileptic Seizures and Syndromes, Edited by Peter Wolf
© 1994 John Libbey & Company Ltd., pp. 231–240

Chapter 29

Benign epilepsy with centrotemporal spikes: do we know all about it?

Charlotte Dravet

Centre Saint-Paul, 300 Boulevard de Sainte-Marguerite, 13009 Marseille, France

Summary

Benign epilepsy with centrotemporal spikes still remains the model of the benign localization-related epilepsies of childhood. However, its EEG and clinical features are variable and many of its aspects can be debated: symptomatology, frequency and severity of the seizures, localization of the focal EEG paroxysms, existence of associated generalized abnormalities, long-term outcome. Other important problems consist of the relationship with other types of epilepsy and the significance of the EEG pattern when it is present in other situations. These questions are discussed by reviewing the literature about this topic.

No one knows everything about a given epileptic syndrome, a given type of epilepsy or a given type of seizure: this limitation of our knowledge is exactly the reason for this book. Concerning benign epilepsy with centrotemporal spikes (BECTS), one could say provocatively, as Loiseau *et al.* said in 1967, that 'it does not exist', because the typical picture described in the books is only rarely encountered in current practice. Nevertheless, BECTS still constitutes the unique model of a truly benign epilepsy.

According to the classification of the International League Against Epilepsy (Commission, 1989), BECTS is one of the three syndromes individualized among the idiopathic localization-related epilepsies (BECTS, childhood epilepsy with occipital paroxysms and primary reading epilepsy); it is also the most frequent and the purest of the three. It is defined as follows: genetic predisposition, male predominance, onset between 3 and 13 years of age, with a peak around age 9, recovery before age 15–16, brief, simple, partial motor hemifacial seizures, often associated with somatosensory symptoms, tending to evolve into usually nocturnal generalized tonic–clonic seizures; on the electroencephalogram (EEG), blunt, high-voltage, centrotemporal spikes, often followed by slow waves, activated by sleep, tending to spread or shift from side to side. Figures 1 and 2 show two examples of the EEG pattern considered characteristic for BECTS.

This description seems to be clear and without ambiguity. However, it appears sometimes difficult to apply in front of a patient. The difficulties can arise from many points: from the symptomatology of seizures, from the frequency or severity of seizures, from the localization of the focal EEG paroxysms, from the association with generalized EEG paroxysms, from the long-term outcome. On

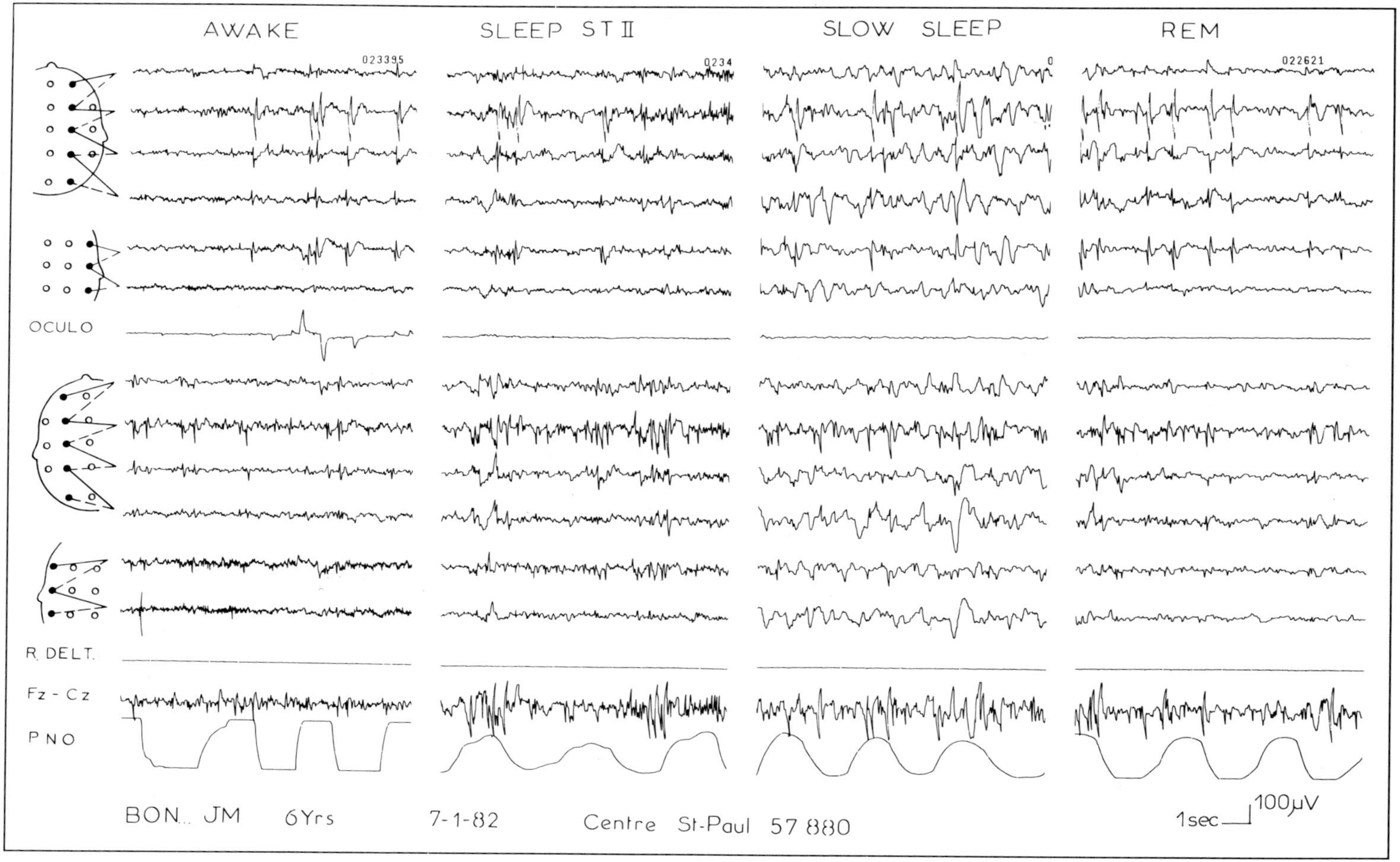

Fig. 1. Left: Awake EEG: high-voltage slow spikes in the right centroanterior temporal area and independent slow spikes, of lower voltage, in the left central area. The three other sets represent sleep EEG records showing the increased number of spikes, without change in their morphology, in stages II, III and REM.

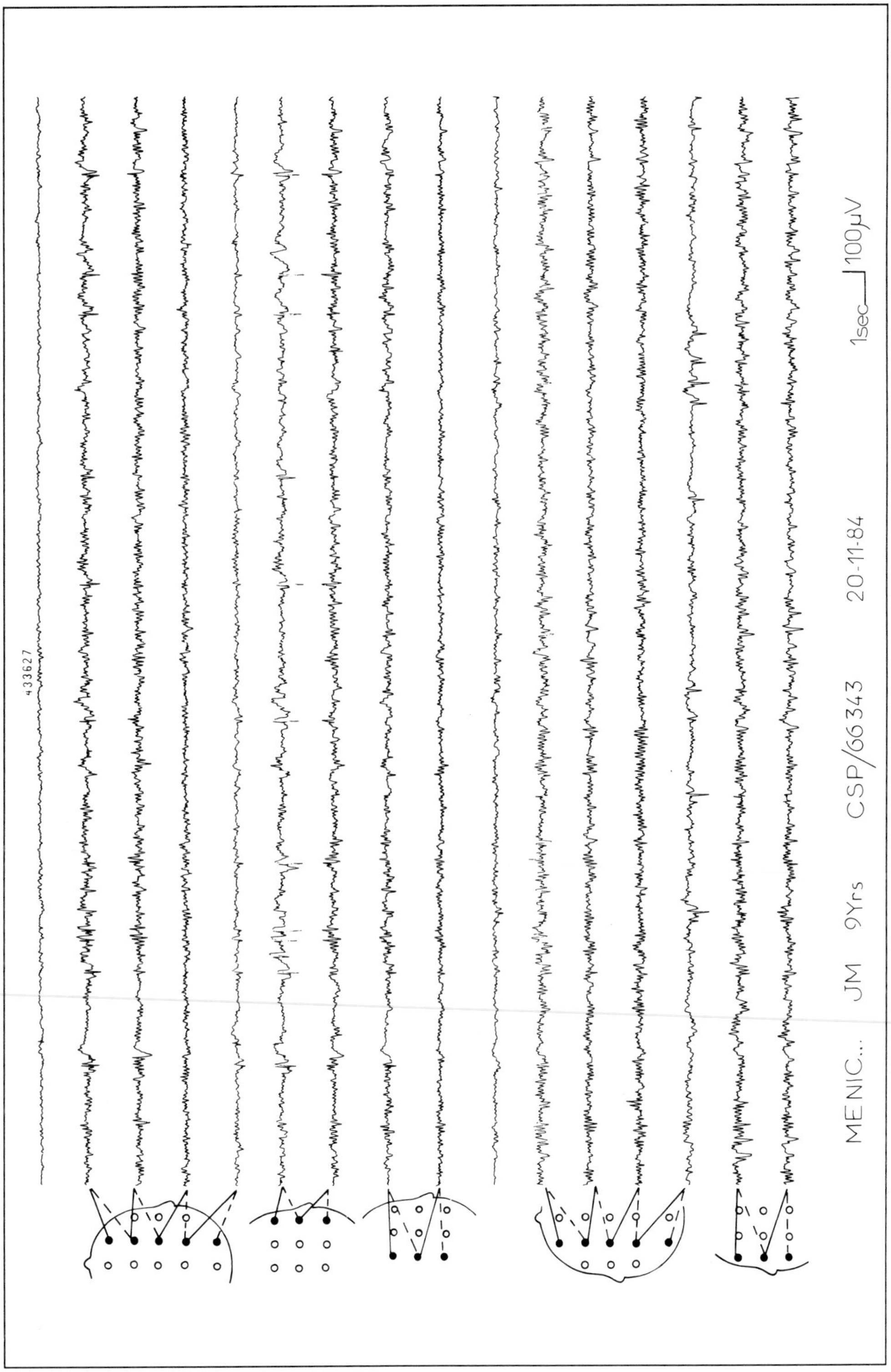

Fig. 2. Association of right centrotemporal and left occipital spikes.

the other hand, the electrographic and clinical picture of BECTS shares common traits with other types of epilepsy, which must be discussed, and the EEG pattern of centrotemporal spikes may be present in other conditions with or without epilepsy. Finally, the genetic components of this syndrome must be considered within the large frame of other genetically determined epilepsies, such as the idiopathic generalized epilepsies.

Symptomatology of seizures

Typical seizures consist of clonic contractions of the hemiface, sometimes preceded by sensations of unilateral paresthesias (pins and needles, electricity, numbness) involving the tongue, lips, gums and inner cheeks; the tonic, clonic or tonic–clonic contractions involve the face, lips and tongue, as well as pharyngeal and laryngeal muscles, causing anarthria or speech arrest and drooling due to sialorrhoea and saliva pooling. Consciousness is preserved but the child has difficulty speaking. The motor seizure can spread to the arm, rarely to the leg, and can also develop into a generalized convulsion, especially when it occurs at night.

In some cases, however, the seizures can show atypical features, as initially noted by Beaussart and Loiseau (1973), and they are not easy to classify, particularly in children under the age of 5: abdominal pain, vertigo, lack of muscular tone, pain in different parts of the body. Morikawa *et al.* (1992) insisted on the existence of non-sylvian seizures, which they found in 11 children among 57, with the same good prognosis. These authors also underlined that typical sylvian seizures can occur in symptomatic focal epilepsies and may also have a good prognosis.

Beydoun *et al.* (1992) studied a group of 41 children with BECTS where they distinguished two patients with complex partial seizures. Dalla Bernardina *et al.* (1992) found 4.3 per cent of patients with complex partial seizures in their group of 162 cases.

The occurrence of typical absence seizures has been emphasized by Beaumanoir *et al.* (1974), who recorded them by long-duration tele-EEG in six of 15 subjects. They were rare in the waking state, never occurring more than twice within 5 h. That may explain why other authors who did not perform the same type of long-term EEG surveillance did not record absence seizures in patients with BECTS.

Frequency and severity of seizures

As a rule seizures are rare, short and without consequences. However, all the authors agree they can be frequent (Loiseau *et al.*, 1967; Blom & Heijbel, 1982). Lerman (1992) indicates they are frequent in 20 per cent of the patients, sometimes occurring in clusters, several times a day, in spite of drug therapy, and becoming troublesome for the child and his/her family. This variability of frequency was studied by Ambrosetto *et al.* (1987) who analyzed the predictive factors of seizure frequency. They found that only two were significant: a convulsive generalized seizure as the first ictal event, and a long interval between the first and the second attacks in the group with rare seizures. The EEG is not useful in determining the risk of recurrence. But Loiseau *et al.* (1988) failed to confirm these findings. For them the only predictive factor is the age at the first seizure: the earlier the onset, the longer the active period.

The occurrence of status epilepticus has been reported in four cases (Fejerman & Di Blasi, 1987; Boulloche *et al.*, 1990; Colamaria *et al.*, 1991). They consisted of partial motor seizures with dysarthria and hypersalivation, without impairment of consciousness, during several hours or days, sometimes resistant to intravenous (IV) diazepam. The awake and sleep EEGs demonstrated continuous spikes and spike waves (SW), diffuse but of higher amplitude in the rolandic areas. In the patient of Colamaria *et al.*, continuous SW during sleep were observed after the end of the status. The long-term outcome of these patients is not known. It is also interesting to consider the case reported by Roulet *et al.* (1989), in which prolonged episodes of drooling and oromotor dyspraxia for several months were correlated with an increased number of rolandic spikes in the EEGs, without associated motor seizures and without recording any ictal EEG pattern.

Localization of focal EEG paroxysms

Typically, the EEG paroxysms are recorded in the centrotemporal areas, either on one side or on both sides. In fact, the possibility of other associated localizations was mentioned as early as 1972 by Beaussart, to be later confirmed by several authors. Morikawa *et al.* (1979) distinguished a group of 31 patients with the association of centrotemporal and extracentrotemporal localizations. The latter were frontal, anterior temporal, midline and occipital. They compared these patients to 41 patients with strictly centrotemporal foci. They found a clear difference between the types of seizures, which were more often non-sylvian in the first group. But they did not find any difference in the prognosis. Holmes (1992) indicated that two patients had frontal spikes and four patients had occipital spikes among his group of 50 patients. Loiseau *et al.* (1992) discussed this problem of extrarolandic location, mainly in the occipital and parieto-postero-temporal region, either in the same recording or in successive recordings during evolution. They concluded that for almost all authors the concept of BECTS is not linked to a specific location of the sharp waves but rather to the typical or suggestive morphology of the sharp waves.

Association of generalized discharges on the EEG

The association of interictal generalized SW has been reported by most authors (Fig. 3). Beaumanoir *et al.* (1974) studied 26 children by standard EEGs, including 15 who were also studied by long-term EEG telemetry for 4–36 h with simultaneous video recording. They found 14 patients who had brief bursts of 3–4/s generalized synchronous or asynchronous spike and slow wave complexes; as a rule, the spike component was most apparent in the frontocentral areas. They were never seen during photic stimulation but were frequently triggered by hyperventilation. In two patients hyperventilation triggered a generalized burst of 3/s spike and slow waves lasting 8 and 9 s, without any apparent clinical concomitant.The tele-EEGs made it possible to record brief generalized bursts of the same type in 11 of the 15 studied patients. Dalla Bernardina and Beghini (1976) recorded them during nocturnal sleep in 40 per cent of patients with epilepsy and in 10 per cent of those without epilepsy. Even if they appeared sometimes only during drowsiness, they never increased during slow sleep, as the focal spikes did. Rose and Duron (1984) compared the generalized SW and the rolandic spikes during sleep and found they had a completely different behaviour, as if they were activated by different mechanisms. Moreover, the generalized SW decreased during antiepileptic treatment while the rolandic spikes were not modified. Degen and Degen (1990) found generalized 3–4/s SW discharges in 65.1 per cent of 43 children with rolandic epilepsies. This association of generalized SW and absence seizures could raise the question of the links between BECTS and idiopathic generalized epilepsies. However, most of the quoted authors did not consider the possible relationship between this EEG pattern and the family history of the patients. Only Degen and Degen (1990) found a high rate of generalized SW (31.9 per cent) in the siblings of their patients. An interesting study is that by Schmitt and Dumermuth (1992), who examined the different types of generalized paroxysms in different types of localization-related epilepsies and found the typical SW at 3/s only in the so-called 'functional' epilepsies, including BECTS.

Long term outcome

The long-term outcome is now better known and it appears that some patients (1–2 per cent) can experience new seizures after a long remission (Beaussart, 1981; Loiseau *et al.*, 1983, 1988; De Romanis *et al.*, 1986). There is no element in their histories or in the EEG and clinical features that makes it possible to predict this recurrence. Seizures recur mostly as isolated or infrequent generalized tonic–clonic seizures (Loiseau *et al.*, 1992), rarely as partial seizures, either of the same type (Ambrosetto *et al.*, 1985) or of a different type (Lerman & Kivity, 1986). It is possible that, after the age of 15–16, the incidence of seizures is not very different between patients who had BECTS and the general population.

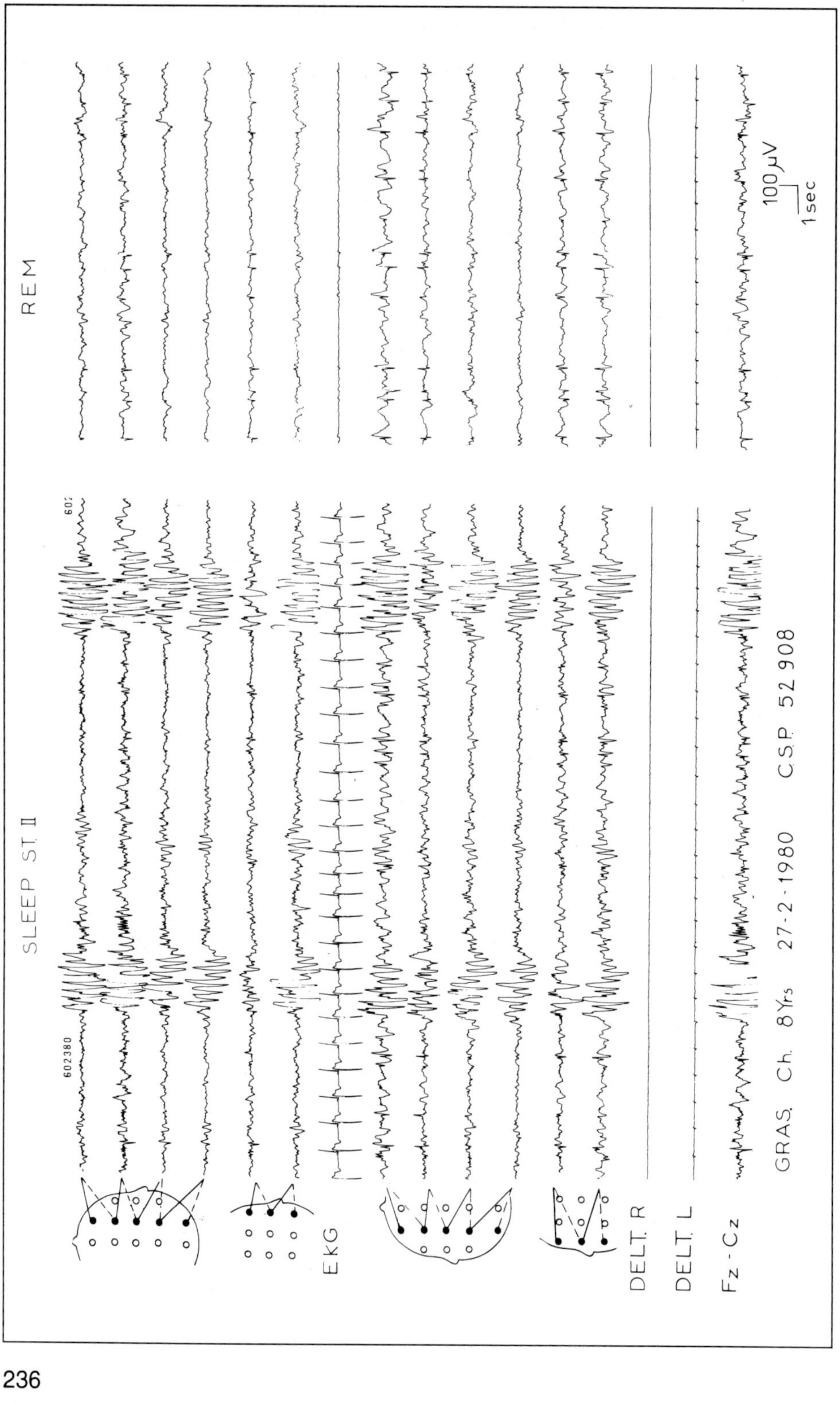

Fig. 3. Left: Existence of generalized SW discharges in sleep stage II. Right: During REM frontocentrotemporal slow spikes predominantly in the left hemisphere.

Relationship with other types of epilepsy

This topic is important enough to deserve a specific chapter (see Genton & Guerrini, Chapter 30). It seems that BECTS constitutes the model of idiopathic localization-related epilepsies in children at a given age, but is only a part of these epilepsies. As underlined by Loiseau *et al.* (1992), the foci have a tendency to migrate with maturation from the posterior to the centrotemporal and, less frequently, to the frontal regions. Probably, different EEG and clinical pictures may also correspond to idiopathic localized epilepsies in infancy (Dravet *et al.*, 1989; Dulac *et al.*, 1989; Watanabe *et al.*, 1990; Vigevano *et al.*, 1992), before the age of 3.

Concerning epilepsy with continuous SW during slow sleep, it has been stated that it can evolve out of an idiopathic localized epilepsy. However, most cases come to our observation some months or years after the onset and it is difficult to give a diagnosis a posteriori. When we have the opportunity to examine the first EEGs, usually we observe some atypical characteristics, such as the high number of the discharges and their tendency to spread widely on one hemisphere or on both hemispheres, these anomalies often appearing diffuse rather than localized. This point needs to be further clarified because it could have consequences in the choice of treatment.

Oller Daurella (1992) has described an epilepsy with unilateral seizures and we think it does exist (Dravet, 1992). In this group some patients share many clinical and EEG features with BECTS, their only particularity being that they have a single type of prolonged unilateral seizures, which can persist after puberty.

In other patients both the clinical and EEG features are more complex and it is not possible to assume the diagnosis of idiopathic localized epilepsy; polymorphous seizures, behavioural disturbances, variable EEG patterns, but the presence of interictal multiple foci activated by sleep lead us to think that the prognosis is probably good for the long term. In the same way, the presence of multiple foci, rolandic and extrarolandic, in patients with signs of brain lesions and epilepsy suggests a rather good long-term prognosis for the seizures (Loiseau & Cohadon, 1981).

Several authors have expressed the hypothesis that BECTS and generalized idiopathic epilepsies could have the same genetic background (Bray & Wiser, 1964, 1965; Beaumanoir *et al.*, 1974; Heijbel *et al.*, 1975). The association of these two types of epilepsy in the same family is not frequent, whereas the association of the two types of EEG pattern has been described in a large number of cases.

Significance of the rolandic-spike EEG pattern

BECTS may occur in patients with brain lesions (Blom *et al.*, 1972; Santanelli *et al.*, 1989; Ambrosetto, 1992; Holmes, 1992). In these cases one can wonder whether (1) it is simply coincidental, (2) the emergence of BECTS is due to a higher level of epilepsy predisposition because of the association of cerebral damage with a genetic condition, or (3) the rolandic epilepsy is the consequence of the lesion. Until now there has been no answer to these questions and, probably, it is different according to the type and the topography of the lesions, as discussed by Ambrosetto (1992). Morikawa *et al.* (1992) have also demonstrated the existence of symptomatic epilepsies with sylvian seizures, rolandic foci and a good outcome.

Rolandic spikes have been described in other situations, such as the Rett syndrome (Niedermeyer & Naidu, 1990), the fragile X syndrome (Musumeci *et al.*, 1988), cerebral tumour (Kraschnitz *et al.*, 1988) and cortical dysplasia with focal cortical myoclonus (Kuzniecky *et al.*, 1988).

Lerman & Kivity (1975) reported the occurrence of focal spikes in 100 children who were referred for an EEG recording at a mean age of 7.7 years, for various symptoms: behaviour problems, minimal brain damage, headache, head trauma, precocious puberty, growth retardation, diabetes mellitus, obesity, nocturnal enuresis, mental retardation, fainting, abdominal pain, febrile convulsions (FC), speech problems, tic, night terrors, somnambulism, febrile delirium and suspected metastases. In 78 cases the focus was centrotemporal, in five cases occipital, in 14 cases centrotemporal and occipital, in three cases centrotemporal with SW discharges. Lerman and Kivity (1992) underlined the fact that such discharges are not related to clinical epilepsy and do not require any antiepileptic treatment. To my knowledge the significance of the rolandic spikes in the EEG of a child who has had FC has not been considered in the literature. Is it predictive for the later appearance of a BECTS? Kajitani (1993) found them in 40 per cent of children with FC and in 28 per cent of clinically healthy near relatives of patients with FC, but he adds that their presence do not necessarily predict a recurrence of FC or later development of epilepsy.

Finally, rolandic spikes have been reported in children without any epileptic manifestation and without any type of brain damage. The first group is represented by the siblings of patients affected by BECTS. Heijbel *et al.* (1975) found this pattern in 34 per cent of siblings submitted to waking and sleep EEG records, Lerman and Apter (1981) in 25 per cent and Degen and Degen (1990) in only 5.8 per cent. The second group is represented by normal healthy children studied in a community. Eeg-Olofsson *et al.* (1971) observed an incidence of 1.2 per cent of rolandic spikes in 743 subjects and Cavazzuti *et al.* (1980) 3.54 per cent in 3726 children.

Dalla Bernardina and Beghini (1976) compared the nocturnal sleep EEG of 10 patients with BECTS and 10 children with rolandic spikes without seizures. They observed differences which they considered important for the differential diagnosis between children with and without epilepsy. They suggest that the risk for epilepsy is higher if, during sleep, rolandic spikes remain unilateral, spike activity continues to be important during rapid-eye-movement (REM) sleep, and generalized SW discharges appear. Other types of neurophysiological studies, including EEG mapping, would be helpful for the distinction between focal abnormalities due to underlying brain lesions and those related to a 'functional' disorder (Lischka & Graf, 1992) and for understanding the physiopathology of BECTS and other conditions associated with rolandic spikes (Gregory & Wong, 1984; Yoshinaga *et al.*, 1992).

In conclusion, that many questions are still without answer is not a reason to doubt of the existence of this syndrome. In our current practice not only do we meet a lot of children who more or less fulfil the criteria for a BECTS but we also meet a number of other children who do not have the typical picture but for which we are able to give a good long-term prognosis because they share some common features with BECTS.

References

Ambrosetto, G. (1992): Opercular macrogyria and benign childhood epilepsy with centrotemporal (rolandic) spikes: report of a case. *Epilepsia* **33** (3), 499–503.

Ambrosetto, G., Tinuper, P. & Baruzzi, A. (1985): Relapse of benign partial epilepsy of children in adulthood: report of a case. *J. Neurol. Neurosurg. Psychiatr.* **48,** 90.

Ambrosetto, G., Giovanardi Rossi, P. & Tassinari, C.A. (1987): Predictive factors of seizure frequency and duration of antiepileptic treatment in rolandic epilepsy: a retrospective study. *Brain Dev.* **9,** 300–304.

Beaumanoir, A., Ballis, T., Varfis, G. & Ansari, K. (1974): Benign epilepsy of childhood with rolandic spikes. *Epilepsia* **15,** 301–315.

Beaussart, M. (1972): Benign epilepsy of children with rolandic (centro-temporal) paroxysmal foci. *Epilepsia* **13,** 795–811.

Beaussart, M. (1981): Crises épileptiques après guérison d'une épilepsie à paroxysmes rolandiques. *Rev. EEG Neurophysiol.* **11,** 489–492.

Beaussart, M. & Loiseau, P. (1973): Evolution et pronostic de l'épilepsie à paroxysmes rolandiques. In: *Evolution and prognosis of epilepsies*, eds. L. Lugaresi, P. Pazzaglia & R. Canger, pp. 215–228. Bologna: Aulo Gaggi.

Beydoun, A., Garofalo, E. & Drury, I. (1992): Generalized spike-waves, multiple loci, and clinical course in children with EEG features of benign epilepsy of childhood with centro-temporal spikes. *Epilepsia* **33** (6), 1091–1096.

Blom, S., Heijbel. J. & Bergfors, P.G. (1972): Benign epilepsy of children with centrotemporal EEG foci: prevalence and follow-up study of 40 patients. *Epilepsia* **13,** 609–619.

Blom, S. & Heijbel, J. (1982): Benign epilepsy of children with centro-temporal EEG foci: a follow-up study on adulthood of patients initially studied as children. *Epilepsia* **23,** 629–632.

Boulloche, J., Husson, A., Le Luyer, B. & Le Roux, P. (1990): Dysphagie, troubles du langage et pointes ondes centro-temporales. *Arch. Fr. Pediatr.* **47,** 115–117.

Bray, F.P. & Wiser, W.C. (1964): Evidence for a genetic aetiology of temporal central abnormalities in focal epilepsy. *N. Engl. J. Med.* **271,** 926–933.

Bray, F.P. & Wiser, W.C. (1965): Hereditary characteristics of familial temporal central focal epilepsy. *Pediatrics* **30,** 207–211.

Cavazzuti, G.B., Cappella, L. & Nalin, A. (1980): Longitudinal study of epileptiform EEG patterns in normal children. *Epilepsia* **21,** 43–55.

Colamaria, V., Sgrò, V., Caraballo, R., Simeone, M., Zullini, E., Fontana, E., Zanetti, R., Grimau-Merino, R. & Dalla Bernardina, B. (1991): Status epilepticus in benign rolandic epilepsy manifesting as anterior operculum syndrome. *Epilepsia* **32** (3), 329–334.

Commission on Classification and Terminology of the International League Against Epilepsy (1989): Proposal for revised classification of epilepsies and epileptic syndromes. *Epilepsia* **30,** 389–399.

Dalla Bernardina, B. & Beghini, G. (1976): Rolandic spikes in children with and without epilepsy (20 subjects polygraphically studied during sleep). *Epilepsia* **17,** 161–167.

Dalla Bernardina, B., Sgrò, V., Fontana, E., Colamaria, V. & La Selva, L. (1992): Idiopathic partial epilepsies in children. In: *Epileptic syndromes in infancy, childhood and adolescence*, 2nd edn., eds. J. Roger, M. Bureau, Ch. Dravet, F.E. Dreifuss, A. Perret & P. Wolf, pp. 173–188. London: John Libbey.

Degen, R. & Degen, H.E. (1990): Some genetic aspects of rolandic epilepsy: waking and sleep EEGs in siblings. *Epilepsia* **31** (6), 795–801.

De Romanis, F., Feliciani, M. & Ruggieri, S. (1986): Rolandic paroxysmal epilepsy: a long term study in 150 children. *Ital. J. Neurol. Sci.* **7,** 77–80.

Dravet, C., Catani, C., Bureau, M. & Roger, J. (1989): Partial epilepsies in infancy: a study of 40 cases. *Epilepsia* **30** (6), 807–812.

Dravet, Ch. (1992): Comments on an epileptic syndrome with unilateral seizures. In: *Epileptic syndromes in infancy, childhood and adolescence*, 2nd edn, eds. J. Roger, M. Bureau, Ch. Dravet, F.E. Dreifuss, A. Perret & P. Wolf, pp. 273–277. London: John Libbey.

Dulac, O., Cusmai, R. & de Oliveira, K. (1989): Is there a partial benign epilepsy in infancy? *Epilepsia* **30** (6), 798–801.

Eeg-Olofsson, O., Peterson, L. & Selleden, U. (1971): The development of the electroencephalogram in normal children from the age of 1 through 15 years: paroxysmal activity. *Neuro-Paediatrie* **4,** 375–404.

Fejerman, N. & Di Blasi, M. (1987): Status epilepticus of benign partial epilepsies in children: report of two cases. *Epilepsia* **28** (4), 351–355.

Gregory, D.L. & Wong, P.K. (1984): Topographical analysis of the centro-temporal discharges in benign rolandic epilepsy of childhood. *Epilepsia* **25,** 705–711.

Heijbel, J., Blom, S. & Rasmuson, M. (1975): Benign epilepsy of childhood with centrotemporal EEG foci: a genetic study. *Epilepsia* **16,** 285–293.

Holmes, G.L. (1992): Rolandic epilepsy: clinical and electroencephalographic features. In: *Benign localized and generalized epilepsies of early childhood (Epilepsy Res.* Suppl. 6), eds. R. Degen & F.E. Dreifuss, pp. 29–43. Amsterdam: Elsevier.

Kajitani, T. (1993): A genetic predisposition to febrile convulsions from an electroencephalographic viewpoint. Proceedings of the 15th Annual Conference on Febrile Convulsions, Tokyo, 19 December 1992. *Brain Dev.* **15,** 390 (abstract).

Kraschnitz, W., Scheer, P., Korner, K., Kratky-Dunitz, M. & Lechner, H. (1988): Rolandic spikes as an electroencephalographic manifestation of an oligodendroglioma. *Pediatr. Padol.* **23,** 313–319.

Kuzniecky, R., Berkovic, S., Andermann, F., Melanson, D., Olivier, A. & Robitaille, Y. (1988): Focal cortical myoclonus and rolandic cortical dysplasia: clarification by magnetic resonance imaging. *Ann. Neurol.* **23,** 317–325.

Lerman, P. (1992): Benign partial epilepsy with centro-temporal spikes. In: *Epileptic syndromes in infancy, childhood and adolescence*, 2nd edn, eds. J. Roger, M. Bureau, Ch. Dravet, F.E. Dreifuss, A. Perret & P. Wolf, pp. 189–200. London: John Libbey.

Lerman, P. & Apter, N. (1981): Familial aspects of BFEC. *Harefuah* **100,** 160–161.

Lerman, P. & Kivity, S. (1975): Benign focal epilepsy of childhood: a follow up of 100 recovered patients. *Arch. Neurol.* **32,** 261–264.

Lerman, P. & Kivity, S. (1986): The benign focal epilepsies of childhood. In: *Recent advances in epilepsy,* Vol. 3, eds. T.A. Pedley & B.S. Meldrum, pp. 136–137. Edinburgh: Churchill Livingstone.

Lerman, P. & Kivity, S. (1992): Focal epileptic EEG discharges in children not suffering from clinical epilepsy. In: *Benign localized and generalized epilepsies of early childhood (Epilepsy Res.* Suppl. 6*)*, eds. R. Degen & F.E. Dreifuss, pp. 99–104. Amsterdam: Elsevier.

Lischka, A. & Graf, M. (1992): Benign rolandic epilepsy of childhood: topographic EEG analysis. In: *Benign localized and generalized epilepsies of early childhood (Epilepsy Res.* Suppl. 6), eds. R. Degen & F.E. Dreifuss, pp. 53–58. Amsterdam: Elsevier.

Loiseau, P. & Cohadon, S. (1981): Les épilepsies à foyers EEG intercritiques multiples. *Rev. EEG Neurophysiol.* **11,** 259–266.

Loiseau, P., Cohadon, F. & Mortureux, Y. (1967): A propos d'une forme singulière d'épilepsie de l'enfant. *Rev. Neurol. (Paris)* **116,** 224–248.

Loiseau, P., Pestre, M., Dartigues, J.F., Commenges, D., Barberger-Gateau, C. & Cohadon, S. (1983): Long term prognosis in two forms of childhood epilepsy: typical absence seizures and epilepsy with rolandic (centro-temporal) EEG foci. *Ann. Neurol.* **13,** 642–648.

Loiseau, P., Duché, B., Cordova, S., Dartigues, J.F. & Cohadon, S. (1988): Prognosis of benign childhood epilepsy with centro-temporal spikes: a follow-up study of 168 patients. *Epilepsia* **29,** 229–235.

Loiseau, P., Duché, B. & Cohadon, S. (1992): The prognosis of benign localized epilepsy in early childhood. In: *Benign localized and generalized epilepsies of early childhood (Epilepsy Res.* Suppl. 6), eds. R. Degen & F.E. Dreifuss, pp. 75–82. Amsterdam: Elsevier.

Morikawa, T., Osawa, T., Ishiara, O. & Seino, M. (1979): A reappraisal of 'benign epilepsy of children with centro-temporal EEG foci'. *Brain Dev.* **1,** 253–265.

Morikawa, T., Seino, M. & Yagi, K. (1992): Is rolandic discharge a hallmark of benign partial epilepsy of childhood? In: *Benign localized and generalized epilepsies of early childhood (Epilepsy Res.* Suppl. 6), eds. R. Degen & F.E. Dreifuss, pp. 59–70. Amsterdam: Elsevier.

Musumeci, S.A., Colognola, R.M., Ferri, R., Gigli, G.L., Petrella, M.A., Sanfilippo, S., Bergonzi, P. & Tassinari, C.A. (1988): Fragile-X syndrome: a particular epileptogenic EEG pattern. *Epilepsia* **29,** 41–47.

Niedermeyer, E. & Naidu, S. (1990): Further EEG observations in children with the Rett syndrome. *Brain Dev.* **12,** 53–54.

Oller Daurella, L. (1992): Is there an epilepsy with unilateral seizures? In: *Epileptic syndromes in infancy, childhood and adolescence*, 2nd edn, eds. J. Roger, M. Bureau, Ch. Dravet, F.E. Dreifuss, A. Perret & P. Wolf, pp. 267–272. London: John Libbey.

Rose, D. & Duron, B. (1984): Valeur prognostique des anomalies EEG observées au cours du sommeil dans l'épilepsie à paroxysmes rolandiques (EPR). *Rev. EEG Neurophysiol.* **14,** 217–226.

Roulet, E., Deonna, T. & Despland, A. (1989): Prolonged intermittent drooling and oromotor dyspraxia in benign childhood epilepsy with centro-temporal spikes. *Epilepsia* **30** (5), 564–568.

Santanelli, P., Bureau, M., Magaudda, A., Gobbi, G. & Roger, J. (1989): Benign partial epilepsy with centro-temporal (or rolandic) spikes and brain lesion. *Epilepsia* **30,** 182–188.

Schmitt, B. & Dumermuth, G. (1992): The value of the EEG in the diagnosis of localized epilepsies in children. In: *Benign localized and generalized epilepsies of early childhood (Epilepsy Res* Suppl. 6), eds. R. Degen & F.E. Dreifuss, pp. 83–94. Amsterdam: Elsevier.

Vigevano, F., Di Capua, M., Fusco, L., Ricci, S., Sebastianelli, R. & Lucchini, P. (1992): Six-month benign familial convulsions. In: *Benign localized and generalized epilepsies of early childhood (Epilepsy Res.* Suppl. 6), eds. R. Degen & F.E. Dreifuss, pp. 127–129. Amsterdam: Elsevier.

Yoshinaga, H., Amano, R., Oka, E. & Ohtahara, S. (1992): Dipole tracing in childhood epilepsy with special reference to rolandic epilepsy. *Brain Topogr.* **4,** 193–199.

Watanabe, K., Yamamoto, N., Negoro, T., Takahashi, T., Aso, K. & Machara, M. (1990): Benign infantile epilepsy with complex partial seizures. *J. Clin. Neurophysiol.* **7,** 409–416.

Epileptic Seizures and Syndromes, Edited by Peter Wolf
© 1994 John Libbey & Company Ltd., pp. 241–256

Chapter 30

Idiopathic localization-related epilepsies: the non-rolandic types

Pierre Genton* and Renzo Guerrini†

**Centre Saint Paul, 13258 Marseille 09, France and †Institute of Child Neurology, Psychiatry and Educational Psychology, University of Pisa, IRCSS Stella Maris, Via dei Giacinti 2, 56018 Calambrone, Pisa, Italy*

Introduction

Following the description of benign childhood epilepsy with centrotemporal spikes (BECTS) (see Dravet, Chapter 29), it was realized that focal epilepsies could be 'idiopathic', i.e. not associated with a brain lesion, and probably genetically determined. It was also soon realized that idiopathic focal epilepsy was one of the most frequent types of epilepsy occurring in children.

It was tempting to find other syndromes of idiopathic focal epilepsy, differing from BECTS from the clinical or neurophysiological point of view, and many such entities were ascribed or added to the exciting new category of 'idiopathic localization-related epilepsies' (ILREs) (Table 1). The field is crowded and opinions diverge on many topics. Several extensive and thoughtful reviews of the ILREs have been published recently (Lüders *et al.*, 1987; Roger & Bureau, 1987; Doose & Baier, 1989; Roger *et al.*, 1990; Dalla Bernardina & Fontana, 1991; Lerman & Kivity, 1991; Loiseau, 1993; Panayiotopoulos, 1993a).

Besides BECTS, however, only two syndromes have been recognized by the latest International Classification of Epilepsies and Epileptic Syndromes (Commission, 1989), i.e. benign epilepsy of childhood with occipital paroxysms (BCEOP) and reading epilepsy. As the latter will be fully discussed in this volume, we will concern ourselves with the former and with other syndromes ascribed to this category or sharing some of the features of ILRE. The main questions we ask ourselves at the outset of our task are the following: (1) how do these syndromes relate to the archetypical BECTS syndrome? and (2) how many distinct clinical, electrophysiological and genetic entities are there in this category of epilepsies?

The criteria of idiopathic localization-related epilepsies

The clinical and electroencephalographic (EEG) features common to ILREs have been summarized by Dalla Bernardina *et al.* (1992a); these criteria beautifully fit the clinical and EEG aspects of BECTS, but need to be discussed in the perspective of other, less typical epileptic syndromes that are both idiopathic and localization-related.

Table 1. Idiopathic and/or benign non-Rolandic, localization-related epileptic syndromes and related disorders described to date, with original authors and year of first publication.

Denomination of syndrome	Authors	Year
(Primary) reading epilepsy	Bickford *et al.*	1956
Landau–Kleffner syndrome	Landau & Kleffner	1957
Epilepsy with continuous spike-waves during slow sleep (ESES)	Patry *et al.*	1971
Benign partial seizures of adolescence	Loiseau & Orgogozzo	1978
Benign psychomotor epilepsy	Dalla Bernardina *et al.*	1980
Benign partial epilepsy with extreme somatosensory evoked potentials	De Marco & Tassinari	1981
Idiopathic epilepsy of childhood with occipital paroxysms	Gastaut	1982
Atypical benign partial epilepsy	Aicardi & Chevrie	1982
Benign frontal lobe epilepsy	Beaumanoir & Nahory	1983
Idiopathic partial epilepsy in infants	Watanabe *et al.*	1987
Idiopathic partial epilepsy in adults	S. Berkovic, unpublished data	1991
Familial infantile convulsions	Vigevano *et al.*	1992a
Continuous localized EEG discharges during sleep (CLEDS)	Galletti *et al.*	1992
Familial frontal lobe epilepsy	Scheffer *et al.*	1993
Idiopathic partial epilepsy with photic-induced occipital seizures	Guerrini *et al.*	1994

Ictal and interictal clinical symptomatology

The absence of neurological deficit, of a lesion of the central nervous system (CNS) and of mental retardation is a major criterion of ILRE. Reports of cases with a cerebral lesion and a typical form of BECTS generally lead to the conclusion that the association is purely coincidental (Santanelli *et al.*, 1989). However, a recent case report of a patient with focal cortical dysplasia and typical BECTS (Ambrosetto, 1993) raises other questions, as this type of lesion is associated with a severe epilepsy in most cases. Other patients with an initial history of BECTS-compatible symptoms and a brain lesion may be diagnosed, at one stage, as having the syndrome of continuous spikes and waves (SW) during slow wave sleep (CSWS; Tassinari *et al.*, 1992), a condition associated with a progressive neuropsychological impairment. Among the patients reported by Gastaut as having BCEOP, as many as 10 per cent had either mental retardation or hemiparesis or both (Gastaut, 1992). It thus appears that ILREs may occur in brain-damaged children. It seems likewise difficult to differentiate, in some cases, a cryptogenic form of focal epilepsy with infrequent seizures and an ILRE.

A benign prognosis (total remission from epileptic seizures without treatment, lack of postictal neuropsychological or neurological deficit) is often considered to be a marker of ILREs. This, however, does not totally hold true for non-rolandic types of ILRE, as many cases of idiopathic occipital lobe epilepsy persist beyond puberty – leading to the statement that, in this type of epilepsy, 'no definite prognosis can be made' (Commission, 1989); moreover, CSWS or Landau–Kleffner syndromes (LKS), in which a significant proportion of cases are considered idiopathic, can leave permanent neuropsychological sequelae (see below).

ILREs are age-dependent conditions that are supposed to begin between the ages of 4 and 8, the maximal range being 18 months to 15 years. Well-demonstrated exceptions seem to be present beyond either extremity. ILREs with onset in infancy have now been described, as familial or sporadic cases (Watanabe *et al.*, 1987, 1990, 1993; Vigevano *et al.*, 1992a, b). A particular, frequent situation is often encountered in adolescents who experience only a single or a single cluster of focal seizures during adolescence (Loiseau & Louiset, 1992). ILREs may even begin in adulthood: twin studies have pointed to the existence of a genetically determined type of localization-related epilepsy with onset in early adulthood (see Berkovic, Chapter 20).

In ILREs, seizures are supposed to be typically infrequent and brief. This is particularly untrue for non-rolandic ILRE, especially for occipital epilepsies, as seizures may be frequent at the onset (Kivity & Lerman, 1992) or even typically have a long duration (Panayiotopoulos, 1989; Kivity & Lerman,

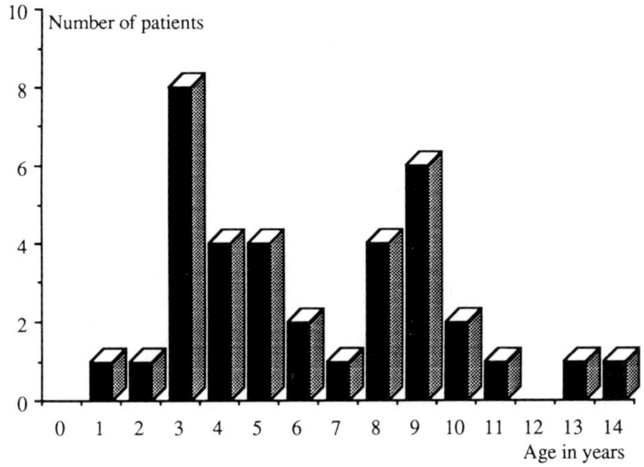

Fig. 1. Distribution of ages at onset of seizures in 36 cases of idiopathic childhood occipital epilepsy. Note the presence of two peaks, at age 3 and at age 9. Although there was no significant segregation of clinical symptomatology or prognosis according to age of onset of seizures, this may point to two different mechanisms with a different age-dependency.

1992). A more common feature is represented by the ictal semiology in ILREs: it appears in all cases that the symptomatology of seizures, even if it may be different from one patient to another, remains stable in a given patient; this may hold true for all the types of ILRE that have been described, although the occurrence of secondary generalization from time to time may give the impression that the patient has two types of seizures.

ILREs typically respond very quickly and completely to antiepileptic drug (AED) therapy. However, AEDs may have little influence on the evolution of seizures in the occipital type of ILRE (Guerrini *et al.*, 1993b); the effects of AED therapy compared with the natural history of ILREs have not been investigated in all syndromes. It appears that, in BECTS, AED therapy has indeed no major influence on the occurrence of seizures during follow-up (Ambrosetto & Tassinari, 1990). Thus, the real common trait of the group of ILREs might be represented by the lack of influence (to some extent) of classical AEDs on the natural course of the epilepsy.

Neurophysiology

ILREs are characterized by a normal background activity and normal cyclic organization of sleep with normal sleep transients. Interictal changes are represented by prominent spikes, slow spikes and SW with a very stable morphology that is unchanged during sleep. It must be noted that interictal changes, although evident in most cases of non-rolandic ILREs, may be absent during long periods in occipital ILRE, appearing only on postictal EEGs (Guerrini *et al.*, 1993b) or randomly (Panayiotopoulos, 1989). It should also be noted that interictal abnormalities are typically absent in the infantile types of ILREs (Watanabe *et al.*, 1990, 1993; Vigevano *et al.*, 1992b).

Sleep produces a major increase of interictal changes in ILREs without change in morphology; this is not found in all cases of occipital ILREs (Gastaut, 1992), where changes may abate during sleep and, in some cases, change their aspect and appear as polyspike waves (Guerrini *et al.*, 1993b).

The presence of discharges of generalized SW has been reported in ILREs, mostly in periods of drowsiness. However, in ILREs these generalized changes are infrequent, brief and subclinical, and they are not increased during sleep or following hyperventilation. There is no apparent overlap between ILREs and generalized idiopathic epilepsies during childhood (Genton & Guerrini, 1993a).

Much attention has been devoted to the computer analysis of interictal changes in ILRE, although most of the studies focus on 'rolandic' spikes. A typical topographic aspect of these consists in a tangential dipole across the central areas of one hemisphere (Wong, 1993). Some studies, however, find it difficult to differentiate between 'functional' (subclinical), 'rolandic' (associated with benign childhood epilepsy) and 'organic' spikes (van der Meij *et al.*, 1993). Morphological analysis of interictal changes has not been performed extensively in other types of ILRE, and the morphology of the sharp anomalies cannot, at the present stage, be used as a firm diagnostic criterion of ILRE, especially in the non-rolandic forms.

Clinical forms of non-rolandic idiopathic localization-related epilepsies

Primary reading epilepsy (Bickford *et al.,* 1956; Wolf, 1992) as well as a benign temporal lobe epilepsy with onset in early adulthood will be discussed elsewhere in this volume (see Berkovic *et al.*, Chapter 31; Wolf *et al.*, Chapter 32). A recently described type of familial frontal lobe epilepsy, with autosomal dominant inheritance, awaits confirmation (Scheffer *et al.,* 1993). Many clinically significant epileptic entities remain to be discussed: the major grouping of patients is represented by the idiopathic occipital lobe epilepsy cases; another important, recently described grouping concerns idiopathic focal epilepsies with onset during infancy. The problems posed by certain EEG aspects with unclear clinical correlations, such as midline spikes (Bagdorf & Lee, 1993), will not be discussed here. Other clinical entities described to date concern, in our opinion, borderline cases of one of the major categories, although the specific problems posed by the syndrome of CSWS and related conditions, such as atypical benign childhood epilepsy and LKS, should be mentioned here.

Idiopathic occipital lobe epilepsies

A clinical and EEG syndrome that differed sharply from BECTS was described by Gastaut (1982, 1992) as 'benign childhood epilepsy with occipital paroxysms' (BCEOP) and was confirmed by other authors (Beaumanoir, 1983; Kivity & Lerman, 1989; Panayiotopoulos, 1989). This entity was characterized by a very striking EEG trait, i.e. the presence of uni- or bilateral occipital SW that disappear when the eyes are opened (Fig. 2). However, the clinical, aetiological and prognostic correlates of BCEOP have been the subject of many controversies.

BCEOP is neither very rare nor very frequent and may represent a significant proportion of childhood-onset occipital lobe epilepsies: in our experience, it represented 4/38 patients with ILRE newly referred to the Centre Saint Paul between 1988 and 1991, *vs.* 14/33 of those referred to the Institute of Child Neurology and Psychiatry of Pisa during the same period (unpublished data); the prevalence varies according to the mode of referral. Gastaut reported on 36 cases of BCEOP in 1982 and found 27 more cases in the following years. Dalla Bernardina *et al.* (1993) found 33 idiopathic *vs.* 12 cryptogenic and 19 symptomatic cases among 64 patients with childhood-onset occipital epilepsy. BCEOP represents 20 per cent of all cases of ILRE in the series of Panayiotopoulos (1989). The sex ratio is close to 1, with a slight preponderance in girls for some authors.

The age at onset of seizures is variable (Fig. 1), with apparently two distinct peaks, around age 3 and around age 9 respectively, within a broad range that begins around age two and reaches into adolescence. The onset of BCEOP may be dramatic, or 'stormy', with frequent and prolonged seizures (Kivity & Lerman, 1992). The age of onset may be correlated with specific clinical traits (Panayiotopoulos, 1989, 1993b): younger patients exhibit a particular pattern of long-lasting, nocturnal seizures with deviation of the eyes, sometimes followed by secondary generalization, while older patients may experience partial seizures, most often characterized by visual hallucinations. Other studies failed to find age-related differences in the ictal symptomatology (Guerrini *et al.*, 1993a, b) and stressed the great variability of seizure patterns between patients (although a single patient tends to experience always the same type of seizure). The ictal features are, in decreasing order of prevalence: tonic deviation of the eyes, secondary generalization, simple partial visual seizures with

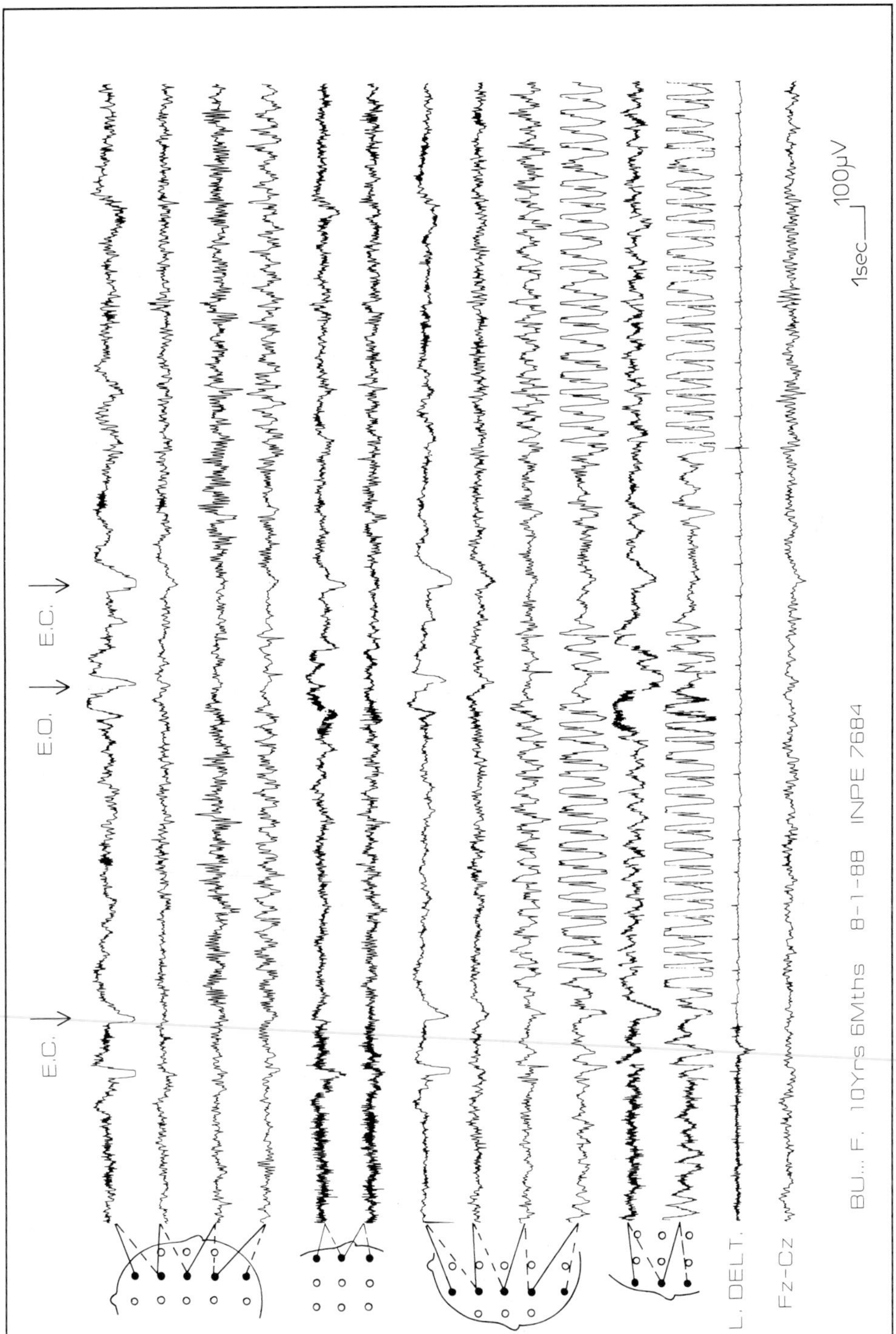

Fig. 2. Idiopathic occipital epilepsy. Boy aged 10 years 6 months with idiopathic occipital epilepsy. An isolated generalized tonic–clonic seizure occurred during sleep 6 months earlier. Left occipitopostero temporal spike waves are activated by eye closure.

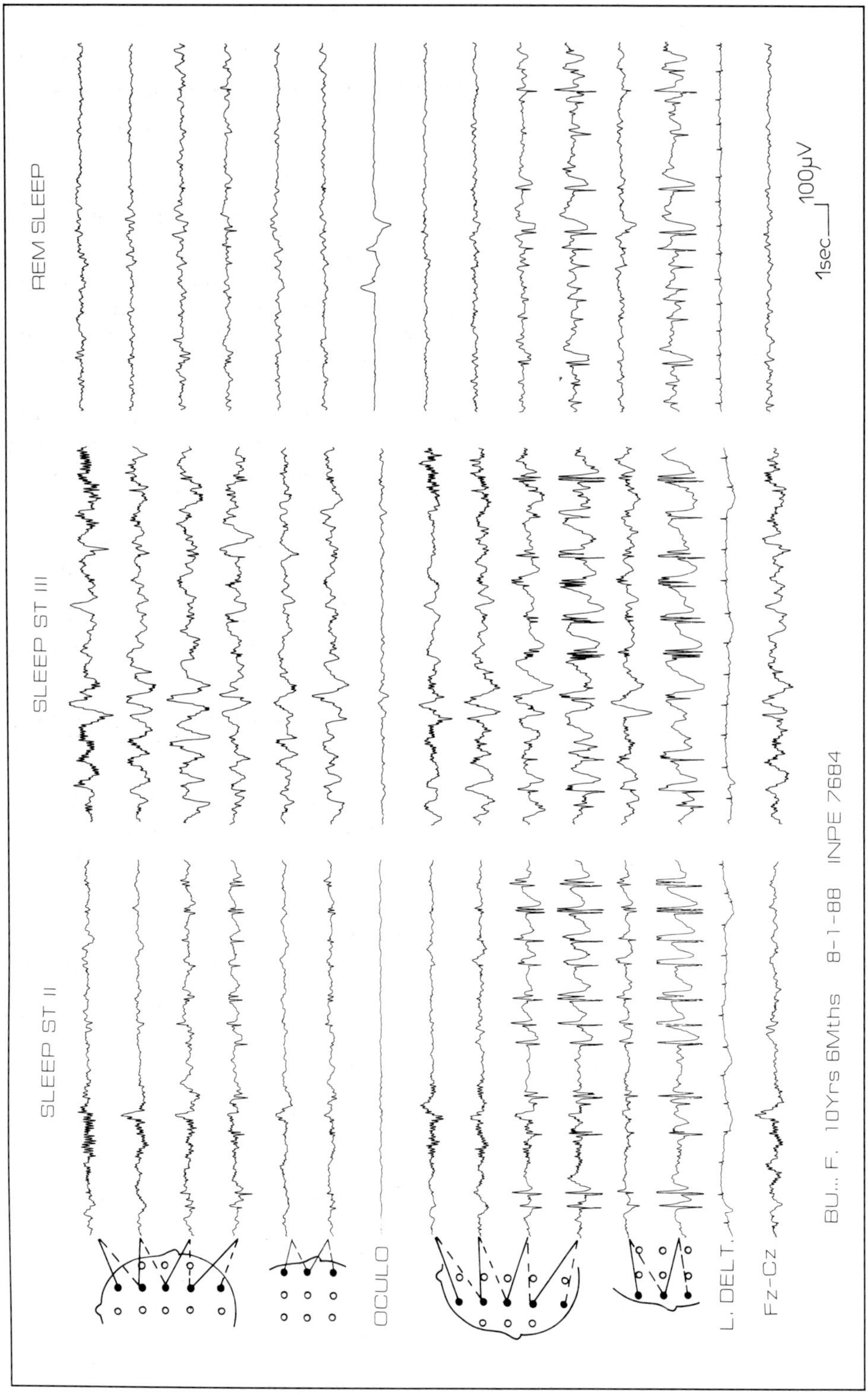

Fig. 3. Idiopathic occipital epilepsy. Same patient as in Fig. 2. Paroxysmal activity is present in all sleep stages. During slow-wave sleep, polyspike waves appear. This morphological variation during sleep did not forecast a bad prognosis in this patient, who was 15 at last follow-up and had sufferred no further seizure since age 10.

hallucinations, headache, vomiting, unilateral motor phenomena, secondary complex partial seizures, dysarthria, oculoclonic seizures and simple partial somatosensory seizures.

All studies have stressed the frequent association with migrainous symptoms, such as vomiting and headache. These symptoms may occur ictally in some patients, postictally in others.

The EEG patterns are also variable. It must be stressed that the typical interictal occipital SW discharges may be found only during short periods in the course of the disease, especially during a few days after a single seizure (Guerrini *et al.*, 1993a, b). They may be absent at the onset of seizures. The morphology of the occipital SW may vary over time, and may change during sleep (Dalla Bernardina *et al.*, 1993) (Fig. 3).

Some patients exhibit a form of idiopathic epilepsy with photic-induced occipital seizures. It is a pure reflex epilepsy, since all seizures are triggered by photic stimuli, a remarkable trait since this phenomenon is mostly found in idiopathic generalized epilepsies (Tassinari *et al.*, 1989; Michelucci & Tassinari, 1993; Guerrini *et al.*, in press). The various seizure types are the same as in other cases of BCEOP, the most frequent being brief or long-lasting seizures with visual symptoms, tonic deviation of the eyes, unresponsiveness and ictal vomiting. In some of these patients, generalized interictal SW discharges may be found in association with occipital spikes. The onset of seizures is around puberty in the majority of patients and there is a strong female predominance. In spite of some similarities with BCEOP, this form seems to represent a distinct entity that is probably underestimated because the triggering role of TV or video games may remain unrecognized in patients with infrequent seizures.

Many patients with a comparable clinical and EEG presentation at the onset have a symptomatic type of occipital epilepsy (Newton & Aicardi, 1983; Cooper & Lee, 1991). Some may have posterior calcifications on the computerized tomography (CT) scan and an intestinal biopsy positive for coeliac disease (Gobbi *et al.*, 1992), and the disease proves to be progressive and severe. Others have various types of brain lesions; Dalla Bernardina *et al.* (1993) studied 16 children with symptomatic occipital epilepsy (porencephalic cyst in five, focal atrophy in seven, focal cortical dysplasia in two and calcifications in two), and found that the clinical and EEG patterns overlapped with those found in cryptogenic and even clearly idiopathic cases of childhood occipital epilepsy. According to these authors, the main features in favour of a symptomatic origin are: a higher prevalence of brief, focal seizures, abnormalities of the background EEG activity, changes in the morphology of SW during sleep. No trait can be considered specific of the idiopathic nature of the occipital epilepsy.

Occipital epilepsy with onset in childhood may thus correspond to a variety of clinical, aetiological and prognostic entities. Some of these patients do have an idiopathic type of epilepsy, but the clinical presentation is very variable even in these cases; the existence of a bimodal distribution of the ages of onset even suggests the possibility of two different clinical entities. The prognosis cannot be ascertained with the same degree of confidence as in BECTS. The genetic background of these idiopathic cases needs further clarification; there are no reports of a genetic overlap with BECTS.

It clearly appears that the classical criteria of ILRE cannot be applied to BCEOP. Given the great variability of clinical and EEG patterns and of prognosis, BCEOP should be called 'idiopathic occipital epilepsy', as the term 'benign' is inappropriate and the reference to the EEG changes may be misleading (Guerrini *et al.*, 1993a). Perhaps there is a subset of patients, as suggested by Panayiotopoulos (1989), that does fulfil the criteria of both idiopathicity and benignity.

Benign psychomotor epilepsy

A large group of patients, with an apparently idiopathic temporal lobe epilepsy manifesting mainly as nocturnal seizures with a strong affective component, was reported in 1980 by Dalla Bernardina *et al.* Their findings were confirmed by another group (Plouin *et al.*, 1990). Seizure onset is between age 2 and 9, with a characteristic pattern of yelling and sudden fright or terror, followed by autonomic symptoms (swallowing, chewing . . .); unresponsiveness may not be total. The seizures occur mostly at sleep onset, but also during waking or sleep. Pavor nocturnus may be a difficult differential diagnosis. The EEG is typical in many but not all cases, showing a normal background activity and high-voltage frontotemporal or parietotemporal spikes that are activated by sleep. The long-term evolution is benign in most cases, although some may still have seizures after age 18 (Dalla Bernardina *et al.*, 1992b).

This category may in fact cover different types of epilepsy that share common clinical (but probably not EEG) findings; some cases may belong to the group of idiopathic focal epilepsies, others may have a cryptogenic type of temporal lobe epilepsy. In a recent review of benign psychomotor epilepsy, Dalla Bernardina *et al.* (1992b) state that 'BPE does not constitute an independent form of idiopathic partial epilepsy, but probably only a relatively rare variant of BECT'.

Benign frontal lobe epilepsy of childhood

Eleven children with frontal lobe epilepsy of good prognosis (all had been seizure-free for at least 5 years) were reported by Beaumanoir and Nahory in 1983; according to Loiseau *et al.* (1991), this type of epilepsy accounts for approximately 11 per cent of all cases of idiopathic focal epilepsies. The seizures had been infrequent, with several types (absence-like, versive, secondarily generalized during sleep) and the EEG findings heterogeneous: some patients exhibited patterns compatible with the diagnosis of BECTS, others had only focal slow activity; the ictal patterns were shifting frontal discharges. This group probably includes both particular forms of BECTS and other, cryptogenic frontal lobe epilepsies with a mild evolution.

Benign epilepsy with giant somatosensory evoked potentials

Unusually ample somatosensory evoked potentials can be elicited by tapping on the sole of a foot in about 1 per cent of all children between the ages of 1 and 13 years (with a peak around age 4–6), more often in males (68 per cent); 30 per cent of these children also have epilepsy (De Marco & Negrin, 1973; De Marco & Tassinari, 1981; Tassinari & De Marco, 1992) (Figs. 4 and 5). Before age 5, the subclinical phenomenon is apparently isolated; later, spontaneous epileptiform EEG changes can appear, first during sleep and then in the waking state, and seizures may occur around age 6. These are mostly of a versive or partial motor type and may be secondarily generalized and occur mostly during the day. Seizures remain infrequent (several per year) and apparently remit spontaneously after 1 year. According to the original authors, the EEG changes are focal or multifocal and resemble those found in BECTS.

However, other authors have shown that the 'extreme' somatosensory evoked potentials are not specific of a given type of epilepsy (Fonseca *et al.*, 1991; Dalla Bernardina *et al.*, 1992a): they can be found in various types of focal epilepsies, including symptomatic cases, and in generalized epilepsies, sometimes with a slightly different morphology. They are found in 5 per cent of all cases of ILRE. Extreme somatosensory evoked potentials are thus considered by these authors to represent a functional, age-dependent phenomenon that bears no particular relationship to any given type of epilepsy.

Atypical benign epilepsy of childhood

This small but significant category of patients was described by Aicardi and Chevrie in 1982 and confirmed by Deonna *et al.* in 1986. Among 32 patients with a clinical picture compatible with the diagnosis of BECTS and intense activation of EEG changes during sleep, seven were singled out with a particular clinical picture (Aicardi & Chevrie, 1982): they had both the typical focal motor or generalized tonic–clonic seizures and atypical seizures, such as absences, jerks or atonic falls. They were drug-resistant but showed no psychomotor deterioration and went into remission at age 9–12. The waking EEG showed focal spikes and SW, with shifting predominance, and the sleep EEG showed 'almost continuous' SW discharges. However, the sleep EEG was recorded only during drowsiness in most patients. Clinically, it was not very clear whether this EEG and clinical condition lasted for a long time, whether or not the falls and episodes of 'sagging' were due to a phenomenon

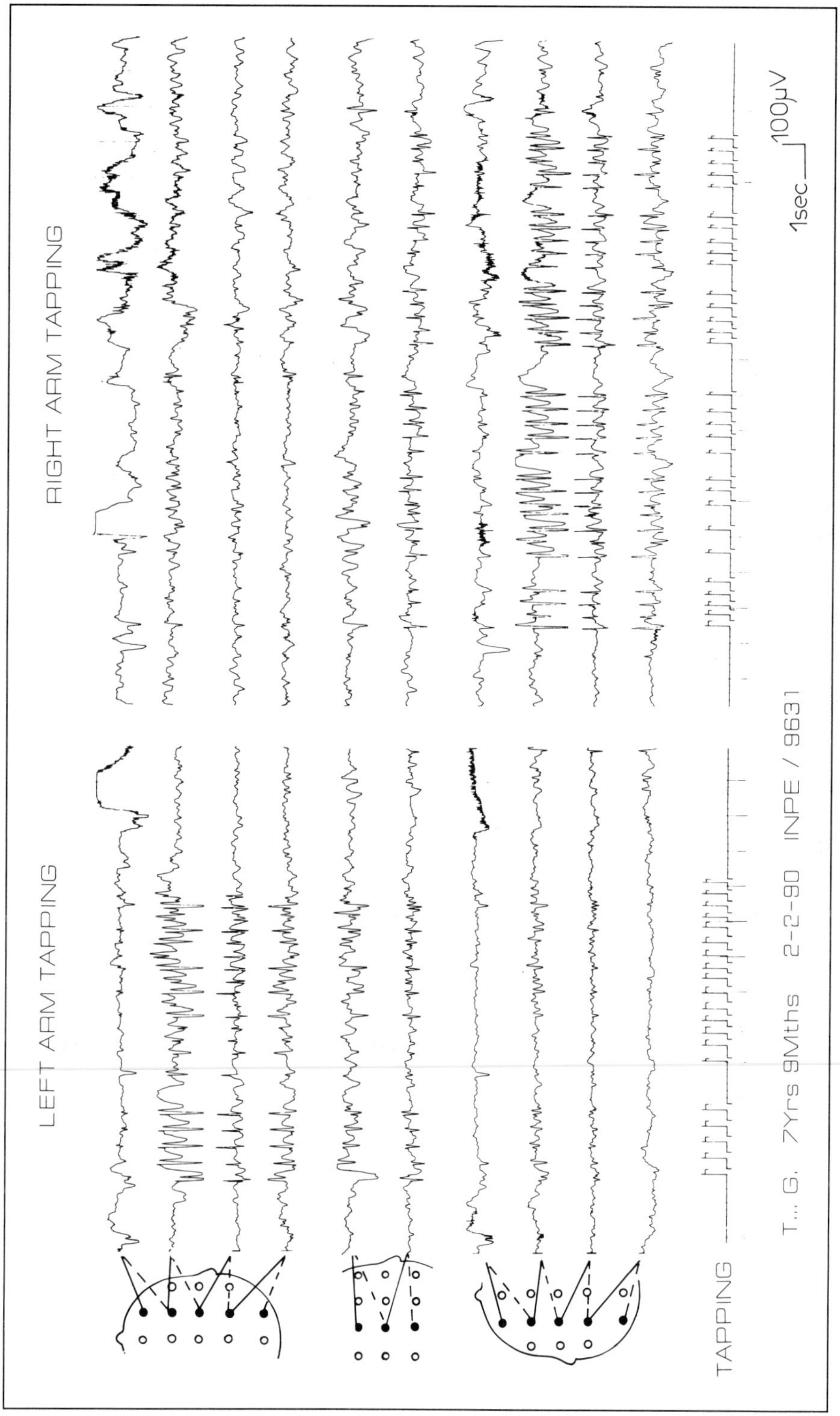

Fig. 4. Epilepsy with extreme somatosensory evoked potentials. Boy aged 7 years 9 months. He presented from age 4 years 6 months on with infrequent, mainly nocturnal, focal clonic seizures involving the left leg and with periods of unsteadiness due to epileptic negative myoclonus involving both legs. The latter phenomenon was easily controlled by antiepileptic medication. This patient is now aged 11 years 6 months and has been seizure-free on valproic acid (VPA) and carbamazepine (CBZ) during the last 3 years. Tapping of the hand palms evokes contralateral spikes with phase reversal over the C3 and C4 electrodes.

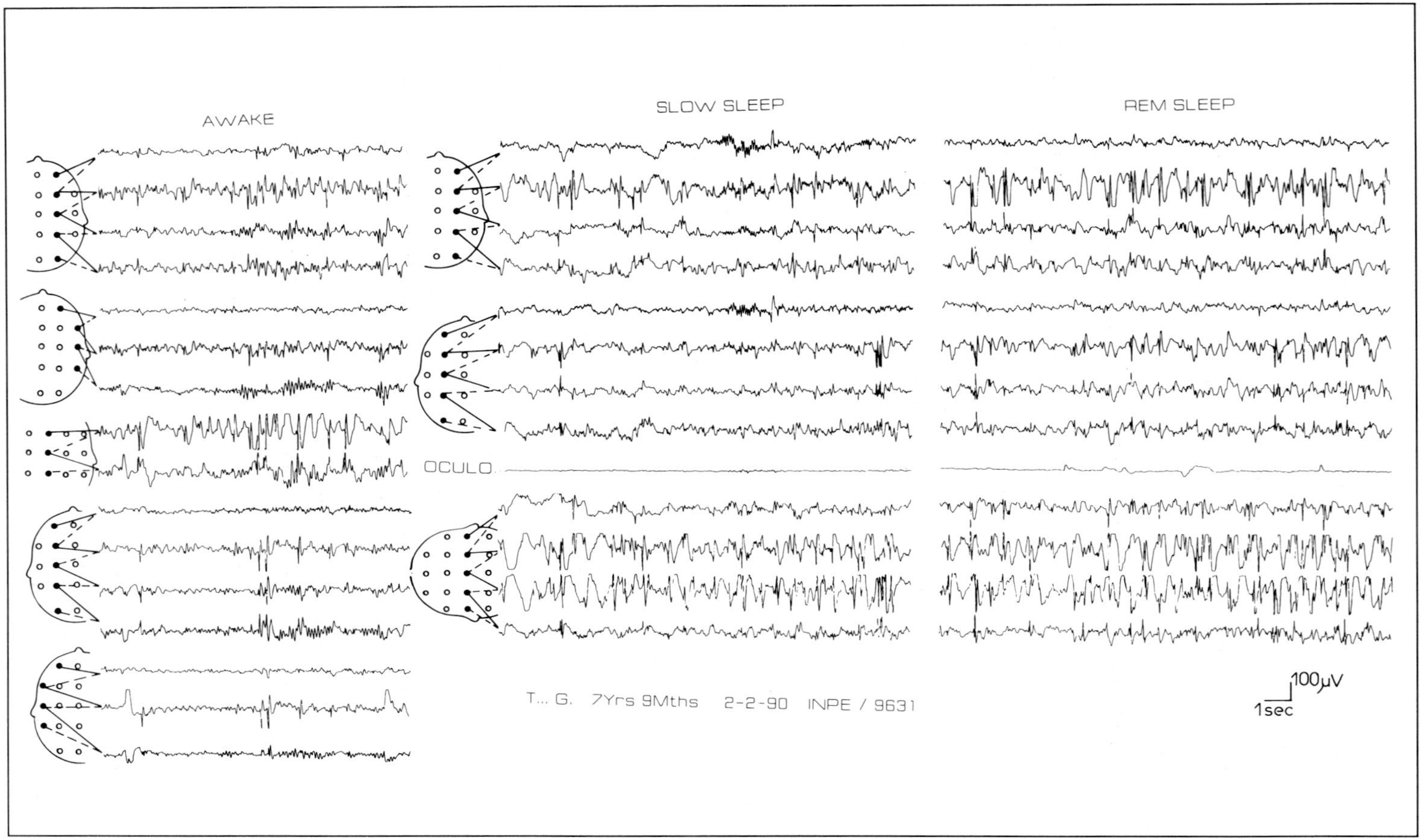

Fig. 5. Epilepsy with extreme somatosensory evoked potentials. Same patient as in Fig. 4. Left: Spontaneous spikes or spike waves are present with phase reversal over the Cz electrode and show equipotentiality over the right centroparietal cortex. Synchronous spikes are present contralaterally. Middle: during slow-wave sleep there is continuous spike–polyspike and wave activity over the vertex. Some of these transients are also found over the centroparietal areas, with right predominance. The activation persists during rapid-eye-movement (REM) sleep.

now better analysed as 'epileptic negative myoclonus' (Guerrini *et al.*, 1993c) and whether the condition was provoked by a given drug. It has been reported that some cases of BECTS may be transiently aggravated, nearly transformed into a syndrome of CSWS following the administration of carbamazepine (Caraballo *et al.*, 1989).

The nosological situation of this entity is thus still unclear, but it is most probable that it represents a subgroup of the larger entity of BECTS, where the activation of EEG changes during sleep (and waking) is extreme and the clinical picture modified accordingly. These changes might be caused by external factors, such as drugs. The prognosis remains excellent.

Continuous focal discharges during sleep

Six cases of apparently idiopathic focal epilepsy were recently reported in which the characteristic finding consisted in continuous lateralized epileptiform discharges during sleep (CLEDS; Galletti *et al.*, 1992). The children were aged 3–7, five out of 6 five out of six had a family history of febrile seizures and all had normal development and normal CT scans. They had a benign type of epilepsy, with predominantly focal motor or unilateral seizures. These findings were contrasted with a similar EEG activation found in patients with brain lesions, mental retardation and neuropsychological deficits attributed to continuous focal EEG discharges during sleep (Pelliccia *et al.*, 1989). However, the EEG pattern these authors report in normal children is consistent with the diagnosis of BECTS, the only particularity being the intense activation profile found during sleep and the absence of typical, orofacial seizures. CLEDS may thus constitute only a variant of the classical form of BECTS.

Epilepsy with continuous spikes and waves during slow-wave sleep (CSWS) and Landau-Kleffner syndrome (LKS)

These entities were described many years ago (Landau & Kleffner, 1957; Patry *et al.*, 1971) and have been the subject of many controversies. The present International Classification (Commission, 1989) ranks both CSWS and LKS among syndromes with both focal and generalized features.

In CSWS, more than 50 per cent of the patients affected have a focal neurological deficit (Tassinari *et al.*, 1992); in LKS, the major clinical symptom is represented by a focal neuropsychological deficit, i.e. verbal agnosia, and many reports have found a symptomatic aetiology in patients with LKS (for a review, see Beaumanoir, 1992). Both syndromes share some of the characters of ILREs:

– the typical EEG features of CSWS and LKS are strongly age-related, covering the same age range as BECTS;
– they are associated, in a majority of patients with LKS and in all patients with CSWS, with epilepsy; various seizure types have been described, some being fairly typical for BECTS, but epilepsy (however severe at the onset and during some stages) constantly remits before age 15;
– typical EEG changes are represented by the association of focal and diffuse paroxysmal discharges that are highly activated during sleep, when they tend to appear as both generalized and continuous, at least during slow-wave sleep.

Apart from BECTS, there is no epileptic entity that is associated with (1) constant remission of seizures around age 15 and (2) a dramatic increase of EEG changes during sleep. Other entities have been discussed here that border on CSWS: CLEDS and atypical benign epilepsy of childhood. The presence or absence of neuropsychological deficits may be related to the duration of the state of continuous discharges during sleep and/or frequent, diffuse discharges during waking. A state of CSWS may be transiently provoked in patients with BECTS by external factors, such as drugs (Caraballo *et al.*, 1989).

There are no data on the genetic background of CSWS or LKS. A male preponderance is noted in CSWS and LKS, as in BECTS. In the present state of our knowledge, we are tempted to think that there is a relationship between these entities but this remains hypothetical. The particular characteristics of CSWS and LKS might be due to interactions between a focal brain lesion and a genetic background that expresses itself as an age-related EEG trait, with marked activation of epileptiform changes during sleep, and a strong tendency towards bilateral synchrony (Dalla Bernardina *et al.*, 1989; Genton & Guerrini, 1993b).

Benign focal seizures of adolescence

Epidemiological data point to a high incidence of epilepsies in adolescents: as a significant proportion of patients had only a single seizure or a cluster of seizures within a very short time, Loiseau & Orgogozzo (1978) were able to individualize a clinical entity they labelled 'benign focal epileptic seizures in teenagers'. In 1992, the same group updated its material and reported on 108 cases (Loiseau & Louiset, 1992). This entity concerns about 25 per cent of all partial seizures with onset during adolescence and is found predominantly in males (71.2 per cent of the sample). There is no significant family or personal history; the seizure(s) are simple partial (14.5 per cent), complex partial (28.5 per cent) or secondarily generalized (57 per cent). The EEG is normal or shows non-focalized slowing if it is performed within 48 h. There is only a single seizure in 80 per cent of the cases, a single cluster of two to five seizures in the others.

This apparently common clinical situation may escape the attention of referral clinicians and may thus be ignored by many epileptologists. It does not seem to bear any relationship to any of the other idiopathic epileptic syndromes (generalized or focal), although more clinical, EEG and genetic data may lead to other conclusions. A history of a single seizure during adolescence may, for instance, be found (without any further information) in family members of patients with a well-defined type of genetically determined epilepsy. Detailed EEG data will be difficult to obtain in such patients, beyond the routine recording performed days after the episode. In our present state of knowledge, however, this particular clinical situation stands apart.

Idiopathic focal epilepsies in infancy

In 1989, Dulac *et al.* reported a group of apparently idiopathic epilepsies with onset of seizures before the age of 3, beginning as early as the eighth day of life. They stressed that no onset of a benign epilepsy was found between the ages of 2 months and 15 months. The early type must thus belong to the group of benign neonatal seizures, while the later type represents an early form of idiopathic focal epilepsy of childhood, even if most children failed to exhibit the typical EEG changes; the interictal EEGs were considered normal in most cases.

However, Watanabe *et al.* (1987, 1990) reported nine infants with complex partial seizures beginning between the ages of 3 and 20 months. The presentation was characteristic, with clusters of seizures recorded in all patients, the site of seizure onset varying between children (temporal, central or frontal). Interictal EEGs were normal. All children had seizures with motion arrest, decreased responsiveness, staring or blank eyes, mostly with automatisms and mild convulsive movements. The prognosis was excellent in all patients at follow-up (age 5–10), with perfect control of seizures using monotherapy carbamazepine (CBZ) or phenobarbital (PB) or without any treatment; four out of nine had a family history of benign seizures (febrile seizures or infantile convulsions). Another grouping of patients was reported recently by the same authors (Watanabe *et al.*, 1993): seven cases with apparently secondarily generalized seizures in clusters during waking or during sleep, with onset at age 3–20 months; the initial ictal symptoms were motion arrest or staring during 5–33 s followed by tonic–clonic generalization. The EEG seizure onset was variable, interictal EEGs were normal, drugs could be discontinued and all patients were seizure-free with follow-ups ranging between 3 and 12 years.

Another clinical setting was recently reported (Vigevano *et al.*, 1992a): seizure onset was between 4 and 7 months, all patients had a family history of similar, benign epilepsy in infancy, mostly in the fathers of probands; focal seizures occurred in clusters, with secondary generalization, the EEG showing shifting onset in central or posterior regions of either hemisphere. The response to antiepileptic treatment was immediate. The interictal EEG remained normal and the prognosis was good in all respects. This new entity, considered to represent 'benign infantile familial convulsions', is genetically distinct from benign neonatal familial convulsions (Vigevano *et al.*, 1992b).

One can thus consider that the occurrence of idiopathic focal epilepsies has been documented in infancy and early childhood. Some of these cases have a clear genetic origin, others not, although a family background of febrile seizures during childhood may be significant. These very early cases share the absence of interictal EEG changes, the shifting ictal EEG patterns, which are prominently present over a very limited region of the scalp, and the lack of postictal EEG depression. The particularities of these features may be due to the developmental stage. The long-term outcome is not known in all, although the family histories point, when given, to very benign conditions. It is not clear, at this stage, whether this entity is a homogeneous one: as in benign familial neonatal convulsions, several distinct genetically determined defects may be responsible for a similar clinical picture that is highly age-dependent.

Conclusions

The group of ILREs is clearly dominated by one syndrome, i.e. BECTS: this type of epilepsy is based on a very frequent, genetically determined anomaly that expresses itself in school-age children and in various disguises (or phenotypes). Several of the syndromes listed in this review are probably clinical variants of BECTS. Other uncommon syndromes may be caused by the interactions between the genetic trait on which BECTS is based and other, acquired or genetic, factors.

However, several types of ILRE bear no relation to BECTS. Idiopathic occipital epilepsy of childhood, however heterogeneous and difficult to diagnose in some cases, is not a by-product of BECTS. Idiopathic (and benign) focal epilepsies with onset during infancy may constitute other entities that are genetically distinct from neonatal convulsions and from BECTS, and there may be several of these. The same is probably true of reading epilepsy and of adult-onset benign partial epilepsy.

It it most unlikely that a single genetic/biochemical anomaly should be responsible for such a spectrum of epileptic conditions, with varying types of age-relationship, of anatomical focal expression and of associated reflex phenomena. Much attention should be devoted, in the near future, to the delimitation of the genetic background of these epileptic entities. Precise observations of the phenotypes (both clinical and EEG) found in patients, in their siblings and in other family members will provide adequate material for molecular genetic studies and elucidate the nosology of this complex field.

For the time being, let us draw some practical conclusions:

– the terms 'idiopathic' and 'benign', when used in the context of focal epilepsies, are not synonymous; only the former should be used to describe such epileptic syndromes, and only with caution in occipital epilepsies of childhood;

– treatment should be very conservative in cases of idiopathic focal epilepsies; the use of drugs may not be necessary at all in many patients, either because the natural course is very benign, or because their efficacy is questionable.

References

Aicardi, J. & Chevrie, J.J. (1982): Atypical benign partial epilepsy of childhood. *Dev. Med. Child Neurol.* **24,** 281–292.

Ambrosetto, G. (1993): Unilateral opercular macrogyria and benign childhood epilepsy with centro-temporal (rolandic) spikes: report of a case. *Epilepsia* **33,** 499–503.

Ambrosetto, G. & Tassinari, C.A. (1990): Antiepileptic drug treatment of benign childhood epilepsy with rolandic spikes: is it necessary? *Epilepsia* **31,** 802–805.

Bagdorf, R. & Lee, Sl. (1993): Midline spikes: is it another benign EEG pattern of childhood? *Epilepsia* **34,** 271–274.

Beaumanoir, A. (1983): Infantile epilepsy with occipital focus and good prognosis. *Eur. Neurol.* **22,** 43–52.

Beaumanoir, A. (1992): The Landau–Kleffner syndrome. In: *Epileptic syndromes in infancy, childhood and adolescence*, 2nd edn, eds. J. Roger, M. Bureau, C. Dravet, F.E. Dreifuss, P. Wolf & A. Perret, pp. 231–243. London: John Libbey.

Beaumanoir, A. & Nahory, A. (1983): Les épilepsies bénignes partielles: 11 cas d'épilepsie partielle frontale à évolution favorable. *Rev. EEG Neurophysiol.* **13,** 207–211.

Bickford, R.G., Wheelan, J.L., Klass, D.W. & Corbin, K.B. (1956): Reading epilepsy: clinical and electroencephalographic studies of a new syndrome. *Trans. Am. Neurol. Assoc.* **81,** 100–102.

Caraballo, R., Fontana, E., Michelizza, B., Zullini, E., Sgrò, V., Pajno Ferrara, F., Dalla Bernardina, B. & Esposito, S. (1989): Carbamazepina, 'assenze atipiche', 'crisi atoniche' e stato di PO continua del sonno (POCS). *Boll. Lega Ital. Epil.* **66/67,** 379–381.

Commission on Classification and Terminology of the International League Against Epilepsy (1989): Proposal for revised classification of epilepsies and epileptic syndromes. *Epilepsia* **30,** 389–399.

Cooper, G.W. & Lee, Sl. (1991): Reactive occipital epileptiform activity: is it benign? *Epilepsia* **32,** 63–68.

Dalla Bernardina, B. & Fontana, E. (1991): Le epilessie parziali idiopatiche. *Ann. Neurol. Psichiatria* **86**(2–4), 103–124.

Dalla Bernardina, B., Bureau, M., Dravet, C., Dulac, O., Tassinari, C.A. & Roger, J. (1980): Epilepsie bénigne de l'enfant avec crises à séméiologie affective. *Rev. EEG Neurophysiol.* **10,** 8–18.

Dalla Bernardina, B., Fontana, E. Michelizza, B., Colamaria, V., Capovilla, G. & Tassinari, C.A. (1989): Partial epilepsies of childhood, bilateral synchronization, continuous spike-waves during slow sleep. In: *Advances in epileptology,* Vol. 17, eds. J. Manelis, E. Bental, J.N. Loeber & F.E. Dreifuss, pp.295–302. New York: Raven Press.

Dalla Bernardina, B., Sgrò, V., Fontana, E., Colamaria, V. & La Selva, L. (1992a): Idiopathic partial epilepsies in children. In: *Epileptic syndromes in infancy, childhood and adolescence*, 2nd edn, eds. J. Roger, M. Bureau, C. Dravet, F.E. Dreifuss, P. Wolf & A. Perret, pp. 173–188. London: John Libbey.

Dalla Bernardina, B., Colamaria, V., Chiamenti, C., Capovilla, G., Trevisan, E. & Tassinari, C.A. (1992b): Benign partial epilepsy with affective symptoms (benign psychomotor epilepsy). In: *Epileptic syndromes in infancy, childhood and adolescence*, 2nd edn, eds. J. Roger, M. Bureau, C. Dravet, F.E. Dreifuss, P. Wolf & A. Perret, pp. 1219–1233. London: John Libbey.

Dalla Bernardina, B., Fontana, E., Cappellaro, O., Zullini, E., Darra, F., Colamaria, V. & Caraballo, R. (1993): The partial occipital epilepsies in childhood. In: *Occipital seizures and epilepsies in children*, eds. F. Andermann, A. Beaumanoir, L. Mira, J. Roger & C.A. Tassinari, pp. 173–181. London: John Libbey.

De Marco, P. & Negrin, P. (1973): Parietal focal spikes evoked by contralateral tactile somatotopic stimulations in four nonepileptic subjects. *Electroencephalogr. Clin. Neurophysiol.* **34,** 308–312.

De Marco, P. & Tassinari, C.A. (1981): Extreme somatosensory evoked potentials (ESEP): an EEG sign forecasting the possible occurrence of seizures in children. *Epilepsia* **22,** 569–575.

Deonna, T., Ziegler, H.L. & Despland, P.A. (1986): Partial epilepsy in neurologically normal children: clinical syndromes and prognosis. *Epilepsia* **27,** 241–247.

Doose, H. & Baier, W.K. (1989): Benign partial epilepsy and related conditions: multifactorial pathogenesis with hereditary impairment of brain maturation. *Eur. J. Pediatr.* **49,** 152–158.

Dulac, O., Cusmai, R. & De Oliveira, K. (1989): Is there a partial benign epilepsy in infancy? *Epilepsia* **30,** 798–801.

Fonseca, L.C., Tedrus, G.M.A. & Odashima, N.S. (1991): Epileptic syndromes in children with somatosensory evoked spikes. *Epilepsia* **32** (Suppl. 1), 88.

Galetti, F., Sturniolo, M.G., Giannotti, F., Cortesi, F. & Brinciotti, M. (1992): Décharges EEG localisées continues pendant le sommeil chez des enfants sans troubles neuropsychiques. *Neurophysiol. Clin.* **22,** 447–457.

Gastaut, H. (1982): L'épilepsie bénigne de l'enfant à pointes-ondes occipitales. *Rev. EEG Neurophysiol.* **12,** 179–201.

Gastaut, H. (1992): Benign epilepsy of childhood with occipital paroxysms. In: *Epileptic syndromes in infancy, childhood and adolescence*, 2nd edn, eds. J. Roger, M. Bureau, C. Dravet, F.E. Dreifuss, P. Wolf & A. Perret, pp. 201–215. London: John Libbey.

Genton, P. & Guerrini, R. (1993a): Lack of association between childhood absence epilepsy and idiopathic partial epilepsy of childhood. *Epilepsia* **34**(Suppl. 2), 176–177.

Genton, P. & Guerrini, R. (1993b): What differentiates Landau-Kleffner syndrome from the syndrome of continuous spikes and waves during slow sleep? *Arch. Neurol.* **50,** 1008–1009.

Gobbi, G., Bouquet, F., Greco, L., Lambertini, A., Tassinari, C.A., Ventura, A. & Zaniboni, M.G. (1992): Coeliac disease, epilepsy and cerebral calcifications. *Lancet* **340,** 439–443.

Guerrini, R., Dravet, C., Vigliano, P., Battaglia, A., Capizzi, G., Bureau, M. & Genton, P. (1993a): Childhood idiopathic occipital epilepsy. *Epilepsia* **34** (Suppl. 2), 178.

Guerrini, R., Battaglia, A., Dravet, C., Bureau, M. & Genton, P. (1993b): Outcome of idiopathic childhood epilepsy with occipital paroxysms. In: *Occipital seizures and epilepsies in children*, eds. F. Andermann, A. Beaumanoir, L. Mira, J. Roger & C.A. Tassinari, pp. 165–171. London: John Libbey.

Guerrini, R., Dravet, C., Genton, P., Bureau, M., Roger, J., Rubboli, G. & Tassinari, C.A. (1993c): Epileptic negative myoclonus. *Neurology* **43,** 1078–1083.

Guerrini, R., Dravet, C., Genton, P., Bureau, M., Bonnani, P. & Roger, J. (1994): Idiopathic partial epilepsy with photic induced occipital seizures, *Epilepsia,* in press.

Kivity, S. & Lerman, P. (1989): Benign partial epilepsy of childhood with occipital discharges. In: *Advances in epileptology,* Vol. 17, eds J. Manelis, E. Bental, J.N. Loeber & F.E. Dreifuss, pp. 371–373. New York: Raven Press.

Kivity, S. & Lerman, P. (1992): Stormy onset with prolonged loss of consciousness in benign childhood epilepsy with occipital paroxysms. *J. Neurol. Neurosurg. Psychiatry* **55,** 45–48.

Landau, W. & Kleffner, F. (1957): Syndrome of acquired aphasia with convulsive disorder in children. *Neurology* **7,** 523–530.

Lerman, P. & Kivity, S. (1991): The benign partial non-rolandic epilepsies. *J. Clin. Neurophysiol.* **8,** 275–287.

Loiseau, P. (1993): Benign focal epilepsies of childhood. In: *The treatment of epilepsy: principles and practice*, ed. E. Wyllie, pp. 503–512. Philadelphia, London: Lea and Febiger.

Loiseau, P. & Louiset, P. (1992): Benign partial seizures of adolescence. In: *Epileptic syndromes in infancy, childhood and adolescence*, 2nd edn, eds. J. Roger, M. Bureau, C. Dravet, F.E. Dreifuss, P. Wolf & A. Perret, pp. 343–345. London: John Libbey.

Loiseau, P. & Orgogozzo, J.M. (1978): An unrecognized syndrome of benign focal epileptic seizures in teenagers. *Lancet* **i,** 1070–1071.

Loiseau, P., Duché, B. & Loiseau, J. (1991): Classification of epilepsies and epileptic syndromes in two different samples of patients. *Epilepsia* **32,** 303–309.

Lüders, H., Lesser, R.P., Dinner, D.S. & Morris, H.H., III (1987): Benign focal epilepsy of childhood. In: *Epilepsy: electroclinical syndromes*, eds. H. Lüders & R.P. Lesser, pp. 303–306. Berlin, Heidelberg: Springer.

Michelucci, R. & Tassinari, C.A. (1993): Television-induced occipital seizures. In: *Occipital seizures and epilepsies in children*, eds. F. Andermann, A. Beaumanoir, L. Mira, J. Roger & C.A. Tassinari, pp. 141–144. London: John Libbey.

Newton, R. & Aicardi, J. (1983): Clinical findings in children with occipital spike wave complexes suppressed by eye opening. *Neurology* **33,** 1526–1529.

Panayiotopoulos, C.P. (1989): Benign childhood epilepsy with occipital paroxysms: a 15 year prospective study. *Ann. Neurol.* **26,** 51–56.

Panayiotopoulos, C.P. (1993a): Benign childhood partial epilepsies: benign childhood seizure susceptibility syndromes. *J. Neurol. Neurosurg. Psychiatry* **56,** 2–5.

Panayiotopoulos, C.P. (1993b): Benign childhood epilepsy with occipital paroxysms. In: *Occipital seizures and epilepsies in children*, eds. F. Andermann, A. Beaumanoir, L. Mira, J. Roger & C.A. Tassinari, pp. 151–164. London: John Libbey.

Patry, G., Lyagoubi, S. & Tassinari, C.A. (1971): Subclinical 'electrical status epilepticus' induced by sleep in children. *Arch. Neurol.* **24,** 242–252.

Pelliccia, A., Galletti, F., Pierantoni, R., Gulotta, E., Ferrara, M., Brinciotti, M. & Benedetti, P. (1989): Décharges EEG localisées continues pendant le sommeil chez l'enfant. *Neurophysiol. Clin.* **19,** 145–154.

Plouin, P., Lerique, A. & Dulac, O. (1990): Etude électroclinique et évolution dans 7 observations de crises partielles complexes dominées par un comportement de terreur chez l'enfant. *Boll. Lega Ital. Epil.* **29/30,** 139–143.

Roger, J. & Bureau, M. (1987): Les épilepsies partielles idiopathiques de l'enfant. *Rev. Neurol.* **143,** 381–391.

Roger, J., Bureau, M., Genton, P. & Dravet, C. (1990): Idiopathic partial epilepsies in the child. In: *Comprehensive epileptology*, eds. M. Dam & L. Gram, pp. 155–170. New York: Raven Press.

Santanelli, P., Bureau, M., Magaudda, A., Gobbi, G. & Roger, J. (1989): Benign partial epilepsy with centrotemporal (or rolandic) spikes and brain lesion. *Epilepsia* **30,** 182–188.

Scheffer, I.E., Bhatia, D., Fish, D.R., Marsden, C.D., Andermann, F., Andermann, E., Manson, J.I., Hopkins, I.J., Harvey, A.S. & Berkovic, S.F. (1993): Autosomal dominant frontal lobe epilepsy: a new xyndrome. *Epilepsia* **34** (suppl. 6), 30.

Tassinari, C.A. & De Marco, P. (1992): Benign partial epilepsy with extreme somato-sensory evoked potentials. In: *Epileptic syndromes in infancy, childhood and adolescence*, second edition, eds. J. Roger, M. Bureau, C. Dravet, F.E. Dreifuss, P. Wolf & A. Perret, pp. 225–229. London: John Libbey.

Tassinari, C.A., Rubboli, G., Plasmati, R., Salvi, F., Ambrosetto, G., Bianchedi, G., Forti, A. & Michelucci, R. (1989): Television-induced epilepsy with occipital seizures: a variety of idiopathic partial occipital epilepsy. In: *Reflex seizures and reflex epilepsies*, eds. A. Beaumanoir, H. Gastaut & R. Naquet, pp. 241–243. Geneva: Editions Médecine et Hygiène.

Tassinari, C.A., Bureau, M., Dravet, C., Dalla Bernardina, B. & Roger, J. (1992): Epilepsy with continuous spikes and waves during slow sleep – otherwise described as ESES (epilepsy with electrical status epilepticus during slow sleep). In: *Epileptic syndromes in infancy, childhood and adolescence*, 2nd edn, eds J. Roger, M. Bureau, C. Dravet, F.E. Dreifuss, P. Wolf & A. Perret, pp. 245–256. London: John Libbey.

van der Meij, W., Wienecke, G.H., van Huffelen, A.C., Schenk-Rootlieb, A.J.F. & Willemse, J. (1993): Identical morphology of the rolandic spik-and-wave complex in different clinical entities. *Epilepsia* **34,** 540–550.

Vigevano, F., Fusco, L., Di Capua, M., Ricci, S., Sebastianelli, R. & Lucchini, P. (1992a): Benign infantile familial convulsions. *Eur. J. Pediatr.* **151,** 608–612.

Vigevano, F., Fusco, L., Sebastianelli, R., Dulac, O., Beck, C., Baldy-Moulinier, M., Labauge, P. & Malafosse, A. (1992b): Le convulsioni infantili familiari benigne: aspetti clinici e genetici. *Boll. Lega Ital. Epil.* **79/80,** 27–28.

Watanabe, K., Yamamoto, N., Negoro, T., Takaesu, E., Aso, K., Furune, S. & Takahashi, I. (1987): Benign complex partial epilepsies in infancy. *Pediatr. Neurol.* **3,** 208–211.

Watanabe, K., Yamamoto, N., Negoro, T., Takahashi, I., Aso, K. & Maehara, M. (1990): Benign infantile epilepsy with complex partial seizures. *J. Clin. Neurophysiol.* **7,** 409–416.

Watanabe, K., Negoro, T. & Aso, K. (1993): Benign partial epilepsy with secondarily generalized seizures in infancy. *Epilepsia* **34,** 635–638.

Wolf, P. (1992): Reading epilepsy. In: *Epileptic syndromes in infancy, childhood and adolescence*, 2nd edn, eds. J. Roger, M. Bureau, C. Dravet, F. E. Dreifuss, P. Wolf & A. Perret, pp. 281–298. London: John Libbey.

Wong, P.K.H. (1993): Stability of source estimates in rolandic spikes. *Brain Topogr.* **2,** 31–36.

Epileptic Seizures and Syndromes, Edited by Peter Wolf
© 1994 John Libbey & Company Ltd., pp. 257–263

Chapter 31

Familial temporal lobe epilepsy: a new syndrome with adolescent/adult onset and a benign course

Samuel F. Berkovic*, R. Anne Howell* and John L. Hopper†

**Department of Neurology, Austin Hospital, Heidelberg, Melbourne, Victoria 3084, Australia and Department of Medicine (Neurology), The University of Melbourne at Austin Hospital, Heidelberg, Melbourne, Victoria 3084, Australia; †The Australian NHMRC Twin Registry, The University of Melbourne, Parkville, Victoria 3084, Australia*

Summary

We describe a new syndrome of familial temporal lobe epilepsy, initially recognized in monozygous twin pairs. Onset is usually early adult life. The seizure pattern is of simple partial seizures suggestive of temporal lobe origin with psychic symptoms of affective and experiential types. Rare complex partial seizures and secondarily generalized tonic–clonic seizures also occur. The latter are often nocturnal and are precipitated by sleep deprivation or stress. Affected individuals typically have no antecedent factors for epilepsy and are of normal intellect. Seizures are easily controlled and mildly affected relatives may remain undiagnosed. The occurrence in monozygous pairs was the key to identifying this new inherited epilepsy but studies in other family members and non-twin pedigrees suggest it is an autosomal dominant disorder with incomplete penetrance.

Introduction

Aetiology of temporal lobe epilepsy

Temporal lobe epilepsy is the best known and probably the commonest form of localization-related epilepsy in adults (Gastaut *et al.*, 1975; Loiseau *et al.*, 1991; Manford *et al.*, 1992). There has been intensive research on refractory temporal lobe epilepsy, stimulated particularly by interest in surgical treatment. Refractory temporal lobe epilepsy is essentially an acquired disorder with a number of recognized causes. These include tumours, vascular malformations, neuronal migration disorders, perinatal insults, post-traumatic lesions, postinfectious lesions and hippocampal sclerosis. Hippocampal sclerosis is the commonest pathological lesion observed; its aetiology is controversial but may often relate to prolonged febrile convulsions or status epilepticus in early childhood. In a minority of cases of surgically treated cases of temporal lobe epilepsy, neither a pathological lesion nor an aetiology can be established (Babb & Brown, 1987; Bruton, 1988).

Genetic factors are thought to have only a minor role in the aetiology of refractory temporal lobe epilepsy. In the studies of Andermann there was no increase in the frequency of seizures in relatives compared with control subjects, although there was a slight increase in the frequency of epileptiform electroencephalographic (EEG) abnormalities. This was interpreted as indicating a small role for genetic factors in the multifactorial aetiology of refractory focal epilepsies (Andermann, 1972, 1982; Andermann & Straszak, 1982). More recently, Andermann's group have shown that, in the subgroup of patients with hippocampal sclerosis associated with febrile convulsions, there is a more important genetic component (Abou-Khalil *et al.*, 1993), confirming earlier observations of Falconer and others (Falconer *et al.*, 1964; Falconer, 1971; Ounsted & Lindsay, 1981). Other investigators have also recently confirmed that genetic factors have a role to play in the aetiology of chronic focal epilepsies (Ottman, 1989; Ottman *et al.*, 1989; Treiman, 1989; Degen *et al.*, 1993).

Non-refractory temporal lobe epilepsy

The frequency of non-refractory temporal lobe epilepsy in the general population is not known. Many reports suggest that only about 30 per cent of all cases of recognized temporal lobe epilepsy enter remission with or without continued antiepileptic medication (Juul-Jensen, 1964; Rodin, 1968; Ounsted & Lindsay, 1981; Pazzaglia *et al.*, 1982; Juul-Jensen & Foldspang, 1983; Mikati & Holmes, 1993). Other studies report remission in 40–62 per cent of cases (Currie *et al.*, 1971; Tsai & Schmidt, 1982) and, based on a review of epidemiological studies, Hauser (1992) estimated that as many as 60–70 per cent of patients with newly identified complex partial seizures can be expected to achieve complete control. Whatever the true proportion of non-refractory cases, it seems likely that this group represents a considerable number of patients with focal epilepsy. Moreover, in many cases, mild temporal lobe epilepsy probably remains undiagnosed; such patients may have rare major seizures, with brief simple focal or complex partial attacks passing unrecognized.

The causes of non-refractory temporal lobe epilepsy have not been fully elucidated. In an epidemiological study of complex partial seizures, febrile seizures, cerebral palsy, head trauma and viral encephalitis emerged as risk factors, but over half the cases had no recognized aetiology (Rocca *et al.*, 1987). Franceschi *et al.* (1989) found abnormalities on magnetic resonance imaging (MRI) in 48 per cent of non-refractory cases; these included findings suggestive of a low-grade tumour or vascular malformation lesion in 10 per cent of cases, and of hippocampal sclerosis in 23 per cent of cases. In comparison, abnormalities are found on visual analysis of MRI in over 80 per cent of refractory cases (Jackson *et al.*, 1990). Thus the known causes or associations of refractory temporal lobe epilepsy are present in some non-refractory cases. Amongst non-refractory cases, however, there is a higher frequency of patients without a recognized aetiology.

Genetic factors have not been identified as a major cause of non-refractory temporal lobe epilepsy. During a twin study of epilepsy, based largely on community ascertained twins, we observed a number of concordant adult monozygous pairs with mild temporal lobe epilepsy. This suggested that genetic factors could be of great importance in non-refractory temporal lobe epilepsy.

Twin study observations

In the Australian study of epilepsy in twins (see Berkovic *et al.*, Chapter 20), we have identified 52 twin pairs with 'symptomatic' localization-related epilepsies. These were operationally defined as those localization-related epilepsies that do not conform to one of the three recognized syndromes of idiopathic localization-related epilepsy where there is a well-known genetic component (Commission, 1989). There were 19 monozygous pairs with symptomatic localization-related epilepsies. Of these, four were concordant for temporal lobe epilepsy that was of late onset and showed a benign course.

Twin family E11 (Fig. 1)

The proband was a female twin who had intense *déjà vu* feelings at the age of 31 and presented with

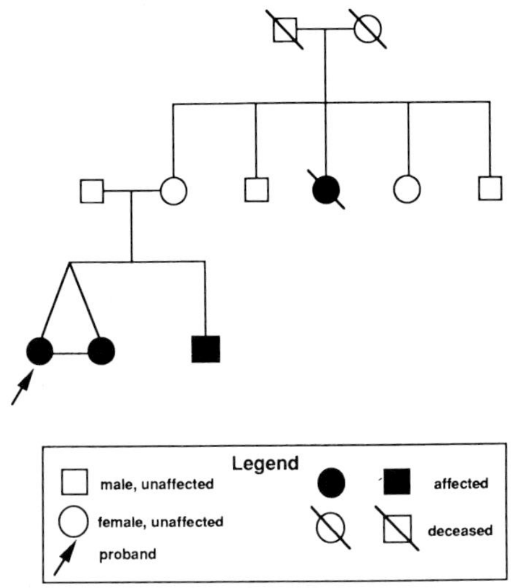

Fig. 1. Pedigree of twin family E11.

a first tonic–clonic seizure at the age of 32. Therapy with phenytoin resulted in a reduction in the frequency of the *déjà vu* feelings, and no further tonic–clonic seizures occurred. Neuroimaging studies were unremarkable and an EEG showed a single right temporal spike during wakefulness. Her monozygous twin sister also had déjà vu since the age of 31 but had had no tonic–clonic seizures when evaluated. An EEG showed theta activity over the right temporal region without epileptiform activity.

Their brother had had *déjà vu* with episodes of loss of awareness between the ages of 15 and 22 and suffered a single nocturnal tonic–clonic seizure at the age of 22 after being sleep-deprived. An aunt in the previous generation was also reported to have had seizures but was deceased and further details were unavailable.

Other twin families

Three other concordant adult-onset monozygous pairs were identified with a similar clinical pattern. They had a history of simple partial seizures with infrequent or no complex partial or secondarily generalized partial seizures. The simple partial seizures comprised psychic symptoms of affective or experiential (dysmnesic, cognitive) types, highly suggestive of temporal lobe origin. Secondarily generalized seizures typically occurred at night and followed a period of sleep deprivation, or excessive physical or emotional stress. Mean (± SD) age of onset of seizures in the four monozygotic pairs was 27 ± 15 years (range 15–63 years). None of the three other monozygous pairs had a more extensive family history of epilepsy. We have also identified a dizygous twin with an unaffected co-twin but an affected mother.

These subjects had a normal neurological examination and a normal intellect. There were no identified antecedents for seizures such as significant perinatal trauma, postnatal head injury, meningitis, encephalitis or febrile convulsions. EEG studies, including sleep recordings, were usually normal or contained minor non-specific and non-localized abnormalities. Localized abnormalities, when present, were relatively sparse, and included temporal slow waves, with rare epileptiform transients (Fig. 2). Epileptiform transients comprised low- to medium-voltage sharp waves with or without aftergoing slow waves. These epileptiform transients lacked distinguishing characteristics such as those observed

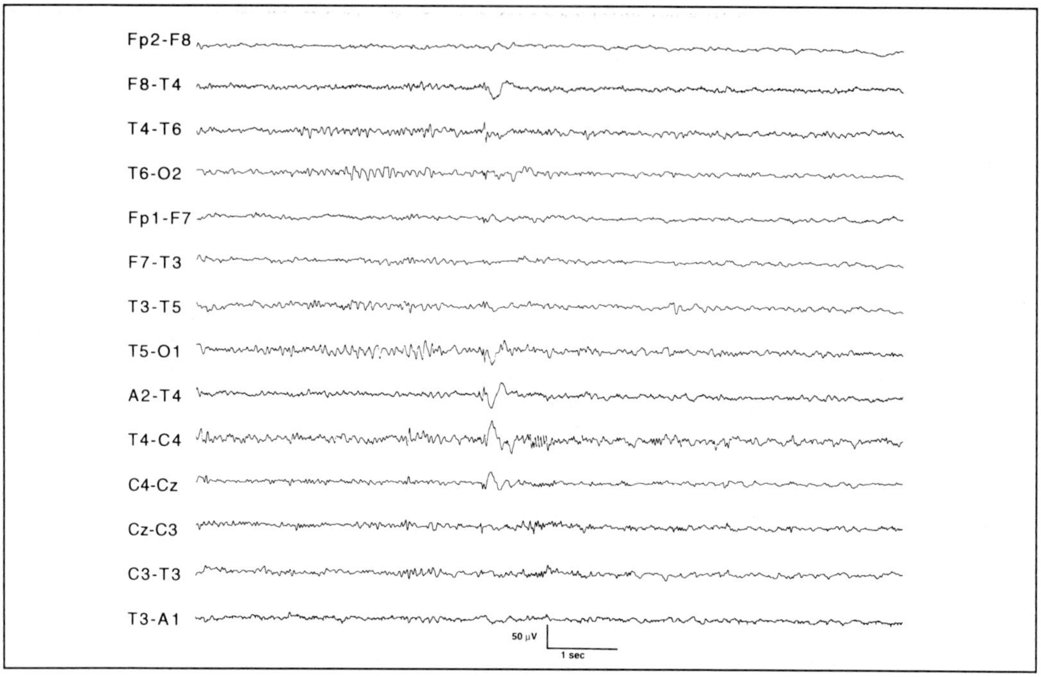

Fig. 2. EEG of an affected monozygotic twin. During drowsing, infrequent right temporal delta waves were seen, sometimes with a preceding low-voltage spike. The delta activity was regarded as a definite lateralized abnormality, but the low-voltage spike was of questionable diagnostic significance.

in benign localization-related epilepsies of childhood. MRI scans of these patients were normal. There was an excellent response to therapy with carbamazepine or phenytoin.

Discussion

Recognition of the syndrome

The clinical features of our monozygous twins with this epilepsy syndrome are shown in Table 1. The twin study observations suggest that this entity may be an important cause of benign temporal lobe epilepsy in the community. We have now also identified similar familial cases of temporal lobe epilepsy, with adult onset and a benign course, in a number of non-twin families (S.F. Berkovic, unpublished). It is important to stress that in many cases the simple partial seizures, of experiential or affective types, were not spontaneously reported; these symptoms were often ignored, or regarded as normal phenomena. Only when a careful history was taken directly from co-twins or other family members was the familial nature of the disorder revealed.

The full clinical extent of this syndrome remains to be explored. Onset of a familial epilepsy in adult life is quite unusual. Although some of our twin and non-twin cases had onset in teenage, it is unclear if this syndrome may sometimes manifest in childhood. The benign nature of the disorder was also striking. Further studies are required to determine if this disorder can also present as a refractory temporal lobe epilepsy. The lack of familial cases of temporal lobe epilepsy (as opposed to a family history of febrile seizures or of generalized epilepsy) amongst intensively studied surgical cases, suggests that this entity is rarely difficult to treat.

Table 1. Clinical features of familial temporal lobe epilepsy.

Onset usually early adult life (range: teenage to elderly)
Simple partial seizures suggestive of temporal lobe origin
Complex partial seizures, rare
Tonic–clonic seizures, rare and often nocturnal
No antecedent factors for epilepsy
Normal intellect
Normal neurological examination
Sparse EEG abnormalities
Seizures easily controlled
Mildly affected relatives often undiagnosed

Why has this syndrome not been previously recognized? There are published cases of 'temporal lobe epilepsy' running in families in the older literature (Gibson, 1959; Rodin & Whelan, 1960; Bray & Wiser, 1964, 1965; Loiseau & Beaussart, 1969). Many, but not all, of these cases are examples of benign localization-related epilepsy of childhood with centrotemporal spikes, and not of true temporal lobe epilepsy. The striking occurrence in a group of monozygotic twins brought this disorder to our attention. The mild and sometimes subtle nature of the epilepsy in family members and the sparsity of EEG abnormalities have obscured recognition of this entity until now.

Genetic aspects

The seizure patterns in affected relatives were similar, although not all patients had tonic–clonic seizures. Unlike the situation in the generalized epilepsies, where phenotypes within families are heterogeneous, in this syndrome the phenotypic pattern appears to 'breed true'.

The pedigree of twin family E11 (Fig. 1) and those of some of our non-twin families (data not shown) suggested autosomal dominant inheritance. Other families, both twin and non-twin, had relatively few affected individuals, indicating that penetrance may be low in many pedigrees. There is now a precedent in the animal literature for an inherited form of temporal lobe epilepsy where seizure onset has been documented from the hippocampus (Rise *et al.*, 1991; Mutoh *et al.*, 1993). This animal model may well be analogous to the human syndrome described here; indeed, a hippocampal origin of the human syndrome is likely, given the types of simple partial seizures reported. Moreover, similar to our preliminary human genetic data, the murine disorder is inherited as a partially dominant trait (Rise *et al.*, 1991).

Conclusion

This syndrome was only detected because of the striking occurrence of an identical seizure pattern in monozygous twins. We suspect that this may be a common cause of temporal lobe epilepsy in the community. It is unusual because it is inherited and of relatively late onset. Recognition of this syndrome may be difficult unless a detailed family history is taken and relatives are questioned about minor symptoms that they may not have believed to be of clinical significance. The occurrence of an animal model of inherited temporal lobe epilepsy raises the exciting possibility of identifying the responsible epilepsy genes for this disorder.

Acknowledgements

Supported by the National Health and Medical Research Council (NHMRC) of Australia, the Australian NHMRC Twin Registry, the Austin Hospital Medical Research Foundation and the Epilepsy Foundation of Victoria.

References

Abou-Khalil, B.,, Andermann, E., Andermann, F., Olivier, A. & Quesney, L.F. (1993): Temporal lobe epilepsy after prolonged febrile convulsions: excellent outcome after surgical treatment. *Epilepsia* **34,** 878–883.

Andermann, E. (1972): Focal epilepsy and related disorders: genetic, metabolic and prognostic studies. PhD thesis, McGill University, Montreal.

Andermann, E. (1982): Multifactorial inheritance of generalized and focal epilepsy. In: *Genetic basis of the epilepsies*, eds. V.E. Anderson, W.A. Hauser, J.K. Penry & C.F. Sing, pp. 129–145. New York: Raven Press.

Andermann, E. & Straszak, M. (1982): Family studies of epileptiform EEG abnormalities and photosensitivity in focal epilepsy. In: *Advances in epileptology: XIIIth Epilepsy International Symposium*, eds. H. Akimoto, H. Kazamatsuri, M. Seino & A. Ward, pp. 105–112. New York: Raven Press.

Babb, T.L. & Brown, W.J. (1987): Pathological findings in epilepsy. In: *Surgical treatment of the epilepsies*, ed. J. Engel, Jr., pp. 511–540. New York: Raven Press.

Bray, P.F. & Wiser, W.C. (1964): Evidence for a genetic etiology of temporal-central abnormalities in focal epilepsy. *N. Engl. J. Med.* **271,** 926–933.

Bray, P.F. & Wiser, W.C. (1965): Hereditary characteristics of temporal-central focal epilepsy. *Pediatrics* **36,** 207–211.

Bruton, C.J. (1988): *The neuropathology of temporal lobe epilepsy.* Oxford: Oxford University Press.

Commission on Classification and Terminology of the International League Against Epilepsy (1989): Proposal for revised classification of epilepsies and epileptic syndromes. *Epilepsia* **30,** 389–399.

Currie, S., Heathfield, K.W.G., Henson, R.A. & Scott, D.F. (1971): Clinical course and prognosis of temporal lobe epilepsy: a survey of 666 patients. *Brain* **94,** 173–190.

Degen, R., Degen, H.E. & Koneke, B. (1993): On the genetics of complex partial seizures: waking and sleep EEGs in siblings. *J. Neurol.* **240,** 151–155.

Falconer, M.A. (1971): Genetic and related etiological factors in temporal lobe epilepsy: a review. *Epilepsia* **12,** 13–31.

Falconer, M.A., Serafetinides, E.A. & Corsellis, J.A. (1964): Etiology and pathogenesis of temporal lobe epilepsy. *Arch. Neurol.* **10,** 233–248.

Franceschi, M., Triulzi, F., Ferini-Strambi, L., Giusti, C., Minicucci, F., Fazio, F., Smirne, S. & Del Maschio, A: (1989): Focal cerebral lesions found by magnetic resonance imaging in cryptogenic non-refractory temporal lobe epilepsy patients. *Epilepsia* **30,** 540–546.

Gastaut, H., Gastaut, J., Goncalves, E., Silva, G. & Fernandes Sanchez, G. (1975): Relative frequency of different types of epilepsy: a study employing the classification of the International League Against Epilepsy. *Epilepsia* **16,** 457–461.

Gibson, W.G. (1959): Temporal lobe epilepsy in two sisters. *Epilepsia* **1,** 316–324.

Hauser, W.A. (1992): The natural history of temporal lobe epilepsy. In: *Epilepsy surgery*, ed. H.O. Lüders, pp. 133–141. New York: Raven Press.

Jackson, G.D., Berkovic, S.F., Tress, B.M., Kalnins, R.M., Fabinyi, G. & Bladin, P.F. (1990): Hippocampal sclerosis can be reliably detected by magnetic resonance imaging. *Neurology* **40,** 1869–1875.

Juul-Jensen, P. (1964): Epilepsy: a clinical and social analysis of 1020 adult patients with epileptic seizures. *Acta Neurol. Scand.* **40** (suppl 5), 1–148.

Juul-Jensen, P. & Foldspang, A. (1983): Natural history of epileptic seizures. *Epilepsia* **24,** 297–312.

Loiseau, P. & Beaussart, M. (1969): Hereditary factors in partial epilepsy. *Epilepsia* **10,** 23–31.

Loiseau, P., Duche, B. & Loiseau, J. (1991): Classification of epilepsies and epileptic syndromes in two different samples of patients. *Epilepsia* **32,** 303–309.

Manford, M., Hart, Y.M., Sander, J.W.A.S. & Shorvon, S.D. (1992): National General Practice Study of Epilepsy: partial seizure patterns in a general population. *Neurology* **42,** 1911–1917.

Mikati, M.A. & Holmes, G.L. (1993): Temporal lobe epilepsy. In: *The treatment of epilepsy: principles and practice*, ed. E. Wyllie, pp. 513–524. Philadelphia: Lea and Febiger.

Mutoh, K., Ito, M., Tsuda, H., Shiraishi, H., Oguro, K., Shirasaka, T., Okuno, T. & Mikawa, H. (1993): Depth EEG in mutant E1 mice: demonstration of secondary generalization of the seizure from the hippocampus. *Electroencephalogr. Clin. Neurophysiol.* **86,** 205–212.

Ottman, R. (1989): Genetics of the partial epilepsies: a review. *Epilepsia* **30,** 107–111.

Ottman, R., Annegers, J.F., Hauser, W.A. & Kurland, W.T. (1989): Seizure risk in offspring of parents wiht generalized versus partial epilepsy. *Epilepsia* **30,** 157–161.

Ounsted, C. & Lindsay, J. (1981): The long-term outcome of temporal lobe epilepsy in childhood. In: *Epilepsy and psychiatry*, eds. E.H. Reynolds & M.R. Trimble, pp. 185–215. Edinburgh: Churchill Livingstone.

Pazzaglia, P., D'Alessandro, R., Lozito, A. & Lugaresi, E. (1982): Classification of partial epilepsies according to the symptomatology of seizures: practical value and prognostic implications. *Epilepsia* **23,** 343–350.

Rise, M.L., Frankel, W.N., Coffin, J.M. & Seyfried, T.N. (1991): Genes for epilepsy mapped in the mouse. *Science* **253,** 669–672.

Rocca, W.A., Sharbrough, F.W., Hauser, W.A., Annegers, J.F. & Schoenberg, B.S. (1987): Risk factors for complex partial seizures: a population-based case-control study. *Ann. Neurol.* **21,** 22–31.

Rodin, E.A. (1968): *The prognosis of patients with epilepsy.* Springfield: Charles C. Thomas.

Rodin, E.A. & Whelan, J.L. (1960): Familial occurrence of focal temporal electroencephalographic abnormalities. *Neurology* **10,** 542–545.

Treiman, D.M. (1989): Genetics of the partial epilepsies. In: *Genetics of the epilepsies*, eds. G. Beck-Mannagetta, V.E. Anderson, H. Doose & D. Janz, pp. 73–82. Berlin: Springer Verlag.

Tsai, J.J. & Schmidt, D. (1982): Long-term seizure prognosis in patients with complex partial seizures. In: *Advances in epileptology: XIIIth Epilepsy International Symposium*, eds. H. Akimoto, H. Kazamatsuri, M. Seino & A. Ward, pp. 43–46. New York: Raven Press.

Epileptic Seizures and Syndromes, Edited by Peter Wolf
© 1994 John Libbey & Company Ltd., pp. 265–281

Chapter 32

Regional manifestation of idiopathic epilepsy

Peter Wolf, Samuel Berkovic, Pierre Genton, Colin Binnie, Victor Elving Anderson and Andreas Draguhn

Introduction

Peter Wolf

Epilepsie-Zentrum Bethel, Klinik für Anfallskranke, Mara I, Maraweg 21, 33617 Bielefeld, Germany

The problem

According to our present knowledge, as it is expressed in the International Classification of Epilepsies and Epileptic Syndromes (Commission, 1989), the idiopathic epilepsies come in two varieties: generalized and localization-related. Recent research, however, leaves some doubt whether these groups are strictly separate or, rather, represent endpoints of a continuum. Patients with idiopathic localization-related epilepsies (ILREs) usually do not have a unilateral epileptic focus but often findings involving corresponding areas of both cerebral hemispheres. In addition, the electroencephalograms (EEGs) may show some amount of 'generalized', i.e. bilateral simultaneous, spike-wave (SW) discharge (Beaumanoir *et al.*, 1974; Wolf, 1992), and it seems that, in their families, both localization-related epilepsies and generalized epilepsies may be found (Wolf, 1992). On the other hand, the concept of generalized epilepsy as it is used today is largely a convention which defines as generalized everything which in the EEG is accompanied by initially bilateral epileptiform discharge. This applies for some seizure types which, clinically, would not prima facie be called generalized, such as absences which interfere with cerebral functions responsible for consciousness and facultatively comprise minimal motor signs or automatisms but nothing more. This is also true for the short, regionally restricted but bilateral jerks of juvenile myoclonic epilepsy (JME). Even the EEG aspect of these seizures, though bilateral, is usually not homogeneously generalized but presents typical regional accentuations, most commonly in the frontal regions. There are, however, important

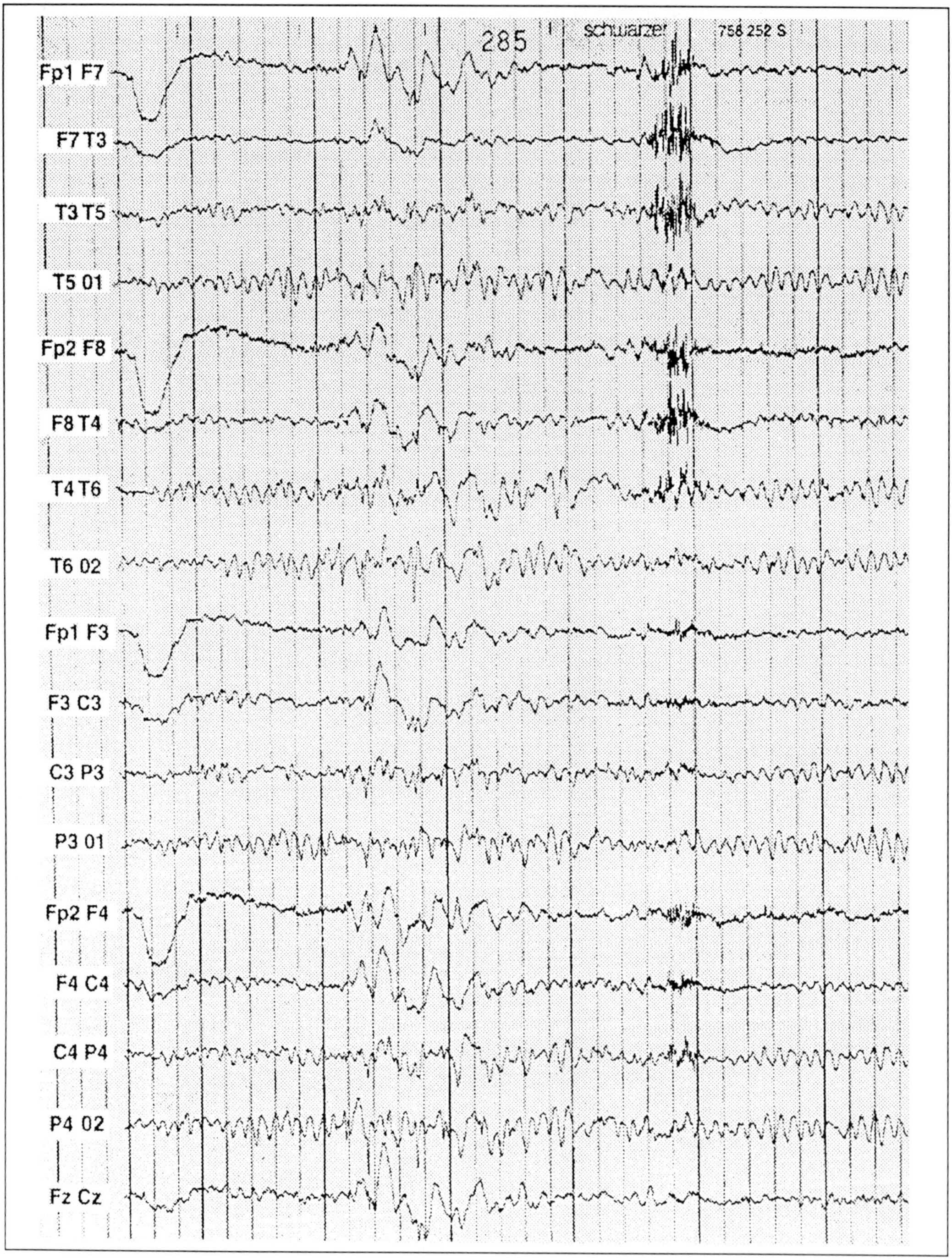

Fig. 1. Spike-wave precipitation within 2 s following eye closure in a 22-year-old female patient with a total of five generalized tonic–clonic seizures since age 14, all precipitated by card and board games or lack of sleep. Unsuccessful treatment with carbamazepine slow-release 600 mg, serum levels 5–6 μg/ml. The occipital accentuation of SW (here asymmetric) is frequently seen with this sensitivity (Fischer, 1989).

subgroups with occipital accentuation, such as in photosensitivity and in eye closure sensitivity (Fig. 1). These sensitivities are again correlated with clinical seizure types. Concerning these, the anatomical connection between eyelid closure (with interruption of vision), occipital discharge and eyelid myoclonus, in eye-closure sensitivity (Guirao Bringas *et al.*, 1987), is more easy to understand than the relation between intermittent light stimuli with occipital discharge and jerks, mostly of the arms but sometimes more expanded. Table 1 summarizes these regional aspects.

Table 1. Regional aspects and modes of precipitation in idiopathic epilepsy

Clinical	Typical EEG pattern	Predominant accentuation	Precipitation
Juvenile myoclonic epilepsy	Bilateral (poly) SW groups	F, C	Sleep deprivation
Photosensitivity	Bilateral (poly) SW groups	O	ILS
Absence	Bilateral SW groups	F, C	Hyperventilation
Absence with eyelid myoclonus	Bilateral SW groups	O	Eye closure, after < 3 s
Childhood epilepsy with occipital paroxysms	Bilateral/unilateral SW runs	O, Tp	Eye closure, after 1–20 s
Benign epilepsy with centro-temporal spikes	Spikes of shifting laterality	C, T	Sleep
Reading epilepsy	Regional sharp waves or single SW L > R	PT or FT	Reading

C = central; F = frontal; ILS = intermittent light stimulation; O = occipital; P = parietal; L = left; R = right; T = temporal; Tp = posterior temporal.

A common feature of all these syndromes and subsyndromes is a strong genetic component which is often syndrome-specific (Berkovic *et al.*, Epilepsy in twins, Chapter 20). Prima facie, the genetic influence would be expected to be 'generalized' in a more proper sense of the word, because the relevant genetic information is present in all nerve cells. Why then is the manifestation regionalized? A chance interaction of exogenous and genetic factors is one possibility but would most probably not result in a small number of well-delimited syndromes. A pathogenetic interplay with increased regional vulnerability as a function of brain maturation is a better possibility but leaves the vulnerability to be defined. In this chapter, yet other possibilities for the regionalization of idiopathic susceptibility will be discussed.

One aspect which appears to be common to most or all of the syndromes to be discussed here deserves to be pointed out in a volume where secondary epileptogenesis is one of the prominent subjects: in these epilepsies, there is no tendency to secondary epileptogenesis.

Regional manifestations of idiopathic epilepsies: an antithesis

Samuel Berkovic

Department of Neurology, Austin Hospital, Heidelberg, Melbourne, Victoria 3084, Australia, and Department of Medicine (Neurology), The University of Melbourne

To present an antithetical view, the following propositions can be made:

– The idiopathic generalized epilepsies (IGEs) and the ILREs are *not* part of a continuum.

– Both groups are polygenic (or multifactorial) disorders, with individual phenotypes being due to a particular grouping of genes.

– Some of these genes are likely to be very common. Such common genes may not necessarily be deleterious mutants but contribute to the expression of the particular phenotype in the presence of abnormal 'epilepsy' genes.

– It is likely that some of these genes can be shared by families with IGE and with ILRE.

The following evidence supports these propositions.

Clinical and family studies

1. The ILREs (centrotemporal and occipital) are clinically distinct from the IGEs, even though generalized SW discharges are seen in many cases of ILRE. The occurrence of absences or myoclonus in these epilepsies is extraordinary, and follow-up studies show that patients with ILREs do not evolve into IGEs.

2. Family studies of ILREs tend to show similar phenotypes although such studies have not been as rigorously done as recent family studies in IGEs.

3. Similarly, patients with regional triggers for IGE (eye closure, photosensitivity, calculation and reading) usually have generalized seizures and not focal attacks. Family studies show other forms of IGEs and not ILREs.

EEG studies

1. Generalized SW discharges are a sensitive but not specific marker for IGEs. They are also seen in cases with neuronal storage, hypothalamic hamartoma (Berkovic *et al.*, 1988), metabolic disorders, secondary bilateral synchrony, etc. (Andermann, 1967; Niedermeyer, 1972). The occurrence of SW discharges in some patients with ILREs is therefore *not* strong evidence of a common link with the IGEs.

2. The fact that generalized SW discharges do not occupy all the cerebrum implies involvement of specific corticothalamic loops. Regional triggers may represent specific local mechanisms (e.g. dopamine for photosensitivity) that entrain those loops. The characteristic single high-voltage discharges in ILREs do not resemble regional fragments of generalized SW discharges.

3. Photosensitivity may be inherited separately (Doose & Baier, 1989).

The conclusion of these propositions is that IGEs are polygenic disorders with phenotypes probably being expressed by a specific combination of genes. Some of these genes must be very common, and might be shared with ILREs.

Discussion 1

During the discussion, Wolf explained that he had no *genetic* continuum in mind between generalized and localization-related epilepsies. Such a continuum would even be difficult to conceptualize. He could perfectly agree with the idea that both groups were polygenic and might share some genes and not share others. His main concern was about a different point. The term generalized was, today, taken too much at its face value, and he suggested going beyond that. Why, for instance, was the typical short volley of jerks in both arms, in JME, called generalized? The jerks not being generalized, there was no reason for that. If the accompanying EEG patterns were not known, nobody would dream of calling these seizures generalized. They were regional in a bilateral synchronous way, and the cerebral region involved remained to be defined. When the ILREs such as benign epilepsy with centrotemporal spikes (BECTS) were considered, there was, again, a bilateral expression of motor seizures, only they manifested not in a synchronous but in a diachronous fashion. This was, perhaps, their only fundamental difference.

Loiseau suggested that this was to some extent a question of semantics. One of the difficulties with the International Classification of Epilepsies was at a semantic level. We too closely stuck to the words. We were unhappy with the term generalized applied to a mild seizure type such as absence seizures. We were unhappy too with the term bilateral because an IGE might be asymmetrical or even present with unilateral signs, for instance, unilateral jerks in JME, or asymmetry in idiopathic grand mal. One must not become confused by such observations. When we are walking by night in shallow waters, we can see around our feet many sparkles due to tiny animals we disturb. When we stop we do not see them any more. They need an external cause to become visible, but they are still present in the water. He figured something similar in idiopathic epilepsies. Most of the cortical sites are prone to discharge, but they spike only when reached by some triggering factor. Such factors might be related with cerebral maturation or whatever other reason, and they might explain some of the phenotypes of idiopathic epilepsies, including the possibility for lateralized manifestations which was being discussed.

Genton went on to review the clinical aspects which the ILREs might contribute to this discussion. He summarized his chapter on the subject (Genton & Guerrini, Chapter 30)

Wolf asked him what he believed made these epilepsies regional.

Genton answered that he was not convinced that they could be called regional. Especially when sleep studies were done, they were, rather, multifocal. The underlying problem was diffused, perhaps a generalized biochemical disorder, but the major presentation was focal, and could change with time.

This question came up again when Loiseau asked Genton whether he agreed that electrographic status epilepticus of sleep (ESES) should be considered as a focal epilepsy because, when seizures were recorded, they were focal.

Genton did agree with this but Wolf objected that, even when the seizures were focal, the term focal epilepsy should remain restricted to conditions where there was one constant focus, without, however, going as far as requiring a focal lesion.

For Loiseau, this concept was too narrow, and he would admit that, in focal epilepsies, focal seizures could originate at various sites. As an example he gave the variability of foci in BECTS.

Wolf replied that this was the very reason why the Commission on Classification and Terminology in his time had suggested the term localization-related, because they wanted to make a terminological difference between conditions with a constant focus and others where focal activity flared up here and there.

Loiseau and Genton then discussed the possible coincidence of an idiopathic syndrome (on a genetic basis) with an epileptogenic lesion. Genton mentioned instances which had begun as symptomatic focal epilepsy in early childhood but later would develop into one of the age-related idiopathic syndromes. There seemed to be, at least intermediately, a phase of overlap of the two conditions but Loiseau would prefer to consider such cases as a succession of independent conditions. In other instances, there could be an association, e.g. when somebody had symptomatic epilepsy together with a genetic marker for benign Rolandic epilepsy, which could then produce Rolandic spikes typical for the latter syndrome. Had this still to be considered as a case of symptomatic epilepsy? Could somebody have two different types of epilepsy? It seemed impossible to establish a general rule for this.

They went on to discuss the possibility that a sibling of a patient with a genetically determined epilepsy had no seizures but the typical EEG pattern for this type of epilepsy, and that there were neuropsychological or behavioural problems which could be aetiologically related to the spike discharge. Should the condition of such a sibling be considered as epileptic? Neither discussant was in favour, and Reynolds warned against the idea that SW activity always implies epilepsy.

An electrophysiological view

Colin D. Binnie

Maudsley Hospital, Denmark Hill, London SE5 8AZ, UK

The distinction between generalized and partial phenomenology is fundamental to concepts of both epileptic seizures and epilepsy syndromes, and is to a considerable degree based on electroencephalographic (EEG) evidence.

When Jasper and Penfield introduced their 'centrencephalic hypothesis' it appeared to provide a unitary physiological basis for generalized epilepsies and for bilaterally synchronous epileptic activity which was thought to arise from a single, deep midline pacemaker. At that time all recognized idiopathic epilepsies were generalized, and all partial epilepsies thought to be lesional.

Several developments over the past quarter-century have called for a total conceptual restructuring, but we create unnecessary problems by clinging to old ideas. We seek to maintain the traditional dichotomies between generalized and partial and between idiopathic and symptomatic, and then have difficulty with the notion of focal abnormalities in epilepsies which are classified as generalized or idiopathic or even both.

The centrencephalic model has now been replaced by Gloor's concept (1968) of the generalized corticoreticular epilepsies. One should perhaps note that reports of its death may be exaggerated, as there remains a body of evidence implicating subcortical epileptogenesis in some experimental models (for instance, the work of Rodin *et al.* (1975) on subcortical effects of bicuculline and pentylene tetrazole in the cat, Gale's work (1985) on the effects of pro- and anticonvulsants in the substantia nigra, and that on lateral geniculate kindling by Shouse and Ryan (1984)).

The corticoreticular model postulates an abnormal, paroxysmal response of hyperexcitable cortex to normal reticular afferents which would ordinarily give rise to spindles. However, this revised model immediately raises the question of whether epileptogenesis is always (or indeed ever) initiated simultaneously throughout the cortex. Generalized discharges can be elicited by unilateral injections of convulsants, and by unilateral lesions or electrical stimulation, particularly in the mesial frontal region. If so-called generalized ictal activity can arise by rapid propagation from a local source, then the distinction between generalized and partial seizures with secondary generalization is reduced to a somewhat arbitrary question of the rate of propagation.

The only direct evidence of localized cortical hyperexcitability in idiopathic generalized epilepsy is provided by the photosensitive baboon (see Binnie, Chapter 7). Here a syndrome, which by any standard is idiopathic, is characterized by epileptogenesis in circumscribed but bilateral areas of the frontorolandic cortex. Above, I suggested that, although human photosensitivity is most often found in idiopathic generalized epilepsy, and although cortical hyperexcitability is not confined to the visual areas – as evidenced by abnormal somatosensory evoked potentials, in this model stimulation of a specific system can elicit partial seizures with rapid generalization. Pattern sensitivity also provides a tool for studying cortical hyperexcitability. Hemifield pattern stimulation demonstrates a markedly asymmetrical threshold for initiating discharges and, by implication, an asymmetry of cortical hyperexcitability, in some 50 per cent of susceptible subjects with idiopathic generalized epilepsy. There is some clinical evidence to be adduced from the ictal phenomenology of that archetypical seizure of idiopathic generalized epilepsy, the absence. Close inspection may reveal features which can be explained only by cerebral dysfunction which is asymmetrical or, indeed, focal. Versive movements have been reported in otherwise clinically and electrographically typical absences which responded selectively to valproate therapy. Stefan (1981), from careful scrutiny of video recordings, describes an asymmetric craniocaudal march of motor activity in some absences.

The neurobiological approach to description of epilepsy proposed by Berkovic and colleagues (Chapter 5) may overcome many difficulties arising from an over-rigorous application of the International League Against Epilepsy (ILAE) classification. However, if we accept, if only as a communication aid, the concept of idiopathic epilepsy as a discrete entity there is no difficulty from the electrophysiological standpoint in accepting that epileptogenesis in idiopathic epilepsies and its EEG manifestations may be localized.

To conclude my discussion of regional manifestations of idiopathic epilepsies, I wish to draw your attention to a fact which has been evident since the studies of Lennox and the Gibbses nearly 60 years ago, and which is so obvious as to be generally ignored. If all cortical regions were equally and synchronously engaged in epileptic discharge, the resulting electrical field would be closed and unrecordable in the EEG, as all areas of the scalp would be equipotential. Bilateral epileptogenesis is, so far as we know, never generalized – and all idiopathic epilepsy is regional.

Regional expression of genes in the brain

Victor Elving Anderson

Epilepsy Clinical Research Program, Genetics and Epidemiology, 400 Church Street S.E., Minneapolis, Minnesota 55455–0341, USA

Since all cells in the brain carry a full complement of genes, it might appear at first glance that a gene mutation would affect all brain cells equally. Yet it is clear that mutations can be quite selective in their action, affecting primarily the liver, bones, connective tissue or other organ systems. The major issue is the regional *expression* of genes.

The human genome contains at least 50,000 genes, and about half of these (some 25,000) are expressed primarily in the brain (Bloom, 1989). This fact alone suggests that genes must play a considerable role in the development and functioning of the brain. A given cell, however, will express only a small fraction of its repertoire at a given time. It is possible (indeed, probable) that most genes are expressed selectively in specific areas of the brain, in specific cell types or even in specific parts of neurones (Struhl, 1991). Furthermore, genes may be expressed at specific points in development or in response to experience (Smeyne *et al.*, 1992).

It would be difficult to detect this regional and temporal variation in gene action by measuring the gene products, since they may be present in only small amounts or may be modified by post-translational events. Therefore attention is often directed toward study of the messenger ribonucleic acid (mRNA). For example, the expression of K^+ channel mRNAs in the rat hippocampus was evaluated in two ways: by *in situ* hybridization to visualize the brain areas and cells involved, and by a quantitative assay of the amount of mRNA produced in the several areas (Tsaur *et al.*, 1992).

The range of possible diversity among individual cells is extended by several additional features of mRNA processing. Sections of the RNA code can be modified by *alternative splicing*, with the result that different mRNAs can be produced from a single gene sequence (Sommer *et al.*, 1990; Luneau *et al.*, 1991). Some receptors, such as the γ-aminobutyric acid (GABA) receptors, are produced by *combinations of subunits*, so that a number of functionally different receptors can result from varying combinations of subunits from a relatively small number of genes (Killisch *et al.*, 1991). Finally, *controlling elements* (promoters, enhancers and silencers) in regions flanking a given gene can regulate the rate at which the mRNA is produced in various areas of the brain (Mori *et al.*, 1992).

Sodium channel genes

Sodium channel genes were first identified in those strains of the fruit fly *Drosophila* that were known to be temperature-sensitive (Ganetzky, 1991). The gene product is inserted in the cell membrane with 24 segments spanning the membrane surrounding a central pore, and including a voltage-sensor mechanism. Five human sodium channel genes have been identified (McKusick, 1992). Mutations in one of these can lead to two different neuromuscular disorders, hyperkalaemic periodic paralysis and paramyotonia congenita (McClatchey *et al.*, 1992), and the other genes appear to function in the brain.

In the rat brain three types of sodium channels have been identified. The mRNA for the type I sodium channel gene is most abundant in the medulla and spinal cord, while type II mRNA is more abundant in the hippocampus, cerebellum, and cerebral cortex. Within neurons, type I is found mainly in neuronal cell bodies and type II in the axons (Mandel, 1992). One mechanism for regional restriction of type II to the brain appears to be a 'silencer', a short DNA sequence that binds to and represses the promoter in other parts of the body (Kraner *et al.*, 1992).

Developmental changes in rat brain sodium channel genes have been demonstrated by Beckh and Pongs (1989). Type I mRNA starts with a low level at birth, increases slowly to 30 days of age and remains at that level thereafter. The level of type II mRNA rises sharply from embryonic day 10 to birth and remains high. In contrast, type III mRNA increases to birth and then falls to a low level by postnatal day 20. The authors postulate that 'the switching of different sodium channel mRNAs could be related with the change from somatic to axonal and dendritic excitability, with the acquisition of complex firing patterns and/or with the progression of myelination'.

Potassium channel genes

The genetic control of potassium channels was also worked out first in *Drosophila* (Adams *et al.*, 1992). By now some 11 genes have been mapped in the human (McKusick, 1992), but as many as 50 different types may actually exist. Beckh & Pongs (1990) studied four members of a potassium channel family and found that both the regional and temporal patterns of mRNA expression are specific for each of the four types studied.

Studies of three potassium channel genes in the adult rat brain showed that mRNA levels for two of them (Kv1.1 and Kv1.2) were relatively high in the hippocampus, thalamus, cerebral cortex and cerebellum (Tsaur *et al.*, 1992). In contrast, a third type (Kv4.2) showed the highest mRNA levels in the cerebellum, intermediate levels in the hippocampus and low levels in the cerebral cortex and thalamus. Within the hippocampus different distributions of these three types were found both in the dentate granule cells and in the hilar cells (interneurones). In a parallel study of subcellular distribution (Sheng *et al.*, 1992) the Kv1.4 protein was found mainly in axons and possibly terminals, while Kv4.2 was concentrated in dendrites and somata. Thus, the expression of potassium channel genes, like the genes for sodium channels, shows complex regional differences.

Regional variation was also seen in rat brains following seizures induced by pentylenetetrazole (Tsaur *et al.*, 1992). The Kv1.2 and Kv4.2 mRNAs were repressed in dentate granule cells, with a maximum effect at 3–6 h after seizures and return to normal by 12 h. This effect was found in dentate granule but not hilar cells. The expression of Kv1.1, on the other hand, showed no changes in mRNA levels in the hippocampus or elsewhere. It may be noted that this *reduction* contrasts with the *increase* seen in c-*fos* and other systems following seizures.

GABA receptor genes

$GABA_A$ receptors with different functional properties are produced by different combinations of subunits, with each subunit being produced by a different gene. Laurie *et al.* (1992) studied the expression of 13 of these subunit genes in the rat brain at seven time points in embryonic and postnatal development. Each transcript exhibited a unique regional and developmental profile of expression. For example, the α_5 gene expression showed a prominent peak in early brain, while γ_2 gene expression mostly remained constant with increasing age.

The observed pattern of change reinforces the view that the role of the perinatal $GABA_A$ system differs substantially from that in the adult brain. The authors conclude that the 'changes appear to coincide with the alteration of GABA's role from putatively excitatory, neurotrophic factor to inhibitory neurotransmitter'.

Conclusion

There is growing evidence for selective regional and temporal expression of genes in the brain that are of interest for epilepsy. If gene mutations are involved in the aetiology of epilepsy, the primary effects most probably will be found in limited brain areas within a limited time frame. Finally, the action of antiepileptic medications and the effect of the seizures themselves on gene expression may be restricted in a similar manner to specific brain areas and to specific developmental ages.

Regional expression of receptors and ion channels

Andreas Draguhn

Institut für Physiologie der Charité, Abteilung Neurophysiologie, Tucholskystr. 2, 10117 Berlin, Germany

Chronic epileptic activity can correspond to alterations on all levels of brain structure and function: development (e.g. migrational disturbances), macroanatomy (e.g. hippocampal sclerosis), microanatomy (e.g. axonal sprouting), synaptic connectivity (e.g. enhanced *N*-methyl-D-aspartate (NMDA)-ergic transmission), ionic environment, etc. Most of these changes occur in circumscribed areas like the hippocampus or frontal lobe and most of them – trivially – will be caused or accompanied by changes in the protein expression pattern of the (surviving) cells. Unfortunately, it is mostly unknown which of the changes are causal for onset or chronification of the various epileptic syndromes or for changes in responsiveness to drugs. According to the complicated and often inconclusive inheritence modi of the different forms of epileptic diseases, it is even uncertain whether genetic alterations will be identified as primary steps in the pathogenesis of many syndromes.

On a more phenomenological basis, however, we can describe epileptic syndromes by their common feature of repetitive neuronal hypersynchronization and thus pinpoint the pathophysiology to the last step in a long chain of events: synaptic transmission and transmembrane ionic currents. This point of view opens the field for an inverted genetic approach, making use of the vast amount of knowledge arising from the molecular neurobiology of transmembrane signal transduction. In this chapter I would like to outline the concept of heterogeneity of receptors and ion channels, which came up – on a genetic level – during the last 10 years, focus on a few new techniques which became or might still become useful for the molecular pathophysiology of epilepsy and finally open the discussion with a few speculative questions concerning the possible application of the receptor/ion channel heterogeneity concept to regional manifestations of epileptic syndromes. For most examples I will focus on the γ-aminobutyric acid A receptor ($GABA_AR$) as *one* representative of the molecules of interest.

Molecular diversity of ion channels and transmitter receptors

The basic elements making neuronal tissue excitable are the same structures that were proposed about 50 years ago by Hodgkin, Huxley and Katz for the neuromuscular junction and the squid giant axon: synapses, releasing highly concentrated packages of low-molecular weight neurotransmitters, postsynaptic transmitter receptors, ion channels coupled to these receptors and voltage-gated ion channels opening upon the initial postsynaptic depolarization. Starting again from pioneering work on the neuromuscular junction, the molecular cloning approach has provided us with the primary structure of most polypeptides involved in signal recognition (receptors) and transduction (mainly, ion channels). During the last 10 years, it has become clear that these key elements of neuronal function are encoded by four groups of genes, each of them building up a big, phylogenetically related *gene family* (Table 2). Three of these groups (with a possible, though not proved, common ancestor) form ion channels which are gated through a built-in sensor: a recognition site for transmitters in the ligand-gated and a intramembraneous voltage-sensor in the voltage-gated ion channels. The fourth group (called '7-TM type' due to the common feature of seven transmembrane segments in each molecule) forms transmitter receptors which are coupled to G proteins (another, huge family of evolutionarily diversified proteins) and activates the plethora of 'second-messenger'-coupled systems. Many neurotransmitters are simply structured molecules and act on receptors of both types (e.g. acetylcholine (ACh), GABA, glutamate (Glu), serotonin).

The genes encoding the subunits of these (often heteromultimeric) molecules proved to be surprisingly 'redundant': for the $GABA_AR$ (probably a pentameric heteromultimer of the AChR type) at least 14 different subunit-encoding complementary DNAs (cDNAs) have been cloned, allowing for more than 1 million (!) different stoichiometries to be constructed. Although few quaternary structures may be energetically favoured, this is a surprising heterogeneity for a molecular switch, supposed to open upon GABA binding and allow chloride anions to flow. The same genetic diversity has been found for most of the other molecules listed in Table 2.

At least five additional groups of genetic and epigenetic cellular mechanisms have to be considered to understand receptor/ion channel heterogeneity: the *expression pattern* of each subunit or receptor subtype is highly regulated by both the cell type and the environmental conditions, including developmental regulation. The archetypic neuromuscular AChR, for example, switches from the 'embryonic' to the 'adult' molecular subunit composition upon innervation of the muscle fibre. The classical concept of regulated temporospatial expression is complicated by the mechanism of *alternative splicing* (e.g. the γ2 $GABA_AR$-subunit can contain or miss a phosphorylation site) and by the newly discovered mechanism of *post-transcriptional* editing: a single exchange of a base in the RNA coding for the glutamate type B receptor (GluR-B)decides whether the resulting receptor/ion channel complex is permeable or impermeable to calcium (Burnashev *et al.*, 1992). This physiologically highly relevant decision mechanism is developmentally regulated. This recent discovery makes it necessary to update many data interpreted in the feeling that the exon parts of a gene and its gene product are equivalent.

Finally, epigenetic events may substantially alter receptor/ion channel function in normal and pathological tissue: *receptor phosphorylation* by protein kinases has been shown to potentiate responses and prevent signal run-down during repetitive receptor activation. And we must not forget that many molecules can be acutely affected by *modulatory substances*. This mechanism appears to be extremely far developed in the $GABA_AR$, which is functionally modulated by many endogenous and exogenous subtances. From a pathophysiological and pharmacological point of view, it is extremely important to notice that the sensitivity towards these modulators (especially benzodiazepines and Zn^{2+}) varies between different molecular receptor subtypes. We should also take into account that the endogenous ligand (if existent) for the benzodiazepine (and problably also for the barbiturate) site is not known.

Table 2. Mechanisms of molecular diversity of receptors and ion channels (with examples)

Multiple genes for different subunits (gene families)

nAChR	GluR	K^+	'7-TM-family'
$GABA_AR$		Na^+	
Glycine		Ca^{2+}	

Regulated expression of subunit combinations (ontogenetic and local)

nAChR: innervation induces adult subtype (γ/ε)
$GABA_AR$: developmental up-regulation of γ2 subunit
$GABA_AR$/GluR: regional expression patterns

Alternative splicing

GluR Flip/Flop
$GABA_AR$ γ2 S/L

'Editing'
GluR-B (R)/(Q)

Phosphorylation
$GABA_AR$: stability of signal (run-down)
possible functional significance of γ2 S/L

Functional regulation by modulatory substances
$GABA_AR$: Benzodiazepines
Barbiturates
Steroids
Zinc
Ca^{2+}

These selected examples should illustrate that the excitable cell membrane contains a highly regulated, dynamic, diverse and specific set of 'communication molecules'. The rapid progress in our understanding of this issue has been largely influenced by new techniques.

New molecular techniques in neurobiology

The basic technology which has opened the field of molecular electrophysiology is *molecular cloning of cDNA* species encoding protein subunits of transmitter receptors and ion channels. Most of our ideas about ion channel structure and function come from the information about primary structure of subunits and heterologous expression experiments (reconstitution of functional receptors/ion channels by RNA-injection in heterologous cells and electrophysiological analysis of the properties). The pioneering work of S. Numa, B. Sakmann and others on the nicotinic AChR should be mentioned here. The discovery of *gene families encoding for multiple subunits* of receptors and ion channels was based on homology screening of cDNA libraries, i.e. searching for additional cDNA species displaying a certain degree of similarity to the probes used. The search for related molecules has proved extremely successful, but it should always be kept in mind that additional regulatory proteins of different evolutionary origin will not easily be detected by this method.

The *polymerase chain reaction* (PCR)has catalysed the possibility to gain an exploding amount of molecular sequence information. The discovery of extremely *rare subunits* (e.g. the retinal $GABA_A$ ρ1 subunit) as well as the analysis of *RNA variants* (alternative splicing, e.g. the protein kinase C (PKC) consensus site missing or containing $GABA_AR$ γ2 short/long subunits; editing of GluR subunit RNA) have been promoted by this technique and it can be expected that the number of different known sequences will increase further within the next few years.

Heterologous expression of various combinations of subunits is providing us with a growing, but far from complete, archive of *functional 'fingerprints'* of the electrical and pharmacological properties of different receptor/ion channel subtypes, which allows the hypothetical correlation of (patho)physiological observations in brains, brain slices or cell cultures to structurally defined members of the extremely widespread family of membrane signalling molecules. This comparative interaction of molecular biology and neuro(patho)physiology will profit from the recent possibility to apply the high-resolution *patch clamp technique to identified cells* in situ *in brain slices* (Edwards *et al.*, 1989). It has even become possible to harvest the cytoplasm after electrophysiological recordings in the patch pipette and analyse the *individual cellular expression pattern* of ion channels by PCR amplification (Lambolez *et al.*, 1992). This is the most advanced method of molecular and functional analysis of nerve cells. However, most information about the highly regulated temporal and spatial expression pattern still comes from the more 'classical' *in situ* hybridization and immunocytochemistry, both with subunit-specific probes. It has become clear during the past few years that most subunits are expressed only in certain regions of the brain, and thus, vice versa, that a given cell population will be functionally defined by the individual set of subunits expressed. The analogous information about developmental regulation of the subunit pattern is less complete for most molecules and regions. However, programmed switches in expression of certain subunits during ontogenesis have already been described (e.g. Laurie *et al.*, 1992). Looking at *in situ* hybridization data we should be aware of the distinction between RNA and protein; the detection of a certain RNA species in a cell population does not exclude the possibility that the functional receptor in the synapse of interest may be assembled by other subunits or that the contribution of a highly abundant RNA to the final set of receptor molecules on protein level is small. Indeed, *subcellular sorting of subunits* has been described with subunit-specific antibodies in the $GABA_AR$.

Together, the new techniques of molecular neurophysiology provide us with tools to analyse receptor and ion channel heterogeneity on both the structural and the functional level.

Perspectives for epilepsy research

How can we apply the newly available concepts and techniques to epilepsy research? If cellular signalling molecules play an important role in the genesis and maintenance of epilepsy, we should look for *specific regional alterations in the expression pattern* of the corresponding subunits. First indications for altered expression patterns of GluR subunits in experimentally induced temporal lobe epilepsy have already been described (Kamphuis *et al.*, 1992).

This approach is especially promising in syndromes with a well-defined regional expression or origin. From *functional alterations* both in human tissue and in animal models (changes in drug susceptibility, changes in ionic conductance specificity (calcium!), changes in biophysical behaviour of excitable cells), electrophysiologists will often be able to make reasonably specific guesses as to which subunits of which receptors or ion channels might be affected. It is then easy to verify these molecular changes with subunit-specific nucleotide or antibody probes.

Given valid animal models or surgically removed epileptic human tissue, we should be able to apply the *combined molecular-electrophysiological approach* to the question, which molecular changes accompagny different epileptic syndromes and what their functional consequences are on a cellular level.

Moreover, the development of new treatment strategies might be brought forward by the increasing knowledge about *different behaviour of cloned and native receptor subtypes towards modulatory substances.* It is uncertain, but feasible, that future work will succeed in influencing experimental or human epileptic syndromes by blocking altered subunit expression with *specific antisense DNA.*

Discussion 2

Panayiotopoulos said that from a clinical point of view it was very important to separate the two conditions, generalized and focal, if not for other then for therapeutic reasons. However, this discussion had considerable theoretical interest. The question raised by Binnie in relation to photosensitivity where a stimulation was given partially, and there was a generalized convulsive response, needed an answer. On the one hand, this was perhaps the best human example of a generalized cortical sensitivity, but, on the other hand, there was an increased susceptibility in the occipital region to normal patterns of stimuli which were occipitally processed. This seemed to imply what Wolf had said about regional epilepsy. As a clinician, he could consider this as an increased cortical excitability with regionally increased sensitivity. Still, this was a subject for research whereas practically and clinically we should still keep the usual dichotomy.

Loiseau addressed Binnie and pointed to the differences in the pattern of epileptiform abnormalities in localization-related and generalized epilepsies. In the former, bland sharp waves were seen instead of real spikes.

Binnie confirmed this but did not have any explanation. On the whole, he found the difference in spike-wave (SW) morphology less important than the difference in spatial distribution and in rhythmicity, whereas Loiseau was positive that, for him, the morphology was more important than the rhythmicity.

Binnie added that he was indeed puzzled by the morphological differences and believed they had to do with the mechanisms which terminate the epileptiform discharge. These could be different in both groups of epilepsies.

Lüders later came back to this issue. He agreed that the benign focal discharges have a very typical waveform which is very constant, and suggested that this indicates that the neuronal pool generating those discharges is stable. He commented on the regional predilections. For this type of discharges, a centrotemporal distribution is extremely characteristic and is probably due to a generator inside the Sylvian fissure. It is also common to find an occipital distribution as well as one around the vertex if the frontal region is involved. In other places such as the mesiotemporal region this type of discharges do not occur. He believed that this had to do with a genetically determined increased epileptogenicity that has its main expression regionally and pointed out that the distribution of the area of increased epileptogenicity may change with maturation, starting occipitally and then migrating anteriorly.

Binnie shared the opinion that the morphology of the rolandic spike had to do with its rather curiously orientated generators. According to him, the view is prevailing that the other variants of idiopathic childhood epilepsy with regional spikes are essentially the same thing. He asked Anderson whether it was likely that a gene is usually expressed at a very specific cerebral site but sometimes, with the same effect, at a different location or whether we had to look for different genetic variants of benign epilepsy in childhood.

Anderson said that there was no answer at the moment but that this was the type of question we had to approach. He hoped that in a year we would know if, in benign epilepsy with centrotemporal spikes (BECTS), it would be easy to find a specific gene or not. If we are lucky, and a gene is mapped, we would have a clue and could move on. His job was to try and find families and encourage the mapping. Although, in this field, many syndromes seem to be multigenic, he hoped that it would be possible to work with syndromes with a single locus. Then one could begin to ask how this gene was expressed in the rat brain, how that information could be translated back to the human, etc. He wasn't sure that this story was now completely in the hands of the geneticists even if this was an exciting thought.

Every time that something had been mapped in the human, such as cystic fibrosis or neurofibromatosis, it had been important to feed back to the clinicians. Finding the gene was only the beginning of the story; then came the questions of its expression, its variation and the possibility of treatment. 'We just have to have a higher order of the interaction between clinicians and geneticists. We have to learn from each other so we can communicate, but none of us will be out of work.'

Draguhn pointed out that most of the genetic facts that had been reported during the meeting were on a phenomenological or a functional basis but, obviously, some molecules were involved in synaptic transmission, excitability and so on. He asked Anderson if he implied that the obviously functionally active genes might not be the best candidates although it might be difficult or a very crude approach to define candidate genes from that phenomenological basis considering the huge multitude of genes which are regulatory and spatially expressed.

Anderson thought it would be possible to find simplifying strategies and get a better feeling as to what kind of gene might be involved.

Draguhn thought that the idiopathic approach would probably be successful if it came from family studies but not if one looked for alterations in proteins which are known to be functionally involved in ion channels. He asked Anderson if he expected that the solution would come from the family studies and genomic mapping.

Anderson confirmed that this would be his approach. Nobody at present has been able to successfully propose a candidate gene for any of the conditions; also one has to be prepared to find that candidate genes have different expressions depending on where in the neuronal network the affected cells are located. At present it is simplest to (1) use phenomenological (or phenotypic) information in families to map a gene for a type of epilepsy to a specific chromosome segment, and then (2) find out what genes identified through molecular studies are linked to the same area.

Berkovic commented briefly that the animal model that came closest to genetic human focal epilepsies was probably a genetic temporal lobe epilepsy in the E1 mouse (Rise *et al.*, 1991).

Janz suggested asking the conventional clinical questions before asking the last questions about genes. He knew of no family studies of idiopathic localization-related epilepsies and, thus, missed the basic information about the type of epilepsy in the families of these patients. He quoted Genton, who had reported an incidence of 30 per cent of such patients having siblings with epilepsy. The types of their epilepsies, however, were not known. He mentioned, from his own study in progress on more than 100 probands with idiopathic generalized epilepsies, having more than 250 family members with some kind of epilepsy, that there were only two cases with some kind of idiopathic 'regional' epilepsy. These were cases of 'rolandic' epilepsy in the second generation of two probands with juvenile myoclonic epilepsy. He therefore agreed with Berkovic that a genetic relation between the two groups of epilepsy was unlikely. He then raised the question of transmission type, suggesting that the absence epilepsies and juvenile myoclonic epilepsy were dominantly inherited, whereas the idiopathic 'regional' epilepsies could have another type of transmission.

In reply to the latter, Anderson said that he saw no way out of this other than careful studies of families. He pointed out that, often, a single family or a few unique families had given a clue as to the mechanisms of gene action so we need not necessarily look for representative or large samples. A breakthrough in the more rare diseases, however, required a clinician who 'is thinking genetically at the family and molecular levels simultaneously to have the hunch that this particular family may be the one that gives us some answer'. He thought that one result from this discussion would be an agreement as to which of the clinical conditions might be strategic in such a way that it related to what we know about the seizures in the mouse, about molecular mechanisms and about patterns of gene expression. One should watch out for places where these overlap. He had the impression that the generalized syndromes appear more promising, but it could very well be that one of the localization-related conditions eventually would give us a strategic insight.

Anderson then asked Draguhn whether he knew of any indication of genes the expression of which changed from one area of brain to another over development.

Draguhn in his answer pointed to the necessity of carefully comparing the time basis and time-scales when talking about this. He agreed that it caused some problems that, in most models, the cortex was handled more or less as an entity. The necessary experiments to elucidate the role of subtle and specific genes which are expressed differentially did not yet seem to have been done in the experimental animals.

In reply to this, Köhr pointed to the findings with alternatively spliced variants of GluRs which are developmentally regulated (Köhr, Chapter 23). They showed a different distribution in the hippocampus during development, and as a response to kindling experiments.

Dalby mentioned the functional differences which the hemispheres obtain during development, and asked if there was any evidence of a differential expression of gene products in the right and left hemispheres.

Anderson found this a wonderful question which confirmed his impression that at this stage we are collecting problems to which we don't yet have the answers.

Wolf added a question which was also meant as a comment on Draguhn's statement that the cortex was usually treated as if it reacted as an entity. In human epilepsies it certainly did not. In the conditionsunder discussion even the motor strip didn't react as an entity. In BECTS, only the hand and face portion of the motor strip was active. Usually, the leg just didn't become involved in this condition. What was the reason for this? One could of course speculate about the phylogenetic development of the human brain where the hand and face representations became much more developed than any other part.

Draguhn explained that he had not been specific enough before; he could add that to his knowledge *in situ* hybridization experiments looking for differential expression of various $GABA_AR$ subunits in local areas of the cortex had been carried out, and maybe there were other examples of ion channels. However, the difference between the methods of molecularity and the clinical problem raised by Wolf was exactly that the cortex behaved much more heterogeneously than the data so far available could explain although the tools were there. In response to Dalby, he wanted to comment that differences between both hemispheres in the expression of genes had been shown for the $\alpha 1$ subunit of the $GABA_AR$ following kindling. If a focus was induced on one side by hippocampal kindling, the expression of the $\alpha 1$ subunit would go down on that side. This was, of course, not a cortical focus, but it was perhaps a starting-point.

Anderson underscored the last point. One can study the detailed structure of the hippocampus, and find evidence that genes are differently expressed there. But the cortex has not been studied with the same intensity. The hippocampus has layers so close together that one could easily study a lot of variation within a relatively small space. It was necessary that someone should point out the right areas for studies of cortical differences. It was highly important to go ahead and ask about the expression of some selected genes in specific areas of the cortex.

References

Adams, L.A., Houamed, K.M. & Tempel, B.L. (1992): Potassium channel genes: genomic complexity, molecular properties and differential expression. In: *Potassium channel modulators*, eds. A.H. Weston & T.C. Hamilton, pp. 14–33. Oxford: Blackwell Scientific Publications.

Andermann, F. (1967): Absence attacks and diffuse neuronal disease. *Neurology* **17,** 205–212.

Beaumanoir, A., Ballis, T., Varfis, G. & Ansari, K. (1974): Benign epilepsy of childhood with rolandic spikes. *Epilepsia* **15,** 301–315

Beckh, S. & Pongs, O. (1990): Members of the RCK potassium channel family are differentially expressed in the rat nervous system. *EMBO J.* **9,** 777–782.

Berkovic, S.F., Andermann, F., Melanson, D., Ethier, R., Feindel, W. & Gloor, P. (1988): Hypothalamic hamartomas and associated ictal laughter: evolution of the characteristic epileptic syndrome and diagnostic value of magnetic resonance imaging. *Ann. Neurol.* **23,** 429–439.

Bloom, F.E. (1989): Strategies for understanding the role of gene defects in the pathogenesis of mental disorders. In: *Genetic approaches in the prevention of mental disorders*, eds. V. Bulyzhenkov, Y. Christen & L. Prilipko, pp. 45–56. Berlin: Springer-Verlag.

Burnashev, N., Monyer, H., Seeburg, P.H. & Sakmann, B. (1992): Divalent ion permeability of AMPA receptor channels is dominated by the edited form of a single subunit. *Neuron* **8,** 189–198.

Commission on Classification and Terminology of the ILAE (1989): Proposal for revised classification of epilepsies and epileptic syndromes. *Epilepsia* **30,** 389–399.

Doose, H. & Baier, W.K. (1989): Generalized spikes and waves. In: *Genetics of the epilepsies*, eds. G. Beck-Mannagetta, V.A. Anderson, H. Doose & D. Janz, pp. 95–103. Heidelberg, Berlin: Springer.

Edwards, F.A., Konnerth, A., Sakmann, B. & Takahashi, T. (1989): A thin slice preparation for patch clamp recordings from neurones of the mammalian central nervous system. *Pflüg. Arch.* **414,** 600–612.

Fischer, R. (1989): Lidschlußempfindlichkeit. Konstanz dieses Phänomens und seine Abhängigkeit von Reizvariationen. Eine klinische Studie. Thesis, University of Witten/Herdecke.

Gale. K. (1985): Mechanisms of seizure control mediated γ-aminobutyric acid: role of the substantia nigra. *Fed. Proc.* **44,** 2414–2424.

Ganetzky, B. (1991): Genetic analysis of ion channels in *Drosophila*. In: *Genetic strategies in epilepsy research*, eds. V.E. Anderson, W.A. Hauser, I.E. Leppik, J.L. Noebels & S.S. Rich, pp. 247–261. Amsterdam: Elsevier.

Gloor, P. (1968): Generalized corticoreticular epilepsies:some considerations on the pathophysiology of generalized bilaterally synchronous spike and wave discharge. *Epilepsia* **9,** 249–263.

Guirao Bringas, I.P., Behl, I. & Wolf, P. (1987): Epileptic discharge after eye closure: relation to epileptic syndromes. In: *Advances in epileptology XVI*, eds. P. Wolf, M. Dam, D. Janz & F.E. Dreifuss, pp. 255–258. New York: Raven Press.

Kamphuis, W., Monyer, H., De Rijk, T.C. & Lopes da Silva, F.H. (1992): Hippocampal kindling increases the expression of glutamate receptor-A Flip and -B Flip mRNA in dentate granule cells. *Neurosci. Lett.* **148,** 51–54.

Killisch, I., Dotti, C.G., Laurie, D.J., Lüddens, H. & Seeburg, P.H. (1991): Expression of $GABA_A$ receptor subtypes in developing hippocampal neurons. *Neuron* **7,** 927–936.

Kraner, S.D., Chong, J.A., Tsay, H.-J. & Mandel, G. (1992): Silencing the type II sodium channel gene: a model for neural-specific gene regulation. *Neuron* **9,** 37–44.

Lambolez, B., Audinat, E., Bochet, P., Crépel, F. & Rossier, J. (1992): AMPA receptor subunits expressed by single Purkinje cells. *Neuron* **9,** 247–258.

Laurie, D.J., Wisden, W. & Seeburg, P.H. (1992): The distribution of thirteen $GABA_A$ receptor subunit mRNAs in the rat brain. III. Embryonic and postnatal development. *J. Neurosci.* **12,** 4151–4172.

Luneau, C.J., Williams J.B., Marshall, J., Levitan, E.S., Oliva, C., Smith, J.S., Antanavage, J., Folander, K., Stein, R.B., Swanson, S., Kaczmarek, L.K. & Buhrow, S.A. (1991): Alternative splicing contributes to K^+ channel diversity in the mammalian central nervous system. *Neurobiology* **88,** 3932–3936.

McClatchey, A.I., Van den Bergh, P., Pericak-Vance, M.A., Raskind, W., Verellen, C., McKenna-Yasek, D., Rao, K., Haines, J.L., Bird, T., Brown, R.H., Jr & Gusella, J.F. (1992): Temperature-sensitive mutations in the III–IV cytoplasmic loop region of the skeletal muscle sodium channel gene in paramyotonia congenita. *Cell* **66,** 769–774.

McKusick, V.A. (1992): *Mendelian inheritance in man: catalogs of autosomal dominant, autosomal recessive, and X-linked phenotypes,* 10th edn. Baltimore: Johns Hopkins University Press.

Mandel, G. (1992): Tissue-specific expression of the voltage-sensitive sodium channel. *J. Membrane Biol.* **125,** 192–205.

Mori, N., Schoenherr, C., Vandenbergh, D.J. & Anderson, D.J. (1992): A common silencer element in the SCG10 and Type II Na^+ channel genes binds a factor present in nonneuronal cells but not in neuronal cells. *Neuron* **9,** 45–54.

Niedermeyer E. (1972): *The generalized epilepsies.* Springfield, IL: Charles C. Thomas.

Rise, M.L., Frankel, W.N., Coffin, J.M. & Seyfried, T.N. (1991): Genes for epilepsy mapped in the mouse. *Science* **253,** 669–673.

Rodin, E., Kitano, H., Wasson, S. & Rodin, M. (1975): The convulsant effects of bicuculline compared with metrazol. *Electroencephalogr. Clin. Neurophysiol.* **38,** 106–107.

Sheng, M., Tsaur, M.-L., Jan, Y.N. & Jan, L.Y. (1992): Subcellular segregation of two A-type K^+ channel proteins in rat central neurons. *Neuron* **9,** 271–284.

Shouse, M.N. & Ryan, W. (1984): Thalamic kindling: electrical stimulation of the lateral geniculate nucleaus produces photosensitive grand mal seizures. *Exp. Neurol.* **86,** 18–32.

Smeyne, R.J., Schilling, K., Robertson, L., Luk, D., Oberdick, J., Curran, T. & Morgan, J.I. (1992): Fos-lacZ transgenic mice: mapping sites of gene induction in the central nervous system. *Neuron* **8,** 12–23.

Sommer, B., Keinänen, K., Verdoorn, T.A., Wisden, W., Burnashev, N., Herb, A., Köhler, M., Takagi, T., Sakmann, B. & Seburg, P.H. (1990): Flip and flop: a cell-specific functional switch in glutamate-operated channels of the CNS. *Science* **249,** 1580–1585.

Stefan H. (1981): Pseudospontanbewegungen bei Patienten mit Petit-mal-Anfällen. *Arch. Psychiatr. Nervenkrankh.* **229,** 277–290.

Struhl, K. (1991): Mechanisms for diversity in gene expression patterns. *Neuron* **7,** 177–181.

Tsaur, M.-L., Sheng, M., Lowenstein, D.H., Jan, Y.N. & Jan, L.Y. (1992): Differential expression of K^+ channel mRNAs in the rat brain and down-regulation in the hippocampus following seizures. *Neuron* **8,** 1055–1067.

Wolf, P. (1992): Reading epilepsy. In: *Epileptic syndromes in infancy, childhood and adolescence,* 2nd edn., eds. J. Roger, M. Bureau, Ch. Dravet, F.E. Dreifuss, A. Perret & P. Wolf, pp. 281–298. London: John Libbey.

Section IV
Symptomatic and cryptogenic epilepsy syndromes

The first chapter in this section highlights some of the difficulties, in symptomatic epilepsies of early childhood, to differentiate between focal and generalized pathology. An update follows of syndromes where classification according to anatomy seems sufficiently established today. At present, the main interest in these of course is related to their accessibility to a surgical approach, and discussions return throughout this section of the epileptogenic focus and the area to be removed. But then questions of high theoretical importance arise, especially concerning mesial temporal lobe epilepsy (MTLE). Even when conservative standards of definition are applied, MTLE seems more frequently to occur bilaterally than epilepsies of other localizations. The reasons for this are little understood; they are discussed in Chapter 38, and this discussion will be taken up again in Section V, especially Chapters 46 and 47.

They are surely different from the Rasmussen syndrome, another syndrome which seems to be unilaterally regional but may not always be as is pointed out in the last papers of the section.

Epileptic Seizures and Syndromes, Edited by Peter Wolf
© 1994 John Libbey & Company Ltd., pp. 285–297

Chapter 33

Lennox–Gastaut syndrome and secondary bilateral synchrony: a comparison

Warren T. Blume

Epilepsy Unit, University Hospital, The University of Western Ontario, 339 Windermere Road, London, Ontario, Canada N6A 5A5

Introduction

The several shared components of these syndromes may impede their distinction and indicate that gradations between them exist. This chapter outlines such components, presents distinguishing features and illustrates the gradations.

Syndrome definitions

Lennox–Gastaut syndrome (LGS)

Lack of a consistent pathological correlate, shared characteristics with several other entities (Fig. 1) and variable associated features among several studies have hampered agreement on the definition of this syndrome. See Aicardi (1986) for review and discussion of several definitions. Without adequate data about its pathogenesis, an encompassing yet descriptive definition is most appropriate at this time, adopting the approach of Aicardi (1986). Thus, LGS consists of: (1) a moderate to severe generalized seizure disorder; and (2) slow spike waves (SSW) on the electroencephalogram (EEG).

Seizures begin in early childhood for most patients with LGS most of whom are or become mentally subnormal. However, neither of these features is requisite as exceptions exist (Bauer *et al.*, 1983).

Secondary bilateral synchrony (SBS)

This electrographic entity has also been subject to several definitions since Penfield & Jasper (1946) first recognized that a focal epileptogenic lesion could produce bilaterally synchronous epileptiform discharges. In 1952, Tukel and Jasper defined SBS as 'bilaterally synchronous discharges which can be shown to arise from a unilateral cortical focus'.

Blume and Pillay (1985) adopted this approach in developing the following definition: sequential focal spikes or sharp waves leading directly to bilaterally synchronous epileptiform paroxysms. Establishment of this association required: (1) the phenomenon to occur at least twice in an EEG, (2) a lead in time of ≥ 2 s, (3) the morphology of triggering spikes should resemble other focal spikes in the same region and differ from that of the bisynchronous epileptiform paroxysms. This definition was more strict than that of other studies, which required only the coexistence of focal spikes or a lesion and bilaterally synchronous discharges. This distinction is physiologically significant, as focal epileptogenic lesions may *indirectly* elicit focal (Lüders *et al.*, 1987), or generalized (Sadler & Blume, 1989), non-lesional EEG abnormalities.

Shared aspects

The bilaterally synchronous discharges of SBS usually repeat at < 3 Hz (Tukel & Jasper, 1952; Blume & Pillay, 1985) and bisynchronous discharges without apparent SBS appear on most EEGs that contain SBS (Blume & Pillay, 1985). Thus, each entity contains bisynchronous SSW. EEGs with SSW of LGS and SBS each may have some 3 Hz spike waves (SW).

The second common element is the presence of moderately severe generalized seizure disorders.

EEGs

Lennox–Gastaut syndrome

The bilaterally synchronous and diffuse SSW is the hallmark of the syndrome, although it may occur in other conditions. The spike either resembles that of 3 Hz SW or its duration extends to 100–200 ms. The 350–500 ms slow wave may partially account for the 1–2.5 Hz repetition rate, as may the occasional pause between each complex of a series. The duration of the prominent electropositive trough between the spike and the wave is also longer than that of 3 Hz spike waves. As with 3 Hz SW, SSW are usually maximally expressed frontally, but instances of parietal-occipital maxima may occur (Blume *et al.*, 1973). A sizeable unilateral lesion would impede their expression giving maximal expression contralaterally (Sorel, 1964; Ohtahara *et al.*, 1976).

These complexes occupy a greater (33–50 per cent) proportion of the awake recording than do 3 Hz SW unless absence status increases the quantity of the latter. Abundance usually decreases with increased age at recording, but SSW quantity has apparently no prognostic value for ultimate seizure control or mental development (Blume *et al.*, 1973).

The interparoxysmal awake EEG always contains excess δ and θ for age; why such components occasionally shift their field and hemisphere of maximum expression is unknown. Persistent unifocal abnormalities are not characteristic of LGS.

Drowsiness and light sleep may augment the abundance of SSW and the single spike may become multiple. Runs of generalized polyspikes or 10–20 Hz waves (epileptic recruiting rhythm (ERR)) (Gastaut & Broughton, 1972) may appear initially in sleep. These may also be seen on awake recordings. In fact, some authors (Zifkin, 1990) consider such rhythms as a criterion for the diagnosis of LGS. As they appear far less abundantly than SSW, a patient with all earmarks of LGS may lack the ERR on one or more recordings (Aicardi & Levy Gomes, 1988).

Unlike 3 Hz spike-waves, SSW may not be associated with a detectable alteration in awareness but subtle absences may pass unnoticed in such patients, most of whom are retarded. Tonic seizures, the most common LGS seizure type, are accompanied by either electrodecremental events or the epileptic recruiting rhythm. Atypical absences are difficult to discern but may occur either with SSW or ERR. High-voltage bisynchronous spikes, superimposed on SSW sequences, may occur with myoclonic seizures. Further discussions are given by Gastaut and Broughton (1972), Gastaut *et al.* (1966b) and Blume (1987).

Secondary bilateral synchrony

As stated, the bisynchronous component of this phenomenon may be 3 Hz SW but they are more likely to repeat at < 3 Hz (Tukel & Jasper, 1952; Blume & Pillay, 1985). Morphology of each SW in a series may vary. Sequential focal spikes or sharp waves immediately precede at least some

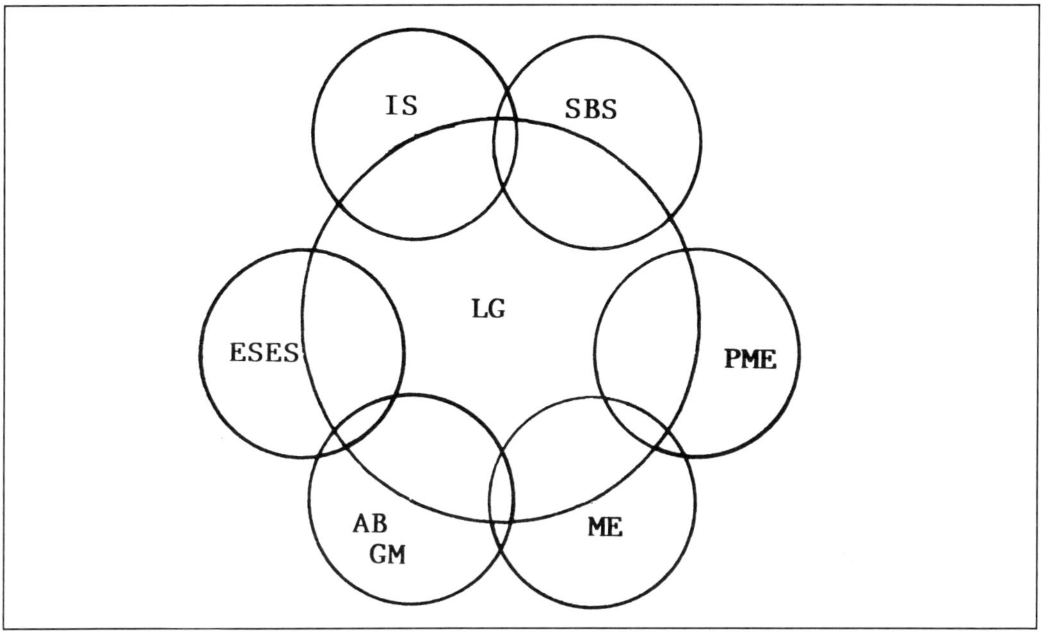

Fig. 1. Concept of syndromes sharing characteristics in varying degrees centring on the Lennox–Gastaut syndrome. LG = Lennox-Gastaut syndrome, IS = infantile spasms, SBS = secondary bilateral synchrony, PME = progressive myoclonic epilepsy, ME = myoclonic epilepsy, AB = absence, GM = grand mal, ESES = electro-

paroxysms. The lack of focal origin for other SW on the EEG does not exclude its presence (Bancaud *et al.*, 1965; Bancaud, 1969). In contrast to SSW with LGS, SBS paroxysms may terminate with a lingering focal discharge (Blume & Pillay, 1985), which is usually ipsilateral to SBS origin.

Again, unlike LGS with SSW, the EEG with SBS will contain focal spikes predominating in one area, which is almost always the SBS triggering zone. This area is usually frontal but temporal or occipital spikes may precipitate bisynchronous paroxysms. Less commonly appearing focal abnormalities include δ and θ; these two also correlate highly with SBS origin (Blume & Pillay, 1985). Finally, multiple spike foci, appearing in almost all patients with SBS, probably facilitate the occurrence of SBS (Blume & Pillay, 1985).

Seizure disorders

Lennox–Gastaut syndrome

The following aspects typify the seizure disorder of the LGS: (1) the seizures are generalized, (2) the patients may fall down during the icti, and (3) antiepileptic drugs (AEDs) do not fully control the attacks. In fact, recurrent seizures are the first sign of neurological illness in the majority of patients with LGS (Gastaut *et al.*, 1966a, b; Chevrie & Aicardi, 1972; Blume *et al.*, 1973). The predominant seizure type depends heavily on the age of seizure onset.

Tonic seizures are the most common type; they occurred in 70 of 100 patients in the Gastaut *et al.* series. For description see Gastaut *et al.* (1966a, b); Gastaut and Broughton (1972); Chatrian *et al.* (1982). Some authors (Zifkin, 1990) consider tonic seizures essential for the diagnosis, while others accept a broader spectrum for the syndrome. Tonic seizures appear among those whose LGS begins at an early age (Table 1) (Chevrie & Aicardi, 1972). It is claimed that 'atypical absence' occurs in about one-third of cases, consisting of gradual onset and offset, mild symmetrical tonic features, colour alterations and salivation. How such attacks are distinguished from mild tonic events is unclear, as the only distinct EEG alteration, the ERR, resembles that of tonic seizures. The abundance of SSW interictally diminishes their specificity as an ictal phenomenon.

Myoclonic seizures and tonic–clonic attacks occur among LGS patients with a later age of seizure onset and therefore form higher proportions of series with an older average age (Table 1) (Chevrie & Aicardi, 1972; Blume *et al.*, 1973). Bauer *et al.* (1983) studied 26 patients with SSW whose seizures began after 6 years and found the following seizure types: generalized tonic–clonic attacks – 25 patients, absence – 24, myoclonic – 16 and tonic – 10. Interestingly, nine had focal seizures, raising the possibility of secondary bisynchrony in some patients.

Table 1. Mean age at the first epileptic seizure (months) in patients with slow spike waves

Type of seizure	Observed	Not observed
Tonic	16.6	31.0
Clonic or tonic–clonic	42.6	17.7
Atypical absences	32.4	22.4
Partial or erratic myoclonias	38.9	23.0
Infantiile spasms	5.7	32.8

Adapted from: Chevrie, J.J. & Aicardie, J. (1972): Childhood epileptic encephalopathy with slow spike-wave: a statistical study of 80 cases. *Epilepsia* **13,** 259–271.

Seizures with secondary bilateral synchrony

Seizures in patients whose EEGs demonstrate SBS may relate directly to the phenomenon itself or may represent associated epileptogenic foci whose discharge may not always become bilaterally synchronous. The former category would include generalized tonic–clonic, atonic, absence, tonic and myoclonic seizures (Blume & Pillay, 1985). The latter would include seizures of the parasagittal region, whose manifestations might be tonic adversive or postural, clonic of a leg or hemiclonic (Tukel & Jasper, 1952). Although frontal foci are more often associated with bisynchronous SW than temporal foci, the latter association may occur (Gabor & Ajmone Marsan, 1969; Blume & Pillay, 1985). Therefore, complex partial seizures may occur at other times in patients with SBS.

Nosology of Lennox–Gastaut syndrome and secondary bilateral synchrony

Shared aspects

Three aspects link these syndromes. The first is a difficult-to-control generalized seizure disorder, while the second is bisynchronous SSW on EEG.

Both aspects are founded on the presence, in each condition, of either a multifocal or diffuse encephalopathy. In the Lennox–Gastaut syndrome this is manifested by mental subnormality and diffuse interparoxysmal EEG abnormalities. Among patients with SBS, evidence of a widespread cerebral disorder includes: mental subnormality in over half such patients, more than one type of seizure in over one-third and multiple spike foci in almost all SBS patients (Blume & Pillay, 1985).

These common aspects lead to gradations between the disorders (below).

Distinguishing aspects

As management of these entities may differ, awareness of dissimilar features will be useful for the clinician.

Although there are several common aetiologies, aspects of the neurological history are more likely to identify an aetiology for SBS than for LGS and that aetiology is likely to involve one part of the cortex more than any other. For SBS, these include trauma, tumour, febrile convulsions with hemiconvulsions, hemiplegia, epilepsy (HHE) syndrome, perinatal factors and regional cortical malformations. None the less, the cause of SBS remains unknown in a substantial proportion of patients.

In contrast to SBS, conditions associated with LGS are more likely to involve the cortex diffusely. Among the minority of LGS patients with associated (causal?) central nervous system conditions, the following have been noted: diffuse cortical malformations including tuberous sclerosis, encephalitis and perinatal hypoxia/ischaemia (Aicardi, 1986; Roger & Gambarelli-Dubois, 1988).

Age of seizure onset is younger and less variable among LGS patients. Studying patients with SSW, Chevrie and Aicardi (1972) found that seizure type correlated with mean age of onset, ranging from 16.6 months for tonic seizures to 42.6 months for clonic or tonic–clonic (Table 1). However, Bauer *et al.* (1983) have documented the less common onset of LGS in patients over 6 years.

Age of seizure onset among patients with SBS has ranged from 1 to 68 years, while the mean ages in these studies have been 10–19 years (Gabor & Ajmone Marsan, 1969; Blume & Pillay, 1985; Gastaut & Zifkin, 1988). Greater difficulty in identifying SBS in the EEG of early childhood may exclude some young patients from the SBS group while slow spike-waves are more likely to be the manifestation of a diffuse encephalopathy in young children than among older patients (Gastaut *et al.*, 1966a, b).

By definition, the EEG of secondary bisynchrony contains a focal onset of the bisynchronous paroxysms, but other indications of such focality will be present. These include focal seizures, or focal components of secondarily generalized seizures, lateralizing features on neurological examination and non-paroxysmal focal features on EEG such as δ or attenuation. All these aspects would be unexpected in the LGS. Gastaut *et al.* (1962) have described patients with primary generalized epilepsy whose grand mal or clonic attacks occasionally predominate unilaterally. In contrast to seizures arising from a cortical focus, proximal portions of limbs are primarily involved in these motor seizures and the laterality shifts among attacks.

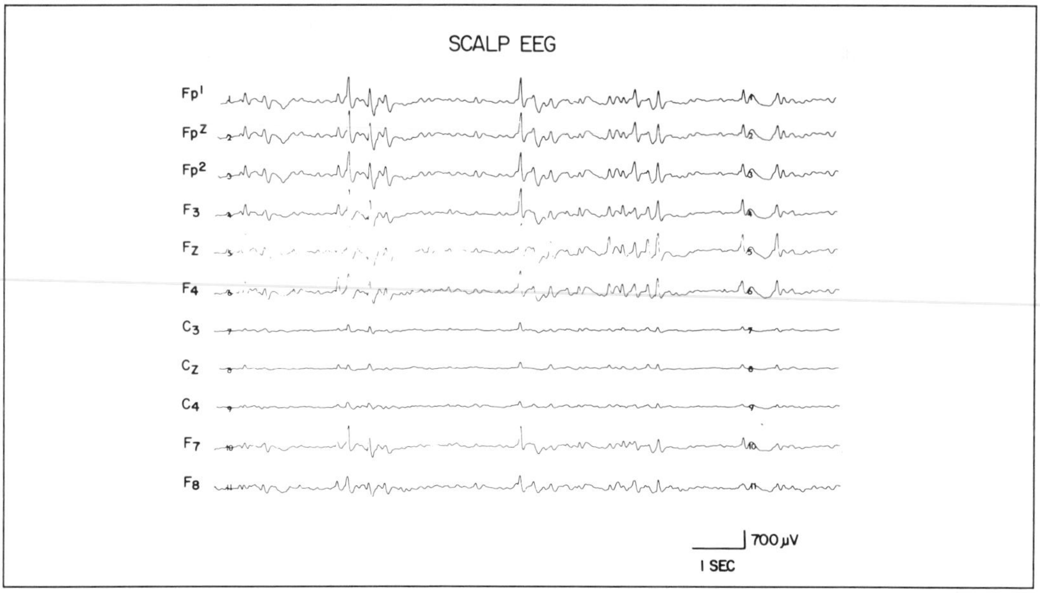

Fig. 2. Bisynchronous bifrontal spikes without visually apparent focus of origin in this recording referred to Pz.

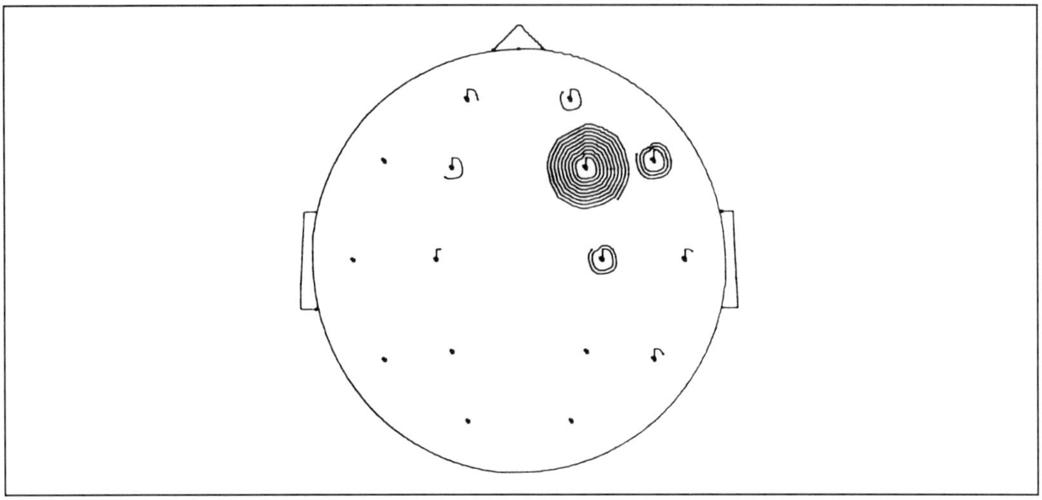

Fig. 3. Automated recognition of earliest onset of bisynchronous spikes (Fig. 2); each circle equals eight spikes originating at site; right superior frontal (F4) origin for most discharges. Same recording methods.

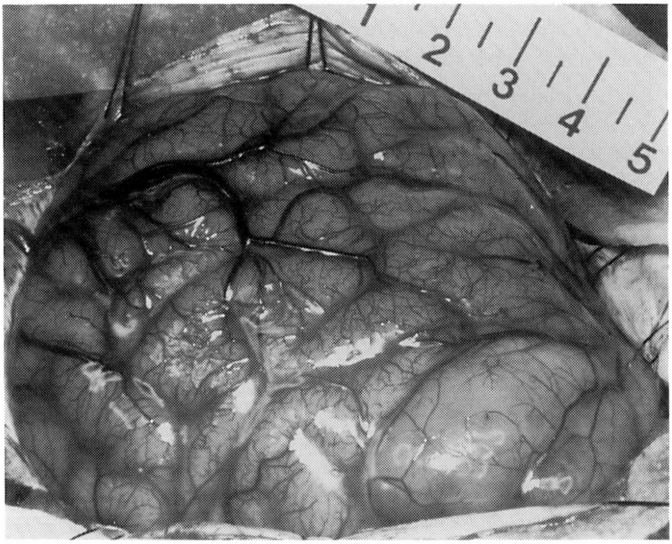

Fig. 4. Right frontal lobe with tumour occupying posterior inferior aspect – right lower portion of photograph. Spikes (Fig. 3) originated just anterior to tumour.

Intermediate conditions

As indicated above, the presence of shared and distinguishing features suggests that gradations between these entities exist. Thus, Gastaut and Gastaut (1976) found computed tomography evidence of focal lesions in 13 of 42 patients with LGS. The following two cases from our epilepsy unit and their EEGs illustrate such intermediate conditions.

Case 1. This 14-year-old boy was neurologically well except for medically refractory seizures of two types since age 3 years. In the first, tonic and then clonic contractions of all limbs would occur, immediately followed by vertigo, loss of consciousness and falls. The second type began with the

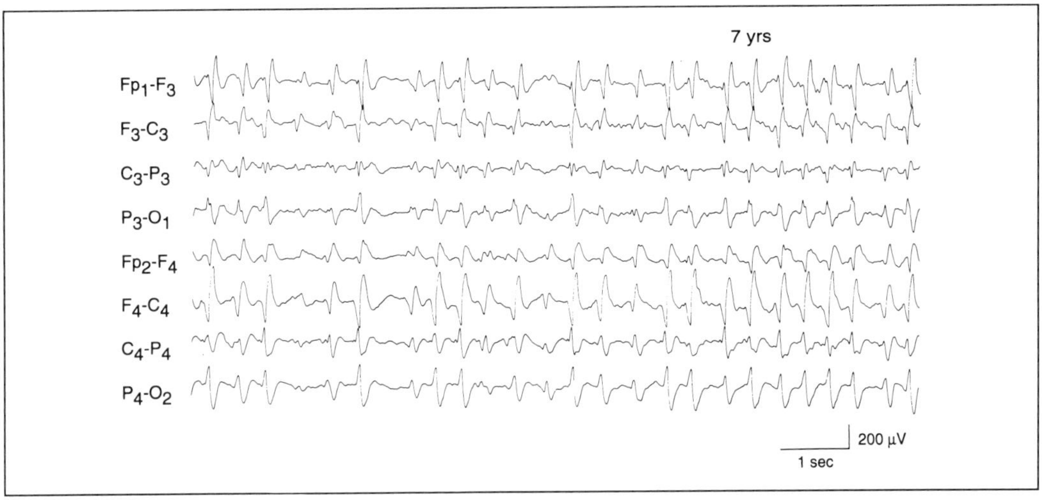

Fig. 5. Continuous bilaterally synchronous and almost symmetrical spikes in a 7-year-old patient with left hemiparesis and right hemisphere pachygyria.

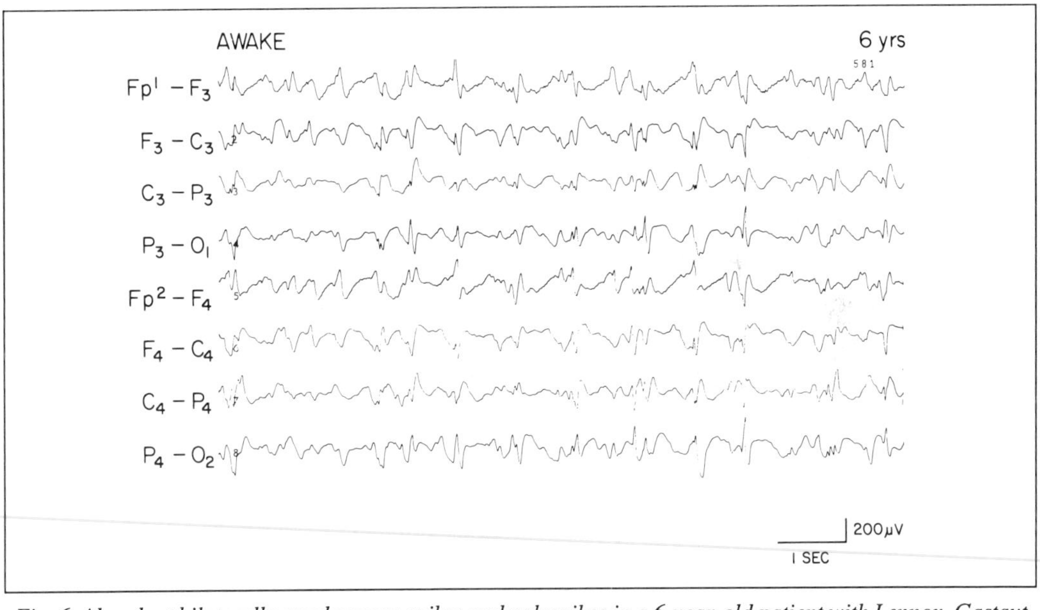

Fig. 6. Abundant bilaterally synchronous spikes and polyspikes in a 6-year-old patient with Lennox–Gastaut syndrome. Note the close resemblance to discharges of Fig. 5.

same vertigo, a sensation that sounds were muffled, staring and apparent confusion. The neurological and mental status examinations were normal. EEGs showed frequent bisynchronous diffuse spikes followed by low-amplitude slow waves (Fig. 2). The medically refractory tonic seizures from early childhood and the abundant, diffuse bisynchronous spikes are all components of LGS. However, some aspects of this clinical picture should raise suspicion that a focal origin, thus SBS, may be lurking: (1) vertigo prior to loss of consciousness in the first type, (2) the initial simple partial features of the second seizure type, and (3) normal mental examination. (This latter feature, while uncommon in LGS, has been reported (Bauer *et al.*, 1983; Aicardi & Levy Gomes, 1988)). Indeed, a spike

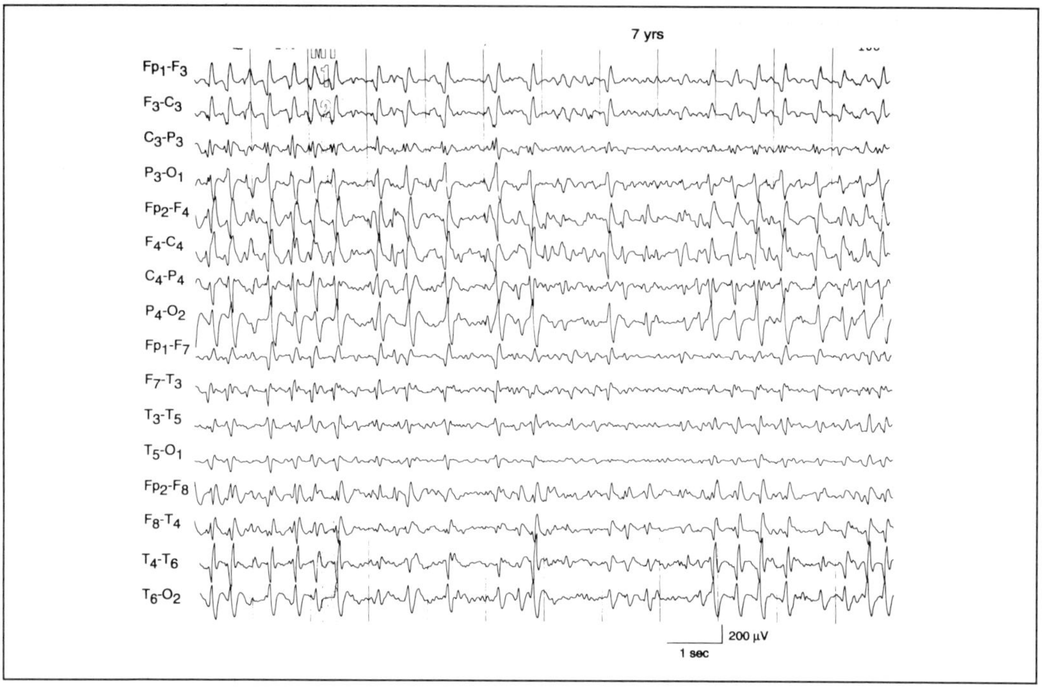

Fig. 7. Same patient as Fig. 5. Greater lateralization of spikes to right hemisphere during another epoch of the same recording.

recognition programme which counted only the earliest of widely synchronous spikes found them to originate in the right frontal region, just anterior to a tumour (Figs. 3 and 4). Resection of the tumour and the epileptogenic area anterior to it stopped the generalized tonic seizures but partial seizures from the right hemisphere began as the tumour slowly infiltrated the right Rolandic and peri-Sylvian regions.

Case 2. The milestones of this 7-year-old right-handed girl were always slightly delayed, e.g. she talked at 24 months and walked at 30 months. By 8 months, a left hemiparesis became apparent. At age 4 years, generalized tonic–clonic seizures began without warning. At age 5 years, myoclonic-atonic seizures first occurred: she would stare, exhibit myoclonus of her periocular muscles, face and arms and then suddenly fall limply. Two global tonic seizures occurred at age 6 years. Episodes of absence status followed by ataxia occurred at this time. Examination at 7 years revealed a mental age of 4 years, a left hemiparesis (with impaired but present fine finger movements) and a bilaterally spastic-ataxic gait.

EEGs showed prolonged sequences of diffuse, almost symmetrical bisynchronous spikes (Fig. 5) closely resembling SSW of a typical LGS patient (Fig. 6). However, on other occasions such discharges predominated over the right hemisphere (Fig. 7), while in still other instances focal spikes leading to bisynchronous spikes, SBS, appeared (Fig. 8). Her magnetic resonance imaging (MRI) scan disclosed diffuse right hemisphere pachygyria; the left hemisphere was structurally normal.

In this patient the early-onset, intractable generalized tonic–clonic, myoclonic, atonic and absence seizures, the abundant bisynchronous spikes and the moderate mental subnormality are all features of LGS. The clinical clue to focal origin of some seizures was the appearance of a left hemiparesis prior to seizure onset. In contrast to this patient, seizures are the initial manifestation of LGS in the majority of patients (Gastaut *et al.*, 1966a, b; Chevrie & Aicardi, 1972; Blume *et al.*, 1973). The

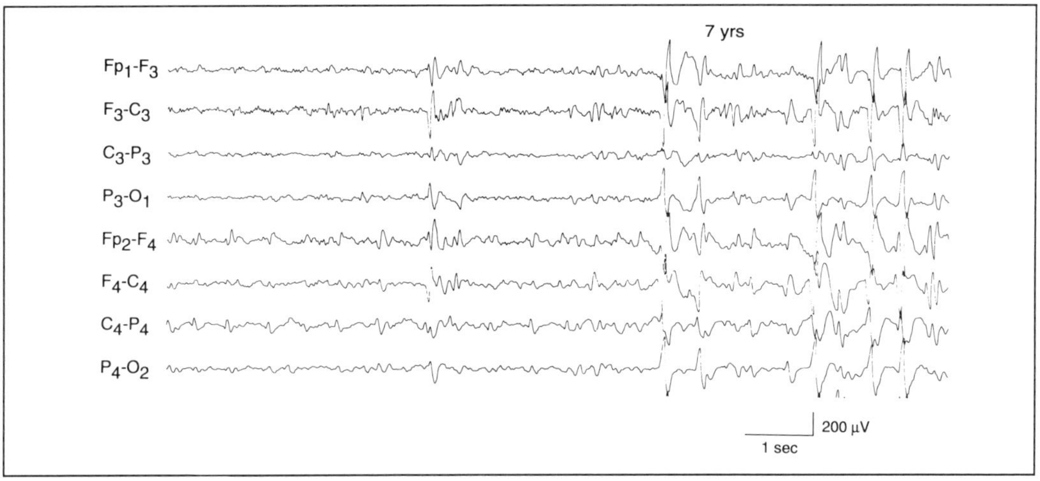

Fig. 8. Right frontal–central (F4–C4) spikes leading to bisynchronous discharges (SBS) in the same recording as Figs. 5 and 7.

diffuse, lateralized and localized EEG features reflect this patient's situation, which shares features of both LGS and SBS.

Possible pathophysiologies of Lennox–Gastaut syndrome and secondary bilateral synchrony

Lennox–Gastaut syndrome

Gastaut *et al.* (1966a, b) ascribed LGS to the reaction of the immature human central nervous system to a chronic diffuse insult. However, the precise mechanism of this reaction has received scant attention experimentally.

Gloor *et al.* (1968) correlated EEG findings in patients with diffuse encephalopathies with their histopathological abnormalities. Patients with diffuse cortical and subcortical grey matter disorders had bilaterally synchronous discharges either as SSW, sharp waves or bursts of δ. Such features rarely occurred in patients with white matter lesions or those involving only cortical grey matter.

Similarly, the feline generalized penicillin epilepsy (FGPE) model has shown that regular spike-wave discharges depend upon interaction between a functional cerebral cortex and a functional thalamus (Gloor *et al.*, 1990). SW appear simultaneously in the cortex and thalamus or slightly earlier in the cortex (Avoli & Gloor, 1982; McLachlan *et al.*, 1984). Both the cortex and thalamus fire action potentials during the spike component and are silent during the wave. This oscillation between bursts of action potentials and virtual silence also begins slightly earlier in the cortex (Gloor *et al.*, 1990). However, during a burst, some thalamocortical neurones reach peak firing slightly ahead of the associated cortical neurones, while thalamic neurones responding to cortical-thalamic input fire a burst of action potentials just after EEG spikes. This burst is followed by an inhibitory pause in the thalamus. This thalamic inhibition may be effected by local thalamic inhibitory neurones and/or the thalamic reticular nucleus. This latter receives collaterals from corticothalamic axons; its γ-aminobutyric acidergic (GABA-)ergic projections to thalamic relay nuclei, hyperpolarizing them, may contribute to the inhibitory pause represented by the wave of the SW complex. Thalamic neurones in this phase may become hyperpolarized into the voltage range in which a low-threshold (calcium) spike (LTS) can be activated. The LTS is activated either synaptically or by direct depolarization from this hyperpolarized state, leading to burst firing of thalamocortical neurones which would excite both cortical neurones and the thalamic reticular nucleus, the latter via collaterals. Thus the cycle would restart.

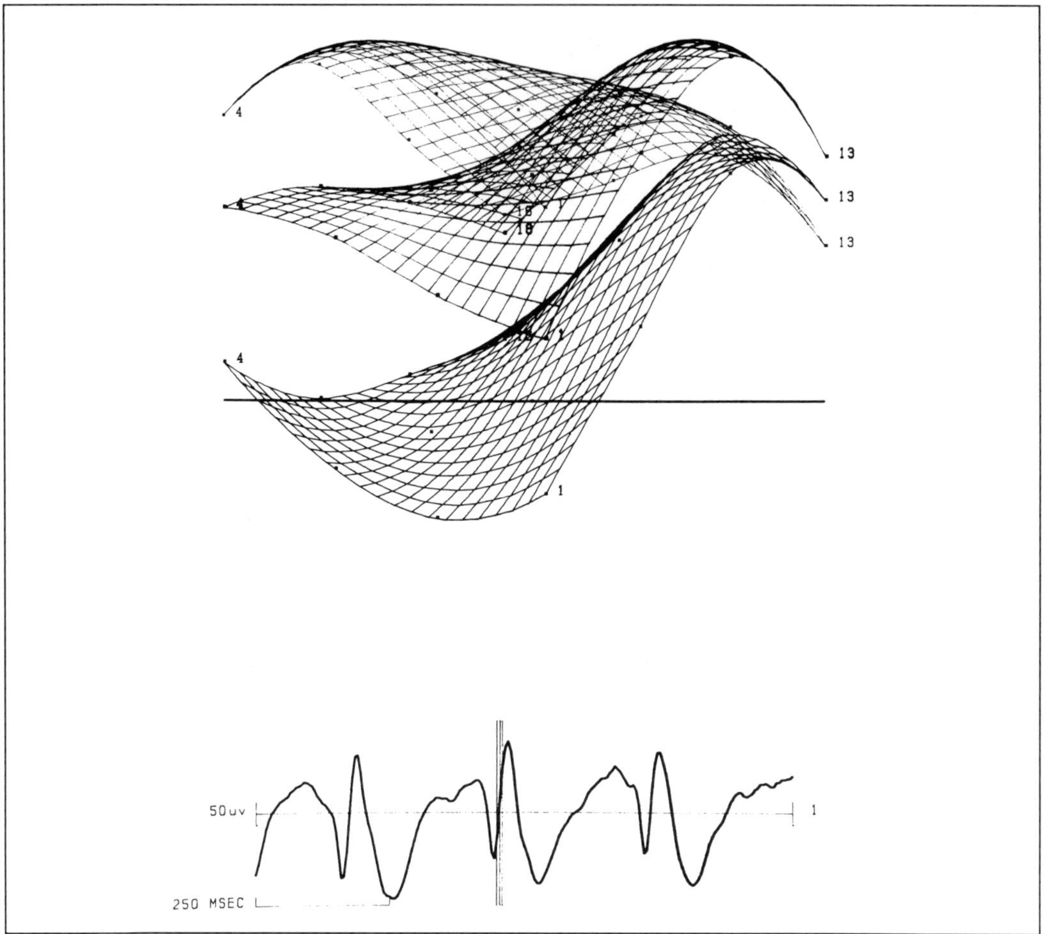

Fig. 9. Frontal view of sequential field potential plots, every 5 ms, of spike of an apparently bilaterally synchronous 3 Hz spike-wave complex. Negative up; left frontal is on right. Dark horizontal line is electrical baseline. Numbers on plots indicate recording electrode positions. Vertical lines in bottom trace depict points of spike-wave complex at which measurements were made. Potential field generally becomes more negative at each 5 ms interval, thus successive plots ascend. Thus, the spike peak is maximum in the left frontal region in the first two plots and then becomes maximum in the right frontal region during the last plot, with a left–right propagation time of about 5–10 ms.

The cellular activities during SSW have not been studied, as no reliable and clinically relevant model has been developed. Cortical SSW have occurred in the FGPE model when thalamocortical interaction has been destroyed or grossly interrupted. Pellegrini *et al.* (1979) accomplished this by severing all thalamic input to the cortex and McLachlan *et al.* (1982) produced a similar effect by systemic hypoxia. I am unaware of any studies which clarify why SW repeat at a slower rate in association with a diffuse encephalopathy – is the thalamus or the cortex primarily responsible for the slower pacing of SW? Does the lower spike synchrony, reflected in the longer-duration spike and trough, produce longer corticothalamic action potential bursts and thus activate the thalamic reticular nuclei or thalamic interneurones for a more prolonged duration leading to a more prolonged inhibition of thalamic relay nuclei?

An additional factor relates to ontogenesis of the nervous system. Among patients with SSW, the type of seizures and ultimate mental evolution correlate strongly with age of seizure onset (Aicardi, 1986). The proportion that age of onset and aetiology each contribute to this correlation is unknown, but the incidence of LGS and SSW declines with age (Blume *et al.*, 1973; Bauer *et al.*, 1983; Aicardi, 1986).

The corpus callosum mediates bisynchrony in experimental and clinical primary generalized epilepsy. Musgrave and Gloor (1980) demonstrated this in the FGPE model. Lemieux and Blume (1986) plotted the sequential potential fields of patients with primary generalized epilepsy and generalized SW. Thirty-five per cent of spikes of 'generalized' SW developed asymmetrically (Fig. 9). The interhemisphere lag times were usually within 15 ms, more consistent with corpus callosal propagation than any other mechanism. We postulated that about one-third of 'generalized' SW develop in one hemisphere and, via rapid callosal propagation, quickly become bisynchronous.

Secondary bilateral synchrony

The mechanism for SBS also remains incompletely understood, but hints arise from conditions favouring its occurrence. Widely synchronous regional spike discharges appear more likely to produce SBS than discrete foci: in a human with depth electrodes, Bickford and Klass (1969) evoked increasingly widely synchronous mesial frontal spikes by augmenting the voltage of electrical stimulation and this culminated in bisynchronous SW. The greater propensity of frontal lobe spikes to develop widely synchronous regional spikes may account for its more common association with bisynchronous SW than discharges from other areas (Gabor & Ajmone Marsan, 1969; Blume & Pillay, 1985). SBS has been reported with mesial frontal lesions or discharge (Tukel & Jasper, 1952; Bancaud *et al.*, 1974) but lesions in other frontal lobe locations may produce SBS.

The abundant callosal connections between the frontal association cortices plays a major role in SBS, probably more than with primary bisynchrony (see above). Corpus callosotomy may abolish SBS and result in either lateralization of the spike discharge or bilaterally asynchronous paroxysms (Williamson, 1992).

A third mechanism facilitating the production of SBS may be the interaction of multiple cortical epileptogenic foci. Blume and Pillay (1985) found at least two spike foci in 96 per cent of SBS patients and three or more foci in 77 per cent as compared with 40 per cent and 35 per cent in patients with spikes but without SBS. Rovit and Swiecicki (1965) found that an experimentally produced epileptic focus produces more frequent discharges when other epileptic foci are present. The presumably increased incidence of discharge in this situation might augment the propensity of bisynchrony.

Intermediate conditions

The significance of positron emission tomography (PET) in elucidating the mechanism of generalized epilepsies such as LGS remains to be established. Chugani *et al.* (1987) found evidence of focal or multifocal hypometabolism by 2-deoxy-2[^{18}F]-fluoro-D-glucose PET scanning in four of 15 LGS patients, all but one of whom were scanned once. Whether areas of hypometabolism paradoxically represent sources of electrographically occult SBS, and thus potentially hypermetabolic zones, remains unknown, but this relationship obtains for partial seizures (Engel, 1989). Do such uneven metabolic rates reflect foci of ictal origin and SBS?

The cellular phenomena of focal and generalized epilepsy differ. Several models of focal epilepsy have produced the paroxysmal depolarization shift – a large-amplitude depolarization associated with a prolonged burst of action potentials and often followed by a long-lasting hyperpolarization (Matsumoto & Ajmone Marsan, 1964; Prince & Connors, 1986). Both synaptic and non-synaptic processes contribute to the depolarization. The following hyperpolarization is mediated primarily by an increase in calcium-mediated potassium conductance. In contrast, the cellular correlate of generalized SW discharges in the FGPE model consists of an alternating sequence of depolarising and hyperpolarizing potentials which resemble normal EPSPs and IPSPs. This IPSP is mediated through $GABA_A$ and possibly $GABA_B$ receptors. While $GABA_A$ inhibition is decreased in focal epileptogenesis, it is preserved in the FGPE model (Avoli *et al.*, 1990).

The mechanism of any transition from focal to generalized epilepsy physiology during SBS has not been elucidated, but the corpus callosum may mediate this conversion. As Schwartzkroin *et al.* (1975) have shown, cellular activity in cortex homotopic to a focal epileptogenic lesion consists of EPSP–IPSP sequences, thereby resembling that of the FGPE model. Such sequences probably elicit cortico-thalamo-cortical excitatory–inhibitory sequences similar to those of SW discharges.

References

Aicardi, J. (1986): *Epilepsy in children.* New York: Raven Press.

Aicardi, J. & Levy Gomes, A. (1988): The Lennox–Gastaut syndrome: clinical and electroencephalographic features. In: The *Lennox–Gastaut syndrome (Neurology and neurobiology*, Vol. 45), eds. E. Niedermeyer & R. Degen, pp. 25–46. New York: Alan R. Liss.

Avoli, M. & Gloor, P. (1982): Interaction of cortex and thalamus in spike and wave discharges of feline generalized penicillin epilepsy. *Exp. Neurol.* **76,** 196–217.

Avoli, M., Gloor, P., & Kostopoulos, G. (1990): Focal and generalized epileptiform activity in the cortex: in search of differences in synaptic mechanisms, ionic movements, and long-lasting changes in neuronal excitability. In: *Generalized epilepsy neurobiological approaches*, eds. M. Avoli, P. Gloor, G. Kostopoulos, & R. Naquet, pp. 213–231. Boston, Massachusetts: Birkhauser Boston.

Bancaud, J. (1969): Physiopathogenesis of generalized epilepsies of organic nature. In: *The physiopathogenesis of the epilepsies*, eds. H. Gastaut, H. Jasper, J. Bancaud & A. Waltregny. Springfield, Illinois: Charles C. Thomas.

Bancaud, J., Talairach, J., Bonis, A., Schaub, C., Szikla, G., Morel, P. & Bordas-Ferer, M. (1965): *La Stéréo-électroencéphalographie dans l'épilepsie*. Paris: Masson.

Bancaud, J., Talairach, J., Morel, P., Bresson, M., Bonis, A., Geier, S., Hemon, E. & Buser, P. (1974): 'Generalized' epileptic seizures elicited by electrical stimulation of the frontal lobe in man. *Electroencephalogr. Clin. Neurophysiol.* **37,** 275–282.

Bauer, G., Aichner, F. & Saltuari, L. (1983): Epilepsies with diffuse slow spikes and waves of late onset. *Eur. Neurol.* **22,** 344–350.

Bickford, R.G. & Klass, D.W. (1969): Sensory precipitation and reflex mechanisms. In: *Basic mechanisms of the epilepsies*, eds. H.H. Jasper, A.A. Ward, Jr & A. Pope, pp. 543-564. Boston: Little, Brown.

Blume, W.T. (1987): Lennox–Gastaut syndrome. In: *Epilepsy electroclinical syndromes*, eds. H. Lüders & R.P. Lesser, pp. 73–92. Berlin: Springer-Verlag.

Blume, W.T. & Pillay, N. (1985): Electrographic and clinical correlates of secondary bilateral synchrony. *Epilepsia* **26 (6),** 636–641.

Blume, W.T., David, R.B. & Gomez, M.R. (1973): Generalized sharp and slow wave complexes: associated clinical features and longterm follow-up. *Brain* **96,** 289–306.

Chatrian, G.E., Lettich, E., Wilkus, R.J. & Vallarta, J. (1982): Polygraphic and clinical observations on tonic–autonomic seizures. *Electroencephalogr. Clin. Neurophysiol.* (Suppl. 35) 100–124.

Chevrie, J.J. & Aicardi, J. (1972): Childhood epileptic encephalopathy with slow spike-wave: a statistical study of 80 cases. *Epilepsia* **13,** 259–271.

Chugani, H.T., Mazziotta, J.C., Engel, J., Jr & Phelps, M.E. (1987): The Lennox–Gastaut syndrome: metabolic subtypes determined by 2-deoxy- 2[18F]-fluoro-D-glucose positron emission tomography. *Ann. Neurol.* **21,** 4–13.

Engel, J., Jr (1989): *Seizures and epilepsy*, p. 328. Philadelphia: F.A. Davis.

Gabor, A.J. & Ajmone Marsan, C. (1969): Co-existence of focal and bilateral diffuse paroxysmal discharges in epileptics: clinical–electrographic study. *Epilepsia* **10,** 453–472.

Gastaut, H. & Broughton, R. (1972): *Epileptic seizures: clinical and electrographic features, diagnosis and treatment,* pp. 37–47. Springfield, Illinois: Charles C. Thomas.

Gastaut, H. & Gastaut, J.L. (1976): Computerized transverse axial tomography in epilepsy. *Epilepsia* **17,** 325–336.

Gastaut, H. & Zifkin, B.G. (1988): Secondary bilateral synchrony and Lennox–Gastaut syndrome. In: *The Lennox–Gastaut syndrome (Neurology and neurobiology, Vol. 45),* eds. E. Niedermeyer & R. Degen, pp. 221–242. New York: Alan R. Liss.

Gastaut, H., Roger, J., Faidherebe, J. & Ouahchi, S. (1962): Non-jacksonian hemiconvulsive seizures: one-sided generalized epilepsy. *Epilepsia* **2,** 56–68.

Gastaut, H., Roger, J., Soulayrol, R., Tassinari, C.A. & Dravet, C. (1966a): L'encéphalopathie épileptique de l'enfant avec pointe-ondes lentes diffuses (alias 'petit mal variant') ou syndrome de Lennox. *Ann. Pediatr.* (Paris) **13,** 2093–2103.

Gastaut, H., Roger, J., Soulayrol, R., Tassinari, C.A., Regis, H., Dravet, C., Bernard, R., Pinsard, N. & Saint-Jean, M. (1966b): Childhood epileptic encephalopathy with diffuse slow spike-waves (otherwise known as 'petit mal variant') or Lennox's syndrome. *Epilepsia* **7,** 139–179.

Gloor, P., Kalabay, O. & Giard, N. (1968): The electroencephalogram in diffuse encephalopathies: electroencephalographic correlates of grey and white matter lesions. *Brain* **91,** 779–802.

Gloor, P., Avoli, M. & Kostopoulos, G. (1990): Thalamocortical relationships in generalized epilepsy with bilaterally synchronous spike-and-wave discharge. In: *Generalized epilepsy neurobiological approaches*, eds. M. Avoli, P. Gloor, G. Kostopoulos & R. Naquet, pp. 190–212. Boston. Massachusetts: Birkhauser Boston.

Lemieux, J.F. & Blume, W.T. (1986): Topographical evolution of spike-wave complexes. *Brain Res.* **373,** 275–287.

Lüders, H., Lesser, R.P., Dinner, D.S. & Morris, H.H., III (1987): Benign focal epilepsy of childood. In: *Epilepsy electroclinical syndromes*, eds. H. Lüders & R.P. Lesser, pp. 303–346. Berlin: Springer-Verlag.

Matsumoto, H. & Ajmone Marsan, C. (1964): Cortical cellular phenomena in experimental epilepsy: interictal manifestations. *Exp. Neurol.* **9,** 286–304.

McLachlan, R.S., Robitaille, Y. & Gloor, P. (1982): Effect of anoxia in feline generalized penicillin epilepsy (FGPE). *Electroencephalogr. Clin. Neurophysiol.* **54,** 39.

McLachlan, R.S., Avoli, M. & Gloor, P. (1984): Transition from spindles to generalized spike and wave discharges in the cat: simultaneous single-cell recordings in cortex and thalamus. *Exp. Neurol.* **85,** 413–425.

Musgrave, J. & Gloor, P. (1980): The role of the corpus callosum in bilateral interhemispheric synchrony of spike and wave discharge in feline generalized penicillin epilepsy. *Epilepsia* **21,** 369–378.

Ohtahara, S., Yamatogi, Y. & Ohtsuka, Y. (1976): Prognosis of the Lennox syndrome – long-term clinical and electroencephalographic follow-up study, especially with special reference to relationship with the West syndrome. *Folia Psychiatr. Neurol. Japan.* **30,** 275–287.

Pellegrini, A., Musgrave, J. & Gloor, P. (1979): Role of afferent input of subcortical origin in the genesis of bilaterally synchronous epileptic discharges of feline generalized penicillin epilepsy. *Exp. Neurol.* **64,** 155–173.

Penfield, W. & Jasper, H.H. (1946): Highest level seizures. *Res. Publ. Assoc. Nerv. Ment. Dis.* **26,** 252–271.

Prince, D.A. & Connors, B.W. (1986): Mechanisms of interictal epileptogenesis. In: *Advances in neurology*, eds. A.V. Delgado-Escueta, A.A. Ward Jr, D.M. Woodbury & R.J. Porter, pp. 275–299. New York: Raven Press.

Roger, J. & Gambarelli-Dubois, D. (1988): Neuropathological studies of the Lennox–Gastaut syndrome. In: *The Lennox–Gastaut syndrome (Neurology and neurobiology, Vol. 45)*, eds. E. Niedermeyer & R. Degen, pp. 73–93. New York: Alan R. Liss.

Rovit, R.L. & Swiecicki, M. (1965): Some characteristics of multiple acute epileptogenic foci in cats. *Electroencephalogr. Clin. Neurophysiol.* **18,** 608–616.

Sadler, R.M. & Blume, W.T. (1989): Significance of bisynchronous spike-waves in patients with temporal lobe spikes. *Epilepsia* **30** (2), 143–146.

Schwartzkroin, P.A., Futamachi, K.J., Noebels, J.L. & Prince, D.A. (1975): Transcallosal effects of a cortical epileptiform focus. *Brain Res.* **99,** 59–68.

Sorel, L. (1964): L'épilepsie myokinétique grave de la première enfance avec pointe-onde lente (petit mal variant) et son traitement. *Rev. Neurol.* **100,** 215–223.

Tukel, K. & Jasper, H. (1952): The electroencephalogram in parasagittal lesions. *Electroencephalogr. Clin. Neurophysiol.* **4,** 481–494.

Williamson, P.D. (1992): Frontal lobe seizures: problems of diagnosis and classification. In: *Advances in neurology*, Vol. 57, eds. P. Chauvel, A.V. Delgado-Escueta, E. Halgren & J. Bancaud, pp. 289–309. New York: Raven Press.

Zifkin, B.G. (1990): The Lennox–Gastaut syndrome. In: *Comprehensive epileptology*, eds. M. Dam & L. Gram, pp. 123–131. New York: Raven Press.

Epileptic Seizures and Syndromes, Edited by Peter Wolf
© 1994 John Libbey & Company Ltd., pp. 299–317

Chapter 34

Supplementary motor area epilepsy: the clinical syndrome

Norman K. So

Department of Neurology, The Cleveland Clinic Foundation, Cleveland, Ohio 44195, USA

Summary

The clinical and other features of seizures arising from the SMA constitute a recognizable syndrome. Seizures may start with a somatosensory aura. The typical seizure is characterized by bilateral, asymmetric, tonic posturing of the extremeties; vocalization, truncal and pelvic movements may also occur. Important historical features that help to identify the syndrome of SMA epilepsy are that seizures are usually quite brief with retained awareness when patients are on antiepileptic drug medication, and that there is a strong pattern of nocturnal predominance in the timing of their occurrence. Seizures can be frequent. Daytime seizures while standing often cause falls. The extracranial EEG frequently shows interictal and ictal abnormalities at the vertex or parasagittal regions. MRI investigation is important to detect a possible structural abnormality in that area.

Introduction

In the 'Proposal for revised classification of epilepsies and epileptic syndromes' (Commission, 1989), supplementary motor seizure is one of the seizure types that make up the frontal lobe epilepsies. It stated that, in supplementary motor seizures, the seizure patterns are postural, focal tonic, with vocalization, speech arrest and fencing postures.

Investigations of the motor functions of the mesial interhemispheric frontal cortex preceded the clinical recognition that seizures may arise from this region. According to Penfield and Welch (1951), Munk (1881) elicited arm movements in monkeys on stimulation of the mesial cortex anterior to the motor leg representation, and was the first to recognize that the movements produced had a different, more diffuse quality than those obtained on stimulation of the primary motor areas. Further experimental work by Horsley & Schäfer (1888) confirmed this finding, and revealed that the characteristic motor response obtained on stimulation of the mesial cortex often caused more proximal than distal limb movement. The area from which these complex proximal postural movements were elicited was designated the mesial extension of area 6aB by Vogt and Vogt (1919).

Foerster (1931) conducted stimulation studies of the human cortex as part of the surgical treatment of post-traumatic epilepsy. He termed area 6aB 'the frontal adversive field', and observed 'rotation of the head, eyes, and trunk to the opposite side and complex synergic movements of flexion or extension of the contralateral arm and leg'. He also noted that epileptic 'attacks of the same type are produced by many different pathological processes involving the area 6aB'.

Penfield and Welch (1949, 1951) explored the functions of the mesial and superior precentral cortex by electrical stimulation. This led Penfield (1950) to introduce the term 'supplementary motor area' (SMA). A rich repertoire of responses were observed on electrical stimulation. Movements were often characterized by the assumption of postures, including the so-called fencing posture, in which the contralateral arm was raised and the head and eyes turned towards that hand. 'The musculature of both sides of the body is employed appropriately so as to bring about the change of position.' Co-ordinate movements such as stepping, or rapid incoordinate movements were also produced by electrical stimulation. Isolated movement of one extremity was less commonly seen. Stimulation could produce repetitive or interrupted vocalization of vowel sounds or multiple syllables. It could also cause partial to complete inhibition of voluntary activity, including speech, without obvious motor effect. Sensory responses included a general body sensation, and epigastric sensation. Autonomic activation resulted in pupillary dilatation. Twenty seizures were produced by electrical stimulation of the supplementary area in 24 patients (Penfield & Welch, 1951). A sensory aura occurred in about a third, and initial inhibitory phenomena often preceded movements. Vocalizations occurred in 15 per cent of the induced seizures. 'These attacks may be considerably more complicated in pattern than simple turning to the opposite side.' Several patients with seizures arising from the SMA who underwent surgery were later described by Penfield and Jasper (1954).

Ajmone-Marsan and Ralston (1957) studied seizures induced by Metrazol injection and classified 14 patients as having SMA seizures on the basis of clinical and electroencephalographic (EEG) findings; whether any underwent confirmatory intracranial EEG study is unknown. An epigastric aura was present in 28 per cent, and a somatosensory aura in 64 per cent. The major motor signs were the conscious M2e posture and conscious head adversion, which each occurred in 72 per cent of the patients. Focal clonic activity was found in 64 per cent. The term M2e as used by Ajmone-Marsan and Ralston (1957) consists of flexion of the elbow of one arm, abduction of the shoulder to 90°, with associated external rotation. The head may look at the postured hand, and the opposite arm may show slight flexion. The leg ipsilateral to the involved arm extends, while the opposite leg flexes at the hip and knee.

According to Penfield and co-workers (Fig. 1), the SMA is situated in the mesial superior frontal cortex, anterior to the primary motor cortex for the lower extremity and above the cingulate gyrus. It may extend superiorly on to the lateral convexity of the hemisphere. Penfield also speculated that there is a supplementary sensory area, posterior to the SMA. The somatotopic organization of the SMA in humans has been recently confirmed (Fried *et al.*, 1991). The anatomical limits of the cortical areas with supplementary motor and sensory functions may be more complex than that originally described by Penfield. The SMA may extend into the cingulate gyrus as sensory responses (Van Buren & Fedio, 1976) and complex motor responses (Talairach *et al.*, 1973) can be obtained by stimulation there. It may also extend beyond the paracentral lobule to the precuneus (S.H. Lim *et al.*, in press).

In the ensuing decades, extensive studies on the physiology of the frontal lobes in motor control were carried out on non-human primates. There has been much debate on the competing models of hierarchical vs. parallel organization amongst the motor centres, of which the SMA is one component. Interested readers are directed to selected reviews on the physiology of the SMA (Wise, 1985; Wiesendanger, 1986; Wiesendanger & Wise, 1992).

Results

In an earlier study from this institution, Morris and co-workers (1988) reported on the characteristic of 11 patients considered to have supplementary motor seizures, three of whom had subdural grid electrodes implanted into the interhemispheric fissure for recording from and stimulation of the SMA. The present study carried on where the last left off, in extending the number of cases, as well as

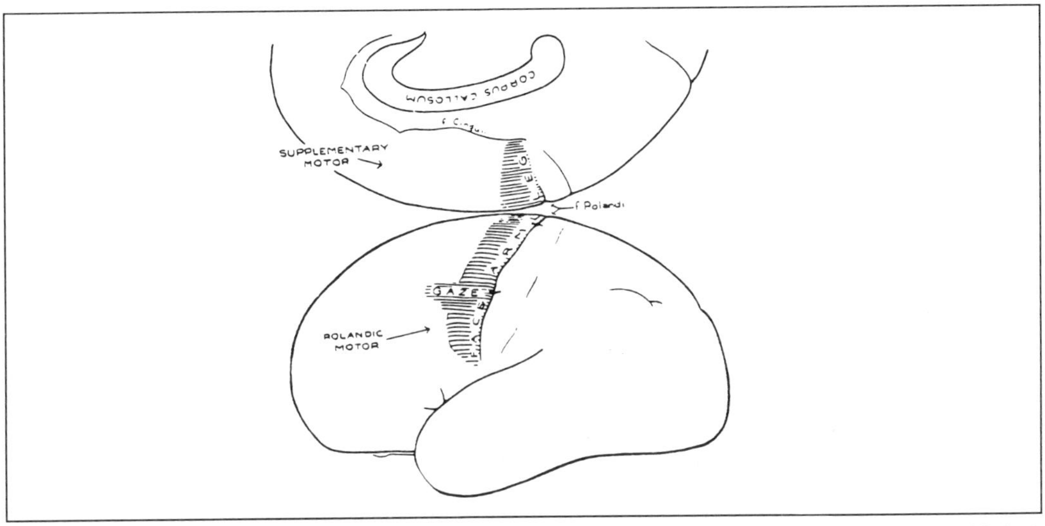

Fig. 1. The location of the SMA in the mesial frontal cortex according to Penfield & Welch (1951) (published with permission: American Medical Association).

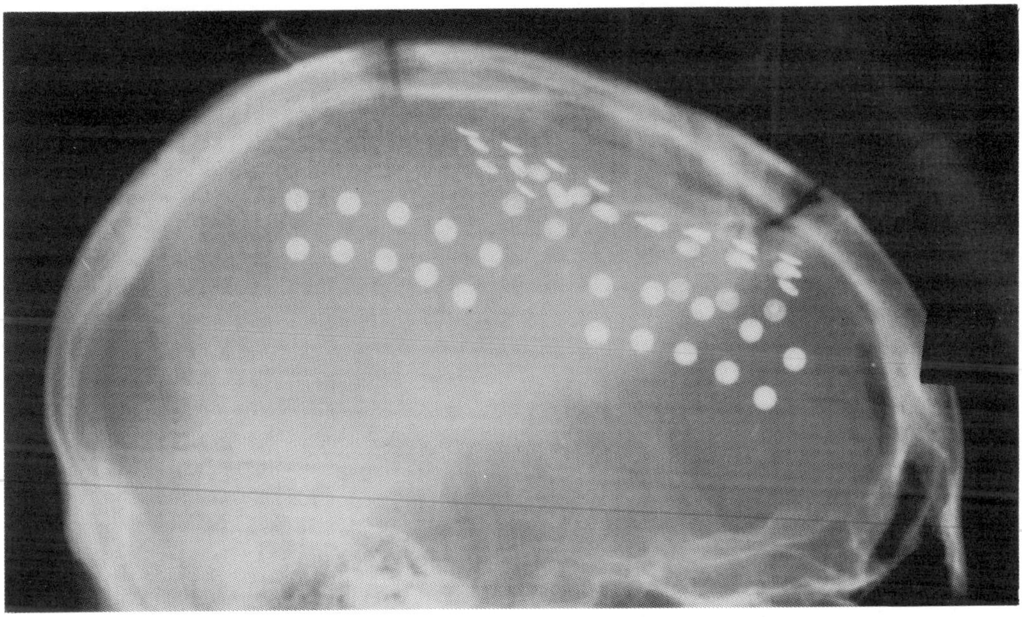

Fig. 2. Case 2. Two bifacial 2 × 5 subdural plates were inserted into the interhemispheric fissure to the right of the falx, with another subdural plate over the parasagittal convexity.

delimiting the criteria of inclusion. Three of the patients in the present study had been included in that prior study.

The study includes 24 patients with seizures confirmed to involve the SMA after investigation by subdural electrode arrays implanted into the interhemispheric fissure up through 1992, whether or not they ultimately received resective surgery. Prior to presurgical evaluation, all patients had demonstrated a poor response to maximal therapy with the major standard antiepileptic drugs.

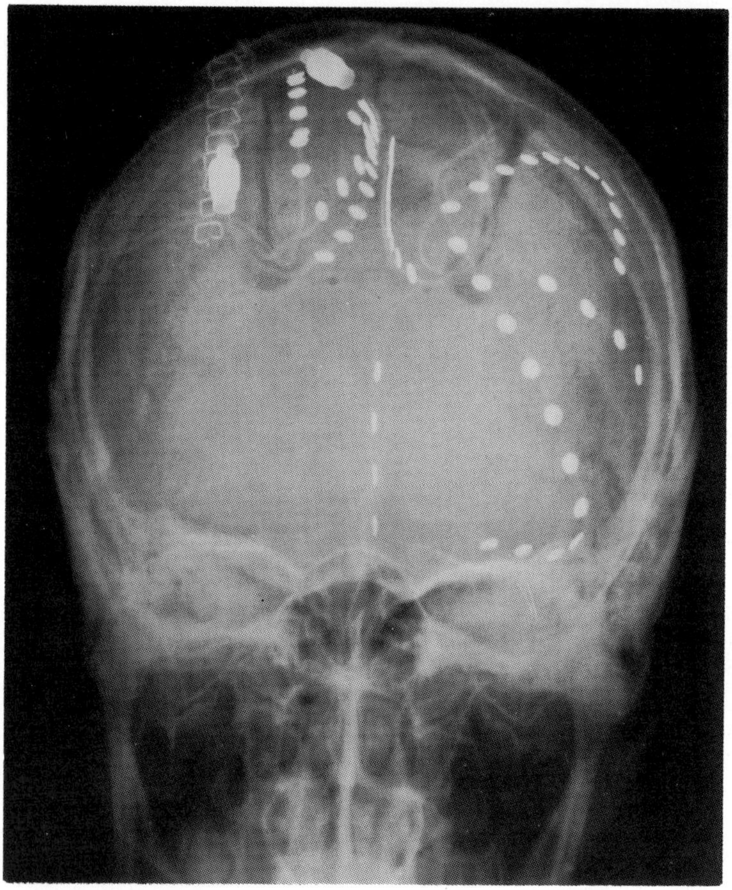

Fig. 3. Multiple subdural strips had been inserted into the interhemispheric fissure on each side of the falx. Additional strips were positioned over the convexities of each hemisphere.

Furthermore, the seizures were judged to be sufficiently socially disabling to warrant surgery. Non-invasive presurgical studies included: prolonged video-EEG monitoring with extracranial electrodes, magnetic resonance imaging (MRI) of the head (in all except one patient), neuropsychological testing, intracarotid amobarbital test, and, from 1990, all patients without a demonstrable structural lesion also underwent positron emission tomography (PET) by the ^{18}F-fluorodeoxyglucose method. The features leading to a suspicion that seizures arise from or near the SMA were based on standard clinical information. A description of the seizures was obtained by history, and by careful review of the videotaped seizures. The scalp EEG features included interictal and ictal epileptiform abnormalities localized to the vertex or adjacent parasagittal regions (see Chapter 35). Preliminary localization is greatly enhanced when a structural lesion is demonstrated on MRI in the frontal interhemispheric region.

Subdural electrode arrays were implanted into the interhemispheric fissure (Lüders *et al.*, 1987) in all patients and frequently also over the the parasagittal convexity. Two general surgical strategies have been used. In the first, a unilateral craniotomy is made at the vertex. Under direct vision, one or two unifacial or bifacial (permitting recording from the two sides) 2 × 5 (10 electrode contacts) subdural plates are inserted into the interhemispheric fissure (Fig. 2). Bifacial interhemispheric electrodes permit subdural recording on the side of craniotomy and epidural recording of the opposite mesial cortex across the falx. The positioning of the subdural plates in the interhemispheric fissure is guided by the pattern of bridging veins draining into the superior sagittal sinus, which must be respected. An additional subdural plate may also be placed across the central sulcus, usually high on the convexity, covering the precentral and postcentral gyri. In the second approach when lateralization to one or the other hemisphere remains uncertain, a midfrontal craniotomy is fashioned to permit introduction of multiple long (up to 11 contacts) subdural strips into the interhemispheric fissure and parasagittal convexity on each side (Fig. 3).

The ictal EEG discharge was confirmed to involve electrode contacts over the SMA in all except two patients. No seizure was recorded in one patient, but localized interictal spikes were found over the supplementary motor cortex. The other patient had subdural electrodes implanted anterior and posterior to a lesion in the SMA seen on MRI; ictal EEG could not be localized, presumably because the electrodes were placed too far away from the lesion. The spatial sampling of subdural electrodes is obviously limited to where they have been placed; thus no claims are made that seizure onsets are confined to the SMA. Supplementary motor cortex is physiologically defined by the results of electrical stimulation through the implanted subdural electrode. SMA responses observed can be grouped under: positive motor responses, negative motor responses, vocalizations and sensory responses. SMA-positive motor responses are distinguished from those of the primary leg area in the paracentral lobule by tonic contraction of one or more body segments as compared with clonic contraction of the leg or foot alone.

Of the 24 patients, 18 proceeded to operation. Six (33 per cent) of the operated patients became seizure-free, or almost seizure-free. Six patients did not receive the operation, because seizure onset involved a wide region of the mesial cortex and overlapped with the primary motor cortex in four patients, and because seizure discharge started in both SMA and could not be lateralized in two patients.

Illustrative case histories

Case 1

This 24-year-old right-handed young woman was first seen at the age of 24 for possible epilepsy surgery. When 18 months old, she had a febrile seizure lasting 5 min with postictal left hemiparesis. Afebrile seizures started at the age of 4, and initially consisted of staring attacks with falls. At age 5, her seizures took a different form and persisted without further change. Seizures mainly occurred in sleep, or shortly after awakening. Sometimes she experienced an aura of light-headedness. She reported preserved awareness, but inability to speak during the attack. She described generalized stiffening of the body, with asymmetric tonic extension of the left side, and sometimes clonic jerks. The seizures were brief, but frequent, occurring up to 10 times each night, with an average of 100–200 per month. Seizures had caused her to fall out of bed at night, and fall to the ground in the daytime with resultant injuries. Her seizures have proved resistant to treatment with all standard as well as experimental antiepileptic drugs.

Examination showed the thumb on the left to be smaller than that on the right. MRI of the head showed abnormal signal in the right posterior frontal parasagittal white matter without gadolinium enhancement (Fig. 4a). ^{18}F-fluorodeoxyglucose PET scan showed an area of hypometabolism in the right posterior frontal parasagittal region. An intracarotid amobarbital test revealed right hemisphere dominance for language and memory. On psychometric testing, the patient had a verbal IQ of 85, performance IQ of 92 and full-scale IQ of 87. There were diminished fine motor speed and manual dexterity bilaterally, with some indication of greater involvement of the left hand. There was also diminished figural fluency relative to word fluency, and impaired performance on the Wisconsin card sorting test. Memory function fell within the expected range. This profile was felt to be consistent with a localized area of dysfunction in the right frontal lobe.

Prolonged extracranial video-EEG monitoring demonstrated sporadic interictal sharp waves at the

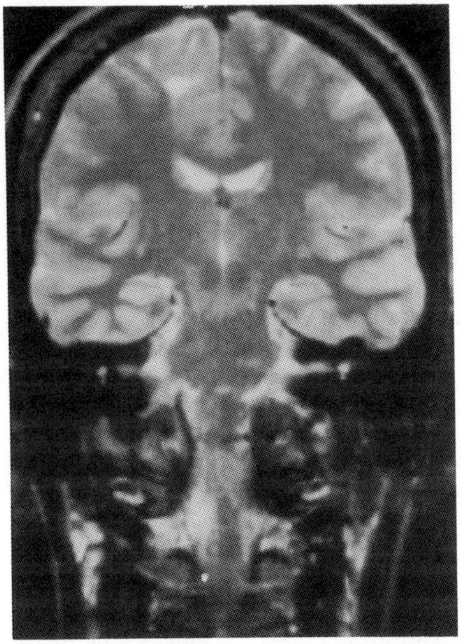

Fig. 4(a). Case 1. Coronal MRI of the head showed an area of abnormal T2 signal increase in the right posterior frontal parasagittal white matter.

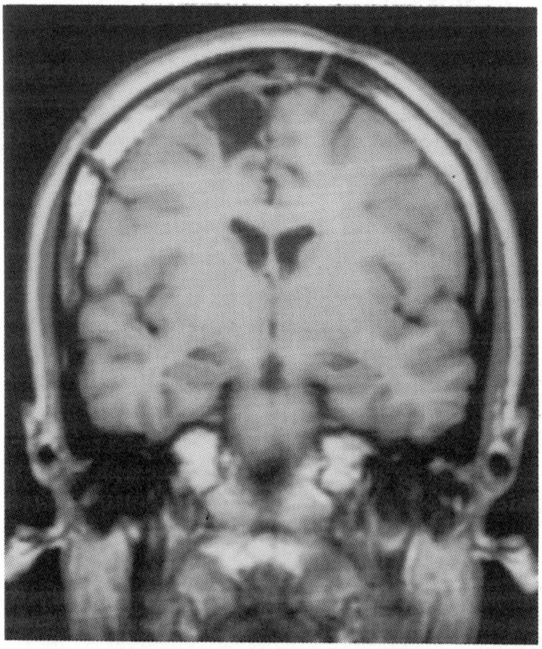

Fig. 4(b). Postresection coronal MRI showing resection of the SMA.

vertex (Cz, FCz). Twenty-nine seizures were recorded in 3 days, predominantly arising from sleep. Video analysis of the seizures showed them to be quite stereotyped (Fig. 5). They started with a brief

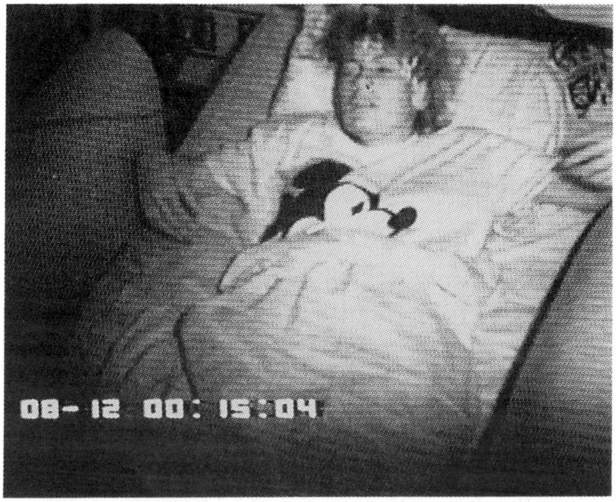

Fig. 5(a). Case 1. Initial motor phenomenon of SMA seizure after arousal from sleep: both arms abducted and elevated, with elbows in flexion; the face tightened to a grimace.

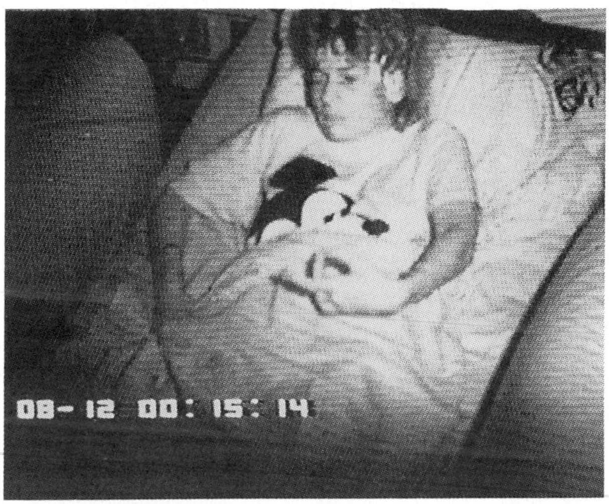

Fig. 5(b). A few seconds later: both arms now extended with the left assuming a more dystonic posture.

period of restlessness, abduction, elevation and then tonic extension of both arms, with the left arm more involved. This was associated with tonic contraction of the face into a grimace. The legs may extend in abduction. Later, there were clonic jerks of the left arm and face, thrashing movements of the trunk and pelvis, and sometimes vocalization. There was no impairment of consciousness by interactive testing. The scalp ictal EEG showed paroxysmal fast activity over the frontocentral region bilaterally, sometimes preceding clinical onset. The seizure discharge evolved into rhythmic, irregular theta activity before it was obscured by muscle artefact.

The patient underwent implantation of convexity and interhemispheric subdural grid electrodes through a right frontal craniotomy. This delineated the ictal and interictal epileptogenic zone in the right mesial interhemispheric region with some extension over the parasagittal convexity. After

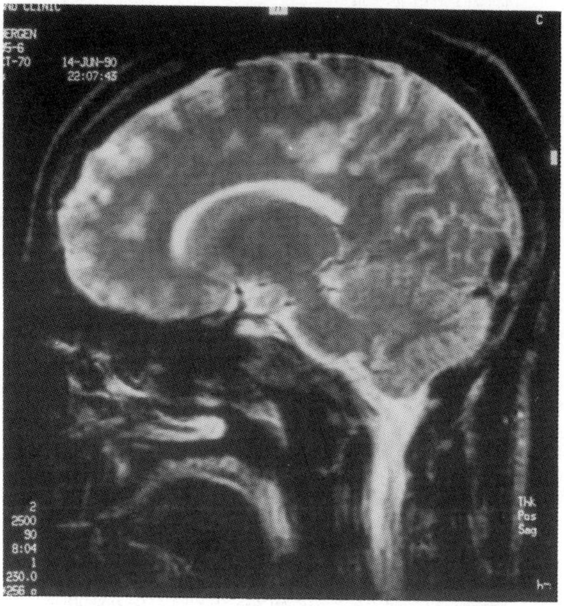

Fig. 6(a). Case 2. MRI of the head showed a lession in the right mesial posterior frontal region. (a) Sagittal scan.

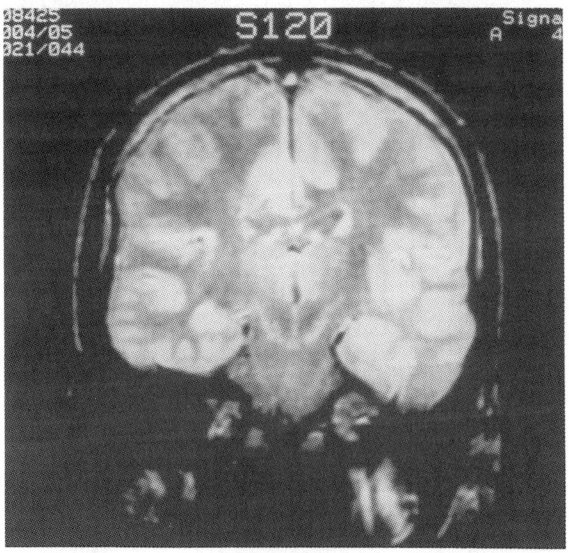

Fig. 6(b). Coronal scan.

functional stimulation, the epileptogenic zone was found to partially overlap with theSMA, and, to a lesser extent, with the primary motor area for leg and arm of the right hemisphere. Resection was then performed just anterior to the primary motor cortex (Fig. 4b), extending 6 cm mesially to include part of the electrically defined SMA, 3 cm along the parasagittal convexity, and subcortically to remove the lesion, which proved to be a ganglioglioma on pathological examination. Postoperatively, the patient had partial paresis of the left leg and, to a lesser degree, of the left arm and hand. This rapidly

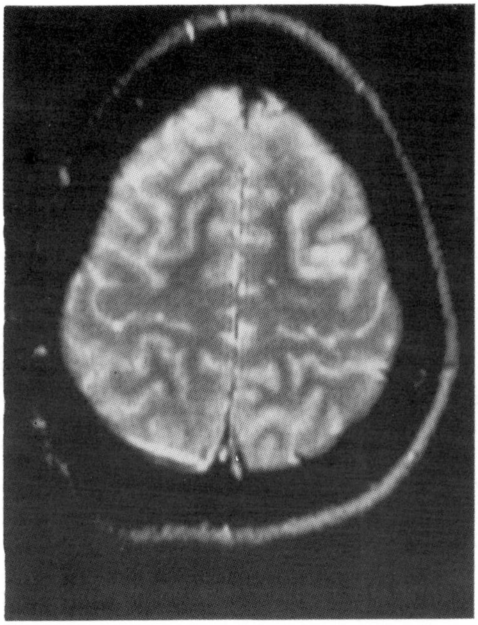

Fig. 7(a).Case 3. MRI of the head showed a discrete lesion in the left middle frontal gyrus. (a) Axial scan.

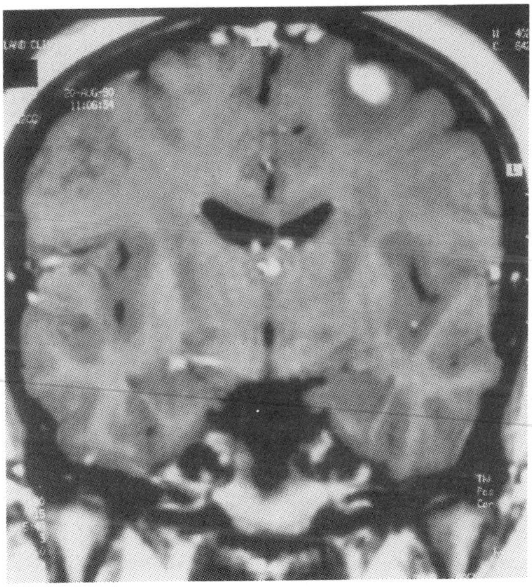

Fig. 7(b). Coronal scan after gadolinium injection.

improved over the first week, and had largely retumed to normal by 2 months. In the postoperative period she has had occasional sensations of light-headedness and dizziness similar to her preoperative auras. She has not experienced any of her habitual SMA seizures in a 1½ year follow-up period on carbamazepine monotherapy. However, she has had four atypical seizures, consisting of shaking of the left side of her body with or without postictal paresis, all occurring in sleep.

Case 2

The patient is a 19-year-old right-handed man who has had seizures since the age of 9. Computerized tomography (CT) and MRI demonstrated a lesion in the right mesial posterior frontal region (Fig. 6). He had no aura. Seizures were reported to consist of stiffening of the arms, sometimes with screaming. Seizures rarely became secondarily generalized. He had two seizures a day on average. Seizures were twice as frequent in daytime wakefulness as in sleep.

The neurological examination was normal. On extracranial video-EEG monitoring, rare interictal spikes were recorded over the left centroparietal region. Analysis of the videotaped seizures showed them to start with abrupt tonic elevation and extension of both arms. The left arm remained extended, while the right arm circled at the shoulder. Screaming sometimes occurred, and there was head version to the left prior to secondary generalization. The scalp ictal EEG showed a slow sharp wave at onset, maximal at the vertex, followed by emergence of rhythmic theta activity through muscle artefact. Two 2 × 5 bifacial subdural arrays were inserted into the interhemispheric fissure on the right, and an 8 × 5 subdural grid positioned over the right parasagittal convexity. Seizures started at right mesial posterior frontal electrodes directly over the lesion. SMA motor responses were obtained by electrical stimulation of some of these electrodes and were situated inferior to the primary motor areas of the foot. A circumscribed removal of the lesion was performed, without resection of SMA cortex. The lesion was a low-grade glioma. At 1 year follow-up, the patient continued to have seizures as before the operation.

Case 3

This right-handed girl eventually had resection of a left frontal ganglioglioma at age 17. Seizures first developed at the age of 7. These were sudden attacks of falling backwards with the hands raised up to the air. She had no aura and no or only brief loss of awareness. Seizures could become secondarily generalized. Before surgery, she was having two to three seizures each day. Seizures in wakefulness were twice as common as those in sleep. The daytime seizures frequently caused falls with resultant head injuries.

MRI revealed a superficial lesion in the left middle frontal gyrus (Fig. 7). An intracarotid amobarbital test demonstrated left hemisphere dominance for language and bilateral memory reserve. The verbal IQ was 98, performance IQ 110 and full-scale IQ 104. Testing also revealed diminished word and design fluency. The pattern suggested dominant frontal lobe dysfunction.

Prolonged extracranial video-EEG monitoring showed frequent sharp waves at the vertex (Cz, Fz, FCz). Ten seizures were recorded in 6 days. Video analysis showed initial bilateral tonic elevation and abduction of the arms until the hands were clearly above the head, with early head turning down and to the left (Fig. 8). There was no demonstrable alteration of memory or awareness when seizures progressed no further. In more prolonged seizures, the patient made waving hand movements while they were elevated. Secondary generalization was marked by head version to the right with tonic deviation of the mouth to the right, right-sided clonic jerks and eventual generalized tonic–clonic seizure activity. The scalp ictal EEG showed a series of sharp waves at the vertex, leading to low-amplitude paroxysmal fast activity, which increased in frequency before the EEG was obscured by electromyographic (EMG) artefact.

The patient then had invasive EEG evaluation with a bifacial 2 × 5 subdural plate in the interhemispheric fissure on the left and a 4 × 11 plate over the left frontoparietal convexity. Ictal EEG activity at onset involved the mesial frontal cortex, including areas defined as supplementary motor cortex by electrical stimulation, as well as a wide region of the convexity defined by electrical stimulation as primary motor and sensory cortex. At operation, only a circumscribed removal of the lesion was performed. This was found to be a ganglioglioma. Postoperatively, the patient suffered no deficits. Seizures have not significantly improved, although there has been some reduction in their intensity.

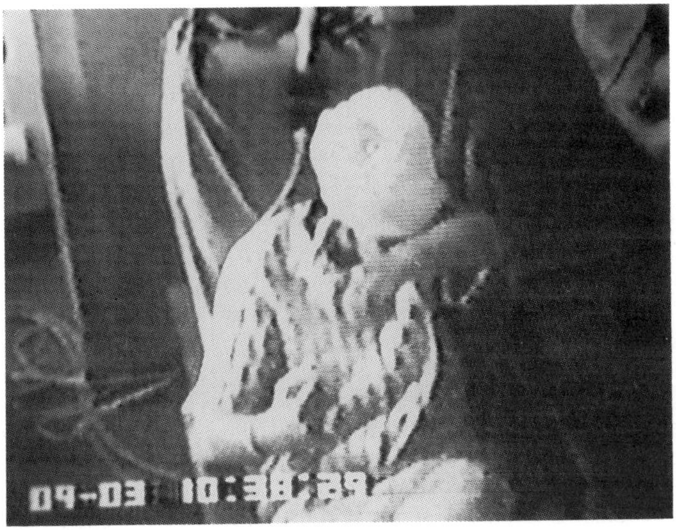

Fig. 8(a). Case 3. Initial phase of SMA seizure showing bilateral tonic elevation and abduction of both arms, with ipsilateral head turning to the left.

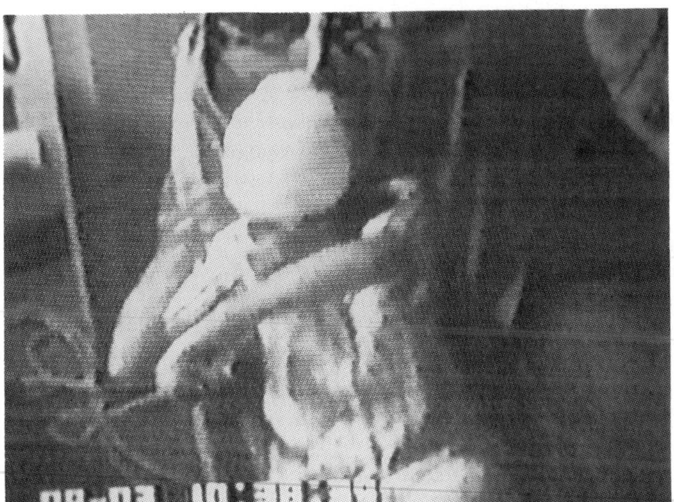

Fig. 8(b). Ten seconds later, there was head version to the right with right-sided clonic jerks leading to a secondarily generalized tonic–clonic seizure.

Case 4

This 28-year-old right-handed man had focal resective surgery for intractable seizures at the age of 28. Seizures first started at the age of 5. No obvious aetiological factor was found prior to operation. He had never experienced an aura. The patient described stiffening of the right arm and body with uncontrollable body movements. He claimed to be aware in some of the seizures. He admitted that he sometimes swore out of frustration during attacks . Seizures were frequent, occurring on average five to six times daily, nearly all while asleep. Occasional seizures also occurred while awake. Frequent nocturnal seizures caused sleep disruption and daytime fatigue.

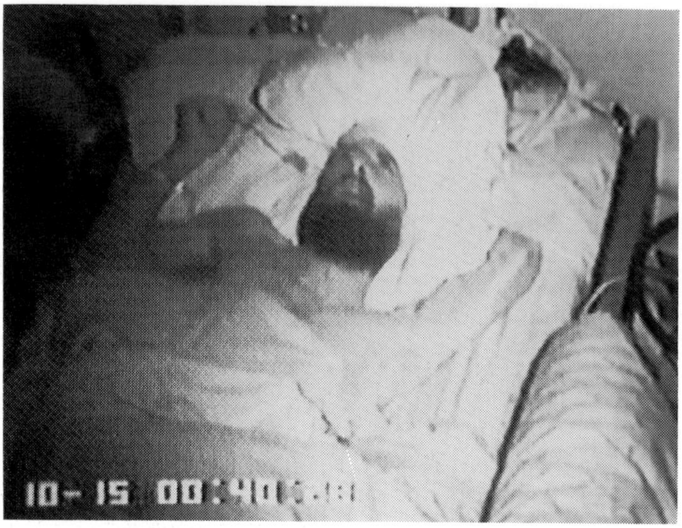

Fig. 9(a). Case 4. Initial arousal from sleep with bilateral arm abduction and elevation.

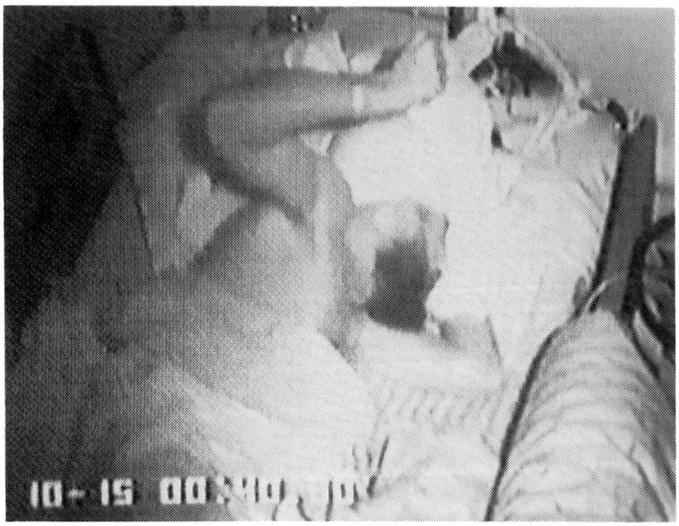

Fig. 9(b). Two seconds later, the patient turned to one side maintaining the posture of the arms.

The neurological examination was normal. CT and MRI of the head were normal. Intracarotid amobarbital tests showed speech in the left hemisphere and poor memory bilaterally. The full-scale IQ was 79, verbal IQ 78 and performance IQ 88. The neuropsychological examination also showed impaired verbal memory and diminished word fluency.

Prolonged video-EEG monitoring with extracranial electrodes recorded no interictal epileptiform discharges. Ictal EEGs were obscured by EMG artefact, although diffuse postictal slowing was present in some seizures. The patient then had evaluation with epidural (Peg) and foramen ovale electrodes. Interictal spikes were seen at both frontal and temporal regions. Ictal EEG was characterized by low-voltage fast activity at the vertex (recorded by an epidural electrode), which started before clinical

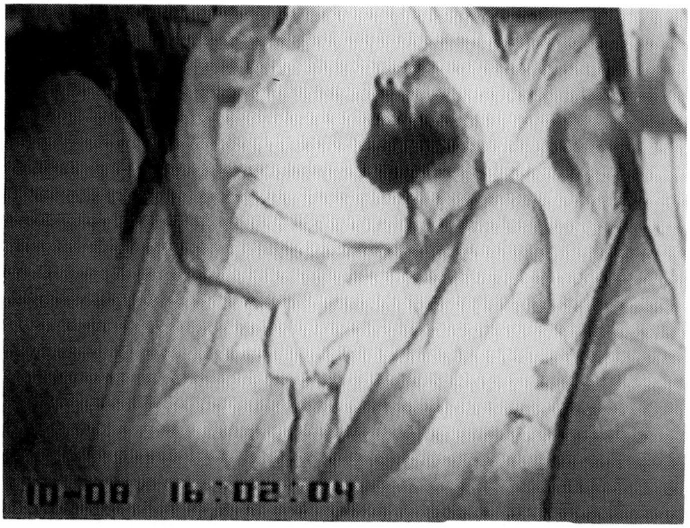

Fig. 9(c).Evolution into a tonic–clonic generalized seizure.

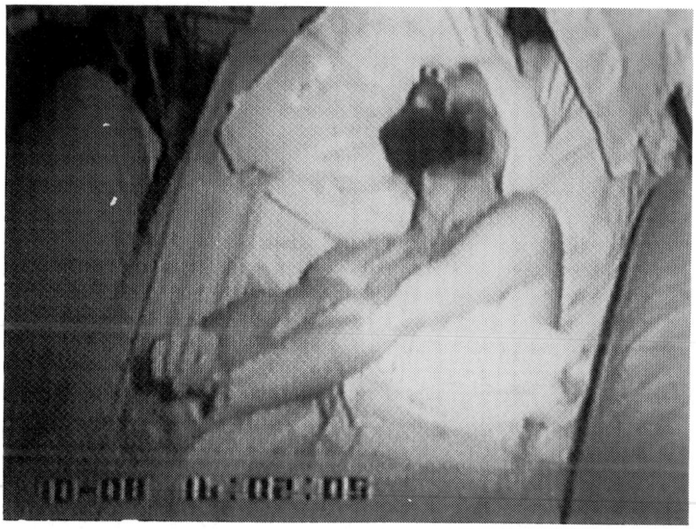

Fig. 9(d). Evolution into a secondarily generalized tonic–clonic seizure.

onset. Two 2 × 5 bifacial subdural arrays were inserted into the interhemispheric fissure on the left, and an 8 × 5 subdural grid was placed over the left frontoparietal convexity. By video analysis (Fig. 9), his habitual seizures started with a phase of arousal from sleep, or a period of quiet staring. He then developed bilateral arm abduction and elevation, with the right side more prominent, and facial grimace. Next followed screaming, thrashing and kicking of all extremeties, and trembling of the body. The patient often crouched on the bed, and sometimes tried to walk away. Towards the end phase of the seizure, the patient often swore profusely. Awareness and memory were preserved in the shorter seizures. More prolonged seizures were accompanied by postictal confusion. The patient also had some secondarily generalized seizures. EEG ictal onset in these seizures developed several seconds before clinical onset at the left anterior mesial frontal electrodes. A few atypical seizures were also recorded late in the evaluation and consisted of twitching of the right side of the mouth, head turning to the right, followed by secondary generalization. Electroencephalographically, these seizures started at the left frontal convexity.

Functional electrical stimulation revealed that the site of seizure onset in the left anterior mesial frontal region was anterior to the functionally defined SMA and primary motor area of the right foot. The patient underwent resection of the left anterior mesial frontal cortex and the first frontal gyrus, sparing the SMA. At operation, a ganglioglioma was found, not previously detected on imaging studies. No neurological deficits developed after operation. The patient has become seizure-free in the last 2 years after operation.

Case 5

This case is of interest in being the only patient found to have independent left and right supplementary motor seizures. The patient was a 32-year-old right-handed man when first seen for evaluation of possible epilepsy surgery. At the age of 3, he was struck on the head by a stone and suffered a depressed right frontal skull fracture that required surgery for removal of bone fragments. Seizures later started at the age of 9. He had a prolonged prodrome of nervousness and irritability before seizures, but no aura. By history, seizures consisted of abrupt bilateral tonic elevation and extension of both arms, and to a lesser extent of the legs, associated with partial or complete loss of awareness and responsiveness. The more prolonged seizures were followed by postictal confusion. Seizures were frequent, three to five per day, predominantly in sleep, but also while awake. Daytime seizures have caused numerous falls. During a seizure, the patient fell into a lawnmower and suffered traumatic amputation of nine digits.

Two years before evaluation at the Cleveland Clinic, the patient had an anterior corpus callosotomy at another institution. Seizures decreased for several weeks but then returned to their usual frequency. Prior to callosotomy, EEGs were reported to show right frontal and right frontotemporal sharp waves, as well as bilateral spike-and-wave discharges. An abnormal area of increased signal in the mesial surface of the right frontal pole was also present in the MRI before callosotomy. Subsequent investigations were as follows: MRI of the head obtained after callosotomy showed an abnormal signal in the parasagittal region of the right frontal lobe and division of the anterior half of the corpus callosum. ^{18}F-fluorodeoxyglucose PET scan revealed right hemisphere hypometabolism maximal over the right frontal region. Intracarotid amobarbital testing showed language to be lateralized in the left hemisphere with bilateral memory representation. Psychometric testing documented a verbal IQ of 86, performance IQ of 75, and full-scale IQ of 79.

Repeat prolonged extracranial video-EEG monitoring showed multifocal independent sharp waves over the right temporal (FT8, F8), right central and vertex (Cz, C4), and left frontal (F3, Fz) regions. There were also frequent bursts of bilateral discharges that seemed to lead from the right hemisphere, as well as independent bursts of multiple spikes from the left and right hemispheres. Twenty-eight seizures were recorded in 5 days, 11 in sleep. The scalp ictal EEG showed either a high-amplitude sharp wave over the right frontocentral region at onset or low-voltage fast activity over the vertex, or it was completely obscured by artefact. The patient had subdural electrodes implanted into the interhemispheric fissure on the right and over the right frontal convexity. Two distinct clinical and electrical seizure patterns were found from the right and left frontal lobes. Right-sided seizures (Fig. 10a) were seen to cause tonic extension of the left arm with flexion of the right arm, which in some cases progressed to clonic jerking of the left side of the face, and eventual head version to the left with generalized convulsive activity. In short seizures, there was rapid recovery of responsiveness. The seizure discharge at onset involved a widespread area of the right frontal lobe, including the right SMA as defined by electrical stimulation, and the right frontal convexity. Left-sided seizures (Fig. 10b) were characterized by sudden head and eye turning to the left, tonic extension of the right arm

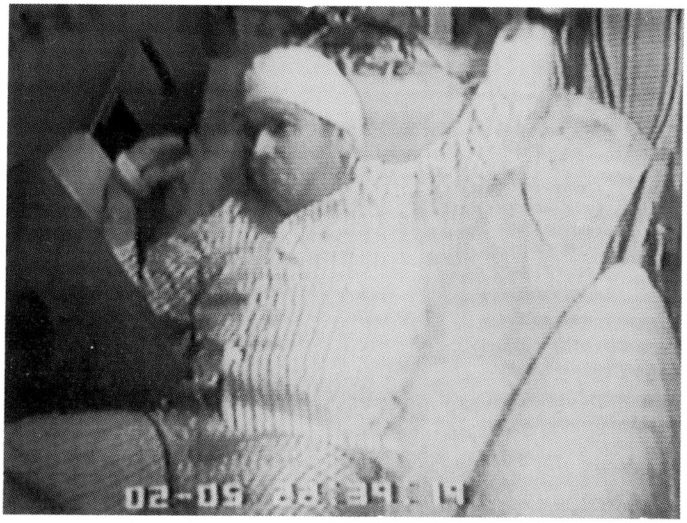

Fig. 10(a). Case 5 . Right SMA seizure associated with tonic extension of the left arm and flexion of the right.

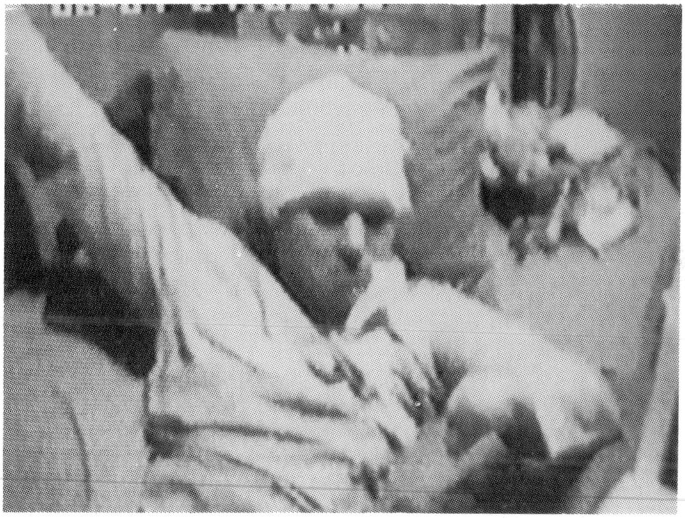

Fig. 10(b). Left SMA seizure associated with tonic extension of the right arm and flexion of the left.

upwards and tonic flexion of the left arm at the elbow. Responsiveness was usually impaired. The ictal EEGs of these left-sided seizures were seen to begin in the left mesial frontal region. An extensive right frontal resection was performed. Pathological examination of the resected specimen revealed subpial gliosis and focal neuronal heterotopia.

Postoperatively the patient continued to have seizures on valproate and phenytoin therapy. Five months after the operation, the patient was found unconscious at the bottom of a flight of stairs. He was presumed to have fallen in a seizure. The patient died from complications of subarachnoid and intraventricular haemorrhage sustained in the fall.

A summary of the main clinical features of all 24 patients follows. The age at onset of seizures ranged from 6 months to 24 years with a median of 8 years. An obvious hemiparesis was present in two patients, and clumsiness in one hand in another two. When aetiological factors are considered, a foreign tissue lesion was ascribed as the cause of epilepsy in seven patients. Five patients had a history of prenatal difficulties, and this seems correlated with the subsequent finding of cortical dysplasia. Remote cerebral injury from abscess, head injury or infarction (porencephaly) was noted in four. The cause of epilepsy remains unknown in eight.

Seizures were usually stereotyped, although a not so clear picture might exist in the first few years when seizures began early in life. Seizures tended to be extremely frequent. Even on maximal antiepileptic drug treatment, the seizure frequency ranged from one every 2 weeks to 25/day. Ninety-six per cent of the patients had daily seizures, averaging four a day. Seizures predominating in sleep or shortly after awakening were characteristic. Eighty per cent of patients showed this nocturnal predominance, while seizures occurred exclusively in sleep in 35 per cent. An aura was present in 10 patients (42 per cent). The most frequent was a somatosensory aura, which could be lateralized to one side of the body in some, but was more commonly a non-lateralized sensation. One patient had a sensation as though 'floating away'. Another had indescribable dizziness and light-headedness. An epigastric aura had not been volunteered in a spontaneous seizure. This was despite having elicited an epigastric sensation in a few patients on electrical stimulation of the mesial frontal cortex. The most frequent (96 per cent) initial motor sign was that of bilateral, often asymmetric, tonic posturing of the extremities. This was most apparent in the upper extremities. The arms frequently elevated and abducted at the shoulders, although not necessarily always rising above the head. One arm could be relatively extended, while the other flexed at the elbow, assuming the 'fencing' posture. The tonic posturing also involved the lower extremities, although this was sometimes overlooked. The legs were typically abducted in semiflexion or extension. It is presumably on this basis that patients often fall when seizures occur in the daytime. Vocalization was seen in about one-third of the patients. This had one of several or mixed qualities. One consisted of forced utterances, which might have been related to involuntary diaphragmatic and laryngeal contractions. Another had an affective component, as though groaning in despair or whining in fear. Third, some patients swore loudly, at the beginning or very end of the seizure; this might represent a conscious reaction in frustration at the events. Responsiveness was often impaired even with retained awareness, possibly from diffuse tonic stiffening that prevented speech and voluntary motor activity, or from motor inhibition. The degree to which consciousness was impaired depended on the intensity and duration of the seizure discharge. Brief seizures lasting 10 to 20 s when patients were on anti-epileptic drug medication often did not cause detectable alteration in awareness or memory. With seizures of increasing severity, there was clouding of consciousness, and secondarily generalized convulsions were obviously accompanied by loss of awareness. Truncal and pelvic movements were seen in about a quarter of the patients. These were unnatural and contorted movements, which should not be confused with a sexual automatism. Focal myoclonic jerks occurred infrequently. When they did, they seemed to represent a fragment of the more developed bilateral tonic seizure. Automatisms were likewise only fragmentary and rare. The only patient who had more complex automatisms had a ganglioglioma in the cingulate gyrus. Her automatisms began after initial tonic posturing, and were thought related to spread of the seizure discharge to mesial temporal structures, as confirmed by intracranial recording with subdural and foramen ovale electrodes. Focal clonic activity occurred mainly in the course of secondary generalization. Lateralized clonic jerks can be a useful lateralizing sign. Head turning was more problematic. Early head turning could be ipsilateral to the SMA of seizure origin. Later head turning when associated with tonic or clonic mouth deviation or lateralized clonic jerks was contralateral to the SMA of seizure onset. Although negative motor or inhibitory phenomena were often demonstrated on electrical stimulation of the anterior mesial frontal cortex, an inhibitory phase could not be discerned in spontaneous seizures, probably owing to its brevity and the difficult operational procedure to establish its existence.

Neuroimaging studies revealed a focal lesion in six of seven patients with a proved tumour, and also revealed abnormalities in three of the five patients with cortical dysplasia. Three had encephalomalacia from remote injury.

Discussion

The syndrome of SMA epilepsy is probably still under-recognized. Many of the patients here have received a number of different diagnoses before the attacks are even accepted as epileptic in nature. They are most commonly mistaken for psychogenic seizures. The unusual tonic posturing, vocalizations, swearing and bilateral movements, often with retained awareness, as well as the subtle scalp EEG ictal changes, are prone to lead the unwary to make a diagnosis of pseudoseizures, even after video-EEG monitoring. However, the stereotopy of the seizure semiology, their brief duration and their predominance in sleep serve to distinguish them from psuedoseizures (Kanner *et al.*, 1990). When in doubt, prolonged video-EEG monitoring with antiepileptic drug withdrawal can be extremely helpful. Medication withdrawal usually leads to increased seizure severity, and eventually a secondarily generalized tonic–clonic seizure. Lateralized clonic activity further aids in the lateralization of the epileptogenic zone.

Since some patients with SMA epilepsy have their seizures exclusively in sleep, they can be mistaken for a sleep disorder. In childhood it is conceivable that SMA seizures can be mistaken for pavor nocturnus. The possibility of a rapid-eye-movement (REM) behaviour disorder is sometimes raised, since the patient can seemingly strike out with tonically extended arms. However, the lack of dream recall, the stereotyped movements and associated generalized convulsions serve to distinguish one from the other. Paroxysmal nocturnal dystonia or hypnogenic paroxysmal dystonia, first described by Lugaresi and Cirignotta in 1981, was originally compared with paroxysmal kinesogenic choreoathetosis and paroxysmal dystonic choreoathetosis (Lance, 1977; Lugaresi *et al.*, 1986). Affected cases had frequent (2–20) attacks arising from NREM sleep characterized by tonic stiffening of one or more limbs, with or without other disorganized movements and vocalization. While attacks by definition should only occur in sleep, some patients also experienced them in wakefulness. More than half had epileptic seizures. The question if these attacks were really epileptic in nature was soon raised (Rajna *et al.*, 1983). More recently, Lugaresi and co-authors reported on evidence that several patients previously diagnosed as having paroxysmal nocturnal dystonia turned out to have frontal lobe epilepsy (Tinuper *et al.*, 1990). It would appear that paroxysmal nocturnal dystonia is none other than SMA epilepsy.

Two other paroxysmal conditions have already been mentioned: paroxysmal kinesogenic choreoathetosis, and paroxysmal dystonic choreoathetosis (Lance, 1977). The published descriptions of these two paroxysmal disorders include a range of dystonic postures, choreoathetosis, and ballistic movements, the individual elements of which may be difficult to distinguish from SMA seizures. However, in paroxysmal dystonic choreoathetosis attacks can last up to 60 min. Attacks are much shorter, usually less than 2 min in duration in paroxysmal kinesogenic choreoathetosis. Unlike SMA epilepsy, attacks nearly all occur in wakefulness, although nocturnal attacks are known to exist. Paroxysmal kinesogenic choreoathetosis is well known, as befits its name, to be triggered by sudden movement. This has not been observed in any patient with SMA seizures. In paroxysmal dystonic choreoathetosis, relaxation and alcohol are common precipitants, but these latter factors can certainly also trigger epileptic seizures. Both paroxysmal disorders are often familial, suggesting autosomal dominant inheritance with incomplete penetrance. In contrast, a symptomatic cause has been identified in a majority of this series of patients with SMA epilepsy: either a foreign tissue lesion or other structural abnormality. All said, the two paroxysmal disorders cannot be completely disentangled from the borderlines of epilepsy. A warning sensation reminiscent of an aura can occur. Some had definite epileptic seizures. In one patient who had EEG recording during an attack of paroxysmal kinesogenic choreoathetosis, the EEG showed 12–15 Hz rhythmic activity over the vertex and hemispheric regions (Perez-Borja *et al.*, 1967).

One limitation of this study is that the patients considered here have been selected because their seizures were sufficiently frequent and disabling to be considered for surgical treatment. Thus the picture that emerges is clearly one extreme in the spectrum that probably exists, and should not be taken to represent the natural history of seizures from the SMA and vicinity. The author and other colleagues at Cleveland Clinic have encountered several patients who have all the clinical characteristics that satisfy the syndrome of SMA epilepsy, often supported by extracranial EEG findings, with or without structural abnormalities in that region on imaging, who have, neverthe less, attained satisfactory seizure control on antiepileptic medications. A few patients became completely seizure-free, while others showed periods of seizure activity alternating with seizure-free months. A group of children with presumed nocturnal SMA seizures starting in the first decade of life with good response to medical treatment have also been described (Vigevano & Fusco, 1993).

In agreement with prior observations on patients with SMA seizures (Penfield & Welch, 1951; Penfield & Jasper, 1954; Ajmone-Marsan & Ralston, 1957; Morris *et al.*, 1988), this study confirms that SMA seizures have a distinct semiology. A somatosensory or other ill-defined sensory aura was present in about half the patients, but unlike Penfield and co-workers, or Ajmone-Marsan and Ralston, we have not encountered an epigastric aura in spontaneous seizures either by history or during prolonged EEG monitoring. This difference may be one that separates spontaneous from induced seizures. Penfield and co-workers' observations were often based on seizures induced by electrical stimulation, while Ajmone-Marsan and Ralston studied seizures induced by Metrazol injection. As emphasized by Penfield and co-workers, motor signs are characterized by the 'assumption of a posture'. However, only a portion of the cases exhibited the 'fencing posture'. The arms may be more or less symmetrically postured and not always rising clear above the head. The head may be turned down or up, and, as already stated, early head turning may be ipsilateral to SMA of seizure origin. A clearly lateralized M2e posture, as described by Ajmone-Marsan and Ralston (1957) was not at all evident. It is possible that such a posture existed as a fragment in the evolution of the seizure, but bilateral, albeit asymmetric, tonic posturing seemed the more important image. Ictal focal clonic activity in the course of seizure progression provided reliable lateralization, as noted by Ajmone-Marsan and Ralston (1957), as did the unilateral tonic facial contraction that accompanied head contraversion with secondary generalization. The uncoordinated and sometimes bizarre truncal and pelvic movements that can occur in 25 per cent of patients have not been noted in the earlier literature. Vocalization occurred in about a third of patients, in agreement with prior observations. It was, however, not possible to demonstrate inhibition of movement in spontaneous seizures, as reported in Penfield's earlier works. This was despite the ability to elicit negative (inhibitory) motor responses by electrical stimulation of the implanted electrodes. The explanation for this discrepancy may again lie in the difference between spontaneous and induced events. While all patients had some seizures in which consciousness was preserved (Morris *et al.*, 1988), consciousness was progressively impaired in proportion to the severity of the seizure.

Acknowledgements

Many thanks to Dr Andrew Bleasel, who abstracted data on many of the patients presented here. Also the study would not have been possible without the collaboration of my colleagues at the Section of Epilepsy and Sleep Disorders, who not only contributed their patients but performed many of their detailed evaluations.

References

Ajmone-Marsan, C. & Ralston, B.L. (1957): *The epileptic seizure: its functional morphology and diagnostic significance.* Illinois: Springfield, Illinois: Charles Thomas.

Commission on Classification and Terminology of the International League Against Epilepsy (1989): Proposal for revised classification of epilepsies and epileptic syndromes. *Epilepsia* **30,** 389–399.

Foerster, O. (1931): The cerebral cortex in man. *Lancet* 309–312.

Fried, I., Katz, A., McCarthy, G., Sass, K.J., Williamson, P., Spencer, S.S. & Spencer, D.D. (1991): Functional organization of human supplementary motor cortex studied by electrical stimulation. *J. Neurosc.* **11,** 3656–3666.

Horsley, V. & Schäfer, E.A. (1888): A record of experiments upon the functions of the cerebral cortex. *Phil. Trsns.* **179,** 1–45.

Kanner, A.M., Morris, H.H., Lüders, H., Dinner, D.S., Wyllie, E., Medendorp, S.V. & Rowan, A.J. (1990): Supplementary motor seizures mimicking pseudoseizues: some clinical differences. *Neurology* **40,** 1404–1407.

Lance, J.W. (1977): Familial paroxysmal dystonic choreoathetosis and its differentiation from related syndromes. *Ann. Neurol.* **2,** 285–293.

Lim, S.H., Dinnit, D.S. Pillay, P.K. *et al.* (1994): Functional anatomy of the human supplementary senssorimotor area: resulkts of exrtraoperative electrical stimulation. *Electroencephalogr. Clin. Neurophysiol.,* in press.

Lüders, H., Lesser, R.P., Dinner, D.S., Morris, H.H., Hahn, J.F. & Friedman, L. (1987): Chronic intracranial recording and stimulation with subdural electrodes. In: *Surgical treatment of the epilepsies,* ed. J. Engel, Jr, pp. 297–321. New York: Raven Press.

Lugaresi, E. & Cirignotta, F. (1981): Hypnogenic paroxysmal dystonia: epileptic seizure or a new syndrome? *Sleep* **4,** 129–138.

Lugaresi, E., Cirignotta, F. & Montagna, P. (1986): Nocturnal paroxysmal dystonia. *J. Neurol. Neurosurg. Psychiatry* **49,** 375–380.

Morris, H.H., Dinner, D.S., Lüders, H., Wyllie, E. & Kramer, R. (1988): Supplementary motor seizures: clinical and electroencephalographic findings. *Neurology* **38,** 1075–1082.

Munk, H. (1881): *Über die Functionen der Grosshirnrinde. Gesammelte Mitteilungen aus den Jahren 1877–1880, mit Einleitung und Anmerkungen.* Berlin: A. Hirschwald.

Penfield, W. (1950): The supplementary motor area in the cerebral cortex of man. *Arch. Psychiatr.* **185,** 670–674.

Penfield, W. & Welch, K. (1949): The supplementary motor area in the cerebral cortex of man. *Trans. Am. Neuroll Association* **74,** 179–184.

Penfield, W. & Welch, K. (1951): The supplementary motor area of the cerebral cortex: a clinical and experimental study. *Arch. Neurol. Psychiatry* **66,** 289–317.

Penfield, W. & Jasper, H. (1954): *Epilepsy and the functional anatomy of the human brain.* Boston: Little Brown.

Perez-Borja, C., Tassinari, C.A. & Swanson, A.G. (1967): Paroxysmal choreoathetosis and seizures induced by movement (reflex epilepsy). *Epilepsia* **8,** 260–270.

Rajna, P., Kundra, O. & Halasz, P. (1983): Vigilance level-dependent tonic seizures: epilepsy or sleep disorder? A case report. *Epilepsia* **24,** 725–733.

Talairach, J., Bancaud, J., Seier, S., Bordas-Ferrer, M., Bonis, A., Szikla, G. & Rusu, M. (1973): The cingulate gyrus and human behaviour. *Electroencephalogr. Clin. Neurophysiol.* **34,** 45–52.

Tinuper, P., Cerullo, A., Cirignotta, F., Cortelli, P., Lugaresi, E. & Montagna, P. (1990): Nocturnal paroxysmal dystonia with short-lasting attacks: three cases with evidence for an epileptic frontal lobe origin of seizures. *Epilepsia* **31,** 549–556.

Van Buren, J.M. & Fedio, P. (1976): Functional representation on the medial aspect of the frontal lobes in man. *J. Neurosurg.* **44,** 275–289.

Vigevano, F. & Fusco, L. (1993): Hypnic tonic postural seizures in healthy children provide evidence for a partial epileptic syndrome of frontal lobe origin. *Epilepsia* **39,** 110–119.

Vogt, C. & Vogt, O. (1919): Allgemeinere Ergebnisse unserer Hirnforschung. *J. Psychol. Neurol.* **25,** 277–462.

Wiesendanger, M. (1986): Recent developments in studies of the supplementary motor area of primates. *Rev. Physiol. Biochem. Pharmacol.* **103,** 1–59.

Wiesendanger, M. & Wise, S.P. (1992): Current issues concerning the functional organization of motor cortical areas in nonhuman primates. *Adv. in Neurol.* **57,** 117–134.

Wise, S.P. (1985): The primate premotor cortex: past, present and preparatory. *Ann. Rev. Neurosci.* **8,** 1–19.

Epileptic Seizures and Syndromes, Edited by Peter Wolf
© 1994 John Libbey & Comany Ltd., pp. 319–330

Chapter 35

Supplementary motor seizures: localization of the epileptogenic zone

Paul C. Van Ness*, Andrew Bleasel* and Ingrid Tuxhorn†

*Section of Epilepsy and Sleep Disorders, Cleveland Clinic Foundation, 9500 Euclid Avenue, Cleveland, OH 44195–1221, USA and †Epilesie-Zentrum Bethel, Maraweg 21, D-33617 Bielefeld, Germany

Introduction

Supplementary motor area (SMA) seizures represent a distinct seizure semiology. Recognition of the condition may lead to appropriate diagnostic testing and medical or surgical treatment.

While medically intractable patients may be over-represented in the tertiary care epilepsy centre population, some patients respond well to antiepileptic drugs. This chapter deals with those cases that were medically intractable and where surgery was considered a treatment option. As of 1993, no well defined, proved best approach to evaluating patients with SMA seizures exists. Determining the localization of the epileptogenic zone when seizures are suspected to arise in or near the SMA is based entirely on experience with patients having other forms of localization-related epilepsy. Anatomical considerations, however, make the application of some techniques rather difficult, particularly when invasive electrodes are involved.

Clinical localization of the epileptogenic zone

The clinical history and physical examination provide useful lateralizing and localizing information in most localization-related epilepsies. SMA seizures are no exception, as outlined (see Chapter 34) by Dr Norman So. Many patients report a somatosensory aura, which usually correctly predicts contralateral lateralization. Subtle sensory or motor abnormalities on clinical examination may also help with lateralization. Head version just prior to a secondarily generalized tonic–clonic seizure, as well as focal clonic activity at the time of secondarily generalized tonic–clonic seizures, may also provide lateralizing information (Chee *et al.*, 1993).

If a careful history of seizure semiology is taken from both the patient and observers, it is clear that many SMA seizure patients have preserved consciousness, even though bilateral movements of the extremities are occurring (Ajmone-Marsan & Ralston, 1957; Waterman *et al.*, 1987). SMA seizures can occasionally be confused with psychogenic seizures. Many of our own patients, however, did exhibit variable loss of consciousness, particularly after drug withdrawal. Postictal confusion was usually minimal. Speech arrest was typical, though vocalizations did occur which were usually more of a repetitive scream. SMA seizures tended to cluster with high frequency in the morning hours and were frequently out of sleep rather than during daytime wakefulness. Thus, some patients are not severely disabled by this form of epilepsy, particularly if daytime seizures do not occur. The seizures can occur during daytime naps, and often going into the room and waking the patient may trigger a seizure. While the semiology is outlined well in Dr So's paper, it bears mentioning again, since the clinical information is of paramount importance in making a diagnosis of SMA seizures.

Structural neuroimaging

Computerized tomography (CT) and magnetic resonance imaging (MRI) scanning have proved useful in evaluating patients with epilepsy. Numerous studies, however, indicate that MRI is superior (Jabbari *et al.*, 1986; Latack *et al.*, 1986; Lesser *et al.*, 1986; Theodore *et al.*, 1986; Schörmer *et al.*, 1987; Heinz *et al.*, 1988; Swartz *et al.*, 1989). High-resolution or turboflash images are often helpful in detailing the anatomy of the mesial hemispheres. Structural lesions producing SMA seizures commonly involve the superior frontal gyrus or occur in the vicinity of the cingulate gyrus. Epileptogenic lesions may be anterior or posterior to the sensorimotor cortex. Lesions may exist in other locations, for example, the middle frontal gyrus. In our experience, these patients had seizures that spread to the SMA and produced the semiology of an SMA seizure.

Functional neuroimaging

The usefulness of functional neuroimaging is certainly well established for temporal lobe epilepsy. In neocortical epilepsies, functional neuroimaging's usefulness is less well documented. The studies of Swartz *et al.* (1989) clearly show that when patients have an MRI lesion they are likely to have positron emission tomography (PET) scan abnormalities. There is no large series of PET scanning in non-lesional extratemporal epilepsy in adults that shows the technique to be useful for localization and helpful for determining prognosis. Nonlesional cases at our own centre generally have uninformative PET scanning.

Single-photon emission computed tomography (SPECT) is another functional neuroimaging test of unproved value for SMA seizures. The technique is tricky since most isotopes have to be injected during the seizure in order to have optimal localizing value. Since SMA seizures are often brief, the scans we have been able to obtain have mostly been postictal and, therefore, often uninformative. It is unlikely that SPECT will ever be useful in SMA seizures unless new isotopes are developed which can be premixed and ready for rapid injection.

Magnetic resonance spectroscopy (MRS) has not been adequately assessed in SMA seizure patients, though the technique holds promise for detecting subtle metabolic abnormalities in the epileptogenic zone (Laxer *et al.*, 1993).

Non-invasive neurophysiology

With the advent of computerized electroencephalographic (EEG) techniques and montage reformatting capabilities, it is now possible to select appropriate montages, filter settings and gains to analyse seizures in many different ways. We recently analysed the scalp interictal and ictal EEGs in a series of patients with SMA seizures recorded at the Cleveland Clinic (Bleasel *et al.*, 1993a). Contrary to earlier reports at our centre (Morris *et al.*, 1988) and other centres (Ajmone-Marsan & Ralston, 1957), every patient had ictal changes seen on scalp EEG. The prototype ictal pattern can be described as an arousal from sleep followed by rhythmic sharp waves, maximal at the vertex or FZ electrodes, followed by low-voltage fast activity and subsequent electromyographic (EMG) artefact (Fig. 1).

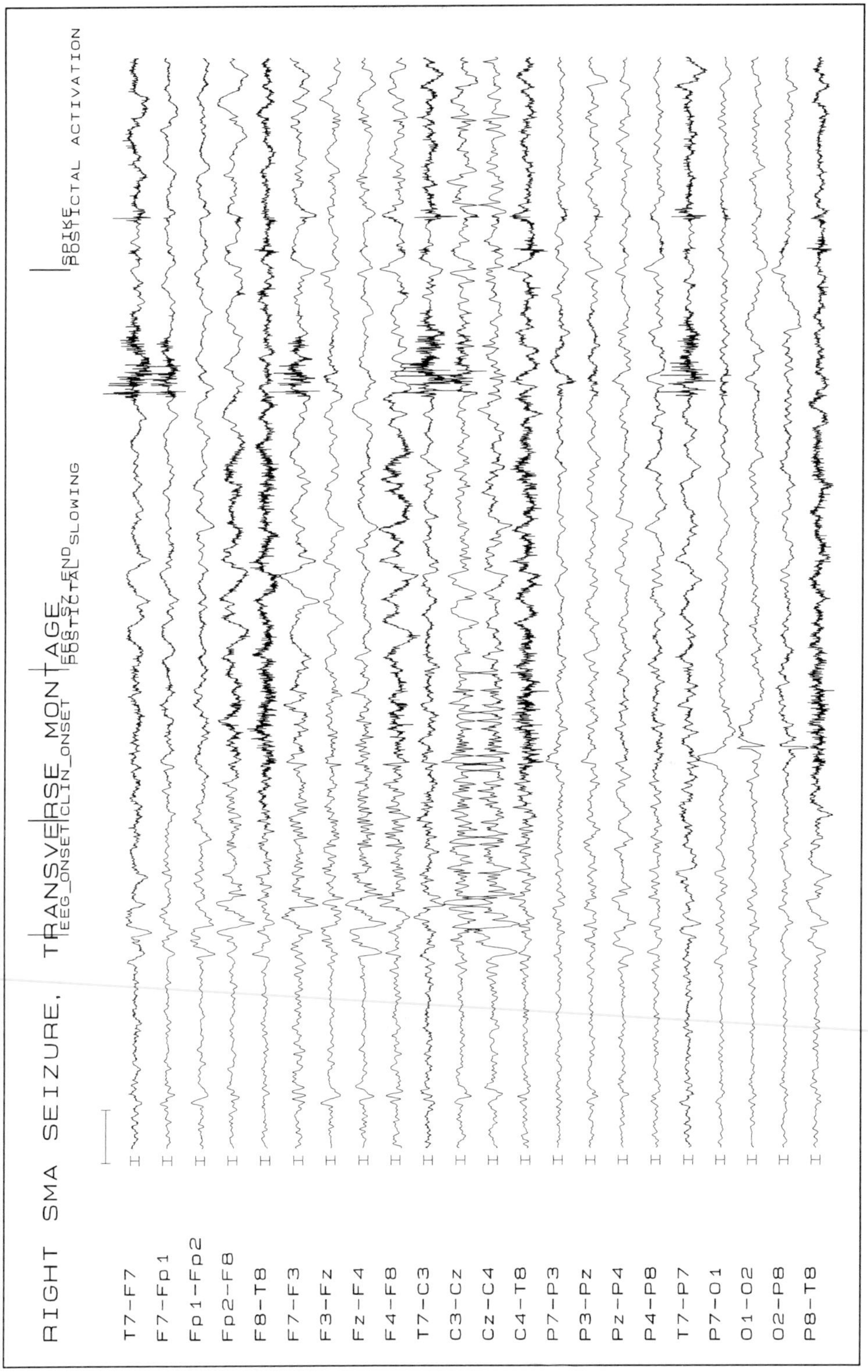

Fig. 1(a). Typical scalp SMA seizure pattern. This is a typical ictal scalp EEG displaying a transverse bipolar montage. Note the postictal spike activation at Cz and postictal slowing.

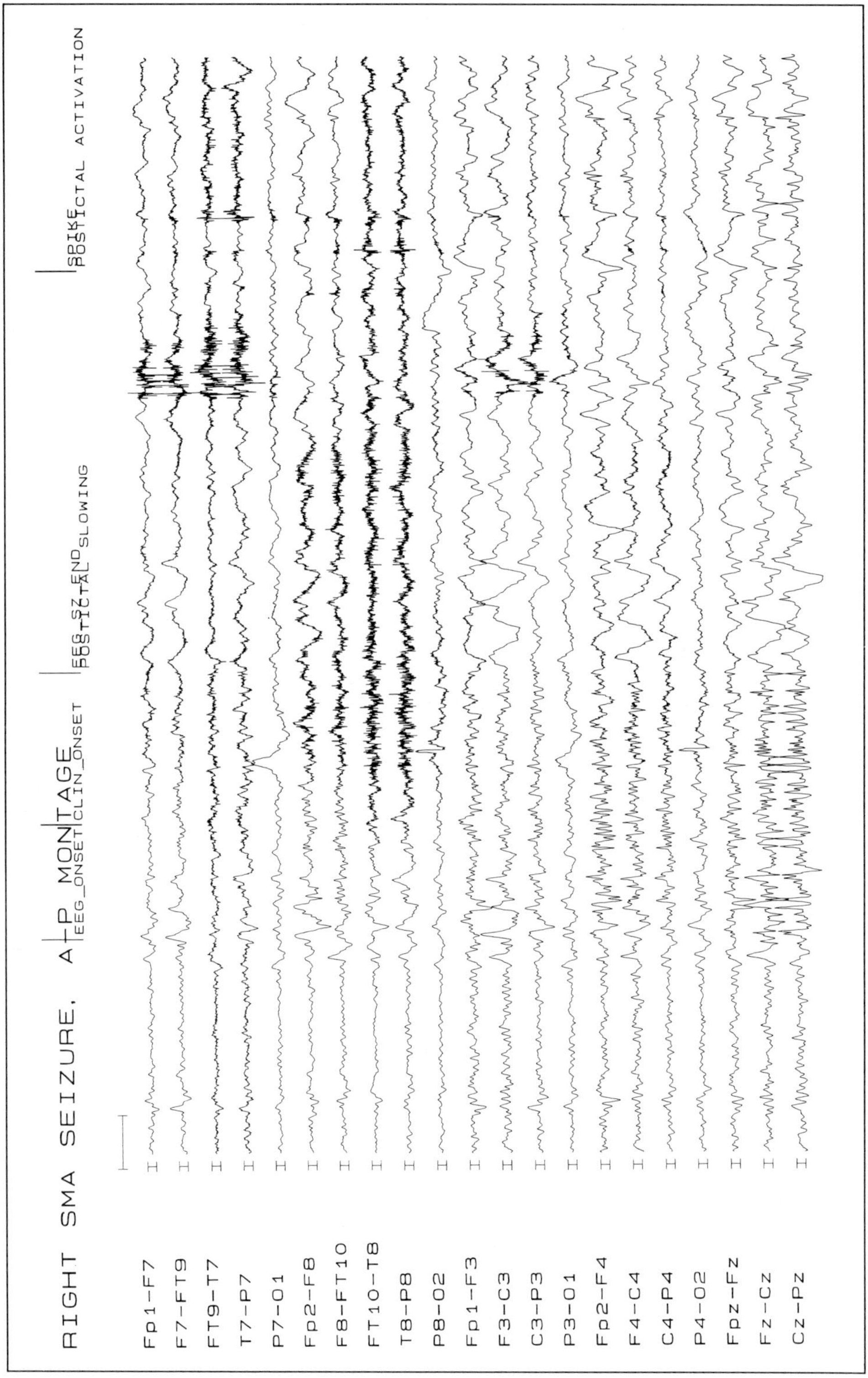

Fig. 1(b). Typical scalp SMA seizure pattern. This is a typical ictal scalp EEG displaying an anteroposterior bipolar montage. Note the postictal spike activation at Cz and postictal slowing. The seizure reveals subtle lateralization to the right side in the anterioposterior montage.

Even with closely spaced electrodes utilizing the 10/10 system, lateralization was often impossible except in a few patients with large lesions.

Interictal EEG was frequently uninformative, though several patients did have midline spikes or sharp waves in wakefulness and sleep and rhythmic midline theta was noted in several cases (Fig. 2). It is important to cautiously interpret midline sharp waves seen exclusively in sleep, since normal vertex waves can occasionally be confused with the spikes and sharp waves of epilepsy, particularly in younger children. Also, not all patients with midline epileptiform discharges and epilepsy will have supplementary motor seizures (Pedley *et al.*, 1981). Secondary bilateral synchrony was not seen in our patients, though Tükel and Jasper (1952) have reported the finding with parasagittal lesions.

Other functional testing

Though not mandatory, other functional testing may provide useful information about patients with SMA seizures. Neuropsychological testing may identify specific lateralized learning disabilities, though localizing value has not been rigorously studied in this patient population. Finding a low IQ, however, may indicate a more diffuse pathology. The intracarotid amytal study may identify memory difficulties in extratemporal cases (Van Ness *et al.*, 1993a), and many patients with epilepsy, particularly those with an early age of seizure onset, may have discordance for language and motor dominance, which may be valuable information for planning surgery (Kosmides *et al.*, 1993).

Invasive EEG monitoring

Non-invasive video-EEG monitoring is an important part of the evaluation of SMA seizures. The lateralizing information gained by observing head version or focal clonic activity prior to a secondarily generalized seizure can be helpful in planning placement of invasive electrodes, and the true nature of the seizure may become apparent. The non-invasive testing of these patients is geared primarily to determining candidacy for further invasive or surgical procedures. While some centres prefer to do lesionectomies and report good results, the philosophy at our epilepsy centre is that resection of the area of ictal onset offers a better opportunity for becoming seizure-free (Van Ness *et al.*, 1990, 1992; Lüders *et al.*, 1992). Certainly large lesions such as tumours may be difficult to evaluate with subdural electrodes and, in these cases, a lesionectomy may be appropriate if the entire lesion is resectable. When a lesion exists and invasive electrodes are planned, it is important to adequately cover the lesion as well as surrounding areas so that ictal onset and early spread of the seizure can be mapped reliably. Lesions of the superior frontal gyrus are optimally covered with interhemispheric and convexity electrodes (Fig. 3). If a stable ictal onset and spread pattern is seen with an adequate seizure sample, the confidence that the epileptogenic zone has been identified is much higher. Variable patterns can be seen when lesions are large and the seizures may exhibit multifocal onsets. If clinical changes occur before the EEG changes are seen, however, the electrode placement must be suboptimal. In well-defined lesional cases we have observed ictal onsets in the medial interhemispheric region or even in superior and lateral portions of the superior frontal gyrus. Seizures can originate in clinically silent areas, producing symptoms only when the seizure reaches an area such as the supplementary motor cortex (Bleasel *et al.*, 1993b).

Chronically implanted subdural electrodes offer an opportunity for detailed functioning mapping that may be difficult to accomplish intraoperatively with stimulation (Lüders *et al.*, 1992). Both techniques, however, are useful in defining the limits of the SMA as well as the somatosensory cortex, which should be spared in any cortical resection where the patient does not have a motor deficit preoperatively. Unfortunately, the presence of eloquent cortex within the epileptogenic zone often limits the resection, making these cases even more challenging.

Non-lesional cases represent the most difficult presurgical situation since seizures may be impossible to lateralize when only partial seizures are observed and the additional problem of anteroposterior localization becomes apparent. While the supplementary motor cortex is usually anterior to the motor

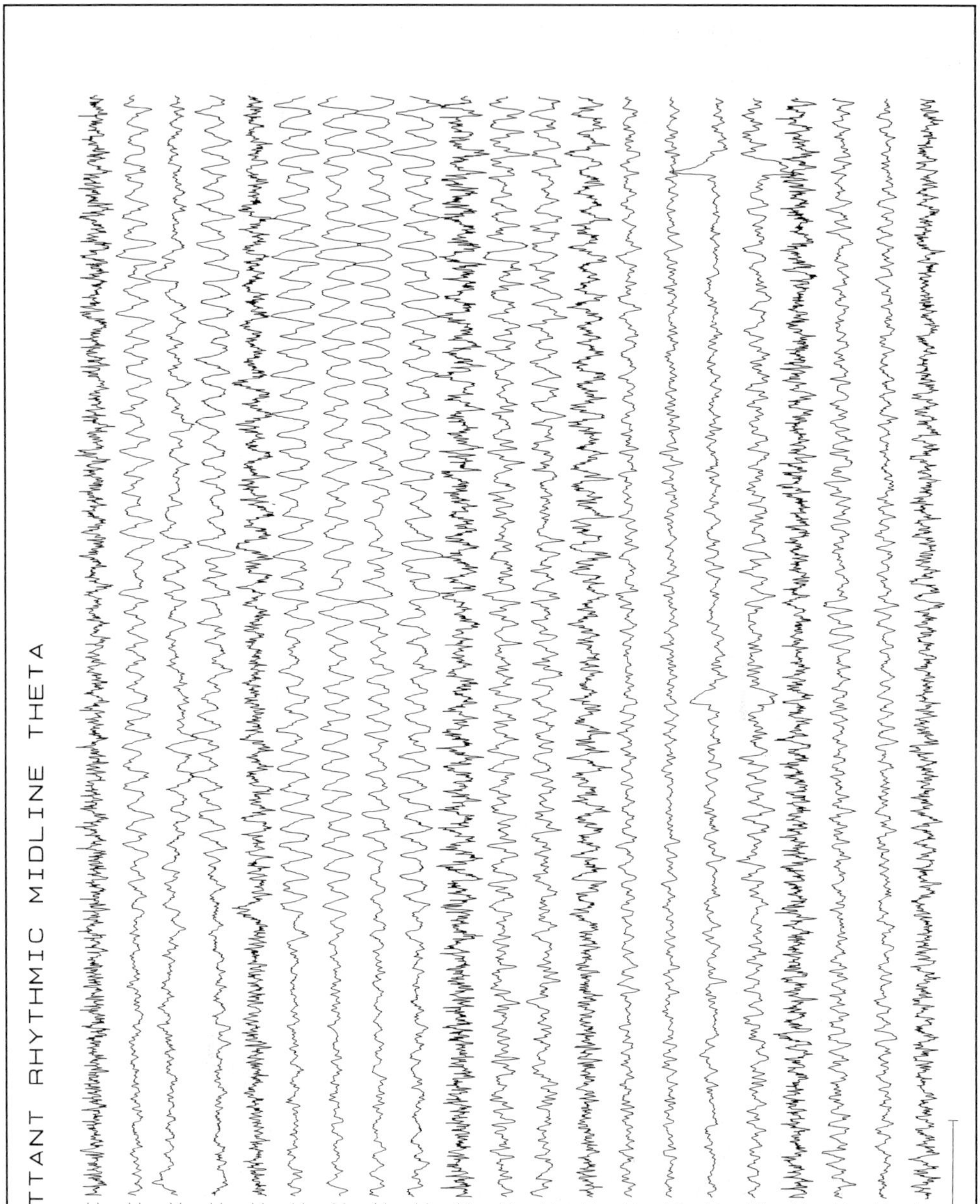

Fig. 2. Midline rhythmic slowing interictally. Rhythmical midline theta, while not considered abnormal specifically, was common in SMA patients.

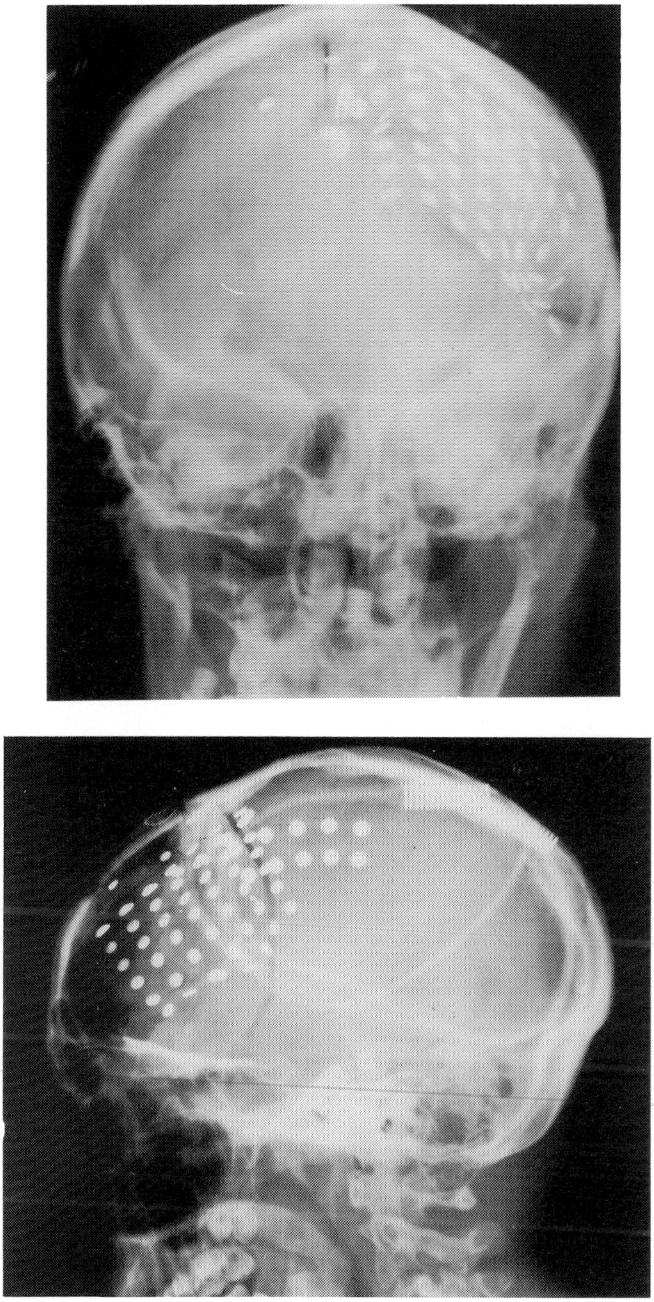

Fig. 3a (top) and b (bottom). Skull X-ray showing interhemispheric and convexity grids.

strip within the interhemispheric area (Penfield & Welch, 1951), recent studies by D.S. Dinner (unpublished) indicate that it may dip below and behind the somatosensory cortex into the mesial parietal region. Several of our patients with SMA seizure semiology did have posterior lesions and ictal onsets.

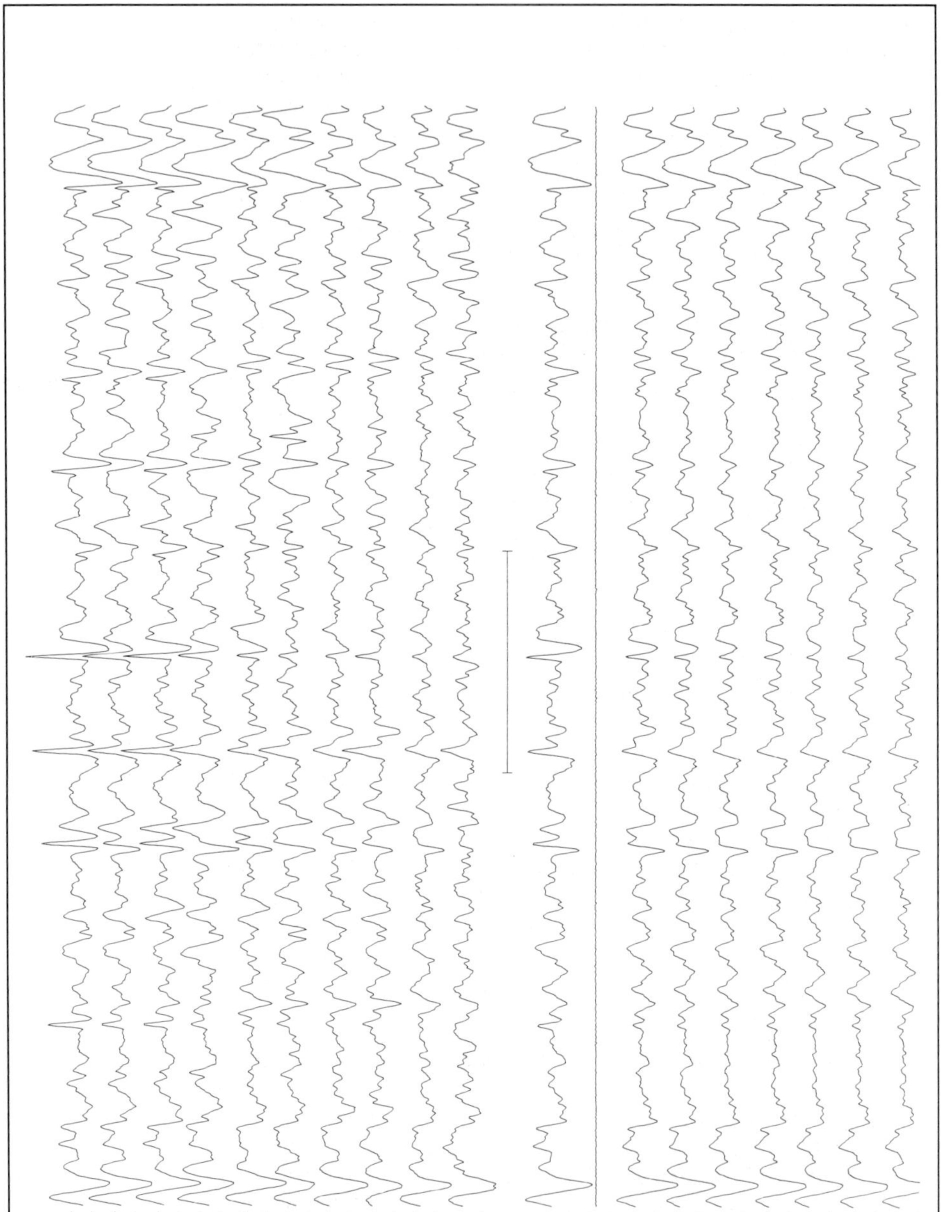

Fig 4. Mesial frontal spike homology. Interictal spiking was recorded with a double-sided grid with C21–C30 contacts subdural and C31–C39 epidural on the falx. Homologous electrodes have the same last digit, i.e. C21 and C31. While the epidural spiking is lower in amplitude, homology is evident. Time bar = 1 s. Amplitude bar = 50 microvolts.

In non-lesional cases, if subdural electrodes are utilized, they should be placed in a widespread area bilaterally. Bancaud and Talairach traditionally used depth electrodes for this purpose (Buser *et al.*, 1992; Talairach *et al.*, 1992), though more centres now utilize subdural grids or strips. At our centre we have utilized double-sided grids with both subdural and epidural (through the falx) recordings. Additionally, it is possible to place strips bilaterally along an anteroposterior axis, providing adequate coverage of the cingulate and SMA. Risks of injuring bridging veins and the superior sagittal sinus are always a concern to the surgeons and may limit electrode placement. Pathology in non-lesional cases is most often microscopic, representing either a cortical dysplasia or other migrational disturbance or gliosis. In one instance we found a ganglioglioma that had escaped detection with a poor-quality MRI.

The principles of localization with subdural grids have been well described elsewhere (Jayakar *et al.*, 1991). The electroencephalographer typically correlates the video and EEG of an ictal event, looking for specific EEG changes prior to the clinical onset. It is helpful to analyse both referentially and with bipolar recordings. Data analysis is particularly enhanced with computerized EEG where reformatting is possible, and it is very helpful to confirm localization by maximal amplitude criteria seen with referential recordings with the phase reversals of bipolar recordings. Subdural and epidural electrode combinations in the same patient usually show lower epidural EEG amplitude (Figs. 4 and 5) thus caution about using amplitude criteria alone for lateralization is advised. It may be possible to record a dipole with both the interictal spikes and the ictal rhythms. Recording a dipole may indicate that the epileptogenic zone is relatively well defined (Sutherling *et al.*, 1990). It may be difficult to differentiate between seizure spread with a phase lag and the existence of a true dipole; thus careful waveform analysis is important.

The supplementary motor cortex rapidly propagates discharges to the opposite hemisphere. Not only has this problem plagued ictal and interictal recordings with subdural electrodes, but it is also a problem with intercerebral depth electrodes, which has been detailed by Buser *et al.* (1992). In their studies of electrical stimulation of the mesial frontal regions, it was clear that propagation occurs rapidly and reliably. In our own studies looking at ictal patterns with invasive electrodes and SMA seizures, Tuxhorn *et al.* (1992) found that even unilateral lesional cases have seizures that are difficult to lateralize because of rapid propagation. Homologous electrodes were often involved synchronously, indicating that the functional anatomy is probably quite homologous between the hemispheres due to callosal connections (Figs. 4 and 5). A standard 200 Hz sampling rate with computerized EEG may make it difficult to analyse 10 ms time differences with propagation patterns; thus at times higher sampling rates may better define the waveforms and determine which are spread by propagation or volume conduction. Localized D/C shifts may also have localizing value.

Not all non-lesional cases were impossible to lateralize, but in our series of 25 patients with subdural electrodes three were non-lateralized and non-localized with the technique. Three had early ictal onset in or near the motor cortex, where surgery was considered too risky, and only 19 of the 25 had actual resections based on the subdural evaluation. In another example of inoperable and yet lateralizable invasive EEG recordings, Williamson (1992) reported 'flip–flop' seizures in a patient, re-evaluated after corpus callosotomy, who had bilateral independent SMA seizures. Adequate seizure sampling is needed to detect bilateral independent ictal onsets.

The most common pathologies in our 19 operated cases were tumours in seven patients and

Fig. 5 (following page). Lateralized referential invasive ictal recording. This 19-year-old male with left mesial frontal cortical dysplasia had a double-sided interhemispheric grid implanted. B21–B30 are right-sided epidural recordings through the falx, while B31–B40 electrodes are subdural over the suspected supplementary motor area. The ictal EEG begins with left-greater than right-sided fast activity progressing to spiking on the left side only and then bilateral, left greater than right, spike-and-wave complexes. Note the lower amplitude and filtering of fast frequencies with the epidural recordings compared to the subdural recordings. The lateralizing findings are minimal, but present. Time bar = 1 s.

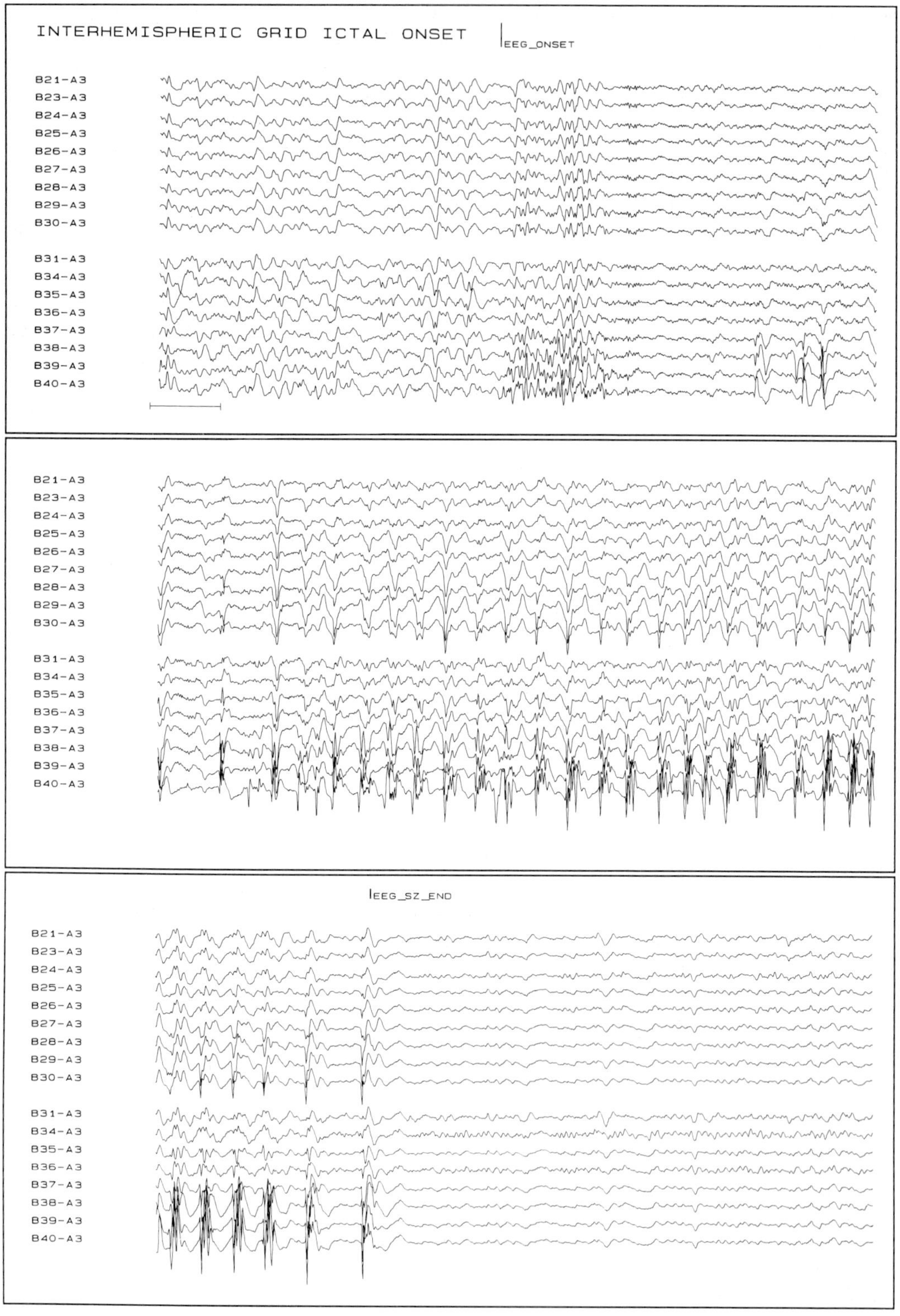
INTERHEMISPHERIC GRID ICTAL ONSET
EEG_ONSET
B21-A3
B23-A3
B24-A3
B25-A3
B26-A3
B27-A3
B28-A3
B29-A3
B30-A3
B31-A3
B34-A3
B35-A3
B36-A3
B37-A3
B38-A3
B39-A3
B40-A3
B21-A3
B23-A3
B24-A3
B25-A3
B26-A3
B27-A3
B28-A3
B29-A3
B30-A3
B31-A3
B34-A3
B35-A3
B36-A3
B37-A3
B38-A3
B39-A3
B40-A3
EEG_SZ_END
B21-A3
B23-A3
B24-A3
B25-A3
B26-A3
B27-A3
B28-A3
B29-A3
B30-A3
B31-A3
B34-A3
B35-A3
B36-A3
B37-A3
B38-A3
B39-A3
B40-A3

migrational abnormalities in 10 patients. Gliosis was seen in four patients and a variety of other pathologies were noted in the remaining cases. Four of the patients had dual pathologies.

Overall seizure outcome in our series indicated that 58 per cent had a good outcome, being either seizure-free or having rare disabling seizures or non-disabling seizures only (Van Ness *et al.*, 1993b). Veilleux *et al.* (1992) reported on eight mesial frontal resections in patients with SMA seizure semiology localized by depth electrodes; four were seizure-free or almost seizure-free with 3–10-year follow-up with use of a 5 cm premotor mesial resection.

Complications may occur even with appropriate functional mapping by subdural electrodes, intraoperative mapping and careful surgery to avoid eloquent cortex. Eight of 20 patients at our centre had a transient hemiparesis or weakness, while three had persistent weakness which was moderate in one and mild in two. Language disturbances were found in four patients transiently and were persistent in two additional cases, even though there was no obvious surgical lesion of a language area (Van Ness *et al.* 1993b). The language disturbances did not represent actual aphasia, but could represent some of the functional consequences of resecting a portion of the supplementary motor cortex.

Patients with lesions were more likely to have a better outcome, though some of the non-lesional cases did do well; thus, at this time, we cannot deny surgery when a structural lesion is not seen on MRI.

Conclusions

SMA seizure semiology is easy to recognize with an appropriate history. Non-invasive EEG evaluation with montages emphasizing the midline electrodes is important to document the seizure type. Invasive EEG is often necessary, particularly in non-lesional cases or in patients with small lesions where the extent of resection will depend on where seizures originate. SMA seizure semiology may occur when seizures originate outside the SMA and spread into it. Invasive neurophysiology may be non-lateralizing because of the normal neurophysiology of rapid propagation to the contralateral supplementary motor cortex. Other data may help with lateralization and the subdural electrodes may still provide localizing information for surgical margins in the anteroposterior direction. Preliminary results indicate that good postoperative seizure outcomes are possible in this group of patients and anecdotal experience indicates that patients can be well controlled postoperataively with antiepileptic medications.

References

Ajmone-Marsan, C. & Ralston, B.L. (1957): *The epileptic seizure: its functional morpholoqy and diagnosis sigificance. A clinical-electrographic analysis of metrazol-induced attacks*, pp. 1–251. Springfield, IL: Charles C. Thomas.

Bleasel, A.F., Van Ness, P.C. & So, N.K. (1993a): Interictal and ictal scalp EEG in patients with supplementary motor seizures. The American EEG Society Meeting, New Orleans, 11–12 October 1993.

Bleasel, A.F., So, N.K., Van Ness, P.C., Comair, Y.G. & Lüders, H.O. (1993): The clinical syndrome of seizures arising from the supplementary motor area. *Epilepsia* **34** (suppl. 6), 54.

Buser, P., Bancaud, J. & Chauvel, P. (1992): Callosal transfer between mesial frontal areas in frontal lobe epilepsies. In: *Frontal lobe seizures and epilepsies*, eds. P. Chauvel, A.V. Delgado-Escueta, E. Halgren & J. Bancaud. *Adv. neurol.* **57,** 589–604.

Chee, M.W.L., Kotagal, P., Van Ness, P.C., Gragg, L., Murphy, D. & Lüders, H.O. (1993): Lateralizing signs in intractable partial epilepsy: blinded multiple observer analysis. *Neurology* **43,** 2519–2525.

Heinz, E.R., Heinz, T.R., Radtke, R. Darwin, R., Drayer, B.P., Fram, E., & Djang, W.T. (1988): Efficacy of MR vs. CT in epilepsy. *AJNR* **9,** 1123–1128.

Jabbari, B., Gunderson, C.H., Wippold, F., Citrin, C., Sherman, J., Bartoszek, D., Daigh, J.D. & Mitchell, M.H. (1986): Magnetic resonance imaging in partial complex epilepsy. *Arch. Neurol.* **43,** 869–872.

Jayakar, P., Duchowny, M., Resnick, T.J. & Alvarez, L.A. (1991): Localization of seizure foci: pitfalls and caveats. *J. Clin. Neurophysiol.* **8,** 414–431.

Kosmides, R.W., Van Ness, P.C. & Turnbull, J. (1993): Clinical correlates of discordance for language and motor dominance determined by the intracarotid amytal test in neocortical focal epilepsies. The American Epilepsy Society Meeting, Miami, FL, 3–9 December 1993 (in press).

Latack, J.T., Abou-Khalil, B.W., Siegel, G.J., Sackellares, J.C., Gabrielsen, T.O. & Aisen, A.M. (1986): Patients with partial seizures: evaluation by MR, CT, and PET imaging. *Radiology* **159,** 159–163.

Laxer, K.D., Rowley, H.A., Novotny, E.J., Gates, J.R., Sato, S., Sutherling, W.W., Elger, C.E., Ebersole, J.S. & Stefan, H. (1993): Experimental technologies. In: *Surgical treatment of the epilepsies,* 2nd edn, ed. J. Engel, Jr, pp. 291–308. New York: Raven Press.

Lesser, R.P., Modic, M.T., Weinstein, M.A., Duchesneau, G.M., Lüders, H., Dinner, D.S., Morris, H.H., Estes, M., Chou, S.M. & Hahn, J.F. (1986): Magnetic resonance imaging (1.5 tesla) in patients with intractable focal seizures. *Arch. Neurol.* **43,** 367–371.

Lüders, H., Awad, I., Burgess, R., Wyllie, E. & Van Ness, P. (1992): Subdural electrodes in the presurgical evaluation for surgery of epilepsy. In: *Surgical treatment of epilepsy* (*Epilepsy Res.* Sup. 5), ed. W.H. Theodore, pp. 147–156. Amsterdam: Elsevier.

Morris, H.H., III, Dinner, D.S., Lüders, H., Wyllie, E. & Kramer, R. (1988): Supplementary motor seizures: clinical and electroencephalographic findings. *Neurology* **38,** 1075–1082.

Pedley, T.A., Tharp, B.R. & Herman, K. (1981): Clinical and electroencephalographic characteristics of midline parasagittal foci. *Ann. Neurol.* **9,** 142–149.

Penfield, W. & Welch, K. (1951): The supplementary motor area of the cerebral cortex. *Arch. Neurol. Psychiat.*ry **66,** 289–317.

Schörmer, W., Meencke, H.J. & Felix, R. (1987): Temporal lobe epilepsy: comparison of CT and MR imaging. *AJR* **149,** 1231–1239.

Sutherling, W.W., Risinger, M.W., Crandall, P.H., Becker, D.P., Baumgartner, C., Cahan, L.D., Wilson, C. & Levesque, M.F. (1990): Focal functional anatomy of dorsolateral frontocentral seizures. *Neurology* **40,** 87–98.

Swartz, B.E., Halgren, E., Delgado-Escueta, A.V., Mandelkern, M., Gee, M, Quinionez, N., Blahd, W.H. & Repchan, J. (1989): Neuroimaging in patients with seizures of probable frontal lobe origin. *Epilepsia* **30,** 547–558.

Talairach, J., Tournoux, P., Musolino, A. & Missr, O. (1992): Stereotaxic exploration in frontal epilepsy. In: *Frontal lobe seizures and epilepsies,* eds. P. Chauvel, A.V. Delgado-Escueta, E. Halgren & J. Bancaud. *Adv. Neurol.* **57,** 651–688.

Theodore, W.H., Dorwart, R., Holmes, M., Porter, R.J. & DiChiro, G. (1986): Neuroimaging in refractory partial seizures: comparison of PET, CT, and MRI. *Neurology* **36,** 750–759.

Tükel, K. & Jasper, H. (1952): The electroencephalogram in parasagittal lesion. *Electroencephalogr. Clin. Neurophysiol.* **4,** 480–494.

Tuxhorn, I., Van Ness, P.C. & Lüders, H.O. (1992): Supplementary motor area seizures: EEG patterns with interhemispheric subdural plate electrodes. *Neurology* **42** (Suppl. 3), 158.

Van Ness, P.C. (1992): Surgical outcome in neocortical (extrahippocampal) focal epilepsy. In: *Epilepsy surgery,* ed. H.O. Lüders, pp. 613–624. New York: Raven Press.

Van Ness, P.C., Awad I.A., Lüders H.O. & Hahn, J.F. (1990): The relationship of epileptogenic zone resection, lesion resection and outcome in 27 cases with neocortical epilepsy. *Ann. Neurol.* **28,** 263.

Van Ness, P.C., Kosmides, R.W. & Turnbull, J. (1993a): Intracarotid amytal test memory abnormalities are common in neocortical focal epilepsies. The American Epilepsy Society Meeting, Miami, FL, 3–9 December 1993 (in press).

Van Ness, P.C., So, N.K., Bleasel, A., Comair, Y.G., Awad, I.A., Morris, H.H., Lüders, H.O. & Tuxhorn, I. (1993b): Epilepsy surgery outcome with supplementary motor seizures. *Ann. Neurol.* **34,** 262.

Veilleux, F., Saint-Hilaire, J.M., Giard, N., Turmel, A., Bernier, G.P., Rouleau, I., Mercier, M. & Bouvier, G. (1992): Seizures of the human medial frontal lobe. In frontal lobe seizures and epilepsies, eds. P. Chauvel, A.V. Delgado-Escueta, E. Halgren & J. Bancaud, *Adv. Neurol.* **57,** 245–255.

Waterman, K., Purves, S.J., Kosuka, B., Strauss, E. & Wada, J.A. (1987): An epileptic syndrome caused by mesial frontal lobe foci. *Neurology* **37,** 577–582.

Williamson, P.D. (1992): Frontal lobe seizures: problems of diagnosis and classification. In: *Frontal lobe seizures and epilepsies,* eds. P. Chauvel, A.V. Delgado-Escueta, E. Halgren & J. Bancaud. *Adv. Neurol.* **57,** 289–309.

Epileptic Seizures and Syndromes, Edited by Peter Wolf
© 1994 John Libbey & Company Ltd., pp. 331–334

Chapter 36

The spectrum of frontal lobe seizures: with a note on frontal lobe syndromatology

Patrick Chauvel[*,†] and Jean Bancaud[†]

[*]*Clinique Neurologique et INSERM CJF 90-12, Hôpital Pontchaillou, 35000 Rennes;* [†]*Service de Neurochirurgie et INSERM U 97, Hôpital Sainte-Anne, 75014 Paris, France*

Jean Bancaud died suddenly on 26 April 1993. The present lines, which summarize an approach to a possible anatomical classification of frontal lobe seizures, are essentially inspired by his teaching. They are dedicated to his memory. P.C.

There remain a number of difficulties in delineating the various syndromes of frontal lobe (FL) epilepsy (FLE). This results, in clinical practice, in frequent misleading identification and classification of their ictal symptoms. With the exception of precentral seizures, the task of establishing correlations between clinical signs and the anatomical/electrical organization of the seizure discharge is usually a complex one. The peculiarity of certain clinical ictal patterns during anterior FL seizures (FLS) can make the differential diagnosis with psychiatric diseases or movement or sleep disorders a difficult one (Broglin *et al.*, 1992).

Individual signs or groups of signs are of little localizing value. Their individual characters are insufficient in themselves to reliably indicate the anatomical origin of the ictal discharge which generates them. Except for the case of primary areas, a given single sign is not necessarily produced by a discharge from a single area. Nor is it possible, by analysing a patient population who have successfully undergone FL surgery, to directly infer the FLS symptomatology from the localization of the cortectomy (Rasmussen, 1983; Talairach *et al.*, 1992).

This is due to the special features of the FLS spread: in the case of a high-frequency discharge, this spread is very fast, within the same lobe, to the contralateral FL, and to the ipsilateral parietal lobe, as well as to the related subcortical structures, and from certain localizations to the temporal lobe. In the case of rhythmic spike-and-wave discharges, the localization seems more stable from the onset, but in this case also tends to be widespread and bilateral (Tükel & Jasper, 1952; Bancaud, 1972).

For the above reasons, the main recent contributions to the anatomical categorization of FLS have come from seizures recorded presurgically with intracerebral electrodes.

There is a general agreement that *posterior FLS* are those basically characterized by motor symptomatology. Recent reports review the distinctive signs of precentral and premotor seizures, while emphasizing the interconnections between these two areas (Ajmone-Marsan & Goldhammer, 1973; Chauvel *et al.*, 1992a). Seizures from the *precentral* area can present several patterns:

– partial myoclonus (uni- or bilateral), predominantly distal
– simple partial motor seizures, tonic–clonic with Jacksonian march (rare)
– tonic postural motor seizures, associated with clonic movements: unilateral, or bilateral and asymmetric
– partial unilateral clonic seizures

Seizures from the *premotor* areas consist of tonic and postural seizures, predominant in upper limbs, with contralateral or ipsilateral adversion. When there is propagation to the primary motor area, this may be associated with unilateral or bilateral, symmetric or asymmetric clonic jerks. For historical reasons, supplementary motor area (SMA) seizures have often been confounded with the result of electrical stimulation of the SMA, and have therefore been artificially distinguished and described separately (Penfield & Welch, 1951). They are mainly postural, with a bilateral (though asymmetric) involvement of limb girdles, adversion of head and eyes, speech arrest or vocalization. In fact, the pure 'classical' SMA seizure is rare (Morris *et al.*, 1988; Chauvel *et al.*, 1992a).

Seizures often arise from the precentral *and* premotor areas (i.e. an epileptogenic zone involving both). The frequency of this situation (approx. 50 per cent) should be underlined.

Seizures from the inferior frontal gyrus in its posterior part are worth special recognition. Because of frequent propagation to the nearby operculoinsular region, motor symptoms are associated with autonomic manifestations. In the non-dominant hemisphere, these seizures are characterized by speech arrest, tonic–clonic facial and brachial movements, facial clonic jerks (contralateral or ipsilateral), brachial postural manifestations, salivation, deglutition and sometimes other autonomic signs (respiratory discomfort, then polypnea; tachycardia, mydriasis). A postictal contralateral facial deficit contributes to the diagnosis. In the dominant hemisphere, the symptomatology is identical to the non-dominant side, except that it can be associated with ictal vocalization or dysarthria, and with postictal aphasia and anarthria.

A very early frontal opercular and insular propagation is generally marked by the presence of gustatory hallucinations or illusions, and by various autonomic signs or symptoms: abdominal-epigastric and pharyngeal sensations, salivation, deglutition, mastication; hyperpnea, a choking sensation, tachycardia or palpitations, cephalic aura, mydriasis.

Seizures originating from the *intermediate FL* (IFLS) are more difficult to localize because of the multidirectional spread of the ictal discharge.

The symptomatology of *dorsolateral* IFLS reflects the specific organization of this region in relation to the frontal eye field (Quesney *et al.*, 1992). The so-called 'forced thinking' subjective phenomena reported by the patients actually are 'eye-orientated' obsessive thoughts, with forced actions directed by the attracted gaze (semipurposeful 'automatisms' involving the upper limbs), and pseudo-compulsive behaviour (with spread to medial IFL). Ictal discharges in this region can also lead to complex visual illusions, often abstract and intellectual, without the specific characteristics of occipital elementary hallucinations or illusions. Tonic deviation of the eyes, preceding head adversion (frontal eye field) are frequently observed, associated or not with complex tonic postural manifestations, which may be bilateral and asymmetric. When autonomic signs occur, they are generally late in the ictal clinical sequence. Secondary tonic–clonic generalization is very frequent in dorsolateral IFLS.

Medial IFLS take the form of two remarkable patterns, which have been described in terms of 'frontal absences' and 'complex motor seizures' (Bancaud & Talairach, 1992).

'Frontal absences' (with spread to lateral IFL) are characterized by speech and movement arrest, alteration of consciousness, mild gestural stereotypes, possible adversion and brisk recovery of contact. 'Complex motor seizures' typically comprise the association of bilateral motor tonic postural signs with gestural automatisms. The alteration of consciousness is variable, and adversion of head and eyes, tonic postural manifestations, autonomic signs (urination), gestural stereotypes and secondary tonic–clonic generalization are associated in various ways. Where there are bilateral tonic discharges, tonic axial and postural seizures with drop attacks (coincident with medial and lateral bilateral discharge) may occur.

Anterior cingulate gyrus (area 24) seizures have been identified mainly from data recorded after direct electrical stimulation of this region (Talairach *et al.*, 1973). The symptomatology described consisted of a facial expression of fear, complex vocalizations, complex gestural sequences or gesticulations, emotional manifestations, various autonomic symptoms and sometimes visual hallucinations, with variable alteration of consciousness.

Seizures originating exclusively in this area seem to be very rare (Wieser *et al.*, 1992). For anatomical reasons, direct evidence for origin in the anterior cingulate gyrus is difficult to obtain. Conversely, this area is frequently involved in seizures originating from limbic frontal and temporal areas, as well as from the adjacent SMA. It therefore represents a common relay for connections with various neocortical areas of the convexity.

The symptomatology of *anterior FLS* has been more recently delineated (Geier *et al.*, 1977). A distinction between polar and orbital seizures has been suggested, a separation which may be artificial, except in terms of their respective aetiological factors.

Seizures of *frontopolar* origin are most often due to trauma. They are characterized by an immediate loss of contact, the face becoming inexpressive and the gaze fixed. There is sudden flexion of the head and sometimes the trunk. A massive loss of tone and sudden fall can follow, with tonic or tonic–clonic motor manifestations. Atypical absences, tonic axial seizures, or complex postural signs can represent other patterns of paroxysmal activation of this region, when it is bilaterally involved in the seizure discharge.

It is still open to debate whether or not the so-called 'complex partial seizures of frontal origin' (Williamson *et al.*., 1985) are actually *orbitofrontal* seizures. Their onset is occasionally marked by an olfactory hallucination, and impairment of consciousness associated with automatisms has been regularly observed. This has been attributed to spread of the ictal discharge to mesial temporal structures (Quesney *et al.*, 1992). In fact, some distinctive characteristics help differentiate complex partial seizures of frontal from those of temporal origin (Wieser *et al.*, 1992). In the former, no early oroalimentary automatisms appear, whereas motor automatisms of the limbs are prominent. The seizures are brief and repetitive, occurring in clusters, with rapid recovery of consciousness between ictal episodes. More or less elaborate patterns of automatism can be observed, from simple, often asymmetrical gestural stereotypes, to complex gestural sequences with bizane gesticulations and shouting, with eupraxic pseudointentional behaviours (Geier *et al.*, 1976). A common trait of these 'automatisms', in exceptional cases reported by the patient, is their apparent organization into 'forced actions'. Some of these seizures are preceded by vague warnings. Others start briskly with a sensation of intense fear, followed by vocalization and violent movements (sometimes aggressive) of the whole body (Waterman *et al.*, 1987), as if the patient were experiencing a frightening hallucination. This emotional or pseudoemotional (with no awareness in most cases) ictal behaviour is generally seen with autonomic signs, such as respiratory changes, facial flushing or pallor, and mydriasis. Perictal urination is typical for involvement of this region.

This attempt to outline the clinical features of seizures of FL origin does not provide a ready-made catalogue of FLS syndromes. In surgical series, most of the FLE cases are symptomatic (63 per cent in Talairach's last series: Talairach *et al.*, 1992). Aetiologies appear to be non-specific for the FL. There is, however, a notably high frequency of post-traumatic and post infectious epilepsies. There is no proof to date of any idiopathic FLE syndrome. However, among the 37 per cent of FLE without identified causes, there are a certain number whose seizures appear to originate from FL limbic or paralimbic areas, which share some evolutive and symptomatological traits. These characteristics may eventually allow the identification of specific syndromes (Chauvel *et al.*, 1992b).

The preceding remarks have essentially given a classical approach to FL 'partial' symptomatology. No extensive discussion of the concepts of 'frontal absences' or 'tonic axial seizures' has been attempted. There is no question, in our opinion, that a large proportion of the syndromes today described under the heading of 'generalized' epilepsies are in fact focal seizures of frontal origin, even though the specific mechanisms of their ictal discharge synchronization are determined by subcortical, thalamic and mesencephalic neuronal networks.

References

Ajmone-Marsan, C. & Goldhammer, L. (1973): Clinical ictal patterns and electrographic data in cases of partial seizures of frontal-central-parietal origin. In: *Epilepsy: its phenomena in man*, ed. M.A.B. Brazier, pp. 235–258. New York/London: Academic Press.

Bancaud, J. (1972): Mechanisms of cortical discharges in 'generalized' epilepsies in man. In: *Synchronization of EEG activity in epilepsies*, eds. H. Petsche & M.A.B. Brazier, pp. 368–381. Vienna: Springer.

Bancaud, J. & Talairach, J. (1992): Clinical semiology of frontal lobe seizures. In: *Adv. Neurol.* **57,** 3–58.

Broglin, D., Delgado-Escueta, A.V., Walsh, G.O., Bancaud, J. & Chauvel, P. (1992): Clinical approach to the patient with seizures and epilepsies of frontal origin. *Adv. Neurol.* **57,** 59–88.

Chauvel, P., Trottier, S., Vignal, J.P. & Bancaud, J. (1992a): Somatomotor seizures of frontal lobe origin. *Adv. Neurol.* **57,** 185–232.

Chauvel, P., Delgado-Escueta, A.V., Halgren, E. & Bancaud, J. (1992b): Frontal lobe seizures and epilepsies. In: *Advances in neurology*, Vol. 57, p. 750. New York: Raven Press.

Geier, S., Bancaud, J., Talairach, J., Bonis, A., Enjelvin, M. & Hossard-Bouchaud, H. (1976): Automatisms during frontal lobe epileptic seizures. *Brain* **99,** 447–458.

Geier, S., Bancaud, J., Talairach, J., Bonis, A., Szikla, G. & Enjelvin, M. (1977): The seizures of frontal lobe epilepsy: a study of clinical manifestations. *Neurology* **27,** 951–958.

Morris, H.H., Dinner, D.S., Lüders, H., Wyllie, E. & Krainer, R. (1988): Supplementary motor seizures: clinical and electroencephalographic findings. *Neurology* **38,** 1075–1082.

Penfield, W. & Welch, K. (1951): The supplementary motor area of the cerebral cortex: a clinical and experimental study. *Arch. Neurol. Psychiatry* **66,** 289–317.

Quesney, L.F., Constain, M. & Rasmussen, T. (1992): Seizures from the dorso-lateral frontal lobe. *Adv. Neurol.* **57,** 233–243.

Rasmussen, T. (1983): Characteristics of a pure culture of frontal lobe epilepsy. *Epilepsia* **24,** 482–493.

Talairach, J., Bancaud, J. & Geier, S. (1973): The cingulate gyrus and human behavior. *Electroencephalogr. Clin. Neurophysiol.* **34,** 644–649.

Talairach, J., Bancaud, J., Bonis, A., Szikla, G., Trottier, S., Vignal, J.P., Chauvel, P., Munari, C. & Chodkiewicz, J.P. (1992): Surgical therapy for frontal epilepsies. *Adv. Neurol.* **57,** 707–732.

Tükel, K. & Jasper, H. (1952): The electroencephalogram in parasagittal lesions. *Electroencephalogr. Clin. Neurophysiol.* **4,** 481–494.

Waterman, K., Purves, S.J., Kosaka, B., Strauss, E. & Wada, J.A. (1987): An epileptic syndrome caused by mesial frontal lobe seizure foci. *Neurology* **37,** 577–582.

Wieser, H.G., Swarz, B.E., Delgado-Escueta, A.V., Bancaud, J., Walsh, G.O., Maldonado, H. & Saint-Hilaire, J.M. (1992): Differentiating frontal lobe seizures from temporal lobe seizures. *Adv. Neurol.* **57,** 267–285.

Williamson, P.D., Spencer D.D., Spencer S.S., Novelly R.A. & Mattson, R.H. (1985): Complex partial seizures of frontal lobe origin. *Ann. Neurol.* **18,** 497–504.

Epileptic Seizures and Syndromes, Edited by Peter Wolf
© 1994 John Libbey & Company Ltd., pp. 335–357

Chapter 37

Analysis of clinical symptomatology during stereo-EEG recorded mesiotemporal lobe seizures

Claudio Munari[*†‡], Laura Tassi[†], Philippe Kahane[*†], Stefano Francione[*§], Matilde Di Leo[†] and Pierpaolo Quarato[†¶]

[*]*INSERM U 318, CHRU de Grenoble, BP 217X, 38043 Grenoble Cedex, France;* [†]*Département des Neurosciences Cliniques et Biologiques de Grenoble BP 217X, 38043 Grenoble Cedex, France;* [‡]*Istituto di Clinica Neurochirurgica, Università di Genova, Ospedale San Martino, Italy;* [§]*Cattedra di Neurofisiopatologia, Università di Genova, Italy;* [¶]*III Clinica Neurologica, Università 'La Sapienza' di Roma, Viale Policlinico, Italy*

Summary

Twenty-five consecutive patients (pts), candidates for surgical treatment for focal epilepsy, were selected on the following criteria:

- temporal origin of all the stereo-EEG-recorded seizures (S);
- surgical intervention on the temporal lobe (TL);
- postoperative follow-up of at least 18 months.

Fifty-seven spontaneous S were recorded in 20 pts: in all of them, at least one S simultaneously started in both mesial and neocortical TL areas (total: 33, as 58 per cent). Initial discharges could only affect: mesial TL structures: 15 S (8 pts); neocortical TL areas: 10 S (5 pts). Clinical symptomatology of MTL limited S was only subjective (mostly an epigastric sensation), without any loss of contact. The most frequent initial electrical change was a low-voltage fast activity. Low-frequency electrical stimulations provoked 11 mesial TLS (6 pts) with identical clinical pattern. The 18 mesial TLS (13 pts) induced by high-frequency electrical stimulation were clinically more complex, whatever the spreading of the discharges might be.

Simultaneous intracerebral recordings of mesial and lateral temporal cortical areas, coupled with intensive direct clinical monitoring, seem able to:

- increase our knowledge on precise anatomo-electro-clinical correlations;
- improve the definition of the epileptogenic area and, consequently, surgical results.

Introduction

Anterior temporal lobectomy is the surgical procedure most frequently performed in patients with severe, drug-resistant, focal epilepsy: respectively 68 per cent and 59 per cent of the interventions carried out before 1985 and between 1986 and 1990 (Engel & Shewmon, 1993). A 'standardized' resection is the most diffuse intervention, but more limited removals have been proposed, of mesial (Yasargil *et al.*, 1985) as well as of lateral neocortical areas (Hardiman *et al.*, 1988), whereas other authors adapt the excision to the individual characteristics of each single patient (Talairach *et al.*, 1974).

In spite of general agreement on the great localizing value of *ictal* recordings (Quesney & Gloor, 1985), it is still unclear if, how and when such data really play a role in the definition of the extent of the surgical removal (Ojemann, 1993; Polkey, 1993). Data obtained during stereo-electroencephalographic (stereo-EEG) investigations (Bancaud *et al.* 1965) could allow the strict correlation between anatomically well localized ictal discharges and ictal clinical symptomatology (Stoffels *et al.*, 1980; Bossi *et al.*, 1984; Tassi *et al.*, 1991;): such information, particularly in temporal lobe (TL) seizures, could improve our knowledge on the anatomo-electro-clinical correlations, and then progressively reduce diagnostic presurgical 'invasive' procedures.

The aim of this study is, first, to verify if ictal electrical discharges *starting and remaining in* mesiotemporal lobe (MTL) structures are frequent. At the same time, we will try to identify the possible ictal clinical features occurring when such discharges are well localized in MTL only.

Materials and methods

Between March 1990 and January 1993, 114 patients suffering from a severe drug-resistant focal epilepsy were operated on in Grenoble. The methodology of investigation was largely derived from that elaborated by J. Bancaud and J. Talairach in Paris (Talairach *et al.*, 1958; Bancaud, 1959), the

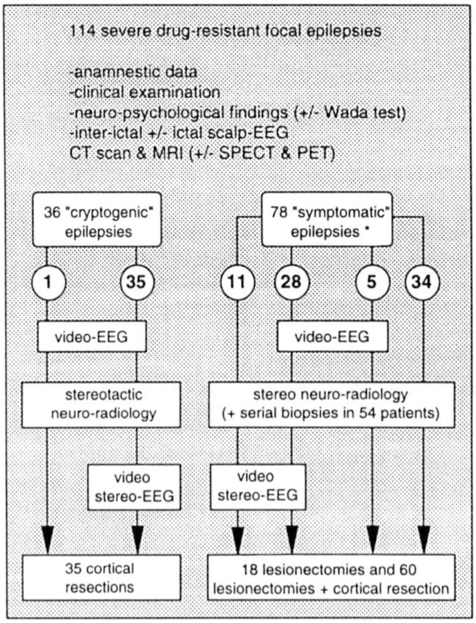

*Fig. 1. Presurgical and surgical strategies used at the Neurosciences Department and INSERM Research Unit U318 of Grenoble Hospital. * One of these patients was operated on twice and only the presurgical and surgical strategies used the second time were considered.*

purpose being to define, on the basis of anatomoelectroclinical correlations, the extent of cortical areas primarily involved by ictal discharges – the 'epileptogenic zone' (EZ) – in order to propose an individually tailored cortical excison (Talairach *et al.*, 1974).

The strategies used were adapted to the particular characteristics of each single patient, as shown in Fig. 1. Schematically, the successive steps of the presurgical evaluation, discussed for each case, combined several clinical, anatomical and neurophysiological data, among which ictal video-EEG recordings were of particular importance (Bancaud *et al.*, 1973; Tassi *et al.*, 1993). This approach then included, in less than two-thirds of the cases, a 'chronic' implantation of multilead intracerebral electrodes (Munari *et al.*, 1993a), the stereotactic placement and number of which were decided not only in order to verify the origin of ictal discharges, but also to appreciate their early spreading (video-stereo-EEG) (Munari & Bancaud, 1985).

Table 1. General characteristics of the 25 patients studied

Pts	Sex	Age	Onset	Duration	Freq/m	ATCD	TLE
1. MC	m	31	14	17	4.5	HT	R
2. PC	m	25	7	18	5	FC	R
3. CBt	f	25	10	15	15	–	R
4. FN	f	36	28	8	20	–	R
5. RD	m	27	18	9	6	–	R
6. MM	m	26	1	25	6	CNS inf	R
7. FF	m	24	2	22	14.5	–	L
8. CBg	f	25	7	18	12.5	FC	R
9. RC	m	26	19	7	14	–	R
10. LP	f	31	6	25	25	FC	R
11. AR	f	24	2	22	120	–	R
12. PF	f	31	19	12	30	–	R
13. EB	f	13	1	12	8	–	R
14. MR	m	38	18	20	4.5	–	R
15. AB	m	21	2	19	17	Perinat	R
16. MG	f	29	1	28	30	FC	L
17. NB	m	10	6	4	100	–	R
18. IP	f	16	10	6	20	FC	R
19. DD	m	17	1	16	30	–	L
20. SA	f	33	31	2	30	–	R
21. JL	m	38	18	20	10	–	R
22. DR	f	46	15	31	30	–	R
23. MN	f	44	12	32	8	CNS inf	R
24. GB	f	28	16	12	15	–	R
25. MV	m	20	4	16	30	–	L

Pts: identification number and initials of patients; m: male; f: female; age at surgery (Age) and at seizure onset (Onset) and epilepsy duration (Duration) are expressed in years; Freq/m: seizure frequency per month; ATCD: antecedents; HT: severe head trauma; FC: febrile convulsions; CNS inf: central nervous system infection; Perinat: perinatal injury; TLE: temporal lobe epilepsy: R: right; L left. Cases 1 to 12 represent the cryptogenic group and cases 13 to 25 the symptomatic one.

Population

For the present study, we selected the 25 operated patients who

- were suffering from a (TLE)
- as defined on the basis of a previously performed *video-stereo-EEG study*
- and whose postoperative *follow-up surpassed 18 months.*

This population (see the general characteristics of each patient in Table 1) has been subdivided into two groups, according to whether an anatomical lesion (AL) had been preoperatively found by magnetic resonance imaging (MRI) or not. The cryptogenic group (CGr) comprises 12 patients without any clear morphological abnormality, while the symptomatic group (SGr) includes the 13 patients for which a signal alteration was found in a TL. There are no statistically significant differences between these two groups (unpaired student's *t*-test) concerning the age, both at surgery and at seizure onset, the epilepsy duration and the seizure frequency (Table 2). The sex ratio was equivalent in CGr and SGr. There were no familial antecedents of epilepsy. Febrile convulsions were reported in 3/12 of CGr and 2/13 of SGr. Neurological and neuropsychological examination was normal in all but one case (left superior quadrantanopia). No major psychiatric disturbances were noted. One patient (no. 2) was left-handed.

Table 2. Comparison between the cryptogenic and the symptomatic groups regarding age at surgery and at seizure onset, epilepsy duration and seizure frequency

	Age	Onset	Duration	Freq/m
CGr + SGr = 25 pts	27.4 ± 8.9 (10–46)	10.7 ± 8.6 (1–31)	16.6 ± 8.1 (2–32)	24.2 ± 27.6 (4.5–120)
CGr = 12 pts	27.6 ± 3.8 (24–36)	11.1 ± 8.5 (1–28)	16.5 ± 6.4 (7–25)	22.7 ± 31.7 (4.5–120)
SGr = 13 pts	27.2 ± 12.0 (10–46)	10.4 ± 9.1 (1–31)	16.8 ± 9.7 (2–32)	25.6 ± 24.4 (4.5–100)

Age at surgery (Age) and at seizure onset (Onset) and epilepsy duration (Duration) are expressed in years, and seizure frequency (Freq/m) in number of fits per month. The mean values are given ± standard deviation (minimum–maximum). CGr: cryptogenic group; SGr: symptomatic group.

The origin of ictal discharges was right-sided in 21/25 patients (11/12 for CGr and 10/13 for SGr). The definition of the 'epileptogenic area' was apparently clear in all patients but one (no. 18), whose 'visual' manifestations were not completely elucidated. In another patient (no. 24), some subjective signs (hypersalivation and pharyngeal wring) evoked a suprasylvian opercular involvement, but we have not been able to document, during stereo-EEG, a suprasylvian early participation.

All patients had a tailored temporal cortical resection including the entire AL in all but one (no. 25) of the symptomatic patients. The removal of the epileptogenic area was voluntarily incomplete in two symptomatic patients: in one (no. 20), since she, a colleague, did not want to miss the anterior part of her epileptic hippocampus, in the other one (no. 25), because the epileptogenic area included speech areas. Specimens of the various removed cortical areas, classified on the basis of stereo-EEG data, underwent histopathological examination and molecular biology research (F. Berger *et al.*, in preparation).

Table 3. Lesion location and pathological diagnosis in the symptomatic group

Pts	Lesion location	Pathological diagnosis
13. EB	R anteromesial	Astrocytoma I
14. MR	R polar	Gangliocytoma I
15. AB	R posteromesial	Gliosis
16. MG	L posteromesial	Ganglioglioma I
17. NB	R polar	Oligodendroglioma II
18. IP	R polar	Ganglioglioma I
19. DD	L anteromesial	Oligodendroglioma I
20. SA	R polar	Cavernous angioma
21. JL	R posteromesial	Astrocytoma I
22. DR	R anteromesial	Astrocytoma I
23. MN	R posterior	Astrocytoma II
24. GB	R external	Astrocytoma I
25. MV	L extended	DNE tumour*

Pts: identification number and initials of patients; R: right; L left. *Dysembryoplastic neuroepithelial tumour.

Morphological data showed diffuse, mesial *and* lateral, gliosis with reduction of the neuronal population in CGr patients, except in one case (no. 12) in which a very small right anteroexternal temporal hamartoma was discovered (B. Pasquier *et al.*, in preparation). In SGr patients low-grade gliomas were mostly found (Table 3).

After more than 18 months' follow-up (M: 28.5 months, SD: 5.5, min: 18, max 37), all the CGr patients (12/12) are seizure-free, as well as 9/13 (69 per cent) of the SGr. Thus, 21 patients (84 per cent) are seizure-free (class IA of Engel's classification, 1987). Three patients (nos. 18, 20, 24) (12 per cent), all in SGr, still have some episodic 'auras' (class IB) similar to those observed preoperatively, even if more rare. The persistence of some subjective manifestations (the term of 'simple partial seizures' would be preferred to 'auras') in these cases could be explained by the deliberately spared hippocampus in one, and by the insufficient presurgical definition of the epileptogenic area in the other two. The possibility of persisting auras was preoperatively announced to two of them (nos. 20, 24). The patient (no. 25) with incomplete removal of both the lesion and the epileptogenic area, had a partial epileptic status 2 weeks after the intervention, lasting 6 days. Seizures have now recurred, after he had remained seizure-free for 16 months.

Methods

The following data were available in all cases: clinical interictal and ictal findings, as described by the patients themselves and their families, neuropsychological evaluation, interictal (and often ictal) scalp EEG recordings and neuroimaging studies (computerized tomography, CT scan; magnetic resonance imaging, MRI).

A video-EEG study was judged necessary in the large majority of cases (23/25), before stereo-EEG investigations, in order to clarify the ictal EEG and clinical symptomatology. In two SGr patients (nos. 19, 24), anatomoelectroclinical features were considered clear enough to plan the strategy of intracerebral electrode implantation.

Following these prestereo-EEG steps, all patients underwent stereotactic stereoscopic neuroradiological investigations (Munari *et al.*, 1987), including serial stereotactic biopsies (Munari & Betti, 1989; Lo Russo & Munari, 1992) in seven. Electrode implantation was performed at a second time. These stereotactic procedures were conducted according to the previously described methodology (Munari, 1987; Munari *et al.*, 1993a), with a technical specificity consisting in the systematic utilization of a computer-driven robot, whose characteristics and advantages have already been described (Benabid *et al.*, 1987, 1992).

Anatomical distribution of the intracerebral electrodes

In the 25 patients, seven to 12 intracerebral electrodes (mean: 10) were stereotactically implanted. Each semirigid electrode (Dixi, Besançon, France) had a diameter of 0.9 mm, and comprised five to 15 leads of 2 mm length, 1.5 mm apart. A lateral orthogonal trajectory (Talairach *et al.*, 1967) was possible in the great majority of cases; an oblique one was judged necessary for 5/247 electrodes. This makes it possible to reach, without any theoretical restriction, anatomical lesions of various locations and almost every cortical or deep brain structure supposed to be involved by the ictal discharges. The possibility to obtain simultaneous information on mesial and lateral structures of different lobes (Table 4) provided a 'three-dimensional' appreciation of ictal discharges. In CGr, three to nine extratemporal cortical sites (mean: seven) were explored; in SGr they varied between one and eight (mean: 4.5/patient). Implantation was unilateral in 23/25 cases, and bilateral but largely asymmetrical for the remaining two (nos 4, 21), one of them being symptomatic.

Video-stereo-EEG recordings

Depth EEG was obtained by bipolar recordings out of contiguous leads. In two patients, the 'acute' exploration lasted 1 day and was conducted in the operative room. In the other 23 cases, procedures were performed in 'chronic' conditions, with a mean duration of about 15 days, allowing an exhaustive evaluation of clinical and EEG features.

We first tried to record spontaneous seizures: this required antiepileptic drug reduction in 32 per cent

Table 4. Anatomical structures explored in the 25 patients

Pts	TP	U	A	H	T1	T2	T3/4	F	Orb	aCG	Op	pCG	P	Occ	LL	PTO	Contra	No. elect
1. MC	1	–	1	2	2	3	–	–	–	–	1	1	1	–	–	–	–	8R
2. PC	–	–	1	1	2	2	–	1	–	1	2	1	3	–	–	–	–	10R
3.CBt	1	–	1	2	1	3	–	2	1	2	–	1	1	–	–	–	–	9R
4. FN	1	–	1	2	1	3	–	1	–	1	1	1	1	–	–	–	A + T2	8R+ 1L
5. RD	1	–	1	2	2	3	–	4	2	2	–	–	–	–	–	–	–	11R*
6. MM	1	–	1	2	2	3	–	2	1	2	1	–	–	–	–	–	–	10R
7. FF	1	–	1	1	1	2	–	1	1	1	1	1	1	–	–	–	–	8L
8. CBg	1	–	1	2	2	3	–	1	2	1	2	–	–	–	–	–	–	11R
9. RC	1	–	1	2	1	3	–	3	2	1	2	–	–	–	–	–	–	11R
10. LP	1	–	1	2	2	4	–	1	1	1	1	1	1	–	1	–	–	11R
11. AR	–	–	1	2	2	3	–	1	1	1	–	2	3	–	–	–	–	10R
12. PF	1	–	1	1	2	3	–	1	1	1	2	1	1	–	1	–	–	12R
13. EB	1	–	1	3	2	4	–	1	–	1	–	1	1	–	–	–	–	9R
14. MR	1	–	1	2	2	3	–	1	1	1	1	–	–	–	–	–	–	9R
15. AB	1	–	1	2	1	3	2	1	–	–	–	1	1	2	1	1	–	10R**
16. MG	1	–	1	2	1	4	–	1	–	1	1	1	1	–	1	–	–	9L
17. NB	1	–	1	2	2	3	–	–	1	0	1	1	1	–	–	–	–	10R
18. IP	1	1	1	1	2	4	–	1	1	1	1	1	1	–	1	1	–	11R
19. DD	1	1	1	1	1	4	–	–	1	–	–	–	–	–	–	–	–	7L
20. SA	1	–	1	2	2	4	2	2	1	2	–	1	1	2	–	–	–	10R
21. JL	–	–	1	2	–	4	1	–	–	–	–	1	1	–	1	–	H + T2	8R + 1L
22. DR	1	–	1	2	2	3	–	1	1	1	2	1	1	–	–	–	–	11R*
23. MN	–	–	1	2	1	4	2	–	–	–	1	1	2	–	1	–	–	10R*
24. GB	1	–	1	2	3	3	2	–	–	–	–	1	1	–	–	–	–	10R
25. MV	1	–	1	2	1	4	–	–	–	–	–	1	1	–	1	–	–	7L

Pts: identification number and initials of patients; TP: temporal pole; U: uncus; A: amygdala; H: hippocampus; T1, T2, T3, T4: first, second, third and fourth temporal convolutions; F: frontal cortex; Orb: orbital cortex; aCG, pCG: anterior and posterior cingulate gyrus; Op: suprasylvian, central opercular region; P: parietal cortex; Occ: occipital cortex; LL: lingual lobule; PTO: parietotemporo-occipital junction; Contra: contralateral explored structures; No.electr: total number of implanted electrodes.

* signifies that one and ** that two electrodes have been introduced using an oblique trajectory.

Cases 1 to 12 represent the cryptogenic group and cases 13 to 25 the symptomatic one.

of the cases (Francione *et al.*, 1992). Then, generally in the second week after implantation, both low- and high-frequency intracerebral electrical stimulation (LFES and HFES) were conducted in the majority of the cases, following our standard clinical and research practice. Electrical stimuli were delivered from a conventional rectangular pulse generator (World Precision Instruments, New Haven, USA) and performed between two contiguous leads, with alternating polarity. The main characteristics of these two types of electrical stimulation (ES) are shown in Table 5. Their operating conditions, advantages and limits have been described elsewhere (Kahane *et al.*, 1993a; Munari *et al.*, 1993b). One of the aims of these stimulations was to reproduce seizures whose clinical features were identical to the patient's known subjective symptoms and objective signs or similar to those observed during the spontaneous fits previously recorded, or both.

All the spontaneous and electrically elicited seizures recorded during stereo-EEG procedures were analysed using a time-synchronized audio-video-EEG system (BMSI, Campbell, USA). We would like to stress the necessity of an associated direct clinical intensive surveillance, in order to perform an ictal and immediately postictal clinical examination, and therefore to obtain precise electro-clinical correlates (Marchini *et al.*, 1989). In these conditions, it was possible:

- to identify the anatomical structures primarily involved by ictal discharges;
- to analyse the type of initial ictal electrical patterns recorded from these structures;
- to know if, how and when ictal discharges spread over different TL or extra-TL areas;
- to observe the initial ictal clinical signs or symptoms, their chronological sequence and their electrical correlates.

Table 5. Main characteristics of low- and high-frequency intracerebral electrical stimulation

	LFES	HFES
Frequency (pulse/s)	1	50
Pulse width (ms)	3	1
Intensity (mA)	0.25–4	0.25–4
Duration (s)	40	5–7

LFES and HFES: low- and high-frequency electrical stimulation. The mean duration of stimulation is given, but ES could become shorter if clinical manifestations occurred, or longer (as for LFES applied during neuropsychological tasks).

Table 6. Electroclinical characteristics of eight spontaneous seizures (six patients) involving only the mesiotemporal lobe structures at the occurrence of ictal clinical symptomatology

A		H		Time interval	Clinical signs	Extra-MTL spreading
^{2}LVFA	———	———	→	5 s	Epig + tach + hpn	No
^{2}LVFA	———	———	→	25 s	Epig + tach + hpn	No
^{19}LVFA	———	———	→	8 s	Ceph	No
^{10}LVFA	→	LVFA	→	7 s	Epig	T2
^{3}LVFA	→	PSp	→	20 s	Epig	No
^{2}Sp	→	Sp	→	9 s	Epig + nausea	No
^{6}LVFA	+	LVFA	→	4 s	Epig	T2
^{7}LVFA	+	LVFA	→	3 s	Epig	TL

A: amygdaloid nucleus; H: hippocampus; LVFA: low-voltage fast activity; PSp: polyspikes; Sp: spikes; Epig: epigastric sensation; tach: feeling of tachycardia; hpn: increase of the respiratory rhythm; Ceph: cephalic sensation; MTL: mesiotemporal lobe; T2: second temporal convolution; TL temporal lobe. Time interval refers to the delay between electrical and clinical onset. Superscript numerals refer to patients' identification numbers.

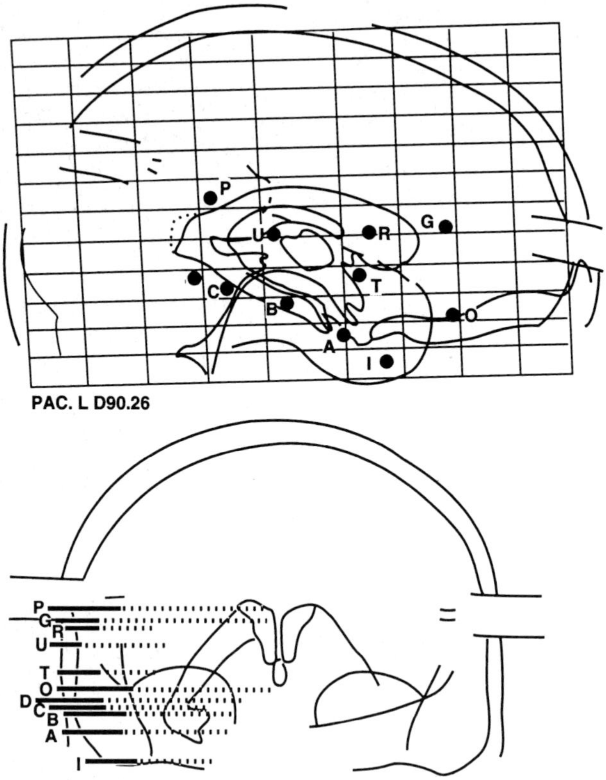

Fig. 2a. Stereotactic scheme (lateral and frontal view) of the patient LP (no.10), showing the location of the 11 intracerebral electrodes. Electrode placement: I: internal and external temporal pole; A: amygdala and anterior T2; B: anterior hippocampus and mid-T2; C: posterior hippocampus and posterior T2; D: gyrus lingualis and posterior T2; T: anterior T1; U: posterior T1; P: posterior parietal cingulate gyrus and parieto-temporal junction; R: precentral opercular region; G: anterior cingulate gyrus and second frontal convolution; O: internal and external posterior orbital cortex.

Results

In the 25 studied patients, 229 clinical seizures were recorded during stereo-EEG procedures, either spontaneous (57 in 20 pts, 1–9/pt) or induced by LFES (45 in 15 pts, 1–7/pt) or by HFES (127 in 24 pts, 1–17/pt).

Spontaneous seizures

In five patients, one (no. 11) in the CGr and four in the SGr (nos. 14, 16, 21, 22), no spontaneous seizures (SS) were recorded.

Among the 57 SS recorded in the remaining 20 patients, a well-localized initial ictal discharge *only* involved:

- MTL structures 15 times (nine patients);
- neocortical areas 9 times (four patients) or lingual lobule and neocortical areas (one patient).

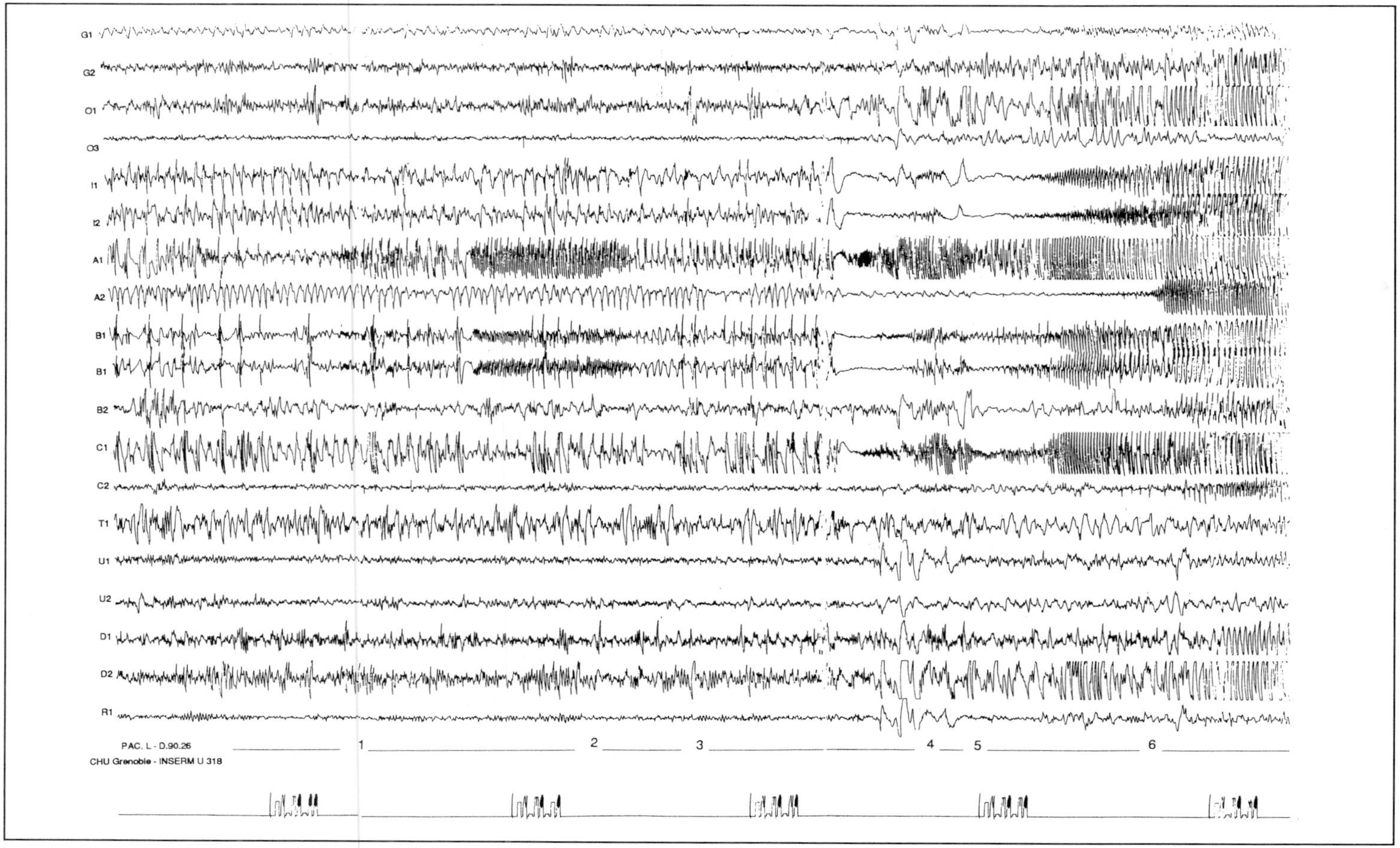

Fig. 2b. Same patient as in Fig. 2a. Example of spontaneous seizure, starting in the mesiotemporal structures. Clinically: 1. the patient looks at the observer; 2. she calls the observer; 3. she says 'I have my sensation' (a rising epigastric feeling); 4. she can denominate; 5. she can execute the given orders 6. she chews. Electrically: the ictal discharge simultaneously starts in anterior mesiotemporal lobe structures (amygdala and anterior hippocampus) (A1–B1) several seconds before the first ictal manifestation; this discharge will involve the other temporal structures (I1, I2, A2, B2, C1) only 25 s later.

In all of these 20 patients we recorded at least one SS (total: 33) with both MTL *and* lateral temporal neocortical areas *simultaneously and initially* involved.

'MTL seizures'

(a) In eight seizures (six patients), the discharge involved only MTL structures when the first clinical signs occurred (Table 6).

The amygdaloid nucleus (A) was always involved:

– three times alone, and there was never secondary extra-MTL cortical spreading;
– three times before the hippocampus (H);
– twice simultaneously with H; the discharges always spread over the temporal neocortex (TNCx) (Fig. 2b).

The more frequently recorded electrical pattern was a low-voltage fast activity (LVFA). The predominant ictal symptomatology was an epigastric sensation. The contact was never impaired during these limited discharges: this explains why patients can describe their subjective symptoms.

Figure 2b shows a well-localized mesiotemporal discharge in a CGr patient (no. 10) (see implantation strategy on Fig. 2a), describing her subjective symptomatology, started before the spreading of the discharge. Figure 2c shows another seizure in the same patient, simultaneously starting in both mesial and lateral temporal areas.

(b) In seven seizures (four patients), discharges primarily involved MTL structures, but the clinical symptomatology only occurred after the extra-MTL spreading (Table 7).

Table 7. Electro-clinical characteristics of seven spontaneous seizures (five patients) involving first the mesiotemporal lobe (MTL) structures but also extra-MTL regions when ictal clinical symptomatology occurred

A		H	Time interval	Extra-MTL spreading	Clinical signs
[8]LVFA	→	Sp	4 s	T1	Epig + nausea +
[19]LVFA	→	Sp	15 s	TP	OAA
		[19]LVFA	1 s	T2	Ceph + aud ill
		[4]LVFA	2 s	TP + T2	Ceph + aud ill
		[2]PSp	24 s	TP + T2	Epig + OAA + GA
		[8]PSp	14 s	TP + T2 + ET	Epig + fear + swall
[4]PSp	+	PSp	15 s	T2	Epig + fear + swall
					Shiver

A: amygdaloid nucleus; H: hippocampus; LVFA: low-voltage fast activity; Sp: spikes; PSp: polyspikes; T1: first temporal convolution; TP: temporal pole; T2: second temporal convolution; ET: extratemporal structures; Epig: epigastric sensation; OAA: oroalimentary 'automatisms'; Ceph: cephalic sensation; aud ill: auditory illusions; GA: gestural 'automatisms'; swall: swallowing. Time interval refers to the delay between MTL and extra-MTL electrical involvement. Superscript numerals refer to patients' identification numbers.

Table 8. Electro-clinical characteristics of five spontaneous seizures (two patients) only involving, without spreading, neocortical areas at the occurrence of clinical manifestations

Extra-MTL	Clinical signs
[1]LVFA T2	Epig
[1]LVFA T2	Epig
[1]LVFA T2	Epig
[1]LVFA T2	Epig
[17]LVFA T2	Funny feeling

Extra-MTL: extramesiotemporal lobe structures; LVFA: low-voltage fast activity; T2: second temporal convolution; Epig: epigastric sensation. Superscript numerals refer to patients' identification numbers.

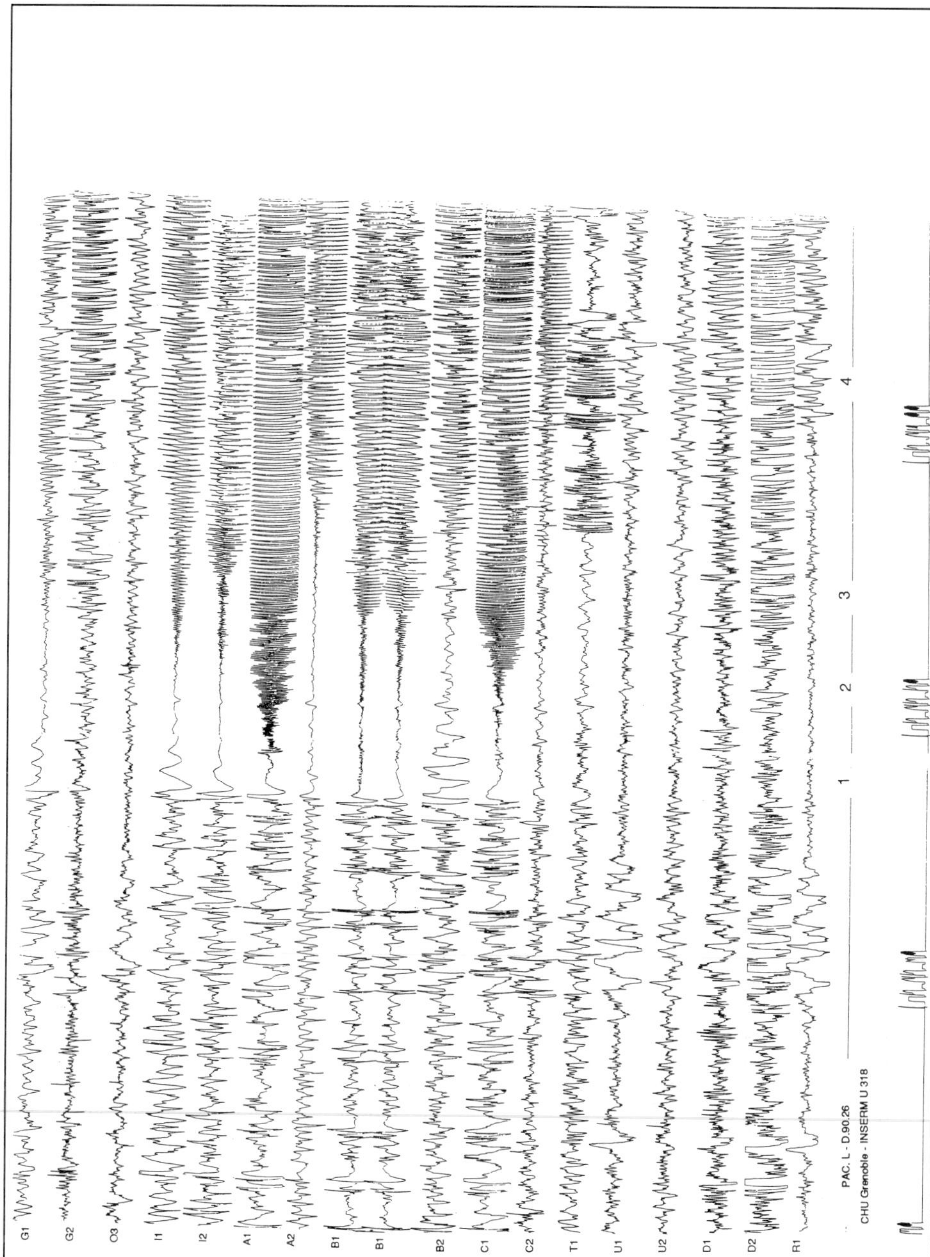

Fig. 2c. Same patient as in Figs. 2a and 2b. Example of a spontaneous seizure in which ictal discharge simultaneously involves external and internal temporal lobe structures from the onset. Clinically: 1. the patient calls the observer; 2. she says 'I have my sensation'; 3. 'The seizure is coming'; 4. she chews. Electrically: the seizure starts with a low-voltage fast activity simultaneously involving I1, I2, A1, A2, B1 and C1.

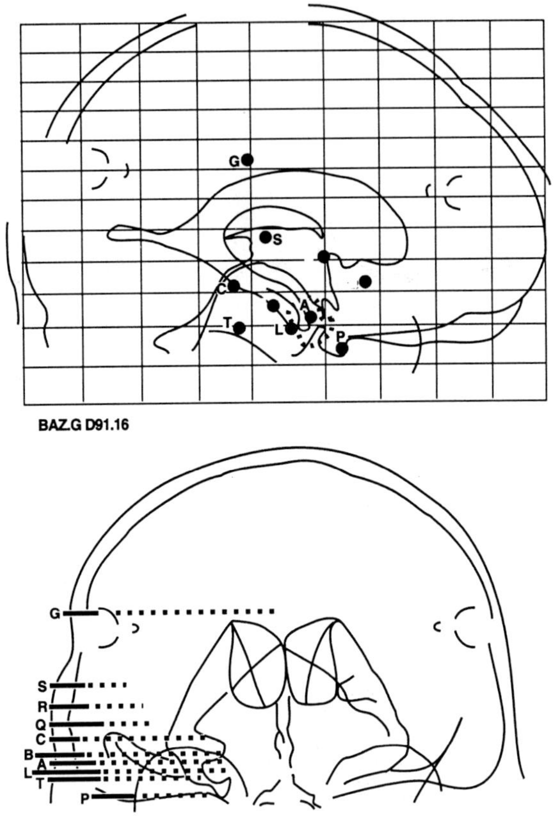

Fig. 3a. Stereotactic scheme (lateral and frontal view) of the patient GB (no. 24), showing the location of the lesion (grade I astrocytoma) and of the 10 intracerebral electrodes. The anteroexternal temporal lesion is represented by the dotted line. Electrode placement: P: uncus and external temporal pole; A: amygdala and anterior T2 (some external leads are intralesional); L: anterior hippocampus and anterior T2 (some external leads are immediately perilesional); B: mid-hippocampus and mid-T2; C: posterior hippocampus and posterior T2; T: T4 and T3; Q: anterior T1; R: mid-T1; S: posterior T1; G: posterior cingulate gyrus and P2.

'TNCx seizures'

The H was always involved, either alone (4 times), after the A (twice) or simultaneously with the A (once).

MTL discharges rarely involved extratemporal areas before the occurrence of ictal clinical signs, the more frequently affected temporal structure being the temporal pole (TP). Ictal symptomatology was more rich. An LVFA was recorded four out of the seven times.

(a) When discharges remained confined to the TNCx (five seizures in two patients), they only involved the second temporal convolution (T2) (Table 8).

(b) In four seizures (four patients) an LVFA first involved the TNCx before spreading over MTL structures (Table 9). Clinical signs were either absent or very slight and they occurred either before or after MTL involvement.

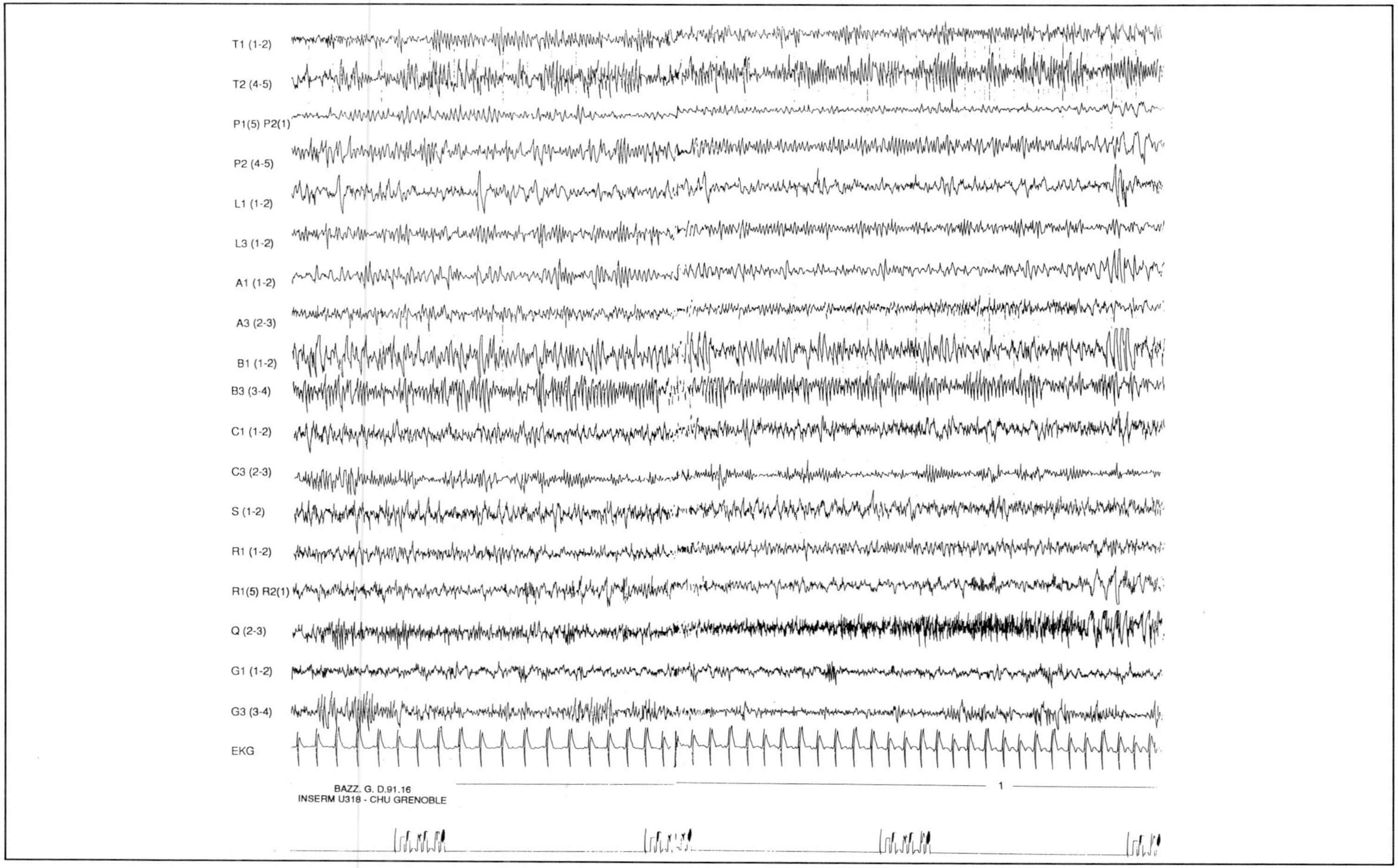

Fig. 3b. Same patient as in Fig 3a. Example of a spontaneous seizure: the ictal discharge is limited to the neocortical region. Clinically: 1. she says 'I have had my sensation' (tachycardia and dispnoea). Electrically: several seconds before the patient's call, low-voltage fast activity only involved the anterior part of T1 (Q 2–3), without clear participation of the lesion.

Figure 3b shows an ictal discharge (imPμ = 2u; Fig 3a), well localized in the anterior part of the first temporal gyrus, relatively distant from the anatomical lesion, located in the white matter. This discharge does not affect the electrode directly exploring the lesion! Figure 3c presents another seizure, in the same patient (no. 24) of the SGr, with a discharge initially involving lateral and rapidly spreading to cortical areas, and including the lesion.

Table 9. Electro-clinical characteristics of four spontaneous seizures (four patients) first involving extramesio-temporal lobe (extra-MTL) structures and secondarily spreading to the MTL structures

Extra-MTL	Clinical signs	Time interval	MTL spreading	Clinical signs
^{24}LVFA T2	No	11 s	H	Eyes opening
^{17}LVFA T2	No	1 s	H	No
^{12}LVFA T1 + T2	Mimicry	15 s	A	No
^{23}LVFA LL → T1 + T2	No	4 s	A + H	No

LVFA: low-voltage fast activity; T2: second temporal convolution; T1: first temporal convolution; LL: lingual lobule; H: hippocampus; A: amygdaloid nucleus. Time interval refers to the delay between extra-MTL and MTL electrical involvement. Superscript numerals refer to patients' identification numbers.

Elicited seizures

We selected only the seizures in which the electrically induced ictal discharges involved only MTL structures at the onset of clinical signs or symptoms.

LFES-elicited seizures

In six patients, 11 'MTL seizures' were recorded by stimulating either the A (three times), the H (seven times), or the TP (once) (Table 10).

In all but one case, ictal discharges always involved both the A and the H. Clinical symptoms were always subjective and mainly characterized by an epigastric sensation. A secondary spreading over both TNCx and extratemporal areas frequently occurred.

Table 10. Electro-clinical characteristics of 11 seizures elicited by low-frequency electrical stimulation (LFES) (six patients) for which ictal discharges were limited to mesiotemporal lobe structures (MTL) when the first clinical symptomatology occurred

LFES site		Involvement	Clinical signs	Spreading
3	^{6}A	A + H	Epig	No
3	^{10}A	A + H	Epig	TP + T2
3	^{22}A	A + H	Rising epig	T + ET
7	^{11}H	H	Epig	T + ET
7	^{9}H	A + H	Ceph	No
7	^{19}H	A + H	Ceph	T + ET
7	^{6}H	A + H	Epig	No
7	^{11}H	A + H	Epig	T + ET
7	^{11}H	A + H	Rising epig	T + ET
7	^{11}H	A + H	Epig + tachy	T + ET
1	^{9}TP	A + H	Epig + warm	No

A: amygdaloid nucleus; H: hippocampus; TP: temporal pole; Epig: epigastric sensation; Ceph: cephalic sensation; tachy: feeling of tachycardia; T2: second temporal convolution; T: temporal; ET: extratemporal structures. Superscript numerals refer to patients' identification numbers.

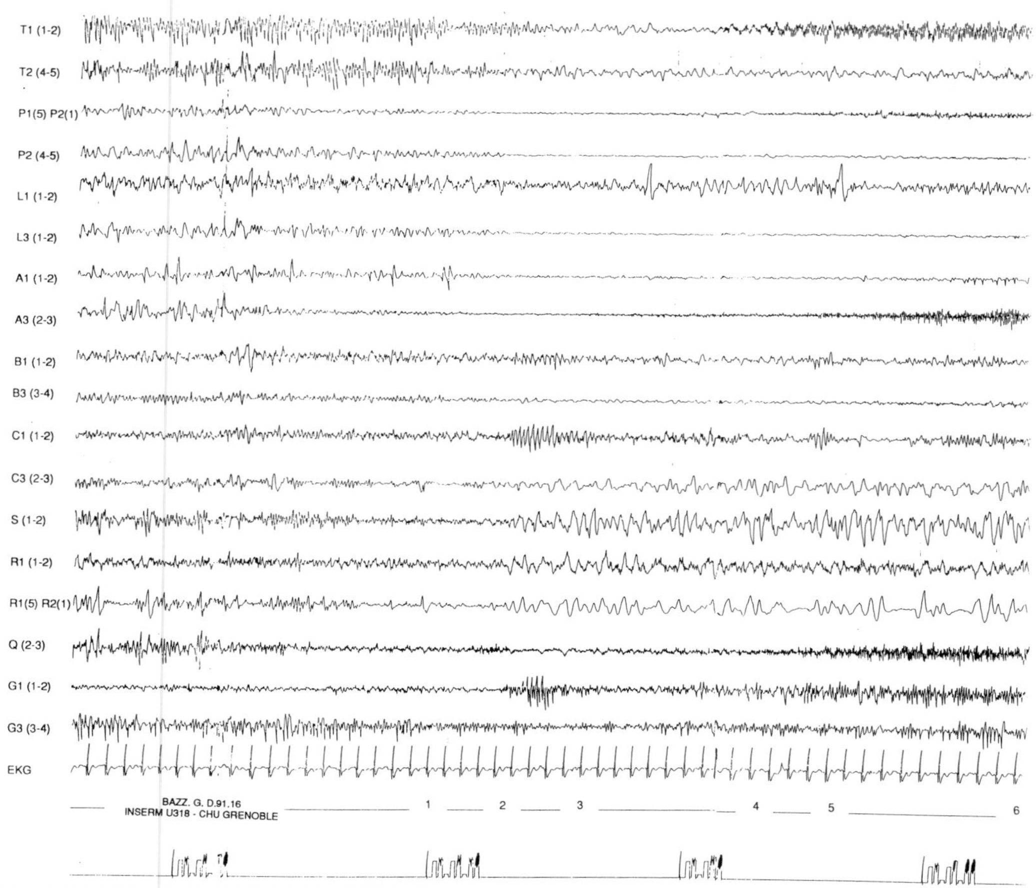

Fig. 3c. Same patient as in Figs. 3a and 3b. Example of a spontaneous seizure in which ictal discharge involves external temporal lobe structures but rapidly spreads to the internal ones. Clinically: 1. she opens and closes her eyes; 2. she opens her eyes; 3. she swallows; 4. she can execute the orders; 5. right lip corner attraction; 6. loss of contact. Electrically: the ictal discharge involves almost simultaneously Q and A3 and only a few seconds later P1, P2, A1, B3 and L3.

HFES-elicited seizures

In 13 patients, 18 'MTL seizures' were induced when ES were applied either in the A (six times), in the H (eight times), in the TP (twice) or in the T2 (twice) (Table 11).

Ictal discharges always immediately involved the H, either alone (four times) or together with the A (14 times). Clinical symptoms were often both subjective and objective (11 times), and rarely isolated (five times). Secondary spreading was rare (four times) but widely extended when present.

Discussion

There are few doubts about the important role that MTL structures can play in the pathogenesis of TL seizures: this hypothesis is supported by many surgical, electrophysiological, pathological and chemical neuroanatomical data.

Table 11. Electro-clinical characteristics of 18 seizures elicited by high-frequency electrical stimulation (HFES) (13 patients) for which ictal discharges were limited to mesiotemporal lobe structures (MTL) when the first clinical symptomatology occurred

	HFES site	Involvement	Clinical signs	Spreading
6	[2]A	A + H	Epig + fear	No
6	[4]A	A + H	Epig + swall	No
6	[11]A	A + H	Rising epig + OAA	No
6	[18]A	A + H	DV + swall	No
6	[21]A	A + H	Strangeness + swall	T + ET
6	[5]A	A + H	Shiver + fear	T + ET
8	[4]H	H	Epig	No
8	[4]H	H	Epig + swall	No
8	[9]H	H	Ceph	No
8	[12]H	H	Strangeness	T + ET
8	[22]H	A + H	Epig + swall	No
8	[1]H	A + H	Epig + flush + fear	No
8	[19]H	A + H	Ceph	T + ET
8	[5]H	A + H	Shiver + fear	No
2	[4]TP	A + H	Epig + swall	No
2	[8]TP	A + H	Tachy + fear	No
2	[3]T2	A + H	Epig	No
2	[19]T2	A + H	Ceph + flush	No

A: amygdaloid nucleus; H: hippocampus; TP: temporal pole; T2: second temporal convolution; Epig: epigastric sensation; swall: swallowing; OAA: oroalimentary 'automatisms'; DV: *déjà-vu* feeling; Ceph: cephalic sensation; Tachy: feeling of tachycardia; T: temporal; ET: extratemporal structures. Superscript numerals refer to patients' identification numbers.

In his recent fascinating and comprehensive historical review, Gloor (1991) raises all the complex questions concerning the respective role of the different anatomical temporal structures. He particularly stresses the similarities between the 'sclerosis' of the hippocampus (Falconer *et al.*, 1964) and the neuronal loss, or gliosis, found in the amygdala when this structure was examined, without forgetting that neuroanatomical and neurochemical changes often concern other neighbouring structures, such as the uncus, the TP and the TNCx too (Gastaut *et al.*, 1959). Then Gloor (1991) discusses the surgical results obtained in two series of 100 patients who underwent a temporal lobectomy, either with major hippocampectomy (Rasmussen & Feindel, 1991) or with amygdalectomy and minimal hippocampal resection (Feindel & Rasmussen, 1991). His conclusion, in agreement with the present authors, is that the removal of the hippocampus could not be very relevant, provided that the excision of the amygdala is as complete as possible, since the results in the two groups are similarly satisfying (i.e. 63 per cent of complete absence or marked reduction of the seizures). However, the completely seizure-free patients (with or without auras?) are 21 per cent in both these series, rising to 39 per cent after some early attacks: this kind of result seems to be somewhat inconclusive for validating the possible role of the amygdala in the pathogenesis of the seizures.

Some other authors believe that 'the anterior hippocampus and/or associated entorrhinal cortex may be all that need be removed to control complex partial seizures caused by a temporal mesiobasal focus' (Goldring *et al.*, 1992). Among the 70 patients operated on in this way, sparing the amygdala, '55 (79 per cent) have benefited from surgery', but patients seizure-free since surgery are only 23 (33 per cent). Also, considering that the extent of the removed hippocampus could play an important role with regard to the surgical results (Siegel *et al.*, 1990), it appears that the removal of the hippocampus *per se* does not necessarily provoke the suppression of the seizures.

Wieser (1988), reporting on a group of 52 non-tumour patients submitted to a selective amygdalo-hippocampectomy (AHE), states that 40 per cent were completely seizure-free, while 11 per cent had 'atypical generalized convulsion' only during drug withdrawal and 4 per cent had only some postoperative seizures. In the discussion of this paper, it appears that in the 50 per cent of patients for whom 'palliative' AHE was insufficient, the subsequent temporal lobectomy had successful outcomes.

In their recent survey of 3992 'limbic resections' (period: 1985–1990), Engel and co-workers (1993) found 68 per cent of seizure-free patients as well after anterior temporal lobectomy as after AHE.

An unprepared reader could be relatively puzzled by the disagreement among different experienced authors. Or he may ingenuously conclude that a more limited intervention can, in general, obtain the same good results as a larger excision, whatever the removed structures are. A good answer is probably suggested by Bonis (1980), who, in a study of a group of 214 consecutive patients (operated on at the Sainte Anne Hospital in Paris), noted that the high success rate (91 per cent) in patients with a preoperatively correct localization of the epileptogenic area dramatically drops to 33 per cent when the localization was estimated to be inadequate. In other words, many cortical areas can be responsible for seizures, but to remove them without previously ascertaining their specific role in each individual patient makes it difficult to correctly assess operative results.

It seems clear that a syndrome of MTL epilepsy (MTLE) must, at least clinically and anatomically, exist, even if its precise definition, recently reattempted by Wieser *et al.* (1993), seems to be relatively difficult to reach.

Unhappily, there are, at present, no convincing studies allowing the presurgical electrical and clinical differentiation between patients who would become seizure-free after an AHE and those who would not! We conclude that the correct clinical indication for obtaining seizure-free patients with only very limited resections is still an entirely open question.

In our experience, both in Paris and in Grenoble (Kahane *et al.*, 1993b), patients presenting with seizures starting only, and always, in MTL areas are rare. This could be largely due to the selection criteria of patients (both by referring neurologists and by ourselves), but we cannot exclude the possibility that it could be, at least partially, explained by the employed presurgical methodology. In other words, in order to record ictal discharges simultaneously affecting both lateral and mesial structures, orthogonally implanted depth electrodes are more informative (Munari, 1987) than anterior or posterior oblique electrodes (Spencer, 1987) or subdural plates (Sperling & O'Connor, 1989), without considering the different indications for electrocorticography (Ojemann, 1993).

Well-limited ictal discharges in the amygdaloid nucleus only seem to be very rare: only 3 per cent of more than 400 temporal lobe seizures (Munari *et al.*, 1984). Wieser's data (1988), using stereo-EEG, were identical: 3 per cent of pure amygdalar seizures. In the present study, pure amygdalar seizures are slightly less rare: 5 per cent. Initial hippocampal discharges represent 7 per cent, but the clinical symptomatology only occurs after their spread (Table 7). Simultaneous amygdalohippocampal discharges are 5 per cent of the total number of spontaneous seizures recorded: two-thirds are rapidly notified by the patients. It appears that discharges, apparently limited to MTL areas, are able to produce a clinical symptomatology in 14 per cent of temporal seizures, whereas localized neocortical temporal seizures are a little more infrequent: 10 per cent. Rasmussen (1982), in 100 patients who were seizure-free after a temporal resection, found that the epileptogenic area was mesial in 28 per cent, lateral in 46 per cent and mesial and lateral in 27 per cent. Conversely, Wieser & Siegel (1991) found that more than 50 per cent (165/320) of seizures originated 'mediobasally'. But these results were obtained with foramen ovale electrodes (Siegfried *et al.*, 1985), and this could explain why these authors are conspicuously silent on discharges simultaneously involving mesial and lateral temporal areas, while they account for 58 per cent of all the spontaneous initial ictal discharges which we recorded. Considering the important differences in the evaluation of both the localization and the extension of the epileptogenic zone, it is astonishing to note that, in a recent paper, theoretically concerning the 'surgically remediable temporal lobe syndrome', only MTLE is discussed by Wieser and co-workers (1993), thus generating the erroneous idea that only MTLE could be surgically remediable.

We separately looked at seizures with clinical signs occurring before the spread of the discharges out of MTL structures in order to better understand the possible localizing value of the directly observed clinical manifestations. This symptomatology was generally very simple, limited to subjective experiences described by the patient during the seizure, and the duration did not exceed 25 s. The relatively short duration of TL seizures without impairment of contact, even with the simultaneous involvement of mesial and lateral temporal areas, is probably correlated with the lack of spread, (Munari *et al.*, 1980a) and is in partial agreement with the report of Wieser & Siegel (1991), who found a mean duration of 61 and 83 s respectively in simple and complex partial seizures. Such limited MTL seizures, without loss of contact, raise the question as to whether it is useful to differentiate partial seizures into simple and complex as function of an impaired contact (not to mention consciousness; Gloor, 1986). This symptom appears to be the consequence of the duration and the extension of the discharges, rather than a localizing ictal phenomenon (Munari *et al.*, 1982).

In seven seizures, the continuous clinical monitoring allowed us to note that the initial mesiotemporal discharges remained perfectly asymptomatic for periods up to 24 s before the extra-MTL spreading: in five out of the seven the seizures started as spikes or polyspikes and waves; in the other two, with LVFA, the delay was less than 2 s. Conversely, an LVFA was recorded in seven out of eight MTL discharges that were symptomatic before the spreading. The possibility that the electrical characteristics of the ictal discharges can modulate both the type and the intensity of the clinical symptomatology is probably not remote.

Initially asymptomatic ictal discharges have been described in the orbital cortex, too (Munari & Bancaud, 1992), strongly suggesting that, at least in some temporal and frontal epilepsies, the 'ictal onset zone' does not necessarily coincide with the 'symptomatogenic zone' (Lüders *et al.*, 1993). But, admitting that the 'ictal onset zone', which is not necessarily symptomatogenic, is an important part of the 'epileptogenic zone', we need to increase our possibilities of identifying it, in neocortical areas as well as in MTL structures: orthogonal, laterally implanted, temporal electrodes seem to be very useful in this respect (Munari *et al.*, 1986).

The discussion concerning the definitions and the possible differences between the different 'zones', first raised by Jasper (Penfield & Jasper, 1954), later renewed by Bancaud (Talairach & Bancaud, 1966) and more recently tackled by Lüders (Lüders & Awad, 1992), is not a purely theoretical one, since it is strictly linked with the question of the limits of the surgical removal. All our reported patients benefited from a both lateral *and* mesial temporal removal, almost always including the temporal pole, stereotactically investigated in 21/25 cases. The posterior limits of the mesial and the lateral cortectomy were defined according to the stereo-EEG ictal data (Talairach *et al.*, 1992; Kahane *et al.*, 1993b) and surgically respected in all but one patient (see above). Complete suppression of the seizures (group IA of Engel, 1987) was obtained in 12/12 cryptogenic patients, whereas 'simple partial' seizures with only subjective symptoms (group IB) persist, in spite of the complete removal of the anatomical lesion, in 3/13 patients (23 per cent) of the symptomatic group, as preoperatively foreseen in two. The one patient in this series who experienced the recurrence of seizures after 15 months is also the only one in which both the removal of the lesion and the excision of the epileptogenic area were incomplete.

Some authors (Awad *et al.*, 1989) include patients with postoperatively persisting auras in the 'seizure-free' group: this way of presenting the results could be accepted in studies concerning the improvement of the quality of life, although it should be borne in mind that even a patient with only 'simple partial' seizures remains epileptic. However, this rating is not useful for a critical evaluation of strategies to localize the 'epileptogenic area'. The same is true for the cases with a greater than 90 per cent reduction in seizure frequency (Wyllie *et al.*, 1987).

The most frequent reasons given for persisting seizures or auras are either an incomplete resection or bilateral discharges (Lieb *et al.*, 1986). In the former case, a temporal reoperation (Polkey *et al.*, 1993) could transform a failure into a success (Penfield & Jasper, 1954; Wieser, 1988; Awad *et al.*, 1991).

There are many studies concerning the clinical symptomatology of TL seizures (Gastaut & Vigouroux, 1967; Daly, 1975; Bancaud, 1981; Bancaud & Talaraich, 1991; Wieser, 1983; Munari *et al.*, 1985; Williamson *et al.*, 1987), but there are only a few papers correlating the clinical symptomatology and the surgical results obtained by removing the cortical areas identified as responsible for the ictal symptoms (Talairach *et al.*, 1974; Delgado-Escueta & Walsh, 1985; Wyllie *et al.*, 1987; Wieser, 1988). Also rare are analytical studies of surgical failures (Van Buren *et al.*, 1975; Munari *et al.*, 1980b; Rasmussen, 1983; Williamson, 1993).

Our results confirm previous anatomo-electro-clinical observations concerning the ictal clinical signs considered as characteristic of temporal lobe seizures (Bancaud *et al.*, 1965, 1973; Bancaud, 1981; Wieser, 1983). They also suggest that most symptoms generally considered as temporal are in fact linked to the spreading of the discharges *out* of MTL to either temporal neocortical, or extratemporal areas, or both. A single ictal clinical sign or symptom, with rare, well-known exceptions, only rarely has high localizing value. However, the occurrence of a clinical symptom (e.g. chewing) in strict chronological relation with a well-localized LVFA (e.g. in the amygdala) does not mean that this symptom represents the function of the activated structure (Bancaud *et al.*, 1966; Munari *et al.*, 1979). It appears that even the most classical and, in this series, the most frequent symptom, the epigastric sensation, should always be considered in the context of all ictal symptoms, paying strong attention to their chronological sequence. There is general agreement on the temporal origin of the epigastric aura. However, an epigastric sensation can also occur at the beginning of frontal dorsolateral seizures (Munari *et al.*, 1990), suggesting, as well as its occasional persistence after a complete temporal lobectomy (Munari *et al.*, 1980b), an insular involvement (Penfield & Rasmussen, 1950).

The usefulness of direct electrical stimulation during electrocorticography for reproducing, in awake patients, their habitual subjective manifestations needs no comment, as the pioneer work of Penfield and Jasper (1954) was later largely confirmed (Olivier, 1983; Ojemann, 1993). Electrical stimulations through depth electrodes (Crandall, 1963), deceptive when they were implanted with a non-rigorous stereotactic methodology (Walker & Ribstein, 1957), can give very important information if included in the stereo-EEG protocol (Bancaud *et al.*, 1973; Munari & Bancaud, 1985). Opinions are, however, divergent since some authors perceive the electrical stimulation as an inaccurate tool for defining the epileptogenic area (Halgren *et al.*, 1983), whereas other studies find more than 90 per cent concordance between spontaneous and electrically induced auras or seizures (Bernier *et al.*, 1990). This study shows a good concordance between the clinical symptomatology of spontaneously recorded seizures and those electrically induced. This concordance is strongly evident when the type, the location and the duration of the discharge are the same, whatever the distance between the stimulated leads and the discharging sites. The results obtained are particularly striking when using low-frequency electrical stimulation (Kahane *et al.*, 1993a), since the intensity of the electrical discharge increases progressively, allowing a more careful clinical analysis (Munari *et al.*, 1993b). Concluding remarks

MTL seizures exist, and can be recorded, even if they are relatively rare. Patients presenting with MTLE exist too, since the surgical removal of mesiotemporal areas allows the suppression of the seizures in a high percentage of patients. A number of patients can present both well-localized MTL seizures and seizures corresponding to largely extended temporal discharges.

Presurgical stereo-EEG investigations in problematic cases can be helpful to:

(a) clarify the differential diagnosis;

(b) obtain satisfactory surgical results;

(c) improve our knowledge on clinical, anatomical and electrical relationships

(d) contribute to the future progressive reduction of indications for stereo-EEG!

The advantages of limited resections, such as AHE, are obvious. However, presurgical investigations should allow patients to have the best chances of becoming seizure-free and not only 'worthwhile improvement', if possible. Further studies concerning strict ictal anatomoelectroclinical correlations in patients rendered completely seizure-free by surgical interventions could improve the diagnostic assessment of MTLE.

References

Awad, I.A., Katz, A., Kong, A.K., Ahl, J. & Lüders, H.O. (1989): Extent of resection in temporal lobectomy for epilepsy: I. Interobserver analysis and correlation with seizure outcome. *Epilepsia* **30,** 756–762.

Awad, I.A., Nayel, M.H. & Lüders, H.O. (1991): Second operation after failure of previous resection for epilepsy. *Neurosurgery* **28,** 510–518.

Bancaud, J. (1959): Apport de l'exploration fonctionnelle par voie stéréotaxique à la chirurgie de l'épilepsie. *Neurochirurgie* **5,** 55–112.

Bancaud, J. (1981): Epileptic attacks of temporal origin in man. *Japan. J. EEG–EMG* (Suppl. Didactic Lectures, Xth ICECN, Kyoto), 61–71.

Bancaud, J. & Talairach, J. (1991): Séméiologie clinique des crises du lobe temporal. In: *Crises épileptiques et épilepsies du lobe temporal*, Vol. 2, Gentilly: Documentation médicale Labaz.

Bancaud, J., Talairach, J., Bonis, A., Schaub, C., Szikla, G., Morel, P. & Bordas-Ferrer, M. (1965): *La stéréo-électro-encéphalographie dans l'épilepsie: informations neuro-physiopathologiques apportées par l'investigation fonctionnelle stéréotaxique.* Paris: Masson.

Bancaud, J., Talairach, J., Morel, P. & Bresson, M. (1966): La corne d'Ammon et le noyau amygdalien: effets cliniques et électriques de leur stimulation chez l'homme. *Rev. Neurol.* **3,** 329–352.

Bancaud, J., Talairach, J., Geier, S. & Scarabin, J.M. (1973): *EEG et SEEG dans les tumeurs cérébrales et l'épilepsie.* Paris: Edifor.

Benabid, A.L., Cinquin, P., Lavallée, S., Le Bas, J.F., Demongeot, J. & De Rougemont, J. (1987): Computer-driven robot for stereotactic surgery connected to CT scan and magnetic resonance imaging. *Appl. Neurophysiol.* **50,** 153–154.

Benabid, A.L., Lavallée, S., Hoffmann, D., Cinquin, P., Demongeot, J. & Danel, F. (1992): Computer-driven robot for stereotactic neurosurgery. In: *Contemporary issues in neurological surgery*, eds. P.J. Kelly & B.A.Kall, pp. 330–342. Boston: Blackwell Scientific Publications.

Bernier, G.P., Richer, F., Giard, N., Bouvier, G., Mercier, M., Turmel, A. & Saint-Hilaire, J.M. (1990): Electrical stimulation of the human brain in epilepsy. *Epilepsia* **31,** 513–520.

Bonis, A. (1980): Long term results of cortical excisions based on stereotactic investigations in severe, drug resistant epilepsies. *Acta Neurochirurg.* **30,** 55–66.

Bossi, L., Munari, C., Stoffels, C., Bonis, A., Bacia, T., Talairach, J. & Bancaud, J. (1984): Somatomotor manifestations in temporal lobe seizures. *Epilepsia* **25,** 70–76.

Crandall, P.H. (1963): Clinical applications of studies on stereotactically implanted electrodes in temporal-lobe epilepsy. *J. Neurosurg.* **20,** 827–840.

Daly, D.D. (1975): Ictal clinical manifestations of complex partial seizures. In: *Advances in neurology*, Vol. 11., eds. J.K. Penry & D.D. Daly, pp. 57–83. New York: Raven Press.

Delgado-Escueta, A.V. & Walsh, G.O. (1985): Type I complex partial seizures of hippocampal origin: excellent results of anterior temporal lobectomy. *Neurology* **35,** 143–154.

Engel, J., Jr (1987): *Surgical treatment of the epilepsies.* New York: Raven Press.

Engel, J., Jr, Van Ness, P.C., Rasmussen, T. & Ojemann, L.M. (1993): Outcome with respect to epileptic seizures. In: *Surgical treatment of the epilepsies*, 2nd edn, ed. J. Engel, Jr , pp. 609–621. New York: Raven Press.

Engel, J., Jr & Shewmon, D.A. (1993): Who should be considered a surgical candidate? In: *Surgical treatment of the epilepsies*, 2nd edn, ed. J. Engel, Jr., pp. 23–34. New York: Raven Press.

Falconer, M.A., Serafetidinis, F.A. & Corsellis, J.A.N. (1964): Etiology and pathogenesis of temporal lobe epilepsy. *Arch. Neurol.* **10,** 233–248.

Feindel, W. & Rasmussen, T. (1991): Temporal lobectomy with amygdalectomy and minimal hippocampal resection: review of 100 cases. *Can. J. Neurol. Sci.* **19,** 603–605.

Francione, S., Dompnier, A., Kahane, P., Tassi, L., Gamblin, E. & Munari, C. (1992): 'Attivazioni' in corso di video-EEG/SEEG in pazienti con epilessia parziale candidati al trattamento chirurgico. Lega Italiana Contro l'Epilessia, Congresso Nazionale, Genoa, 16–19 December, 1992. Abstract Book, pp. 54–55.

Gastaut, H. & M. Vigouroux, M. (1967): Electroclinical correlations in 500 cases of psychomotor seizures. In: *Temporal lobe epilepsy*, eds. E. Baldwin & P. Bailey, pp. 118–128. Springfield: Charles C. Thomas.

Gastaut, H., Toga, M., Roger, J. & Gibson, W.C. (1959): A correlation of clinical, electroencephalographic and anatomical findings in nine autopsied cases of 'temporal lobe epilepsy'. *Epilepsia* **1,** 56–85.

Gloor, P. (1986): Consciousness as a neurological concept in epilepsy: a critical review. *Epilepsia* **27**(suppl.), 514–527.

Gloor, P. (1991): Mesial temporal sclerosis: historical background and overview from a modern perspective. In: *Epilepsy surgery*, ed. H.O. Lüders, pp. 689–703, New York: Raven Press.

Goldring, S., Edwards, I., Haring, G.W. & Bernard, K.L. (1992): Results of anterior temporal lobectomy that spares the amygdala in patients with complex partial seizures. *J. Neurosurg.* **77,** 185–193.

Halgren, E., Wilson, C.L., Squires, N.K., Engel, J., Jr, Walter, R.D. & Crandall, P.H. (1983): Dynamics of the hippocampal contribution to memory: stimulation and recording studies in man. In: *The molecular, cellular and behavioral neurobiology of the hippocampus*, ed. W. Seifert, pp. 529–571. New York: Academic Press.

Hardiman, O., Burke, T., Phillips, J., Murphy, S., O'Moore, B, Staunton, H. & Farrel, M.A. (1988): Microdysgenesis in resected temporal neocortex incidence and clinical significance in focal epilepsy. *Neurology* **38,** 1041–1047.

Kahane, P., Tassi, L., Francione, S., Hoffmann, D., Lo Russo, G. & Munari, C. (1993a): Manifestations électro-cliniques induites par la stimulation electrique intra-cérébrale par 'chocs' dans les épilepsies temporales. *Neurophysiol. Clin.* **22,** 305–326.

Kahane, P., Francione, S., Tassi, L., Hoffman, D., Lo Russo, G., Garrel, S., Feuerstein, C., Perret, J., Benabid, A.L. & Munari, C. (1993b): Traitement chirurgical des épilepsies partielles graves pharmaco-résistantes: approches diagnostiques et thérapeutiques. *Epilepsia* **5,** 179–204.

Lieb, J.P., Engel, J. Jr & Babb, T.L. (1986):. Interhemispheric propagation time of human hippocampal seizures: relationship to surgical outcome. *Epilepsia* **27,** 286–293.

Lo Russo, G. & Munari, C. (1992): Stereotaxic approach to intracranial lesions. *Ital. J. Neurol. Sci.* **13,** 17–44.

Lüders, H.O. & Awad, I. (1992): Conceptual considerations. In: *Epilepsy surgery*, ed. H.O. Lüders, pp. 51–62. New York: Raven Press.

Lüders, H.O., Engel, J. Jr & Munari, C. (1993): Non invasive preoperative evaluation: general principles. In: *Surgical treatment of the epilepsies*, Vol. 2, ed. J. Engel, Jr, pp. 137–154. New York: Raven Press.

Marchini, M., Munari, C., Parietti, L., Broglin, D., Giallonardo, A.T. & Bancaud, J. (1989): Contribution of the direct clinical observation to the ictal semiology knowledge: stereo-EEG and videotape study of 57 frontal lobe seizures. *Boll. Lega Ital. Epil.* **66/67,** 115–123.

Munari, C. (1987): Depth electrode implantation at hospital Sainte Anne, Paris. In: Surgical treatment of the epilepsies, ed. J. Engel, Jr, pp. 583–588. New York: Raven Press.

Munari, C. & Bancaud, J. (1985): The role of the stereo-EEG in the evaluation of partial epileptic seizures. In: *The epilepsies,* eds. P.L. Morselli & R.J. Porter, pp. 267–306. London: Butterworths.

Munari, C. & Bancaud, J. (1992): Electroclinical symptomatology of partial seizures of orbital frontal origin. In: *Advances in neurology*, Vol. 57, Part 12, eds. P. Chauvel, A.V. Delgado-Escueta, H. Halgren & J. Bancaud, pp. 257–265. New York: Raven Press.

Munari, C. & Betti, O.O. (1989): The stereotactic biopsy of brain lesions: a critical review. In: *Cerebral Gliomas* (Excerpta Medica International Congress Series No. 828), eds. G. Broggi & M.A Gerosa, pp. 179–206. Amsterdam: Elsevier.

Munari, C., Bancaud, J., Bonis, A., Buser, P., Talairach, J., Szikla, G. & Philippe, A. (1979): Rôle du noyau amygdalien dans la survenue de manifestations oro-alimentaires au cours des crises épileptiques chez l'homme. *Rev. EEG Neurophysiol.* **9** (3), 236–240.

Munari, C., Bancaud, J., Bonis, A., Stoffels, C., Szikla, G. & Talairach, J. (1980a): Impairment of consciousness in temporal lobe seizures: a stereo-electro-encephalographic study. In: *Advances in epileptology, XIth Epilepsy International Symposium,* eds. R. Canger, F. Angeleri & J.K. Penry, pp. 111–114. New York: Raven Press.

Munari, C., Talairach, J., Bonis, A., Szikla, G. & Bancaud, J. (1980b): Differential diagnosis between temporal and 'perisylvian' epilepsy in a surgical perspective. *Acta Neurochirurg.* **30,** 97–101.

Munari, C., Stoffels, C., Bossi, L., Brunet, P., Bonis, A. Bancaud, J. & Talairach, J. (1982): Partial seizures with elementary or complex symptomatology: a valid classification for temporal lobe seizures? In: *Advances in epileptology: XIIIth Epilepsy International Symposium,* eds. H. Akimoto, H. Kazamatsuri, M. Seino & A. Ward, pp. 25–27. New York: Raven Press.

Munari, C., Bonis, A., Musolino, A., Bancaud, J., Buser, P., Brunet, P., Talairach, J. & Chodkiewicz, J.P. (1984): Amygdaloid nucleus involvement during temporal lobe seizures in man: physiopathological and surgical implications. In: *Advances in epileptology: XVth Epilepsy International Symposium,* ed. R.J. Porter pp. 463–468. New York: Raven Press.

Munari, C., Soncini, M., Brunet, P., Musolino, A., Chodkiewicz, J.P., Talairach, J. & Bancaud, J. (1985): Sémiologie électroclinique des crises temporales subintrantes. *Rev. EEG Neurophysiol. Clin.* **15** (3), 289–298.

Munari, C., Musolino, A., Blond, S., Brunet, P., Giallonardo, A.T., Chodkiewitz, J. P. & Bancaud, J. (1986): Stereo-EEG exploration in patients with intractable epilepsy: topographic relations between a lesion and epileptogenic areas. In: *Intractable epilepsy: experimental and clinical aspects,* eds. D. Schmidt & P.L. Morselli, pp. 129–146. New York: Raven Press.

Munari, C., Giallonardo, A.T., Musolino, A., Brunet, P., Chodkiewicz, J.P., Bancaud, J. & Talairach, J. (1987): Specific neuroradiological examinations necessary for stereotactic procedures. In: *Methods of presurgical evaluation of epileptic patients,* eds. H.G. Wieser & C.E. Elger, pp. 141–145. Berlin: Springer Verlag.

Munari, C., Tassi, L., Lo Russo, G., Canevini, M. P. & Hamasaki, T. (1990): La terapia chirurgica delle epilessie parziali: schematizzazione metodologica o approccio personalizzato? *Boll. Lega. Ital. Epil.* **70/71,** 61–67.

Munari, C., Hoffmann, D., Francione, S., Kahane, P., Tassi L., Lo Russo, G. & Benabid, A.L. (1993a): Stereo-electro-encephalo-graphy methodology: advantages and limits. *Acta Neurol. Scand.* **152,** 56–67.

Munari, C., Kahane, P., Tassi, L., Francione, S., Hoffmann, D., Lo Russo, G. & Benabid, A.L. (1993b): Intracerebral low frequency electrical stimulation: a new tool for the definition of the 'epileptogenic area'? *Acta Neurochirurg.* **58** (suppl.), 181–185.

Ojemann, G.A. (1993): Intraoperative tailoring of temporal lobe resections. In: *Surgical treatment of the epilepsies,* 2nd edn, ed. J. Engel, Jr, pp. 481–488. New York: Raven Press.

Olivier, A. (1983): Surgical management of complex partial seizures. In: *Epilepsy: an update on research and therapy,* eds. G. Nistico, R. Di Perri & H. Meinardi, pp. 309–324. New York: Alan R. Liss.

Penfield, W. & Jasper, H. (1954): *Epilepsy and the functional anatomy of the human brain.* Boston: Little, Brown.

Penfield, W. & Rasmussen, T. (1950): *The cerebral cortex of man,* 248 pp. New York: Macmillan.

Polkey, C.E. (1993): Preoperative tailoring of temporal lobe resections. In: *Surgical treatment of the epilepsies,* 2nd edn, ed. J. Engel, Jr, pp. 473–480. New York. Raven Press.

Polkey, C.E., Awad, I.A., Tanaka, T. & Wyler, A.R. (1993): The place of the reoperation. In: *Surgical treatment of the epilepsies,* 2nd edn, ed. J. Engel, Jr, pp. 663–667. New York: Raven Press.

Quesney, L.F. & Gloor, P. (1985): Localization of epileptic foci. *Electroencephalogr. Clin. Neurophysiol* **37,** 165–200.

Rasmussen, T. (1982): Localizational aspects of epileptic seizure phenomena. In: *New perspectives in cerebral localization,* eds. R. Thompson & G. Green, pp. 177–203. New York: Raven Press.

Rasmussen, T. (1983): Surgical treatment of complex partial seizures: results, lessons, and problems. *Epilepsia* **24** (suppl. 1), S65–S76.

Rasmussen, T. & Feindel, W. (1991): Temporal lobectomy: review of 100 cases with hippocampectomy. *Can. J. Neurol. Sci.* **18,** 601–602.

Siegel, A.M., Wieser, H.G., Wichmann, W. & Yasargil, M.G. (1990): Relationships between MR-imaged total amount of tissue removed, resection scores of specific mediobasal limbic subcompartments and clinical outcome following selective amygdalohippocampectomy. *Epilepsy Res.* **6,** 56–65.

Siegfried, J., Wieser, H.G. & Stodiek, S.G.R. (1985): Foramen ovale electrodes: a new technique enabling presurgical evaluation of patients with mesiobasal temporal lobe seizures. *Appl. Neurophysiol.*, **48,** 408–417.

Spencer, D.D. (1987): Depth electrode implantation at Yale University. In: *Surgical treatment of the epilepsies*, ed. J. Engel, Jr, pp. 603–607. New York: Raven Press.

Sperling, M.R. & O'Connor, M.J. (1989): Comparison of depth and subdural electrodes in recording temporal lobe seizures. *Neurology* **39,** 1497–1504.

Stoffels, C., Munari, C., Bonis, A., Bancaud, J. & Talairach, J. (1980): Manifestations génitales et 'sexuelles' lors des crises épileptiques partielles chez l'homme. *Rev. EEG Neurophysiol.* **10** (4), 386–392.

Talairach, J. & Bancaud, J. (1966): Lesions, irritative zone and epileptogenic focus. *Confin. Neurol.* **27,** 91–94.

Talairach, J., David, M. & Toumoux, P. (eds.) (1958): *L'exploration chirurgicale stéréotaxique du lobe temporal dans l'épilepsie temporale.* Paris: Masson.

Talairach, J., Szikla, G., Tournoux, P., Prossalentis, A., Bordas-Ferrer, M., Covello, L., Iacob, M. & Mempel, E. (eds.) (1967): *Atlas d'anatomie stéréotaxique du télencéphale: études anatomo-radiologiques.* Paris: Masson.

Talairach, J., Bancaud, J., Szikla, G., Bonis, A. & Geier, S. (1974): Approche nouvelle de la neurochirurgie de l'épilepsie: méthodologie stéréotaxique et résultats thérapeutiques. *Neurochirurgie* **20** (suppl. 1), 1–240.

Talairach, J., Bancaud, J., Bonis, A., Szikla, G, Trottier, S., Vignal, J.P., Chauvel, P., Munari, C. & Chodkiewicz, J.P. (1992): Surgical therapy for frontal epilepsies. In: *Advances in neurology*, Vol. 57, Part 46, eds. P. Chauvel, A.V. Delgado-Escueta, H. Halgren & J.Bancaud, pp. 707–732. New York: Raven Press.

Tassi, L., Kahane, P., Francione, S., Lo Russo, G., Hoffmann, D., Mayanrd, R., Lorenzi, A., Perret, J. & Munari, C. (1991): Etude SEEG des manifestations dysmnésiques spontanées: rôle respectif des structures néocorticales et amygdalo-hippocampiques. *Neurophysiol. Clin.* **21,** 325–326.

Tassi, L., Francione, S., Kahane, P. & Munari, C. (1993): Semeiologia elettro-clinica delle crisi parziali. In: *Le epilessie oggi,* 3rd edn, ed. R. Canger, pp. 167–185. Milano: Masson.

Van Buren, J.M., Ajmone Marsan, C. & Matsuga, N. (1975): Temporal lobe seizures with additional foci treated by resection. *J. Neurosurg.* **43,** 596–607.

Walker, A.E. & Ribstein, M. (1957): Chronic depth recording in focal and generalized epilepsy: an evaluation of the technique. *Arch. Neurol. Psychiatry* **78,** 44–45.

Wieser, H.G. (1983): *Electroclinical features of the psychomotor seizure.* Stuttgart, New York: Gustav Fischer.

Wieser, H.G. (1988): Selective amygdalo-hippocampectomy for temporal lobe epilepsy. *Epilepsia* **29** (suppl. 2), 100–113.

Wieser, H.G. & Siegel, A.M. (1991): Analysis of foramen ovale electrode-recorded seizures in correlation with outcome following amygdalohippocampectomy. *Epilepsia* **32,** 838–850.

Wieser, H.G., Engel, J., Jr, Williamson, P.D., Babb, T.L. & Gloor, P. (1993): Surgically remediable temporal lobe syndromes. In: *Surgical treatment of the epilepsies*, 2nd edn, ed. J. Engel, Jr, pp. 49–63. New York: Raven Press.

Williamson, P.D. (1993): Postscript: lessons from failures. In: *Surgical treatment of the epilepsies*, 2nd edn, ed. J. Engel, Jr, pp. 587–591. New York: Raven Press.

Williamson, P.D., Wieser, H.G. & Delgado-Escueta, A.V. (1987): Clinical characteristics of partial seizures. In: *Surgical treatment of the epilepsies*, ed. J. Engel, Jr., pp. 101–120. New York: Raven Press.

Wyllie, E., Lüders, H., Morris III, H.H., Lesser, R.P., Dinner, D.S., Hahn, J., Estes, M.L., Rothner, A.D., Erenberg, G., Cruse, R. & Friedman, D. (1987): Clinical outcome after complete or partial cortical resection for intractable epilepsy. *Neurology* **37,** 1634–1644.

Yasargil, M.G., Teddy, P.J. & Roth, P. (1985): Selective amygdalohippocampectomy: operative anatomy and surgical technique. *Adv. Tech. Stand. Neurosurg.* **12,** 93–123.

Epileptic Seizures and Syndromes, Edited by Peter Wolf
© 1994 John Libbey & Company Ltd., pp. 359–368

Chapter 38

Bilateral temporal lobe epilepsy

Jerome Engel

Departments of Neurology and Anatomy and Cell Biology and the Brain Research Institute, UCLA School of Medicine, 710 Westwood Plaza, Los Angeles, California 90024–1769, USA

Introduction

The term *temporal lobe epilepsy* has been used extensively in the literature for many years (Baldwin & Bailey, 1958; Penry & Daly, 1975; Lindsay *et al.*, 1979a, b, c), but there is no generally accepted definition of this disorder. In the broadest sense, temporal lobe epilepsy is characterized by recurrent simple and complex partial seizures, the principal symptoms of which are generated predominantly by mesial temporal lobe limbic structures. At least three forms of temporal lobe epilepsy are recognized, and the reasons for bilateral abnormalities may differ among them.

1. Chronic epileptic disorders due to epileptogenic regions in distant temporal or extratemporal neocortex can have preferential initial spread of ictal discharge to mesial temporal lobe limbic areas. In these conditions, the earliest ictal symptoms may reveal the likely site of ictal onset (e.g. vertiginous or auditory auras suggesting lateral temporal neocortex; visual auras suggesting more posterior neocortex), while ictal onset in so-called 'silent areas' may provide no clinical clues to the location of the epileptogenic region. In either case, once the ictal discharge has propagated to mesial temporal limbic structures, the subsequent signs and symptoms are indistinguishable from those of other forms of temporal lobe epilepsy. The incidence and character of bilateral abnormalities depends on the location and nature of the primary epileptogenic lesion, since the density of commissural projections from neocortex is variable (Reeves & Roberts, 1993) and some pathological substrates tend to be multifocal.

2. Chronic epileptic disorders due to specific structural epileptogenic lesions in, or immediately adjacent to, mesial temporal lobe limbic areas (e.g. hamartomas, gliomas, dysplasias, vascular malformations, or scars, in or near amygdala, hippocampus or parahippocampal gyrus) are characterized by seizures that only have the clinical features of mesial temporal ictal events. Bilateral abnormalities with these disorders are more common with primary epileptogenic lesions that are often multifocal.

3. A specific chronic epileptic disorder associated with hippocampal sclerosis is regarded as a discrete syndrome, referred to as *mesial temporal lobe epilepsy* (MTLE) (Engel, 1992; Wieser *et al.*, 1993). Seizures originate in the sclerotic hippocampus (Babb *et al.*, 1984) and are clinically indistinguishable from those caused by other mesial temporal lesions.

However, there are several unique aspects of this condition, as shown in Table 1. The aetiology of hippocampal sclerosis is unknown, but there is evidence to suggest some genetic predisposition in addition to one or more acquired insults that cause hippocampal cell loss and neuronal reorganization conducive to epileptogenesis (Engel, 1992). Despite the well-localized pathophysiological substrate, it is clear that the epileptogenic region is more extensive than one temporal lobe, since auras often persist following anterior temporal lobectomy (Vickrey *et al.*, 1992). Bilateral disturbances in this disorder are common and it is unknown to what extent they can be attributed to bilateral insults initially (Babb & Brown, 1987) or to some progressive process. Although direct commissural connections between hippocampi in the human are sparse or non-existent (Wilson *et al.*, 1987) and contralateral ictal spread from mesial temporal limbic areas is characteristically slow (Lieb *et al.*, 1986), bilateral mesial temporal ictal discharges are usually necessary for complex partial seizures to occur. Therefore, frequent contralateral involvement in these ictal events could cause enduring neuronal disturbances.

Table 1. The syndrome of mesial temporal lobe epilepsy (MTLE)

A. History

1.Increased incidence of complicated febrile convulsions.
2. Increased incidence of a family history of epilepsy.
3. Onset in latter half of first decade of life.
4. Auras are common and occur in isolation.
5. Secondarily generalized seizures occur frequently.
6. Seizures often remit for several years until adolescence or early adulthood.
7. Seizures often become medically intractable.
8. Interictal behavioural disturbances can occur (most commonly depression).

B. Clinical seizure

1. Aura is usually present – most common is epigastric rising, often other autonomic or psychic symptoms, with emotion (e.g. fear), can be olfactory or gustatory sensation (several seconds).
2. Complex partial seizure – often begins with arrest and stare, oroalimetary automatisms and complex automatisms common. Posturing of one upper extremity may occur contralateral to thc ictal discharge (1 to 2 min).
3. Postictal phase – usually includes disorientation, reccnt memory deficit, amnesia for the event and dysphasia if seizures begin in the language-dominant hemisphere (several minutes).

C. Neurological examination

1. Usually normal.
2. May have recent memory deficit.

D. EEG

1. Unilateral or bilateral independent anterior temporal spikes, maximum amplitude in basal electrodes.
2. May be inermittent or continuous rhythmic slowing in one mesial temporal area.
3. Extracranial ictal activity appears only with complex partial symptoms, usually initial or delayed focal onset pattern of 5–7/s rhythmic activity maximum amplitude in one basal temporal derivation.
4. Depth electrode ictal onset most often high-amplitude rhythmic spikes or sharp waves, less commonly low-voltage fast or suppression.
5. Propagation to contralateral side is slow (> 5 s, but may be minutes) or does not occur at all.

E. Focal functional deficits

1. Usually temporal lobe hypometabolism on interictal FDG-PET, often involves ipsilateral thalamus and basal ganglia.
2. Usually temporal lobe hypoperfusion on interictal SPECT and characteristic pattern of hyper- and hypoperfusion on ictal SPECT.
3. Usually material-specific memory disturbances on neuropsychological testing and amnesia wih contralateral intracarotid sodium amobarbital injection.
4. Mesial temporal EEG slowing and attenuation of normal rhythms can be seen with scalp/sphenoidal electrodes, but more common with depth electrodes; exacerbated by IV pentothal test.

F. Structural imaging
1. May have small hippocampus on one side (on MRI).
2. May have small temporal lobe on one side.
3. May have enlarged temporal horn on one side.

G. Pathophysiology
1. Hippocampal sclerosis (> 30 % cell loss with spccific patterns).
2. Sprouting of dentate granule cell mossy fibres.
3. Selective loss of certain hilar neurones (somatostatin and NPY-containing cells).
4. Hamartomas and heterotopias may occur as 'dual pathology'.
5. Microdysgenesis common.
6. Seizures may originate in sclerotic hippocampus but much larger area appears to be included in the epileptogenic region.

H. Features that place diagnosis in doubt
1. History of severe head trauma, encephalitis or other specific causal events.
2. Focal motor or specific sensory symptoms at seizure onset or postictally.
3. Interictal focal neurological deficits.
4. Marked cognitive impairment on neuropsychological testing.
5. Bilaterally synchronous, generalized or extratemporal focal EEG spikes.
6. Diffuse or extratemporal focal EEG slowing.
7. Cerebral lesion other than hippocampal sclerosis on MRI.

FDG-PET: Fleurodioxyglucose-positron emission tomography; SPECT: single photon emission computed tomography; IV: intravenous; NPY: neuropeptide Y. From Engel (1993), with permission.

MTLE is by far the most common form of temporal lobe epilepsy (Babb & Brown, 1987), but hippocampal sclerosis may also coexist with other temporal or extratemporal lesions (Levesque *et al.*, 1991). In this situation, it is unclear when: (1) the hippocampal sclerosis is the actual primary epileptogenic lesion while the other structural abnormality is unrelated; (2) the hippocampal sclerosis is merely a marker for a predisposition to epilepsy; or (3) the hippocampal sclerosis is a consequence of repeated epileptic seizures. Clearly, hippocampal damage can be caused by profound systemic insults that produce cerebral hypoxia or hypoglycaemia, but the pattern of cell loss in these situations does not have the characteristic anatomical distribution of epileptogenic hippocampal sclerosis (Babb & Brown, 1987). Recently identified patterns of axonal sprouting and synaptogenesis (Sutula *et al.*, 1989; Babb *et al.*, 1991; de Lanerolle *et al.*, 1992 and de Lanerolle *et al.*, Chapter 46), as well as selective loss of specific cell types (de Lanerolle *et al.*, 1992), may be unique features of the hippocampal sclerosis responsible for MTLE.

Manifestations of bilateral temporal lobe epilepsy

Bilateral interictal EEG spikes

The most commonly encountered evidence of bilateral temporal lobe dysfunction among patients with temporal lobe epilepsy is the occurrence of independent bilateral mesial temporal interictal electroencephalographic (EEG) spikes. In patients with medically refractory complex partial seizures who have undergone extensive evaluation as potential candidates for surgical treatment, some degree of independent bilateral mesial temporal interictal epileptiform discharges are the rule rather than the exception. Although a majority of patients with such bilateral independent interictal EEG spikes have a clear predominance on the side that ultimately is determined to be the site of habitual seizure generation, a significant number show no clear preponderance on one side, and in 10–15 per cent the preponderance is contralateral to what is considered to be the primary epileptogenic region (Engel *et al.*, 1984). Patients with bilateral independent interictal spikes can usually be shown to have a single primary epileptogenic region (So *et al.*, 1989), and there is as yet no convincing evidence to justify consideration of bilateral spikes in this patient population as a poor prognostic sign.

Some patients with temporal lobe epilepsy have bilaterally synchronous, usually frontally predominant, interictal spikes in addition to unilateral or independent bilateral mesial temporal spikes. In contrast to independent bilateral mesial temporal spikes, synchronous bilateral spikes do have a poor prognosis for outcome following anterior temporal lobectomy (Engel *et al.*, 1975). It is now generally assumed that this EEG finding is more likely to indicate complex partial seizures of frontal lobe, rather than mesial temporal lobe, origin. Before the advent of magnetic resonance imaging (MRI) scans, functional imaging and chronic intracranial electrode recordings, such patients were likely to be subjected to anterior temporal lobectomy based on seizure semiology and the presence of interictal mesial temporal spikes, with poor results because the primary frontal epileptogenic region was left *in situ* (Engel *et al.*, 1975). It should be noted that extratemporal interictal spikes, either bilateral or unilateral, suggest that the primary epileptogenic region is not in the temporal lobes. On the other hand, some patients with temporal lobe epilepsy may also have a benign 3/s spike-and-wave trait (Metrakos & Metrakos, 1966), which presumably should not influence surgical outcome.

Bilateral ictal EEG onsets

It is not unusual during extensive presurgical evaluation of patients with medically refractory complex partial seizures who are candidates for anterior temporal lobectomy to record spontaneous seizures originating independently from both mesial temporal areas. Most commonly there is one side that generates the habitual seizures, while one or a few atypical seizures arise from the contralateral side. Although atypical contralateral seizures may in some patients be a consequence of drug withdrawal or irritation from depth electrodes (Engel & Crandall, 1983), this appears to be a rare occurrence (Marciani & Gotman, 1986; Spencer *et al.*, 1981; Marks *et al.*, 1991). Sometimes the atypical contralateral seizure appears after a series of habitual seizures, perhaps because the primary epileptogenic region has undergone profound postictal inhibition or even exhaustion. None of these contralateral seizure types appear to have any prognostic significance for postoperative outcome, so it is important to recognize them as atypical events. Family and friends can help by reviewing the videotape to ascertain that these are not the habitual seizures causing disabilities outside the hospital. This phenomenon, however, demonstrates that contralateral epileptogenicity, more commonly evidenced by interictal spikes, is also associated, at least in some patients, with a lowered threshold for generation of spontaneous seizures.

A more disturbing problem, when surgical treatment is being considered, is presented by the patient who generates spontaneous seizures from both sides of the brain when no unusual precipitating factors can be identified (Morrell, 1989; Hirsch *et al.*, 1991a, b). For such patients, it is important to try to identify ictal and postictal clinical features that could allow the patient or observers to keep track of each seizure type independently. Usually this requires video monitoring and chronic bilateral invasive EEG recording, the most effective approach being depth electrodes. Even though seizures of one type, beginning from one side, may predominate during the in-patient intracranial evaluation, this represents an artificial condition and may not accurately reflect what is happening at home. Rather than base a surgical decision on some magic ratio between the two types of seizures captured in the hospital, it is more reasonable to ask the patient and others to keep a record of when, and under what circumstances, the two types of seizures occur outside the hospital. Then, if one is clearly more frequent or more disabling, there are no other conflicting findings (e.g. contralateral focal functional deficits or lesions) and the patient is willing to accept the possibility that the other type of seizure may remain postoperatively, surgical treatment is a reasonable option.

Occasionally, patients have spontaneous habitual seizures that arise independently from both sides of the brain, with no distinguishing features. When invasive recordings reveal that such seizures occur with equal frequency from each side in the hospital, nothing more can be done. If one side clearly predominates, surgery may still be offered, but obviously the risk of a less than satisfactory outcome is considerable. In this situation, the decision to recommend surgery is aided by the presence of a congruent lesion on MRI, or other lateralizing evidence of temporal lobe functional deficits, such as material-specific memory disturbances on neuropsychological testing, localized interictal hypometabolism on positron emission tomography (PET) and global amnesia with contralateral intracarotid amobarbital injections. Ictal single-photon emission computed tomography (SPECT) is obviously of no value here because it offers no information about persistent deficits and does not contribute to an understanding of the frequency of seizure generation from each side of the brain.

Given that there is no evidence of contralateral non-epileptic functional deficit, the worst outcome to be expected following anterior temporal lobe resection in a patient with bilateral ictal onsets is that the seizures generated contralateral to the resection persist at the same frequency as before. Interestingly, however, contralateral seizures in many patients cease following surgery, or run down and either eventually stop or recur less frequently than preoperatively (Morrell, 1985; Hirsch *et al.*, 1991b). There is some evidence to suggest that contralateral seizure persistence postoperatively depends on duration of the seizure disorder or frequency of seizures prior to surgery, or both (Morrell, 1989).

Bilateral non-epileptic dysfunction

Patients with medically refractory complex partial seizures often show evidence of bilateral temporal dysfunction independent of interictal or ictal epileptiform abnormalities on EEG. Bilateral EEG slowing or attenuation of fast activity, particularly as recorded with depth electrodes implanted into mesial temporal structures, and bitemporal hypometabolism with PET or hypoperfusion with SPECT occur, but are difficult to assess because there are not adequate standards for determining when contralateral temporal function is minimally abnormal. For instance, most PET and SPECT studies are based on temporal lobe asymmetries, rather than on absolute measures of cerebral metabolism or cerebral perfusion. The more commonly encountered evidence of bitemporal dysfunction comes from neuropsychological evaluation, particularly material-specific memory disturbances referable to both hemispheres. Resection of the epileptogenic mesial temporal structures usually results in improvement in contralateral memory function and an average 10 point increase in IQ (Rausch & Crandall, 1982), indicating that this deficit is potentially reversible.

The extent to which contralateral functional deficits reflect a degree of epileptogenicity is unclear; however, thresholds for electrical stimulation-induced after-discharge are commonly lower in the hippocampus contralateral to ictal onset (Cherlow *et al.*, 1977), providing further evidence of increased epileptogenicity in this area. No attempts have been made to correlate reduced hippocampal after-discharge thresholds or interictal spike occurrence and seizure generation in the contralateral temporal lobe with evidence of contralateral material-specific memory deficit, or to correlate postoperative improvement in contralateral memory function with decrease or disappearance of EEG spikes or seizures of contralateral mesial temporal origin. Such data would be useful in determining whether contralateral epileptic and non-epileptic dysfunction reflect similar mechanisms, or whether they are discrete phenomena that respond independently to elimination of the primary epileptogenic region.

Bilateral structural disturbances

Yet another manifestation of bilateral temporal lobe epilepsy is bilateral structural disturbance. This is unusual in the case of alien tissue lesions such as tumours and vascular malformations, but is well known to occur with the most common pathological substrate of temporal lobe epilepsy, hippocampal sclerosis (Margerison & Corsellis, 1966; Babb & Brown, 1987). Autopsy studies of hippocampi from patients with *long-standing* temporal lobe epilepsy revealed that the degree of cell loss is usually asymmetrical, but present, to some degree, on both sides in the majority of patients (Babb & Brown, 1987). As many as 25 per cent of patients in one study had symmetrical damage (Margerison & Corsellis, 1966), but these were institutionalized patients who died after a long history of chronic epilepsy, and it is uncertain whether such observations would apply to a much younger population of potential surgical candidates.

The cause of hippocampal sclerosis remains unknown, as is the reason why this structural defect should so often be asymmetrical or unilateral. Many investigators believe that the hippocampal sclerosis characteristic of MTLE has a specific pattern of cell loss (for instance, relative sparing of the CA_2 region) that is different from the more nonspecific hippocampal damage associated with hypoxia, toxic exposure and other insults that cause diffuse brain damage (Babb & Brown, 1987). More recently, investigators have also described selective loss of particular cell types, such as hilar neurones containing somatostatin and neuropeptide Y (NPY) as well as dentate granule cell mossy fibre sprouting (Sutula *et al.*, 1989; Babb *et al.*, 1991; de Lanerolle *et al.*, 1992) which may also be specific for mesial temporal lobe epilepsy. There are no studies to date that indicate whether hippocampal damage contralateral to primary epileptogenic hippocampal sclerosis is relatively non-specific, or whether it can demonstrate those features believed to be characteristic of epileptogenic hippocampal sclerosis. There is also no evidence yet reported in the literature concerning whether patients with bilateral mesial temporal interictal spikes, ictal onsets or focal functional disturbances are more likely to have contralateral hippocampal sclerosis, and whether this hippocampal sclerosis is of a specific or non-specific type. Such information would be important for determining whether bilateral temporal lobe epilepsy in patients with hippocampal sclerosis reflects bilateral consequences of the initial epileptogenic insult, or whether a primary epileptogenic hippocampus can induce functional and structural changes in the contralateral hippocampus. High-resolution MRI can now identify bilateral hippocampal atrophy (Jack *et al.*, 1992), making some *in vivo* correlations between function and structure possible, but atrophy is not necessarily the same as hippocampal sclerosis.

Causes of bilateral temporal lobe epilepsy

Some types of epileptogenic lesions are more likely to occur bilaterally than others. For instance, glial tumours and vascular malformations are more likely to be unilateral, while damage due to trauma, generalized infectious processes such as herpes encephalitis, or metabolic disturbances such as hypoxia are more likely to produce bilateral lesions. Multiple propagation patterns from a single extratemporal lesion may also, rarely, give rise to seizures that appear to originate independently from each mesial temporal lobe (Hirsch *et al.*, 1991a). Of considerable interest with respect to human epilepsy, however, is the possibility that an epileptogenic area of brain can itself induce distant, perhaps contralateral, functional and structural disturbances. Although such secondary epileptogenesis involving contralateral structures has clearly been demonstrated in experimental animals in the form of the mirror focus phenomenon (Morrell, 1959/60) and kindling (Goddard *et al.*, 1969), the relevance of these observations to human epilepsy remains controversial (Goldensohn, 1984). The obvious implication that some forms of human epilepsy may be progressive is difficult to definitively prove, since medical intervention invariably alters the natural history of the disease process.

Given that it takes days to kindle a rat, weeks to kindle a cat and many months to kindle a rhesus monkey (Wada *et al.*, 1978), it is likely that any similar effect in the human brain would take a long time to develop, even without antiepileptic drug treatment. Nevertheless, it is likely that the human brain differs quantitatively but not qualitatively from lower mammalian brains, and that similar functional, if not structural, effects of repeated epileptic seizures do occur in some patients, and do have clinical importance. This may not necessarily be the establishment of a secondary epileptogenic region capable of initiating spontaneous seizures in the opposite hemisphere, but could be reflected merely as increased epileptogenicity, making seizures more severe, more frequent or more difficult to treat, and it may also underlie the appearance of contralateral focal functional deficits, which clearly disrupt memory, and may also be reflected as interictal behavioural disturbances (Engel *et al.*, 1991).

Although by no means definitive, there is ample evidence for epileptic seizure-induced disruption of contralateral mesial temporal lobe function in patients with temporal lobe epilepsy. It can be argued that the typical course of the MTLE syndrome reflects progression, with seizures that begin in the first decade of life and are initially easy to treat, but then often become medically refractory during adolescence or early adulthood (Engel, 1992; Wieser *et al.*, 1993). The late appearance of contralateral memory deficits and interictal behavioural disturbances may also be considered evidence of progression in this disorder. At least one large EEG study has documented an increase in bilateral interictal temporal spikes, over time, of approximately 1 per cent per year (Hughes, 1985). An investigation of patients with temporal lobe epilepsy due to glial tumours, lesions that are unlikely to occur bilaterally, revealed evidence of spontaneous contralateral seizure generation in 15 per cent of patients (Morrell, 1985). In this study, failure of seizures of contralateral origin to disappear after surgical resection of the primary epileptogenic region correlated with both duration of the epileptic disorder and frequency of epileptic seizures preoperatively. A report of another surgical series, limited to those patients who did well postoperatively, noted that patients with the shortest duration of epilepsy prior to anterior temporal lobectomy were most likely to become seizure-free; those with an intermediate duration of epilepsy were most likely to continue to have auras; while those with the longest preoperative duration of epilepsy were most likely to continue to have occasional complex partial seizures (Engel & Cahan, 1986). No attempt was made in this last study, however, to correlate these findings with the presence of epileptogenicity in the contralateral temporal lobe, as opposed to residual epileptogenic properties on the side of surgery.

Patients with hippocampal sclerosis often continue to experience their habitual auras after anterior temporal lobe resection (Vickrey *et al.*, 1992), but the origin of these ictal events remains unknown. Clearly the epileptogenic region in these patients is much larger than the mesial temporal structures where seizures appear to begin, and indeed larger than the entire anterior temporal lobe, indicating some recruitment of distant tissue into the epileptogenic process; however, this could include ipsilateral limbic structures such as the insula and more posterior hippocampus, as well as contralateral mesial temporal lobe limbic areas. It is important to note here that patients with temporal lobe epilepsy commonly have hypometabolism on PET that extends to the ipsilateral thalamus and extratemporal cortical regions (Henry *et al.*, 1990), and that residual seizures following temporal lobectomy most commonly originate from the side of surgery (Polkey *et al.*, 1993).

The concept of secondary epileptogenesis in human temporal lobe epilepsy and the possibility that this condition might reflect a progressive disturbance are of extreme clinical importance, because they imply that early surgical intervention would yield much better outcomes. Clearly, this is the case with respect to psychosocial rehabilitation (Rausch & Crandall, 1982), which supports, but by no means proves, a view that there is progressive non-epileptic dysfunction, presumably involving contralateral structures, which ultimately becomes irreversible. Further studies are needed to substantiate published reports that clinically significant epileptiform abnormalities in the contralateral mesial temporal lobe can also be avoided if surgery is performed early in the course of the disorder. If permanent contralateral epileptic or non-epileptic disturbances can be induced in the human brain by recurrent complex partial seizures of temporal lobe origin, it remains unknown which types of epileptogenic disturbances are capable of inducing such changes, and what periods of time are necessary before such changes become irreversible. Although there is a suspicion that patients with MTLE are particularly susceptible to this form of progression, more data are needed as a basis for determining when early surgical intervention is justified, and which patients who already have evidence of bilateral temporal lobe epilepsy will benefit from surgical resection of one temporal lobe.

Conclusions

The term 'bilateral temporal lobe epilepsy' is not used in a consistent fashion in the literature. It is generally presumed that mesial temporal structures must be bilaterally involved for the impaired consciousness that characterizes complex partial seizures. Obviously, involvement of the contralateral mesial temporal limbic structures in the habitual complex partial ictal event is not sufficient to justify considering a patient to have bilateral temporal lobe epilepsy. There is usually some degree of postictal confusion following complex partial seizures, and this also presumably reflects bilateral mesial temporal dysfunction, which can last for variable periods of time. This transient involvement of the contralateral hemisphere also is not sufficient to warrant a diagnosis of bilateral temporal lobe epilepsy. In some patients, however, the postictal disturbances may be persistent, and evidence of prolonged contralateral dysfunction, such as material-specific memory deficit, may be considered evidence of bilateral temporal involvement in the underlying disease process. The fact that this contralateral material-specific memory dysfunction usually disappears following successful surgical removal of the primary epileptogenic region, however, indicates a reversible functional disturbance, which, in itself, also would not warrant a diagnosis of bilateral temporal lobe epilepsy.

Bilateral independent mesial temporal interictal spikes are commonly encountered and certainly provide evidence for enduring bilateral epileptogenicity, and patients with this finding might be considered by some to have bilateral temporal lobe epilepsy. This observation alone, however, is not considered to be a contraindication to anterior temporal lobe surgery, and does not appear to influence postoperative outcome. Consequently, contralateral interictal spikes might also reflect reversible functional disturbances rather than permanent contralateral epileptogenicity.

The term 'bilateral temporal lobe epilepsy' might most appropriately be applied to patients for whom bilateral independent temporal lobe ictal onsets have clearly been demonstrated. Some seizures originating contralateral to the primary or predominant epileptogenic region, however, are induced only by unusual circumstances, such as irritation from depth electrode implantation, drug withdrawal or postictal suppression of the primary epileptogenic region, and are considered to be atypical events. If there is no evidence that contralateral temporal structures generate seizures spontaneously outside the hospital, then this also need not be considered bilateral temporal lobe epilepsy. Among those patients with habitual spontaneous seizures that are generated from both temporal lobes, who would inarguably be said to have bilateral temporal lobe epilepsy, surgical cures can still be achieved by resection of the more active epileptogenic anterior temporal lobe, again indicating a reversible functional disturbance of the contralateral hemisphere. This leaves only a few patients with irreversible contralateral independent temporal lobe seizures, many of whom have bilateral structural disturbances as well. Although some of these patients have had initial epileptogenic insults capable of producing bilateral brain damage, others have not; thus, further clinical research is needed to examine whether and, if so, the circumstances under which a primary epileptogenic region can induce distant structural or functional disturbances, or both, specifically sclerosis of the contralateral hippocampus.

Temporal lobe epilepsy, particularly MTLE, presents a number of paradoxes with respect to contralateral disturbances and possible progressive symptoms. Bilateral mesial temporal epileptic and non-epileptic abnormalities appear to be much more common in this condition than bilateral neocortical abnormalities in the non-limbic epilepsies, and yet commissural connections between the hippocampi in the human are few or absent. On the other hand, it is a generally held clinical impression that bilateral independent neocortical interictal EEG spikes are associated with a much poorer surgical outcome than bilateral independent mesial temporal interictal EEG spikes, suggesting that the latter are more likely to represent reversible functional disturbances.

A better understanding of the mechanisms that underlie these phenomena will permit more rational decisions regarding the timing of surgical intervention in individual patients.

Acknowledgements

Original research reported by the author was supported in part by Grants NS-02808, NS-15654 and GM-24839, from the National Institutes of Health, and Contract DE-AC03-76-SF00012 from the Department of Energy.

References

Babb, T.L. & Brown, W.J. (1987): Pathological findings in epilepsy. In: *Surgical treatment of the epilepsies*, ed. J. Engel, pp. 511–540. New York: Raven Press.

Babb, T.L., Kupfer, W.R., Pretorius, J.K., Crandall, P.H. & Levesque, M.F. (1991): Synaptic reorganization by mossy fibers in human epileptic fascia dentata. *Neuroscience* **42,** 351–363.

Babb, T.L., Lieb, J.P., Brown, W.J., Pretorius, J. & Crandall, P.H. (1984): Distribution of pyramidal cell density and hyperexcitability in the epileptic human hippocampal formation. *Epilepsia* **25,** 721–728.

Baldwin, M. & Bailey, P. (1958): *Temporal lobe epilepsy.* Springfield, Ill.: Charles C. Thomas.

Cherlow, D.G., Dymond, A.M., Crandall, P.H., Walter, R.D. & Serafetinides, E.A. (1977): Evoked response and after-discharge thresholds to electrical stimulation in temporal lobe epileptics. *Arch. Neurol.* **34,** 527–531.

de Lanerolle, N.C., Brines, M.L., Kim, J.H., Williamson, A., Philips, M.F. & Spencer, D.D. (1992): Neurochemical remodeling of the hippocampus in human temporal lobe epilepsy. In: *Molecular neurobiology of epilepsy (Epilepsy Res. Suppl. 9)*, eds. J. Engel, Jr, C. Wasterlain, E.A. Cavalheiro, U. Heinemann & G. Avanzini, pp. 205–220. Amsterdam: Elsevier.

Engel, J. Jr (1992): Recent advances in surgical treatment of temporal lobe epilepsy. *Acta Neurol. Scand.* **86** (Suppl 5), 71–80.

Engel, J., Jr (1993): Update on surgical treatment of the epilepsies. *Neurology* **43,** 1612–1617.

Engel, J. Jr, Bandler, R., Griffith, N.C. & Caldecott-Hazard, S. (1991): Neurobiological evidence for epilepsy-induced interictal disturbances. In: *Advances in neurology*, Vol. 55, pp. 97–111. New York: Raven Press.

Engel, J. Jr & Cahan, L. (1986): Potential relevance of kindling to human partial epilepsy. In: *Kindling 3*, ed. J. Wada, pp. 37–51. New York: Raven Press.

Engel, J. Jr & Crandall, P.H. (1983): Falsely localizing ictal onsets with depth EEG telemetry during anticonvulsant withdrawal. *Epilepsia* **24,** 344–355.

Engel, J. Jr, Driver, M.V. & Falconer, M.A. (1975): Electrophysiological correlates of pathology and surgical results in temporal lobe epilepsy. *Brain* **98,** 129–156.

Engel, J. Jr, Sutherling, W.W., Cahan, L., Crandall, P.H., Kuhl, D.E. & Phelps, M.E. (1984): The role of positron emission tomography in the surgical therapy of epilepsy. In: *Advances in epileptology: XV*, eds. R.J. Porter, R.H. Mattson, A.A. Ward & M. Dam, pp. 427–432. New York: Raven Press.

Goddard, G.V., McIntyre, D.C. & Leech, C.K. (1969): A permanent change in brain function resulting from daily electrical stimulation. *Exp. Neurol.* **25,** 295–330.

Goldensohn, E.S. (1984): The relevance of secondary epileptogenesis to the treatment of epilepsy: kindling and the mirror focus. *Epilepsia* **25** (Suppl 2), S156–S173.

Henry, T.R., Mazziotta, J.C., Engel, J., Jr, Christenson, P.D., Zhang, J.-X., Phelps, M.E. & Kuhl, D.E. (1990): Quantifying interictal metabolic activity in human temporal lobe epilepsy. *J. Cerebral Blood Flow Metab.* **10,** 748–757.

Hirsch, L.J., Spencer, S.S., Spencer, D.D., Williamson, P.D. & Mattson, R.H. (1991b): Temporal lobectomy in patients with bitemporal epilepsy defined by depth electroencephalography. *Ann. Neurol.* **30,** 347–356.

Hirsch, L.J., Spencer, S.S., Williamson, P.D., Spencer, D.D. & Mattson, R.H. (1991a): Comparison of bitemporal and unitemporal epilepsy defined by depth electroencephalography. *Ann. Neurol.* **30,** 340–346.

Hughes, J.R. (1985): Long-term clinical and EEG changes in patients with epilepsy. *Arch. Neurol.* **42,** 213–223.

Jack, C.R., Sharbrough, F.W., Cascino, G.D., Hirschorn, K.A., O'Brien, P.C. & Marsh, W.R. (1992): Magnetic resonance image-based hippocampal volumetry: correlation with outcome after temporal lobectomy. *Ann. Neurol.* **31,** 138–146.

Levesque, M.F., Nakasato, N., Vinters, H.V. & Babb, T.L. (1991): Surgical treatment of limbic epilepsy associated with extrahippocampal lesions: the problem of dual pathology. *J. Neurosurg.* **75,** 364–370.

Lieb, J.P., Engel, J. Jr & Babb, T.L. (1986): Interhemispheric propagation time of human hippocampal seizures. I. Relationship to surgical outcome. *Epilepsia* **27,** 286–293.

Lindsay, J., Ounsted, C. & Richards, P. (1979b): Long-term outcome in children with temporal lobe seizures. I. Social outcome and childhood factors. *Dev. Med. Child Neurol.* **21,** 285–298.

Lindsay, J., Ounsted, C. & Richards, P. (1979b): Long-term outcome in children with temporal lobe seizures. II. Marriage, parenthood and sexual indifference. *Dev. Med. Child Neurol.* **21,** 433–440.

Lindsay, J., Ounsted, C. & Richards, P. (1979a): Long-term outcome in children with temporal lobe seizures. III. Psychiatric aspects in childhood and adult life. *Dev. Med. Child Neurol.* **21,** 630–636.

Marciani, M.G. & Gotman, J. (1986): Effects of drug withdrawal on location of seizure onset. *Epilepsia* **27,** 423–431.

Margerison, J.H. & Corsellis, J.A. (1966): Epilepsy and the temporal lobes: a clinical, electroencephalographic and neuropathological study of the brain in epilepsy, with particular reference to the temporal lobes. *Brain* **89,** 499–530.

Marks, D., Katz, A., Scheyer, R. & Spencer, S.S. (1991): Clinical and electrographic effects of acute anticonvulsive withdrawal in epileptic patients. *Neurology* **41,** 508–512.

Metrakos, J.D. & Metrakos, K. (1966): Childhood epilepsy of subcortical ('centrencephalic') origin: some questions and answers for the pediatrician. *Clin. Pediatr.* **5,** 537–542.

Morrell, F. (1959/60): Secondary epileptogenic lesions. *Epilepsia* **1,** 538–560.

Morrell, F. (1985): Secondary epileptogenesis in man. *Arch. Neurol.* **42,** 318–335.

Morrell, F. (1989): Varieties of human secondary epileptogenesis. *J. Cllin. Neurophysiol.* **6,** 227–275.

Penry, J.K. & Daly, D.D. (eds.) (1975): *Complex partial seizures and their treatments (advances in neurology, Vol. 11).* New York: Raven Press.

Polkey, C.E., Awad, I.A., Tanaka, T. & Wyler, A.R. (1993): The place of reoperation. In: *Surgical treatment of the epilepsies,* 2nd edn, ed. J. Engel, Jr, pp. 663–667. New York: Raven Press.

Rausch, R. & Crandall, P.H. (1982): Psychological status related to surgical control of temporal lobe seizures. *Epilepsia* **23,** 191–202.

Reeves, A.G. & Roberts, D.W. (1993): In: *Epilepsy and the corpus callosum,* Vol. 2. New York: Plenum Press.

So, N., Gloor, P., Quesney, L.F., Jones-Gotman, M., Olivier, A. & Andermann, F. (1989): Depth electrode investigations in patients with bitemporal epilepiform abnormalities. *Ann. Neurol.* **25,** 423–431.

Spencer, S.S., Spencer, D.D., Williamson, P.D. & Mattson, R.H. (1981): Ictal effects of anticonvulsant medication withdrawal in epileptic patients. *Epilepsia* **22,** 297–307.

Sutula, T., Cascino, G., Cavazos, J., Parada, I. & Ramirez, L. (1989): Mossy fiber synaptic reorganization in the epileptic human temporal lobe. *Ann. Neurol.* **26,** 321–330.

Vickrey, B.G., Hays, R.D., Graber, J., Rausch, R., Engel, J. Jr & Brook, R.H. (1992): A health-related quality of life instrument for patients evaluated for epilepsy surgery. *Med. Care* **30,** 299–319.

Wada, J.A., Mizoguchi, T. & Osawa, T. (1978): Secondarily generalized convulsive seizures induced by daily electrical stimulation in rhesus monkeys. *Neurology* **28,** 1026–1036.

Wieser, H.G., Engel, J. Jr, Williamson, P.D., Babb, T.L. & Gloor, P. (1993): Surgically remediable temporal lobe syndromes. In: *Surgical treatment of the epilepsies,* 2nd edn, ed. J. Engel, Jr, pp. 49–63. New York: Raven Press.

Wilson, C.L., Isokawa-Akesson, M., Babb, T.L., Engel, J. Jr, Cahan, L.D. & Crandall, P.H. (1987): A comparative view of local and interhemispheric limbic pathways in humans: an evoked potential analysis. In: *Fundamental mechanisms of human brain function,* eds. J. Engel, Jr, G.A. Ojemann, H.O. Lüders & P.D. Williamson, pp. 27–38. New York: Raven Press.

Epileptic Seizures and Syndromes, Edited by Peter Wolf
© 1994 John Libbey & Company Ltd., pp. 369–374

Chapter 39

A note on temporal lobe epilepsy in preadolescent children with respect to epilepsy surgery

Elaine Wyllie

Pediatric Epilepsy Program, The Cleveland Clinic Foundation, Desk S51, 9500 Euclid Avenue, Cleveland, Ohio 44195–5221, USA

Summary

Temporal lobe epilepsy is a well-defined epilepsy syndrome in adolescents and adults, but few data based on video-EEG are available for infants and children. Age-related differences have been reported in studies of very young patients, while children over 4 or 5 years old appear to have seizures similar to those in adults except that the automatisms in children tend to be more simple and bland. EEG findings may be complex in children with temporal lobe epilepsy due to low-grade tumours, and surgical strategy is focused mainly on resection of the tumours and surrounding cortex. Some children with mesial temporal sclerosis have had EEG findings similar to those in adults, but few cases have been reported and more data are needed.

Introduction

Temporal lobe epilepsy has been well characterized in adults, based on results of video-electroencephalography (EEG) in thousands of epilepsy surgery candidates over the last few decades (Delgado-Escueta *et al.*, 1982; Theodore *et al.*, 1983; Wieser, 1983; Kotagal, 1993; Quesney, 1986; Williamson, 1986; Bancaud, 1987; Maldonado *et al.*, 1988; Kotagal, 1991). However, very little is known about this problem in infants and children. Only recently have limited data become available about temporal lobe epilepsy in early childhood, based on observations from video-EEG (Holmes, 1984; Duchowny, 1987; Yamamoto *et al.*, 1987; Wyllie *et al.*, 1993). Previously the only available information was retrospective, obtained historically from adolescents or adults with temporal lobe epilepsy who had seizures beginning earlier in life.

Clarification of the clinical and EEG features of temporal lobe epilepsy in children is critical to the development of accurate criteria for identification of paediatric surgical candidates. As increasing numbers of patients are referred earlier for consideration of epilepsy surgery, this issue assumes practical as well as scientific importance.

Video-EEG studies of complex partial seizures in childhood

The typical manifestations of temporal lobe epilepsy – complex partial seizures – were studied in children with videotape observation by Holmes (1984) and Duchowny (1987). Holmes (1984) noted that automatisms occurred at some time during complex partial seizures in 87 per cent of 38 children who were 5–19 years of age, and that the automatisms were similar to those in adults, including chewing, lip smacking, thrashing, fumbling with objects, gesturing, facial grimacing or walking. However, in the younger patients studied by Duchowny (1987), the automatisms tended to be more often alimentary than gestural. Duchowny noted that 66 per cent of babies 0–2 years old had grimacing, lip smacking, chewing or eyelid fluttering during complex partial seizures, but none had gestural automatisms.

The studies from Holmes (1984) and Duchowny (1987) added significantly to our understanding of complex partial seizures in infants and children. However, their series included patients with seizures starting from temporal or extratemporal regions. Therefore, their observations were not strictly focused on the features of temporal lobe epilepsy in early childhood.

Video-EEG studies of temporal lobe epilepsy in childhood

Two recent studies were based on video-EEG observation of infants and children specifically with temporal lobe epilepsy. Patients in these series were selected by unilateral temporal EEG seizure pattern (Jayakar & Duchowny, 1990) or seizure-free outcome after temporal lobectomy (Wyllie *et al.*, 1993).

Jayakar and Duchowny (1990) studied 26 patients with ictal EEG showing a unilateral temporal seizure pattern, and found age-related differences in behaviours during seizures. Infants 0–2 years old typically had seizures beginning with motor phenomena (28 per cent of 11 patients), while children 6–12 years old typically had seizures beginning with staring (90 per cent of eight patients). Automatisms were common in seizures from children of all ages (71–88 per cent), but tended to be simpler in younger children.

The work of Jayakar and Duchowny (1990) provided important new information about the semiology of complex partial seizures in infants and children with temporal lobe epilepsy. However, a limitation of the study was that by selecting patients based on EEG criteria, the EEG features of the epilepsy could not be analysed as an independent variable. In an effort to explore both the EEG and clinical features of temporal lobe epilepsy in childhood, we studied children selected by seizure-free outcome after temporal lobectomy (Wyllie *et al.*, 1993).

The 14 children selected because of seizure-free outcome by Wyllie and colleagues (1993) were 16 months to 12 years old. The series was weighted toward children over 5 years old, and so was unable to add to the observations in very young children reported by Jayakar and Duchowny (1990). Results in these predominantly school-aged children were similar to those from Holmes (1984), with oral or gestural automatisms noted in almost all patients. In all these patients the automatisms tended to be simpler and blander than those typically seen in adolescents and adults. The children studied by Wyllie and colleagues (1993) usually only had chewing movements and quiet fingering of nearby objects during their complex partial seizures.

The children studied by Wyllie *et al.* (1993) included two main groups: those with intractable temporal lobe epilepsy due to otherwise asymptomatic low-grade temporal lobe tumours, and those with non-neoplastic aetiologies such as cortical dysplasia or mesial temporal sclerosis. The children with tumours typically had complex EEG findings: eight of the nine children had prominent extratemporal interictal sharp waves, poorly defined EEG seizure onset or false lateralization of EEG seizure patterns (Figs. 1 & 2). Despite these complex EEG features, all nine patients had a seizure-free outcome after resection only of the tumour and surrounding temporal lobe. In these children with tumours, the main value of the video-EEG evaluation was not localization of the epileptogenic zone, which failed in almost every case, but confirmation that the reported behaviours were indeed epileptic seizures with semiology typical of temporal lobe onset.

The complicated findings on scalp/sphenoidal EEG led to further study with invasive electrodes in one-third of the tumour patients in the series from Wyllie *et al.* (1993). However, in each case the invasive techniques failed to further clarify the location of seizure onset. The only benefit from invasive recording in this group was for a child with a left posterior temporal tumour. In this child, the cortical stimulation studies with subdural electrodes helped define the posterior extent of resection. Except when extraoperative functional location studies were required, however, invasive electrodes appeared to be unimportant in the presurgical evaluation of children with complex partial seizures due to a temporal lobe tumour. Regardless of scalp/sphenoidal or invasive EEG results, the strategy was resection of the temporal tumour and surrounding cortex. Some patients had resection of mesial temporal structures and others did not, so this study was unable to shed new light on whether the hippocampus and amygdala should be removed.

Five children studied by Wyllie *et al.* (1993) had a non-neoplastic aetiology for the temporal lobe epilepsy. Although cortical dysplasia was a common pathological substrate in the paediatric temporal lobectomy series from Duchowny and colleagues (1992), it was the pathological diagnosis in only one of the patients from Wyllie *et al.* (1993). Four children in the series from Wyllie *et al.* (1993) had presumed mesial temporal sclerosis with unilateral hippocampal atrophy on magnetic resonance imaging (MRI) and unilateral temporal hypometabolism on positron emission tomography (PET). Three of the four children had a history of febrile convulsions in infancy prior to onset of complex partial seizures, compared with none of the patients with tumours or cortical dysplasia ($P = 0.01$). Unfortunately, pathological confirmation of mesial temporal sclerosis was not possible, because mesial temporal structures were not removed *en bloc* and specimens were inadequate for examination. However, the children clearly fitted the clinical syndrome of mesial temporal sclerosis as described by Wieser and colleagues (1993). Each of the four children had EEG features typical of those seen in mesial temporal epilepsy in adolescents and adults, with EEG seizures and interictal sharp waves maximal at sphenoidal or anterior/inferior temporal scalp electrodes on the side with hippocampal atrophy and PET hypometabolism.

A limitation of the study by Wyllie *et al.* (1993) was that the patient group was skewed toward those children with temporal lobe epilepsy who were more likely to receive epilepsy surgery: children usually outside of infancy with temporal tumours or more severe epilepsy. Another limitation was that only patients with tumours were operated in the face of worrisome or atypical EEG findings. It is likely that other infants and children with early mesial temporal sclerosis remained unrecognized and were rejected from surgical candidacy, because of atypical electroclinical features. Prospective studies are in progress to better characterize the early findings of mesial temporal sclerosis on EEG and neuroimaging and to better characterize the diagnostic features of this disorder in young children.

Identification of surgical candidates

The exact percentage of children with temporal lobe epilepsy who are refractory to medication is unknown. However, in children with persistent complex partial seizures despite adequate drug trials, epilepsy surgery should be considered. With careful selection of candidates for operation, seizure-free outcome after surgery can be expected for the majority of children (Wyllie *et al.*, 1988, 1993; Duchowny *et al.*, 1992; Falconer, 1970; Jensen, 1976; Green, 1977; Jensen & Vaernet, 1977; Rasmussen, 1977; Polkey, 1980; Goldring & Gregorie, 1984; Lindsay *et al.*, 1984; Meyer *et al.*, 1986).

Adverse effects of temporal lobectomy in adults have included asymptomatic superior homonymous quadrantanopsia, language dysfunction and decreased scores on postoperative memory testing (Katz *et al.*, 1989). Language and memory changes are usually mild and have predominantly been reported

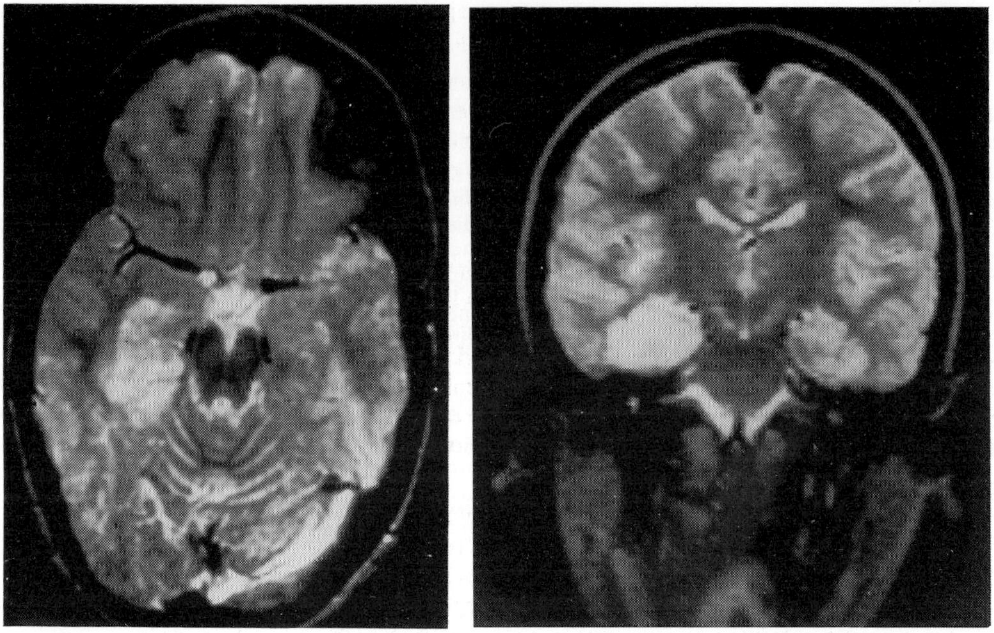

Fig. 1. MRI from an 8-year-old girl showing a right temporal ganglioglioma. Complex partial seizures began at 3 years old and occurred an average of three times per week despite aggressive treatment with antiepileptic medication.

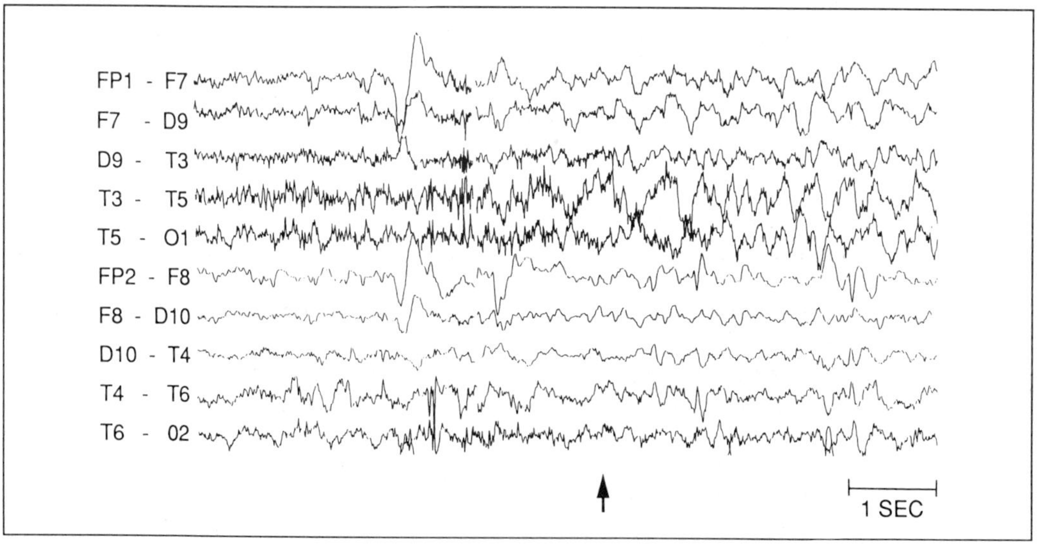

Fig. 2. EEG from the same child during a typical complex partial seizure. At the arrow, 8 s after clinical onset, the EEG seizure pattern became apparent over the left temporal lobe, even though the tumour was on the right. EEG seizures were also left temporal when recorded with foramen ovale electrodes. Interictal sharp waves were predominantly seen over the left temporal area, maximal at the left sphenoidal electrode. Only rare interictal sharp waves were seen over the right temporal lobe. Despite these falsely lateralizing ictal and interictal EEG features, the child remained seizure-free 3 years after resection of the right temporal lobe and tumour.

after left temporal lobectomy (Chelune *et al.*, 1991; Wyllie *et al.*, 1991). Cognitive effects of temporal lobectomy have not yet been studied in large series of children, and prospective studies are in progress.

A concern about early surgery in children has been that they may grow out of the seizures spontaneously later in life. However, it has not been clearly demonstrated that children with temporal lobe epilepsy are more likely to have spontaneous remission than are adults. Few follow-up studies have examined children selected by EEG findings diagnostic of temporal lobe epilepsy (Harbord & Manson, 1987; Kotagal *et al.*, 1987), but in these studies the rate of spontaneous remission has been low.

In children with temporal lobe tumours, the rate of spontaneous remission of complex partial seizures is probably close to zero. In addition, these children bear the potential risk of eventual malignant degeneration of their tumour, although the true incidence of this phenomenon is unknown. For these reasons, this author feels that early surgery is appropriate for children with complex partial seizures and a potentially neoplastic lesion on MRI. The strategy would be resection of the tumour and surrounding temporal lobe, even if EEG findings are complex. In these children, the main value of video-EEG may be to clarify that the reported behaviours are indeed complex partial seizures with semiology typical of temporal lobe onset.

In children without a neoplastic aetiology for the temporal lobe epilepsy, the optimal timing for consideration of epilepsy surgery in children is controversial. However, this author feels that surgery should be considered for any patient who had medically refractory, disabling complex partial seizures and a clear diagnosis of unilateral temporal lobe epilepsy based on results of video-EEG, MRI, PET and neuropsychological testing. Occasionally, these criteria will be met in preadolescent children.

References

Bancaud, J. (1987): Sémiologie clinique des crises épileptiques d'origine temporale. *Rev. Neurol.* **143,** 392–400.

Chelune, G.J., Naugle, R.I., Luders, H. & Awad, I.A. (1991): Prediction of cognitive change as a function of preoperative ability status among temporal lobectomy patients seen at 6-month follow-up. *Neurology* **41,** 399–404.

Delgado-Escueta, A.V., Bascal, F.E. & Treiman, D.M. (1982): Complex partial seizures on closed-circuit television and EEG: a study of 691 attacks in 79 patients. *Ann. Neurol.* **11,** 292–300.

Duchowny, M.S., Levin, B., Jayakar, P., Resnick, T., Alvarez, L., Morrison, G. & Dean, P. (1992): Temporal lobectomy in early childhood. *Epilepsia* **33,** 298–303.

Duchowny, M.S. (1987): Complex partial seizures of infancy. *Arch. Neurol.* **44,** 911–914.

Falconer, M. (1970): Significance of surgery for temporal epilepsy in childhood and adolescence. *J. Neurosurg.* **33,** 233–252.

Goldring, S. & Gregorie, E.M. (1984): Surgical management using epidural recordings to localize the seizure focus: review of 100 cases. *Neurosurgery* **60,** 457–466.

Green, J.R. (1977): Surgical treatment of epilepsy during childhood and adolescence. *Surg. Neurol.* **8,** 71–80.

Harbord, M.G. & Manson, J.I. (1987): Temporal lobe epilepsy in childhood: Reappraisal of etiology and outcome. *Pediatr. Neurol.* **3,** 263–268.

Holmes, G.L. (1984): Partial complex seizures in children: an analysis of 69 seizures in 24 patients using EEG FM radiotelemetry and videotape recording. *Electroencephalogr. Clin. Neurophysiol.* **57,** 13–20.

Jayakar, P. & Duchowny, M.S. (1990): Complex partial seizures of temporal lobe origin in early childhood. *J. Epilepsy* **3,** 41–45.

Jensen, I. (1976): Temporal lobe epilepsy. *Acta Neurol. Scand.* **53,** 335–357.

Jensen, I. & Vaernet, K. (1977): Temporal lobe epilepsy: follow-up investigation of 74 temporal lobe resected patients. *Acta Neurochirurg.* **37,** 173–200.

Katz, A., Awad, I.A., Kong, A.K., Chelune, G.J., Naugle, R.I., Wyllie, E., Beauchamp, G. & Lüders, H. (1989): Extent of resection in temporal lobectomy for epilepsy. II. Memory changes and neurologic complications. *Epilepsia* **30,** 763–771.

Kotagal, P. (1991): Seizure symptomatology of temporal lobe epilepsy. In: *Epilepsy surgery*, ed. H. Lüders, pp. 143–156. New York, NY: Raven Press.

Kotagal, P. (1993): Psychomotor seizures: clinical and EEG findings. In: *The treatment of epilepsy: principles and practice*, ed. E. Wyllie, pp. 378–492. Philadelphia, PA: Lea & Febiger.

Kotagal, P., Rothner, A.D., Erenberg, G., Cruse, R. & Wyllie, E. (1987): Complex of childhood onset: a five-year follow-up study. *Arch. Neurol.* **4487,** 1177–1180.

Lindsay, J., Ounsted, C. & Richards, P. (1984): Long-term outcome in children with temporal lobe seizures. V: Indications and contraindications for neurosurgery. *Dev. Med. Child Neurol.* **26,** 25–32.

Maldonado, H.M., Delgado-Escueta, A.V., Walsh, G.O., Swartz, B.E. & Rand, R.W. (1988): Complex partial seizures of hippocampal and amygdalar origin. *Epilepsia* **29,** 420–433.

Meyer, F.B., Marsh, W.R., Laws, E.R. & Sharbrough, F.W. (1986): Temporal lobectomy in children with epilepsy. *J. Neurosurg.* **64,** 371–376.

Polkey, C.E. (1980): Selection of patients with intractable epilepsy for resective surgery. *Arch. Dis. Child.* **55,** 841–844.

Quesney, L.F. (1986): Clinical and EEG features of complex partial seizures of temporal lobe origin. *Epilepsia* **27**(suppl. 2), S27–S45.

Rasmussen, T.B. (1977): Surgical aspects. In: *Topics in child neurology*, ed. G. Wise, pp. 143–153. Inglewood Cliffs, NJ: Spectrum Publications.

Theodore, W.H., Porter, R.J. & Penry, J.K. (1983): Complex partial seizures: clinical characteristics and differential diagnosis. *Neurology* **33,** 1115–1121.

Wieser, H.G. (1983): *Electroclinical features of the psychomotor seizure.* London, England: Butterworths.

Wieser, H.G., Engel, J., Jr, Williamson, P.D., Babb, T.L. & Gloor, P. (1993): Surgically remediable syndromes of infancy and early childhood. In: *Surgical treatment of the epilepsies*, Vol. 2, ed. J. Engel, Jr, pp. 49–64. New York, NY: Raven Press.

Williamson, P.D. (1986): Intensive monitoring of complex partial seizures: diagnosis and subclassification; In: *Advances in neurology*, Vol. 46, *Intensive neurodiagnostic monitoring,* ed. R.J. Gumnit, pp. 69–84. New York, NY: Raven Press.

Wyllie, E., Lüders, H., Morris, H.H., Lesser, R.P., Dinner, D.S., Hahn, J., Estes, M.L., Rothner, A.D., Erenberg, G., Cruse, R. & Friedman, D. (1988): Subdural electrodes in the evaluation for epilepsy surgery in children and adults. *Neuropediatrics* **19,** 80–86.

Wyllie, E., Naugle, R., Awad, I., Chelune, G., Lüders, H., Dinner, D., Skibinski, C. & Ahl, J. (1991): The intracarotid amobarbital procedure (Wada test): I. Prediction of decreased modality-specific memory scores after temporal lobectomy. *Epilepsia* **32,** 865–869.

Wyllie, E., Chee, M., Granstrom, M.L., DelGiudice, E., Estes, M., Comair, Y., Pizzi, M., Kotagal, P., Bourgeois, B. & Lüders, H. (1993): Temporal lobe epilepsy in early childhood. *Epilepsia* **34,** 859–868.

Yamamoto, N., Watanabe, K., Negoro, T., Takaesu, E., Aso, K., Furune, S. & Takahashi, I. (1987): Complex partial seizures in children: ictal manifestations and their relation to clinical course. *Neurology* **37,** 1979–1982.

Epileptic Seizures and Syndromes, Edited by Peter Wolf
© 1994 John Libbey & Company Ltd., pp. 375–382

Chapter 40

Lateral (neocortical) temporal lobe epilepsy

Alois Ebner

Epilepsie-Zentrum Bethel, Klinik Mara I, Maraweg 21, D-33617 Bielefeld, Germany

Summary

In this study, two groups of patients with psychomotor seizures were compared with regard to auras and ictal clinical symptoms. The first group consisted of 14 patients with circumscribed lesions affecting the temporal neocortex as revealed by MRI (neocortical temporal lobe epilepsy group: nTLE). The second group consisted of 18 patients who were seizure free after temporal lobectomy (mesial temporal lobe epilepsy group: mTLE). Significant differences were found in auditory/visual auras and epigastric auras; auditory/visual auras were more frequent in the nTLE and epigastric auras were more frequent in the mTLE. There was no difference between the two groups regarding other auras (memory illusions, fear, gustatory or none) or ictal symptoms (alteration of consciousness, automatisms, staring, vocalization, agitation or autonomic changes). This finding is explained by the mostly non-overlapping character of the ictal onset zone and the symptomatogenic zone, meaning that clinical symptoms in neocortical epilepsy are already expressions of the spread of seizure activity arising frequently in clinically silent cortical areas.

Introduction

The term lateral posterior temporal lobe epilepsy (TLE) was included in the Proposal for an International Classification of Epilepsies and Epileptic Syndromes of 1985 (Dreifuss *et al.,* 1985). This epileptic syndrome is one of the four TLEs subdivided by Wieser (1983), who based his classification on ictal EEGs with regard to onset and propagation patterns. The division into these separate seizure types based on functional interrelationships was recently criticized by Gates and Gumnit (1990). These authors state that these divisions should be interpreted cautiously since after a mean follow-up of 6 years only 57 per cent of the patients were seizure-free. Therefore, Gates and Gumnit argue that the purity of the ictal localization is, at best, suspect.

In the revised version of the International Classification (Dreifuss *et al.,* 1989) two forms of TLE were included: mesial and lateral TLE. The latter is 'characterized by auras of auditory hallucinations, visual perceptual hallucinations, or language disorder in case of a dominant hemisphere focus. These are followed by dysphasia, disturbed orientation or prolonged auditory hallucinations, head movement to one side, and sometimes staring automatisms'. There is only one other report dealing with the subdivision of TLEs based on a cluster analysis of clinical symptoms (Kotagal *et al.,* 1988). The results of that study showed that a subdivision in different forms of TLE could not be supported.

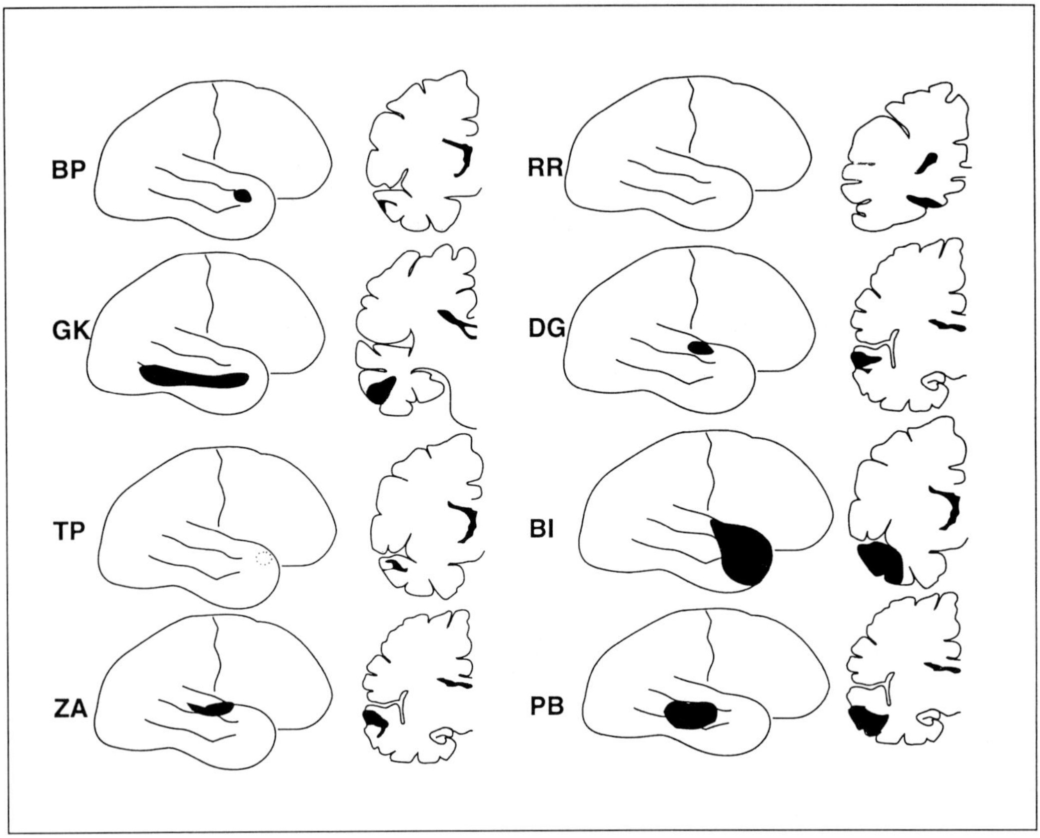

Fig. 1a. Right-sided neocortical temporal lobe lesions traced after the MRIs in a lateral and coronal view of eight patients.

In this contribution, ictal clinical symptoms of a group of patients with neocortical TLE (nTLE) are compared with the clinical semiology of a group of patients with mesial TLE (mTLE).

Methods

Among 66 consecutive patients with the diagnosis TLE based on the usual preoperative work-up of clinical examination, intensive video-EEG monitoring, magnetic resonance imaging (MRI), positron emission tomography (PET) and neuropsychological tests, including the Wada test, 14 patients were found to have a circumscribed lesion affecting the neocortex of the temporal lobe. Site and extension of the lesions found in the MRI scans are shown in Figs. 1a and 1b. The average age of this nTLE group is 27 years, ranging from 12 to 51 years. There were four females and 10 males. The average epilepsy duration was about 11 years, the range 5 to 27 years. Three patients had surgery with resection of the lesion and the mesial structures. Two patients are seizure-free, one still has seizures. Three patients had only neocortical resections including the lesion and have remained seizure-free.

The control group with mTLE consisted of 18 patients who became seizure-free after temporal lobectomy. The average age was 27 years, range 13–51 years. There was again a preponderance of males compared with females. The mean epilepsy duration was about 19.4 years, ranging from 3 to 45 years.

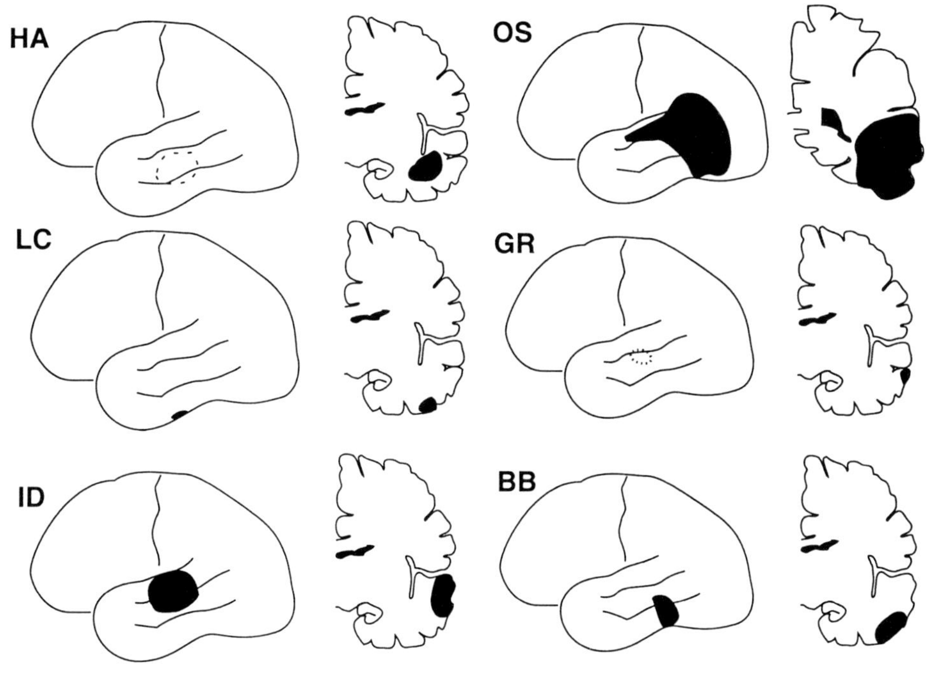

Fig. 1b. Left sided neocortical temporal lobe lesions traced after the MRIs in a lateral and coronal view of six patients.

All patients underwent an intensive video-EEG monitoring of several days. A total of 85 seizures were recorded in the nTLE group and 125 seizures in the mTLE group.

The ictal symptoms of the psychomotor seizures as described in the patients' charts were retrospectively reviewed and compared between the two groups. Only auras and psychomotor signs and symptoms but not motor symptoms, such as dystonic posturing, clonus or secondarily generalized tonic–clonic seizures, indicating spread to extratemporal areas, were included in the analysis.

Results

Figure 2a shows the results regarding the auras. There was a slightly significant difference in epigastric auras, which were more frequent in the mTLE, group with almost 90 per cent compared with 50 per cent in the neocortical group. The opposite was the case in the visual or auditory auras, in which illusions and hallucinations of the same modality were included. One patient only of the mesial temporal group had a visual aura. This patient had a mesially located hamartoma extending posteriorly to the occipitotemporal junction. Other auras such as memory illusions, fear or gustatory auras, were rare and not significantly different. Only a small percentage of the patients did not experience any aura at all.

Location and extent of the lesions of the five patients with visual or auditory auras are shown in Fig. 3. The three patients with auditory auras all had lesions in or close to the superior temporal gyrus. The patient with visual illusions had a lesion at the occipitotemporal junction and the patient who described the colourful lights on the left had a rather extensive lesion at the anterior part of the right temporal lobe. This patient continues to have seizures since removal of the lesion together with the

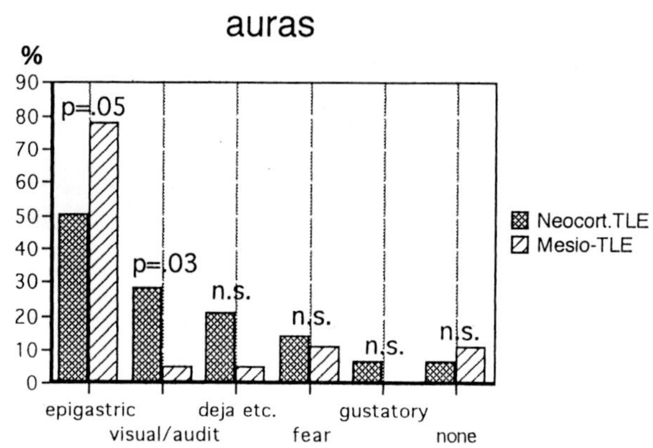

Fig. 2a. Comparison of the frequency of auras reported in the mesial and neocortical TLE groups. Only epigastric and visual/auditory auras showed a significant difference (Fisher's exact test).

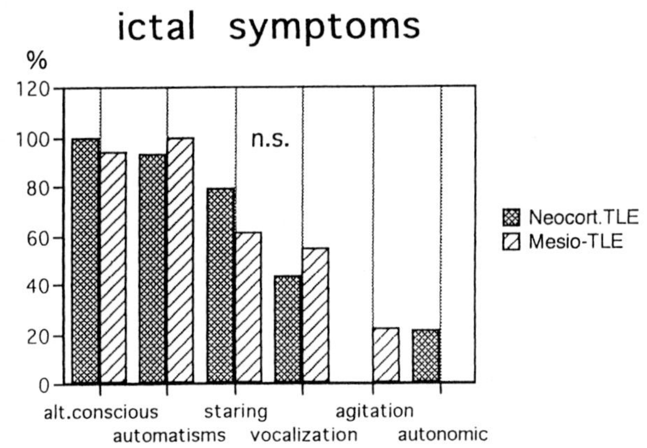

Fig. 2b. Comparison of the frequency of ictal symptoms observed in the mesial and neocortical TLE groups. There is no significant difference between the two groups (Fisher's exact test).

mesial structures, indicating that his epileptogenic zone is apparently more extended, as was probably indicated by the visual aura.

Figure 2b shows the results with regard to ictal symptoms immediately following the auras. Alteration of consciousness, oroalimentary automatisms, behaviour arrest and staring, vocalization, agitation and autonomic signs showed no difference in the two groups.

To summarize, except for epigastric and visual/auditory auras, there was no difference in the clinical semiology of psychomotor seizures arising from either neocortical temporal or mesiotemporal areas.

Illustrative case ZA (see Figs. 1 and 4). This is an 18-year-old man with a history of psychomotor seizures since the age of 13. He experienced an aura of hearing voices of former familiar friends followed by an epigastric aura, then shook his head several times, began staring and became unresponsive. After evaluation with surface, epidural and foramen ovale electrodes, he underwent phase II evaluation with a subdural grid covering the lesion and strip electrodes lying over the basal temporal areas (Fig. 4a).

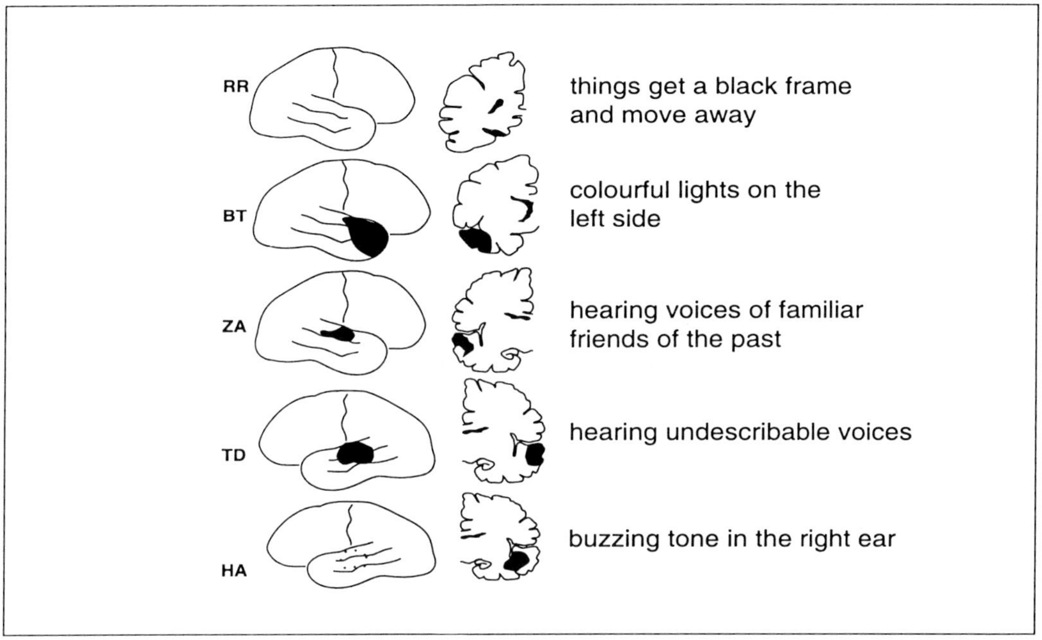

Fig. 3. Location and extent of the temporal lesions of the five patients reporting visual/auditory auras. On the right side the description of the patient for his/her aura is given.

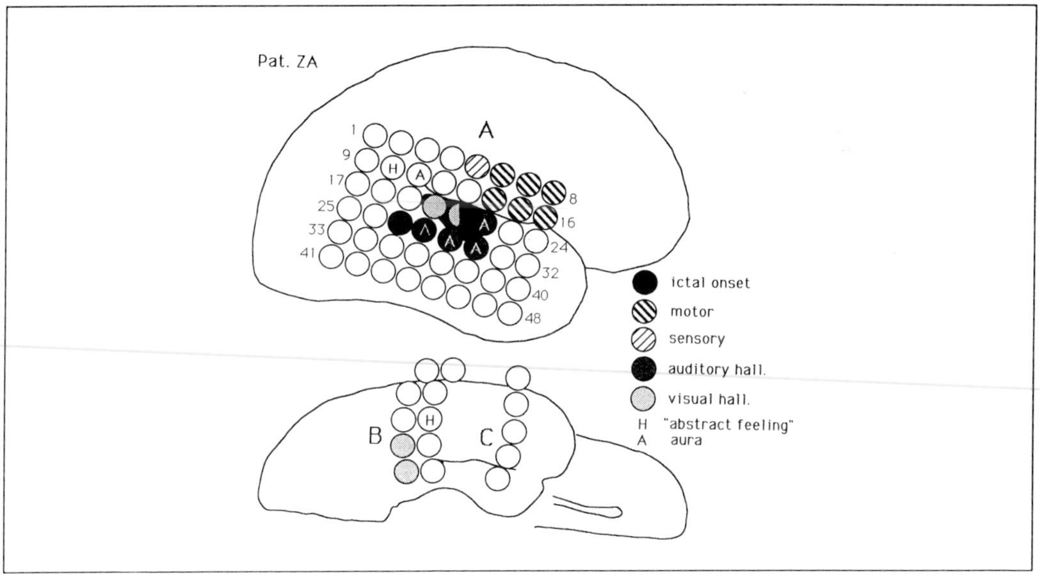

Fig. 4a. Focal onset of EEG seizure (black circles, electrodes 27, 28) and results of extraoperative electrical stimulation producing motor (electrodes 6–8 and 14–16) and sensory responses (electrode 5) as well as auditory (electrodes 21, 22, 28–30) and visual (electrodes 20, 21; two electrodes at the B plate) phenomena. A stands for the habitual aura and H for a hallucination the patient described as 'abstract feeling' produced by electrical stimulation.

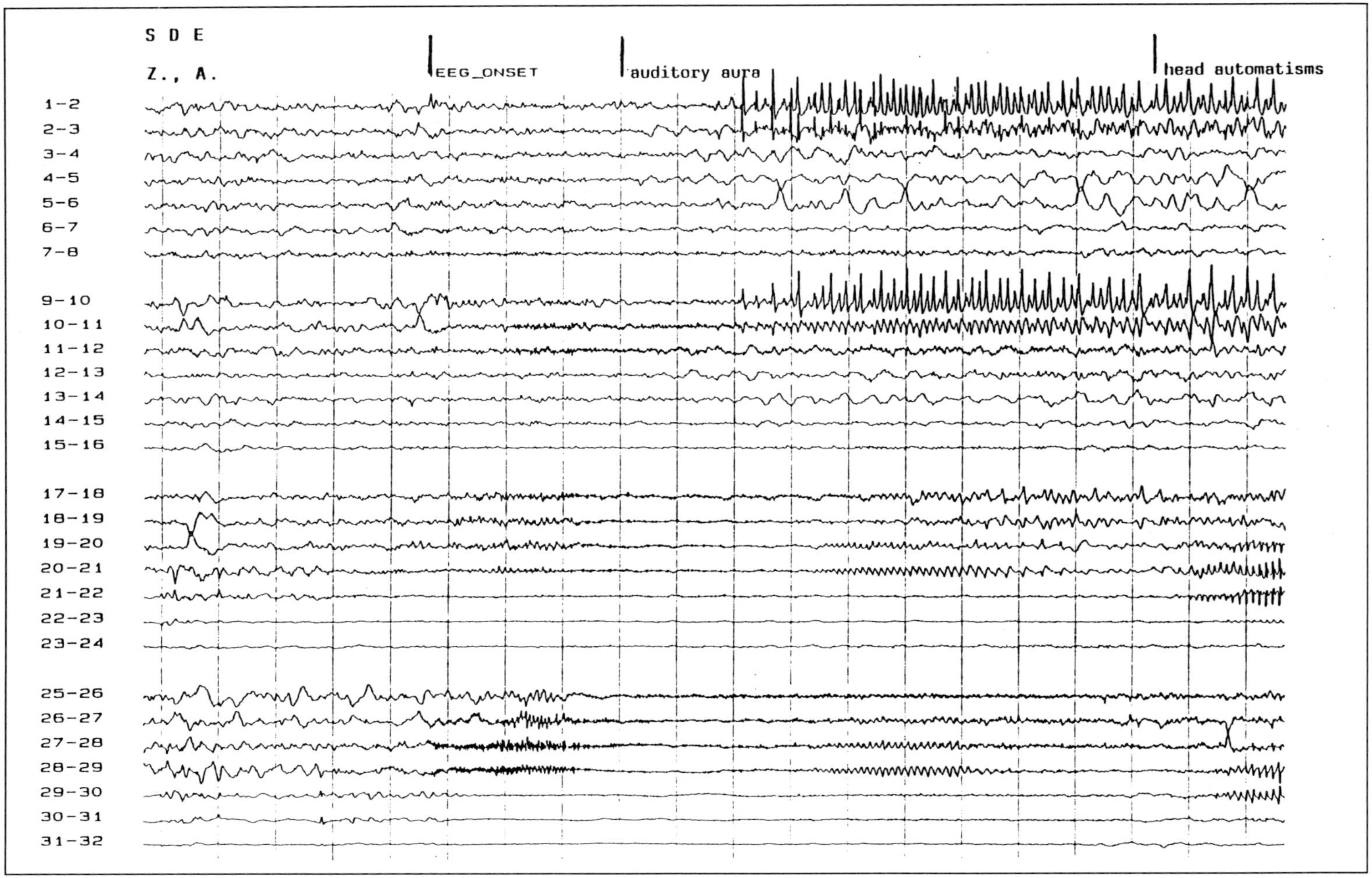

Fig. 4b. Focal EEG seizure onset at electrodes 27 and 28. Three seconds later the patient indicates his habitual aura, followed by automatisms 10 s later. The electrodes 1–32 of the A plate (cf. Fig. 4a) are shown in a bipolar montage.

All 13 seizures recorded invariably started focally from two electrodes (Fig. 4b). These two electrodes were lying posteriorly and inferiorly to the lesion. Three seconds after EEG seizure onset, the patient experienced his habitual aura followed by the highly stereotyped sequence of ictal symptoms.

Electrical stimulation of the subdural electrodes lying in the vicinity of the lesion elicited the patient's habitual auras and seizures (Fig. 4a).

The patient underwent a lesionectomy including the ictal onset zone as defined by the subdural electrodes. Unfortunately, the lesion was a hamartoma histologically extended with a small string into the basal ganglia and therefore could not be resected completely. In the 7 months follow-up, the patient had two secondary generalized seizures in the immediate postoperative phase. Since then he has only experienced his habitual auras two to three times per week.

Discussion

In this study, a comparison of the ictal semiology of psychomotor seizures in a group of patients with nTLE and with mTLE was made. The mTLE group was defined as a group of patients being seizure-free after temporal lobectomy, indicating that the epileptogenic zone was correctly determined and resected. The nTLE was defined by the presence of circumscribed lesions in the temporal neocortex as revealed by MRI scans. The question is whether it is justified to call this a neocortical temporal epilepsy. In favour of this assumption is Gloor's statement from 1987: 'if a brain lesion can be demonstrated in a patient with seizures, the likelihood that the seizures are in some way the consequence of this lesion is high'.

It should be emphasized, however, that an ideal nTLE group would be one being seizure-free after resection of the epileptogenic area of the temporal neocortex including the lesion if present. The only difference found in the two groups was a slightly significant higher frequency of epigastric auras in the mTLE, although still 50 per cent of the patients of the nTLE group also experienced epigastric auras, and there were significantly more auditory/visual auras in the nTLE group (5 *vs.* 1). The patient with a visual aura and mTLE had a hamartoma which extended posteriorly to the medial temporo-occipital junction. Other auras, such as memory illusions (*déjà vu*, etc.), fear/anxiety or gustatory auras, as well as psychomotor symptoms (alteration of consciousness, automatisms, staring, vocalization, autonomic signs), showed no significant difference. It is remarkable that only one patient in the nTLE and two patients in the mTLE group experienced no aura.

How can this close overlapping of mesial and lateral TLE symptoms be explained?

In a case with a circumscribed lesion in the superior temporal gyrus and an auditory aura there is no problem in making a diagnosis of nTLE. But what about those cases with lateral temporal lesions whose seizure semiology and EEG are indistinguishable from mTLE?

It is important to keep in mind that the initial sensation of an aura or any other initial ictal symptom is related to the first functional area activated by the seizure that has access to consciousness (So, 1993). But this may not be the site of seizure origin. Psychomotor seizures may arise in silent neocortical areas lying in the extratemporal as well as in the temporal cortex (Engel, 1992).

Neocortical seizures actually most often arise in silent areas. This assumption is based on the results of electrical cortical stimulation revealing that most of the neocortex is electrically not excitable. This also holds true for the temporal neocortex. Penfield & Jasper (1954) originally thought that electrical stimulation of the temporal cortex produces specific recollection or a temporary alteration of the interpretation of visual and auditory stimuli.

Later studies, however, using extraoperative depth electrode stimulation of the mesial structures instead of the intraoperative electrical stimulation of the neocortex, could produce very similar results. Thus experiential phenomena, as they were called by Penfield and Jasper, are not specific for the lateral temporal neocortex. Rather, as was proposed by Gloor (1990), reciprocal connections between the limbic structures and the temporal isocortex have to be activated in order to get these phenomena.

several reports of fairly large series of well-documented occipital lobe epilepsy (Blume & Whiting, 1991; Salanova *et al.*, 1992; Williamson *et al.*, 1992a). There is remarkable agreement of the observations and conclusions in the two most recent reports. Although the other report differed in emphasis, examination of the listed data demonstrates considerable agreement also.

Occipital lobe seizures can be divided into early and subsequent clinical manifestations. The early manifestations are thought to reflect seizure activity in the occipital lobe, while subsequent clinical features are the result of seizure spread beyond the occipital lobe. These concepts can be applied to many types of partial seizures but, as will be apparent, they are particularly important when considering occipital lobe epilepsy.

Early clinical seizure manifestations

Elementary visual hallucinations

Elementary visual hallucinations are the most frequent initial symptoms in all three of the recent studies (Blume & Whiting, 1991; Salanova *et al.*, 1992; Williamson *et al.*, 1992a) and have been a well-recognized sign of occipital lobe epilepsy for many years (Gowers, 1879; Holmes, 1927; Penfield & Jasper, 1954; Ajmone-Marsan & Ralston, 1957). These hallucinations commonly consist of flashing bright spots with a greenish luminescence (phosphenes) or steady and flashing monochromic or multichromic coloured lights. Crude geometric forms are also described.

It is quite possible that parietal or neocortical posterior temporal lobe seizures could spread posteriorly and produce elementary visual hallucinations (Russell & Whitty, 1955; Ludwig & Ajmone-Marsan, 1975), but this would be uncommon. Elementary visual hallucinations, either in isolation or as an initial part of a more elaborate seizure, should always suggest occipital lobe epilepsy.

Ictal amaurosis

Complete or partial loss of vision has long been recognized as a symptom of occipital lobe epilepsy (Gowers, 1879; Harris, 1897; Holmes, 1927; Penfield & Jasper, 1954), and yet it is often not appreciated. Hysteria has been diagnosed in some patients with this epileptic symptom (Williamson *et al.*, 1992a). Ictal blindness was the second most common symptom in both the Yale and the Montreal series (Salanova *et al.*, 1992; Williamson *et al.*, 1992a). It is usually a blackout but occasionally is described as a whiteout. In some patients, both elementary visual hallucinations and ictal blindness occur in the same or different seizures. Prolonged ictal blindness has been reported as a type of status epilepticus (Barry *et al.*, 1985). Theoretically, ictal blindness could occur from posterior spread from a more anterior focus. This was documented in one patient with parietal lobe epilepsy (Williamson *et al.*, 1992b).

Ictal hemianopic deficits do occur but are reported much less frequently. Perhaps such deficits would not be noticed. When testing is possible, transient postictal hemianopia can be demonstrated in some patients. As discussed below, static visual field deficits are common in patients with occipital lobe epilepsy.

Eye movement sensation

Pulling or moving sensations in the eyes without detectable movement have been reported repeatedly in patients with occipital lobe seizure origin (Holtzman & Goldensohn, 1977; Salanova *et al.*, 1992; Williamson *et al.*, 1992a). This occurs early in the seizure, usually as an initial symptom, and is thought to reflect seizure activity in the extracalcarine occipital cortex. It is an uncommon symptom, but awareness of it can lead to the correct diagnosis of occipital lobe epilepsy.

Blinking

Eye blinking is such a ubiquitous sign in patients having seizures that its diagnostic significance must be viewed with caution. Blinking, however, has been repeatedly reported as an early sign in occipital lobe epilepsy (Penfield & Jasper, 1954; Bancaud, 1969; Takeda *et al.*, 1970; Olivier *et al.*, 1982; Munari *et al.*, 1984; Salanova *et al.*, 1992; Williamson *et al.*, 1992a). In the author's experience, this type of ictal blinking has a forced quality or may consist of eyelid flutter. As such, it can be distinguished from the more casual blinking associated with many other seizure types.

Head/eye deviation

Head or eye deviation or both have controversial localizing significance for seizures in general (Robillard *et al.*, 1983; Ochs *et al.*, 1984). Head and eye deviation, when present at the beginning of occipital lobe seizures, are reported to be almost always contralateral to the side of seizure origin (Munari *et al.*, 1984; Salanova *et al.*, 1992). One of the recent reports, however, casts some doubt on the high degree of lateralizing reliability of this finding (Williamson *et al.*, 1992a). In patients with occipital lobe epilepsy, head and eye deviation is usually contralateral to the side of seizure origin, but cannot be considered an absolutely reliable lateralizing sign.

Subsequent seizure manifestations

Occipital lobe seizures may not progress beyond the initial phase of occipital lobe seizure discharge. These simple partial seizures without altered consciousness would consist of some or all of the findings described above. Most of the occipital lobe seizures described in contemporary reports, however, have clinical features consistent with spread beyond the occipital lobe. Indeed, the spread patterns of occipital lobe epilepsy are responsible for the dramatic and often complicated clinical features of these seizures. Over 35 years ago, Ajmone-Marsan and Ralston (1957) predicted that occipital lobe seizures could spread via many different pathways: medial, lateral, above and below the sylvian fissure. Furthermore, the clinical manifestations would reflect the different spread patterns. These predictions and observations have now been conclusively documented with intracranial electrode recording and results of surgery (Bancaud, 1969; Takeda *et al.*, 1970; Blume & Whiting, 1991; Salanova *et al.*, 1992; Williamson *et al.*, 1992a). The following relationships among spread patterns and clinical characteristics have been observed:

Medial inferior spread via occipital temporal projections

This type of spread can produce signs and symptoms typical of medial temporal lobe epilepsy with visceral sensations, experiential phenomena and automatisms. Occipital temporal spread is one of the most frequently documented spread patterns (Bancaud, 1969; Takeda *et al.*, 1970; Williamson *et al.*, 1981, 1987, 1992a; Olivier *et al.*, 1982; Williamson, 1986; Blume & Whiting, 1991; Salanova *et al.*, 1992). Failure to recognize or appreciate the early signs and symptoms of occipital lobe seizure origin commonly results in the incorrect diagnosis of temporal lobe epilepsy.

Lateral occipital temporal neocortical spread

This type of spread is reported to be responsible for complex visual or auditory hallucinations (Penfield & Perot, 1963). The involvement of medial limbic structures in complex hallucinations has been stressed by several authors (Halgren *et al.*, 1978; Gloor *et al.*, 1982; Wieser, 1982). Possibly both medial and lateral temporal lobe seizure spread is necessary. Although the issue of localization and complex formed hallucinations has not been resolved, it is generally agreed that their occurrence indicates spread outside the occipital lobe in patients with occipital lobe seizure origin. Although relatively uncommon, complex visual hallucinations and experiences have been reported in patients with occipital lobe epilepsy (Penfield & Perot, 1963; Blume & Whiting, 1991; Salanova *et al.*, 1992; Williamson *et al.*, 1992a). They usually occur after the initial signs and symptoms of occipital lobe seizure origin. In turn, they can be followed by medial temporal involvement with signs and symptoms typical of medial temporal lobe epilepsy.

Lateral suprasylvian spread

Spread of the occipital lobe seizure laterally and superiorly would produce focal sensory-motor activity (Blume & Whiting, 1991; Salanova *et al.*, 1992; Williamson *et al.*, 1992a).

Medial suprasylvian spread

Spread to the medial surface of the hemisphere can produce a variety of clinical manifestations. One of the more common types of seizures reported with occipital lobe epilepsy is asymmetrical tonic seizures (Munari *et al.*, 1984; Salanova *et al.*, 1992; Williamson *et al.*, 1992a). This might take the form of head deviation or complex postures. The complex tonic postures, similar to those described in seizures beginning in the supplementary motor area, are presumably due to spread to that main region. Opportunities to document this hypothesis have been rare (Williamson *et al.* 1992b).

Contralateral spread

Spread to the contralateral occipital lobe has been demonstrated during bilateral occipital lobe depth electrode recording (Williamson *et al.*, 1992a). This is presumably the cause of ictal blindness (Salanova *et al.*, 1992; Williamson *et al.*, 1992a). Spread to the opposite occipital lobe would also set the stage for all of the possible spread patterns described above for ipsilateral seizure discharge. This latter possibility has been documented, helping to explain some of the extremely complicated clinical features seen in patients with occipital lobe epilepsy (Williamson *et al.*, 1992a).

Determinants of spread

What determines different spread patterns is largely conjectural. Certainly, logic would dictate that the exact localization of the original epileptic discharge; above or below the calcarine fissure, medial, or lateral occipital lobe would have some bearing on subsequent spread patterns (Ajmone-Marsan & Ralston, 1957). Many patients with occipital lobe epilepsy have demonstrable lesions (Blume & Whiting, 1991; Salanova *et al.*, 1992; Williamson *et al.*, 1992a). It may be that different seizures in the same patients might begin in different regions of the epileptogenic brain surrounding the lesion. This was clearly demonstrated in one patient (Williamson *et al.*, 1992a) and may explain the observation of many different seizure types in the same patients.

Other findings

Visual field deficits

Many patients with occipital seizure origin have static visual field deficits (Williamson *et al.*, 1992a). These can be very subtle, requiring formal testing for detection.

Surface electroencephalography (EEG)

Blume *et al.* (1991) found ictal and interictal scalp EEG to be helpful in localizing the region of seizure origin in the majority of patients with seizures beginning in the 'posterior cortex'. Review of their EEG data, however, indicates that most EEG localization was posterior temporal or temporal occipital. None had exclusively occipital abnormalities, and some had anterior temporal paroxysmal activity. The two recent reports on occipital lobe epilepsy did not find scalp EEG particularly helpful (Salanova *et al.*, 1992; Williamson *et al.*, 1992a). The most common localization of scalp EEG abnormalities was posterior temporal in both studies, and occipital abnormalities were very uncommon.

It can be concluded that precise occipital localization of scalp EEG abnormalities in patients with occipital lobe epilepsy is an uncommon occurrence. However, since the vast majority of patients with medial temporal lobe epilepsy have anterior temporal scalp EEG abnormalities (Williamson *et al.*, 1993b), localization of paroxysmal abnormalities in the posterior temporal region should suggest extratemporal, possibly occipital lobe, seizure origin. This possibility would be strongly reinforced if the patient's seizures contained findings suggesting occipital lobe seizure origin.

Neuroimaging

Lesions detectable by modern neuroimaging were present in most patients in all three recent reports. (Blume & Whiting, 1991; Salanova *et al.*, 1992; Williamson *et al.*, 1992a). Although low-grade glial tumours were the single most common lesion in two series, porencephaly and gliosis or both were the most frequent finding in the large Montreal series. This latter study excluded patients with neoplasms prior to 1985 (Rasmussen, 1983; Salanova *et al.*, 1992), thus explaining the low incidence of mass lesions.

Surgical results

Surgical techniques varied among the three centres recently reporting on occipital lobe epilepsy. Overall, good results occurred in 65–80 per cent of patients regardless of the type of surgery performed. Selecting those patients with circumscribed occipital lobe lesions who had lesion resection, 50–88 per cent became seizure-free. Only rarely did patients not improve following lesion resection. Some patients underwent temporal lobectomy, either because of failure to recognize occipital lobe seizure origin, or in an attempt to remove the part of the brain thought responsible for most of the clinical seizure manifestations. Surprisingly, about half of these patients experienced good results, with a few even becoming seizure-free (Salanova *et al.*, 1992; Williamson *et al.*, 1992).

Parietal lobe epilepsy

Very little has been written about parietal lobe epilepsy. Over 25 years ago, Bancaud and colleagues (Bancaud & Talairach, 1965) commented that there was a wealth of information concerning the effects of destructive lesions in the parietal lobes, but few data about seizures originating there. Until recently, little has changed, with only two older reports discussing parietal lobe epilepsy (Ajmone-Marsan & Goldhammer, 1973; Geier *et al.*, 1977). Recently, there have been two reports on parietal lobe epilepsy (Williamson *et al.*, 1992a; Cascino *et al.*, 1993). Both studied similar patients and both reported similar results.

In order to be consistent with the discussion of occipital lobe epilepsy, parietal lobe epilepsy will be examined in terms of initial signs and symptoms and subsequent findings.

Early clinical seizure manifestations

Elementary somatosensory sensations

Simple partial somatosensory seizures do occur, but much less frequently than might be expected. Of 21 patients from two different studies with documented parietal lobe seizure origin, only five had contralateral somatosensory aura (Williamson *et al.*, 1992b; Cascino *et al.*, 1993).

Other early symptoms

Of the other early signs described in parietal lobe epilepsy, most would suggest spread beyond the parietal lobe, such as ictal amaurosis or abdominal visceral sensations. One patient in the report by Cascino *et al.* (1993) had 'scrambled vision' as an aura, but it is not clear what that means. A patient from the Yale series reported that seizures often occurred while attempting to open containers, suggesting seizures were precipitated by a complex somatosensory input. This latter phenomenon was repeatedly documented during video monitoring. Language disturbances, vertigo and complex sensory auras are possible, but they must be uncommon, since they were not described in the two recent reports.

Considering known parietal lobe function, the absence of specific auras should not be surprising. As suggested by Niedermeyer (1974), except for the primary sensory area, the parietal lobe is probably clinically silent in terms of seizure symptomatology. Conversely, special testing during localized parietal lobe seizures might be required. Since parietal lobe seizures tend to spread rapidly, such testing would usually be logistically impossible.

Early signs

There are no early signs that identify parietal lobe origin. Disturbances of language could conceivably accompany parietal seizure activity in the language dominant hemisphere. This would have lateralizing but not localizing significance. Language dysfunction was not reported as a part of parietal lobe seizures in any patient from the more recent series (Williamson *et al.*, 1992b; Cascino *et al.*, 1993). The reason there are no early signs again relates to parietal lobe function. There are no parietal lobe functions that would produce objective findings.

Subsequent seizure manifestations

As with occipital lobe epilepsy, subsequent seizure clinical characteristics will depend upon variable spread patterns, but the options are slightly different. Posterior spread into the occipital lobe has been documented (Williamson *et al.*, 1992b). This spread pattern produced ictal amaurosis. Spread anteriorly over the convexity results in clonic motor activity, while medial spread to the interhemispheric surface could produce asymmetrical tonic posturing. This latter possibility has been documented with intracranial recording. In addition to tonic posturing, automatisms have been reported consistently in some patients with parietal lobe epilepsy (Geier *et al.*, 1977; Williamson *et al.*, 1922b; Cascino *et al.*, 1993). A remarkable patient from the Yale series with a small unilateral parietal glioma appeared to have bilateral independent hippocampal seizure origin during depth electrode recording (Williamson *et al.*, 1992b).

Other findings

Surface EEG

Although a lateralized parietal focus would suggest parietal lobe seizure origin, in practice this finding is uncommon in patients with documented parietal lobe epilepsy. Both recent studies of parietal lobe epilepsy reported that scalp ictal and interictal changes were unreliable markers in most cases of parietal lobe epilepsy (Williamson *et al.*, 1992b; Cascino *et al.*, 1993).

Neuroimaging

All patients in the two recent studies had parietal lobe lesions detected with computerized tomography (CT) or magnetic resonance imaging (MRI) (Williamson *et al.*, 1992b; Cascino *et al.*, 1993). Some patients had been evaluated prior to lesion detection, and parietal lobe seizure origin had not been demonstrated during intracranial recording. Pathology was available for 20 patients, and low-grade gliomas were the most common finding (60 per cent).

Surgical results

Both of the recent studies clearly showed that, when surgery was aimed at lesion resection plus removal of limited surrounding brain, surgical results in terms of seizure control were excellent. This was true in patients who had previous inappropriate surgery due to inaccurate or failed localization, as well as those whose initial surgery was directed at the responsible lesion. The surgical results also demonstrated that lesions can be safely resected from either parietal lobe without producing unacceptable neurological deficits.

Conclusions

There is converging evidence in the recent and past literature that occipital lobe seizures can be correctly identified on the basis of clinical seizure characteristics in the majority of patients whose seizures originate in the occipital lobe. Since seizures among patients or within patients may not be uniform or stereotyped, a precise, strictly defined syndrome cannot be established. This observation in itself should serve to alert the investigator to the possibility of occipital lobe seizure origin in some patients with particularly complicated presentations that suggest multiple different seizure types. The fact that most patients with occipital lobe epilepsy will have causative lesions detectable with neuroimaging underlies the importance of this technology in the evaluation of all patients with localization-related epilepsy.

In contrast to the positive findings when investigating patients with occipital lobe epilepsy, the results of studies of patients with parietal lobe seizure origin are less encouraging. Neither clinical seizure characteristics nor surface EEG served to correctly identify the majority of patients with parietal lobe seizure origin. Although all patients in the two recent series had MRI lesions, the lesions served to identify and not confirm probable parietal lobe seizure origin. Parietal lobe seizure origin must be considered in those patients being evaluated for surgery whose preoperative findings do not clearly demonstrate the region of seizure origin.

References

Ajmone-Marsan, C. & Goldhammer, L. (1973): Clinical ictal patterns and electrographic data in cases of partial seizures of frontal-central-parietal origin. In: *Epilepsy, its phenomena in man*, ed. M.A.B. Brazier, pp. 235–258. New York: Academic Press.

Ajmone-Marsan, C. & Ralston, B.L. (1957): *The epileptic seizure: its functional morphology and diagnostic significance*, pp. 211–215. Springfield, Illinois: Charles C. Thomas.

Bancaud, J. (1969): Les crises épileptiques d'origine occipitale (étude stéreo-électroencéphalographique). *Rev Oto-neuro-ophthalmol.* **41**, 299–315.

Bancaud, J. & Talairach, J. (1965): L'épilepsie de l'aire motrice supplémentaire: un diagnostic particulièrement difficile chez l'enfant. *Rev. Neuropsychiatr. Infant.* **13**, 483–498.

Barry, E., Sussman, N.M., Bosley, T.M. & Harner, N.E. (1985): Ictal blindness and status epilepticus amaurotics. *Epilepsia* **26**, 557–584.

Blume, W.T. & Whiting, S.E. (1991): Epilepsy surgery in the posterior cortex. *Ann. Neurol.* **29**, 638–645.

Cascino, G.D., Hulihan, J.F., Sharbrough, F.W. & Kelly, P.J. (1993): Parietal lobe lesional epilepsy: electroclinical correlation and operative outcome. *Epilepsia* **34**, 522–527.

Commission on Classification and Terminology of the International League Against Epilepsy (1985): Proposal for classification of epilepsies and epileptic syndromes. *Epilepsia* **26** (suppl. 3), 268–278.

Delgado-Escueta, A.V., Swartz, B., Maldonado, H., Walsh, G.O., Rand, R.W. & Halgren, E. (1987): Complex partial seizures of frontal lobe origin. In: *Presurgical evaluation of epileptics: basics, techniques, implications*, eds. H.G. Wieser & C.E. Elger, pp. 268–299. Berlin, Heidelberg, New York: Springer-Verlag.

French, J.A., Willamson, P.D., Thadani, V.M., Darcey, T.M., Mattson, R.H., Spencer, S.S. & Spencer, D.D. (1993): Characteristics of medial temporal lobe epilepsy I. Results of history and physical examination. *Ann. Neurol.* **34**, 774–780

Geier, S., Bancaud, J., Talairach, J., Bonis, A., Hossard-Boucharud, H. & Enjelvin, M. (1977): Ictal tonic postural changes and automatisms of the upper limb during epileptic parietal lobe discharges. *Epilepsia* **18**, 517–524.

Gloor, P., Olivier, A., Quesney, L.F., Andermann, F. & Horowitz, S. (1982): The role of the limbic system in experiential phenomena of temporal lobe epilepsy. *Ann. Neurol.* **12**, 129–144.

Gowers, W.R. (1879): Cases of cerebral tumour illustrating diagnosis and localisation. *Lancet* **i**, 363–365.

Halgren, E., Walter, R.D., Cherlow, D.G. & Crandall, P.H. (1978): Mental phenomena evoked by electrical stimulation of the human hippocampal formation and amygdala. *Brain* **101**, 83–117.

Harris, W. (1897): Hemianopia, with especial reference to its transient varieties. *Brain* **20**, 308–364.

Holmes, G. (1927): Savill memorial oration on local epilepsy. *Lancet* **i**, 957–962.

Holtzman, R.N.N. & Goldensohn, E.S. (1977): Sensations of ocular movement in seizures originating in occipital lobe. *Neurology (Minneapolis)* **27**, 554–556.

Ludwig, B.I. & Ajmone-Marsan, C. (1975): Clinical ictal patterns in epileptic patients with occipital electroencephalographic foci. *Neurology* **25,** 463–471.

Morris, H.H., Dinner, D.S., Lüders, H., Wyllie, E. & Kramer, R. (1988): Supplementary motor seizures: clinical and electroencephalographic findings. *Neurology* **38,** 1075–1082.

Munari, C., Bonis, A., Kochen, S., Pestre, M., Brunet, P., Bancaud, J., Chodkiewicz, J.P. & Talairach, J. (1984): Eye movements and occipital seizures in man. *Acta Neurochirurg.* **33,** 47–52.

Niedermeyer, E. (1974): *Compendium of the epilepsies*. Springfield, Illinois: Charles C. Thomas.

Ochs, R., Gloor, P., Quesney, L.F., Ives, J. & Olivier, A. (1984): Does head-turning during a seizure have a lateralizing or localizing significance? *Neurology* **34,** 884–890.

Olivier, A., Gloor, P., Andermann, F. & Ives, J. (1982): Occipitotemporal epilepsy studied with stereotaxically implanted depth electrodes and successfully treated by temporal resection. *Ann. Neurol.* **11,** 428–432.

Penfield, W. & Jasper, H. (1954): *Epilepsy and the functional anatomy of the human brain*. London: J & A Churchill.

Penfield, W. & Perot, P. (1963): The brain's record of auditory and visual experience. *Brain* **86,** 595–596.

Rasmussen, T. (1975): Surgery for epilepsy arising in regions other than the temporal and frontal lobes. In: *Neurosurgical management of the epilepsies*, Vol. 8, eds. D.P. Purpura, J.K. Penry & R.D. Walter, pp. 207–226. New York: Raven Press.

Rasmussen, T. (1983): Characteristics of a pure culture of frontal lobe epilepsy. *Epilepsia* **24,** 482–493.

Robillard, A., Saint-Hilaire, J.M., Mercier, M. & Bouvier, G. (1983): The lateralizing and localizing value of adversion in epileptic seizures. *Neurology (Cleveland)*, **33,** 1241–1242.

Russell, W.R. & Whitty, C.W.M. (1955): Studies in traumatic epilepsy. 3. Visual fits. *J. Neurol.* **18,** 79–96.

Salanova, V., Andermann, F., Olivier, A., Rasmussen, T. & Quesney, L.F. (1992): Occipital lobe epilepsy: electroclinical manifestations, electrocorticography, cortical stimulation and outcome in 42 patients treated between 1930 and 1991. *Brain* **115,** 1655–1680.

Spencer, S.S. & Spencer, D.D. (1991): *Surgery for epilepsy*. Boston: Blackwell Scientific Publications.

Takeda, A., Bancaud, J., Talairach, J., Bonis, J. & Bordas-Ferrer, M. (1970): Concerning epileptic attacks of occipital origin. *Electroencephalogr. Clin. Neurophysiol.* **28,** 644–649.

Waterman, K., Purves, S.J., Kosaka, B., Strauss, E. & Wada, J.A. (1987): An epileptic syndrome caused by mesial frontal lobe foci. *Neurology* **37,** 577–582.

Wieser, H.G. (1982): Zur Frage der lokalisatorischen Bedeutung epileptischer Halluzinationen. In: *Halluzination bei Epilepsien und ihre Differentialdiagnose*, ed. K. Karbowski, pp. 67–92. Berne: Huber.

Williamson, P.D. (1986): Intensive monitoring of complex partial seizures: diagnosis and subclassification. In: *Intensive neurodiagnostic monitoring*, ed. R.J. Gumnit, pp. 69–84. New York: Raven Press.

Williamson, P.D., Spencer, S.S., Spencer, D.D, & Mattson, R.H. (1981): Complex partial seizures with occipital lobe onset. *Epilepsia* **22,** 247–248.

Williamson, P.D., Spencer, D.D., Spencer, S.S., Novelly, R.A. & Mattson, R.H. (1985): Complex partial seizures of frontal lobe origin. *Ann. Neurol.* **18,** 497–504.

Williamson, P.D., Wieser, H.G. & Delgado-Escueta, A.V. (1987): Clinical characteristics of partial seizures. In: *Surgical treatment of the epilepsies*, ed. J. Engel, Jr, pp. 101–120. New York: Raven Press.

Williamson, P.D., Thadani, V.M., Darcey, T.M., Spencer, D.D., Spencer, S.S. & Mattson, R.H. (1992a): Occipital lobe epilepsy: clinical characteristics, seizure spread patterns and results of surgery. *Ann. Neurol.* **31,** 3–13.

Williamson, P.D., Boon, P.A., Thadani, V.M., Darcey, T.M., Spencer, D.D., Spencer, S.S., Novelly, R.A. & Mattson, R.H. (1992b): Parietal lobe epilepsy: diagnostic considerations and results of surgery. *Ann. Neurol.* **31,** 193–201.

Williamson, P.D., French, J.A., Thadani, V.M., Kim, J.H., Novelly, R.A., Spencer, S.S., Spencerr, D.D. & Mattson, R.H. (1993): Characteristics of medial temporal lobe epilepsy II. Interictal and ictal scalp electroencephalography, neuropsychological testing, neuroimaging, surgical results and pathology. *Ann. Neurol.* **34,** 781–787.

Epileptic Seizures and Syndromes, Edited by Peter Wolf
© 1994 John Libbey & Company Ltd., pp. 391–394

Chapter 42

Why is Rasmussen's encephalitis unilateral?

Olivier Dulac

Hôpital Saint Vincent-de-Paul, 82 Avenue Denfert Rochereau, F-75674, Paris Cedex 14, France

The very particular clinical condition described by Rasmussen consists of the combination of intractable focal epilepsy, progressive focal neurological dysfunction, focal cortical atrophy, and inflammation predominantly in the cortical grey matter of one cerebral hemisphere (Rasmussen *et al.*, 1958; Bancaud, 1985; Andermann, 1991). Most virological studies have failed to show that a virus was involved, but Poland *et al.* (1991) were able to demonstrate the presence of cytomegalovirus (CMV) gene by polymerase chain reaction, thus suggesting but not demonstrating that CMV is involved in the pathophysiology of the disease. The reason why it involves one hemisphere remains unclear, since both the aetiology and the pathophysiology that probably determine this major asymmetry also remain unclear.

The clinical and electroencephalographic (EEG) pattern is that of focal discharges involving multiple independent foci within a wide epileptogenic zone, and discharging in a subcontinuous fashion. The clinical seizures consist of clonic fits of one limb or the face lasting less or slightly more than a minute (Dulac *et al.*, 1983; Oguni *et al.*, 1991). Occasionally there may be secondary generalization of focal seizures with Jacksonian march, but this mainly involves periods of worsening. The EEG demonstrates disorganization of the basic rhythm on the abnormal hemisphere and discharges of rhythmic theta activity or sharp waves of low amplitude lasting 10–60 s over one lobe, and then within another part of the hemisphere (So & Gloor, 1991). Polygraphy shows that there is often a lack of clinical and EEG correlations (Dulac *et al.*, 1983). Over one-half of the patients exhibit epilepsia partialis continua (EPC) without EEG correspondence (Oguni *et al.*, 1991). Long video-EEG recordings show that EPC persists during sleep and that there is no major modification of seizure frequency by the sleep/wake cycle (Dulac *et al.*, 1983). Electrocorticography recordings disclosed multiple independent foci that shed light on the clinical and scalp EEG findings. Over a period of a few months or years, the part of the body that is involved by the clinical discharges increases (So & Gloor, 1991).

Until the first seizures, the onset age of which ranges from 1 to 15 years, the patient has normal development and cognitive functions and the radiological investigations, including magnetic resonance imaging (MRI) are normal (Tampieri *et al.*, 1991). After a few months of evolution, a focal motor defect appears and worsens progressively, and the patient is left with hemiplegia, mental deterioration and various focal neurological defects. Several cases of precocious puberty, suggesting hypothalamic lesions and therefore widespread brain involvement, have been reported (Dulac *et al.*,

1983; Oguni *et al.*, 1991). There is no evidence of correlation between seizure severity and neurological defects, in contrast with conditions following status epilepticus. The ictal motor manifestations finally disappear in the most defective part of the body.

After a few months of seizure activity most patients exhibit radiological abnormalities. They consist of cortical atrophy that predominates in the perisylvian area, with dilatation of the ventricles involving the same side but later the contralateral one. The white matter appears normal on computerized tomography (CT) but MRI discloses high T_2 signal intensity in the area corresponding to the most atrophic region of the cortex. This hypersignal area is partly reversible following prolonged steroid administration (Chinchilla *et al.*, in press). Repeat radiological investigations show progressive worsening of intensity and extension or cortical atrophy that involves the frontal lobe after a few months of the disease.

Histology has mainly been studied on biopsy, focal cortical resection or hemispherectomy samples. It shows both necrosis and inflammation. Necrosis consists of cavitation of the cortex, producing severe and extensive atrophy, and scattered areas of neuronal cell loss. Inflammation comprises microglial nodules and patchy areas of perivascular cuffs of round cells following the Virchow–Robin spaces. The inflammation mainly involves the periphery of the lesion, whereas the necrotic areas are devoid of inflammatory infiltration. This suggests that the necrosis is a consequence of inflammation that extends progressively in a centrifugal manner (Robitaille, 1991).

There are very few full brain neuropathological studies. Of eight available cases, two showed clearly bilateral involvement of the inflammatory signs (Gupta *et al.*, 1984; Robitaille, 1991; Chinchilla *et al.*, in press). This suggests that the disease may be bilateral, or become bilateral at some stage of the evolution. Indeed, most reported series were produced by neurosurgical units to which the patients had been referred for surgical treatment, including hemispherectomy, a generally accepted procedure for patients who have become hemiplegic. Two series were collected by neuropaediatric centres, the Centre Saint Paul, Marseille, and the Hôpital Saint Vincent de Paul, Paris (Dulac *et al.*, 1983, Chinchilla *et al.*, in press): there was EPC on both sides and focal neurological defects and cortical atrophy also involved both sides. In all cases, however, the disease was initially unilateral and the contralateral involvement seems to have been somewhat delayed.

In a few cases with bilateral neuropathological study, inflammatory abnormalities were disclosed in the supposedly normal hemisphere, although there was no previous clinical evidence of such an involvement. Therefore, the inflammation seems to precede the occurrence of seizures. In addition, even in patients becoming seizure-free after hemispherectomy, neuropsychological deterioration obviously exceeds the expected consequences of functional exclusion of a single hemisphere (Taylor, 1991).

The overall evolution of the disease is characterized by its progressive stabilization at a stage of major atrophy of one hemisphere with severe motor and cognitive defect. High-dose steroids (Chinchilla *et al.*, in press) and immunoglobulins (Walsh, 1991) have occasionally helped to stabilize the disease at an early stage. Focal resection produces no long-term improvement of seizure frequency and discharges recur at the edge of the resection (Olivier, 1991). Callosotomy only prevents secondary generalization in very few patients who experience this type of seizures (Spencer & Spencer, 1991). Multiple subpial transection may prevent for 1–2 years progressive worsening of cognitive functions in conjunction with the cessation of seizure discharges in the transected area (Morrell *et al.*, 1991). Only hemispherectomy has been followed by persistent relief of seizures in all cases submitted to this procedure. To my knowledge no case has been reported of recurrence of either intractable epilepsy or progressive neurological defect in the contralateral hemisphere following hemispherectomy, although a small proportion of patients do exhibit a few seizures postoperatively (Villemure *et al.*, 1991). However, very few data are available with regard to the type of seizures and the corresponding EEG discharge observed in such conditions. They may correspond to incomplete disconnection and still be produced by the atrophic hemisphere, or they may be produced by the remaining hemisphere, either due to ongoing inflammation of the latter or to a 'mirror focus'. One patient I followed clearly had seizures produced by the remaining hemisphere.

The disease is therefore characterized by inflammation involving mainly the cortex in a patchy although focal manner, mainly in the perisylvian area. This inflammation starts in the first decade with a peak between 3 and 6 years of age. It produces progressive necrosis and atrophy in the centre of the damaged area and grows centrifugally. It produces seizure activity that is mainly characterized by multiple independent foci and is subcontinuous, behaving as if these foci were more or less independent from the functional activity of the rest of the brain. Whether seizure activity contributes to the extension of the inflammation and necrosis centrifugally remains unknown. However, it may be so, since multiple subpial transection seems to reduce progressive worsening of neurological defect. Poland *et al.* (1991) suggested that 'epileptic' neurones or cortex could promote regional accentuation of viral gene expression, and thus establish a vicious circle, by activation of protein kinase C.

One hypothetical mechanism of progressive worsening, involving in most cases a single hemisphere, could therefore be that continuous seizure activity disturbs the blood–brain barrier, increasing permeability to inflammatory cells and various circulating substances toxic to the brain. In addition, it would trigger viral gene expression. Viral genes, or accumulation of toxic substances, or both, would trigger inflammation. Inflammation, in turn, would cause neuronal disconnection, continuous seizure activity and necrosis.

A number of questions remain open:

– What triggers inflammation in the grey matter? Is it a virus or an autoimmune phenomenon, or both, one following the other?
– Why does it occur exclusively at an early age? Is there a role played by the permeability of the blood–brain barrier that is still increased at this age?
– Why does it involve particularly the perisylvian area? Is there at the age range of onset increased vulnerability of the blood vessels or of the blood–brain barrier in this region of the brain?

References

Andermann, F. (1991): *Chronic encephalitis and epilepsy: Rasmussen's syndrome,* pp. 1–295. Boston: Butterworth-Heinemann.

Bancaud, J. (1985): Kojewnikow's syndrome (epilepsia partialis continua) in children. In: *Epileptic syndromes in infancy, childhood and adolescence,* eds. J. Roger, C. Dravet, M. Bureau, F.E. Dreifuss and P. Wolf, pp. 286–298. London: John Libbey.

Chinchilla, D., Dulac, O., Robain, O., Plouin, P., Ponsot, G., Pinnel, J.F. & Graber, D. (1994). A reappraisal of Rasmussen syndrome with special emphasis on high dose steroid treatment. *J. Neurol. Neurosurg. Psychiatry* in press.

Dulac, O., Dravet, C., Plouin, P., Bureau, M., Ponsot, G., Gerbaut, L., Roger, J. & Arthuis M. (1983): Aspects nosologiques des épilepsies partielles continues chez l'enfant. *Arch. Fr. Pediatr.* **40,** 689–695.

Gupta, P.C., Rapin, I., Houroupian, D.S., Roy, S., Llena, J. & Tandon, P.N. (1984): Smoldering encephalitis in children. *Neuropediatrics* **15,** 191–197.

Morrell, F., Whisler, W.W. & Smith, M.C. (1991): Multiple subpial transection in Rasmussen's encephalitis. In: *Chronic encephalitis and epilepsy: Rasmussen syndrome,* ed. F. Andermann, pp. 219–233. Boston: Butterworth-Heinemann.

Oguni, H., Andermann, F. & Rasmussen, T.B. (1991): The natural history of the syndrome of chronic encephalitis and epilepsy: a study of the MNI series of forty-eight cases. In: *Chronic encephalitis and epilepsy: Rasmussen syndrome,* ed. F. Andermann, pp. 7–25. Boston: Butterworth-Heinemann.

Olivier, A. (1991): Cortical resection for diagnosis and treatment of seizures due to chronic encephalitis. In: *Chronic encephalitis and epilepsy: Rasmussen syndrome,* ed. F. Andermann, pp. 205–211. Boston: Butterworth-Heinemann.

Poland, S., Power, C., Blume, W.T., Girvin, J.P. & Rice, G.P.A. (1991): Herpesviruses as etiologic candidates in Rasmussen's encephalitis. In: *Chronic encephalitis and epilepsy: Rasmussen syndrome,* ed. F. Andermann, pp. 159–165. Boston: Butterworth-Heinemann.

Rasmussen, T., Olszewski, J. & Lloyd-Smith, D. (1958): Focal seizures due to chronic localized encephalitis. *Neurology* **8,** 435–445.

Robitaille, Y. (1991): Neuropathologic aspects of chronic encephalitis. In: *Chronic encephalitis and epilepsy: Rasmussen syndrome*, ed. F. Andermann, pp. 79–110. Boston: Butterworth-Heinemann.

So, N. & Gloor, P. (1991): Electroencephalographic and electrocorticographic findings in chronic encephalitis of Rasmussen type. In: *Chronic encephalitis and epilepsy: Rasmussen syndrome*, ed. F. Andermann, pp. 37–45. Boston: Butterworth-Heinemann.

Spencer, S.S. & Spencer, D.D. (1991): Corpus callosotomy in chronic encephalitis. In: *Chronic encephalitis and epilepsy: Rasmussen syndrome*, ed. F. Andermann, pp. 213–218. Boston: Butterworth-Heinemann.

Tampieri, D., Melanson, D. & Ethier, R. (1991): Imaging of chronic ecephalitis. In: *Chronic encephalitis and epilepsy: Rasmussen syndrome*, ed. F. Andermann, pp. 47–60. Boston: Butterworth-Heinemann.

Taylor, L.B. (1991): Neuropsychologic assessment of patients with chronic encephalitis. In: *Chronic encephalitis and epilepsy: Rasmussen syndrome*, ed. F. Andermann, pp. 111–121. Boston: Butterworth-Heinemann.

Villemure, J.G., Andermann, F. & Rasmussen, T.B. (1991): Hemispherectomy for the treatment of epilepsy due to chronic encephalitis. In: *Chronic encephalitis and epilepsy: Rasmussen syndrome*, ed. F. Andermann, pp. 235–241. Boston: Butterworth-Heinemann.

Walsh, P. (1991): Treatment of Rasmussen's syndrome with intravenous gammaglobulin. In: *Chronic encephalitis and epilepsy: Rasmussen syndrome*, ed. F. Andermann, pp. 201–204. Boston: Butterworth-Heinemann.

Epileptic Seizures and Syndromes, Edited by Peter Wolf
© 1994 John Libbey & Company Ltd., pp. 395–398

Chapter 43

Progress in the semiology of Rasmussen's encephalitis: adolescent or adult onset and double pathology

Yvonne Hart[*], David Fish[†], Yves Robitaille[‡] and Frederick Andermann[§]

[*]*Department of Neurology, Atkinson Morley's Hospital, Copse Hill, London SW20 0NE, UK;* [†]*National Hospital for Neurology and Neurosurgery, Queen Square, London WC1N 3BG, UK;* [‡]*Hôpital Sainte-Justine, 3175 Chemin de la Côte Saint-Catherine, Montreal, Quebec, Canada;* [§]*Montreal Neurological Institute and Hospital, 3801 University Street, Montreal, Quebec, Canada H3A 2B4*

The original description of chronic encephalitis and epilepsy by Rasmussen and colleagues (1958) was of three young children who developed a syndrome of focal seizures, progressive hemiparesis and a deterioration in cognitive abilities, in two cases following a minor infective episode. More than 100 cases have been reported in the literature since, the majority resembling those originally described (Gupta *et al.*, 1974; Piatt *et al.*, 1988; Rasmussen & Andermann, 1991). However, in recent years it has become clear that a significant proportion of patients with chronic encephalitis and epilepsy, though broadly falling into the description given above, show either clinical or pathological features which are in some way atypical (Gray *et al.*, 1987; McLachlan *et al.*, 1993). It may be that through the study of these atypical cases some light may be shed on the aetiology of Rasmussen's syndrome, the nature of which is as yet unknown. We have identified nine patients in whom the onset of symptoms occurred in adolescence or adulthood, and three patients in whom, although the clinical presentation and course were characteristic of chronic encephalitis and epilepsy, pathological examination revealed both encephalitic changes and a second pathology.

Chronic encephalitis and epilepsy developing in adolescence or adulthood

The mean age of onset of chronic encephalitis and epilepsy in most series is between 5 and 6 years of age, and its development above the age of 12 is unusual. However, nine patients were identified from three centres (Montreal, São Paulo and London (UK)) in whom the onset of the condition occurred in adolescence or adulthood. The clinical, radiological and pathological features were reviewed.

The patients fell readily into three groups. The first of these comprised four patients who developed the condition in adulthood, between the ages of 21 and 40 years, but whose clinical features were in many other respects similar to those found in the childhood form of the disease.

Illustrative clinical history

This right-handed housewife first developed symptoms at the age of 40, when, following an operation for spinal fusion, she noted that she was tending to use the wrong words.

This symptom resolved after several days. A few months later she had an influenza-like illness, followed 1 week later by a generalized tonic–clonic seizure preceded by jerking of the right arm. Postictally she was aphasic for several hours. Thereafter she continued to have intractable motor and sensory seizures, sometimes with secondary generalization, and followed by numbness and weakness of the right arm. These were accompanied by the insidious development of persistent poverty of movement of this limb, and a progressive deterioration in her speech and reading abilities.

Neurological examination was normal at the onset of her seizure disorder, but later confirmed mild pyramidal weakness of the right upper limb and expressive dysphasia. Routine haematology and biochemistry were normal, and autoantibodies, treponemal serology and human immunodeficiency virus (HIV) tests negative. Cerebrospinal fluid (CSF) examination showed the presence of oligoclonal bands. Computerized tomography (CT) and magnetic resonance imaging (MRI) scans were normal, but electroencephalograms (EEGs) repeatedly showed diffuse slow activity interrupted by frequent sharp and slow wave discharges over the left hemisphere, with shifting localization.

Trials of high-dose steroids and intravenous immunoglobulins failed to halt the progression of her symptoms. Stereotactic biopsy was therefore carried out and showed the presence of chronic inflammatory changes, typical of chronic encephalitis.

Two of the other patients in this group also had a course typical of the childhood form of Rasmussen's encephalitis, their ages at onset being 22 and 31 years. However, both had early clinical and/or electrographic evidence of occipitotemporal epileptic involvement. This, particularly the occipital symptomatology, is very uncommon at the onset of the childhood form. Both had progressive hemiparesis and intellectual impairment. The former developed seizures early in her first pregnancy, while in the latter symptoms occurred shortly after an upper respiratory tract infection. This patient was treated by a right occipitotemporal resection. She had only occasional seizures afterwards, but later went on to develop hemiparesis of the right, opposite, side of the body in addition to the left, evidence for bilateral involvement. The fourth patient, who also had bilateral involvement, developed focal seizures with secondary generalization at the age of 21, followed by a progressive dementing illness. Extensive investigation failed to reveal the cause of this, and the diagnosis of chronic encephalitis and epilepsy was made at post-mortem examination.

The EEG in each of these patients showed a diffuse or focal slow-wave abnormality, accompanied in three of the cases by focal epileptiform transients, features similar to those found in the childhood form of the disease. Radiological changes were much less marked than those commonly seen in children. Two patients had normal MRI scans. One had signal changes in the left occipital and medial temporal region, while the other had a small degree of ventricular enlargement on pneumoencephalography (this patient was investigated before the days of modern neuroimaging and an MRI scan was not performed). CSF examination was normal in two of the patients, while oligoclonal bands were isolated from the other two, again similar to the situation in children, in whom oligoclonal bands have been reported in approximately 50 per cent (Dulac *et al.*, 1991). In two of the patients, tissue was examined for the presence of cytomegalovirus but none found.

The second group included three patients developing their first symptoms in adolescence (between the ages of 14 and 16 years), but in whom the clinical features were otherwise very similar to those found in the childhood form of the disease. All three had partial, predominantly motor, seizures, a slowly progressive hemiparesis, and some degree of deterioration in cognitive abilities, which was unusually mild in one. Two of these patients, unlike those developing seizures in adult life, had epilepsia partialis continua. One had early seizures of occipital origin, an unusual localization in children, sometimes with secondary generalization. Two were treated with focal surgical resections and had a rather benign course afterwards, one having occasional seizures only and the other having no seizures since 5 years following operation (total follow-up 25 years).

The third group consisted of two patients who presented acutely with the development of partial and secondarily generalized tonic–clonic seizures at the ages of 25 and 48 years. The radiological investigations then available (pneumoencephalography and angiography) suggested the presence of a frontal space-occupying lesion in each case. Early surgery was therefore performed, but, although there was some focal swelling, no discrete mass was found, and pathological examination showed changes of chronic encephalitis. One of these patients was lost to follow-up after several months: she had no seizures or hemiparesis at the time of her last visit, but she was moderately depressed and had some evidence of cognitive deterioration. The other patient also had only rare seizures following surgery, but developed mild hemiparesis and dysphasia.

Unfortunately both of these patients were seen before the advent of modern neuroimaging techniques. Their pathological changes were typical of encephalitis of Rasmussen's type, and clinically both had some evidence of progressive intellectual or neurological deterioration, albeit mild. They are thus different from some other patients who have been reported (Jensen & Klinken, 1976), who did not have a progressive course, but in whom similar changes of chronic encephalitis were found following temporal lobectomy for seizures. However, in view of the fact that these two patients may represent a distinct entity, it is reasonable to consider them separately.

The other seven patients had clinical presentations similar to those seen in children, although in one hemiparesis did not develop, despite marked deterioration in cognitive abilities. Occipital involvement appeared to be more common in these patients, occurring in three out of seven, compared with only three of 42 children in the Montreal series of patients developing the condition under the age of 12 years (Oguni *et al.*, 1991). The course of the seizures was variable, but in general was more benign than that seen in children, and showed a better response to focal resection. There was a tendency for those patients with a milder seizure disorder to have less marked intellectual deterioration. Two patients had evidence suggestive of bilateral disease, which is uncommon in children. Two of the three patients with adolescent or adult onset reported by McLachlan *et al.* (1993) also had bilateral involvement, another important, though still unexplained, clinical difference.

It remains unclear whether such patients represent part of the spectrum of the same disease that occurs in children, or whether they are different clinical entities with similar presentations both clinically and pathologically. We have noticed that the pathological changes are sometimes less florid in adults, and it may be that they represent a later stage of a disease process which is less malignant from the outset, although this is not a universal finding and at least one adult developing chronic encephalitis and epilepsy leading to death in 2 years has been described (Gray *et al.*, 1987). Further study, with intensive virological and immunological investigation, is needed to clarify this point.

Double pathology in Rasmussen's encephalitis

In a series of 48 patients, three were identified as having clinical features suggestive of chronic encephalitis, but were shown on pathological examination to have an additional pathology.

Illustrative clinical history

This child had a difficult delivery and delayed developmental milestones. She had a febrile seizure at the age of 2 years, and later developed generalized tonic–clonic seizures, drop attacks and focal motor seizures involving the left face and arm: by the age of 8 she had up to 20 seizures per day. By age 7 she had developed a mild left hemiparesis. General examination showed her to have two *café-au-lait* spots and a depigmented macule with typical 'ash-leaf' configuration. CT scan showed atrophy of the left cerebral hemisphere. No periventricular calcified lesions were found.

Right frontal resection was performed. Pathological examination showed changes of both typical chronic encephalitis and tuberous sclerosis, with large dysplastic pyramidal cells disorientated within cortical columns and in ectopic positions, diffuse reactive gliosis and occasional microscopic clusters of large gemistocytic astrocytes in subpia and cortex. Her seizures continued and she later underwent hemispherectomy.

In contrast to this patient, in whom chronic encephalitic changes were seen in association with tuberous sclerosis, the other two patients had vascular abnormalities. One, a boy who developed visual, sensory and secondarily generalized seizures at the age of 12, had a left occipital lobectomy at age 19. He was found to have a remote subdural haematoma and evidence of an old intracerebral haemorrhage. Microscopically, a chronic inflammatory infiltrate, with lymphocytes, plasma cells, histiocytes and rare multinucleated giant cells, was present: in addition there was evidence of endarteritis obliterans, areas of neuronal loss and gliosis, and flecks of calcified neurites. Clusters of large vessels resembling cavernous angiomas were also found.

The other patient was a girl with visual and olfactory symptoms, and occasional secondarily generalized seizures, who subsequently developed persistent dysphasia and right hemiparesis. Neuro-imaging showed the presence of left hemispheric atrophy. Left temporal lobectomy was carried out: at operation, large thrombosed veins were present on the cerebral surface. Microscopic examination showed features of chronic encephalitis and an organizing vasculitis predominating in small arteries and veins, with surrounding multiple cavernous angiomas. Occipital localization, as seen in these last two patients is unusual in the classical childhood form of the disease and its presence should make one suspect that the underlying process may not be typical.

The presence of a separate pathology in association with chronic encephalitis in these patients is of some aetiological interest. There is a possibility that these are chance findings: however, none of them are common conditions, and their occurrence together would be an unusual coincidence. Other possible explanations would be that the structural lesion may have caused an alteration in the blood–brain barrier, increasing the likelihood of viral infection, or that it may in some way have provoked a non-specific chronic autoimmune response. Less likely is the possibility of an idiosyncratic encephalitic reaction to drug therapy used for epilepsy caused by the underlying lesion.

References

Dulac, O., Robain, O., Chiron, C., Plouin, P., Pinel, J.F., Vigevano, F., Raynaud, C. & Ponsot, G. (1991): High-dose steroid treatment of epilepsia partialis continua due to chronic focal encephalitis. In: *Chronic encephalitis and epilepsy: Rasmussen's syndrome*, ed. F. Andermann, pp. 193–199. Boston: Butterworth-Heinemann.

Gray, F., Serdaru, M., Baron, H., Daumas-Duport, C., Loron, P., Sauron, B. & Poirier, J. (1987): Chronic localised encephalitis (Rasmussen's) in an adult with epilepsia partialis continua. *J. Neurol. Neurosurg. Psychiatry* **50,** 747–751.

Gupta, P.C., Roy, S. & Tandon, P.N. (1974): Progressive epilepsy due to chronic persistent encephalitis: report of 4 cases. *J. Neurol. Sci.* **22,** 105–120.

Jensen, I. & Klinken, L. (1976): Temporal lobe epilepsy and neuropathology. *Acta Neurol. Scand.* **54,** 391–414.

McLachlan, R.S., Girvin, J.P., Blume, N. T. & Reichman, H. (1993): Rasmussen's chronic encephalitis in adults. *Arch. Neurol.* **50,** 269–274.

Oguni, H., Andermann, F. & Rasmussen, T.B. (1991): The natural history of the syndrome of chronic encephalitis and epilepsy: a study of the MNI series of forty-eight cases. In: *Chronic encephalitis and epilepsy: Rasmussen's syndrome*, ed. F. Andermann, pp. 7–35. Boston: Butterworth-Heinemann.

Piatt, J.H., Jr, Hwang, P.A., Armstrong, D.C., Becker, L.E. & Hoffman, H.J. (1988): Chronic focal encephalitis (Rasmussen syndrome): six cases. *Epilepsia* **29,** 268–279.

Rasmussen, T. & Andermann, F. (1991): Rasmussen's syndrome: symptomatology of the syndrome of chronic encephalitis and seizures. 35-year experience with 51 cases. In: *Epilepsy surgery*, ed. H. Lüders, pp. 173–182. New York: Raven Press.

Rasmussen, T., Olszweski, J. & Lloyd-Smith, D.L. (1958): Focal seizures due to chronic encephalitis. *Neurology* **8,** 435–455.

Epileptic Seizures and Syndromes, Edited by Peter Wolf
© 1994 John Libbey & Company Ltd., pp. 399–404

Chapter 44

The medical treatment of chronic encephalitis and epilepsy

Yvonne Hart[*], Frederick Andermann[†], David Fish[‡], Miguel Cortez[§], Paul Hwang[§], Kenneth Silver[¶], Natalio Fejerman[**] and Allan Sherwin[†]

[*]*Department of Neurology, Atkinson Morley's Hospital, Copse Hill, London SW20 0NE, UK;* [†]*Montreal Neurological Institute and Hospital, 3801 University Street, Montreal, Quebec, Canada H3A 2B4;* [‡]*National Hospital for Neurology and Neurosurgery, Queen Square, London WC1N 3BG, UK;* [§]*Division of Neurology, The Hospital for Sick Chioldren, 555 University Avenue, Toronto, Ontario, Canada M5G 1X8;* [¶]*Montreal Children's Hospital, 2300 Tupper Street, Montreal, Quebec, Canada H3H 1P3;* [**]*Hospital de Pediatria 'Prof. Juan P. Garrahan', Combate de los Pozos 1881, Buenos Aires 1245, Argentina*

Despite much research, the cause of Rasmussen's encephalitis (chronic encephalitis and epilepsy), first described in 1958 (Rasmussen *et al.*), remains unknown. This rare condition, which usually has its onset in childhood, develops after a minor infective episode such as an upper respiratory tract infection in about 50 per cent of cases (Rasmussen & Andermann, 1992). This is followed by the onset of focal seizures, often with secondary generalization, and in about half the children epilepsia partialis continua (EPC) later ensues. The symptoms are accompanied by the development of a progressive hemiparesis and a gradual deterioration in cognitive abilities. Pathologically, the changes of chronic encephalitis range from a florid inflammatory picture, with abundant microglial nodules and lymphocytic perivascular cuffing, to a more remote picture in which neuronal loss and gliosis are the predominant features (Robitaille, 1991).

The major contender for the underlying aetiology in chronic encephalitis of this nature is a viral infection (Poland *et al.*, 1991), the possibilities including chronic infection or acute infection leading to a local immune response. Factors supporting an underlying viral aetiology include the frequency of a preceding infective episode, the similarities between this condition and Russian spring–summer encephalitis, the association which sometimes occurs with ipsilateral uveitis, the results of cerebrospinal fluid examination, the pathological findings and the occasional reported identification of cytomegalovirus in pathological specimens. Another possibility is that chronic encephalitis is the result of an independent autoimmune process (Grenier *et al.*, 1991).

The seizures in chronic encephalitis are refractory to conventional antiepileptic drugs (Dubeau & Sherwin, 1991), and focal surgical resection is rarely of lasting benefit. Hemispherectomy may succeed in stopping the seizures (Honovar *et al.*, 1992) but inevitably produces a neurological deficit if one is not already present. There is thus a pressing need for the development of alternative treatments to prevent the otherwise inexorable deterioration and obviate the need for destructive surgical

Table 1. Summary of clinical features of patients and results of investigations

Pt	Age (years)	Sex	Age at sz (years)	Sz types	EPC	Bx	Time until Rx (years)	Regime	Outcome
1	13	M	6	SPS, GTC	No	No	6.5	IVIG 400 mg/kg/day for 3 days, then 400 mg/kg in single dose at monthly intervals for 5 months	Condition stabilized
2	7	M	6	GTC, SPS, myoclonus	Yes	Yes	0.5	IVIG 400 mg/kg/day for 3 days, repeated every 3 weeks for 6 months	SPS controlled, still some myoclonus, hemiparesis improved
3	8.5	M	5	SPS, GTC, tonic, myoclonic	Yes	No	2	IVIG 400 mg/kg/day for 3 days, repeated every 20 days for 1 year. Pr 1 mg/kg/day for same period	Myoclonus persisited, other sz reduced by 75%. Marked improvement in hemiparesis after 1 month (able to walk again)
4	10.5	F	5.5	SPS, GTC	No	Yes	3.5 till steroids, 4 till IVIG	MP 400 mg/m^2 IV alt days for 3 days – 3 courses at 6-weekly intervals. IVIG 200 mg/kg – 12 courses at 1-month intervals	No improvement with MP. > 50% decrease in sz and slight improvement in hemiparesis with IVIG
5	13	M	9	SPS, GTC	No	Yes	< 0.5 till Pr. 1.5 to IVIG. 2 to 2nd steroids	Pr 80 mg/day for 2 months, then 60 mg alt days for 4 months. Then IVIG 0.5 g/kg/day for 2 days, x28 at monthly intervals. Steroids added – MP 400 mg/m^2 IV alt days for 3 days, then Pr 2 mg/kg daily, reducing over 1 year	50% improvement in sz for several months then relapsed but no further progression
6	43	F	40	SPS, GTC	No	Yes	2	MP 0.5 g/day for 3 days, 5 courses + Pr 10–20 mg daily for 1 year. IVIG 400 mg/kg over 3 days, 3 courses at monthly intervals	Sz frequency reduced for few days after each course of MP. No effect of IVIG
7	24	M	7.5	CPS, GTC	Yes	Yes	15.5	MP 400 mg/m^2 IV alt days for 3 days, then Pr 2 mg/kg/day for 10 days, then tapered	EPC stopped but steroid psychosis occurred
8	14	M	6	SPS, CPS	No	Yes	5	Pr 2 mg/kg/day tapered over 2 months	50% decrease in sz
9	11	M	4	CPS, GTC	No	Yes	3	Pr 5 mg/kg/day for 3 days, tapering to 15 mg alt days for 1 year	No improvement. Behavioural problems
10	14	M	12	SPS, CPS	Yes	No	1	Pr 2 mg/kg/day tapered over 3 months	25% decrease in sz
11	10	M	4	SPS, GTC	Yes	Yes	5.5	Pr 2 mg/kg/day tapered over 6 months	No improvement
12	9	F	4	SPS, GTC	Yes	Yes	4	Pr 2 mg/kg/day tapered over 5 months	50% improvement in sz – maintained since (6 months)
13	12.5	F	4	SPS, CPS, GTC	No	Yes	5.5	Pr 2 mg/kg/day for 2 months, then tapered	25% improvement in sz
14	7.5	F	5	SPS, GTC	Yes	Yes	< 0.5	Pr 2 mg/kg/day tapered over 6 months	No improvement

Pt	Age (years)	Sex	Age at sz (years)	Sz types	EPC	Bx	Time until Rx (years)	Regime	Outcome
15	Died aged 27	F	21	SPS, CPS, GTC	No	Yes	2	Pr 60 mg/day for 2 months, then tapered	No improvement
16	14	F	8.5	SPS, CPS, GTC	Yes	Yes	1.5	ACTH injections over 4 weeks	No sz for 2 weeks; fluid retention

GTC = generalized tonic–clonic seizures; SPS = simple partial seizures; CPS = complex partial seizures; EPC = epilepsia partialis continua; IVIG = intravenous immunoglobulins; Pr = prednisolone; MP = methylprednisolone; ACTH = adrenocorticotrophic hormone; Bx = biopsy; Rx = treatment; Sz = seizures; alt = alternate.

procedures. Various medical treatments have been proposed in the light of the putative aetiologies, including high-dose steroids, intravenous immunoglobulins (IVIG), and antiviral agents such as acyclovir and gancyclovir.

The rationale for using IVIG lies in their capacity to modulate the immune system, which they do by various means, including the neutralization of autoantibody by the formation of an idiotype–anti-idiotype dimer, the binding and down-regulation of B cell antigen receptors by anti-idiotypic antibodies, and the recognition of anti-idiotypic antibody by regulatory T cells (Ballow, 1991). They have been used with some success in a number of neurological conditions in which autoimmune processes are suspected or known to play a part, including Guillain–Barré syndrome, chronic inflammatory demyelinating neuropathy, myasthenia gravis and multiple sclerosis (Dwyer, 1992). Their use in herpes simplex encephalitis has also been reported (Berlit, 1988). Steroids have been used in a similar range of neurological diseases because of their immunosuppressant effect. In addition, both immunoglobulins and steroids have been used in the treatment of epilepsy *per se* (Dreifuss *et al.*, 1986; Echenne *et al.*, 1991), steroids particularly having a role in the management of infantile spasms. There thus appears to be ample justification for assessing these drugs in patients with chronic encephalitis and epilepsy. The results of immunoglobulin and/or high-dose steroid treatment in 16 patients treated at four centres (Montreal, Toronto, Buenos Aires and London) are presented in this chapter.

All the patients were diagnosed as having chronic encephalitis and epilepsy on the basis of clinical and radiological findings, and in all but three patients biopsy confirmation was also available. Their seizures were intractable to conventional antiepileptic drugs, but their neurological deficits were such that hemispherectomy was not yet considered appropriate. Treatment with either high-dose steroids or immunoglobulins, or, in a few patients, both drugs concomitantly, was given. The protocols varied, both due to the fact that several centres were involved, and because of changing opinion regarding the most effective regime: they are summarized in Table 1. Fourteen patients were treated with high-dose steroids and five with immunoglobulins.

The patients included nine males, seven females. Two (both with pathologically confirmed disease) developed the condition in adult life (at the ages of 21 and 40 years): the others were children, their mean age at onset being 6.2 years. In addition to seizures, 12 had mild hemiparesis and three of the other four evidence of intellectual deterioration. Eight patients had EPC. The patients were followed for a mean of 2.0 years (range 0.5–4.0 years).

Six of the 14 patients treated with high-dose steroids showed no improvement in their seizure frequency. Six had a decrease in seizure frequency of at least 50 per cent, while the other two had a reduction in seizure frequency of the order of 25 per cent. However, except in the case of two patients, there was an acute deterioration in seizure control within days or weeks of the steroids being tapered and then withdrawn. Only one patient showed a significant reduction in hemiparesis as a result of steroid treatment: although some other patients showed some improvement, this appeared to be related to seizure control and deterioration again occurred with recurrence of the seizures. The improvement in seizure control tended to be greatest in patients taking the highest doses of steroids for the longest periods of time. There did not appear to be any major association between the effect of steroids and the duration of disease, there being, for example, no response in one patient having the condition less than 6 months, while another who had developed it more than 15 years earlier, showed a reduction in seizure frequency, albeit at the expense of a steroid-induced psychosis. Neither patient with adult-onset disease showed any improvement. Side-effects, mainly minor, were common, but one patient developed a psychosis, and another was noted as developing behavioural problems.

Four of the five patients treated with IVIG (two of whom received concomitant steroid therapy) showed a lessening in their seizure frequency while receiving treatment. The fifth showed no reduction in seizure frequency, but did have stabilization of his symptoms. The treatment was stopped after 5 months, and 2 months later he had an acute increase in seizure frequency. There were no apparent adverse effects as a result of immunoglobulin treatment in this group of patients.

Although the effect of treatment in some patients was encouraging, this was not always the case, and the place of these drugs in the management of Rasmussen's encephalitis remains unclear. The condition is very uncommon, and it would be unlikely that one centre would gain sufficient experience to provide an answer: ideally a disease registry should be set up, using standardized protocols. This is particularly the case in view of a number of confounding issues which complicate assessment. They include spontaneous variations in the activity of the condition (and it has been suggested that in some patients chronic encephalitis may have a relapsing and remitting course (Dulac *et al.*, 1992)) and a lack of reliable parameters for measuring disease activity. Seizure frequency is often very variable, the relationship of magnetic resonance imamging (MRI) and electroencephalographic (EEG) abnormalities to disease activity unclear, and changes in cerebrospinal fluid (CSF) inconsistent. Magnetic resonance spectroscopy (MRS) may prove to be helpful in the future (Peeling & Sutherland, 1993) but further assessment is needed and the technique is not yet widely available.

The knowledge that a diagnosis of Rasmussen's encephalitis implies a relentless neurological deterioration makes it imperative that, in addition to symptomatic antiepileptic medication, treatment aimed at ameliorating the disease course be instituted at an early stage. Such treatment at present is of necessity given on an empirical basis, and the following protocol, drawn up in association with O. Dulac, will need to be revised in the light of new developments. Our current practice is to start patients on treatment with IVIG, given by infusion at a dose of 400 mg/kg/day on 3 successive days. In making the diagnosis of chronic encephalitis and epilepsy, we demand the presence of EPC and either progressive neurological deficit, progressive hemispheric atrophy on computerized tomography (CT) or MRI scan, the presence of oligoclonal or monoclonal banding on CSF examination, or biopsy evidence of chronic encephalitis. If biopsy confirmation of the condition is available in the presence of focal seizures, the child need not have EPC, provided he or she has other evidence of progressive disease.

If no improvement is seen within 1 month of IVIG therapy, we start treatment with high-dose steroids. The patient is given three infusions of intravenous methylprednisolone (each dose 400 mg/m^2 of body surface) on alternate days. One month later he or she is given a further infusion of intravenous methylprednisolone, 400 mg/m^2 body surface, in a single dose, repeated at monthly intervals for the first year, 2-monthly intervals for the second year, and 3-monthly intervals for the third year, unless serious side-effects occur. We give concomitant treatment with oral prednisolone, starting at a dose of 2 mg/kg/day, and reducing the dose very gradually over the following months, according to the clinical response. The duration of the oral prednisolone treatment is usually of the order of at least 1–2 years. We consider that comparison of results based on this protocol represents a step forward toward optimal rational therapy. Controlled trials, particularly when the cause of the disease is more firmly established, should then be considered.

References

Ballow, M. (1991): Mechanisms of action of intravenous immunoglobulin therapy and potential use in autoimmune connective tissue diseases. *Cancer* **68,** 1430–1436.

Berlit, P. (1988): Prognosis and long-term course of viral encephalitis. *J. Neuroimmunol.* **20,** 117–125.

Dreifuss, F., Farwell, J., Holmes, G., Joseph, C., Lackman, L., Madsen, J.A., Minarcik, C.J., Rothner, A.K. & Shewmon, D.A. (1986): Infantile spasms: comparative trial of nitrazepam and corticotropin. *Arch. Neurol.* **43,** 1107–1110.

Dubeau, F. & Sherwin, A.L. (1991): Pharmacologic principles in the management of chronic encephalitis. In: *Chronic encephalitis and epilepsy: Rasmussen's syndrome*, ed. F. Andermann, pp. 179–192. Boston: Butterworth-Heinemann.

Dulac, O, Chinchilla, D. Plouin, P., Pinel, J.F. & Robain, O. (1922): Follow up of Rasmussen syndrome treated by high dose steroids. *Epilepsia* **33** (suppl. 3), 128 (abstract).

Dwyer, J.M. (1992): Manipulating the immune system with immune globulin. *N. Engl. J. Med.* **326,** 107–116.

Echenne, B., Dulac, O., Parayre-Chanex, M.J., Chiron, C., Taillebois, L., Cognot, C., Andary, M., Clot., J. & Baldy-Moulinier, M. (1991): Treatment of infantile spasms with intravenous gamma-globulins. *Brain Dev.* **13,** 313–319.

Grenier, Y., Antel, J.P. & Osterland, C.K. (1991): Immunologic studies in chronic encephalitis of Rasmussen. In: *Chronic encephalitis and epilepsy: Rasmussen's syndrome*, ed. F. Andermann, pp. 125–134. Boston: Butterworth-Heinemann.

Honovar, M., Janota, I. & Polkey, C.E. (1992): Rasmussen's encephalitis in surgery for epilepsy. *Dev. Med. Child Neurol.* **34,** 3–14.

Peeling, J. & Sutherland, G. (1993): ^{1}H magnetic resonance spectroscopy of extracts of human epileptic neocortex and hippocampus. *Neurology* **43,** 589–594.

Poland, S., Power, C., Blume, W.T., Girvin, J.P & Rice, G.P.A. (1991): Herpesviruses as etiologic candidates in Rasmussen's encephalitis. In: *Chronic encephalitis and epilepsy: Rasmussen's syndrome*, ed. F. Andermann, pp. 159–165. Boston: Butterworth-Heineman.

Rasmussen, T. & Andermann, F. (1992): Update on the syndrome of 'chronic encephalitis and epilepsy'. *Cleveland Clin. J. Med.* **56** (suppl. 2), S181–S184.

Rasmussen, T., Olszewski, J. & Lloyd-Smith, D. (1958): Focal seizures due to chronic localized encephalitis. *Neurology* **8,** 435–445.

Robitaille, Y. (1991): Neuropathologic aspects of chronic encephalitis. In: *Chronic encephalitis and epilepsy: Rasmussen's syndrome*, ed. F. Andermann, pp. 79–110. Boston: Butterworth-Heinemann.

Section V

Epileptogenesis and ictogenesis: epilepsy as a dynamic process

Epileptogenesis refers to the processes which cause a brain to produce epileptic seizures, and ictogenesis to the mechanisms causing an individual seizure to occur. In this section, the importance of exchange between clinicians and theoreticians becomes most palpable.

Secondary epileptogenesis is still a controversial matter. Theoreticians often seem to take its clinical relevance for granted. But authors from several large epilepsy centres (Chapter 45a–d) found little evidence for it in a longitudinal comparison of seizure semiology in individual patients. Then, in a book where benign idiopathic epilepsies are discussed at some length, it may be pointed out that there are large patient groups where secondary epileptogenesis does not occur. If the definition of Lothman is followed (Chapter 51), secondary epileptogenesis can only be considered in terms of focal epileptogenesis. Could it explain, as the findings of Cavalheiro (Chapter 52) seem to indicate, TLE following febrile convulsions? The answer, as Holthausen (Chapter 47) explains, is 'perhaps'. Could it partly account for bilateral mesiotemporal epilepsies (see Chapter 38)? De Lanerolle *et al.* (Chapter 46) describe differences between cryptogenic and tumour-related TLEs concerning a variety of findings in temporal lobe tissues of operated patients. They seem to indicate that the 'cryptogenic' group may indeed represent an idiopathic epilepsy syndrome with its own pathogenesis and development, but, probably, different again from the genetically determined idiopathic syndromes. It would be premature to relate these findings to the problem of temporal lobe epileptic bilaterality (Chapter 38), which, however, will not fail to come to mind.

Sprouting of mossy fibres, one of the findings of de Lanerolle *et al.*, was observed by Represa and Ben-Ari (Chapter 53) secondary to kainate and to kindling. So, if secondary epileptogenesis occurs at all in clinical epilepsy, would it be explained by a kindling process? Garant and Moshé (Chapter 50), like, indeed, most authors of this book, would not jump to any rapid conclusions. Then, in spite of bilateral findings on glutamate receptors following kindling, as reviewed above by Köhr (Chapter 23), kindling is still considered as a merely focal model whereas a view of epilepsy as a process (see Chapter 59) comes more to mind in relation to the onset of epilepsy with generalized tonic–clonic seizures, especially grand mal on awakening (see Chapter 27).

The last-mentioned examples point to the relevance of single seizures at the onset of epilepsy and provide, thus, a link between ictogenesis and epileptogenesis. Seizure precipitation, as discussed in Section II is another clinical aspect of ictogenesis. The four concluding chapters (54–57) of this section report highly interesting new findings concerning ictogenesis, which may remind us that, in clinical epilepsy, this aspect deserves to receive more attention, just like its counterpart, the prevention of seizure generation (see Chapter 66).

Epileptic Seizures and Syndromes, Edited by Peter Wolf
© 1994 John Libbey & Company Ltd., pp. 407–430

Chapter 45

Longitudinal evolution of epileptic syndromes: a video workshop

Masakazu Seino

National Epilepsy Center, Shizuoka Higashi Hospital, 668 Urushiyama, Shizuoka 420, Japan

Introduction

It is a well-known fact that West's syndrome is followed by other types of epilepsy in 50–60 per cent of the sufferers. Lennox–Gastaut syndrome or other secondary generalized epilepsies are the most common types (Jeavons & Livet, 1992). Similarly, early infantile epileptic encephalopathy with suppression bursts (Ohtahara *et al.*, 1992) may evolve to West's syndrome, although only a limited number of the cases evolve further to Lennox–Gastaut syndrome (Ohtahara *et al.*, 1992). However, benign localization-related epilepsy in childhood with centrotemporal electroencephalographic (EEG) foci, and childhood absence epilepsy, which represent the most comparable forms of idiopathic epilepsies, are clearly distinct and even mutually exclusive in terms of phenotype and probably of genotype. No case has been reported of idiopathic localization-related epilepsy which has evolved into one of the syndromes of idiopathic generalized epilepsy (Genton, 1993).

In idiopathic generalized epileptic syndromes with age-related onset in childhood and adolescence – childhood absence epilepsy, juvenile absence epilepsy, juvenile myoclonic epilepsy and epilepsy with grand mal on awakening – the therapeutic response is almost always favourable and the course of these syndromes is usually benign. The differences between these disorders mostly concern the seizure types and ictal EEGs, and the age at seizure onset. Hence, there is a good possibility that these four syndromes constitute one disease which takes various clinical forms according to their onset age. For practical purposes, it seems a reasonable solution to differentiate classification according to a patient's earliest seizure type (Wolf, 1992). The close relationship between these syndromes has been discussed mainly in terms of cross-sectional aspects of their clinical features instead of the longitudinal course of evolution of the disorders. Epilepsy with myoclonic absences, for example, though having bisynchronous spike-waves at about 3 Hz, may be associated with a particular evolution characterized by the disappearance of myoclonic absences while subclinical and clinical generalized tonic seizures appear. These features suggest that the syndrome evolves toward a cryptogenic or symptomatic epileptic syndrome similar to Lennox–Gastaut syndrome (Tassinari *et al.*, 1992). Although the existence of 'frontal absences' is often discussed in the context of a bioelectrical mechanism of secondary bilateral synchrony (Bancaud & Talairach, 1992), I have not observed a single case of idiopathic generalized epilepsy with typical absences evolving to any frontal epileptic syndrome.

This chapter summarizes a video workshop which was planned to elucidate the modes of longitudinal evolution of clinical and EEG seizure manifestations occurring in individual epileptic syndromes. The workshop was expected to provide substantial information on the mode of evolution of seizures and syndromes, which might also give us some knowledge on the extent to which a given case remains within the same taxonomic category or shifts from one syndrome to the other during a long-term course of epilepsy. This, in turn, may answer the question as to what extent the International Classification of Epilepsies and Epileptic Syndromes (Commission, 1989) is usable in terms of recognition and prediction of the long-term outcome of the condition, which is still a subject of controversies in today's clinical epileptology.

In this workshop, participants were required to present a closed-circuit television/EEG videotape illustrating at least three seizure events representative of a given patient in a chronological order. The clinical course had to be followed up for longer than 5 years in childhood-onset epileptic syndromes and for 10 years in adulthood-onset syndromes. Ancillary information to be presented included interictal and ictal EEGs of diagnostic significance, neuroimages if worth while, interictal neuropsychological findings and response to antiepileptic drugs or other therapeutic measures.

In spite of the fact that we could recruit only a limited number of participants in the workshop, resulting in more limited information than we had anticipated, we hope that the longitudinal evolution of epileptic syndromes will be more elucidated by the use of CCTV/EEG videotape in the future. As they say 'seeing is believing.'

Longitudinal evolution of frontal lobe complex partial seizures: a progressive seizure syndrome?

Walter van Emde Boas

Department of Clinical Neurophysiology, Instituut voor Epilepsiebestrijding 'Meer & Bosch'de Cruquiushoeve', Achterweg 5, 2103 SW Heemstede, The Netherlands

Although the classification of epileptic seizures (Commission on Classification, 1981) does not yet describe individual types of complex partial seizures according to the area of the brain where the seizures have their origin, it is now generally accepted that complex partial seizures will indeed show varying and yet highly specific clinical characteristics, depending on the area of seizure onset. Accordingly, in the International Classification of Epilepsies and Epileptic Syndromes, it is suggested that symptomatic localization-related seizure syndromes should be classified anatomically, i.e. as temporal lobe, frontal lobe, parietal lobe or occipital lobe epilepsies (Commission on Classification, 1989). Delineation of such an individual syndrome primarily requires the recognition of a highly characteristic seizure semiology which can be proved to correlate with certain specific electroencephalographic (EEG) features and other findings, all associated with a specific and restricted anatomical localization of the epileptogenic zone within one lobe of the brain. In addition, however, it requires the identification of specific and typical elements in the medical and seizure history and in the evolutional pattern of the seizures.

The proposed syndrome of mesial temporal lobe epilepsy (Engel, 1992) is a good example of such an anatomically defined seizure syndrome. For most of the seizure types that can be attributed to specific areas of the brain, including frontal lobe complex partial seizures, however, little is known about the evolution of these individual types of seizures over time. Typically, in a recent and very comprehensive book on frontal lobe seizures and epilepsies, a great number of chapters deal with the different semiologies associated with different anatomical areas, but very little is written about the temporal evolution of these seizures (Chauvel *et al.*, 1992). Probably this reflects the fact that, for the recognition, identification and detailed follow-up of these individual syndromes, the history of the patient, as given by the patient, the parents or others, although indispensable, usually will not be sufficient or reliable, especially not regarding the exact semiology of the individual seizures. Prolonged interictal and ictal EEG and video monitoring is therefore indispensable, not only for the establishment of the diagnosis of these difficult-to-recognize seizure syndromes, but also for the detailed documentation of the evolution of the seizure semiology.

Long-term EEG and CCTV monitoring, however, constitutes an expensive and time-consuming procedure with limited availability, which, for that reason, should be applied selectively and for specific indications only (Mattson, 1986). Accordingly, repeated seizure recordings in the same patient over the years are rare. Two patients with frontal lobe complex partial seizures are presented who were followed over a period of 11 years and in whom repeated ictal seizure monitoring was performed during this period. In both patients the evolution of the seizure disorder suggested a progressive epileptic syndrome. Whether this is typical of frontal lobe complex partial seizures in general or reflects a negative bias of patients selected for repeated seizure monitoring has yet to be established.

Patients

The clinical data of the two patients are summarized in Table 1. In both patients the medical history up to the onset of seizures was essentially negative.

Table 1. Patient characteristics

	Patient 1	Patient 2
Sex	Male	Female
Year of birth	1969	1971
History		
Family history	Negative	Negative
Pregnancy and birth	Normal	Normal
Development	Normal	Normal
Febrile convulsions	Negative	?
Onset of seizures	5 years	3 years (10 years?)
Diagnosis of epilepsy	10 years	10 years
Start of AED treatment	10 years	10 years
Findings (period)	1981–1992	1981–1992
Physical status	Normal	Normal
Neurological status	Normal	Normal
Neuroimaging (CT, MRI)	Negative	R. frontal lesion; stable (cryptic angioma)
Neuropsychology	Normal (1992)	Slight frontal lobe dysfunction

In patient 1 a few occasional seizures were noticed during early childhood; in patient 2 a single convulsion occurred at age 3, not preceded but followed by onset of a febrile episode some hours after the seizure. In both patients recurrent seizures became manifest around the end of the first decade.

Physical and neurological findings were negative and only in patient 2 could an aetiological lesion be established on computerized tomography (CT) and magnetic resonance imaging (MRI). Since this lesion, a cryptic angioma, proved to be stable over a period of 11 years, the slight neuropsychological frontal lobe dysfunction documented recently in this patient most probably reflects the progressive epileptic disturbance rather than the anatomical lesion.

EEG findings

The EEG findings are summarized in Table 2. In both patients the interictal EEG findings over the years have been largely non-contributory. The background activity over the years was either normal or showed some slight diffuse excess of irregular slow activity, possibly reflecting antiepileptic drug (AED) treatment rather than specific brain dysfunction.

Local intermittent or paroxysmal slowing was present in most records in both patients, shifting from more posterior localizations in earlier records to more anterior frontal and temporal areas in later records and with consistent lateralization and localizing predominance (right frontal) only in patient 2, consistent with the existing lesion in that patient. In neither patient were specific epileptiform abnormalities documented, despite a great number of EEG studies, including sleep recordings. Even repeated ictal recordings did not reveal specific epileptiform discharges during the seizures in either patient. In both, however, there were consistent slow-wave abnormalities either preceding (patient 1) or during the seizure (patient 2) suggesting a left frontal onset in patient 1 (Fig. 1) and a right frontal onset in patient 2 (Fig. 2).

Table 2. EEG findings

EEG	Patient 1	Age	Patient 2	Age
Background	Normal or mild diffuse Slow (AEDs)	10–32	Nornal or mild diffuse Slow (AEDs)	10–21
Local slowing	Posterior R > L	10	Posterior R >> L	10
	Centroparietal R > L	13	Posterior R >> L but less	11–12
	Posterior R	19	Frontal/frontotemporal R >> L	14–21
	Frontotemporal L	21		
	Frontotemporal R > L	32		
Epileptiform discharges	None	10–32	None	10 –21
Ictal onset	Left frontal	22, 32	Right frontal	18, 20, 21

Longitudinal evolution of the seizures

The evolution of the seizure disorder over the years is summarized in Tables 3 and 4.

Patient 1 experienced nocturnal seizures only. Initially these consisted of occasional brief sudden turning movements, apparently triggered by arousals and without further clinical signs or sequelae. From the age of 10 years on the seizure pattern became more elaborate: an initial sudden stretching or bending movement would then be followed by turning of the body to the left, forward bending of head and trunk and a tonic flexion of the left arm in front of the chest and head, followed by some movements of the legs and then awakening. The duration of the seizures remained limited to less than 20 s and there was no postictal confusion. Sometimes, however, the patient would fall out of his bed, resulting in occasional injuries, since the patient at that time worked as a sailor and slept in a high bunk above a steel floor. Over the years the seizure frequency varied but in general tended to increase. Moreover, during the third decade his seizures became more severe and prolonged, with predominant thrashing and kicking movements of the body and legs now following the original early symptoms and with some confusion apparent after the seizures, which now lasted half a minute or more.

Over the years the patient was treated with adequate dosages of phenobarbitone, phenytoin, carbamazepine, sodium valproate, ethosuximide, clobazam and vigabatrine, either as monotherapy or in various combinations, but without consistent efficacy. Overall, phenytoin appeared to be the most effective drug but, with the exception of two periods of 10–12 months at age 16 and 19 years, the patient never became seizure-free.

Table 3. Seizure history: patient 1

Age (years)	Seizure frequency	Seizure type and severity
5–10	Occasional seizures	Nocturnal seizures only (brief abrupt motor behaviour) on arousal only; no consistent awakening
10–20	Varying: from 1–2/night, 0–3 nights/month to 4–10/night every night	Spontaneous; 13–16 s; falls out of bed, wakes up; no confusion
20–32	Varying as before but in general more frequent	Spontaneous, 30–40 s; more pronounced motor behaviour; some confusion
16 and 19	10–12 months seizure-free (on AEDs)	
20	One single generalized seizure following abrupt withdrawal of all AEDs	

Table 4. Seizure history: patient 2

Age (years)	Seizure frequency	Seizure type and severity
3	Single seizure (febrile?)	'Generalized'
10–14	Occasional seizures	Generalized with partial (L) onset (provoked by sleep deprivation?)
14–17	Increasing from 1–2/day, 0–3 days/month to 1–3/day, 0–20 days/month	Spontaneous complex partial seizures (loss of consciousness without or with some automisms with left arm or both and some vocalizations); occasional generalized seizures with partial onset
17–21	Increasing further to 3–8/day most days	Spontaneous complex partial seizures (loss of consciousness usually with quite elaborate automatisms and vocalizations; urinary incontinence); subtle nocturnal partial motor seizures; occasional generalized seizures with partial onset
14–21	No true seizure-free periods (at present seizure-free following partial R frontal lobectomy; 6 months follow-up)	

In patient 2 not only the severity but also the type of seizures changed over the years. The first episode, at the age of 3 years and followed, not preceded, by a febrile illness, was described as a generalized convulsion but the initial symptoms may well have been unobserved. Between 10 and 14 years there occurred a few occasional generalized tonic–clonic seizures, all apparently provoked by sleep deprivation or jet lag and all with signs of partial onset, the left arm being stretched up as the initial sign of the seizure. More of these seizures with partial onset and secondary generalization would occur occasionally during the remainder of the second decade, always triggered by either long air travel or inconsistent use of AED therapy. From the age of 14 years on, however, the patient started to experience absence-like episodes, often limited to a short-lasting clouding of consciousness, but

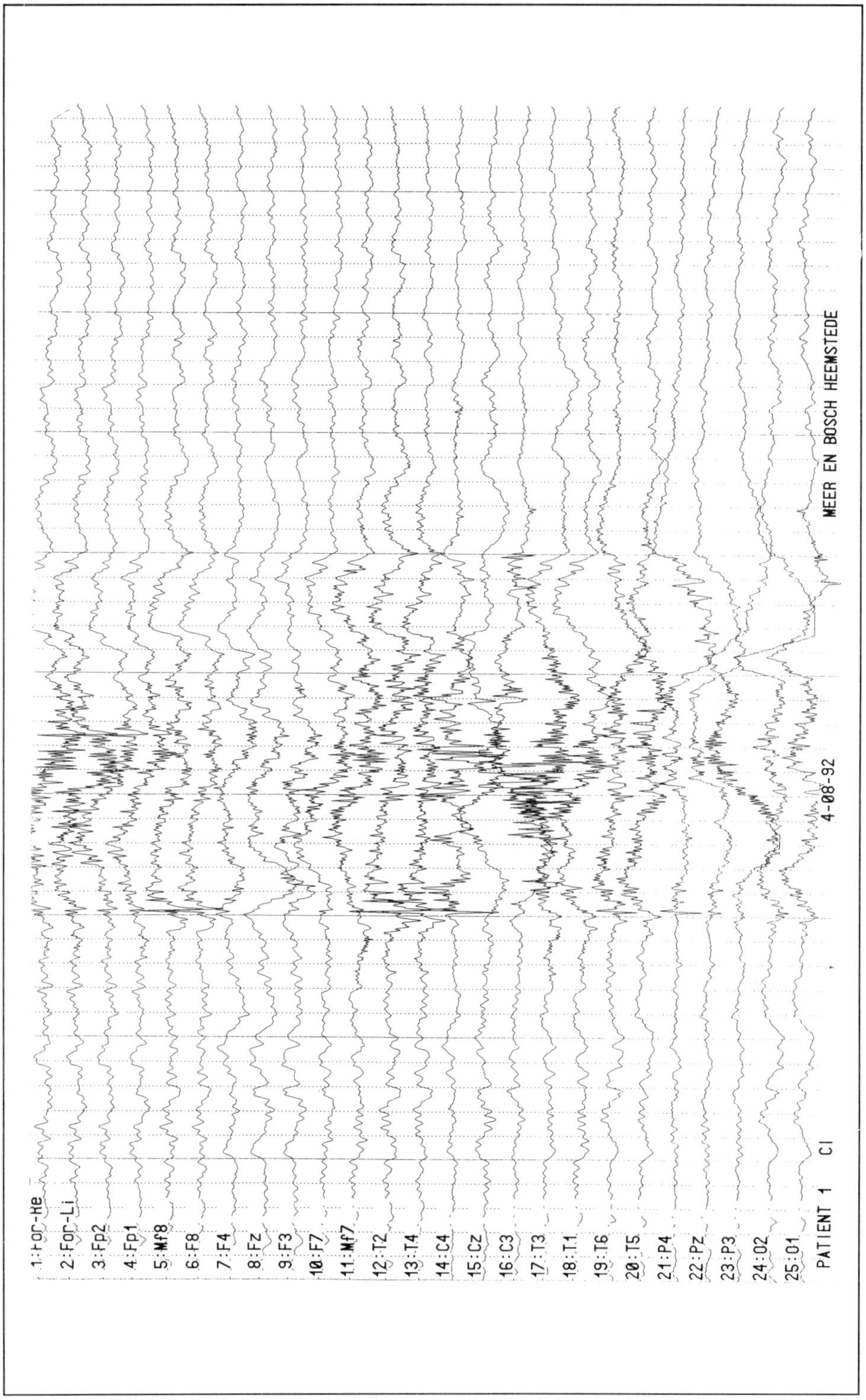

Fig. 1. Brief nocturnal episode (abortive seizure) in patient 1. Left frontal slow wave preceding motor behaviour and a single sharp wave at the end of the episode. (For = fronto-orbital electrode; Mf = inferior frontal electrode. Common average recording.)

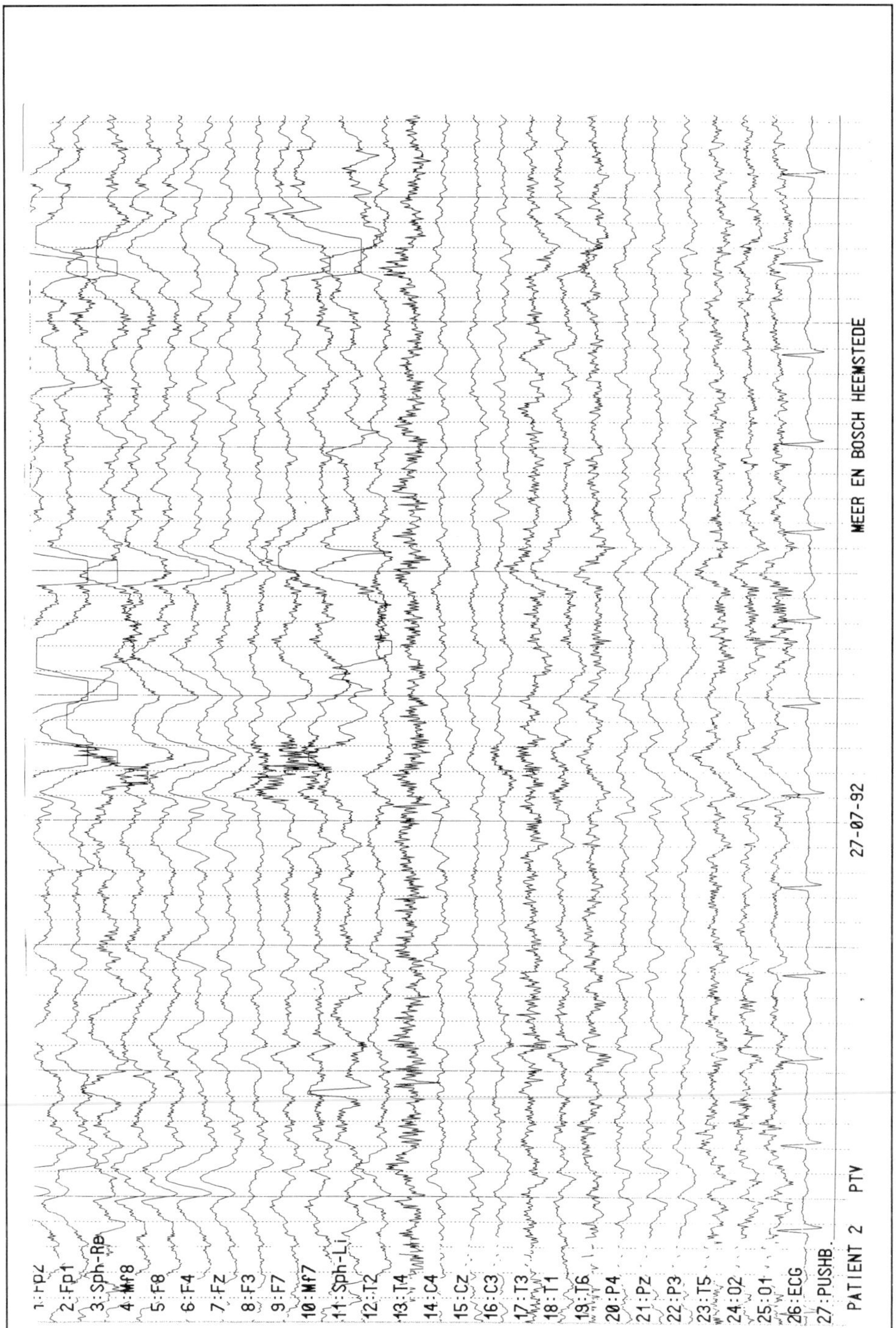

Fig. 2. Accentuation of right frontal delta wave paroxysms during –not preceding – a complex partial seizure in patient 2. (Sph = sphenoidal electrode; Mf = inferior frontal electrode. Common average recording.)

sometimes accompanied by slight vocalizations or some automatisms, mostly waving with the arms, left more than right.

The frequency of these seizures tended slowly but consistently to increase over the years and as from age 17 the severity and average duration of the seizures also increased, the vocalizations and the motor automatisms becoming more elaborate and with urinary incontinence accompanying some of the episodes. Moreover, during this period the patient also started to have subtle nocturnal seizures with short motor automatisms of the left arm, without further symptoms and without awakening.

Phenytoin, carbamazepine, sodium valproate and vigabatrine in adequate dosages and either alone or in various combinations showed no consistent effect on either seizure frequency or severity and, although carbamazepine overall appeared to be the most effective drug, there were no true seizure-free periods between ages 14 and 21.

Following a partial right frontal lobectomy, including the lesion, in December 1992, the patient is at present seizure-free but a more extended period of follow-up is needed to assess the long-term result of surgery in her case.

Discussion

In both patients presented here a diagnosis of frontal lobe epilepsy could be established on the basis of the seizure semiology, the (ictal) EEG findings and, in patient 2, the associated epileptogenic lesion in the affected frontal lobe.

Patient 1 showed the typical nocturnal complex partial seizures, associated with the fronto-orbital and anterior cingulate cortex (Williamson *et al.*, 1985), while in patient 2 the seizure semiology, notably the absence-like episodes, appeared to suggest an epileptogenic zone inferior to the lesion, in the intermediate frontal region, with secondary invasion of neighbouring frontal areas during the more elaborate seizures (Bancaud & Talairach, 1992).

Despite this difference in the apparent area of onset, the patients' histories show a number of similarities. Following one or a few occasional seizures during early childhood, recurrent seizures became apparent around the end of the first decade and after that became gradually more frequent, more severe and more prolonged and elaborate. In both patients the seizure disorder proved to be medically therapy-resistant and more or less progressive in severity. This appears to be in accordance with the fact that much of the recent literature on frontal lobe epilepsy is based on patients investigated for possible surgery (Chauvel *et al.*, 1992), an indication of the severe and therapy-resistant character of these seizures. Whether this is really typical for frontal lobe seizure syndromes in general, however, remains unclear.

In principle, the longitudinal evolution of a seizure syndrome will be characterized by a number of parameters concerning the actual seizures as well as by 'secondary' parameters concerning predominantly the mental or physical status of the patients. Seizure parameters are: frequency, duration, severity (or complexity) and the number of different seizure types in the same patient, all of which could over time either become better, remain stable or become worse.

In Table 5 these different evolutional patterns are listed and the patterns identified in patients 1 and 2 as well as other patients, taken from our data base of frontal lobe seizure patients, are shown.

Table 5. Possible evolution of seizures

		Identified in	Reliability for establishing evolutionary pattern	
Seizures	Evolution	patient 1, 2 or others	History	EEG/CCTV
Frequency	Increase	1, 2		
	No change	*	++	+/–
	Decrease			
Duration	Increase	1		
	No change	2	+/–	++
	Decrease			
Severity and complexity	Increase	1, 2		
	No change	*	+/–	++
	Decrease			
Number of types	Increase	1		
	No change	2	+/–	++
	Decrease			

* indicates that this pattern has been identified in one or more patients other than patient 1 or patient 2. Other patients showing the same evolution as patient 1 or patient 2 are not indicated.

It is clear that in our material no patients have been identified who showed real improvement on any of the four parameters, even though they may have remained stable for some of them. It should be realized, however, that our impression of the evolution of the seizure syndrome in these patients is based on the findings during repeated EEG and CCTV monitoring and that repeated monitoring is not likely to be performed in a patient who does well on therapy. On the other hand, patients who show signs of deterioration or changes in the seizure semiology or who are investigated for possible surgical treatment will be monitored more often.

This bias appears indeed to be reflected in the material of over 1000 patients, collected during more than 12 years of long-term EEG and CCTV monitoring at the Instituut voor Epilepsiebestrijding at Heemstede, since patients with documented frontal lobe complex partial seizures in whom comparable repeated EEG and CCTV studies were performed covering a time period of 2 years or more represent less than 2 per cent (10–15 patients) of our material. In other patients we performed repeated monitoring only within a shorter period of time, usually during presurgical evaluation and with reduction of AED therapy. Most patients with frontal lobe seizures, however, were re-referred to the treating neurologist, once that the diagnosis was established and thus were lost to follow-up.

The fact that the majority of these patients with proved frontal lobe complex partial seizures are not referred back to a specialized epilepsy centre, actually suggests that the prognosis of frontal lobe seizure syndromes in general, following correct diagnosis and treatment, may be rather good and that patients like the two presented here, with signs of a progressive seizure disorder, do indeed reflect a negative selection bias. Specific follow-up studies, requiring close co-operation between specialized epilepsy centres and general neurologists who take care of the day-to-day treatment of these patients, are needed to establish the overall evolution of frontal lobe seizure syndromes and for the early identification of those patients in whom a possibly progressive seizure disorder should be treated aggressively, possibly with an early surgical intervention.

Acknowledgements

Patients 1 and 2 gracefully and readily gave permission to show the video images of their seizures to the public audience in Bielefeld and, although remaining anonymous, must be gratefully mentioned here for their co-operation.

The author also thanks D.N. Velis for his careful reading and useful suggestions during the preparation of this text.

Longitudinal evolution of seizure semiology of supplementary motor area origin

Ulrich Specht

Epilepsie-Zentrum Bethel, Klinik Mara I, Maraweg 21, 33617 Bielefeld, Germany

Although seizures with onset in the supplementary motor area were first described more than 30 years ago (Penfield & Jasper, 1954; Ajmone-Marsan & Ralston, 1957), little is known about change in seizure semiology over time. A case history is presented with a follow-up over a period of 11 years, including ictal recordings with closed-circuit television (CCTV)-electroencephalography (EEG).

Case history

KH was born in November 1962. A brother and a grandmother of his father had epilepsy of unknown type. Pregnancy, delivery and psychomotor development were normal and he had no severe illness. His first seizures occurred at the age of 6. In a medical report in 1969, these seizures were described as follows: 'The head and the eyes, sometimes the trunk too, were turning to the left and the left arm was stretched out. The boy was unconscious. The seizures lasted up to 30 s and occurred several times a day, with a maximum of 30.' Under the initial medication of primidone and ethosuximide, he was seizure-free for 15 months, which has been the only seizure-free period until now. At the age of 15, he started falling during the seizures. This has led to numerous minor head injuries.

In 1981 he was first an in-patient at Klinik Mara I, Epilepsy-Centre Bethel. Stereotyped seizures very similar to the ones described above were observed: sudden unconscious tonic deviation of head and eyes to the left, with a mild anteroflexion of the head, and an asymmetric elevation and abduction of the arms, the left arm stretched and the right semiflexed. A groaning vocalization frequently appeared. Very rarely, these tonic seizures with a duration between 5 and 30 s, were followed by mild and brief automatisms (e.g. fumbling movements of the hands) before consciousness was recovered. The patient reported no aura. The seizures occurred randomly over day and night, with a frequency of 1 to 6 per day and rare days without seizures. Two habitual fits were recorded with CCTV-EEG.

After two additional stays in 1982 and 1983, he came back in 1992. Now he mentioned an indescribable aura which, he said, had preceded his seizures since the beginning of his epilepsy. Again stereotyped tonic-postural seizures with a frequency of one to five (maximum 10) per day and many associated falls could be observed. During the seizures he was unresponsive and amnesic. Compared with our observations in 1981, seizure semiology was nearly identical. In addition, generalized tonic–clonic seizures with a frequency of 0–1/ month occurred. During an intensive monitoring with CCTV-EEG the patient showed his habitual tonic-postural seizures (Fig. 1) evolving to left-sided clonic and generalized clonic seizures. Such seizures had never before been described during the course of his epilepsy and were probably caused by the reduction of the antiepileptic drugs. The left-sided clonias were considered as a lateralizing sign to the right hemisphere.

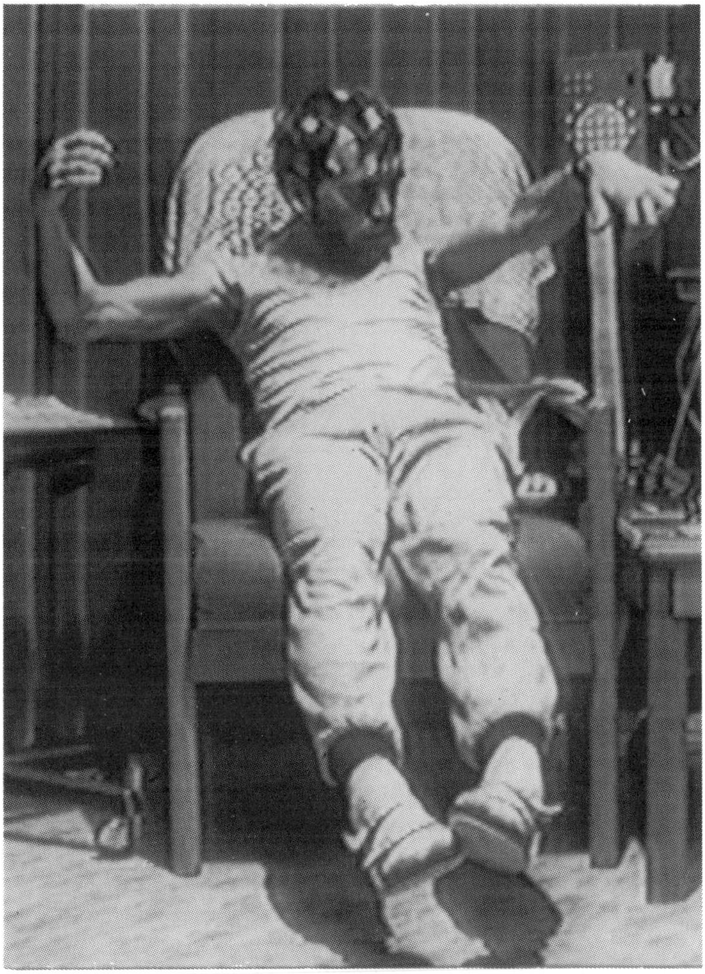

Fig. 1. A typical tonic-postural seizure of K.H., recorded in 1992.

The general physical examination was normal and the neurological examination showed a slight slowing of alternating movements of the left hand. A psychological assessment in 1981 revealed a psychomotor slowing, which probably could be ascribed to the medication. The Wechsler IQ was 115 (verbal: 118, performance: 110). The patient showed substantial emotional disturbances, which led to several psychiatric interventions between 1979 and 1986. Afterwards he finished a vocational education and now he has been employed since 1990. During the years, no decline in cognitive function was observed. The magnetic resonance imaging (MRI) in 1992 showed a mild cerebellar atrophy, but no focal lesion.

The patient had received numerous antiepileptic drugs, mostly in polytherapy. The only positive effect was seen with high-dose monotherapies of carbamazepine or phenytoin (Table 1). A further increase of the dose led to intolerable side-effects of the respective drug.

EEG descriptions prior to the first stay in the Epilepsy Centre mentioned a background slowing of 7 Hz as the only constant finding. Several mild focal changes were seen in different areas of both hemispheres, mostly intermittent slowing, rarely spikes. A typical spike-and-wave pattern was mentioned twice, once accompanied by what was called a petit mal seizure, which unfortunately was not described.

Table 1. Antiepileptic therapy

AED	Poly-/ Mono- therapy	Maximum serum level in mg/l (dose in mg)	Year	Anti- epileptic effect	Side-effects
CBZ	M	17	1992	+	Diplopia, ataxia
	P		1976–81		
PHT	M	30–46	1992	+	(Ataxia, nystagmus)
	P		1976–92		
PRM	P	(750)	1969–76	–	
PHB	P	56	1982	–	Sedation
VPA	P	111 (3000)	1982	–	
MSM	P	20* (600)	1982	–	Hiccup
ESM	P	60	1983	–	

AED: antiepileptic drug ; CBZ: carbamazepine; PHT: phenytoin; PRM: primidone; PHB: phenobarbitone; VPA: valproate; MSM: methsuximide; ESM: ethosuximide; *: *N*-desmethyl-methsuximide; +: reduction of seizure frequency; –: no effect.

Intensive EEG recordings in the Epilepsy-Centre were performed in 1981, 1983 and 1992.

In 1981 rare interictal left temporal sharp transients were found, but no typical epileptiform activity. Ictal recordings showed inconstant findings: diffuse fast activity, sometimes brief rudimentary generalized slow spikes and waves at the beginning of the seizure, and sometimes no changes. In 1983 again no epileptiform activity was recorded interictally. Diffuse flattening and inconstant diffuse fast activity were the ictal findings.

In 1992 – as mentioned above – intensive CCTV-EEG monitoring with surface and sphenoidal electrodes was performed. This revealed an interictal intermittent slowing plus rare sharp waves in the right frontocentral region. The seizures were accompanied by a diffuse flattening, with an ictal pattern of bilateral frontocentral diffuse fast activity as an inconstant finding. There was no lateralization from the EEG viewpoint.

Comment

In conclusion emphasis must be laid on two points:

1. During the whole course of epilepsy over a period of 24 years the seizures showed a very stereotyped semiology.

2. In contrast, this frontal lobe epilepsy was accompanied by various, inconstant and thus puzzling EEG changes, which led to a variety of diagnoses (Table 2).

Table 2. Evolution of and changes in diagnosis

1969	Adversive absences
1970	Adversive seizures
1976	Pyknoleptic adversive petit mal
1982	Secondary generalized seizures: atypical absences (starting tonic-versive) and tonic(-psychomotor) seizures
1985	Symptomatic epilepsy + pseudoseizures
1986	Mixed seizure disorder + pseudoseizures
1992	Cryptogenic focal epilepsy with tonic-postural seizures originating in the right (?) supplementary motor area

The present diagnosis of cryptogenic epilepsy of the supplementary motor area is based on intensive monitoring with ictal recordings which, however, did not pinpoint an epileptic EEG focus. Thus, some doubts remain concerning the classification. Unlike the evolution of the two previous cases with frontal lobe epilepsy, this is an example of a non-evolutionary long-term course in spite of drug resistancy with numerous seizures over the years.

Persistent epileptic spasms of infancy onset

Hideo Shigematsu

National Epilepsy Center, Shizuoka Higashi Hospital, Urushiyama 886, Shizuoka (420), Japan

Infantile spasms, if arrest of psychomotor development and hypsarrhythmia coexist, are taken as pathognomonic for West syndrome. It is generally agreed that infantile spasms are age-dependent in their onset and disappear by about age 5 years (Jeavons, 1985). Nevertheless, epileptic spasms that mimic infantile spasms are not uncommon in patients with symptomatic generalized epilepsy who have an alleged history of West syndrome. The epileptic spasms consist of a sudden and transient contraction of muscles of the neck, trunk and limbs. They are differentiated from tonic seizures or myoclonic seizures by their clinical and electroencephalographic (EEG) features. Two patients who have shown persistent epileptic spasms are reported. In both, the spasms occurred in early infancy and have continued to recur over 10 years.

Patients

Patient 1 is a 15-year-old boy. There were no contributory disorders in his personal history, but in the family history one cousin had febrile convulsions. Before the seizure onset, his development was normal. At present, he has no gross motor abnormalities but has severe mental retardation. The initial seizures occurred at age 15 months. The seizures were prone to occur on awakening. In a supine posture, the arms were lifted up abruptly with accompanying flexion of the elbows and a facial expression of displeasure. In a sitting position, if the neck muscles were involved, only head nods occurred. When the seizures were more intense, the legs were elevated with flexion of the knees. Muscle hypertonicity involved the proximal ends of the extremities as well as of the body axis. He was brought to our hospital at age 16 months, and adrenocorticotropic hormone therapy was tried several times, but without improvement of seizures. A computed tomographic scan of the head showed no specific finding.

An interictal EEG at age 17 months showed transient paroxysmal waves resembling hypsarrhythmia (Fig. 1). Ictal EEGs at age 16 months and at ages 2 and 5 years showed only high-voltage slow waves followed by an electrodecrementation coinciding with each spasm (Fig. 2a–c). The spasms persisted until the age of 15 years. When sitting, he nodded forward repeatedly with or without shrugging of the shoulders and abduction of both arms. When the seizures were more intense, he bent his head forward and downward and fell suddenly to the ground. The falling spells were occasionally followed by atypical absence-like episodes or obtundation of consciousness accompanied by a burst of bisynchronous slow spike-and-wave discharges on the EEG. This particular type of fall is classified as flexor spasms type by Ikeno *et al.* (1985). An ictal EEG at age 10 years demonstrated an overall electrodecrementation followed by a short run of alpha-like rhythm (Fig. 2d). We could not recognize any change in the clinical and EEG manifestations between age 1 year and age 10 years (Fig. 3). Besides the spasms, generalized tonic seizures also occurred from age 2 years to the present time (Fig. 4a–b), and atypical absences and myoclonic seizures were noted at age 5 years (Figs. 5 and 6).

Patient 2 is an 11-year-old boy. His personal history was non-contributory, but in the family history one cousin had febrile convulsions. Until the seizure onset, his development was normal. At present, he has no gross motor abnormalities, but has moderate mental retardation. The initial seizures occurred at age 5 months. He nodded forward repeatedly on awakening, with a facial expression of displeasure

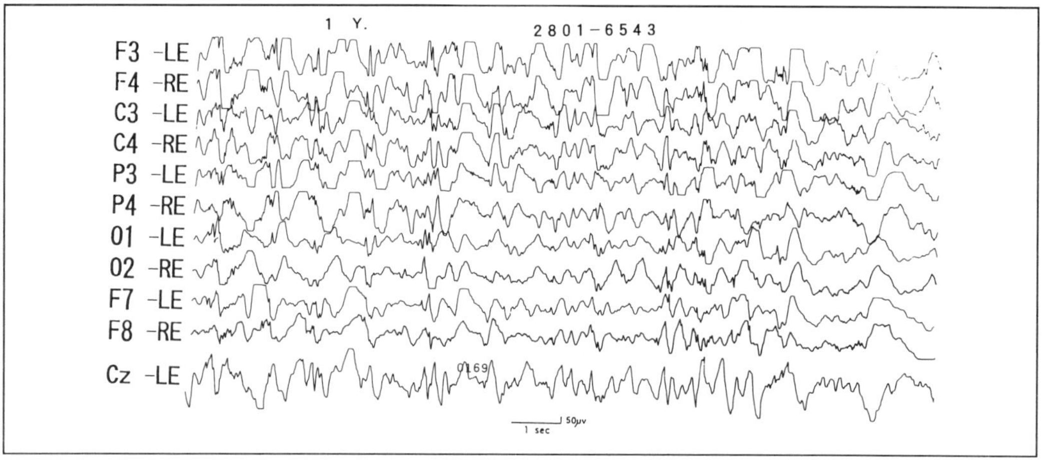

Fig. 1. Interictal EEG during waking from patient 1 at age 17 months. A burst of bilateral diffuse and often asymmetrical high-voltage slow-wave activity is intermingled with multifocal spikes or sharp waves.

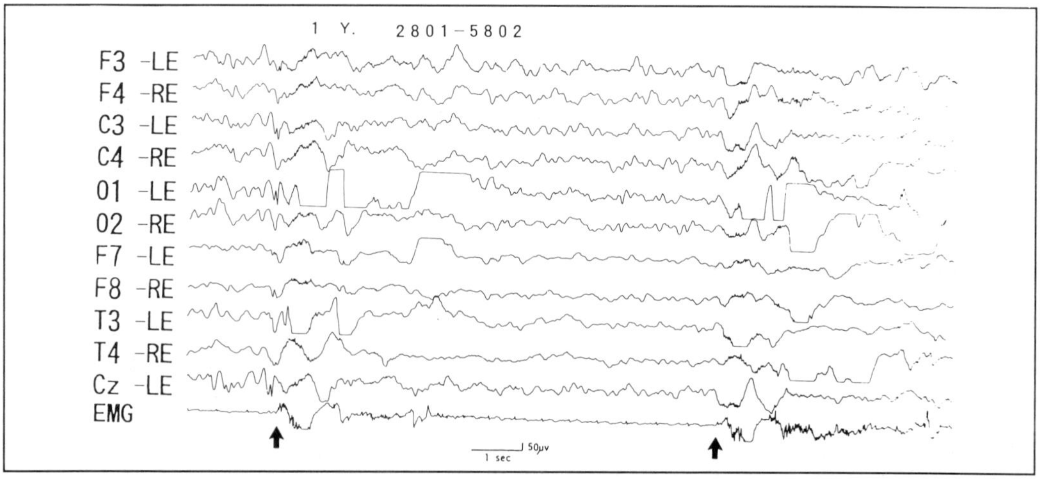

Fig. 2 (a). Ictal EEG from patient 1. At age 16 months an electrodecrementation coincides with each spasm. Arrows indicate the onset of epileptic spasms.

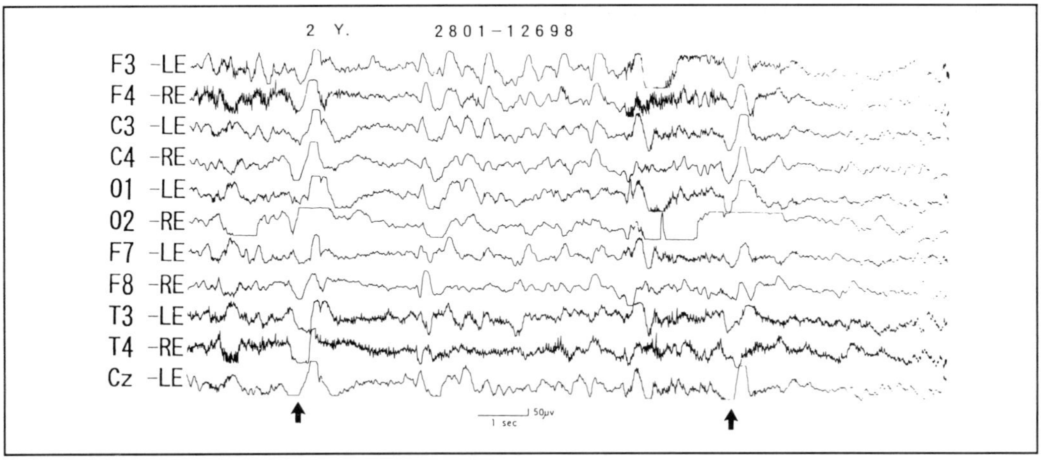

Fig. 2(b). Ictal EEG from patient 1. At age 2 years an overall electrodecrementation is associated with each spasm. High-voltage baseline deflection is probably a movement artefact. Arrows indicate the onset of epileptic spasms.

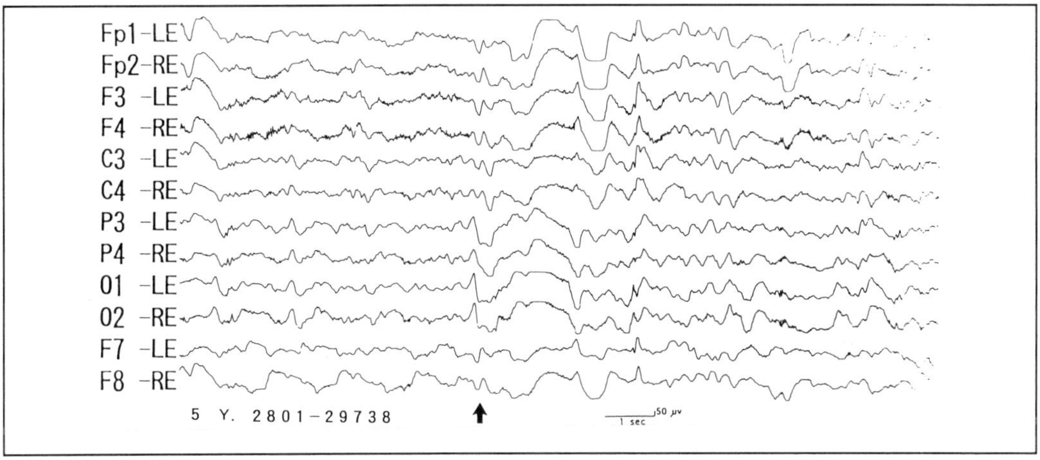

Fig. 2 (c). Ictal EEG from patient one. At age 1 years a run of slow waves occurs predominantly on the posterior head followed by overall flattening. Arrows indicate the onset of epileptic spasms.

and abrupt shrugging of the shoulders; abduction of both arms occurred without apparent hypertonicity at the distal ends of the arms. He was brought to our hospital at age 9 months. Adrenocorticotropic hormone therapy was tried several times, but was only transiently effective. A computed tomographic scan of the head showed only mild cortical atrophy.

An interictal EEG at age 9 months showed paroxysmal waves resembling hypsarrhythmia (Fig. 7). Ictal EEGs at age 10 months and at ages 2 and 7 years demonstrated generalized flattening of the background activity associated with the spasm (Fig. 8a–c). The spasms persisted until the age of 11 years. Besides the spasms, generalized tonic seizures were observed, mainly during sleep, from age 3 years (Fig. 9). An interictal EEG at age 10 years showed bisynchronous and diffuse irregular sharp and slow waves (Fig. 10). A generalized tonic seizure during waking also occurred with an abrupt increase of tonicity of the extremities lasting for a few seconds (Fig. 11). We could not recognize any clinical or EEG changes in the seizures between age 10 months and age 7 years (Fig. 12).

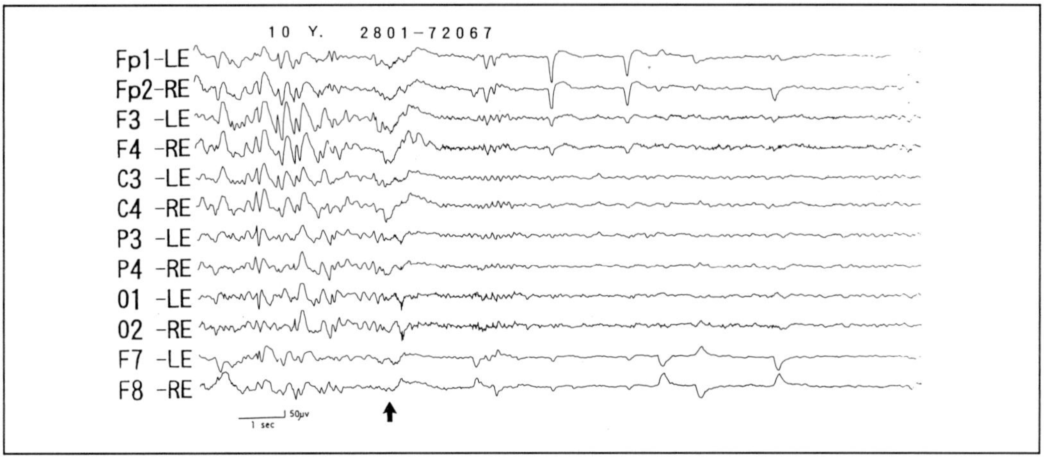

Fig. 2 (d). Ictal EEG from patient 1. At age 10 years an overall electrodecrementation is followed by a short run of alpha-like rhythm. Arrows indicate the onset of epileptic spasms.

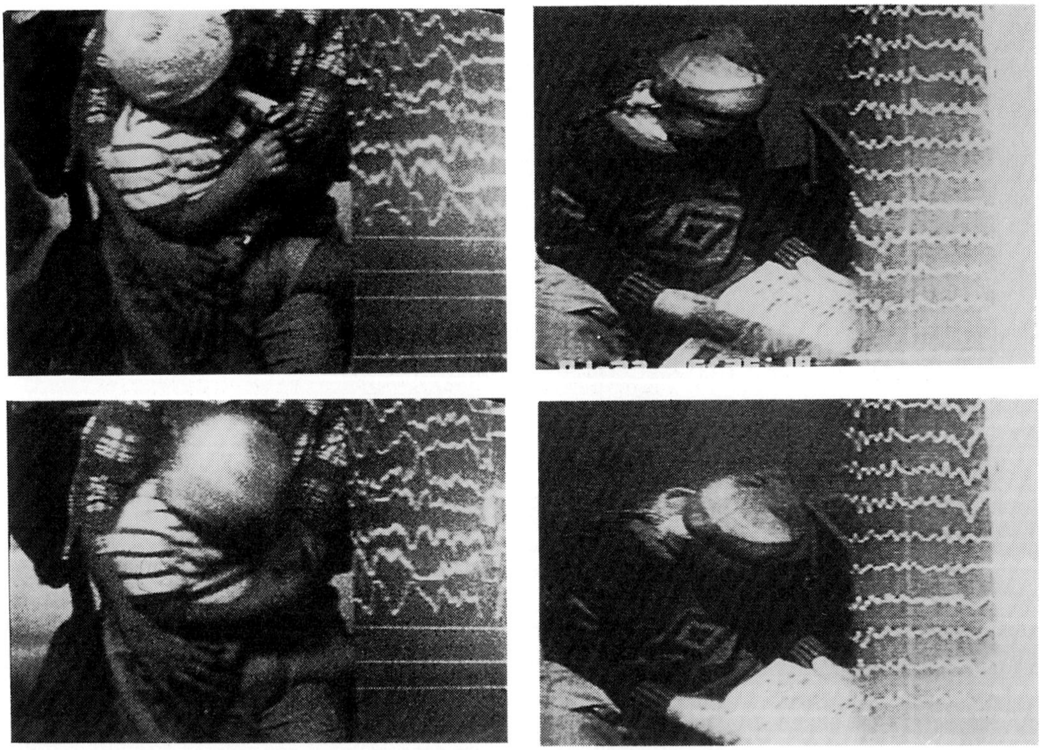

Fig. 3. Simultaneously recorded seizures and EEGs from patient 1. When sitting, at age 2 years, he nodded forward repeatedly, and abrupt shrugging of the shoulders and abduction of both arms occurred. With more intense seizures, he bent his head forward and downward, striking the table (left). While handling a book in a sitting position, at age 10 years, he flexed his head abruptly forward and downward with shrugging of the shoulders (right). There was no definite hypertonicity of the distal ends of the arms at either age. The seizures were prone to repeat on awakening.

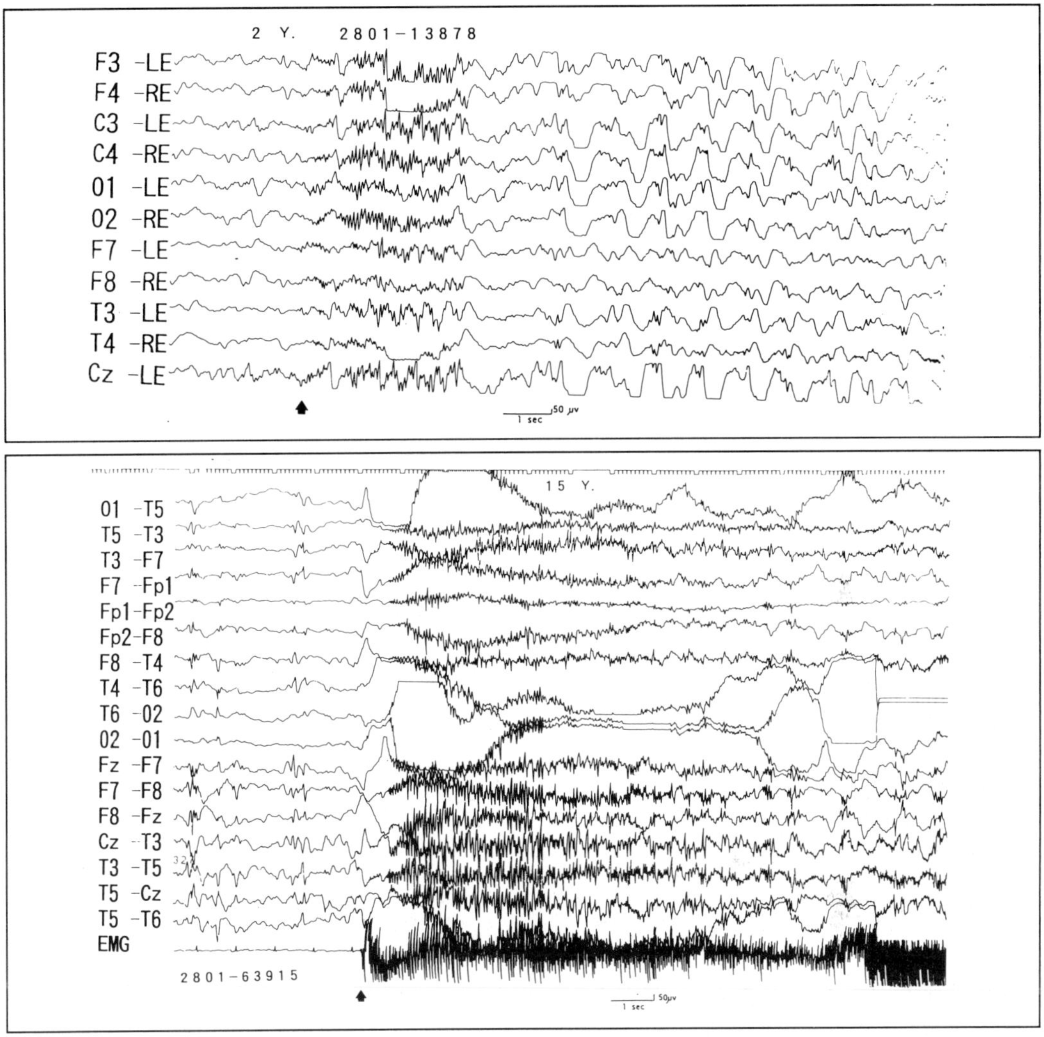

Fig. 4. Ictal EEGs from patient 1. At age 2 years and 9 months, during an axial tonic seizure, a change of respiration rate and eye opening were associated with bisynchronous but asymmetrical and diffuse fast rhythm lasting for several seconds (a, above). At age 15 years, a generalized axorhizomelic tonic seizure accompanied a burst of bisynchronous, nearly symmetrical fast rhythm (b, below). Arrows indicate the onset of generalized tonic seizures.

Discussion

The case histories of two patients describe the longitudinal evolution of ictal EEGs and clinical seizures characterized by head nods or epileptic spasms. The spasms, which have persisted for the past 15 years in one patient and 11 years in the other one, were the initial seizure manifestation. Apart from the head nods or spasms, both patients developed generalized tonic seizures of varying severity. In both cross-sectional and longitudinal observations, the spasms were not regarded as a partial sign of the tonic seizures.

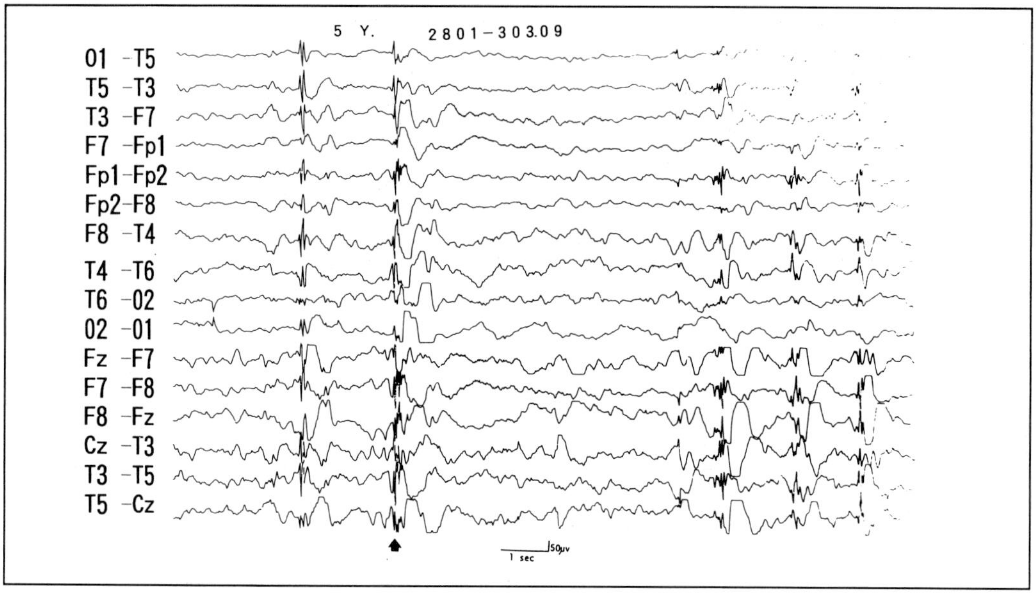

Fig. 5. Ictal EEG from patient 1 at age 5 years. Myoclonic jerks coincide with bisynchronous but diffuse polyspikes and waves. Arrow indicates the onset of myoclonic seizure.

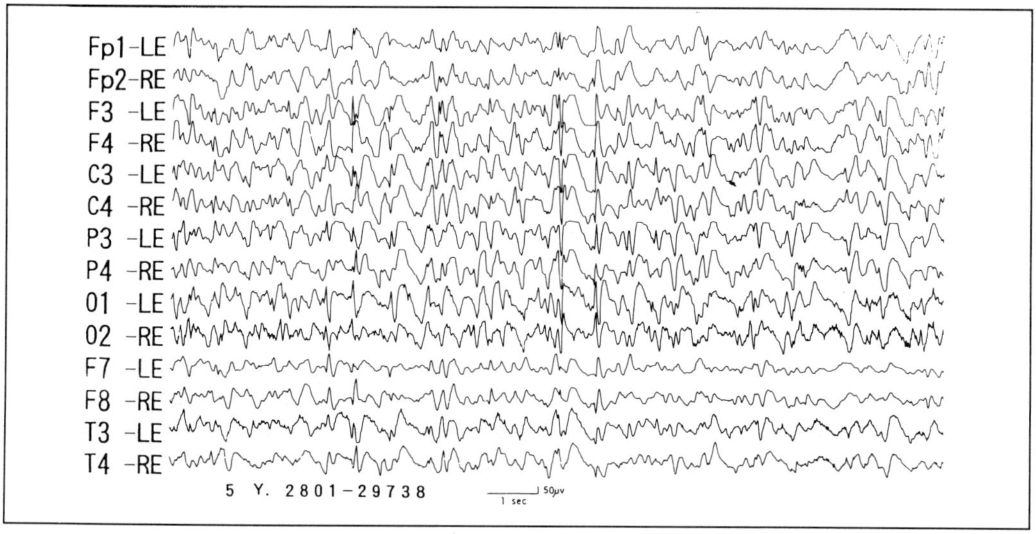

Fig. 6. Ictal EEG from patient 1 at age 5 years during atypical absence-like episodes. Bilateral and diffuse, very irregular, high-voltage slow-wave activity is often intermingled with bisynchronous but asymmetrical spikes or sharp waves.

Both patients, as they grew up, fulfilled the diagnostic criteria of Lennox–Gastaut syndrome, especially in terms of EEG and clinical seizure types. There are many reports on the possible evolution of West syndrome to Lennox–Gastaut syndrome, in individual patients (Gastaut *et al.*, 1966; Lombroso, 1983). Patients with Lennox–Gastaut syndrome may have seizures mimicking infantile spasms with similar EEGs (Shigematsu *et al.*, 1987; Donat & Wright, 1991). The difference between

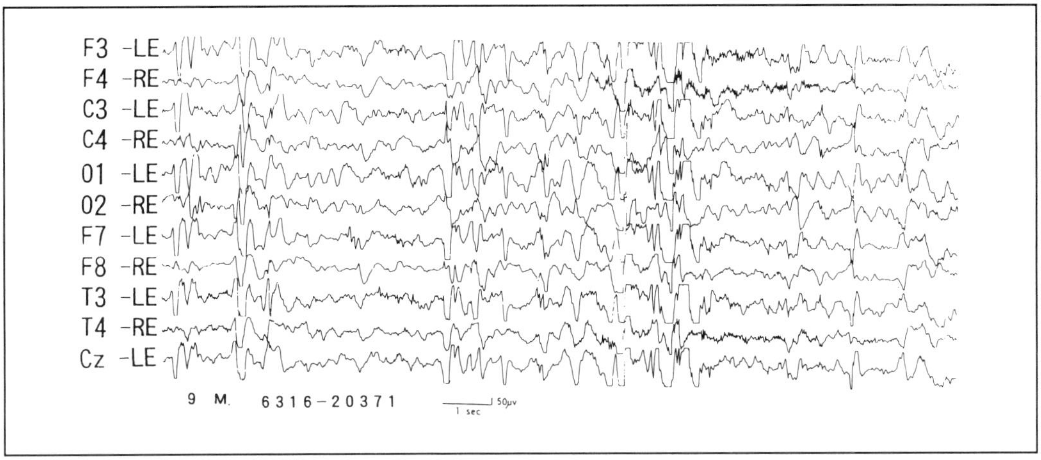

Fig. 7. Interictal EEG during waking from patient 2 at age 9 months. A burst of bilateral but asymmetrical, diffuse high-voltage slow-wave activity is intermingled with asynchronous spikes or sharp waves.

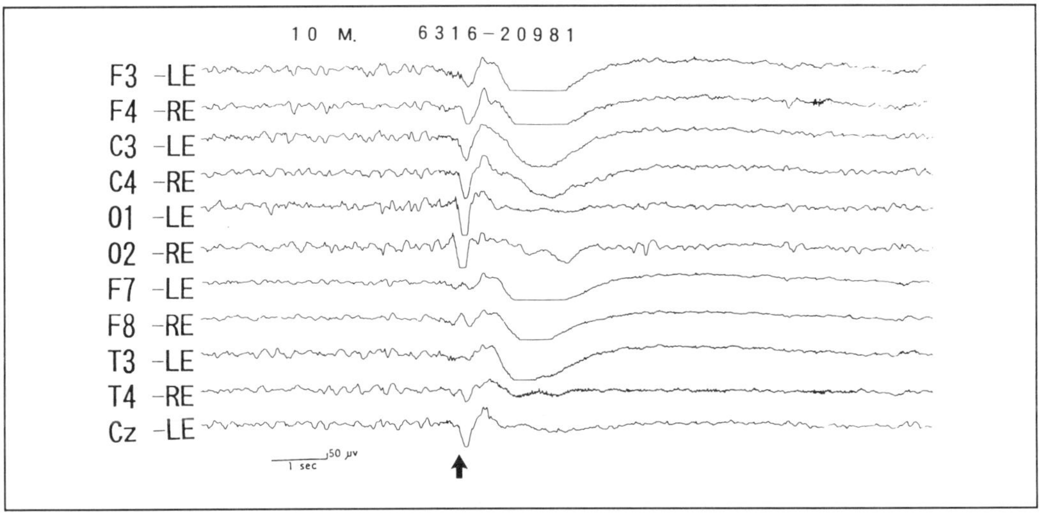

Fig. 8. (a) Ictal EEG from patient 2. At age 10 months, generalized flattening of the background activity is associated with the spasm. Arrows indicate the onset of epileptic spasms.

late West syndrome and the atypical form of early Lennox–Gastaut syndrome is controversial (Gastaut, 1982), but it is generally agreed that West syndrome is an age-dependent epileptic encephalopathy with the triad of infantile spasms, hypsarrhythmia and mental retardation. At least at their onset, the clinical features of our patients agreed with the diagnostic criteria of West syndrome. However, while infantile spasms never persist until 5 years of age, according to Jeavons (1985), it is obvious that, here, the spasms continued until the second decade of life. Therefore, it is likely that they did not have West syndrome but, rather, Lennox–Gastaut syndrome from the onset. Recognition of the longitudinal outcome, instead of cross-sectional observation, is particularly important in West syndrome, as is true in other infantile epileptic syndromes. It is usually, though not alway, necessary to follow up the electroclinical seizure events for at least 5 years.

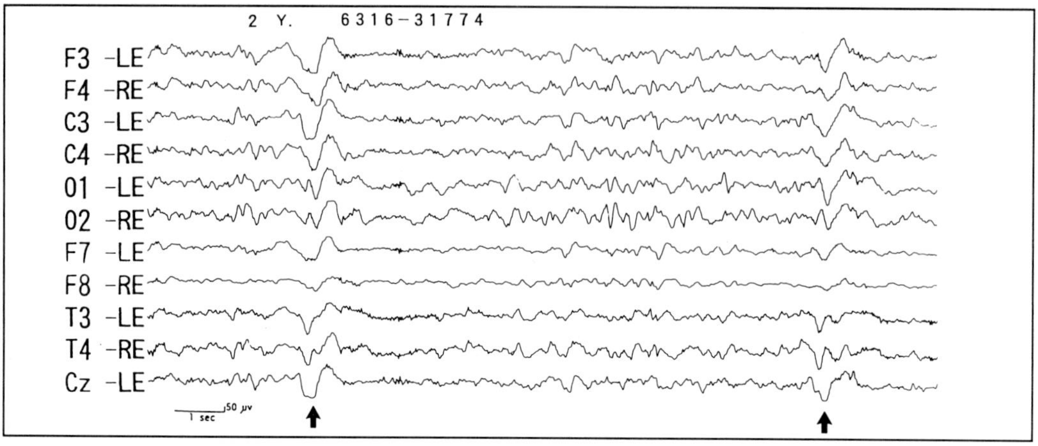

Fig. 8. (b) Ictal EEG from patient 2. At age 2 years, an overall amplitude decrement is intermixed with low-voltage fast activity at the time of the spasm. Baseline deflection is probably a movement artefact. Arrows indicate the onset of epileptic spasms.

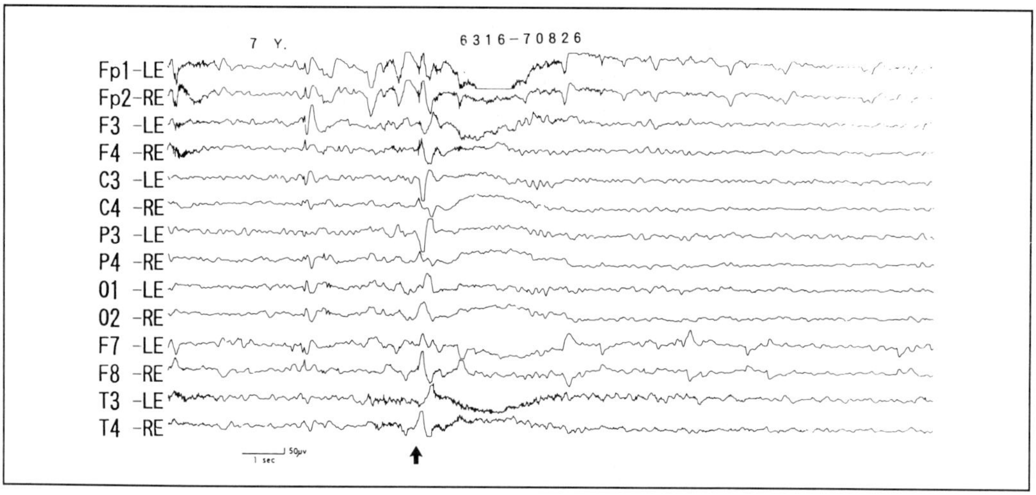

Fig. 8. (c) Ictal EEG from patient 2. At age 7 years, the EEG consists of overall flattening and movement artefact. Arrows indicate the onset of epileptic spasms.

We might question whether or not the head nods or spasms are a part of the mild tonic seizures. Gobbi *et al.* (1987) reported that periodic spasms were an unusual form of epileptic seizure, but our patients did not demonstrate a common set of clinical and EEG focal signs. Gastaut *et al.* (1963) reported that infantile spasms evolved to tonic seizures, but the interictal and ictal EEGs of our patients clearly showed that generalized tonic seizures of varying degrees existed independently of the seizures characterized by head nods or spasms. Thus, the spasms seem to form their own taxonomic group among the category of generalized seizures. We might also ask whether or not the head nods or spasms are of an epileptic nature (Lombroso & Fejerman, 1977; Dravet *et al.*, 1986; Brunquell *et al.*, 1990). In our patients, the majority of the ictal EEGs showed either flattening of the background activity or electrodecrementation from the onset of seizures in infancy to the present time of adolescence. We

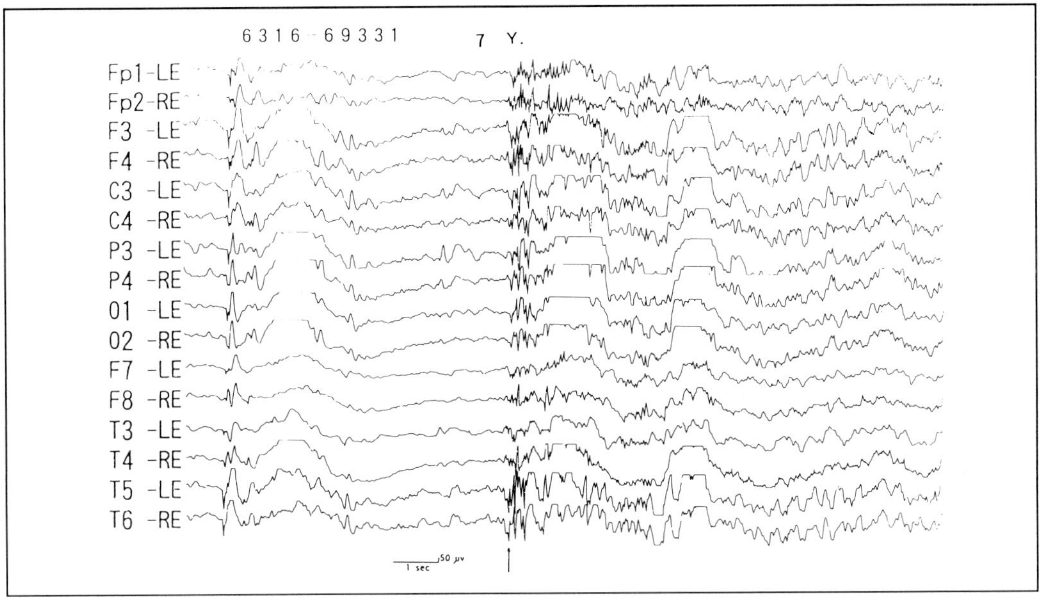

Fig. 9. Ictal EEG from patient 2 at age 7 years during a generalized tonic state first observed during sleep at age 3 years. Eye opening and increased tonicity of the arms coincided with bisynchronous diffuse spikes. Arrow indicates the onset of a generalized tonic seizure.

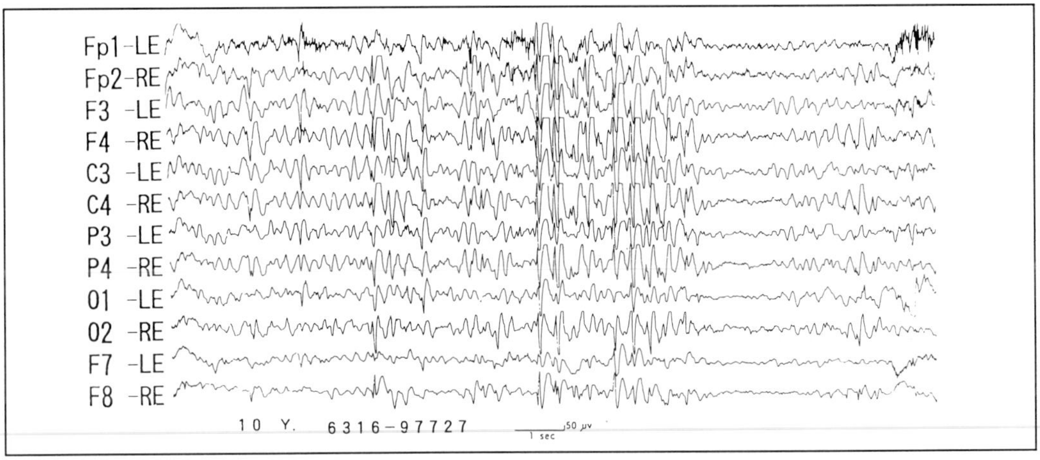

Fig. 10. Interictal EEG during waking from patient 2 at age 10 years. Bisynchronous but asymmetrical, diffuse high-voltage slow-wave activity often occurs with intense synchronization.

therefore conclude that the head nods or spasms are of an epileptic nature. Further, and more importantly, the patients drop or fall suddenly to the ground when the spasms are intense enough. In addition, the spasms are occasionally followed by atypical absence-like episodes or obtundation of consciousness accompanied by a burst of bisynchronous slow spikes and waves.

In fact, what we called infantile spasms has persisted until adolescence in both of our patients. Therefore, we prefer the term 'epileptic spasm' to infantile spasms, which will be proposed in 1993

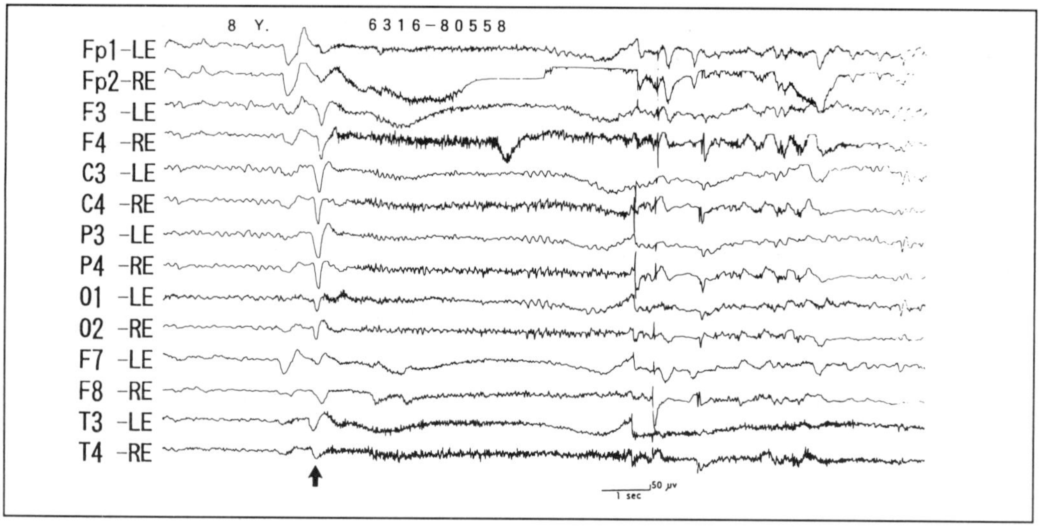

Fig. 11. An ictal EEG from patient 2 at age 8 years. A generalized tonic seizure observed during waking is associated with bisynchronous but apparently asymmetrical fast waves. Arrow indicates the onset of a generalized tonic seizure.

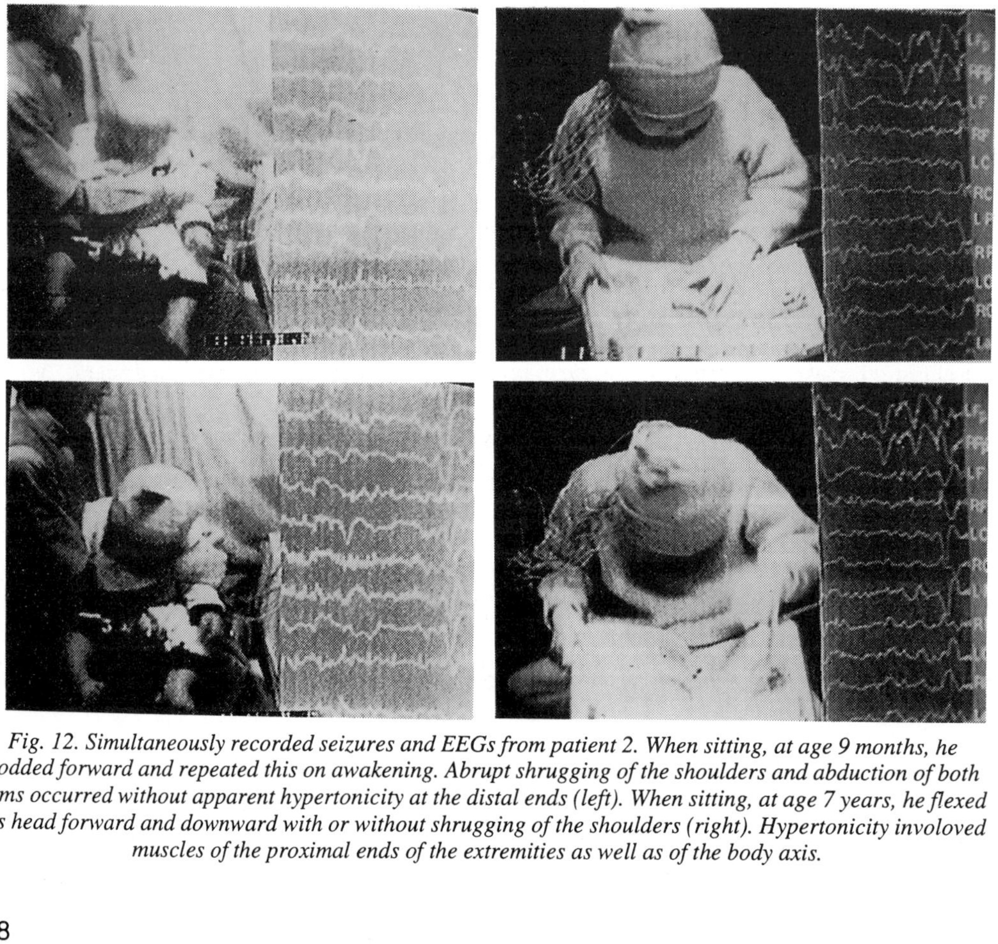

Fig. 12. Simultaneously recorded seizures and EEGs from patient 2. When sitting, at age 9 months, he nodded forward and repeated this on awakening. Abrupt shrugging of the shoulders and abduction of both arms occurred without apparent hypertonicity at the distal ends (left). When sitting, at age 7 years, he flexed his head forward and downward with or without shrugging of the shoulders (right). Hypertonicity involoved muscles of the proximal ends of the extremities as well as of the body axis.

by the Commission on Classification of the International League Against Epilepsy. Epileptic spasms thus defined are not necessarily age-dependent and may persist until the second decade of life.

References

Ajmone-Marsan, C. & Ralston, B.L. (1957): *The epileptic seizure, its functional morphology and diagnostic significance,* pp. 1–251. Springfield, Ill.: Thomas.

Bancaud, J. & Talairach, J. (1992): Clinical semiology of frontal lobe seizures. In: *Frontal lobe seizures and epilepsies (Advances in neurology,* Vol. 57), eds. P. Chauvel, A.V. Delgado-Escueta, E. Halgren & J. Bancaud, pp. 3–58. New York: Raven Press.

Brunquell, P., Keever, M.M. & Russman, B.S. (1990): Differentiation of epileptic from nonepileptic head drops in children. *Epilepsia* **31,** 401–405.

Chauvel, P., Delgado-Escueta, A.V., Halgren, E. & Bancaud, J. (eds.) (1992):*Frontal lobe seizures and epilepsies (Advances in neurology,* Vol. 57). New York: Raven Press.

Commission on Classification and Terminology of the International League Against Epilepsy (1981): Proposal for revised clinical and electroencephalographic classification of epileptic seizures. *Epilepsia* **22,** 489–501.

Commission on Classification and Terminology of the International League Against Epilepsy (1989): Proposal for revised classification of epilepsies and epileptic syndromes. *Epilepsia* **30,** 389–399.

Donat, J.F. & Wright, F.S. (1991): Seizures in series: similarities between seizures of the West and Lennox–Gastaut syndromes. *Epilepsia* **32,** 504–509.

Dravet, C., Giraud, N., Bureau, M. & Roger, J. (1986): Benign myoclonus of early infancy or benign non-epileptic infantile spasms. *Neuropediatrics* **17,** 33–38.

Engel, J., Jr (1993): Recent advances in surgical treatment of temporal lobe epilepsy. In: *Future research in epileptology,* eds J. Overweg, A.P. Aldenkamp & H.M. de Boer. *Acta Neurol. Scand.* **86** (Suppl. 140), 71–80.

Gastaut, H. (1982): 'Benign' or 'functional' (versus 'organic') epilepsies in different stages of life: an analysis of the corresponding age-related variations in the predisposition to epilepsy. In: *Henri Gastaut and the Marseilles school's contribution to the neurosciences,* ed. R.J. Broughton, pp. 17–44. Amsterdam: Elsevier.

Gastaut, H., Roger, J., Ouahchi, S., Timsit, M. & Broughton, R. (1963): An electro-clinical study of generalized epileptic seizures of tonic expression. *Epilepsia* **4,** 15–44.

Gastaut, H., Roger, J., Soulayrol, R., Tassinari, C.A., Régis, H. & Dravet, C. (1966): Childhood epileptic encephalopathy with diffuse slow spike-waves (otherwise known as 'petit mal variant') or Lennox syndrome. *Epilepsia* **7,** 139–179.

Genton, P. (1993): Relationship between idopathic generalized and idiopathic partial epilepsies. International workshop, idiopathic generalized epilepsies: clinical, experimental and genetic aspects. Abstract Part 1.

Gobbi, G., Bruno, L., Pini, A., Rossi, P.A. & Tassinari, C.A. (1987): Periodic spasms: an unclassified type of epileptic seizure in childhood. *Dev. Med. Child Neurol.* **29,** 766–775.

Ikeno, T., Shigematsu, H., Miyakoshi, M., Ohba, A., Yagi, K. & Seino, M. (1985): An analytic study of epileptic falls. *Epilepsia* **26,** 612–621.

Jeavons, P.M. (1985): West syndrome: infantile spasms. In: *Epileptic syndromes in infancy, childhood and adolescence,* eds. J. Roger, C. Dravet, M. Bureau, F.E. Dreifuss & P. Wolf, pp. 42–50. London: John Libbey.

Jeavons, P.M. & Livet, M.O. (1992): West syndrome: infantile spasms. In: *Epileptic syndromes in infancy, childhood and adolescence,* 2nd edn, eds. J. Roger, M. Bureau, Ch. Dravet, F.E. Dreifuss, A. Perret & P. Wolf, pp. 53–66. London: John Libbey.

Lombroso, C.T. (1983): A prospective study of infantile spasms: clinical and therapeutic correlations. *Epilepsia* **24,** 135–158.

Lombroso, C.T. & Fejerman, N. (1977): Benign myoclonus of early infancy. *Ann. Neurol.* **1,** 138–143.

Mattson, R.H. (1986): Intensive neurodiagnostic monitoring: strategy for optimal use. In: *Intensive neurodiagnostic monitoring (Advances in neurology,* Vol. 46), ed. R.J. Gumnit, pp. 281–290. New York: Raven Press.

Ohtahara, S., Ohtsuka, Y., Yamatogi, Y., Oka, E. & Inoue, H. (1992): Early-infantile epileptic encephalopathy with suppression- bursts. In: *Epileptic syndromes in infancy, childhood and adolescence*, 2nd edn, eds. J. Roger, M. Bureau, Ch. Dravet, F.E. Dreifuss, A. Perret & P. Wolf, pp. 25–34. London: John Libbey.

Penfield, W. & Jasper, H. (1954): *Epilepsy and the functional anatomy of the human brain.* Boston: Little, Brown.

Shigematsu, H., Yagi, K. & Seino, M. (1987): A peculiar minor seizure characterized by flexor spasms in Lennox–Gastaut syndrome evolved from West syndrome. *Japan. J. Psychiatry Neurol.* **41,** 457–458.

Williamson, P.D., Spencer, D.D., Spencer, S.S., Novelly, R.A. & Mattson, R.H. (1985): Complex partial seizures of frontal lobe origin. *Ann. Neurol.* **18,** 497–504.

Wolf, P. (1992): Juvenile myoclonic epilepsy. In: *Epileptic syndromes in infancy, childhood and adolescence*, 2nd edn, eds. J. Roger, M. Bureau, Ch. Dravet, F.E. Dreifuss, A. Perret & P. Wolf, pp. 313–328. London: John Libbey.

Epileptic Seizures and Syndromes, Edited by Peter Wolf
© 1994 John Libbey & Company Ltd., pp. 431–448

Chapter 46

Adaptive changes of epileptic human temporal lobe tissue: properties of neurones and glia

Nihal C. de Lanerolle, Subu N. Magge, Matthew F. Philips, Paul Trombley, Dennis D. Spencer and Michael Brines*

*Section of Neurosurgery and *Neuroendocrinology Program, Yale University School of Medicine, 333 Cedar Street, New Haven, Connecticut 06510, USA*

Summary

Temporal lobe epilepsy (TLE) is an important seizure syndrome that has been well studied. A significant proportion of patients with TLE are medically intractable and treated surgically for seizure control. Temporal lobe tissue (including the hippocampus) removed from such patients has been examined by a variety of neurobiological techniques, and shows that, in hippocampi which are seizure foci, along with principal cell loss there is also selective loss of hilar interneurones containing somatostatin, neuropeptide Y and substance P. Additionally, there is evidence of 'sprouting' of neural systems containing dynorphin, somatostatin, neuropeptide Y and substance P, and reorganization in the distribution of several neurotransmitter receptor systems and the sodium pump.

Primary cell cultures established from neocortical seizure foci show that glial cells (astrocytes) at these foci show many adaptive changes, which include differences in the proportions of flat and fibrous astrocytes, the release and uptake of glutamate by these astrocytes, their calcium responses and electrophysiology. These studies on resected human tissue reflect upon the subclassification of temporal lobe seizure syndromes.

Introduction

The manifestation of various types of seizures and seizure syndromes is usually the result of an underlying epileptogenic neural substrate. The definition of these neural substrates may provide additional means for more precisely classifying seizures and seizure syndromes. Temporal lobe epilepsy (TLE) is an important seizure syndrome that has been much studied (Wieser *et al.*, 1993). A significant proportion of patients with TLE are medically intractable and treated surgically for seizure control (Spencer & Spencer, 1991). The neural tissue removed through surgery from patients with TLE has been examined by a number of neurobiological techniques to define its properties and the adaptive changes that the central nervous system (CNS) has undergone. In this chapter, we will review such studies that we have carried out on a population of about 100 patients. We hope to show that such studies provide additional insight into the nature of temporal lobe seizure syndromes.

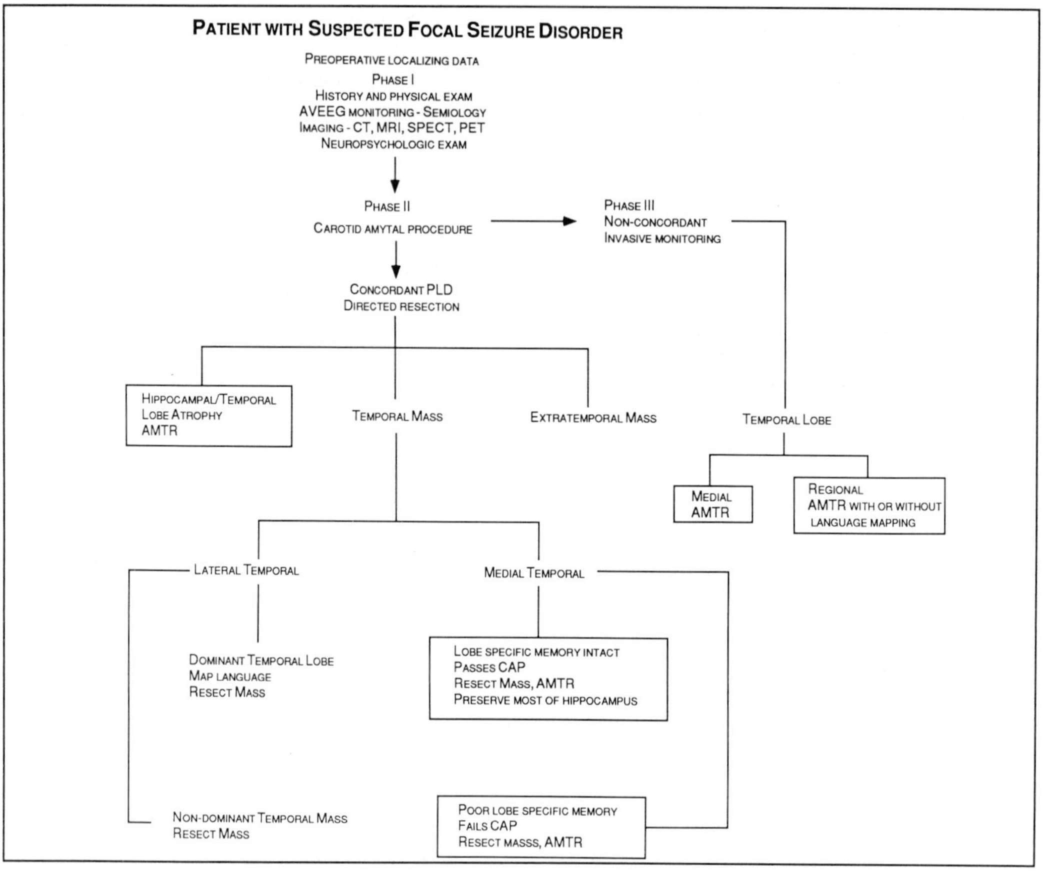

Fig. 1. A decision tree (courtesy of Dr Dennis Spencer) showing the phased evaluation of patients that results in neurosurgery. This tree lists the preoperative localizing data (PLD) necessary to offer a patient a specific form of temporal lobe resection either without (concordant) or with (non-concordant) invasive electrode monitoring. Points in the tree that are boxed represent surgical procedures from which hippocampal tissue was obtained for the studies reported in this chapter. Abbreviations: AMTR, anteromedial temporal lobectomy with appropriate amounts of hippocampectomy; AVEEG, audiovisual EEG; CAP, carotid amytal procedure; CT, computerized tomography; MRI, magnetic resonance imaging; SPECT, single-photon emission computerized tomography; PET, positron emission tomography.

Tissue selection for study

The decision tree adopted at the Yale–West Haven Veterans Administration Epilepsy Program for the phased evaluation of patients with intractable TLE is shown in Fig. 1. This table shows the situations in which neural tissue is removed in the surgical treatment of epilepsy. All patients undergo a preoperative phase I evaluation (Fig. 1). They then undergo the carotid amytal procedure (Wada test) in phase II. If the results of these procedures are concordant in localizing the seizure focus, the patients undergo directed resection. In such directed resections, hippocampal tissue is removed in three circumstances: (1) as a result of anteromedial temporal lobe resection (AMTR) with hippocampectomy in patients with hippocampal/temporal lobe atrophy; (2) as a result of AMTR with hippocampectomy in patients with a medial temporal lobe mass (also resected) and poor temporal lobe-specific memory; (3) as a result of AMTR with partial hippocampectomy in patients with a medial temporal lobe mass (also resected) and intact lobe-specific memory. If the preoperative localizing data are non-concordant, patients are studied with depth electrode monitoring, and if a hippocampal seizure focus is detected, they subsequently undergo AMTR with hippocampectomy (Fig. 1). The hippocampal tissue obtained through the above four procedures was studied by a variety of neuroanatomical procedures – cell counts, immunohistochemical localization of neuroactive substances, receptor autoradiography and electron microscopy. These studies will be discussed below to demonstrate the adaptive changes observed in *neurones* and *neural systems* in patients with TLE.

Neural tissue resected from patients with neocortical masses (low-grade gliomas) were used to make primary tissue cultures of glia. In the removal of such neocortical seizure foci, the tissue was divided into three regions based on intraoperative electrocorticographic recordings – (1) the lesion itself, (2) adjacent hyperexcitable cortex, and (3) a zone of normal cortex to ensure tumour-free margins. The three zones were cultured separately. Glial cells in primary culture from these tissues were used to study their properties. These studies will be discussed below to demonstrate the adaptive changes observed in glia in patients with intractable epilepsy.

Adaptive changes in neuronal systems – hippocampus

Much of our work on hippocampal tissue removed from patients with medically intractable TLE has been described in previous reviews (de Lanerolle *et al.*, 1992a, b). Therefore, in this chapter we will only summarize this work in order to examine its relevance to understanding seizure syndromes.

Our studies have revealed several forms of reorganization in the hippocampus of patients with TLE. These changes fall into several categories: (1) loss of principal neurones – granule cells and pyramidal neurones; (2) selective loss of hilar (CA4) interneurones; (3) change in chemical phenotype of neurons; (4) neuronal plasticity as evidenced by 'sprouting' of chemically defined neurones, and redistribution of neurotransmitter receptors; (5) increase in levels of second-messenger systems and sodium pump.

Loss of principal neurones

Neuronal cell counts (Kim *et al.*, 1990) in the subfields of the hippocampi removed from patients and compared with counts from autopsy samples from neurologically normal subjects revealed three patterns of cell loss. In a majority (85 per cent) of patients in whom the hippocampus was shown to be atrophied on imaging and evaluated to be the focus of seizure initiation, there is significant (> 50 per cent) loss of dentate granule cells and pyramidal cells in most areas of Ammon's horn (CA fields). Along with these general trends in neuronal loss, there is also individual variability. This variability is expressed in the dentate by cases with little granule cell loss, to cases in which the granule cell layer is reduced to almost a single layer of cells (de Lanerolle *et al.*, 1992b). In area CA1 the pattern of cell loss can vary from a small focal loss of cells in the proximal region of CA1, to cases with extensive loss of neurones throughout CA1. This group of patients has traditionally been described as having hippocampal sclerosis and referred to in our publications as cryptogenic temporal lobe epilepsy (CTLE) patients.

Within the category of patients from among whom the above group was identified is another group of patients (about 15 per cent) where neuronal loss was much less significant, being reduced by about 25 per cent in the dentate gyrus and all CA fields. Visual inspection alone of Nissl-stained sections of the hippocampus of these patients does not reveal this small degree of neuronal loss. These hippocampi do not show the neurochemical reorganization observed in the other members of the CTLE group. This group of patients has been referred to by us as atypical CTLE patients.

The hippocampi removed from patients along with a temporal lobe mass also show a small (25 per cent) reduction in neuronal numbers in all hippocampal fields. These hippocampi also do not show the neurochemical reorganization seen in the dentate and hilus of CTLE patients. This group of patients is referred to in our publications as tumour-related temporal lobe epilepsy (TTLE) patients.

Neurone counts in the subiculum in all three groups showed no significant cell loss compared with autopsy controls.

Selective loss of hilar (CA4) interneurones

The hilus of the normal human hippocampus contains a variety of neuronal types. These include pyramidal cells, mossy cells, large aspinous and sparsely spinous cells (Seress & Mrzljak, 1992) and a variety of interneurones. The interneurones form a band of cells in the subgranular zone of the hilus, referred to as the polymorphic zone, as well as scattered in the deeper parts of the hilus. Immunohistochemical staining of hippocampi from TTLE and atypical CTLE patients revealed that these

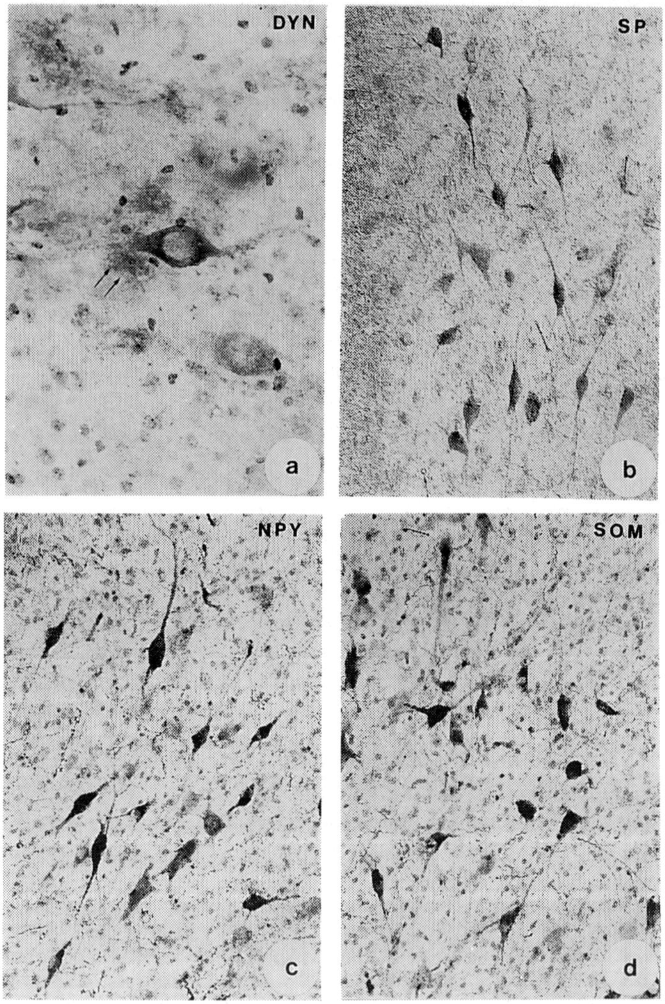

Fig. 2. Photomicrographs of peptidergic neurones in the dentate hilus localized by immunocytochemistry. (a) A dynorphin (DYN) immunoreactive neurone in the hilus of a CTLE hippocampus. Arrows indicate DYN immunoreactive mossy fibre endings on proximal dendrite excrescences of the labelled cell, suggesting that this neurone may be a mossy cell. (b) Substance P- (SP) immunoreactive neurones in the subgranular polymorphic zone of the hilus of a TTLE hippocampus. (c) Neuropeptide Y- (NPY) immunoreactive neurones in the subgranular polymorphic zone of the hilus of a TTLE hippocampus. (d) Somatostatin- (SOM) immunoreactive neurones in the subgranular polymorphic zone of the hilus of a TTLE hippocampus.

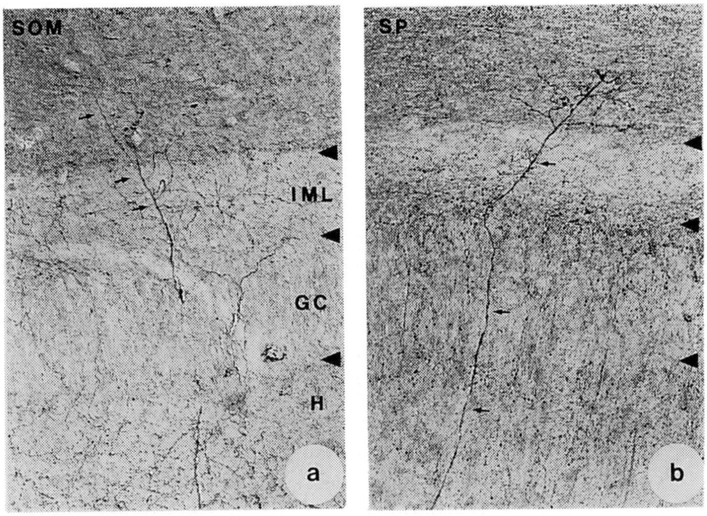

Fig. 3 (a). A photomicrograph of the dentate gyrus of a TTLE hippocampus showing somatostatin- (SOM) like immunoreactive profiles. Arrows point out an immunoreactive dendrite of a hilar SOM neurone that passes through the granule cell layer and inner molecular layer and into the middle molecular layer. (b) Substance P- (SP) like-immunoreactive elements in the dentate gyrus of a TTLE hippocampus. Arrows point to an SP-immunoreactive dendrite that passes from the hilus into the middle molecular layer. The dendrite gives off several branches in the IML and the middle ML. Abbreviations: GC, granule cell layer; H, hilus; IML, inner molecular layer. The arrow heads indicate the boundaries between H, GC and IML.

interneurones contain a variety of neuropeptides, which include neuropeptide Y (NPY), somatostatin (SOM) and substance P (SP) (Fig. 2) (de Lanerolle *et al.*, 1992a, b). The pattern of staining in these groups is the same as in hippocampi of neurologically normal autopsy specimens. Some of the SOM and SP neurones in the subgranular zone have dendrites that extend through the dentate granule cell layer into the molecular layer (ML), in addition to extending in the hilus (Fig. 3). In comparison with the above two patient groups, the hilus of the CTLE group shows a significant loss of SOM-, NPY- and SP-immunoreactive neurones, particularly in the subgranular polymorphic zone. The loss of these neurones may be detectable, occasionally, even in the relative absence of principal cell (granule and pyramidal) loss (e.g. patient IH139, KA).

In some animal models of epilepsy (Sloviter, 1987) an additional population of large hilar interneurones referred to as mossy cells, are also reported to be lost. In the rodent, the mossy cells are a very abundant cell type in the hilus. They are large and have prominent excrescences on their proximal dendrites, on which mossy fibre terminals from granule cells synapse. In the human, mossy cells are not an abundant cell type in the hilus, nor are they the largest neurones (Seress & Mrzljak, 1992). It is not clear yet if this subpopulation is selectively lost in the CTLE hilus, even though this has been suggested (Babb *et al.*, 1989). Clearly in CTLE cases where there is extensive hilar neurone loss, mossy cells would be among the neurones lost. As best as we can determine, the interneurones immunoreactive for SOM, NPY and SP do not appear to possess an essential phenotype of mossy cells, i.e. proximal dendrite excrescences (Fig. 2). In the section below we report that at least some mossy cells are preserved in CTLE hippocampi.

Change in chemical phenotype of neurones

In animal models, hippocampal neurones express new neuroactive substances after seizures. In rats induced to seizure by kainic acid (KA) treatment, the dentate granule cells express NPY, a protein

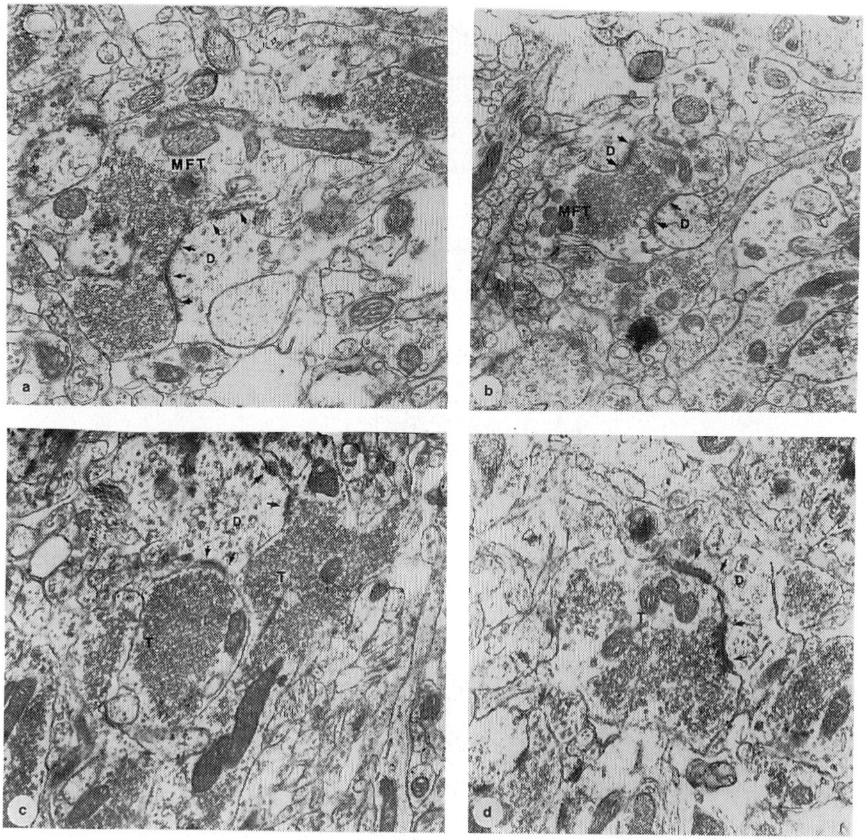

Fig. 4 (a) and (b). Electron micrographs of mossy fibre terminals (MFT) forming asymmetrical synapses on dendrites (D) in the dentate hilus of a TTLE hippocampus. The mossy fibre terminals are characterized by their large size and densely packed vesicles. (c) and (d) are electron micrographs of terminals closely resembling those in (a) and (b) and thus presumptive MFTs but found in the inner molecular layer of a CTLE hippocampus. Such terminals are not seen in the inner molecular layer of TTLE.

not normally expressed by them. In the hippocampi of human TLE patients, NPY expression in granule cells is not observed. However, in many CTLE patients, there are surviving neurones in the hilus that atypically express the opioid peptide dynorphin (DYN) (Fig. 2a). At least a subpopulation of these DYN-immunoreactive neurones may be inferred to be mossy cells, as immunoreactive clumps resembling the excrescences on mossy cells can be seen associated with the proximal dendrites of these DYN-immunoreactive neurones (see de Lanerolle *et al.*, 1992a, Fig. 3f). Such DYN-immunoreactive hilar neurones are not found in the TTLE or atypical CTLE hippocampi. Neurones resembling large aspinous hilar neurones are reported to be immunoreactive for tyrosine hydroxylase in TLE patients with sclerosis, and not found in normal hippocampi (Zhu *et al.*, 1990). The functional significance of these abnormal expression patterns of neuroactive substances in hilar neurones remains to be elucidated.

Evidence of neuronal plasticity

Sprouting

Regrowth and modification of neurons surviving brain injury is a well-established observation. The hippocampus of animal models of epilepsy (Cronin & Dudek, 1988; Sutula *et al.*, 1989) and

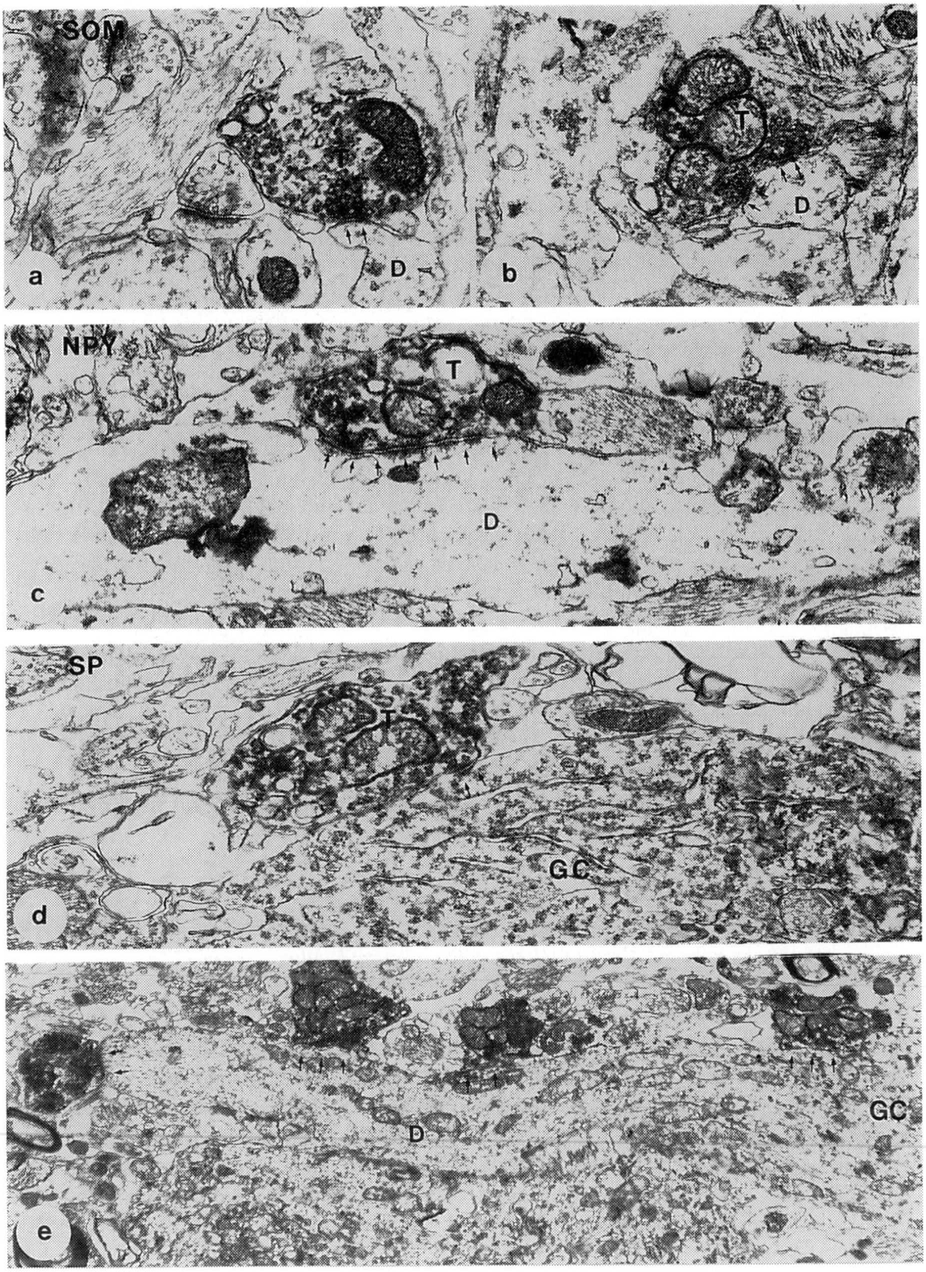

Fig. 5(a). Electron micrograph of a somatostatin-immunoreactive (SOM) terminal forming a synapse on a dendritic spine in the outer molecular layer of a TTLE hippocampus. (b) SOM-immunoreactive terminal forming a synapse on a dendrite in the inner molecular layer of a CTLE hippocampus. (c) A neuropeptide Y-immunoreactive (NPY) terminal forming an asymmetrical synapse in the proximal part of the apical dendrite of a dentate granule cell in the inner molecular layer of a CTLE hippocampus. (d) Electron micrograph of a substance P- immunoreactive (SP) terminal forming a synapse (arrows) on a granule cell soma in a CTLE hippocampus. (e) Large SP-immunoreactive terminals forming synapses (arrows) along the length of the proximal part of a granule cell apical dendrite in a CTLE hippocampus.

hippocampi after lesions of afferents to it (Tauck & Nadler, 1985) are reported to show this phenomenon. Evidence of 'sprouting' or new growth of neuronal processes is also seen in hippocampi of CTLE patients, mainly in the dentate gyrus, but is absent in TTLE and atypical CTLE groups.

Four chemically defined neural systems show sprouting in CTLE hippocampi. DYN is an opioid-like neuropeptide found in dentate granule cells and their mossy fibre axons in all groups of hippocampi. In the CTLE, in addition to this there is a dense band of DYN immunoreactivity in the inner molecular layer (IML) of the dentate. It is thought that this immunoreactivity is due to recurrent collaterals from remaining granule cell mossy fibre axons. In support of this, our electron microscopic analysis of these hippocampi has revealed synaptic terminals in the IML with a characteristic mossy fibre terminal morphology, making asymmetrical synaptic contact with granule cell apical dendrites in CTLE (Philips, 1993) (Fig. 4). Such mossy fibre terminals were not found in the IML of other groups. Babb *et al.* (1992) have also shown such terminals with vesicular zinc, characteristic of mossy fibres, in the IML of sclerotic hippocampi.

The next most striking example of sprouting is in relation to NPY-immunoreactive fibres. In TTLE and atypical CTLE, NPY-immunoreactive fibres are at high density in the hilus. In the ML NPY fibres are sparse in the IML, moderately dense in the middle ML, where the fibres are mostly orientated perpendicular to the granule cell layer, and most dense in the outer ML, where their orientation is parallel to the granule cell layer. Electron microscopic examination of the ML revealed NPY immunoreactivity to be in axons and axon terminals. These terminals are mostly round vesicle-containing asymmetrical terminals, and form synapses on granule cell dendrites in the IML (Fig. 5), as well as on smaller dendrites (of unidentified origin) in the IML and outer ML (Philips *et al.*, 1992b; Philips, 1993). In the ML of CTLE hippocampi there is a much higher density of NPY-immunoreactive fibres which fill both the IML and the outer ML. These fibres, which appear to be orientated mostly perpendicular to the granule cell layer, form a network in the ML. Electron microscopic studies reveal that, as in the other two groups, in CTLE NPY is confined to axons and axon terminals, which are more numerous in CTLE than in the other groups (Philips *et al.*, 1992b).

The distribution of SOM-immunoreactive fibres in the area dentata is similar to NPY in the TTLE and atypical CTLE group. In the CTLE hippocampi there is an increase in SOM-immunoreactive fibres throughout the ML, as with NPY, but less abundant. Electron microscopic studies of the dentate ML reveal that in TTLE and atypical CTLE hippocampi immunoreactivity is contained in dendrites running through the molecular layer and in asymmetrical terminals synapsing in the outer molecular layer (Fig. 5a). In CTLE by comparison, there are extremely few or no immunoreactive dendrites in the ML, but an increase in SOM-immunoreactive axons and terminals in the IML as well as the outer ML. In the inner ML the SOM terminals formed synapses with granule cell apical dendrites (Fig. 5b).

SP-immunoreactive processes have a distinct distribution in area dentata of TTLE and atypical CTLE. In these two groups, the most striking feature is that SP axons and terminal-like processes form a dense band on either side of the granule cell layer, with some fibres passing between these bands through the granule cell layer (Fig. 6). Additionally, SP-immunoreactive fibres form a network throughout the hilus and a dense plexus in the outer ML. Electron microscopic analysis of these groups revealed small substance P-like immunoreactive (SPLI) asymmetrical and symmetrical terminals synapsing on to both proximal dendrites of granule cells, and other small unidentified dendrites in the IML and outer ML (Philips *et al.*, 1992a).

In contrast to the above two groups, in the CTLE patients the band of SPLI along the hilar border of the granule cell layer was lost. The supragranular band of immunoreactivity was preserved but appeared to extend its territory from the granule cell/IML border somewhat into the IML (Fig. 6). Electron microscopic studies indicated that in this supragranular region, in addition to the SPLI terminal types seen in TTLE and atypical CTLE, there were new synaptic formations, with a greater proportion of small SPLI terminals directly synapsing on granule cell somata (Fig. 5d). Also in the IML were large SPLI terminals which studded the proximal dendrites of granule cells (Fig. 5e). Thus in CTLE, there is a new synaptic input closer to the granule cell bodies.

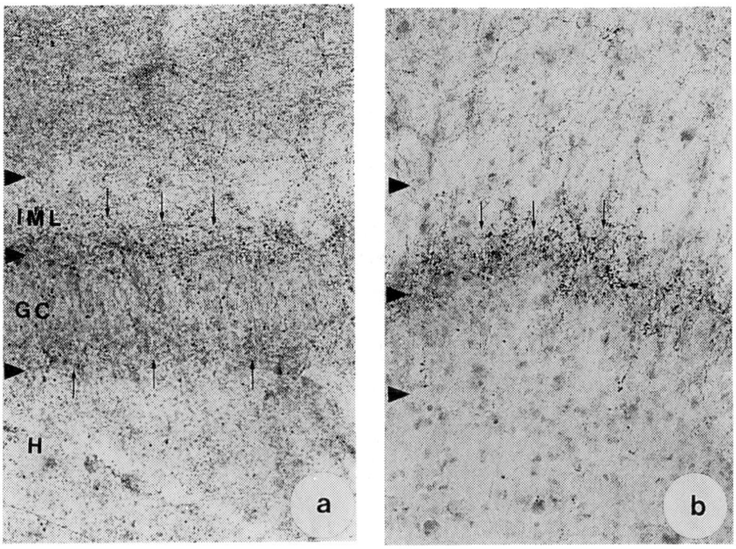

Fig. 6. Photomicrographs of the dentate gyrus of (a) TTLE and (b) CTLE hippocampus showing substance P-(SP) like immunoreactivity (black dots and rows of dots). In TTLE (a) SP immunoreactivity forms bands of immunoreactivity on either side of the granule cell (GC) layer (indicated by fine arrows). In CTLE (b) the band of immunoreactivity on the border of the hilus is lost, whereas the band of immunoreactivity on the molecular layer edge of the GC persists and spreads into the inner molecular layer (IML) (fine arrows). The arrow heads mark the boundaries between the hilus (H), the GC, the IML and the outer ML.

Redistribution of neurotransmitter receptors

In reflection of the wide array of neurotransmitters and neuromodulator substances distributed in the hippocampus, there are a variety of neurotransmitter/modulator related receptors as well. We have studied the distribution of many receptor systems using receptor autoradiography (de Lanerolle *et al.*, 1989, 1990a, b, in press; Johnson *et al.*, 1992a, b). The distribution of these neuroreceptor systems in surgically removed hippocampi reflect some common patterns. Often receptors are reduced in regions where there is cell loss, suggesting that the receptors are located on the neurones lost. In other instances, receptor density is increased in areas of cell loss, indicating the possibility of receptor up-regulation on surviving neurones, or their expression on glia. Space does not permit us to discuss here all these changes observed. However, a feature most striking in the CTLE hippocampi, compared with the autopsy, TTLE or atypical CTLE hippocampi, is the expression of several new patterns of receptor distribution, especially in the area dentata. These new patterns of distribution are seen for SOM, NPY, vasoactive intestinal polypeptide (VIP), dopamine D2 and KA receptors.

SOM receptors, localized with radioiodinated SOM, are found throughout the dentate ML in CTLE compared with its confinement to the IML in the other groups. Ligand binding was also increased in the hilus (Robbins *et al.*, 1991). NPY receptors localized with [^{125}I] Bolten–Hunter labelled NPY are found to be dense in the hilus and IML of CTLE. In contrast NPY receptor density in the ML is very low in the other groups (de Lanerolle *et al.*, 1989). VIP receptors, localized with 3-[^{125}I] iodotyrosol VIP, show high levels of ligand binding in the ML and low levels on granule cells of the non-CTLE groups. In CTLE there is greater VIP-binding in the hilus and on the granule cell bodies, with levels similar to the other groups in the ML (de Lanerolle *et al.*, in press). Dopamine D2 receptors, localized with [^{125}I]iodosulpiride, are found in high density on granule cell bodies and in the IML, and in slightly lower density in the subgranular polymorphic zone of CTLE. In the other groups the levels of D2 receptor are very low in the IML but high in the middle ML. However, the density here is not as great

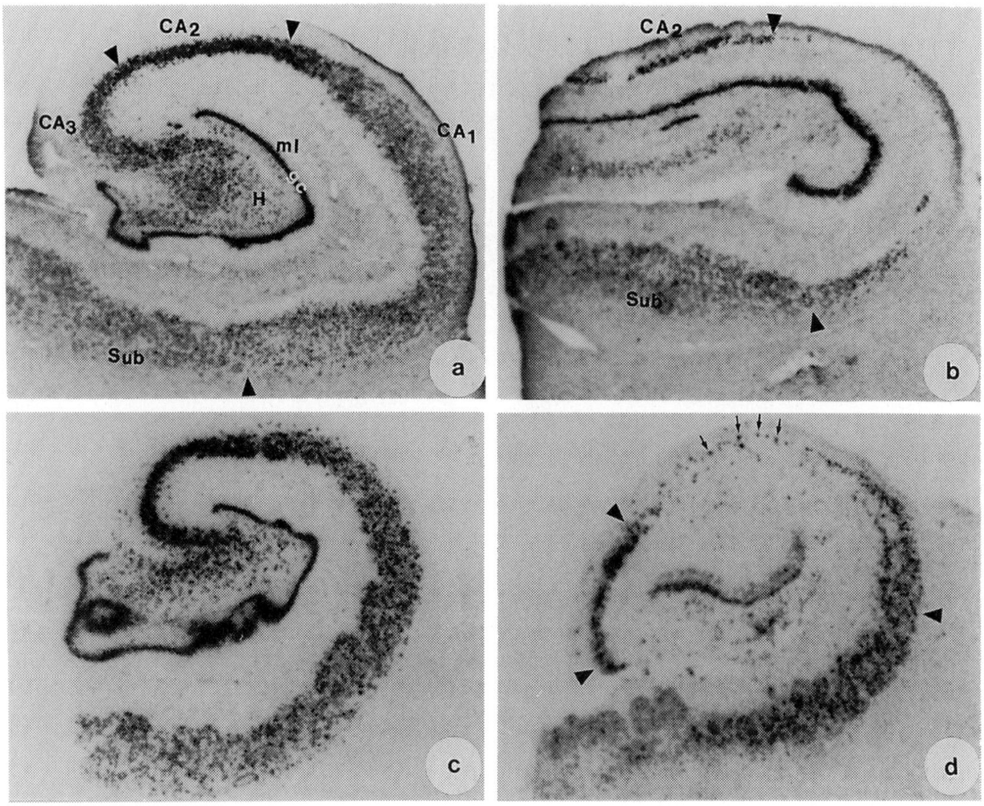

Fig. 7(a) and (b). Photomicrographs of autoradiograms of the distribution of mRNA for the α1 isoform of Na^+,K^+-ATPase (sodium pump) localized by in situ hybridization in a TTLE and CTLE hippocampus respectively. In situ localization of the enzyme mRNA is seen as black dots, and is restricted to neurones in the granule cell layer and neuronal somata in Ammon's horn. In the CTLE case (b) note the reduced labelling in regions of neuronal loss, especially in CA1 and the hilus. (c) and (d) show the localization of mRNA for the α3 isoform of Na^+,K^+-ATPase in a TTLE and CTLE case respectively. Note that α3 is more heavily expressed in the CA3 and CA1 area compared to α1. In CTLE the interneurones that survive in CA1 preferentially express the α3 isoform (arrows) and little α1 (compared with b). mRNA for the α2 isoform is at very low levels in all principal neurones alone (not shown).

as in the IML of CTLE (de Lanerolle *et al.*, 1990b). The most distinctive difference in the distribution of KA receptors is that in TTLE and atypical CTLE cases receptors are dense only in the IML, whereas CTLE is characterized by a more diffuse distribution extending into the middle ML (de Lanerolle *et al.*, 1990a).

Increase in levels of second-messenger systems and sodium pump

[^{3}H]phorbol-12, 13-dibutyrate (PDBU) was used to study the protein kinase C (PKC) and [^{3}H]forskolin to study the adenylate second-messenger systems respectively (Sundaresan *et al.*, 1990). The results of these studies show that there is a clear increase in PKC in the ML of the CTLE hippocampus and particularly on granule cell bodies (as well as in the CA fields) when compared with autopsy controls. In TTLE there is increased PDBU binding only in the ML. When binding levels are adjusted for the number of surviving neurons, there is a significant increase in PDBU binding in all areas of the CTLE hippocampus compared to TTLE. Similarly, when adjusted for neurone counts, [^{3}H]forskolin binding was also increased in the ML and all CA fields (Sundaresan *et al.*, 1990).

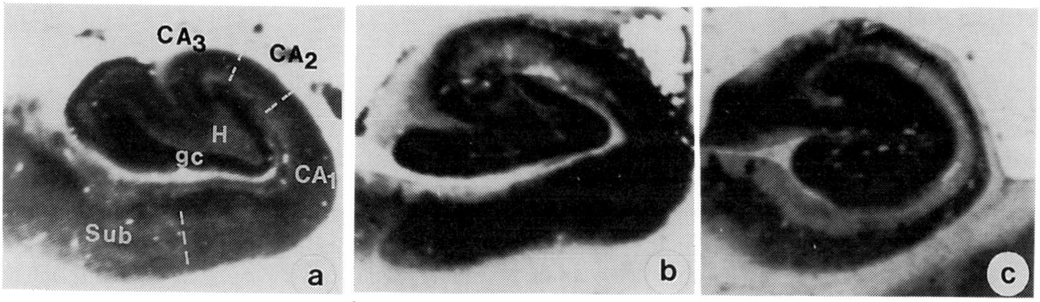

Fig. 8(a), (b) and (c) are autoradiograms showing the distribution of total ^{3}H-ouabain binding in an autopsy, TTLE and CTLE hippocampus respectively. Non- specific binding was undetectable (not shown). In TTLE and CTLE cases, ouabain binding is higher throughout the hippocampus than in autopsy controls, with the molecular layer of the dentate showing the greatest binding. Note that somata, especially notable in the granule cell layer, possess relatively low levels of ^{3}H-ouabain binding. While matter is characterized by binding at background levels. Note that a band of dense binding occurs in CA1 in spite of heavy principal neurone loss (panel c), corresponding to the interneurones visualized by the α3 mRNA pattern (Fig. 7d). Abbreviations: CA1 to CA3, areas of Ammon's horn; H, hilus; gc, granule cell layer; Sub, subiculum.

The enzyme Na^+,K^+-adenosine triphosphatase (ATP)ase (Na^+ pump) is a family of highly homologous isoforms, of which the α2 and α3 isoforms are differentially expressed in the CNS. This enzyme family is crucial for brain function as it establishes the transmembrane gradient which underlies electrical excitability. Changes in Na^+ pump capacity have been hypothesized to play a role in human epilepsy (Grisar & Delgado-Escueta, 1986; Grisar *et al.*, 1992) and critically buffers the excitotoxic potential of glutamate *in vitro* (Brines & Robbins, 1992). It may therefore be an important factor in human epilepsy. Mapping of sodium pump distribution in autopsy human hippocampus, as compared with CTLE and TTLE tissue, has been accomplished at the transcriptional level, utilizing *in situ* hybridization histochemistry for the catalytic alpha subunit isoforms (Fig. 7) (M.L. Brines, unpublished observations), and at the translational level, using ^{3}H-ouabain *in vitro* autoradiography (Brines *et al.*, in prep.), which binds to mature protein (Fig. 8).

In TTLE and atypical CTLE-specific binding of ^{3}H-ouabain is very high throughout the hippocampus, such that neurones express very high levels of Na^+ pump while glia do not (Fig. 8). Somata are relatively unlabelled, consistent with prior study of the rat (Brines *et al.*, 1991) as well as a study utilizing histochemical sodium pump assays (Stahl & Baskin, 1990). The highest levels of ^{3}H-ouabain binding (consistent with mature, functional Na^+ pump) occurs in regions of high synaptic density, especially the dentate ML (Fig. 8). White matter exhibits very low Na^+ pump density. CTLE hippocampus is characterized by a marked principal neurone cell loss, especially in CA1, the hilus and CA3 subfields. This neuronal drop-out is also accompanied by a co-ordinate reduction in the messenger ribonucleic acid (mRNA) for all three catalytic subunit isoforms (Fig. 7b, d) and the specific binding of ^{3}H-ouabain (Fig. 8c). A narrow band of binding is retained in the CA1 subfield, however. These findings are consistent with the concept that Na^+ pump expression is very high in neurones and low in glia, since as the neurones are lost, the amount of Na^+ pump diminishes markedly. These observations are consistent with those observed in *in vitro* model systems (Brines & Robbins, 1993).

However, because Na^+ pump is an integral membrane protein, changes in distribution patterns may merely result from neuronal losses. To assess for this, we determined total protein *in situ*, using a Coomassie blue staining procedure (Miller *et al.*, 1988) applied to specimens from which ^{3}H-ouabain binding was obtained. No differences were observed between autopsy and TTLE tissue throughout the hippocampus. The highest protein content was measured in the dentate ML, CA1 pyramidal layer and the subiculum, which ranged from 271 ng protein/mm^2 in dentate ML to 284 ng/mm^2 in the subiculum. The findings are significant for a very marked reduction in regional protein content for CTLE, with a 35 per cent reduction in the CA1 and hilar subfields, while CA2 and the dentate ML were relatively spared (6 per cent reduction). Interestingly, a narrow band of dense protein staining was observed for CTLE hippocampus in a region, morphologically identical to the region labelled using ^{3}H-ouabain. This protein presumably corresponds to that within the membranes of interneurones in stratum orions (particularly those expressing SOM and/or NPY), which we have previously described (de Lanerolle *et al.*, 1992b) within this region. Interestingly, the neurones which remain in this severely sclerotic hippocampal region are enriched in $\alpha3$ mRNA (Fig. 7d) (M.L. Brines, unpublished observations). The significance of these findings is unknown. Changes in protein content and ^{3}H-ouabain binding were limited to the hippocampus, as measurements of adjacent cortical tissue did not differ significantly in protein content for any group.

When expressed as ^{3}H-ouabain-bound/unit protein, both epilepsy groups are characterized by significant increases in Na^+ pump in the ML, CA2 and subicular regions (~15 per cent increase compared with autopsy). Further, CTLE cases exhibited moderate increases in [^{3}H]-ouabain binding (compared with TTLE and autopsy) in CA4 and CA3 subfields. Deep cortex bound ^{3}H-ouabain identically in all groups. We conclude that changes in cell number do not explain the observed changes in Na^+ pump protein for the epilepsy patients and that the observed increases are real. Whether this is a primary or secondary effect (due to the chronically increased electrical activity which in turn requires increased function of Na^+ pump protein) remains to be elucidated.

Significance of neuronal adaptation for hippocampal excitability

In the face of the above range of neuronal adaptation, an obvious question of importance is how these changes affect hippocampal excitability. Slice electrophysiological studies have confirmed that CTLE hippocampi are functionally hyperexcitable (Masukawa *et al.*, 1989; de Lanerolle *et al.*, 1992b). Our observations of increased levels of sodium pump activity and second-messenger systems also suggest a higher degree of neuronal activity in this tissue.

How then might the specific adaptive changes in chemically defined neuronal systems influence hippocampal excitability? Are all the changes observed of importance to hyperexcitability? Some exclusions can be made. First, it could be argued that CA1 cell loss is not important in and of itself, for patients with end folium sclerosis (where CA1 is intact) still have intractable seizures (Margerison & Corsellis, 1966; Bruton, 1988). Also, in our series of over 100 patients we had one case (IH139, KA) where there was no significant principal cell loss but all the other reorganizational changes described above. Thus, in theory, all the reorganizational changes other than principal cells loss may be of importance for hyperexcitability. What might these changes do to influence the excitability of granule cells?

Considering a surviving granule cell, the mossy axon DYN-positive recurrent collateral to the proximal part of the apical dendrite of granule cells has been suggested to provide a new excitatory input to granule cells (Babb *et al.*, 1992). Assuming that the physiological effects of neurotransmitters on granule cells are similar to those in other areas of the hippocampus and brain, certain deductions could be made. Specifically, SOM and NPY have been reported to function as inhibitory neuromodulators by some workers (Pittman & Siggins, 1981; Colmers *et al.*, 1988; Jacquin *et al.*, 1988). If true, increased SOM and NPY synaptic inputs more proximal to the granule cell somata and the increase in their receptors in the ML, would probably produce an increased inhibition of the granule cells. If, on the other hand, these substances produced excitation (Mueller *et al.*, 1986; Scharfman & Schwartzkroin, 1988), then a further excitation of granule cells would be expected. SP is also shown to be an excitatory substance, and thus increased innervation of granule cells by SP-containing terminals would be presumed to also enhance excitation. The increase in KA receptor likewise may result in glutamate-mediated excitation. However, dopamine D2 receptors have been reported to mediate hyperpolarization and thus inhibition (Vallar & Meldolesi, 1989). The strong increase in D2

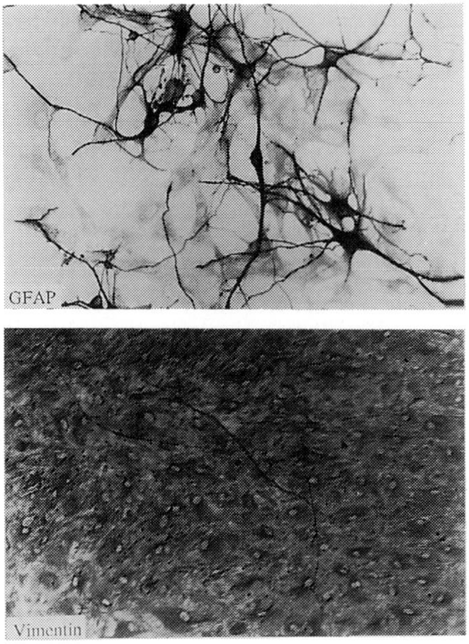

Fig. 9. Upper panel shows a portion of a human glial cell culture prepared from human neocortex immunostained for glial fibrillary acidic protein (GFAP). Note that the fibrous glial astrocytes are strongly positive for GFAP (dark in colour), whereas the flat cells are very weakly stained or not stained at all. The lower panel shows that the flat cells, however, stain strongly for vimentin, whereas the fibrous cells stain only weakly.

receptors in the IML and hilus would argue for mechanisms increasing inhibition on the dentate granule cells. It thus appears that the adaptive responses of neurone systems in the area dentata of CTLE patients may produce enhancement of both presumptive excitatory and inhibitory mechanisms in place of normal control mechanisms. Thus the hyperexcitability of these neurones may lie in an imbalance in these mechanisms favouring excitation, and thus seizures from time to time. Physiological confirmation of such mechanisms is lacking at present.

Changes in glia – neocortical seizure foci

The neocortical seizure foci studied were removed from the temporal lobe, frontal lobe and parietal lobe of patients with a long history of complex partial seizures. Primary cultures (3 weeks) of glia dissociated from tissue obtained from the three regions associated with each lesion (tumour, hyperexcitable cortex, normal cortex) were characterized by a number of techniques (Magge, 1993).

Characterization of glial cell types in culture

By about 5–7 days in culture, two distinct types of glia are distinguishable in culture. One population consists of polymorphic flat cells, which are generally phase-dark. The other population consists of fibrous process-bearing cells possessing phase-bright cell bodies and phase-dark processes. Immunohistochemical staining for glial fibrillary acidic protein (GFAP), a marker for astrocytes, shows that the fibrous cells are strongly GFAP-positive. In contrast, flat cells are very weakly GFAP-positive or GFAP-negative, but stain very intensely for vimentin, a marker for immature glial cell types (Fig. 9). The fibrous cells also preferentially express the $\alpha 1$ isoform of Na^+,K^+-ATPase. The cells in these cultures did not stain for neuronal markers, such as neurofilament, microtubule-associated protein (MAP) or growth cone-associated protein 34 (GAP 34). The treatment of the cultures with 1.0 MM dibutyryl cyclic adenosine monophosphate (AMP) for about 4 h caused the flat cells to convert to a process-bearing form (Moonen *et al.*, 1976) and become more strongly GFAP-positive. On the basis of these results, these two populations of cells can be considered astrocytes.

Estimation of the proportion of flat and fibrous astrocytes in the cultures from the three groups of tissue for each patient reveal significant differences. The fibrous cell density per total cells in the culture is greatest in tumour cultures, least in normal cultures and intermediate in cultures from hyperexcitable tissue.

Electrophysiology of flat and fibrous cells

Flat and fibrous astrocytes also have distinct electrophysiological properties (Magge *et al.*, 1992b). Two-week-old flat and fibrous cells from cultures derived from normal cortex were examined using whole-cell clamp recording. Fibrous cells studied under current clamp conditions are capable of generating action potentials at as little as 150 pA depolarizing current. These action potentials could be reversibly blocked with 1 μM tetrodotoxin (TTX). In contrast, all flat cells examined were non-excitable and did not generate action potentials. In whole-cell voltage clamp recordings, depolarizing voltage steps elicited a rapid inward current followed by a sustained outward current. The outward current is reversibly blocked by 1 μM TTX. This suggests that the observed inward current is due to a transmembrane flux of sodium ions through voltage-sensitive channels.

HPLC studies of glutamate released from astrocyte cultures

Glutamate released by astrocytes in culture was examined by high-performance liquid chromatography (HPLC) (Magge *et al.*, 1992a; Magge, 1993). Seven-day-conditioned media contain millimolar concentrations of glutamate (range 0.16–6.03 mM), compared with micromolar concentrations in unconditioned media. When glutamate concentrations are adjusted for total protein, a statistically significant gradation in glutamate levels is seen with tumour > hyperexcitable > normal. Therefore, these tumour glia synthesize large amounts of glutamate.

Glutamate uptake in astrocyte cultures

To investigate the possibility that the extremely high (millimolar) quantities of glutamate observed in conditioned media (see above) were the result of decreased glutamate transporter function, the uptake of glutamate from the medium was studied by following the time-dependent uptake of 50 nM [^{3}H]-glutamate added to the culture medium (Magge *et al.*, 1992a; Magge, 1993). Glutamate is taken up rapidly via a sodium-dependent mechanism from the medium with maximum velocity at 2.5 to 5.0 min. When uptake at 5 min was compared for glia from tumour, hyperexcitable and normal tissue, a gradation of uptake capacity was seen, with uptake being highest in glia from tumour, less in hyperexcitable and least in normal tissue. Thus, the glutamate uptake mechanisms are enhanced, not reduced, in tumour glia.

Calcium responses in glia

We have also asked whether the astrocytes derived from epilepsy cases are hyper-responsive. To accomplish this, time-lapse scanning confocal laser microscopy was used to examine astrocytic responses to glutamate (Cornell-Bell *et al.*, 1991; de Lanerolle *et al.*, 1991; Gunel *et al.*, 1991). Glial cultures were perfused with saline or glutamate receptor agonists and imaged using the fluorescent calcium indicator Fluo-3AM. Definitive and reproducible differences in calcium levels between cultures were observed before and after exposure to glutamate. Large increases in intercellular calcium and changes in oscillation rate were seen in cell cultures from normal, hyperexcitable and tumour regions. Exposure to 100 μM glutamate caused normal astrocytes to increase their calcium levels and oscillate at a higher rate (mean period 5.1 ± 0.3 s–2.8 ± 0.1 s). At baseline (saline alone), hyperexcitable cultures exhibited a significantly higher rate of oscillation than normal or tumour-derived cultures (0.94 ± 0.09 s). Exposure to glutamate produced a slight increase in the otherwise rapid oscillation rate (0.85 ± 0.1 s). Cells from tumour cultures displayed a baseline oscillation rate similar to that of normal cells (4.4 ± 0.08 s), which was observed mainly in the flat astrocytes in these cultures. In contrast, the fibrous cells did not oscillate. The flat cells increased intracellular calcium after glutamate exposure, followed by a return to baseline and a drop in oscillation frequency (6.0 ± 0.8 s). The fibrous cells did not oscillate after a glutamate- induced spike.

Summary

The above studies on neuroglia from neocortical seizure foci suggest that these cells have undergone several distinctive changes, which may be of relevance to seizure initiation. The high concentration of fibrous astrocytes in the tumour and hyperexcitable region, with the ability to generate neurone-like action potentials, may indicate that glia themselves may serve to initiate waves of depolarizaton at such seizure foci. In hyperexcitable regions, the property of glia to display rapid and repetitive oscillations of intracellular calcium and an increased ability to propagate intercellular calcium waves, suggests that astrocytes at some seizure foci may have the capability of signal transduction normally attributed to neurones. Furthermore, the ability of astrocytes at seizure foci to release enhanced quantities of glutamate into the extracellular space, thus creating a pool of high glutamate around which neurones may be highly excited, would be yet another potential mechanism of epileptogenesis in neocortical seizure foci.

Relevance of findings for classification of seizures and seizure syndromes

In a recent review of surgically remediable temporal lobe syndromes (Wieser *et al.*, 1993), it has been suggested that, if a syndromatic subclassification is attempted, probably two epilepsies of the temporal lobe could be distinguished. These two syndromes have been described as (1) a surgically remediable TLE syndrome called mesial temporal lobe epilepsy (MTLE) and (2) a neocortical epilepsy with lesions outside the limbic system and ictal discharges that rapidly propagate into the limbic system causing an identical ictal semiology. The authors note that in this second condition the lesions are not necessarily limited to the temporal lobe, but may occur in other areas of neocortex, where the seizures originate and rapidly propagate to the hippocampal formation to produce an ictal pattern that resembles 'limbic seizures' without noticeable initial symptoms that might suggest a frontal, parietal or occipital onset (Wieser *et al.*, 1993). Further, they define the essential pathological substrate of MTLE as hippocampal sclerosis with a marked loss of neurones in the CAl region and some loss in the end folium (CA3/CA4) and relative sparing of the CA2 region. The patients identified as showing the MTLE syndrome are also predicted to have a good outcome following limited temporal lobe resections.

The population of patients defined as having MTLE, on the basis of clinical history, seizure pattern and other features (Wieser *et al.*, 1993), is very similar to the group of patients described in our study as CTLE patients. However, while it is the case that a majority of our CTLE patients show hippocampal sclerosis of the pattern described for MTLE, it is our contention that this is not the essential defining pathological state of this group. Three important observations lead us to this conclusion. First, patients with end folium sclerosis (loss of hilar and CA3 neurones, but no loss in CA1) in our series as well as in others (Margerison & Corsellis, 1966) indicate that CAl cell loss is not an essential condition in this syndrome. Second, in a few patients in our series ($n = 3$) the degree of CA1 cell loss was minimal, being confined to only a small area in the proximal region of CA1. Third, we have observed in one patient (KA) no significant loss of principal neurones (granule cells or pyramidal cells), cell counts being similar to neurologically normal autopsy hippocampi. However, in these exceptional patients, as well as in all other patients with CA1 sclerosis, the invariant observation was the selective loss or a significant reduction in the populations of subgranular hilar interneurones containing SOM, NPY and SP. This loss is accompanied by increased NPY and SOM fibre staining in the ML and DYN staining in the IML.

The syndromatic subclassification of 'neocortical epilepsy' (Wieser *et al.*, 1993) seems to apply to the patients defined as TTLE by our group. In the TTLE group, as with the other neocortical lesions,

Scharfman, H.E. & Schwartzkroin, P.A. (1988): Further studies of the effects of somatostatin and related peptides in area CA1 of rabbit hippocampus. *Cell. Mol. Neurobiol.* **8,** 411–429.

Seress, L. & Mrzljak, L. (1992): Postnatal development of mossy cells in the human dentate gyrus: a light microscopic Golgi study. *Hippocampus* **2,** 127–142.

Sloviter, R. (1987): Decreased hippocampal inhibition and selective loss of interneurons in experimental epilepsy. *Science* **235,** 73–76.

Spencer, S.S. & Spencer, D.D. (1991): *Surgery for epilepsy.* Oxford: Blackwell Scientific Publishers.

Stahl, W.L. & Baskin, D.G. (1990): Histochemistry of ATPases. *J. Histochem. Cytochem.* **38,** 1099–1122.

Sundaresan, S., de Lanerolle, N.C., Brines, M.L. & Spencer, D.D. (1990): Second messengers in the hippocampus in human temporal epilepsy. *Soc. Neurosci. Abstr.* **16,** 308.

Sutula, T., Xiao-Xian, H., Cavazos, J. & Scott, G. (1989): Synaptic reorganization in the hippocampus induced by abnormal functional activity. *Science* **239,** 1147–1150.

Tauck, D. & Nadler, J. (1985): Evidence of functional mossy fibre sprouting in hippocampal formation of kainic acid treated rats. *J. Neurosci.* **5,** 1016–1022.

Vallar, L. & Meldolesi, J. (1989): Mechanisms of signal transduction at the dopamine D2 receptor. *Trends Pharmacol. Sci.* **10,** 74–77.

Wieser, H.-G., Engel, J., Williamson, P., Babb, T.L. & Gloor, P. (1993): Surgically remediable temporal lobe syndromes. In: *Surgical treatment of the epilepsies*, 2nd edn, ed. J. Engel, pp. 49–63. New York: Raven Press.

Zhu, Z.Z., Armstrong, D., Grossman, R. & Hamilton, W. (1990): Tyrosine hydroxylase immunoreactive neurons in the temporal lobe in complex partial seizures. *Ann. Neurol.* **27,** 564–572.

Epileptic Seizures and Syndromes, Edited by Peter Wolf
© 1994 John Libbey & Company Ltd., pp. 449–467

Chapter 47

Febrile convulsions, mesial temporal sclerosis and temporal lobe epilepsy

Hans Holthausen

Epoilepsie-Zentrum Bethel, Klinik Mara I, Maraweg 21, 33617 Bielefeld, Germany

Definition

'A febrile seizure is an event in infancy or childhood usually occurring between 3 months and 5 years of age, associated with fever but without evidence of intracranial infection of defined cause. Seizures with fever in children who have suffered a previous nonfebrile seizure are excluded. Febrile seizures are to be distinguished from epilepsy, which is characterized by recurrent nonfebrile seizures.'

Consensus statement on febrile seizures, National Institute of Health Consensus Development Conference Summary, 1981.

Introduction

For decades a discussion has been going on as to whether febrile convulsions (FCs) are risk factors for the development of temporal lobe epilepsy (TLE). Besides theoretical considerations paediatricians would like to know if prophylactic anticonvulsant medication can prevent TLE in a subgroup of children with FCs. They are puzzled by many conflicting data from the literature, with figures as high as a 79 per cent incidence of FCs in patients with TLE in one publication (Falconer, 1976) and statements like 'temporal lobe epilepsy – not a consequence of childhood febrile convulsions in Denmark' (Lee *et al.*, 1981).

Obviously methodological and statistical aspects play a major role in the interpretation of the data. In addition, there are many other questions not yet fully answered which to some extent may explain the difficulties one has with investigations on the association between FC and TLE:

- Do seizures cause brain damage?
- What causes mesial temporal sclerosis (MTS) and Ammon's horn sclerosis (AHS)?
- What is MTS?
- Are there kindling processes in man?

MTS is the pathological substrate usually found in patients with TLE and a history of FCs. How are FCs, MTS and TLE related to each other?

Theoretically there are three possibilities (see Table 1):

1. Hypothesis: FCs cause MTS, and these changes are responsible for the TLE.
2. Hypothesis: there is no relation: a child may have FCs; MTS develops independently, which causes TLE,
3. Hypothesis: there is a pre-existing pathology which is responsible both for the child's FC (with focal signs) and for the MTS (being responsible for the occurrence of TLE).

Table 1. Febrile convulsions, mesial temporal sclerosis (MTS) and temporal lobe epilepsy (TLE)

1. Hypothesis	Febrile convulsions (with focal signs)	→MTS → TLE
2. Hypothesis	(a)Febrile convulsions	
	(b)— —	→MTS →TLE
3. Hypothesis	Pre-existing pathology in mesial temporal structures	→Febrile convulsions (with focal signs) →MTS → TLE

Epidemiological studies on children with FCs

That FCs might be a risk factor for TLE has been argued for a long time by various authors. Lennox (1953) compared the seizure types following FCs in 272 children with the seizure types of 1900 'office patients' of whom only 16 per cent had a history of an FC, and found psychomotor seizures as the only seizure type in 17.1 per cent of the FC group compared with 5.9 per cent in the 'office patients' group – a statistically significant difference. From this and from his investigations on TLE (Lennox, 1950), he assumed that 'febrile seizures of early childhood may in certain cases cause injury to the temporal lobe'.

There is a countless number of publications on FCs differing in many aspects of investigation, and methodology. Major reviews of the literature on the risk of epilepsy following FCs have been done by Millichap (1968) and Wallace (1988) (Table 2). They found incidences of epilepsy following FC as low as 2.6 per cent and as high as 100 per cent.

Table 2. The risk of seizures and epilepsy following febrile convulsions.

Author	Source of subjects	No. of studies	Unprovoked seizures (%)	Epilepsy (%)	Author's comment
Millichap, 1968	Various	31	3–81	2.6–100	No selection or categorization
Wallace, 1988	(a) Hospital	10	7–18*		
	(b) Hospital	3		20–40	'Severe constitutional illness or very prolonged initial seizures'
Wallace, 1988	Hospital	10†		1.5–5	'Have reflected the situation in the general population more accurately'

*Seizures and/or epilepsy; †1940–1980.

It doesn't need further explanation that outcome figures are different when study design and applied statistics are different. Wallace (1988) compared the results of studies on children with 'severe constitutional illnesses or very prolonged seizures' who were referred to centres known for their skills in treatment of severe seizure disorders with the results of studies which were also hospital-based but 'have reflected the situation in the general population more accurately'. Purely as a consequence of this type of selection 7 per cent–40 per cent of the children in the 'first group of studies' had seizures or epilepsy following FC, compared with the much lower figure of 1.5 per cent–5 per cent in the second group of studies.

The studies listed in Table 3 are either 'cohort' studies (National Collaborative Perinatal Project

(NCPP), National Child Development Study (NCDS), Child Health and Education Study (CHES)) or community-based and are done prospectively.

Table 3. Longitudinal studies of children with febrile convulsions (FCs)

Author	Source of subjects	No. of children	Length of follow-up	% of children with epilepsy following FCs	Author's comment
Nelson & Ellenberg, 1978	NCPP	1706	Up to age 7 years	< 2%	
Annegers *et al.*, 1979	Community	666	8291 person-years	6%	
Ross *et al.*, 1980	NCDS	372	11 years	0.5%	Treated at home
				12%	Treated in hospital
Verity *et al.*, 1985	CHES	289	5 years	7%	Afebrile seizures
Annegers *et al.*, 1987	Community	687	10145 person-years	7%	

CPP = National Collobarative Perinatal Project; NCDS = National Child Development Study; CHES = Child Health and Education Study (GB)

How selection influences outcome can be seen from the Great Britain NCDS (Ross *et al.*, 1980). Of children with FC treated at home 0.5 per cent only developed epilepsy by the age of 11 years compared with 12 per cent of those who were treated in hospitals.

In a 10-year follow-up report on the cohort of 16,004 children born in one week in Great Britain, the incidence of epilepsy following FCs is still very low. Information was available on 14,676 children. Of the 382 children with FCs, 13 had one or several afebrile seizures. At highest risk were children with focal signs during FCs – five of 17 developed epilepsy (Verity & Golding, 1991).

The very low figure of less than a 2 per cent risk for epilepsy following FCs in Nelson & Ellenberg's (1987) study needs to be commented on because it is the study referred to whenever there is a discussion on the issue of FCs and TLE. Nelson and Ellenberg reported the risk of afebrile seizures (2.2 per cent) separate from the risk of epilepsy (1.3 per cent). From a methodological point of view, this might be correct but it doesn't take into consideration that children with FCs and subsequent afebrile seizures may have a higher cumulative risk for epilepsy. Moreover, children with FC were followed up to the age of 7 years only. It is well known that the onset of TLE occurs many times at the end of the first decade, in the second decade of life or even later. In a study on epilepsies following status epilepticus or FCs, Fujiwara *et al.* (1979) were able to demonstrate that in the majority of cases onset of complex partial seizures (CPS) occurred in the second decade of life (Table 4), and Hauser (1992) stated that there is an increased risk for epilepsy following FCs well through the third decade of life.

Table 4. Interval between initial status epilepticus and onset of subsequent epilepsies.

Type of seizure	< 2 years	2–5 years	6–9 years	> 10 years	Total
Secondary generalized	22	3	2	0	27
Simple partial	12	3	5	1	21
Complex partial	1	7	14	9	31
Total	35	13	21	10	79

From Fujiwara *et al.*, 1979.

Only children with complicated FCs have a higher risk for epilepsy. Wallace's review of the literature on risk factors (1988) is listed in Table 5. The type of subsequent seizures depends on different complex features of the FCs. Almost all studies show that there is an increased risk for complex partial seizures when FCs are lateralized, particularly for lateralized seizures of long duration (Aicardi & Chevrie, 1976, 1983, Aicardi, 1987; Wallace, 1982), whereas recurrent simple FCs and a family history of epilepsy are risk factors for later generalized epilepsy (Annegers *et al.*, 1987) (Table 6).

Table 5. Predisposing factors for later non-febrile seizures.

Factor	No. of publications: factor relevant yes/no
Family history of epilepsy	5/6
Perinatal factors	3/3
Age at onset of FCs (age of onset < 1 year)	11/1
Long duration of FCs	7/1
Repetitive FCs during the course of one illness	3/0
Lateralized and focal seizures	9/0

From Wallace, 1988.

Table 6. Epilepsy following febrile convulsions (FCs).

1. Lateralized FCs	→	Complex partial seizures
2. Recurrent generalized (tonic–clonic?) FCs	→	Generalized epilepsy
3. Onset within the first year of life	→	Increased risk of recurrence (of FCs)
4. Family history of FCs	→	Increased risk of recurrence (of FCs)
5. Family history of epilepsy	→	Increased risk of epilepsy

Wallace, 1988, and Annegers *et al.*, 1987.

Consequences of prolonged FCs in reports on childhood status epilepticus

For the discussion on the association between TLE and FCs, the investigation of Aicardi & Chevrie (1970) on the consequences of childhood status epilepticus is of great importance. The result that CPS occurred in a very high percentage of children with a previous history of status epilepticus (children with prolonged FCs included) but with seizure semiology during status epilepticus different from their later CPS suggests that TLE indeed could be a consequence of prolonged seizures (Table 7). Similar results have been reported by Gastaut *et al.* (1960), Roger *et al.* (1974) and Fujiwara *et al.* (1979). All these studies have in common that for the vast majority of cases the initial status epilepticus was the first convulsive event and that CPS as the main seizure type were present in a very high percentage of these children later on.

Table 7. Classification of seizures during and following status epilepticus.

Classification of seizures during status epilepticus	*n*	Classification of seizures following status epilepticus	*n*	*n**
Generalized (clonic or tonic–clonic)	102	Generalized clonic	43	16
Unilateral clonic	94	Unilateral	16	5
Generalized tonic	19	Partial motor	16	8
Unilateral tonic	2	**Psychomotor**	30	18
Partial motor	11	Lennox–Gastaut syndrome	16	11
			10	6
Erratic (newborn)	11	Infantile spasms	15	6
		Status		
Total	239		146	70

*One seizure type only. From Aircardi & Chevrie, 1970.

In Aicardi and Chevrie's (1970) study, 67 of 239 children with status epilepticus who were mentally and neurologically normal prior to status epilepticus presented with fever (children with meningitis and encephalitis excluded). Almost all 67 children belonged to the age-group > 6 months, < 3 years.

The initial episode was usually associated with a common upper respiratory infection. Aicardi and Chevrie (1970) felt that these children with 'cryptogenic febrile status epilepticus' had the most severe expression of idiopathic FCs. About 25 per cent of these previously normal children were mentally or neurologically impaired following (febrile) status epilepticus. The number of children out of this interesting subgroup having temporal lobe seizures only is unknown, which is unfortunate as this is just the group we are interested in.

In contrast to these studies on the consequences of status epilepticus in children from the 1950s, 1960s, and 1970s, Maytal *et al.* (1989) reported a very low morbidity and mortality. Of the 46 children with FCs lasting more than 30 min (out of 193 children with status epilepticus), only two who were neurologically abnormal prior to the status epilepticus had unprovoked seizures later on. But the short mean follow-up duration of 13.2 months for the children with FCs does not allow conclusions to be drawn from this material. In contrast to the older studies, only a small minority of the children (five out of 46) had FCs lasting more than 1 h. This is most probably due to the fact that children with status epilepticus are treated more vigorously now.

FCs in temporal lobectomy series

The incidence of FC in Jensen's report (Jensen, 1976) on 74 temporal lobectomies was 9 per cent; in Green's report (Green, 1967) on 88 patients it was 16 per cent. In Paillas's series (Paillas, 1958), 28 per cent of the patients had a history of 'convulsions of infancy'. The typical pathological substrate in patients with TLE and a history of FC is unilateral MTS. There are no reports in the literature of patients with TLE and a history of prolonged FCs who do not have MTS! In Lindsay's publication on developmental aspects of 50 children with TLE finally undergoing temporal lobectomy (Lindsay *et al.*, 1984), MTS was found in 20 patients, of whom 19 had a history of prolonged seizures in infancy, 'frequently associated with fever', followed by a silent interval before the onset of their habitual focal seizures. In contrast, only one of 17 patients with tumours had a history of early convulsions. In a series of 30 children operated by Falconer (Falconer, 1974), 20 children had MTS; 'of these 15 (75 per cent) had a history of severe febrile convulsion during infancy, whereas only one of 10 children with other lesions had a febrile convulsion'. But MTS was found in association with lesions like hamartomas when 'early prolonged seizures supervened' (Falconer *et al.*, 1964).

In a report on 71 patients undergoing temporal lobectomy with MTS or non-specific pathology, nine had a history of transient hemiparesis following a febrile convulsion (Darkins & Polkey, 1985). None of the nine patients had 'gross evidence of additional brain damage' and their outcome with respect to seizure control did not differ from the 62 patients without this history.

Because most centres publish the incidences of FCs in their series of TLE within the context of their neuropathology reports, more figures are given in the section on MTS in temporal lobectomy series.

History of FCs in population-based studies on patients with CPS

The analysis of the Rochester, Minnesota, linkage system on epilepsy between 1935 and 1979 has given strong evidence of an association between FCs and CPS. A history of FCs was found in 20 per cent ($n = 16$) of patients with CPS but only in 2 per cent of control subjects (Rocca *et al.*, 1987). FCs were complicated in 14 of the 16 cases. The authors felt, however, that their material does not answer the question whether CPS and FCs are causally related or just have a common underlying cause ('pre-existing pathology'), or whether FCs could be an early manifestation of CPS.

History of FCs in 'medical' series of patients with CPS

In three paediatric series (Table 8), one-third of children with CPS had a history of FC. We cannot conclude that this figure represents the situation in all children with CPS. It rather reflects our experience that CPS are difficult to treat medically when there is a history of FC. For the low figure of 9 per cent in the report of Schmidt *et al.* (1985) on adult patients, we can assume that events in early life like FCs might have been forgotten or that witnesses (e.g. parents) who could be asked are not alive any more.

Table 8. Medical patients with complex partial seizures.

Author	Patients	No. of subjects	% of febrile seizures	Author's comment
Ounsted *et al.*, 1966	Children	100	32	Prolonged
Hassan *et al.*, 1966	Children	34	38	
Schmidt *et al.*, 1985	Adults	155	9*	Complicated FC
Kotagal *et al.*, 1987	Children	30	33	

*Seizure control: patients with FC = 29%; patients without FC = 65%

FC in neuroimaging series of patients with TLE

In a series of 50 consecutive cases selected for temporal lobectomy (Berkovic *et al.*, 1991), 10 patients (20 per cent) had a history of prolonged FCs (see Table 9). Magnetic resonance imaging (MRI) of these 10 patients showed atrophy of one hippocampus with an increased signal on T2-weighted images. In six of these 10 patients FCs were not only prolonged but also lateralized. In these six cases the side of the hippocampal atrophy was contralateral to the side of the convulsions during the FC. Histological examination revealed hippocampal sclerosis. Eight of the 10 patients (80 per cent) became seizure-free following temporal lobectomy, confirming that patients with TLE and a history of FC are excellent candidates for epilepsy surgery.

Table 9. Side of hippocampal atrophy on MRI in patients with TLE and a history of prolonged unilateral FCs

n	
50	Consecutive cases of temporal lobectomies reviewed
↓	
10	Cases selected because of the history of prolonged febrile convulsions
↓	
10	Atrophy of one hippocampus with increased signal on T2 weighted images
↓	
6	Patients had lateralized prolonged febrile convulsions
↓	
6	Side of hippocampal atrophy in accordance with lateralization of the febrile convulsions

From Berkovic *et al.*, 1991.

In a study comparing the diagnostic value of positron emission tomography (PET) vs. single-photon emission computed tomography (SPECT) in a selected group of patients with TLE six out of 20 patients had a history of FCs (Ryvlin *et al.*, 1992).

From our own first 97 consecutive cases in which TLE was confirmed by means of presurgical evaluation (Wohlrab *et al.*, 1993), 30 patients (33 per cent) had radiological signs typical for hippocampal sclerosis, e.g. atrophy of the hippocampal formation visible on T1-weighted MRI images or an increased signal on T2-weighted MRI images, or both. Eleven of the 30 patients (37 per cent) with MRI signs of hippocampal sclerosis had a history of FC. Eight of them have meanwhile had a temporal lobectomy and are seizure-free (follow-up of at least 6 months). Neuropathology revealed MTS in all cases. Nine out of 42 patients (21 per cent) with TLE with no definite neuroimaging diagnosis had a history of FC as well. In contrast, none of our 25 patients with lesions other than hippocampal sclerosis (usually benign and dysontogenetic tumours) had a history of FCs. This result is in accordance with the reports of Lindsay *et al.* (1984) and of McMillan *et al.* (1987). In about half of our non-MTS lesional cases with TLE the lesions involved mesial structures like amygdala, hippocampus and gyrus parahippocampalis. These findings are strong arguments against the hypothesis that a pre-existing pathology of any kind may be responsible both for FCs and for the development of MTS.

FCs, TLE and MTS

Introductory remarks

There are countless publications from many different fields of research dealing with the question whether changes like AHS or MTS are the cause or the consequence of seizures. Although at first it seems a hopeless undertaking to try to find the answer to this question, the discussion on the association between FC and TLE would be incomplete if we did not include considerations on possible mechanisms which could cause AHS or MTS. These changes are the pathological substrate in patients with TLE and a history of prolonged and lateralized FCs.

Definition

'Mesial temporal sclerosis (MTS) is Ammon's horn sclerosis plus changes in other structures of the mesial part of the temporal lobe such as the amygdala and uncus' (Falconer *et al.*, 1964).

MTS in temporal lobectomy series

The percentage of MTS in series of temporal lobe resections for drug-resistant TLE is around 50 per cent, sometimes even higher (Meencke & Veith, 1991; Table 10). Percentages of FCs in this subgroup of patients with TLE and MTS vary within a range of 18–80 per cent (Table 11).

Table 10. Frequency of hippocampal sclerosis (HS) in temporal lobe resections

	n	HS	%
Falconer *et al.*, 1964	100	49	49
Meyer *et al.*, 1954	12	7	58
Earle *et al.*, 1953	153	100	63
Brown, 1973	29	19	65
Cavanagh & Meyer, 1956	27	19	70
Mathieson, 1975	184	140	76
Brown & Babb, 1986	114	73	64

Adapted from Meencke & Veith, 1991 (with modification).

Table 11. Incidences of febrile convulsions in neuropathology reports of patients with mesial temporal sclerosis

Author	Patients with MTS	% of febrile convulsions	Comment
Falconer *et al.*, 1964	47	40	Adults
Falconer & Taylor, 1968	47	30	Adults
Davidson & Falconer, 1975	24	79	Children
Mathieson, 1975	140	18	
Bruton, 1984	107	79	

What are the reasons for this very high variability of the incidences of FC in the surgical series with MTS? In Falconer's two series of adult patients (Falconer *et al.*, 1964; Falconer & Taylor, 1968), comprising 100 patients each, the incidence of MTS was 50 per cent. The rate of 'severe and prolonged' FCs in the cases with MTS was 40 per cent in the first study; in the second series, when only FCs lasting longer than 30 min were taken into account, the rate was 30 per cent (Table 11).

Falconer felt that these figures were too low because adults might have forgotten that they had FCs but that the high figure of 79 per cent of FCs in his paediatric series (Davidson & Falconer, 1975) was most probably too high and the result of selection, because more children were referred for epilepsy surgery when physicians and parents became aware of the good postoperative prognosis in patients with TLE and a history of FCs. For Falconer it was no question that 'severe FCs are an important cause of the lesion (MTS) which then matures into an epileptogenic one'.

Because 'AHS' is frequently found at autopsies of patients who had never experienced a single seizure, this causative view has not been accepted in general. The fact that various kinds of hippocampal damage in association with different aetiologies have been reported under terms like AHS or hippocampal sclerosis might have led to some of the confusions and misunderstandings we have been dealing with until very recently (Gloor, 1991).

However, according to Babb and Brown (1987), who used more precise quantitative methods to determine neuronal loss in the various regions of the hippocampus, there is a unique pattern of hippocampal sclerosis in human TLE that is evidently quite different from 'hippocampal sclerosis' in other conditions. Illustrations of several kinds of hippocampal damage caused by aetiologies like perinatal anoxia, kernicterus, etc. are shown in this publication to explain the differences compared with the changes in TLE in terms of the distribution and the amount of cell loss.

In their group of patients studied with depth electrodes, seizure onset was 'anterior focal' when neuronal loss was found predominantly in the anterior part of the Ammon's horn and 'regional' when the damage was equally distributed over the anterior and the posterior part of the hippocampus. Hence, the authors concluded that most probably synaptic reorganization near the site of the hippocampal damage causes seizures.

There was no correlation between the amount of cell loss and age of TLE onset, duration of epilepsy and frequency of seizures, but they did find a significant decrease of granule cells in the fascia dentata when generalized seizures occurred early in life. From this and from their review of the literature, Babb and Brown (1987) support the concept that hippocampal sclerosis occurs early in life, that it is not a progressive disease, but that synaptic reorganization takes place over time, creating epileptogenic connections which will eventually cause TLE.

Sagar and Oxbury's article (1987), on the correlation of hippocampal neurone loss in association with early childhood convulsions in 32 patients who had a temporal lobectomy for medically refractory seizures is a landmark in the field of research on the association between FCs and TLE. Although not mentioned, it is very likely that the majority of the early childhood convulsions were FCs. The amount of cell loss was significantly correlated with a history of convulsions before the age of 4 years. The majority of patients with convulsions in the < 4 years age-group had prolonged seizures (> 30 min) or repetitive seizures during the first day; in half of them the seizures were unilateral or there was unilateral postictal weakness contralateral to the side of the temporal lobe removed later on for the relief of seizures. Moreover, the histological picture in patients with a history of convulsions who were older than 4 years at the time of the convulsions or in patients with no history of convulsions in childhood was different from the findings in the group with early childhood convulsions. Classical AHS as it has been delineated, e.g. by Margerison and Corsellis (1966), that is, loss of pyramidal cells in the H1-field (Sommer's sector) plus pyramidal cell loss in the end folium, plus loss of granule cells in the dentate gyrus, was present in the early childhood convulsion group but not in the other group, with the exception of one patient. This latter group had what the authors called 'non-specific hippocampal sclerosis', e.g. neurone loss in the H1 field or in the endfolium alone – never granule cell loss in the dentate gyrus. Sagar and Oxbury (1987) stated that 'it seems highly probable that a severe convulsion in early childhood is responsible for the profound neuron loss in AHS, and that milder forms of nonspecific neuron loss may arise from epilepsy over a long period of time'. They suggested that neuropathological results should be reported with regard to these two types of changes (AHS *vs.* non-specific neurone loss) instead of combining both findings under the term MTS.

The difference between the two groups is not limited just to the degree of cell loss and its distribution over the Ammon's horn formation but includes a number of changes like synaptic reorganization, expression of neurotransmitters, distribution of receptors, etc. An excellent overview with respect to these changes is given by de Lanerolle *et al.* (Chapter 46).

Neuropathology reports on MTS

Historical overview

'Mesial temporal sclerosis . . . is a process which essentially involves usually one but sometimes both temporal lobes. During the past century and a half many post mortem studies of the brains of chronic epileptics who died a natural death have demonstrated its presence in more than half of them. The lesion is thus frequent and also is clearly of anoxic origin with its main brunt following on the Ammon's horn (hippocampus) . . . where there is selective loss in the Sommer sector (h1) and in the end-folium (h3, h4, h5) with preservation of cells in the "resistant" sector (h2). However, it also often involves the amygdala as well. Sometimes it is the only lesion present in the brain in epilepsy, and post mortem studies suggest that whenever it is present it is unilateral in 80 per cent of instances. No one has yet fully explained why it is so often unilateral' (Falconer, 1976).

Up to now we still don't know why MTS in association with FCs occurs predominantly unilaterally. Recent results of modern neurochemical methods in neuroanatomy, however, have provided a fundamental understanding of the peculiar distribution of nerve cell loss usually found in AHS. It has been a long way from Bouchet and Cazauvieilh in 1825, who were the first to describe this type of lesion in the temporal lobe, to some of the recent indications of its possible aetiological mechanisms.

Toward the end of the last century neuropathologists from German speaking countries have done major contributions to the research on the association between brain pathology and epilepsy. Meynert reported in 1868 that Ammon's horn sclerosis is a frequent finding in patients with epilepsy and that this lesion was found predominantly unilaterally. ('Ungleichheit der Durchmesser des Querschnittes beider Ammons-hörner der Epileptiker, bedingt durch die vorangehende Atrophie des einen von ihnen, welche mit schwieliger bis knorpelartiger Härte und solenner Anämie derselben einhergeht, nicht selten mit einem wachsartigen Glanze und durchscheinendem Ansehen auf dem Querschnitt.') AHS was left-sided in 11, right-sided in five and bilateral in only four of the 20 reported cases; mental retardation was present in eight patients.

Meynert's findings were confirmed by Pfleger in 1880, who found AHS in 27 cases out of 300 autopsies. Twenty-five of the 27 had epilepsy. AHS was unilateral in 22 of the 25 patients (88 per cent).

Sommer (1880) discussed for the first time a histological picture of the AHS (report on 50 patients with 'genuine epilepsy'); the Ammon's horn was normal in 25 patients; the right side was affected in 11 patients, the left side in 13 patients; both sides were affected in one patient only.

A precise picture of the peculiar type of changes characteristic of AHS was given by Bratz as early as 1899. As confirmed later by authors like Corsellis and Bruton (1983), Babb and Brown (1987) and Mouritzen-Dam (1980), Bratz demonstrated that pyramidal cell loss was most prominent in the Sommer sector (CA1 region of Lorente de Nó) and was less dramatic but still evident in the CA3 and CA4 region, and that there was a 'resistant sector', the CA2 region, in between. Further details are mentioned, such as the preservation of the cell population in the subiculum, the oblique border to the area of destruction in the adjacent CA1 region and the preservation of 'spindle cells', most probably γ-aminobutyric acidergic (GABA-ergic) neurones as we now know. Half a century before Cavanagh and Meyer (1956), Bratz pointed out that the destruction was not limited to the Ammon's horn formation but extended to parts of the parahippocampus and sometimes even to large adjacent temporal neocortical areas. Most interesting for our discussion was his early observation that AHS was found contralateral to the side of the convulsion in infancy in three patients and that there was a time lag until the onset of the 'genuine epilepsy', which in many cases, according to Bratz, had a subtle symptomatology at its onset with signs like 'dizziness', and only later severe convulsions and a mental decline. He did not find differences in the pattern of AHS when comparing older patients with children. There were no hints of an early process within the Ammon's horn; the vascularization of the Ammon's horn formation was well preserved. As a conclusion to his work he raised the previously unanswered question whether this type of pathology occurs due to an intrinsic process within the Ammon's horn or due to processes in remote areas of the brain causing secondary changes in the Ammon's horn formation. Because eight patients in his series with 'genuine epilepsy' but a focal lesion in extratemporal areas did not have AHS, he concluded that seizures *per se* would not cause this type of cell damage.

In an attempt to explain the peculiar type of the distribution of nerve cell losses in AHS, O. Vogt (1925) introduced the term 'pathoclisis', assuming that morphologically different cell populations within the Ammon's horn must have specific chemical properties – a hypothesis fully confirmed now with modern neurochemical methods. In contrast, Spielmeyer's hypothesis (1925, 1927), that AHS is a consequence of vasospasms occurring during seizures, did not stand the test of time.

Stauder (1935) in his investigation on 53 patients with a so-called 'genuine epilepsy' was the first to report that those patients in which AHS was present at autopsy had suffered from ictal signs and symptoms (e.g. olfactory and gustatory sensations, sensory aphasia, 'dreamy states', etc.) similar to patients with seizures because of well-defined lesions (like tumours) in the temporal lobe. None of his patients with a 'genuine epilepsy' and a normal hippocampus had those 'temporal lobe symptoms'. But despite his findings Stauder did not question the old concept of 'genuine epilepsy', which at that time was thought to be a hereditary disease. Surprisingly he discussed seriously the possibility that AHS is a secondary change because of the frequent head traumas which patients with 'genuine' epilepsy would experience, although there were no data to support this hypothesis. In this publication the percentage of times that AHS was unilateral is not mentioned.

Earle *et al.* (1953) were convinced that AHS occurs due to temporal compression (herniation) during delivery, which might affect blood supply to the hippocampal formation. In their view AHS, or 'incisural sclerosis' as they called the changes, is the cause and not the consequence of seizures. The time delay between the damaging event and the onset of seizures would be explained by a process for which they used the term 'ripening'.

Scholz (1963) tried to combine the different views of O. Vogt and of W. Spielmeyer with his theory that the characteristic feature of AHS – selective neuronal loss in certain sections of the hippocampus – could be explained by the assumption that 'topistic units' would suffer anoxic damage during seizures ('local consumption' theory). This concept has not been confirmed.

Peiffer (1963) found AHS to be present in 39.6 per cent of 362 brains from patients with epilepsy; in 50 per cent it was bilateral. Neurone loss was more severe with a longer duration of the epilepsy and with a higher frequency of tonic–clonic seizures. Peiffer was convinced at that time that neuronal loss occurs as a consequence of seizures in a kind of chain reaction via hypoxia, metabolic changes, brain oedema, herniation, compression of bigger vessels, etc.

Veith (1970, 1982), who dedicated a great part of his research to the question of whether seizures would cause selective parenchymal necrosis, found AHS in 160 of 450 brains (35.5 per cent) of patients with epilepsy; it was present on both sides in 50 per cent of the cases presenting with epilepsy after the first year of life and in 67 per cent of the cases who had seizures starting within the first year of life.

For the great majority of patients in his series all kinds of pre- existing pathology or peri- and postnatal complications were known. More than half of the patients were mentally retarded. From this and the fact that he frequently found AHS in young children who died from inborn malformations or perinatal complications but did not have seizures, Veith firmly stated that AHS is not a consequence of seizures but that epilepsy and AHS may have a common underlying pathomechanism. Veith did not report an observation he made which might be of interest: when AHS was unilateral, the amygdala was usually abnormal as well, compared with bilateral AHS, where the amygdala were more often normal (G. Veith, 1993, pers. comm.).

Hanefeld and Crome's investigation (1979) of 127 brains of children with epilepsy is similar to Veith's work. Only five of the 127 children had normal intelligence, and different kinds of brain pathology besides AHS were present in most cases. Fifty-nine children (46 per cent) had AHS; it was bilateral in 51 (86 per cent). Because AHS was as frequent in the 'control group' of mentally retarded children without epilepsy, these authors also concluded that seizures cannot be the sole cause for this type of brain pathology and that pre- and perinatal damage in particular may play an essential role.

Mouritzen-Dam (1980) in her quantitative study found a decreased number of neurones in the hippocampus of 20 patients with epilepsy compared with controls; atrophy of the hippocampus was bilateral in 18 patients. All 20 patients had generalized tonic–clonic (GTC) seizures. Twelve had simple partial and seven complex partial seizures, in addition to GTC seizures. The two patients with unilateral atrophy had suffered from complex partial seizures. The amount of cell loss was correlated with the duration of the epilepsy, with the frequency of seizures but not with seizure types and not with a history of status epilepticus. Like the studies of Veith and Hanefeld, most of the patients in Mouritzen-Dam's investigation were disabled by their epilepsy and had been institutionalized.

The degree of vulnerability of hippocampus cells is most probably age-dependent, as was shown by Corsellis and Bruton in 1983. They looked for acute changes in the brains of 20 patients with epilepsy who died in status epilepticus. Severe cell loss in both hippocampi (and, to a lesser degree, in the cerebellum, thalamus, striatum and neocortex) was present in six children age 3 years and younger; it was not present in two children who died at the ages of 12 and 13 years and it was present in only three out of 13 adult patients. These acute changes are, of course, different from classical AHS.

In their quantitative study DeGiorgio *et al.* (1992), compared the findings in the hippocampal formation of five patients with epilepsy who died after an episode of 'sustained generalized convulsive status epilepticus' but where there was at least a week between the occurrence of status epilepticus and the time of death, with the findings in five normal controls and in five controls matched for age, hypoxia, ischaemia, previous epilepsy and alcohol abuse.

They demonstrated that status epilepticus causes selective cell loss in the Sommer sector and in the CA3 region, as in 'classical AHS'. There was no selective cell loss in normal controls but they could not find a statistical difference from the second control group matched for epilepsy, hypoxia and ischaemia. The standard deviation, however, was extremely high in the status epilepticus group but not in the second 'control group'. The figures are too small to draw fundamental conclusions.

Death after prolonged infantile FCs where no other reason is found is an extremely rare event. Four such cases were studied by Fowler in 1957. There was no unique picture of cerebral damage. In one child with a hemiclonic symptomatology, hippocampal and amygdaloid cell loss was unilateral (in addition to unilateral frontal and bilateral temporal neocortical damage). In two cases both temporal lobes, neocortical and hippocampal areas and both frontal lobes were mostly affected, but in one case both hippocampi were normal.

What can be concluded from this short review of the extensive work of so many neuropathologists on the association between seizures and AHS? It is obvious that many of the investigations were done on populations very different from the group of patients suffering from TLE and having a history of prolonged FCs. The vast majority of patients in the pathological series were mentally retarded and institutionalized. Many of them had perinatal complications, were handicapped or had seizures from early on in life. In contrast, most patients with TLE, MTS and a history of FCs are not mentally retarded. Indeed, they are viewed by most epilepsy surgery centres as excellent candidates for epilepsy surgery (Wieser *et al.*, 1993). Patients with TLE and MTS have almost consistently a better outcome following epilepsy surgery compared with patients with other kinds of pathology in the resected temporal lobe (Davidson & Falconer, 1975; Falconer, 1976; Lindsay *et al.*, 1984; McMillan *et al.*, 1987). The fact that patients with TLE, MTS and a history of FCs who become seizure-free after removal of the mesial temporal structures tend to be seizure-free in follow-up studies 5 years and 10 years later (Engel, 1987; Wieser, 1991) could be an argument against the assumption that MTS is a bilateral disease with one side more affected than the other one.

Moreover, all previous neuropathology series on the consequences of seizures for the brain have one major disadvantage in common: the classification of seizures and epilepsies of the subjects studied were poorly based on history. This shortcoming did not seem to play a role as long as 'systemic' factors, vascular or metabolic changes following seizure activity were blamed for the sequelae.

Interestingly, AHS was found to be predominantly unilateral in the older neuropathology series – 80 per cent in Meynert's report (1868), 96 per cent in Bratz's publication (1899) – but not in the series from the 1940s to the 1960s. One is inclined to assume that this difference is due to the fact that anticonvulsant medication was not available in the last century and therefore many patients with TLE and unilateral MTS had a far less favourable course, sometimes with rapid deterioration and death, compared with what can be achieved for this group of patients nowadays. This view is supported by the case histories in Bratz's paper in particular. On the other hand, after the invention of anticonvulsant drugs, studies on institutionalized patients with epilepsy might not have been done on the 'target group' of patients with TLE.

In the light of recent results that seizures *per se* can cause nerve cell loss, at least in the hippocampus, only those studies seem today to be suitable for scientific investigation where it has been documented that the brain areas available for histological studies were involved during the seizure activity. This is emphasized by findings from our hemispherectomy series. One child with hypomelanosis Ito and a large right-sided cortical dysplasia extending from the frontal to the parieto-occipital area had daily seizures from the second day of life for about 20 months. The girl had experienced an estimated 20,000 seizures prior to the time of the functional hemispherectomy; the seizures were focal clonic–tonic or focal tonic–clonic, and many times with cyanosis usually lasting several minutes. Presurgical evaluation revealed a centroparietal seizure origin. The hippocampal formation and its neighbouring structures of the resected temporal lobe were virtually unchanged!

In contrast, severe AHS was seen after a functional hemispherectomy in a boy age 10 years with a large central suprasylvian porencephalic cyst, whose seizures were arising from neocortical areas around the lesion, but where regular seizure spread into the mesiotemporal structures could be demonstrated by means of investigation with foramen ovale and epidural electrodes. Seizure onset was within the fourth year of life and there were several documented episodes with hemiclonic convulsions lasting 1 h and more.

For many reasons the ideal situation for study purposes will never take place: that a child who never had an unprovoked seizure will present with his/her first prolonged FC when fully hooked up to an electroencephalograph (EEG) and that the same patient will have a temporal lobectomy later on in life because of medically intractable TLE.

TLE and MTS after meningitis and encephalitis

Marks *et al.* (1992) published their data on 38 patients with a history of meningitis (n = 16) or encephalitis (n = 22) who had been evaluated for epilepsy surgery because of medically intractable partial seizures. The vast majority from the meningitis group had clinical, EEG and neuroimaging evidence of mesial TLE. In seven of eight patients who had a temporal lobectomy, neuropathology showed MTS. The postoperative outcome was excellent.

In contrast, MTS in the encephalitis group was present only when the encephalitis had occurred before the age of 4 years. Because most children in the meningitis group had the disease before age 4, the authors hypothesized that the occurrence of MTS was more dependent on the time of the central nervous system (CNS) insult than on the damaging event. Unfortunately, this publication does not give an answer to the question whether MTS is the sequela of the infection or of seizures at the time when the patients had meningitis or encephalitis, because the incidence of seizures during the time of the illness was not known and correlations therefore could not be done. Seizures are common with encephalitis (Rantala *et al.*, 1991) and with meningitis (Rosman *et al.*, 1985; Pomeroy *et al.*, 1990) and it seems possible that seizures in the acute phase of meningitis or encephalitis are FCs (Rosman et al., 1985). In the Rochester study on risk factors for complex partial seizures (Rocca *et al.*, 1987), four patients out of 82 had a history of encephalitis; two of them had seizures at that time. But it is not known whether these two differ from the two patients without seizures in terms of localization of the epileptogenic focus and in terms of the presence of MTS.

Two patients of Ounsted *et al.* (1985) who developed drug-resistant TLE 9 and 8 years after acute meningitis in childhood, but have been otherwise entirely normal, had severe convulsions during the time of the CNS infections. Neuropathology showed classical AHS after anterior temporal lobectomy. Both patients have been seizure-free postoperatively.

Animal experiments, slice investigation and kindling

During the last 25 years, with the invention of modern research techniques, many of the controversies on the association between certain types of seizures and brain damage have been solved; some important questions remain open though. A new era of research on the impact of seizures on the brain began with the work of Meldrum and his co-workers. In a series of experiments with baboons they demonstrated first that prolonged convulsions led to severe changes of 'systemic factors', such as blood-pressure, blood gases, cerebral blood flow and body temperature (Meldrum & Brierly, 1973; Meldrum & Horton, 1973), and that neurone loss occurred when these changes passed certain limits.

More importantly, they showed in subsequent experiments that seizure activity itself causes nerve cell damage; neurone loss very similar to the pattern found in humans after status epilepticus was present when 'systemic factors' were excluded – e.g. by paralysation, artificial ventilation, etc. (Meldrum *et al.*, 1973). Neuronal damage under this condition was less severe, though, compared with the findings in experiments where systemic factors played a role. Widespread lesions occurred with seizures lasting several hours. With a series of seizures of short duration induced by allylglycin, a pattern of nerve cell loss similar to hippocampal sclerosis of patients with TLE was present 1 to 6 weeks after induction (Meldrum *et al.*, 1974). Animals with this type of lesion, however, did not have spontaneous temporal lobe seizures later on (Meldrum, 1983).

It appears that the mechanism by which seizure activity causes nerve cell loss independently from systemic factors is the excessive depolarization produced by excitatory neurotransmitters like glutamate and aspartate. This was shown for the first time by Olney *et al.* (1971), who suggested the concept of excitatory amino acid toxicity (Olney, 1978). The same authors were the first to report the neurotoxicity of kainic acid, which is an analogue of glutamate (Olney *et al.*, 1974). Pyramidal neurones of the CA3 region and the dentate granule cells are most vulnerable to kainic acid (Nadler *et al.*, 1980).

Kainic acid was used by Ben-Ari and his co-workers to create a model for TLE in rodents (Ben-Ari *et al.*, 1980a, b; Ben-Ari, 1985). This model is of the utmost interest. In a series of experiments the Ben-Ari group was able to demonstrate that kainic acid had a neurotoxic effect not only at the site of injection but also on limbic structures 'distant' from the site of injection. Injection of kainic acid into the amygdala produces 'initially limbic motor seizures' in rats. There is rapid spread of epileptiform activity from the injected amygdala to the ipsilateral Ammon's horn and to the contralateral amygdala. Antagonizing of limbic seizures did not prevent the local damage at the site of injection in the amygdala but prevented nerve cell loss in the hippocampus.

It is hypothesized that the 'distant' effect is most probably caused by epileptiform activity and 'its associated convulsions', whereas the local damage occurs most probably due to a direct toxic effect of kainic acid. There is further evidence for this hypothesis in the different pattern of cell damage of the two affected sites: massive proliferation of microglia is seen early at the site of injection (the amygdala) whereas the 'distant' changes in the Ammon's horn are less pronounced and are not seen until 4–6 days after the injection into the amygdala. The histological picture of the cell damage in the hippocampus very closely resembles AHS in human TLE: the earliest changes in the hippocampus are seen in the CA3 region, the hilus and the CA1 region are affected, but the CA2 region is spared (for review see Ben-Ari, 1985).

The same 'distant' changes in the hippocampus (of rats) can be seen after sustained electrical stimulation of the perforant path (Sloviter, 1983). The perforant path from the entorhinal cortex to the dentate gyrus is the common pathway for all the inputs to the hippocampal formation from various parts of the brain, including the amygdala. The mossy fibres which are the axons of the dentate granule cells project to neurones in the CA3 region. Synaptic reorganization of mossy fibres, which might be functionally excitatory (Tauck & Nadler, 1985), occurs in the Ammon's horn formation of kainic acid-treated rats. Mossy fibre reorganization is seen also with electrical kindling of the entorrhinal cortex, amygdala or olfactory bulbs (Sutula *et al.*, 1988, 1990) and also after pentylenetetrazole-induced seizures (Galurai *et al.*, 1988).

These changes in kindled animals are of interest because axonal sprouting and mossy fibre synaptic reorganization has been shown to occur in the hippocampus of patients who have had a temporal lobectomy for drug-resistant temporal lobe seizures (Sutula *et al.*, 1989). In eight of 10 hippocampi of patients with TLE, mossy fibre reorganization was associated with hippocampal sclerosis, but in two specimens synaptic reorganization was the only finding (Babb *et al.*, 1988). So far, typical hippocampal sclerosis like that in human TLE has not developed in the kindled animals. There is loss of polymorphic neurones in the hilus of the dentate gyrus, in addition to mossy fibre reorganization, but not the characteristic pattern with severe cell loss in the CA1, CA3 and CA4 region, (Cavazos & Sutula, 1990). But structural changes in the hilus induced by abnormal functional activity may just be the first step in a process that creates local circuits of increased excitability.

Synaptic reorganization of interneurones of the hilus seems to be characteristic for the 'cryptogenic' human temporal lobe cases (see de Lanerolle, Chapter 46).

Although it is far too early to state that the cause and consequence of human mesial temporal lobe seizures have been explained by the abundant data from animal studies, some conclusions may be allowed as far as the issue of FCs and TLE is concerned:

- Prolonged seizures *per se* may cause structural changes in the hippocampal formation.
- These structural changes seem first to be of minor degree, as with mossy fibre reorganization. This could create a neuronal network which is functionally hyperexcitable.
- With severe (and frequent?) seizures AHS may develop.
- Remote lesions may cause changes in the hippocampal formation via propagation of abnormal activity spreading into the hippocampus.

The latter observation is of particular interest because, if one is looking for a pre-existing pathology in patients with TLE, MTS and a history of FCs, this hypothetical pathology could be located 'remote' from the mesial temporal structures.

Although less important for the investigation on the association between FCs, MTS and TLE, it should be mentioned that the specific distribution of nerve cell loss in AHS seems to be well understood now. Nerve cell death due to excessive activation (burst firing) occurs due to an increase in intracellular Ca^{2+} when the capacity of calcium-buffering proteins of these cells is limited (Meldrum *et al.*, 1973; Schanne *et al.*, 1979; Griffiths *et al.*, 1984). Calcium-buffering proteins are not present in the CA3 region (which is rich in kainate receptors) or in the CA1 region (which is rich in *N*-methyl-D-aspartate (NMDA) receptors) (Sloviter, 1989). In the CA4 region the calcium buffering protein calbindin is present in the dentate granule cells but not in the hilar interneurones or the mossy cells (Sloviter *et al.*, 1991).

Results of animal experiments have possibly given the answer to the question why there are no reports on the association between neonatal convulsions and MTS or convulsions at an age younger than 3 months. Peterson *et al.* (1989) reported that because receptors were not developed at a young age hippocampal neurones of newborn rats were resistant to the neurotoxic effect of NMDA. Sperber *et al.* (1990) could show that with kindling in rat pups no synaptic reorganization could be observed, in contrast to adult rats; they concluded that the immature CNS may be resistant to the development of 'epileptic damage'.

Concluding remarks

The lesion most often found in TLE is MTS. There is strong evidence that this structural abnormality is the cause of 'limbic' psychomotor seizures for the vast majority of patients with TLE.

MTS is predominantly unilateral in patients with 'mesial TLE'. Several damaging factors are known to produce MTS or AHS.

There is no doubt that children with long-lasting lateralized FCs are at risk for TLE. Children with FCs must be followed up for at least 20 years before outcome figures on the association with TLE become reliable. Patients with mesial TLE and a history of prolonged lateralized FCs have MTS contralateral to the side of the convulsion in childhood.

In the light of recent results in different fields of research on the possible aetiology of mesial TLE the following assumptions may therefore be allowed:

1. Neuronal populations within the Ammon's horn formation may be involved in lateralized FCs. Cell death may occur with prolonged lateralized FCs, due to excessive intracellular Ca^{2+} influx.
2. Functionally hyperexcitable synaptic reorganization takes place over time, creating a network which might after several years be powerful enough to exhibit 'limbic' seizures. In that sense MTS would be the consequence of FCs and the cause of TLE.

But this view is still a hypothetical one. As long as we do not know the cause and the mechanism of action of prolonged lateralized FCs, a different explanation may be found later on. Prospective MRI studies on children with prolonged and lateralized FCs could be helpful. This type of investigation would most probably reveal if hippocampal asymmetry develops over time or if differences are already present at the time of the FCs.

So far, there are no data to support the idea that FCs with focal signs are just the first manifestation of TLE or that a pre-existing pathology is responsible both for the prolonged FCs and for the later TLE.

As far as prevention of TLE is concerned, no one knows if antiepileptic medication given to children with FCs with risk factors can actually prevent later epilepsy because these studies haven't been conducted. The incidence of TLE following FCs in recent prospective studies is low. The figures of children with long-lasting FCs (of more than 30 min duration) in these studies are also low. The hemiconvulsion–hemiplegia syndrome is now almost non-existent. One is inclined to believe that these facts are achievements due to advances in the field of modern intensive care for young children at risk.

References

Aicardi, J. (1987): Status epilepticus in infants and children: consequences and prognosis. *Int. Pediatr.* **2,** 189–195.

Aicardi, J. & Chevrie, J.J. (1970): Convulsive status epilepticus in infants and children – a study of 239 cases. *Epilepsia* **11,** 187–197.

Aicardi, J. & Chevrie, J.J. (1976): Febrile convulsions: neurological sequelae and mental retardation. In: *Brain dysfunction in infantile febrile convulsions,* eds. M.A.B. Brazier & F. Coceani, pp. 247–257. New York: Raven Press.

Aicardi, J. & Chevrie, J.J. (1983): Consequences of status epilepticus in infants and children. In: *Status epilepticus (Advances in Neurology,* 34), eds. A.V. Delgado-Escueta, C.G. Wasterlain, D.M. Treiman & R.J. Porter, pp. 115–125. New York: Raven Press.

Annegers, J.F., Hauser, W.A., Elveback, L.R. & Kurland, L.T. (1979): The risk of epilepsy following febrile convulsions. *Neurology* **29,** 297–303.

Annegers, J.F., Hauser, W.A., Shirts, S.B. & Kurland, L.T. (1987): Factors prognostic of unprovoked seizure after febrile convulsions. *N. Engl. J. Med.* **316,** 493–498.

Babb, T.L. & Brown, W.J. (1987): Pathological findings in epilepsy. In: *Surgical treatment of the epilepsies,* ed. J. Engel, Jr, pp. 511–540. New York: Raven Press.

Babb, T.L., Kupfer, W.R. & Pretorius, J.K. (1988): Synaptic reorganization of mossy fibres into the inner molecular layer in human epileptic fascia dentata. *Soc. Neurosci. Abstr.* **14,** 881.

Ben-Ari, Y. (1985): Limbic seizure and brain damage produced by kainic acid: mechanisms and relevance to human temporal lobe epilepsy. *Neuroscience* **14** (2), 375–403.

Ben-Ari, Y., Tremblay, E. & Ottersen, O.P. (1980a): Injections of kainic acid into the amygdaloid complex of the rat: an electrographic, clinical and histological study in relation to the pathology of epilepsy. *Neuroscience* **5,** 515–528.

Ben-Ari, Y., Tremblay, E., Ottersen, O.P. & Meldrum, B.S. (1980b): The role of epileptic activity in hippocampal and 'remote' cerebral lesions induced by kainic acid. *Brain Res.* **91,** 79–97.

Berkovic, S.F., Andermann, F., Olivier, A., Ethier, R., Melanson, D., Robitaille, Y., Kuzniecky, R., Peters, T. & Feindel, W. (1991): Hippocampal sclerosis in temporal lobe epilepsy demonstrated by magnetic resonance imaging. *Ann. Neurol.* **29,** 175–182.

Bouchet, C. & Cazauvieilh, V. (1825): De l'epilepsie concideree dans ses rapports avec la l'alienation mentale. *Arch. Gen. Med.* **9,** 510–542.

Bratz E. (1899): Ammonshornbefunde bei Epileptischen. *Arch. Psychiatr. Nervenkr.* **32,** 820–835.

Brown, W.J. (1973): Structural substrates of seizure foci in the human temporal lobe. In: *Epilepsy: its phenomena in man,* ed. M.A.B. Brazier, pp. 339–374. New York: Academic Press.

Brown, W.J. & Babb, T.L. (1986): Central pathological considerations of complex partial seizures. In: *Epilepsy,* ed. A. Hopkins. Chapman and Hall.

Bruton, C.J. (1984): Neuropathology of temporal lobectomy. MD thesis, University of London.

Cavanagh, J.B. & Meyer, A. (1956): Aetiological aspects of Ammon's horn sclerosis associated with temporal lobe epilepsy. *Br. Med. J.* **2,** 1403–1407.

Cavazos, J. & Sutula, T. (1990): Progressive neuronal loss induced by kindling: a possible mechanism in mossy fibre reorganization and hippocampal sclerosis. *Brain Res.* **527,** 1–6.

Consensus statement on febrile seizures. (1981): In: *Febrile seizures,* eds. K.B. Nelson & J.H. Ellenberg, pp. 301–306. New York: Raven Press.

Corsellis, J.A.N. & Bruton, C.J. (1983): Neuropathology of status epilepticus in humans. In: *Status epilepticus (Advances in neurology,* 34), eds. A.V. Delgado-Escueta, C.G. Wasterlain, D.M. Treiman & R.J. Porter, pp. 129–139. New York: Raven Press.

Darkins, A. & Polkey, C.E. (1985): The relationship of transient hemiparesis following febrile convulsions in infancy to subsequent temporal lobectomy for intractable seizures. *J. Neurol. Neurosurg. Psychiat.ry* **48** (6), 551–555.

Davidson, S. & Falconer, M.A. (1975): Outcome of surgery in 40 children with temporal-lobe epilepsy. *Lancet* **i,** 1260–1263.

DeGiorgio, C.M., Tomiyasu, U., Gott, P.S. & Treiman, D.M. (1992): Hippocampal pyramidal cell loss in human status epilepticus. *Epilepsia* **33** (1), 23–27.

Earle, K.M., Baldwin, M. & Penfield, W. (1953): Incisural sclerosis and temporal lobe seizures produced by hippocampal herniation at birth. *Arch. Neurol. Psychiat.ry (Chigago)* **69,** 27–42.

Engel, J., Jr (ed.) (1987): *Surgical treatment of the epilepsies.* New York: Raven Press.

Falconer, M.A. (1974): Mesial temporal (Ammon's horn) sclerosis as a common cause of epilepsy – etiology, treatment, and prevention. *Lancet* **ii** 767–770.

Falconer, M.A. (1976): Surgical treatment of sequelae of severe febrile convulsions. In: *Brain dysfunction in infantile febrile convulsions,* eds. M.A.B. Brazier & F. C'oceani, pp. 307–326. New York: Raven Press.

Falconer, M.A. & Taylor, D.C. (1968): Surgical treatment of drug-resistant epilepsy due to mesial temporal sclerosis. *Arch. Neurol.* **18,** 253–261.

Falconer, M.A., Serafetinides, E.A. & Corsellis, J.A.N. (1964): Etiology and pathogenesis of temporal lobe epilepsy. *Arch. Neurol.* **10,** 233–248.

Fowler, M. (1957): Brain damage after febrile convulsions. *Arch. Dis. Child.* **32,** 67–76.

Fujiwara, T., Ishida, S., Miyakoshi, M., Sakuma, N., Moriyama, S., Morikawa, T., Seino, M. & Wada, T. (1979): Status epilepticus in childhood: a retrospective study of initial convulsive status and subsequent epilepsies. *Folia Psychiatr. Neurol. Japan* **33** (3), 337–344.

Gastaut, H., Poirier, F., Payan, G., Salamon, G., Toga, M. & Vigouroux, M. (1960): HHE syndrome: hemiconvulsions, hemiplegia, epilepsy. *Epilepsia* **1,** 418–447.

Gloor, P. (1991): Mesial temporal sclerosis: historical background and an overview from a modern perspective. In: *Epilepsy surgery,* ed. H. Lüders, pp. 689–703. New York: Raven Press.

Golarai, G., Parada, I. & Sutula, T. (1988): Mossy fiber synaptic reorganization ainducerd by repetitive pentylenetetrazol seizures. *Soc. Neurosci. Abstr.* **14,** 882.

Green, J.R. (1967): Temporal lobectomy, with special reference to selection of epileptic patients. *J. Neurosurg.* **26,** 584–594.

Griffiths, T., Evans, M.C. & Meldrum, B.S. (1984): Intracellular calcium accumulation in rat hippocampus during seizures induced by bicuculline or L-allylglycine. *Neuroscience* **10,** 385–395.

Hanefeld, F. & Crome, L. (1979): Beziehungen zwischen Epilepsie und neuropathologischen Befunden im Kindesalter. In: *Epilepsie* (1978), eds. H. Doose & G. Groβ-Selbeck, pp. 66–77. Stuttgart: Thieme Verlag.

Hassan, A.H., El-Banhawy, A., El-Gengaihy, T. & El- Gengaihy, E. (1966): A study of Egyptian epileptics with temporal lobe focus. *J. Egypt. Med. Assoc.* **49,** 529–541.

Hauser, W.A. (1992): Seizure disorders: the changes with age. *Epilepsia* **33** (suppl. 4), 6–14.

Jensen, I. (1976): Temporal lobe epilepsy – etiological factors and surgical results. *Acta Neur. Scand.* **53,** 103–118.

Kotagal, P., Rothner, A.D., Erenberg, G., Cruse, R.P. & Wyllie, E. (1987): Complex partial seizures of childhood onset – a five-year follow-up study. *Arch. Neurol.* **44,** 1177–1180.

Lee, K., Diaz, M. & Melchior, J.C. (1981): Temporal lobe epilepsy – not a consequence of childhood febrile convulsions in Denmark. *Acta Neurol. Scand.* **63,** 231–236.

Lennox, W.G. (1950): Phenomena and correlates of psychomotor triad. *Neurology* **1,** 357.

Lennox, W.G. (1953): Significance of febrile convulsions. *Pediatrics* **11,** 341–357.

Lindsay, J., Glaser, G., Richards, P. & Ounsted, C. (1984): Developmental aspects of focal epilepsies of childhood treated by neurosurgery. *Dev. Med. Child Neur.* **26,** 574–587.

McMillan, T.M., Powell, G.E., Janota, I. & Polkey, C.E. (1987): Relationship between neuropathology and cognitive functioning in temporal lobectomy patients. *J. Neurol. Neurosurg. Psychiat.ry* **50,** 167–176.

Margerison, J.H. & Corsellis, J.A.N. (1966): Epilepsy and the temporal lobes. *Brain* **89,** 499–530

Marks, D.A., Kim, J., Spencer, D.D. & Spencer, S.S. (1992): Characteristics of intractable seizures following meningitis and encephalitis. *Neurology* **42,** 1513–1518.

Mathieson, G. (1975): Pathology of temporal lobe foci. In: *Advances in Neurology,* Vol. 11, eds. J.K. Penry & D.D. Daly, pp. 163–185. New York: Raven Press.

Maytal, J., Shinnar, S., Moshe, S.L. & Alvarez, L.A. (1989): Low morbidity and mortality of status epilepticus in children. *Pediatrics* **83** (3), 323–329.

Meencke, H.J. & Veith, G. (1991): Hippocampal sclerosis in epilepsy. In: *Epilepsy surgery,* ed. H.O. Lüders, pp. 705–715. New York: Raven Press.

Meldrum, B.S. (1983): Metabolic factors during prolonged seizures and their relation to nerve cell death. In: *Status epilepticus (Advances in Neurology,* 34), eds. A.V. Delgado-Escueta, C.G. Wasterlain, D.M. Treiman & R.J. Porter, pp. 261–275. New York: Raven Press.

Meldrum, B.S. & Brierley, J.B. (1973): Prolonged epileptic seizures in primates: ischaemic cell change and its relation to ictal physiological events. *Arch. Neurol.* **28,** 10–17.

Meldrum, B.S. & Horton, R.W. (1973): Physiology of status epilepticus in primates. *Arch. Neurol.* **28,** 1–9.

Meldrum, B.S., Vigouroux, R.A. & Brierley, J.B. (1973): Systemic factors and epileptic brain damage. *Arch. Neurol.* **29,** 82–88.

Meldrum, B.S., Horton, R.W. & Brierley, J.B. (1974): Epileptic brain damage in adolescent baboons following seizures induced by allylglycine. *Brain* **97,** 417–428.

Meyer, A. Falsoner, N.A. & Beck, E. (1954): Pathological findings in temporal lobe epilepsy. *J. Neurol. Neurosurg. Psychiatry* **17,** 276–285.

Meynert, T. (1868): Studien über das pathologisch-anatomische Material der Wiener Irren-Anstalt. *Vierteljahresschrift für Psychiatrie in ihren Beziehungen zur Morphologie und Pathologie, Statistik und gerichtliche Medicin,* Vol. 2, pp. 381–402.

Millichap, J.G. (1968): Definition and statistics. In: *Febrile convulsions,* ed. J.G. Millichap, pp. 1–16. New York: Macmillan.

Mouritzen Dam, A. (1980): Epilepsy and neuron loss in the hippocampus. *Epilepsia* **21,** 617–629.

Nadler, J.V., Perry, B.W., Gentry, C. & Cotman, C.W. (1980): Degeneration of hipppocampal CA3 pyramidal cells induced by intraventricular kainic acid. *J. Comp. Neurol.* **192,** 333–359.

Nelson, K.B. & Ellenberg, J.H. (1978): Prognosis in children with febrile seizures. *Pediatrics* **61** (5), 720–727.

Olney, J.W. (1978): Neurotoxicity of excitatory amino acids. In: *Kainic acid as a tool in neurobiology,* eds. E.G. McGeer, J.W. Olney, P.L. & McGeer, pp. 95–121. New York: Raven Press.

Olney, J.W., Ho, O.C. & Rhee, V. (1971): Cytotoxic effects to acidic and sulphur containing amino acids on the infant mouse central nervous system. *Exp. Brain Res.* **14,** 61–76.

Olney, J.W., Rhee, V. & Ho, O.L. (1974): Kainic acid: a powerful neurotoxic analogue of glutamate. *Brain Res.* **77,** 507–512.

Ounsted, C., Glaser, G.H., Lindsay, J. & Richards, P. (1985): Focal epilepsy with mesial temporal sclerosis after acute meningitis. *Arch. Neurol.* **42** (11), 1058–1060.

Paillas, J.E. (1958): Aspects cliniques de l'épilepsie temporale. In: *Temporal lobe epilepsy,* eds. M. Baldwin & R. Bailey, pp. 411–439. Springfield: C.C. Thomas.

Peterson, C., Neal, J.H. & Cotman, C.W. (1989): Development of *N*-methyl-D-aspartate excitotoxity in cultured hippocampal neurons. *Dev. Brain Res.* **48,** 187–195.

Pfeiffer, J. (1963): Morphologische Aspekte der Epilepsien. In: *Pathologische, Pathologisch-anatomische und klinische Probleme der Epilepsien,* Vol. 100, eds. M. Müller, H. Spatz & P. Vogel. Berlin, Göttingen, Heidelberg: Springer Verlag.

Pfleger, L. (1880): Beobachtungen über Schrumpfung und Sclerose des Ammonshorns bei Epilepsie. *Allg. Zeitschr. Psych.* **36,** 359–365.

Pomeroy, S.L., Holmes, S.J., Dodge, P.R. & Feigin, R.D. (1990): Seizures and other neurologic sequelae of bacterial meninigtis in children. *N. Engl. J. Med.* **323** (24), 1651–1657.

Rantala, H., Uhari, M., Uhari, M., Saukkonen, A.L. & Sorri, M. (1991): Outcome after childhood encephalitis. *Dev. Med. Child Neurol.* **33,** 858–867.

Rocca, W.A., Sharbrough, F.W., Hauser, W.A., Annegers, J.F. & Schoenberg, B.S. (1987): Risk factors for complex partial seizures: a population-based case-control study. *Ann. Neurol.* **21,** 22–31.

Roger, J., Lob, H. & Tassinari, C.A. (1974): Status epilepticus. In: *Handbook of clinical neurology: the epilepsies,* Vol. 15, eds. P.J. Vinken & G.W. Bruyn, pp. 145–188. Amsterdam: North-Holland.

Rosman, N.P., Peterson, D.B., Kaye, E.M. & Colton, T. (1985): Seizures in bacterial meningitis: prevalence, patterns, pathogenesis, and prognosis. *Pediatr. Neurol.* **1,** 278–285.

Ross, E.M., Peckham, C.S., West, P.B. & Butler, N.R. (1980): Epilepsy in childhood: findings from the National Child Development Study. *Br. Med. J.* **1,** 207–210.

Ryvlin, P., Philippon, B., Cinotti, L., Froment, J.C., Le Bars, D. & Mauguière, F. (1992): Functional neuroimaging strategy in temporal lobe epilepsy: a comparative study of ^{18}FDG-PET and ^{99}TC-HMPAO-SPECT. *Ann. Neurol* **31,** 650–656.

Sagar, H.J. & Oxbury, J.M. (1987): Hippocampal neural loss in temporal lobe epilepsy: correlation with early childhood convulsions. *Ann. Neurol.* **22,** 334–340.

Schanne, F.A.X., Kane, A.B., Young, E.E. & Forber, J.L. (1979): Calcium dependence of toxic cell death: a final common pathway. *Science* **206,** 700–702.

Schmidt, D., Tsai, J.-J. & Janz, D. (1985): Febrile seizures in patients with complex partial seizures. *Acta Neurol. Scand.* (Short Comm.) **72,** 68–71.

Scholz, W. (1963): 'Topistic' lesions. In: *Selective vulnerability of the brain in hypoxaemia*, eds. J.P. Schadé & W.H. McMenemey, pp. 257–267. Oxford: Blackwell Scientific Publications.

Sloviter, R.S. (1983): Epileptic brain damage in rats induced by sustained electrical stimulation of the perforant path. I. Acute electrophysiological and light microscopic studies. *Brain Res. Bull.* **10,** 675–698.

Sloviter, R.S. (1989): Calcium-binding protein (Calbindin-D28KO) and parvalbumin immunocytochemistry: localization in the rat hippocampus with specific reference to the selective vulnerability of hippocampal neurons to seizure acitivity. *J. Comp. Neurol.* **280,** 183–196.

Sloviter, R.S., Sollas, A.L., Barbaro, N.M. & Laxer, K.D. (1991): Calcium-binding protein (Calbindin-D28K) and parvalbumin immunocytochemistry in the normal and epileptic human hippocampus. *J. Comp. Neurol.* **308,** 381–396.

Sommer, W. (1880): Erkrankung des Ammonshorns als Atiologisches Moment der Epilepsie. *Arch. Psychiatr. Nervenkr.* **10,** 631–675.

Sperber, E.F., Sutula, T.P. & Moshé, S.L. (1990): Synaptic sprouting following kindled seizures is age related. *Epilepsia* **31** (5), 633.

Spielmeyer, W. (1925): Zur Pathogenese örtlich elektiver Gehirnveränderungen. *Ztschr. Neurol. Psychiatr.* **99,** 756–776.

Spielmeyer, W. (1927): Die Pathogenese des epileptischen Krampfes. *Histopathologischer Teil. Ztschr. Neurol. Psychiat.* **109,** 501–519.

Stauder, K.H. (1935): Epilepsie und Schläfenlappen. *Arch. Psychiatr.* **104,** 181–212.

Sutula, T.P. (1990): Experimental models of temporal lobe epilepsy: new insights from the study of kindling and synaptic reorganization. *Epilepsia* **31** (3), 45–54.

Sutula, T., Xuiao-Xian, H., Cavazos, J. & Scott, G. (1988): Synaptic reorganization in the hippocampus induced by abnormal functional activity. *Science* **239,** 1147–1150.

Sutula, T., Cascino, G., Cavazos, J., Parada, I. & Ramirez, L. (1989): Mossy fibre synaptic reorganization in the epileptic human temporal lobe. *Ann. Neurol.* **26,** 321–330.

Tauck, D.L. & Nadler, J.V. (1985): Evidence of functional mossy fiber sprouting in hippocampal formation of kainic acid-treated cats. *J. Neurosci.* **5,** 1016–1022.

Taylor, D.C. & Ounsted, C. (1971): Biological mechanisms influencing the outcome of seizures in response to fever. *Epilepsia* **12,** 33–45.

Veith, G. (1970): Anatomische Studie über die Ammonshornsklerose im Epileptikergehirn. *Dtsch. Z. Nervenheilk.* **197,** 293–314.

Veith, G. (1982): *Ergebnisse morphologischer Epilepsieforschung: mit Beitrügen zur umstrittenen Pathogenese zerebraler Parenchymschadigungen und deren klinischer Bedeutung.* Gesellschaft fur Epilepsieforschung, Verlag Bodelschwinghsche Anstalten Bielefeld.

Verity, C.M. & Golding, J. (1991): Risk of epilepsy after febrile convulsions: a national cohort study. Br. Med. J. **303,** 1376–1383.

Verity, C.M., Butler, N.R. & Golding, J. (1985): Febrile convulsions in a national cohort followed up from birth. II – Medical history and intellectual ability at 5 years of age. *Br. Med. J.* **290,** 1311–1315.

Vogt, O. (1925): Der Begriff der Pathoklise. *J. Psychol. Neurol.* (Leipzig) **31,** 245–255.

Wallace, S.J. (1982): Prognosis after prolonged unilateral febrile convulsions. In: *Advances in epileptology, XIIIth Epilepsy International Symposium,* eds. H. Akimoto, H. Kazamatsuri, M. Seino, pp. 97–100. New York: Raven Press.

Wallace, S.J. (1988): Prognosis for non-febrile seizures. In: *The child with febrile seizures*, ed. S.J. Wallace, pp. 109–126. London: Butterworth.

Wieser, H.G. (1991): Selective amygdalohippocampectomy: indications and follow-up. *Can. J. Neurol. Sci.* **18,** 617–627.

Wieser, H.G., Engel, J., Jr, Williamson, P.D., Babb, T.L. & Gloor, P. (1993): Surgically remediable temporal lobe syndromes. In: *Surgical treatment of the epilepsies*, 2nd edn, ed. J. Engel, Jr, pp. 49–63. New York: Raven Press.

Wohlrab, G., Holthausen, H., Moch, A., Tuxhorn, I. & Fortenbacher, I. (1993): Temporallappenepilepsie und frühe mentale Retardation. Posterpräsentation auf der Jahrestagung der Deutschen Gesellschaft für Neuropädiatrie, Dresden.

Epileptic Seizures and Syndromes, Edited by Peter Wolf
© 1994 John Libbey & Company Ltd., pp. 469–480

Chapter 48

Age dependency of seizure-induced hippocampal dysfunction

Ellen F. Sperber

Albert Einstein College of Medicine, Departments of Neurology and Neuroscience, 316 Rose F. Kennedy Center, 1410 Pelham Parkway S., Bronx, New York 10461, USA

Summary

Mesial temporal sclerosis and temporal lobe epilepsy in adulthood have been attributed to seizure-induced damage in early life. However, clinical studies suggesting that seizures induce damage in children are inconclusive. In the present report, the question of whether seizures produce age-related changes in the hippocampus is studied by determining whether seizures produce damage in developing rats. Several seizure models were employed to induce seizures in immature and adult rats including: kainic acid, flurothyl and kindling. Hippocampal damage was determined neuroanatomically by assessing cell loss and mossy fibre sprouting and electrophysiologically by the *in vitro* slice preparation. Results indicate that seizures produce hippocampal damage in adult rats but not in developing rats. Several possible explanations for the greater resistance to seizure-induced hippocampal damage in immature rats are discussed.

Introduction

Temporal lobe epilepsy is the most frequent form of epilepsy in adults. Approximately 40–60 per cent of newly diagnosed epileptic cases are classified as temporal lobe epilepsy (Hauser & Kurland, 1975; Granieri *et al.*, 1983; Joensen, 1986). The seizures are associated with a partial or complete loss of consciousness, lack of responsiveness to external stimuli, presence of automatisms and some degree of anterograde or retrograde amnesia. Hippocampal tissue obtained at autopsy or from patients with intractable seizures following anterior lobectomy reveals a specific type of hippocampal damage referred to as mesial temporal sclerosis. Mesial temporal sclerosis is characterized by extensive cell loss in the CA3 pyramidal neurones (hippocampal endblades) and often CA1 (Sommer sector). In contrast, pyramidal cells of the small transitional zone between CA1 and CA3 (CA2 area or resistant sector) and the granule cells of the dentate gyrus, subiculum and fibres *en passage* remain intact (Margerison & Corsellis, 1966; Bruton, 1988). The extent of the sclerosis appears to be correlated with the severity of the seizure disorder (Margerison & Corsellis, 1966).

The primary hippocampal afferent is the entorhinal cortex, which terminates on granule cells in the dentate gyrus. Under normal conditions, the axons of these granule cells, mossy fibres, form synapses with the diverse polymorphic neurones in the hilar region and the pyramidal neurones in the CA3 region of the hippocampus. The Timm–Haug silver sulphide histochemical procedure has become a valuable tool in visualizing mossy fibre terminals and their synaptic reorganization. The Timm stain detects zinc, which is particularly abundant in the mossy fibre synaptic boutons (Timm, 1958; Haug, 1967). This stain has recently been used to demonstrate the formation of aberrant mossy fibre terminals following damage of the hilar and CA3/4 pyramidal cells. Loss or damage of these cells may occur following seizures. Therefore, the presence of mossy fibre synaptic reorganization in the dentate gyrus can be used as a marker of hilar and CA3/4 pyramidal cell loss. Tissue obtained from temporal lobe epileptic patients reveals synaptic reorganization of mossy fibre terminals in the supragranular layer of the dentate gyrus (Babb *et al.*, 1988; Sutula *et al.*, 1989; Houser *et al.*, 1990). Therefore, it appears that temporal lobe epilepsy is associated with a specific pattern of hippocampal cell loss, mesial temporal sclerosis and aberrant mossy fibre synapses in the dentate gyrus.

There has been much debate regarding the relationship between temporal lobe epilepsy and seizures early in life. The question has been repeatedly raised, 'Is the hippocampal sclerosis a consequence of convulsions early in life?' or 'Is the sclerosis a result of an injury that becomes epileptogenic'? Two different approaches suggest that seizures in infancy result in mesial temporal sclerosis and this damage predisposes the child to adult chronic epilepsy. The first approach is based on autopsied brains of children that died following status epilepticus. Corsellis and Bruton (1983) observed hippocampal changes in children who died during or following status epilepticus. However, because the aetiology is unknown, it cannot be determined if the damage was present prior to status epilepticus or a result of status epilepticus. Zimmerman (1938) demonstrated that hypoxia and asphyxia in infants with or without convulsions can produce damage similar to mesial temporal sclerosis with a greater involvement of the CA1 area. These findings suggest that the damage is a function of hypoxia and asphyxia and not the result of the convulsion. In fact, Represa *et al.* (1989) report an absence of hippocampal lesions in children who experienced seizures. Based on autopsy studies, it is therefore difficult to establish whether seizures do indeed produce hippocampal damage in young children.

The second approach which suggests that seizures early in life result in epilepsy at a later age is reports of adult patients with intractable temporal lobe epilepsy and mesial temporal sclerosis who had anterior temporal lobectomy. These studies found a high incidence of convulsions (especially febrile) or status epilepticus early in life (Falconer, 1971; Sagar & Oxbury, 1987), thereby suggesting that temporal lobe epilepsy and its concomitant pathological changes (mesial temporal sclerosis) are the result of seizure early in life (Aicardi & Chevrie, 1970; Ellenberg *et al.*, 1984). However, it is impossible to determine from these retrospective clinical studies the actual age when seizures produced the damage, whether hippocampal damage was present prior to the onset of the seizures and the effect of hippocampal damage on seizure occurrence. None the less, Falconer *et al.* (1964, 1971) proposed that most infantile (especially febrile) seizures were responsible for the development of mesial temporal sclerosis and temporal lobe epilepsy in adults. Based on the findings of these retrospective studies, the prevailing view of the 1960s and 1970s was that seizures and status epilepticus in infancy produced mesial temporal sclerosis and subsequently temporal lobe epilepsy in adulthood.

These retrospective findings are in contrast to more recent prospective studies, which do not indicate a causal relationship between childhood seizures and subsequent temporal lobe epilepsy. Nelson and Ellenberg (1976) found that only a small percentage of children with febrile seizures develop temporal lobe epilepsy later in life. Similarly, Shinnar *et al.* (1990) and Berg and Shinnar (1991) report that the risk of seizure recurrence in children following one unprovoked idiopathic seizure is low. The age of the initial seizure or seizure severity and duration did not effect the likelihood of recurrence, whereas aetiology of the seizure was one of the most important predictors. These studies indicate that children with evidence of a brain lesion, injury or malformation were more likely to experience repeated seizures. This suggests that there may be a relationship between seizure recurrence and the presence of previous damage. Several additional studies (Dunn, 1988; Maytal *et al.*, 1989; Maytal & Shinnar, 1990; Shinnar *et al.*, 1992) report that status epilepticus in children without an antecedent injury does not result in brain damage or recurrent seizures later in life. Thus, these prospective studies suggest that seizures in childhood are not associated with clinical sequelae unless a brain insult is already present. Furthermore, recent studies of epileptic children who underwent temporal lobe resectioning indicate that mesial temporal sclerosis is infrequently observed in children under 12 years of age and, when present, is significantly less severe (Dunn, 1988; Duchowny *et al.*, 1992) and often associated with other abnormalities, such as cortical dysplasias or hamartomas.

In this chapter, we are addressing the question, 'Is seizure-induced damage age-related'? Temporal lobe epilepsy is associated with mesial temporal sclerosis in adults. However, it is not clear at what age the damage occurs. Several studies indicate that status epilepticus and seizures have the highest incidence and onset during infancy (Hauser, 1983, 1990). In fact, Maytal *et al.* (1989) demonstrate that, regardless of the aetiology of the seizure, the highest incidence of status epilepticus is between 1 and 3 years of age, particularly for febrile status epilepticus. This suggests that the immature brain is more susceptible to status epilepticus and seizures than the mature brain. None the less, this does not necessarily indicate that young children are more susceptible to seizure-induced hippocampal damage.

The above studies highlight some of the problems inherent in clinical research, including: obtaining biopsies soon after the seizure, controlling for the age of onset of initial seizure, number of subsequent seizures and presence of prior brain damage. Since animal studies are not limited by such factors, animal models were used to determine whether seizures early in life result in hippocampal damage and whether the presence of damage increases the likelihood of seizures and damage later in life.

Kainic acid, an analogue of the excitatory amino acid neurotransmitter, glutamate, is a potent excitotoxin (Olney *et al.*, 1974; Schwarcz *et al.*, 1978; Shinozaki & Koniski, 1980). Regardless of the route of administration, kainic acid results in characteristic behavioural and electrographic seizures that parallel temporal lobe epilepsy in humans. Similar to temporal lobe epilepsy: kainic acid produces partial seizures with secondary generalization involving limbic structures (Menini *et al.*, 1980; Schwob *et al.*, 1980; Ben-Ari *et al.*, 1981; Lothman & Collins, 1981; Tanaka *et al.*, 1982); at high doses, kainic acid produces status epilepticus (Nadler *et al.*, 1978; Ben-Ari *et al.*, 1981; Albala *et al.*, 1984; Holmes & Thompson, 1988; Sperber *et al.*, 1991c) and recurrent spontaneous seizures (Kleinrok *et al.*, 1980; Pisa *et al.*, 1980; Cavalheiro *et al.*, 1983a; Thompson *et al.*, 1990); kainic acid seizures are blocked by the same anticonvulsants (Nadler *et al.*, 1986) and is associated with a similar pattern of hippocampal damage (Nadler *et al.*, 1978; Lothman & Collins, 1981; Nitecka *et al.*, 1984).

Kainic acid seizure-induced changes in adult rats

Kainic acid, when administered to adult rats (15 mg/kg, intraperitoneally (IP)), results in status epilepticus lasting 30 min or longer. At least 2 weeks following the seizure, the brains were examined for neuroanatomical and neurophysiological changes. Neuroanatomical assessment included light microscopy, using cresyl violet histology to assess neuronal loss and Timm histochemistry to identify mossy fibre synaptic reorganization. Histological results demonstrate dramatic cell loss, particularly in the hilus and CA3/4 hippocampal area of adult rats (Fig. 1a). The remaining hippocampal subfields, fibres *en passage*, dentate gyrus and subiculum were intact. This pattern of damage following kainic acid treatment in adult rats has been reported by others (Nadler *et al.*, 1978; Lothman & Collins, 1981; Nitecka *et al.*, 1984) and parallels the hippocampal damage that is characteristic of temporal lobe epileptic patients (Earle *et al.*, 1953; Cavanagh & Meyer, 1956; Gastaut *et al.*, 1958; Falconer *et al.*, 1964; Margerison & Corsellis, 1966; Mathieson, 1975; Babb *et al.*, 1988; Bruton, 1988).

Kainic acid seizure, in adult rats, resulted in extensive positive Timm staining in the supragranular layer of the hippocampal dentate gyrus. This indicates the presence of synaptic sprouting and reorganization of the mossy fibre terminals in this area (Fig. 1c). The labelling of synaptic terminals was dense and extended in a continuous band between the blades and throughout the crest of the dentate gyrus. A similar pattern of mossy fibre terminal reorganization following kainic acid seizures

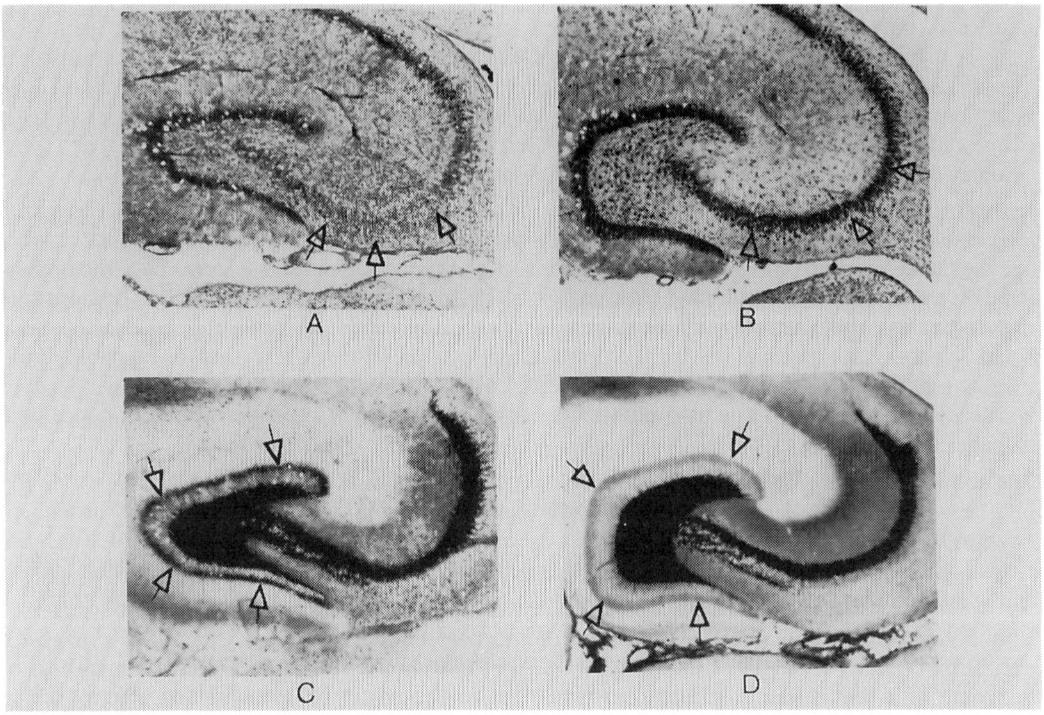

Fig. 1. Kainic acid seizure results in age-related hippocampal damage. In adult rats, kainic acid seizure-induced damage is indicated by extensive cell loss in the hippocampal CA3/CA4 area (A) and mossy fibre sprouting in the supragranular layer of the dentate gyrus (C). In contrast, in rat pups following kainic acid seizure, no cell loss (B) or synaptic reorganization (D) is apparent. (thionin stain, A and B; Timm–Haug silver sulphide histochemistry, C and D; horizontal sections).

in adult rats has been observed by others (Tauck & Nadler, 1985; Cronin & Dudek, 1988), in addition to that observed in tissue specimens from human adults with temporal lobe epilepsy (Babb *et al.*, 1988; Sutula *et al.*, 1989; Houser *et al.*, 1990).

Reorganization of mossy fibre terminals and newly formed synapses may alter the levels of excitation or inhibition in the dentate granule layer (Tauck & Nadler, 1985). To determine if these newly sprouted fibres have functional significance, we examined the response of the aberrant mossy fibre synapses in the dentate supragranular layer to perforant path stimulation by using *in vitro* slice preparation. Hippocampal slices from rats treated with kainic acid were stimulated in the perforant path, using an orthodromic paired-pulse paradigm. Population spikes were recorded from the dentate granule cell layer. The percentage change in amplitude of the second population spike (test pulse) to the initial population spike (conditioning pulse) at various interstimulus intervals from 10 to 10,000 ms was calculated. Results indicate a triphasic profile in slices from the control rats: initial fast inhibition, followed by facilitation and a long inhibition. Slices from kainic acid-treated adult rats showed an enhanced inhibition (Fig. 2a). A similar pattern of enhanced inhibition in slices from adult rats exposed to seizures has been demonstrated by several others (King *et al.*, 1985; Oliver & Miller, 1985; Sloviter, 1991), while increased excitation has been reported using a different paired-pulse paradigm (Tauck & Nadler, 1985).

Lack of kainic acid seizure-induced changes in immature rats

The next series of experiments were conducted to determine if seizure-induced neuroanatomical and

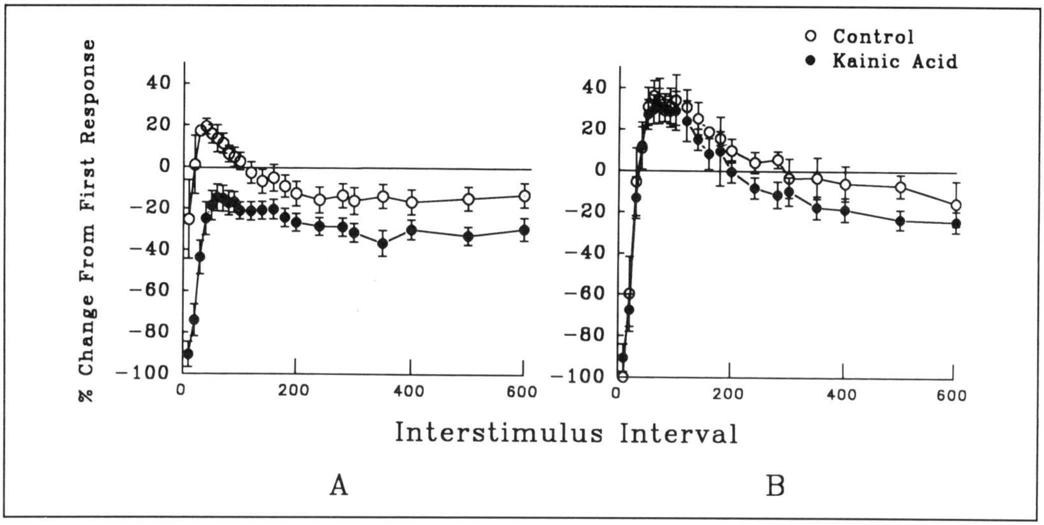

Fig. 2. Kainic acid seizure-induced age-related changes in hippocampal granule cell response to perforant stimulation. Slices from adult rats following kainic acid seizure (A) resulted in an initial inhibition (0–20 ms) followed by facilitation (25–200 ms) and an enhanced inhibition at 200–600 ms, as compared with slices from adult controls. Stimulation profile of slices from 15-day-old rats exposed to kainic acid seizure (B) did not show the enhanced inhibition and appear to be no different from adult or 15-day-old control animals.

electrophysiological changes were age-related. The above experiments were repeated with 5- and 15-day-old rats. Initial observations suggested that, in comparison with adult rats, rat pups that were administered kainic acid (2.5 and 5 mg/kg, respectively, IP) experienced more severe seizures. The seizures had a shorter onset, consisting of continuous forelimb clonus followed by the rats remaining in a prone position with increased axial tonus. In contrast, in adult rats, seizures consisted of bouts of clonus, rearing and jumping in the absence of tonic seizures. These results demonstrate age-related changes in seizure susceptibility to kainic acid seizures and are similar to those reported by Albala *et al.* (1984). In this earlier study, 16- and 35-day-old and adult rats were exposed to increasing doses of kainic acid (2.5–20 mg/kg, IP). Results demonstrated that a greater percentage of 16-day-old pups had generalized convulsions and status epilepticus and they had significantly higher mortality rates at significantly lower doses.

Immature rats appear to be more sensitive to kainic acid and have more severe seizures than adult rats. Therefore, it was expected that immature rats would be more sensitive to the neurotoxic effects of kainic acid. However, this was not the case. Immature rats exposed to kainic acid seizures at 5- and 14 days of age were sacrificed at least 2 weeks later and examined for neuropathological changes (using cresyl violet staining and Timm histochemistry) in the hippocampus. In contrast to adult rats, histological examination of tissue from immature rats did not reveal any cell loss in the hilus or CA3/4 hippocampal area (Fig. 1b). These results are consistent with our previous studies, in which 15-day-old rats and adults were exposed to kainic acid seizures and examined for histological changes after 5 days (Albala *et al.*, 1984) or 45 days (Okada *et al.*, 1984). In the latter study, neuronal loss was assessed by cell counts in the CA1 and CA3 pyramidal cell layer. Results indicate neuronal loss and degeneration in both hippocampal subfields in adult rats treated with kainic acid but not in 15-day-old rats. Several other studies have confirmed the finding that kainic acid-induced hippocampal damage in rats is age-dependent and cannot be observed before approximately 3–4 weeks postnatally (Nitecka *et al.*, 1984; Wolf & Keilhoff, 1984; Holmes & Thompson, 1988).

Results of Timm histochemistry and electrophysiological studies of 5- and 15-day-old rats exposed to kainic acid seizures were consistent with the absence of neuronal damage. Neither synaptic reorganization of the mossy fibres in the dentate gyrus (Fig. 1d) nor changes in perforant path stimulation profiles (Fig. 2b) were found in developing rats at least 2 weeks following kainic acid seizure. These results from rat pups exposed to seizures were in marked contrast to those we observed in adult rats. Adult rats demonstrated a dramatic increase in mossy fibre sprouting in the dentate gyrus and enhanced inhibition in perforant path stimulation profiles.

Why is kainic acid seizure-induced damage age-related?

The present findings indicate that, in adult rats, kainic acid seizures result in extensive neuronal damage in the hilus and CA3/4 area, reorganization of mossy fibre terminals in the supragranular layer of the dentate and enhanced inhibition following perforant path stimulation. In contrast, kainic acid seizures in immature rats did not produce changes in the hippocampus. There are several explanations as to why kainic acid seizures produce age-related neuroanatomical and electrophysiological changes. These include: seizures are not propagated by the hippocampus; developmental differences in the density of the kainic acid receptor; specificity of the kainic acid model; seizure-induced alterations which subsequently determine whether damage occurs.

The first possibility is that seizure activity in rat pups is not propagated by the hippocampus. In this case, we would not expect seizure-induced hippocampal damage. However, this does not seem plausible since several studies indicate that kainic acid induces prolonged electrographic discharges in the hippocampus of immature rats (Okada *et al.*, 1984), although in some cases cortical seizure discharges precede the onset of hippocampal discharges (Cavalheiro *et al.*, 1983b; Cherubini *et al.*, 1983). Hippocampal involvement in the immature brain during kainic acid seizures has been demonstrated by comparing changes in glucose metabolism in 15- and 35-day old and adult rats during status epilepticus (Albala *et al.*, 1984). Autoradiograms demonstrate age-specific changes in glucose metabolism. Despite these differences, an increase in glucose metabolism was observed in the hippocampus of all three age-groups. These results confirm our electroencephalographic (EEG) findings and demonstrate hippocampal involvement in seizure activity in mature rats, as well as immature rats.

The second possible explanation for the lack of kainic acid-induced hippocampal damage in developing rats may be that there are developmental differences in the density of kainic acid receptors. The presence of fewer kainate receptors in the immature brain could attenuate the effects of kainic acid damage. However, this does not appear to be likely since Miller *et al.* (1990) measured the density of the kainate receptor throughout ontogeny (1–28 days of age). They demonstrated that the density of the ^{3}H-kainic acid binding at 14 days of age was similar to the adult level. These results appear to contradict previous studies which report that the kainate receptors develop at a later age. These differences may be attributed to procedural differences, such as the fact that the earlier studies measured binding of only high-affinity receptor sites while Miller and Insel (1990) measured both high- and low-affinity components. In addition, the earlier reports were done on whole hippocampus or striatum while the more recent study compared developmental changes in binding of CA1, CA3 and dentate gyrus. Despite these differences, there is agreement that the kainic acid receptors are present in substantial numbers at 14 days of age and reach adult levels after 28–30 days of age. This indicates that the lack of kainic acid seizure-induced damage in the young animal cannot be attributed to a developmental difference in the density of kainate receptors.

The kainate receptors appear to be present in adult numbers at 15 days of age, the age at which we exposed our rats to kainic acid seizures; however, it cannot be concluded from binding studies that the kainate receptors are functionally or structurally mature at this age. In fact, *in situ* hybridization studies (Pellegrini-Giampietro *et al.*, 1991) indicate developmental changes in the kainate/a-amino-3-hydroxy-5-methyl-4-isoxazol propionic acid (AMPA) receptor subunits. Pellegrini-Giampietro *et al.* (1991) compared messenger ribonucleic acid (mRNA) expression of glutamate receptors Glu-R1,

2 and 3 during ontogeny in the CA1, CA3 and dentate gyrus. The results indicate that each receptor subunit has a unique developmental pattern of mRNA expression. This suggests that the Glu-R subunits may have a unique function in the immature brain in terms of excitotoxic effects. It is possible that the observed age-related differences following kainic acid seizures may be specific to kainic acid activity at the receptor and not to the effects of kainic acid seizure activity *per se.* To rule out this possibility, it was necessary to establish the specificity of our results for the kainic acid model by repeating these experiments using additional seizure models, such as flurothyl and kindling.

Similar to kainic acid seizures, flurothyl can produce status epilepticus. However, unlike kainic acid status epilepticus, flurothyl is a model of generalized seizures from onset. To induce status epilepticus, 14-day-old rats and adults were placed in a sealed chamber and continuously exposed to flurothyl vapours. After 45 min of status epilepticus, the rats were removed. Animals recovered from the seizure within a few minutes. The brains were later examined for neuroanatomical and neurophysiological changes (after 2–4 weeks). Unfortunately, as a result of the flurothyl-induced status epilepticus, adult rats did not survive. However, other studies have reported that, in adult rats, flurothyl-induced status epilepticus produces lesions in the hippocampal CA4 area (Nevander *et al.*, 1985).

In the immature rats, the results of flurothyl-induced status epilepticus were similar to those observed following kainic acid. Hippocampal pyramidal cell loss was not observed in 5- or 15-day-old rats exposed to flurothyl. These results are also consistent with those of Wasterlain (1976) in 4-day-old rat pups. In addition, flurothy- induced status epilepticus did not result in mossy fibre sprouting in the dentate gyrus (Sperber *et al.*, 1991a, b) or changes in perforant path stimulation profiles (Haas *et al.*, 1992).

Similar to kainic acid seizures, kindling is a model of partial seizures with secondary generalization. However, in contrast to kainic acid seizures, kindling is not excitotoxic and only infrequently does it result in spontaneous seizures (Pinel & Rovner, 1978; Kleinrok *et al.*, 1980; Pisa *et al.*, 1980; Kajima *et al.*, 1983). For the kindling experiments, two groups of rats (15-day-old and adult rats) were kindled from the amygdala. The adult rats were stimulated until they had three stage 5 seizures and the pups were stimulated at 15 min intervals until they had several severe seizures (stage 6 and 7) (Haas *et al.*, 1990; Sperber *et al.*, 1990). In the adult kindled rats, Timm histochemistry revealed mossy fibre terminal sprouting and reorganization in the supragranular layer of the dentate gyrus. However, the labelling was substantially less than that observed following kainic acid status epilepticus. This suggests a correlation between seizure severity and extent of reorganization of the mossy fibre pathway in the hippocampal dentate gyrus. Since positive Timm staining is a reliable marker for hilar and CA3/CA4 damage, there also appears to be a correlation between seizure severity and extent of subsequent damage. Adult rats treated with kainic acid had more severe seizures, dramatic Timm staining and marked CA3/CA4 neuronal loss. In contrast, kindled adult rats had less severe seizures and fewer Timm-stained mossy fibre synapses and cell loss was not apparent by light microscopy. A similar parallel between seizure severity and extent of hippocampal damage has been suggested in temporal lobe epileptic patients (Margerison & Corsellis, 1966).

The results of the *in vitro* slice preparation from adult kindled rats confirm our kainic acid data. Paired-pulse stimulation from the perforant path produced a triphasic profile in slices from adult kindled rats in comparison with slices from adult control. The response was characterized by an initial inhibition at short interstimulus intervals, followed by an enhanced inhibition at longer interstimulus intervals. Also consistent with our kainic acid and flurothyl findings, perforant path stimulation of slices from 15–16-day-old kindled rat pups and control pups were identical. This further demonstrates that seizures altered the response of dentate granule cells to perforant path stimulation in adult kindled rats but not immature kindled rats.

Similar results were obtained with three different seizure models: kainic acid, flurothyl and kindling. This suggests that our findings of age-related seizure-induced damage are not specific for kainic acid seizures and indicates that seizures produce age-related hippocampal damage independent of the seizure model. This conclusion is further substantiated by studies of others using additional seizure models. For instance, pilocarpine-induced status epilepticus results in hippocampal damage of adult rats but not immature rats (Cavalheiro *et al.*, 1987), while bicuculline induced status epilepticus produced damage in adolescent baboons (Meldrum & Brierley, 1973) but not immature (2-week-old) monkeys (Soderfeldt *et al.*, 1990).

Finally, it is possible that the apparent age-related differences in seizure-induced damage is a result of age-related alterations in the brain, which may subsequently determine whether damage is incurred. That is, seizure *per se* may activate different receptor subunits in the mature and immature brain, and this may affect seizure susceptibility or excitoxicity. To test this hypothesis, we conducted *in situ* hybridization studies to examine changes in the gene expression of the kainic acid receptor subtypes, Glu-R1, 2 and 3 in the hippocampus (Friedman *et al.*, 1991, 1993). Fifteen-day-old rats and adults were exposed to kainic acid seizures. Results indicate age-related differences in gene expression of mRNA for all three kainate receptor subunits. Hippocampal tissue from adult rats following kainic acid seizures demonstrated an increase in mRNA expression for Glu-R2 and 3 in the dentate gyrus. In contrast, tissue from 15-day-old rat pups exposed to kainic acid seizures demonstrated an up-regulation of mRNA expression for Glu-R1 and 2 in the dentate gyrus. These results indicate that seizures produced age-related hippocampal changes in the production of mRNA. Perhaps the increase in Glu-R1 or the increase in Glu-R1 in combination with Glu-R2 in pups is associated with some protective mechanism for seizure-induced damage.

Is hippocampal sclerosis a consequence of convulsions early in life?

The results of the present studies indicate that hippocampal damage is not produced by seizures early in life. This raises the question, at what age do seizures result in adult patterns of hippocampal sclerosis? We have repeated these experiments in rats older than 14 days of age and our findings, in addition to those of others (Nitecka *et al.*, 1984; Wolf & Keilhoff, 1984; Holmes & Thompson, 1988), suggest that kainic acid seizure-induced damage is apparent at approximately 3 weeks of age in the rat. Unfortunately, it is difficult to equate ages across species since the brains of different species do not develop completely in parallel or have identical developmental time courses. To relate our findings to human children, more accurate correlates of developmental milestones are needed. However, in general, a 2-week-old rat approximates a human child of 1–3 years of age.

It is possible that neuronal damage is present in developing rats exposed to seizures, but the pathology cannot be easily detected by the light microscopy techniques employed. In fact, Sutula *et al.* (1988), initially reported a lack of cell loss in adult kindled rats and only by using more sophisticated cell-counting techniques later confirmed the presence of a hilar lesion (Cavazos & Sutula, 1990). As a result, cell loss may be present in the developing hippocampus, but it is not readily apparent. On the other hand, the lack of Timm staining of the mossy fibre granules in the supragranular layer suggests that no lesion is present. In addition, the lack of hippocampal glial cell proliferation in the rat pup further suggests that neuronal damage is not present. Finally, in a previous study Okada *et al.* (1984) counted cells in 15-day-old rats and found no cell loss. These results confirm our hypothesis that seizure-induced damage is age-specific by demonstrating a decrease in hippocampal cell numbers in adult rats treated with kainic acid but not in immature rats.

The present research has addressed the issue of seizure-induced damage in developing rats by using a very specific and limited definition of damage. Damage has been defined as the presence of hippocampal sclerosis in the hilar CA3/CA4 areas, mossy fibre synaptic reorganization in the dentate gyrus and changes in response of dentate granule cells to perforant path stimulation. According to our definition, seizure-induced hippocampal damage has not been observed in developing rats in our studies (Haas *et al.*, 1991, 1992; Sperber *et al.*, 1991a, b, c; Sperber, 1992; Sperber & Haas, 1992) and those of others (Nitecka *et al.*, 1984; Wolf & Keilhoff, 1984; Cavalheiro *et al.*, 1987; Holmes & Thompson, 1988;). However, other indices of damage have been observed in immature rats following seizures. For instance, several studies indicate that seizures may produce deficits in brain DNA, RNA, proteins, protein synthesis, cholesterol, weight and number of cells in the immature brain (Wasterlain, 1976; Fando *et al.*, 1979; Wasterlain & Dwyer, 1983; Dwyer & Wasterlain, 1984; Dwyer *et al.*, 1986). These effects are not permanent and they dissipate by adolescence. Although these changes were not associated with hippocampal neuronal loss (Wasterlain 1975, 1976; Wasterlain & Dwyer, 1983), these studies indicate that seizures may result in changes in the immature brain other than those we have examined.

Is the sclerosis a result of an injury that becomes epileptogenic?

It is already known that lesions, even in very young rats, will result in mossy fibre sprouting (Zimmer, 1973, 1974; Laurberg & Zimmer, 1980, 1981). Therefore, the absence of sprouting that we observed in immature rats is not the result of an inability to sprout, but rather a lack of sprouting in response to seizures *per se*. We are now addressing the question of whether this lesion will result in age-related differences in the propensity for seizures. Clinical evidence suggests that the likelihood of recurrent seizures is low in children with no other underlying pathology; however, in the presence of an already compromised brain, the probability increases substantially (Maytal *et al.*, 1989; Maytal & Shinnar, 1990; Shinnar *et al.*, 1990). This suggests that an initial insult may become epileptogenic and produce seizures later in life. This is the question we are currently addressing by producing hippocampal lesions at various ages and exposing the animal to seizures.

Acknowledgements

The author wishes to express her thanks to K.Z. Haas for his technical expertise and assistance and Dr P.K. Stanton for the use of his electrophysiology equipment. This research was supported by a grant from the American Epilepsy Foundation.

References

Aicardi, J. & Chevrie, J.J. (1970): Convulsive status epilepticus in infants and children. *Epilepsia* **11,** 187–197.

Albala, B.J., Moshé, S.L. & Okada, R. (1984): Kainic-acid-induced seizures: a developmental study. *Dev. Brain Res.* **13,** 139–148.

Babb, T.L., Kupfer, W.R. & Pretorius, J.K. (1988): Recurrent excitatory circuits by 'sprouted' mossy fibers into the fascia dentata of human hippocampal epilepsy. *Epilepsia* **29,** 674.

Ben-Ari, Y., Tremblay, E., Riche, D., Ghilini, G. & Naquet, R. (1981): Electrographic, clinical and pathological alterations following systemic administration of kainic acid, bicuculline or pentetrazole: metabolic mapping using the deoxyglucose method with special reference to the pathology of epilepsy. *Neurosci.ence* **6,** 1361–1391.

Berg, A.T. & Shinnar, S. (1991): The risk of seizure recurrence following a first unprovoked seizure: a quantitative review. *Neurology* **41,** 965–972.

Bruton, C.J. (1988): *The neuropathology of temporal lobe epilepsy,* pp. 1–158. New York: Oxford University Press.

Cavalheiro, E., Richie, D. & Le Gal La Salle, G. (1983a): Long term effect of intrahippocampal kainic acid in rats: a method of inducing spontaneous recurrent seizures. *Electroencephalogr. Clin. Neurophysiol.* **54,** 603–613.

Cavalheiro, E.A., De Feo, M.R., Mecarelli, O. & Ricci, G.F. (1983b): Intracortical and intrahippocampal injections of kainic acid developing rats: an electrographic study. *Electroencephalogr. Clin. Neurophysiol.* **56,** 480–486.

Cavalheiro, E.A., Silva, D.F., Turski, W.A., Calderazzo-Filho, L.S., Bartolotto, Z. & Turski, L. (1987): The susceptibility of rats to pilocarpine-induced seizures is age dependent. *Dev. Brain Res.* **37,** 43–58.

Cavanagh, J.B. & Meyer, A. (1956): Aetiological aspects of Ammon's horn sclerosis associated with temporal lobe epilepsy. *Br. Med. J.* **2,** 1403–1407.

Cavazos, J.E. & Sutula, T.P. (1990): Progressive neuronal loss induced by kindling: a possible mechanism for mossy fiber synaptic reorganization and hippocampal sclerosis. *Brain Res.* **527,** 1–6.

Cherubini, E., De Feo, M.R., Mecarelli, O. & Ricci, G.F. (1983): Behavioral and electrographic patterns induced by systemic administration of kainic acid in developing rats. *Dev. Brain Res.* **9,** 69–77.

Corsellis, J.A.N. & Bruton, C.J. (1983): *Neuropathology of status epilepticus in humans.* New York : Raven Press.

Cronin, J. & Dudek, F.E. (1988): Chronic seizures and collateral sprouting of dentate mossy fibers after kainic acid treatment in rats. *Brain Res.* **474,** 181–184.

Duchowny, M., Lewin, B., Jaykar, P., Resnick, T., Alvarez, L., Morrison, G. & Dean, P. (1992): Temporal lobectomy in early childhood. *Epilepsia* **33,** 298–303.

Dunn, W.D. (1988): Status epilepticus in children: etiology, clinical features and outcome. *J. Child. Neurol.* **3,** 167–173.

Dwyer, B.E. & Wasterlain, C.G. (1984): Selective focal inhibition of brain protein synthesis during generalized bicuculline seizures in newborn marmoset monkeys. *Brain Res.* **309,** 109–121.

Dwyer, B.E., Wasterlain, C.G., Fujikawa, D. & Yamada, L. (1986): Brain protein metabolism in epilepsy. In: *Advances in neurology: status epilepticus*, eds. A.V. Delgado-Escueta, A.A.J. Ward, D.M. Woodbury & R.J. Porter, pp. 903–918. New York: Raven Press.

Earle, K.M., Baldwin, M. & Penfield, W. (1953): Incisural sclerosis and temporal lobe seizures produced by hippocampal herniation at birth. *Arch. Neurol. Psychiatry* **69,** 27–42.

Ellenberg, J.H., Hirtz, D.H. & Nelson, K.B. (1984): Age at onset of seizures in young children. *Ann. Neurol.* **15,** 127–134.

Falconer, M.A. (1971): Genetic and related aetiological factors in temporal lobe epilepsy: a review. *Epilepsia* **12,** 13–31.

Falconer, M.A., Serafetinides, E.A. & Corsellis, J.A.N. (1964): Etiology and pathogenesis of temporal lobe epilepsy. *Arch. Neurol.* **10,** 233–248.

Fando, J.F., Conn, M. & Wasterlain, C.G. (1979): Brain protein synthesis during neonatal seizures: an experimental study. *Exp. Neurol.* **63,** 220–228.

Friedman, L.K., Pelligrini-Giampietro, D.E., Sperber, E.F., Bennet, M.V.L., Moshé, S.L. & Zukin, R.S. (1991): Glutamate receptor gene expression in neonate and adult rats following flurothyl- and kainate-induced seizures. *Soc. Neurosci. Abstr.* **17,** 794.

Friedman, L.K., Pelligrini-Giampietro, D.E., Sperber, E.F., Bennet, M.V.L., Moshé, S.L. & Zukin, R.S. (1993): Kainate-induced status epilepticus alters glutamate and GABA-A receptor gene expression. *J. Neurosci.* **14,** 2697–2707.

Gastaut, H., Vigouroux, M. & Fischer-Williams, M. (1958): Partial epilepsies with localized expression (still called 'Jacksonian') and those with diffuse expression (still called 'psychomotor'). In: *Temporal lobe epilepsy*, eds. M. Baldwin & P. Bailey, pp. 13–22. Springfield, IL: Charles C. Thomas.

Granieri, E., Rosati, G. & Tola, R. (1983): A descriptive study of epilepsy in the district of Lopparo, Italy, 1964–1978. *Epilepsia* **24,** 502–514.

Haas, K., Sperber, E.F. & Moshé, S.L. (1990): Kindling in developing animals: expression of severe seizures and enhanced development of bilateral foci. *Dev. Brain Res.* **56,** 275–280.

Haas, K.Z., Sperber, E.F., Stanton, P.K. & Moshé, S.L. (1991): Age-specific changes in hippocampal paired-pulse inhibition following kindling. *Proceedings Focus on Epilepsy Symposium IBRO Satellite Meeting.* Quebec, Canada.

Haas, K.Z., Sperber, E.F., Moshé, S.L. & Stanton, P.K. (1992): Dentate gyrus paired-pulse physiology after flurothyl-induced status epilepticus in the immature rat. *Electroencephalogr. Clin. Neurophysiol.* **83,** 68.

Haug, K.M.S. (1967): Electron microscopical localization of the zinc in hippocampal mossy fiber synapses by a modified sulfide silver procedure. *Histochem.istry* **8,** 355–368.

Hauser, W.A. (1983): Status epilepticus, frequency, etiology and neurological sequelae. In: *Advances in neurology*, Vol. 34: *Status epilepticus,* eds. A.V. Delgado-Escueta, D.M. Treiman & R.J. Porter, pp. 3–14. New York: Raven Press.

Hauser, W.A. (1990): Status epilepticus: epidemiologic considerations. *Neurology* **40,** 9–13.

Hauser, W.A. & Kurland, L.T. (1975): The epidemiology of epilepsy in Rochester, Minnesota, 1935–1968. *Epilepsia* **1,** 1–66.

Holmes, G.L. & Thompson, J.L. (1988): Effects of kainic acid on seizure susceptibility in the developing brain. *Dev. Brain Res.* **39,** 51–59.

Houser, C.R., Miyashiro, J.E., Swartz, B.E., Walsh, G.O., Rich, J.R. & Delgado-Escueta, A.V. (1990): Altered patterns of dynorphin immunoreactivity suggest mossy fiber reorganization in human hippocampal epilepsy. *J. Neurosci.* **10,** 267–282.

Joensen, P. (1986): Prevalence, incidence, and classification of epilepsy in the Faroes. *Acta Neurol. Scand.* **76,** 150–155.

Kajima, M.T., Tanaka, S., Ohgami, S. & Yonemasu, Y. (1983): Rapid hippocampal kindling following intraamygdaloid injection of quisqualic acid in cats. *No To Shinkai* **35,** 569–574.

King, G.L., Dingledine, R., Giacchino, J.L. & McNamara, J.O. (1985): Abnormal neuronal excitability in hippocampal slices from kindled rats. *J. Neurophysiol.* **54,** 1295–1304.

Kleinrok, Z., Czuczwar, S.J., Turski, L. & Zarkowski, A. (1980): Effect of intracerebroventricular injection of kainic acid on electrically and chemically induced convulsions in mice. *Pol. J. Pharmacol. Pharm.* **32,** 261–264.

Laurberg, S. & Zimmer, J. (1980): Lesion-induced rerouting of hippocampal mossy fibers in developing but not in adult rats. *J. Comp. Neurol.* **190,** 627–650.

Laurberg, S. & Zimmer, J. (1981): Lesion-induced sprouting of the hippocampal mossy fiber collaterals to the fascia dentata in developing and adult rats. *J. Comp. Neurol.* **200,** 433–459.

Lothman, E.W. & Collins, R.C. (1981): Kainic acid induced limbic seizures: metabolic, behavioral, electroencephalographic and neuropathological correlates. *Brain Res.* **218,** 299–318.

Margerison, J.H. & Corsellis, J.A.N. (1966): Epilepsy and the temporal lobes. *Brain* **89,** 499–530.

Mathieson, G. (1975): Pathology of temporal lobe foci. In: *Advances in neurology*, Vol. 11, ed. J.K. Penry & D.D. Daly, pp. 163–185. New York: Raven Press.

Maytal, J. & Shinnar, S. (1990): Febrile status epilepticus. *Pediatrics* **86,** 611–616.

Maytal, J., Shinnar, S., Moshé, S.L. & Alvarez, L.A. (1989): The low morbidity and mortality of status epilepticus in children. *Pediatrics* **83,** 323–331.

Meldrum, B.S. & Brierley, J.B. (1973): Prolonged epileptic seizures in primates: ischemic cell change and its relation to ictal physiological events. *Arch. Neurol.* **28,** 10–17.

Menini, C., Meldrum, B.S., Richie, D., Silva-Conte, L. & Stutemann, J. (1980): Sustained limbic seizures induced by intra-amygdaloid kainic acid in the baboon: symptomology and neuropathological consequences. *Ann. Neurol.* **8,** 501–509.

Miller, L.P., Johnson, A.E. & Gelhard, R.E. & Inset, T.R. (1990): The ontogeny of excitatory amino acid receptors in the rat forebrain– II. Kainic acid receptors. *Neuroscience* **35,** 45–51.

Nadler, J.V., Perry, B.W. & Cotman, C.W. (1978): Intraventricular kainic acid preferentially destroys hippocampal pyramidal cells. *Nature* **271,** 676–677.

Nadler, J.V., Okazaki, M.M., Gruenthal, M., Ault, B. & Armstrong, D.R. (1986): Kainic acid seizures and neuronal cell death: insights from studies of selective lesions and drugs. *Adv. Exp. Med. Biol.* **203,** 673–686.

Nelson, K.B. & Ellenberg, J.H. (1976): Predictiors of epilepsy in children who have experienced febrile seizures. **295,** 1027–1033.

Nevander, G., Ingvar, M., Auer, R. & Siesjø, B.K. (1985): Status epilepticus in well-oxygenated rats causes neuronal necrosis. *Ann. Neurol.* **19,** 281–290.

Nitecka, L., Tremblay, E., Charton, G., Bouillot, J.P., Berger, M.L. & Ben-Ari, Y. (1984): Maturation of kainic acid seizure–brain damage syndrome in the rat. II. Histopathological sequelae. *Neuroscience* **13,** 1073–1094.

Okada, R., Moshé, S.L. & Albala, B.J. (1984): Infantile status epilepticus and future seizure susceptibility in the rat. *Dev. Brain Res.* **15,** 177–183.

Oliver, M.W. & Miller, J.J. (1985): Alternations of inhibitory processes in the dentate gyrus following kindling- induced epilepsy. *Exp. Brain Res.* **57,** 443–447.

Olney, J.W., Rhee, V. & DeGubareff, T. (1974): Kainic acid: a powerful neurotoxic analogue of glutamate. *Brain Res.* **77,** 507–512.

Pellegrini-Giampietro, D.E., Bennett, M.V. & Zukin, R.S. (1991): Differential expression of 3 glutamate receptor genes in developing rat brain: an *in situ* hybridization study. *Proc. Nat. Acad. Sci. USA* **88,** 4157–4161.

Pinel, J.P.J. & Rovner, L.I. (1978): Experimental epileptogenisis: kindling induced epilepsy in rats. *Exp. Neurol.* **58,** 190–202.

Pisa, M., Sanberg, P.R., Corcoran, M.E. & Fibiger, H.C. (1980): Spontaneously recurrent seizures after intracerebral injections of kainic acid in rat: a possible method of human temporal lobe epilepsy. *Brain Res.* **200,** 481–487.

Represa, A., Robain, O., Tremblay, E. & Ben-Ari, Y. (1989): Hippocampal plasticity in childhood epilepsy. *Neurosci. Lett.* **99,** 351–355.

Sagar, H.J. & Oxbury, J.M. (1987): Hippocampal neuron loss in temporal lobe epilepsy: correlation with early childhood convulsions. *Ann. Neurol.* **22,** 334–340.

Schwarcz, R., Scholz, D. & Coyle, J.T. (1978): Structure–activity relations for neurotoxicity of kainic acid derivatives and glutamate analogues. *Neuropharmacology* **17,** 145–152.

Schwob, J.E., Fuller, T., Price, J.L. & Olney, J.W. (1980): Widespread patterns of neuronal damage following systemic or intracerebral injections of kainic acid: a histological study. *Neuroscience* **5,** 991–1014.

Shinnar, S., Berg, A.T., Moshé, S.L., Petix, M., Maytal, J., Kang, H., Goldensohn, E.S. & Hauser, W.A. (1990): The risk of seizure recurrence following a first unprovoked seizure in childhood: a prospective study. *Pediatrics* **85,** 1076–1085.

Shinnar, S., Maytal, J., Krasnoff, L. & Moshé, S.L. (1992): Recurrent status epilepticus in children. *Ann. Neurol.* **31,** 598–604.

Shinozaki, H. & Koniski, S. (1980): Actions of several antihelminthics and insecticides on rat cortical neurons. *Brain Res.* **24,** 368–371.

Sloviter, R.S. (1991): Permanently altered hippocampal structure, excitability, and inhibition after experimental status epilepticus in the rat: the 'dormant basket cell' hypothesis and its possible relevance to temporal lobe epilepsy. *Hippocam.* **1,** 41–66.

Soderfeldt, B., Fujikawa, D.G. & Wasterlain, C.G. (1990): Neuropathology of status epilepticus in the neonatal marmoset monkey. In: *Neonatal seizures*, eds. C.G. Wasterlain & P. Vert, pp. 91–98. New York: Raven Press.

Sperber, E.F. (1992):Developmental profile of seizure-induced hippocampal damage. *Epilepsia* **33,** 44.

Sperber, E.F. & Haas, K.Z. (1992): Resistance to seizure induced hippocampal damage following kainic acid seizures in 5 day old rats. *Soc. Neurosci. Abstr.* **18,** 553.

Sperber, E.F., Haas, K. & Moshé, S.L. (1990): Mechanisms of kindling in developing animals. In: *Kindling 4*, ed. J.A. Wada, pp. 157–168. New York: Plenum Press.

Sperber, E.F., Haas, K.Z., Stanton, P.K. & Moshé, S.L. (1991a): Resistance to damage of the immature hippocampus to flurothyl-induced status epilepticus. *Epilepsia* **32,** 47.

Sperber, E.F., Stanton, P.K., Haas, K.Z., Shinnar, S. & Moshé, S.L. (1991b): Resistance of the immature brain to hippocampal damage following flurothyl induced status epilepticus. *Ann. Neurol.* **30,** 495.

Sperber, E.F., Has,K.Z., Stanton, P.K. & Moshé, S.L. (1991c): Resistance of the immature to seizure-induced synaptic reorganization. *Dev. Brain Res.* **60,** 88–93.

Sutula, T., Xiao-Xian, H., Cavazos, J. & Scott, G. (1988): Synaptic reorganization in the hippocampus induced by abnormal functional activity. *Science* **239,** 1147–1150.

Sutula, T., Cascino, G., Cavazos, J. & Parada, I. (1989): Mossy fiber synaptic reorganization in the epileptic human temporal lobe. *Ann. Neurol.* **26,** 321–330.

Tanaka, T., Kajiima, M., Daita, G., Oghani, J., Yonemasu, S. & Riche, D. (1982): Electroclinical features of induced status epilepticus in freely moving cats: microinjection to the dorsal hippocampus. *Electroencephalogr. Clin. Neurophysiol.* **54,** 288–300.

Tauck, D.L. & Nadler, J.V. (1985): Evidence of functional mossy fiber sprouting in hippocampal formation of kainic acid-treated rats. *J. Neurosci.* **5,** 1016–1022.

Thompson, J.L., Stafstrom, C.E., Chronopoulos, A., Thurber, S. & Holmes, G.L. (1990): Effect of age on seizure susceptibility following kainic acid induced status epilepticus. *Epilepsia* **31,** 634.

Timm, F. (1958): Zur Histochemie der Schwermetalle. Das sulfid-silber Verfahren, *Dt.sch Z. Ges. Gerichtl. Med.* **46,** 706–711.

Wasterlain, C.G. (1975): Developmental brain damage after chemically induced epileptic seizures. *Eur. Neurol.* **13,** 495–498.

Wasterlain, C.G. (1976): Effects of neonatal status epilepticus on rat brain development. *Neurology* **26,** 975–986.

Wasterlain, C.G. & Dwyer, B.E. (1983): Brain metabolism during prolonged seizures in neonates. In: *Advances in neurology: status epilepticus*, eds. A.V. Delgado-Escueta, C.G. Wasterlain, D.M. Treiman & R.J. Porter, pp. 241–260. New York : Raven Press.

Wolf, G. & Keilhoff, G. (1984): Kainate and glutamate neurotoxicity in dependence on the postnatal development with special reference to hipppocampal neurons. *Dev. Brain Res.* **14,** 15–21.

Zimmer, J. (1973): Changes in the Timm sulfide silver staining pattern of the rat hippocampus and fascia dentata following early postnatal deafferentation. *Brain Res.* **64,** 313–326.

Zimmer, J. (1974): Proximity as a factor in the regulation of aberrant axonal growth in postnatally deafferented fascia dentata. *Brain Res.* **72,** 137–142.

Zimmerman, H.M. (1938): The histopathology of convulsive disorders in children. *J. Pediatr.* **13,** 859–890.

Epileptic Seizures and Syndromes, Edited by Peter Wolf
© 1994 John Libbey & Company Ltd., pp. 481–488

Chapter 49

Neuronal hyperexcitability due to transient down–regulation of the GABA-ergic system following neocortical lesions

Heiko J. Luhmann*, Thomas Mittmann*, Rainald Schmidt-Kastner†, Ulf T. Eysel† and Uwe Heinemann*

**Institute of Neurophysiology, University of Cologne, Robert-Koch-Str. 39, D-50931 Cologne, Germany*
†Department of Neurophysiology, Institute of Physiology, Ruhr-University Bochum, Universitätsstr. 150, D-44801 Bochum, Germany

Summary

The effects of a focal cortical heat lesion on the structural and functional properties of the neocortex were studied in adult rats with neuroanatomical, immunohistochemical and *in vitro* electrophysiological techniques. In the vicinity of the 2–3 mm large lesions, pronounced neuronal damage and astrocytic reaction were detected. After survival times of 2–5 days and at distances between 2 and 4 mm from the centre of the lesion, extra- and intracellularly recorded responses to orthodromic stimulation of the afferents revealed a prominent neuronal hyperexcitability consisting of long-latency and multiphasic epileptiform synaptic responses. These long-lasting responses were reversibly blocked by the *N*-methyl-D-aspartate (NMDA) receptor antagonist D-aminophosphonovaleric acid (D-APV), indicating that they were generated within the neocortical network by activation of NMDA receptors. In addition, prolonged burst discharges were observed in supragranular regular spiking cells upon stimulation of the afferent pathway. The analysis of the inhibitory GABA-ergic system by measuring the peak conductances of stimulus-evoked fast (f-) and late (l-) inhibitory postsynaptic potentials (IPSPs) revealed a significant down-regulation in the efficacy of intracortical inhibition. These results indicate that the lesion causes a functional impairment of the GABA-ergic system with a subsequent increase in NMDA receptor-mediated excitation. This lesion-induced hyperexcitability may provoke long-term modifications in the neocortical synaptic network.

Introduction

A focal lesion, arising from mechanical injury to the brain or, for example, a tumour, may substantially alter the functional properties of the nervous tissue. Seizure activity, as one of the more severe consequences, often occurs during the first days after brain injury. These early post-traumatic seizures are probably the direct result of the lesion. In addition, long-term epileptic disorders have been observed in a substantial number of patients suffering from brain damage. It is a matter of discussion if these late traumatic seizures result from the initial lesion or whether they are caused by the early post-traumatic hyperexcitability (Meldrum, 1978; Söderfeldt *et al.*, 1981). For pharmacological intervention, and in order to prevent the establishment of permanent pathophysiological activity, it is necessary to understand the mechanisms underlying the early post-traumatic seizures. The *in vitro* technique offers several advantages for the analysis of lesion-induced functional modifications at the cellular and network level. The excitatory and inhibitory input on to single neurones can be studied in detail and manipulations of the external bathing solution allow a pharmacological analysis. In the following report, the short-term consequences of a focal cortical heat lesion were investigated with intra- and extracellular recording techniques in adult rat neocortical slices. In addition, neuroanatomical and immunohistochemical methods were applied to characterize the structural properties of the lesion.

Methods

Adult (> 2 months) Wistar rats were anaesthetized with pentobarbital sodium (50 mg/kg body weight intraperitoneally (IP) and a local cortical heat lesion was induced in the frontal or parietal cortex by photocoagulation with a high-intensity xenon light (Eysel & Schmidt-Kastner, 1991). After survival times of 1 to 9 days, neocortical slices of 400 μm thickness were prepared from the lesioned and the untreated contralateral hemispheres. Slices were either immediately immersion-fixed in 4 per cent paraformaldehyde and 0.01 per cent glutaraldehyde in phosphate-buffered saline (pH 7.6) or selected for electrophysiological examination. The methods for maintaining and analysing the slices were similar to those reported in a previous study (Luhmann & Heinemann, 1992). In brief, slices were transferred to an incubation or interface-type recording chamber and maintained at 34–35°C. The bathing solution contained (in mM) 124 NaCl, 3 KCl, 1.25 NaH_2PO_4, 1.8 $MgSO_4$, 1.6 $CaCl_2$, 26 $NaHCO_3$ and 10 glucose and when saturated with 95 per cent O_2/5 per cent CO_2 had a pH of 7.4. Slices were incubated for leastl h before recording began. Extracellular field potential (FP) responses in layers II/III to electrical stimulation (200 μs duration, < 0.1 Hz) of the afferent pathway were analysed in their duration, amplitude, onset latency and presence of multiple components. In neocortical slices obtained from lesioned animals, the expression of epileptiform activity was investigated at various distances from the lesion. Intracellular recordings were performed in layers II/III with sharp microelectrodes (60–120 MΩ) filled with 2 M potassium acetate. After obtaining a stable intracellular recording, neurones were analysed for their intrinsic membrane properties (resting membrane potential V_m, neuronal input resistance R_N, spike frequency accommodation, discharge rates, cell type) and synaptic input (presence of synaptic bursts or multiphasic components, excitatory and inhibitory postsynaptic potentials (EPSPs and IPSPs, respectively)). A pharmacological manipulation was achieved by local drop application of the *N*-methyl-D-aspartate (NMDA) receptor antagonist D-aminophosphonovaleric acid (D-APV; SIGMA, Basle/Switzerland) with a broken micropipette on the slice surface near the recording site at a concentration of 100 μM.

For later anatomical and immunohistochemical examination of the tissue, fixed slices were resectioned at 50 μm on a freezing microtome. Nissl staining was performed on mounted and defattened sections with cresyl violet. For immunohistochemistry, sections were reacted free-floating, using the peroxidase–antiperoxidase (PAP) method (Schmidt-Kastner *et al.*, 1991). After elimination of endogenous peroxidase with 3 per cent H_2O_2, sections were exposed to 1 per cent normal serum from pig or rabbit. Sections were incubated in one of the following primary antibodies overnight: antiglial fibrillary acidic protein (anti-GFAP, 1 : 2000; DAKO, Hamburg, Germany), mouse monoclonal antivimentin (clone V9, 1 : 250; DAKO), mouse monoclonal antiparvalbumin (1 : 2000; SIGMA) or rabbit antimicrotubule-associated proteins (anti-MAP, 1 : 500; SIGMA). Rabbit antisera were detected by swine antirabbit (1 : 100 for 30 min) and rabbit PAP complex (1 : 200 for 60 min). Mouse monoclonals were visualized with rabbit antimouse immunoglobulin G (IgG) (1 : 100) or goat antimouse (1 : 100) and subsequent monoclonal mouse PAP complex (1 : 200) (all from DAKO). Diaminobenzidine was used as the chromogen.

Results

Anatomy

The lesion was located in the parietal and partly in the frontal cortex, had a diameter of 2–3 mm and reached ventrally into the infragranular layers. Nissl-stained sections showed condensed dark-stained neuronal somata in the immediate vicinity of the lesion. A pattern of focal or laminar damage surrounding the coagulated tissue could not be detected. When compared with the contralateral untreated hemisphere (Fig. 1a and c), antibodies to MAP revealed loss of neuronal elements and fragmentation of dendritic processes near the lesion (Fig. 1b and d). Labelling for parvalbumin was insufficiently preserved to permit any detailed conclusion on the effect of the lesion on the structure of inhibitory interneurones. Immunostaining for GFAP revealed a dense pattern of reactive astrocytes in the tissue surrounding the lesion and a moderate increase in astrocytes in the entire neocortical slice from the lesioned hemisphere (Fig. 1f and h). The contralateral unlesioned cortex showed only weak GFAP labelling (Fig. 1e and g). Immunolabelling for vimentin was augmented in reactive vascular structures close to the lesion.

Physiology

The *in vitro* electrophysiological analysis revealed a time- and space-dependent expression of epileptiform activity in neocortical slices obtained from lesioned animals. After 1 day's survival time, stimulus-evoked FP responses in layers II/III showed a relatively normal pattern, consisting of a short-latency biphasic component of 15–30 ms in duration and > 1 mV in amplitude (Fig. 2a1). Between postlesion days 2 and 5 and at distances of 2–3 mm from the centre of the lesion, low-threshold stimulation of the afferents often evoked a long-lasting multiphasic FP response with variable onset latency (Fig. 2a2). The FP responses could last for more than 100 ms and varied considerably in shape from stimulus to stimulus suggesting that they were generated in a polysynaptic network. The duration of the FP responses were markedly reduced after local application of 100 μM D-APV, indicating that this prolonged discharge was mediated by activation of NMDA receptors. A decline in the FP duration could be observed at increasing distances form the lesion centre (Fig. 2b). At distances of ≥ 2.8 mm, the FP responses showed the normal duration and pattern. In addition, after survival times of 6 days, orthodromic stimulation revealed normal short-lasting FP responses even close to the lesion site (Fig. 2a3).

The intracellular analyses of synaptic responses in slices from lesioned animals confirmed the extracellular observations. Whereas neurones recorded in untreated control cortex responded to subthreshold stimulation of the afferents with a short-latency (2–5 ms) monophasic EPSP of 50–80 ms in duration (Fig. 3a1), EPSPs recorded in lesioned cortex often revealed multiple components and were characterized by their longer duration, exceeding 100 ms (Fig. 3b1). In addition, synaptic bursts consisting of up to seven action potentials could be occasionally observed in regular spiking cells recorded in lesioned cortex. A prominent difference between control and lesioned cortex could be detected in the efficacy of the inhibitory γ-aminobutyric acidergic (GABA-ergic) system. Whereas suprathreshold synaptic stimulation of the afferent pathway evoked a fast IPSP (f-IPSP) and late IPSP (l-IPSP) in every neurone recorded in control slices (Fig. 3a2), a large number of cells in lesioned cortex did not reveal a distinct l-IPSP (Fig. 3B2). Furthermore, the peak conductances (G) of the IPSPs in control cortices ($G_{f\text{-}IPSP}$= 138.7 nS, $G_{l\text{-}IPSP}$ = 24.9 nS) was larger as compared with the IPSPs recorded in lesioned tissue ($G_{f\text{-}IPSP}$ = 47.5 nS, $G_{l\text{-}IPSP}$ = 9.6 nS). With increasing survival time, a marked increase in the peak conductance of the l-IPSP could be observed in neurones recorded in lesioned cortex, suggesting a gradual recovery in GABA-ergic function.

In addition to these lesion-induced modifications in the synaptic network properties, supragranular neocortical neurones from lesioned animals were characterized by marked alterations in their intrinsic membrane properties. The resting membrane potential was different in cells recorded in lesioned (–73.5 mV) and control cortex (–80.1). Furthermore, the neuronal input resistance was larger in

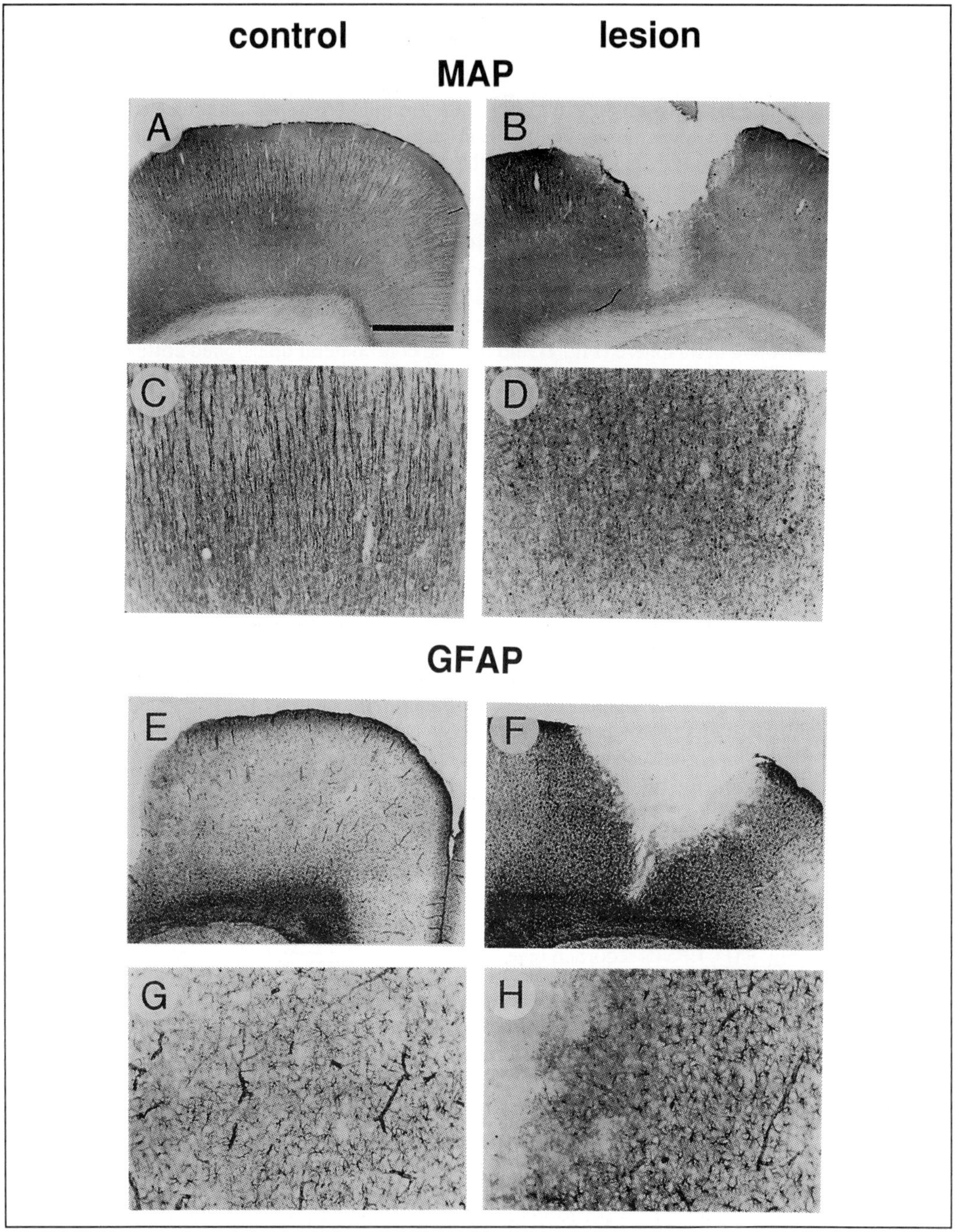

Fig. 1. Anatomy of the focal heat lesion in the frontal cortex of an adult rat after 3 days' survival time. Photographs of coronal sections from the untreated control hemisphere (left column) and the contralateral lesioned hemisphere (right column). Sections were reacted for microtubule-associated protein (MAP, A–D) and for glial fibrillary acidic protein (GFAP, E-H) and are shown at two different magnifications. Scale bar in A represents 1 mm for A, B, E, F and 250 µm for C, D, G, H, respectively.

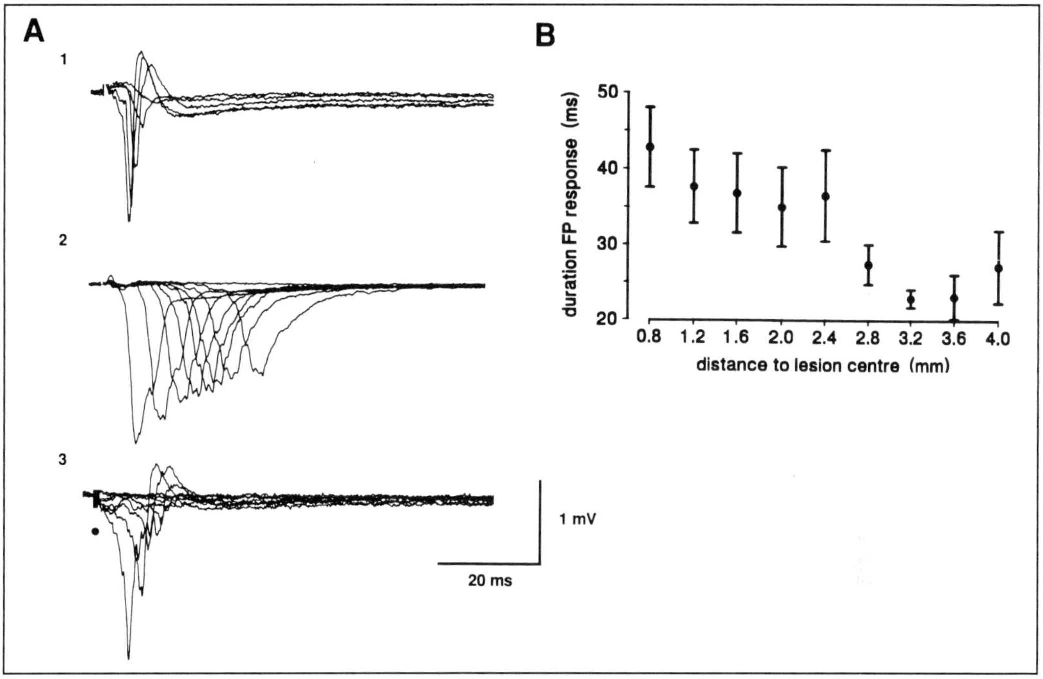

Fig. 2. Field potential (FP) responses to synaptic stimulation of the afferent fibres in neocortical slices obtained from animals with focal cortical heat lesion with different survival times. A: Representative examples of FP responses after 1 (A1), 4 (A2) and 8 (A3) days' survival time postlesion. Stimulus intensity was gradually increased and negativity is downward in all three recordings. Note variable onset latency of the responses shown in A2. B: Changes in the duration of the FP response at increasing distances from the centre of the heat lesion. Bars on filled circles indicate standard error of the mean. Total number of FPs analysed for this parameter n = 206.

neurones analysed in slices with focal lesions (42.3 MΩ) as compared with controls (35.2 MΩ). Intrinsic burst firing responses to intracellular injection of depolarizing current pulses were never observed in lesioned or control cortices.

Discussion

A tumour or a focal ischaemic lesion causes prominent alterations in the anatomical and physiological properties of the injured tissue (for a detailed description of the structural modifications see also de Lanerolle *et al.*, Chapter 46). Reactive astrocytosis and structural damage of neuronal processes and somata represent the acute immediate responses of the tissue to the lesion. Possible long-term consequences include reorganization of axonal connections (Ben-Ari, Chapter 53), disinhibition with subsequent hyperexcitability (Franck *et al.*, 1988; Meier *et al.*, 1992) and changes in the properties or composition of the glutamate receptor subunits (Köhr, Chapter 23). Our observations on the short-term functional effects of a local cortical heat lesion indicate a pronounced down-regulation in the efficacy of the GABA-ergic system. The peak conductance of the f- and l-IPSP was significantly smaller in neocortical slices obtained from lesioned animals as compared with age-matched untreated controls. Similar results have been reported in the hippocampus of kainate-lesioned rats (Franck *et al.*, 1988; Cornish & Wheal, 1989; Meier *et al.*, 1992). *In vitro* analyses of the CA1 area demonstrated a decrease of GABA-ergic inhibition, particularly of the f-IPSP, and pronounced hyperexcitability persisting for more than 500 days (Meier *et al.*, 1992). Functional impairment of GABA-ergic

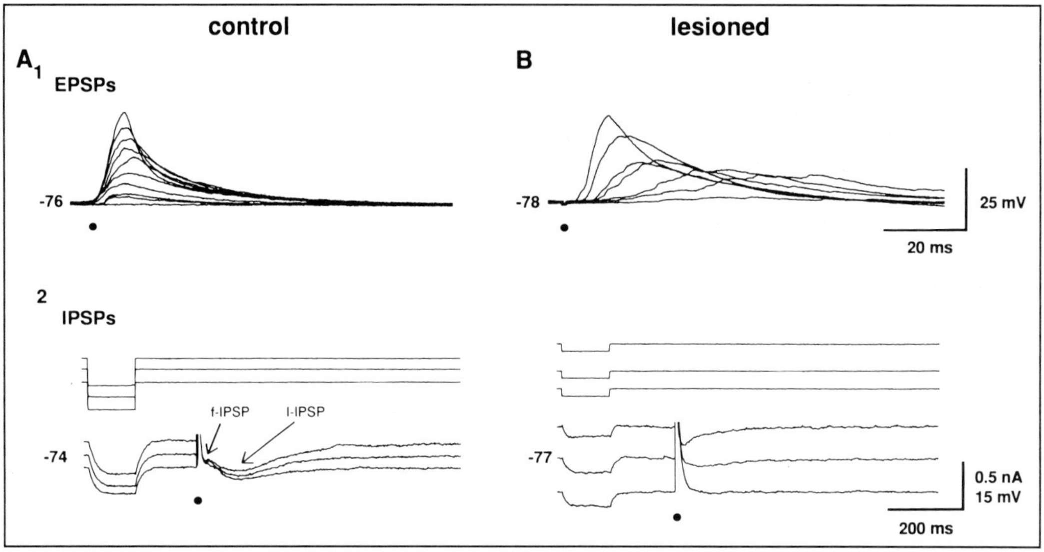

Fig. 3. Intracellular recordings from supragranular neurones in untreated control cortex (A) and in the lesioned cortex 6 days postlesion (B). Subthreshold stimulation of the afferent pathway at increasing intensity evokes a monophasic excitatory postsynaptic potential (EPSP) in the control cell (A1) and a long-latency multiphasic EPSP in the neurone recorded in the lesioned cortex (B1). Increasing the stimulus intensity to double the threshold to elicit an action potential reveals a biphasic inhibitory postsynaptic potential (IPSP) in the control cell (A2) and only a small fast (f-) IPSP in the neurone recorded from the lesioned animal (B2). Current protocol is shown in the upper traces and corresponding voltage responses are documented below. Resting membrane potentials are indicated by numbers left of each trace. Peak conductance of the f-IPSP and l-IPSP in A2 (control) amounts to 221 and 38 nS, respectively. Peak conductance of the f-IPSP in B2 (lesioned) is 20 nS.

inhibition ('dormant basket cell' hypothesis) may account for recurrent seizure activity in human temporal lobe epilepsy (Lothman, Chapter 51). Intracellular recordings in neocortical slices obtained from tissue removed from patients with pharmacoresistant seizures also indicate a prominent reduction in GABA-ergic inhibition, which is at least partly mediated by a loss of somatostatin-like immunoreactivity (Strowbridge *et al.*, 1992b). One of the functional consequences of this impairment in intracortical inhibition is the expression of prolonged synaptic excitation and burst discharges in human epileptic tissue (Strowbridge *et al.*, 1992a). Long-lasting hyperactivity and burst responses have also been observed under *in vivo* conditions in the cat visual cortex, which was heat-lesioned in a similar way to that described in this study (Eysel & Schmidt-Kastner, 1991). Our data suggest that these bursts are not generated by certain intrinsic membrane properties but rather by a down-regulation of inhibitory mechanisms with a subsequent increase in NMDA receptor-mediated excitation. It has been shown in rat neocortical slices that even a minor reduction in GABA-ergic inhibition induces epileptiform activity (Chagnac-Amitai & Connors, 1989) and unmasks NMDA receptor-mediated excitation (Luhmann & Prince, 1990a, b). A suppression of inhibitory mechanisms can also be observed under acute hypoxic conditions *in vivo* and *in vitro*. A selective susceptibility of the GABA-ergic system has been described in the hippocampus (Fujiwara *et al.*, 1987; Leblond & Krnjevic, 1989; Krnjevic *et al.*, 1991) and the neocortex (Luhmann & Heinemann, 1992; Rosen & Morris, 1993) and in both regions inhibitory dysfunction results in enhanced NMDA receptor-mediated excitation (Krnjevic, 1990). Postlesion hyperactivity involving activation of NMDA receptors may cause irreparable structural and functional deficits and lead to manifestation of epileptiform activity (Meyer, 1989; Morimoto & Sato, 1992).

In addition to these lesion-induced modifications in the synaptic network properties, brain injury also alters the membrane characteristics of single neurones. In agreement with recent observations in the chronically injured cortex (Prince & Tseng, 1993), the neuronal input resistance was significantly higher in lesioned cortex as compared with untreated control. These results suggest that the lesion causes changes in the cell's passive membrane properties which may influence spike initiation, firing pattern and membrane excitability (Titmus & Faber, 1990). Increases in membrane time constant and input resistance have been described in axotomized cat motoneurones (Yamuy *et al.*, 1992) and recently in the 'undercut cortex' (Prince & Tseng, 1993). These changes would also lead to enhanced excitation due to amplification and prolongation of EPSPs, which would consequently be more likely to cause activation of NMDA receptors.

Acknowledgements

We are most grateful to Ute Neubacher and Marianne Scheid for superior technical help. This study was supported by grants from the Deutsche Forschungsgemeinschaft to U.T.E. and R.S.-K. (Ey8/13) and to H.J.L. (SFB 194/B4), and a grant from the Ministerium für Wissenschaft und Forschung NRW to H.J.L. (400 410 90).

References

Chagnac-Amitai, Y. & Connors, B.W. (1989): Horizontal spread of synchronized activity in neocortex and its control by GABA-mediated inhibition. *J. Neurophysiol.* **61,** 747–758.

Cornish, S.M. & Wheal, H.V. (1989): Long-term loss of paired pulse inhibition in the kainic acid-lesioned hippocampus of the rat. *Neuroscience* **28,** 563–571.

Eysel, U.T. & Schmidt-Kastner, R. (1991): Neuronal dysfunction at the border of focal lesions in cat visual cortex. *Neurosci. Lett.* **131,** 45–48.

Franck, J.E., Kunkel, D.D., Baskin, D.G. & Schwartzkroin, P.A. (1988): Inhibition in kainate-lesioned hyperexcitable hippocampi: physiologic, autoradiographic, and immunocytochemical observations. *J. Neurosci.* **8,** 1991–2002.

Fujiwara, N., Higashi, H., Shimoji, K. & Yoshimura, M. (1987): Effects of hypoxia on rat hippocampal neurones *in vitro. J. Physiol. (Lond.)* **384,** 131–151.

Krnjevic, K. (1990): Anoxia and NMDA receptors. *Adv. Exp. Med. Biol.* **268,** 475–479.

Krnjevic, K., Xu, Y.Z. & Zhang, L. (1991): Anoxic block of GABAergic IPSPs. *Neurochem. Res.* **16,** 279–284.

Leblond, J. & Krnjevic, K. (1989): Hypoxic changes in hippocampal neurons. *J. Neurophysiol.* **62,** 1–14.

Luhmann, H.J. & Heinemann, U. (1992): Hypoxia-induced functional alterations in adult rat neocortex. *J. Neurophysiol.* **67,** 798–811.

Luhmann, H.J. & Prince, D.A. (1990a): Control of NMDA receptor-mediated activity by GABAergic mechanisms in mature and developing rat neocortex. *Dev. Brain Res.* **54,** 287–290.

Luhmann, H.J. & Prince, D.A. (1990b): Transient expression of polysynaptic NMDA receptor-mediated activity during neocortical development. *Neurosci. Lett.* **111,** 109–115.

Meier, C.L., Obenaus, A. & Dudek, F.E. (1992): Persistent hyperexcitability in isolated hippocampal CA1 of kainate-lesioned rats. *J. Neurophysiol.* **68,** 2120–2127.

Meldrum, B. (1978): Physiological changes during prolonged seizures and epileptic brain damage. *Neuropädiatrie.* **9,** 203–212.

Meyer, F.B. (1989): Calcium, neuronal hyperexcitability and ischemic injury. *Brain Res. Rev.* **14,** 227–243.

Morimoto, K. & Sato, M. (1992): NMDA receptor complex and kindling mechanisms. In: *Molecular neurobiology of epilepsy*, eds. J. Engel, C. Wasterlain, E.A. Cavalheiro, U. Heinemann & G. Avanzini, pp. 297–305. Amsterdam, London, New York, Tokyo: Elsevier.

Prince, D.A. & Tseng, G.-F. (1993): Epileptogenesis in chronically injured cortex: *in vitro* studies. *J. Neurophysiol.* **69,** 1276–1291.

Rosen, A.S. & Morris, M.E. (1993): Anoxic depression of excitatory and inhibitory postsynaptic potentials in rat neocortical slices. *J. Neurophysiol.* **69,** 109–117.

Schmidt-Kastner, R., Heim, C. & Sontag, K.-H. (1991): Damage of substantia nigra pars reticulata during pilocarpine-induced status epilepticus in the rat: immunohistochemical study of neurons, astrocytes and serum-protein extravasation. *Exp. Brain Res.* **86,** 125–140.

Söderfeldt, B., Kalimo, H., Olsson, Y. & Siesjö, B. (1981): Pathogenesis of brain lesions caused by experimental epilepsy: light- and electron-microscopic changes in the rat cerebral cortex following bicuculline-induced status epilepticus. *Acta Neuropathol. (Berl.)* **54,** 219–231.

Strowbridge, B.W., Masukawa, L.M., Spencer, D.D. & Shepherd, G.M. (1992a): Hyperexcitability associated with localizable lesions in epileptic patients. *Brain Res.* **587,** 158–163.

Strowbridge, B.W., Bean, A.J., Spencer, D.D., Roth, R.H., Shepherd, G.M. & Robbins, R.J. (1992b): Low levels of somatostatin-like immunoreactivity in neocortex resected from presumed seizure foci in epileptic patients. *Brain Res.* **587,** 164–168.

Titmus, M.J. & Faber, D.S. (1990): Axotomy-induced alterations in the electrophysiological characteristics of neurons. *Prog. Neurobiol.* **35,** 1–51.

Yamuy, J., Engelhardt, J.K., Morales, F.R. & Chase, M.H. (1992): Passive electrical properties of motoneurons in aged cats following axotomy. *Brain Res.* **570,** 300–306.

Epileptic Seizures and Syndromes, Edited by Peter Wolf
© 1994 John Libbey & Company Ltd., pp. 489–503

Chapter 50

Developmental models of secondary epileptogenesis

Douglas S. Garant*† and Solomon L. Moshé*†‡

*Laboratory of Developmental Epilepsy and Epilepsy Management Center, Departments of *Neurology, †Neuroscience and ‡Pediatrics, Montefiore Medical Center and Albert Einstein College of Medicine, 1300 Morris Park Avenue, Bronx, New York 10461, USA*

Introduction

Epidemiological evidence overwhelmingly demonstrates that epileptogenesis is much more pronounced in children than in adults (Gibbs & Gibbs, 1963; Hauser & Kurland, 1975; Woodbury, 1977). The period of greatest susceptibility to seizures encompasses the first few years of life (Nelson & Ellenberg, 1978).

There is great concern among paediatric epileptologists that seizures early in life may lead to a chronic seizure disorder, that, because of the plastic and vulnerable nature of development, participation of an otherwise healthy brain in an aberrant discharge may condemn a child to a life of epilepsy. Whether there exists sufficient evidence to support this concern is a matter of continuing controversy (see Hauser; Holthausen, this volume).

These concerns obviously loom large in clinical decisions about medication and intervention. However, only by identifying the pathological changes induced by seizures can rational decisions be made concerning the institution of age-appropriate treatments. Because seizures are the most frequent manifestation of central nervous system dysfunction in the newborn and young child, their recognition and the understanding of their significance are critical for prompt diagnosis and treatment.

In this chapter, we shall discuss some of the information gathered from developmental studies of animal models of epileptogenesis. In particular, we are most interested in those findings which might elucidate mechanisms of enhanced secondary epileptogenesis in the immature brain, and which might bear on issues of clinical research and therapeutic intervention in paediatric epilepsy.

What is secondary epileptogenesis?

The topic of secondary epileptogenesis always generates intense debate. Much of this debate, however, concerns the definition of the term. Those who feel it is of limited significance in human epilepsy apply the strict criterion of the creation of an independent secondary focus capable of generating clinical seizure discharges even after the primary focus is removed (Goldensohn, 1984). While there are clinical reports validating this 'strict' interpretation, they are rare (see Hiyoshi &

Wada, 1992). Others argue that even the existence of a mirror spike focus is sufficient evidence of secondary epileptogenesis to warrant serious concern (Morrell *et al.*, 1983, 1984, 1985, 1989, 1991b; Engel & Cahan, 1986; Morrell & de Toledo-Morrell, 1986; Engel & Shewmon, 1991).

For the purpose of this review, we will establish the following working definition: secondary epileptogenesis is the process by which previously non-epileptic brain becomes capable of sustaining or initiating epileptiform activity as a consequence of repeated invasion by ictal discharges.

Developmental considerations

In any discussion of ontogenesis, it must be appreciated that the immature brain is not merely a simpler, smaller version of what it will become in the adult (Moshé, 1987). During development the brain undergoes a panoply of significant changes, during which cells arise, migrate, make and remake contacts and often die. These formative processes are the substrates of neuronal plasticity, and yet can also support changes in excitability resulting from, or even leading to, seizures (Garant *et al.*, 1992). Developmental changes in seizure susceptibility are therefore unlikely to be simple, linear processes. Indeed, clinical and experimental studies reveal 'developmental windows' of increased epileptogenicity, bracketed by periods of relative seizure resistance (Pinel & Rovner, 1978; Moshé, 1989). Moreover, because brain areas mature on different schedules (Moshé *et al.,* 1991), the structures likely to support and to be influenced by seizures will vary as the brain develops.

Despite gross anatomical differences, the early brain development of various mammals is surprisingly consistent (Davison & Dobbing, 1968; Carey, 1982). A critical point to be kept in mind when making age comparisons across species, however, is that there are limits to the correspondences which can be made. Not only do rates of development differ, but the ultimate mature states are often different, and such differences are unlikely to be consistently maintained among all the systems comprising an organism. None the less, correlative ontogenic studies indicate that the developmental status of the brain of a 5–10-day-old rat may be equivalent in many respects to that of a newborn human infant (Gottlieb *et al.,* 1977; Benjamin & McKhann, 1981; Moshé, 1987).

Animal models

In this chapter we are concerned with the processes of epileptogenesis, both primary and secondary. It would obviously be best to be able to observe the evolution of spontaneous recurrent seizures in animals. Unfortunately, animal models involving epileptogenesis and spontaneous seizures are much rarer than are models of acute reactive seizures. In turn, models of secondary epileptogenesis are even more rare, and developmental studies in these models are rarer still.

Neocortical epileptogenesis

The propensity of cortex to generate seizure discharges has been demonstrated to be greatest during the second postnatal week (Hablitz & Heinemann, 1987, 1989; Luhmann & Prince, 1990). Simple partial seizures have been modelled in animal neocortex by the topical application of convulsant drugs such as penicillin or pentylenetetrazole, which induce acute epileptiform discharges evolving and persisting up to several hours; by mechanical damage to or freezing of the cortex, which induces longer-lasting foci; or by application of metals, including cobalt and aluminium, which can result in discharges persisting weeks to years. The seizure activity induced in these models stands in basic agreement with human foci (Ward, 1969).

The only model of simple partial seizures studied to any extent in the immature brain, however, has been penicillin-induced foci. These foci can be induced very early in development, at a stage of cortical developmental corresponding to the intrauterine phase in humans (Wright & Bradley, 1968; Mareš, 1973a). Unfortunately, in contrast to what one would predict from the clinical experience and from the basic studies presented above, penicillin foci in immature cortex exhibit significantly lower neuronal synchronization than is observed in adult animals (Prince & Gutnick, 1972), and the projection of focal discharges to other cortical regions also matures slowly (Mareš, 1973a, b).

Limbic epileptogenesis

Complex partial seizures in humans often originate from limbic foci predominantly comprised of the archi- and palaeocortex of the amygdala and hippocampus. Animal models of complex partial seizures therefore involve seizure discharges localized to these structures.

In contrast with the findings from models of neocortical focal seizures, limbic after-discharges (ADs) can be induced in animals at very early stages of development using electrical stimulation parameters effective in adult rats (i.e. 60 Hz sine wave current for 1 s) (Marešová & Mareš, 1988; Baram *et al.*,1993). In younger animals (7–15 days old), the AD threshold is higher than in adult rats (Moshé *et al.*, 1981; Stark *et al.*, 1986; Velíšek & Mareš, 1991; Baram *et al.*, 1993). In 21–39-day-old (prepubescent and pubescent) rats, however, the AD threshold is lower than in younger or older rats (Moshé *et al.*, 1981; Gilbert & Cain, 1982). The most common form of automatism observed in the rat during limbic ADs is the 'wet dog shake', which can be evoked as early as the first postnatal week (Mareš & Zouhar, 1988; Marešová & Mareš, 1988), and which bears some resemblance to certain clinical manifestations of partial complex seizures observed in humans (Engel & Cahan, 1986). They accompany both amygdala and hippocampal ADs (Lerner-Natoli *et al.*, 1984): whereas in the amygdala wet dog shakes occur throughout the duration of the AD, in the hippocampus wet dog shakes are associated with the termination of the AD (Squillance *et al.*, 1980).

A widely studied model of complex partial seizures employs the excitatory amino acid analogue kainic acid (Olney *et al.*, 1974), which can produce electrographic and behavioural seizures when injected systemically or intracerebrally (Ben-Ari *et al.*, 1981; Lothman & Collins, 1981). There are several important parallels between kainic acid seizures and human complex partial seizures (Sperber, this volume). The behavioural seizures induced by kainic acid are similar to those that can be elicited by direct stimulation of limbic sites and are similarly age-specific (Albala *et al.*, 1984; Okada *et al.*, 1984).

Another chemically-induced model of limbic epilepsy involves the combined administration of lithium and the cholinergic agonist pilocarpine (Turski *et al.*, 1986; Cavalheiro, this volume). Ontogenic study of this model has revealed developmental seizure differences similar to those obtained with kainic acid (Cavalheiro *et al.*, 1987). Thus, results from both these models indicate that developing rats are more susceptible to chemically-induced seizures: in other words, epileptogenesis is greater in the immature brain.

Our concern here, however, is whether these models can enlighten us about ontogenic differences in *secondary* epileptogenesis. Significantly, rats may go on to develop spontaneously recurring seizures long after either kainic acid (Kleinrok *et al.*, 1980; Pisa *et al.*, 1980; Cavalheiro *et al.*, 1982; Thompson *et al.*, 1990) or lithium/pilocarpine seizures (Leite *et al.*, 1990; Cavalheiro, this volume), although this important epileptogenic process has only rarely been studied, no doubt due to the infrequency both of the phenomenon and the seizures themselves. The incidence of spontaneous seizures appears to be age-dependent: rats younger than 30 days rarely develop spontaneous seizures (Thompson *et al.*, 1990). Because these younger rats do not exhibit the hippocampal neuronal loss and mossy fibre sprouting that adults show after kainic acid or lithium/pilocarpine seizures (Cavalheiro, this volume; Sperber, this volume), it is difficult to determine how much the development of these spontaneous seizures is due to induced damage. If one believes that these spontaneously recurring seizures reflect secondary epileptogenesis, however, these studies must be interpreted as indicating that the process is unlikely to be a significant factor in the immature brain.

The kindling model

Kindling has become an established model of epilepsy that is valuable for understanding the basic mechanisms of progressive epileptogenesis. Kindling, once established, appears to be permanent (Goddard *et al.*, 1969; McIntyre & Racine, 1986) and is extremely difficult to extinguish, demonstrating its robustness (Handforth, 1982; Hiyoshi & Wada, 1990).

As a rule, the triggering of ADs is required in order for kindling to occur (Racine, 1972a; Racine *et al.*, 1972). The induction of repeated ADs can be considered as an initial stage of kindling (Mareš & Marešová, 1989). While the subthreshold for AD stimulation can gradually decrease the AD threshold (defined as the lowest current intensity capable of eliciting an AD), the repeated failure to induce an AD usually indicates that the site cannot be kindled. Thus, the determination of the AD threshold can be considered as an index of the epileptogenicity of the stimulated site, although the AD threshold does not accurately predict the speed with which generalized kindled seizures will emerge (Zaide, 1974; Racine *et al.*, 1977; Moshé *et al.*, 1981).

During the course of kindling, the ADs increase in amplitude and duration and propagate to other brain sites. In amygdala-kindled animals, the ADs occur in other ipsilateral limbic sites and in the contralateral amygdala (McIntyre, 1975; McCaughran *et al.*, 1977; McCaughran *et al.*, 1978; Nobrega & Gaito, 1978). Eventually, ADs spread to the basal ganglia, including the substantia nigra and other subcortical structures, which correlates with the emergence of generalized seizures (Wada *et al.*, 1975; Bonhaus *et al.*, 1986). The metabolic activity of brain areas as measured by 2-deoxyglucose autoradiography (Ackermann, *et al.*, 1986) corresponds well with the AD propagation recorded on the electroencephalograph (EEG) (Engel *et al.*, 1978). EEG studies in cats, monkeys and baboons indicate that the patterns of kindled seizure propagation appear to be the same in all species (Wada & Sato, 1974; Wada *et al.*, 1975, 1978).

The behavioural manifestations of kindled seizures depend on the stimulated site and the animal species. The motor phenomena occurring during amygdala and hippocampal kindling in rats are best described by five-point scale designed by Racine (1972b). By the time unilateral clonic seizures of the forelimb occurs, which involve forebrain and midbrain structures (Browning, 1985; Gale, 1988), the seizure activity has propagated to involve the ipsilateral hemisphere. The most severe seizures normally evoked are characterized by bilateral clonus and falling, which involve further generalization of epileptiform activity to the lower brainstem (Browning, 1985; Browning & Nelson, 1986). Although bilateral clonus and falling are commonly considered to be the end-points of kindling, Pinel & Rovner (1978) proceeded with stimulations to demonstrate more severe seizures, including tonic–clonic convulsions and eventually spontaneous seizures after 350 or more stimulations. The induction of spontaneous seizures satisfies the important criterion necessary to establish kindling as a key animal model of epilepsy (McNamara *et al.*, 1986; Wada, 1986). Spontaneous seizures have also been observed in cats (Wada *et al.*, 1974).

Lesion studies have revealed that the major trans-synaptic changes in limbic kindling occur within the ipsilateral hemisphere and propagate downstream to brainstem structures (McIntyre, 1975; McCaughran *et al.*, 1977, 1978; Nobrega & Gaito, 1978). The forebrain commissures do not appear to be critical for the development of generalized convulsions but may play a significant role in 'transferring' the epileptiform activity to homotopic sites of the contralateral hemisphere (McCaughran *et al.*, 1978). The term 'transfer' is used to describe the observation that the establishment of kindling at a primary site results in fewer stimulations required to establish kindling in a secondary site (Goddard *et al.*, 1969). Transfer has been documented among various structures within the same hemisphere, including amygdala and neocortex (Seidel & Corcoran, 1986) or hippocampus (Aihara *et al.*, 1982), and prepiriform cortex and amygdala (Zhao & Moshé, 1987), as well as to contralateral, usually homotopic structures (Goddard *et al.*, 1969; McIntyre & Goddard, 1973; Zhao & Moshé, 1987). Destruction of the kindled focus does not reduce the epileptogenicity of the secondary site (Goddard *et al.*, 1969), which is now capable, upon stimulation, to support kindled seizures on its own, utilizing the kindling network already established (McIntyre & Goddard, 1973). Thus, the degree of kindling transfer to a secondary brain area can be considered a quantifiable measure of the secondary epileptogenesis affecting that area. Transfer has been proposed to be the substrate for the development and persistence of both experimental and clinical mirror foci, secondary foci that have been induced by and become completely independent of the original epileptogenic focus (Morrell, 1969; Morrell & de Toledo-Morrell, 1986).

Developmental aspects of kindling

The propensity for the development of kindling is age-related and there are ontogenic differences in every aspect of kindling, which have been reviewed recently (Velíšek *et al.*, 1993). The current literature on kindling in developing animals deals predominantly with electrical kindling in rats and cats (Moshé *et al.*, 1981; Holmes & Weber, 1986; Lee *et al.*, 1986; Holmes & Thompson, 1988; Shouse *et al.*, 1990). The only study which has attempted to induce chemical kindling with kainic acid in rat pups failed (Holmes & Thompson, 1988).

Amygdala kindling can be produced in 7–18-day-old pups using frequent stimulations, e.g. every 15 min (Moshé & Albala, 1983; Moshé *et al.*, 1983; Lee *et al.*, 1986; Stark *et al.*, 1986; Holmes & Thompson, 1987; Michelson *et al.*, 1989; Haas *et al.*, 1990; Baram *et al.*, 1993). In adults, this type of stimulation either significantly retards or fails to induce kindling (Goddard *et al.*, 1969; Racine *et al.*, 1973; Peterson *et al.*, 1981; Moshé & Albala, 1983). Immature rats have short refractory periods to kindling stimuli during and after the establishment of kindling (Moshé & Albala, 1983, 1984). Consequently, they are more sensitive to the development of repetitive seizures and status epilepticus than adults. With maturation, the intensity of postictal refractoriness increases to adult levels, irrespective of any previous history of kindled convulsions (Moshé & Albala, 1984). The age-related change in postictal refractoriness probably reflects the immaturity of seizure-suppressing systems, including subcortical nuclei (Moshé & Sperber, 1990), and are evidence of increased epileptogenesis early in development.

Another indication of greater epileptogenicity is that rat pups tend to develop kindled seizures more rapidly than do adults, as measured by the number of stimuli, delivered at an optimal interval, required to reach a given seizure severity (Moshé *et al.*, 1983). Indeed, in the immature rat, the second and third weeks of postnatal life represent a period of increased sensitivity to seizures, although the AD threshold is much higher than in adult rats. Prepubescent pups (21 days old) require a greater number of stimulations to kindle than other age-groups, even though their AD threshold is lower (Moshé *et al.*, 1981), and neonatal rats (5–7 days old) are even more resistant to kindling (Michelson & Lothman, 1991; Velíšek & Mareš, 1991; Baram *et al.*, 1993).

Spontaneous seizures in rat pups have been reported after many fewer stimuli than are required in the adult, but they are still rare (Sperber *et al.*, 1991a). The most in-depth investigation to date (Shouse *et al.*, 1990) describes the development of persistent epilepsy in kittens kindled while still immature: the younger the animal at the time of initial kindling, the higher the probability of subsequent appearance of spontaneous seizures. Although these spontaneous seizures exhibited multifocality (Shouse *et al.*, 1990), it is not clear whether spontaneous seizures, observed in any model, *originate* from a site anatomically distinct from the locus of stimulation; that is, whether they satisfy the 'strict' interpretation of secondary epileptogenesis.

Kindling in immature animals persists into adulthood, despite the continuing maturation of the brain. Rats kindled as pups are more susceptible to the development of kindled or chemically-induced seizures as adults (Moshé & Albala, 1982; Holmes & Weber, 1983). In adulthood, kindled seizures can be easily elicited not only from the previously kindled amygdala (Moshé & Albala, 1982), but also from the contralateral amygdala (Moshé & Albala, 1983) or ipsi- or contralateral hippocampus (Haas *et al.*, 1990, 1992), requiring fewer stimulations than similar transfer in rats kindled as adults. This acceleration suggests that transfer of epileptogenicity to other structures occurred during kindling in infancy and remained unaltered through maturation. The persistence of kindling occurs in the absence of any changes in AD threshold, indicating again that the relationship between kindling rate and AD threshold is not linear.

In contrast to transfer, in adult rats the phenomenon of 'kindling antagonism' has been described (Burchfiel *et al.*, 1982), in which concurrent kindling of two limbic foci by alternating stimulations results in the suppression of generalized seizures from one or both sites. Rat pups, in contrast, do not demonstrate kindling antagonism to the development of generalized seizures when stimulated between amygdala and ipsi- or contralateral hippocampus, or between the two amygdala (Haas *et al.*, 1990; Sperber *et al.*, 1991). Indeed, there is a 'kindling synergy' in pups, in that the rate of kindling with alternating stimulations exceeds what one would expect from simple, 'additive' transfer (Moshé & Albala, 1982, 1983; Haas *et al.*, 1990, 1992). This idea of synergistic foci suggests that the concept of an epileptogenic *network* may be a better way to imagine the kindling process than the interaction of isolated seizure foci (Moshé *et al.*, 1981; Applegate *et al.*, 1986, 1987; Applegate & Burchfiel, 1990; Konkol *et al.*, 1990), though this questions the definition of secondary epileptogenesis.

Thus a history of seizures during immaturity can permanently alter the seizure susceptibility of the brain. The persistence of kindling into adulthood appears to require as few as four seizures of mild symptomatology in rat pups (Moshé & Albala, 1982). While this is certainly the case for early kindling, kainic acid seizures induced in 12- or 18-day-old pups have been reported *not* to have an enhancing effect on subsequent kindling (Holmes & Thompson, 1988). These results suggest that the precise developmental stage of the brain the number of seizures it experiences may be important variables in assessing future seizure susceptibility.

Kindling and synaptic plasticity

What neuronal changes are responsible for the different course of kindling in immature animals? To date, there is no evidence demonstrating that the local kindling changes are due either to loss of normally present synapses or to formation of new ones. The enhancement of seizures in adulthood following postnatal kindling is not due to neuronal loss or glial scarring (Moshé & Albala, 1982, 1983), nor is it associated with synaptic reorganization in the dentate gyrus (Sperber *et al.*, 1991b), as is kindling in the adult (Cavazos & Sutula, 1989; Cavazos *et al.*, 1991). However, a stable increase in the efficacy of *pre-existing* synapses can be elicited by high-frequency stimulation of a number of neuronal pathways in the central nervous system: this phenomenon is known as long-term potentiation, or LTP (Bliss & Lømo, 1973), and has been implicated as a possible substrate for learning and memory. The range of high-frequency trains which generate LTP, when applied repeatedly, can lead to kindling in both immature and adult animals. Kindling, which involves the progressive growth in amplitude and frequency of ADs, has been proposed to be associated with structural modification of pre-existing synapses similar to those induced when LTP is established (McNamara *et al.*, 1986; Mody & Heinemann, 1987; Morrell, 1991a).

On the face of it, the similarity between LTP and kindling suggests that a similar mechanism may underlie these two phenomena. Such a commonality would be welcome, because the substantial literature regarding LTP could be drawn upon to extend our understanding of secondary epileptogenesis. Unfortunately, many observations argue against the existence of a common mechanism. Structures prone to kindling often provide no LTP for target sites, whereas the neocortex and hippocampus kindle slowly despite showing strong LTP; kindling appears to require the elicitation of ADs, and yet LTP can be induced without evoking ADs; and LTP decays with time, while kindling is permanent (McIntyre & Racine, 1986).

None the less, ontogenic studies of synaptic plasticity suggest that the two phenomena may at least have similar developmental timetables. Several reports demonstrate that the ability to induce LTP in hippocampal slices appears only after the first week of life (Baudry *et al.*, 1981; Harris & Teyler, 1984). It has also been shown that *N*-methyl-D-aspartate (NMDA) receptor mechanisms, presynaptic plasticity, calcium regulation and synaptic inhibition all change markedly between 7 and 15 days of age in rats (Muller *et al.*, 1989). In an important recent communication (Velíšek *et al.*, in press), the ability of synaptic stimulation to elicit LTP and its converse, long-term depression (LTD; Stanton, 1991), was studied in hippocampal slices from 15-, 30- and 60-day-old rats. No developmental differences were reported in the incidence of NMDA receptor-dependent LTP. When NMDA receptors were blocked, however, only slices from 15-day-old rat pups exhibited an additional, NMDA-independent component of LTP; slices from this age-group also exhibited the greatest incidence of LTD. These results demonstrate a significantly increased capacity for synaptic plasticity in rats younger than 30 days of age. Although their importance to normal developmental processes in the rat is obvious, it is noteworthy that all these changes occur during the aforementioned 'critical period' for seizure susceptibility, and may be expected also to contribute to the increased epileptogenicity of the immature brain.

Clinical implications

The data presented above demonstrate that most of the information available from animal studies concerning secondary epileptogenesis is derived from kindling experiments. Consequently, this section will address the possible clinical implications of kindling and kindling related processes in terms of human evidence for secondary epileptogenesis.

The possible occurrence of kindling in humans is the nightmare of clinical epileptologists. The evidence that kindling occurs in humans, however, is controversial (Morrell *et al.*, 1983; Goldensohn, 1984; Engel & Cahan, 1986; Moshé & Ludvig, 1988; Morrell, 1989, 1991b; Engel & Shewmon, 1991). Reports of kindling occurring in adult humans are few (Monroe, 1970; Sramka *et al.*, 1977; Dhuna *et al.*, 1991). Certainly, these rare occurrences are not sufficient to allow for a positive answer to the question of whether human kindling occurs, or if it is more prevalent in the young.

Does secondary epileptogenesis, defined as a secondary epileptic focus capable of initiating seizures even after the primary focus is removed, occur in humans? In the kindling studies, the observed seizures result from the application of an external stimulation, so it can be argued that kindling is not an analogous situation to human epileptic disorders. However, it should be pointed out that triggering factors in most human epilepsies are not known. Morrell has reported four cases in which secondary foci occurred in humans with seizures whose primary focus had a tumour located in a discrete brain area, and speculated that in these very few cases the propensity for the development of such secondary foci is directly related to the duration of the epileptic illness and inversely related to the patient's age (Morrell, 1985; Morrell & de Toledo-Morrell, 1986); these correlations are similar to those evident in developmental kindling studies in animals (Moshé & Albala, 1982, 1983). Furthermore, others have argued that it is unclear whether these secondary foci in humans are truly capable of initiating a seizure after the primary focus has been removed (Torres & Jacome, 1982; Goldensohn, 1984). In this respect, human secondary epileptogenesis may differ from that observed in lower mammals. At the present time, the consensus of the epilepsy community is that secondary epileptogenesis, if it occurs at all, is a very uncommon event in human epilepsies (Moshé & Shinnar, 1993).

If kindling were to occur in humans, then one would predict from the animal studies that infants and young children would be more susceptible. This increased susceptibility would affect primary epileptogenesis as well as secondary epileptogenesis in terms of the creation of secondary foci. The 'synergism' and 'positive transfer' that were observed during alternating kindling of developing animals (Haas *et al.*, 1990, 1992) may further enhance the development of multiple seizure foci. Additional but closely related risks may include the increased risk of progressive worsening of established epilepsy, and the risk that these changes may in the process adversely affect the function of affected or neighbouring brain, or cause brain damage outright. Therefore, one would conclude that children may require better control of their seizures than adults because of the increased risk of secondary epileptogenesis.

Epidemiological studies suggest that the immature brain is more susceptible to seizures than is the mature brain. There is a clear increased risk of children developing epilepsy in response to extrinsic triggers, e.g. febrile seizures. However, prospective studies (Hauser, this volume) indicate that the risk of subsequent epilepsy is relatively low in the absence of underlying brain disease. In the case of febrile seizures, the underlying pathological condition can be manifested as a pre-existing developmental abnormality or delay (Nelson & Ellenberg, 1976, 1978); partial or lateralized febrile seizures, which indicate the existence of a region of increased epileptogenesis (i.e. a structural abnormality); or afebrile seizures, which indicate an established epileptogenic process (Hauser, this volume).

This dilemma has been well delineated in the recent 10-year follow-up to the British National Childhood Encephalopathy Study (Madge *et al.*, 1993), in which the authors entertain two competing, though not necessarily mutually exclusive, hypotheses to explain the increased risk of seizures in children. The first is the hypothesis we have presented above regarding kindling and secondary epileptogenesis, that seizures beget seizures (Gowers, 1881). An alternative explanation is that seizures are only *associated* with other seizures, but that each seizure is independently determined by an underlying abnormality or trauma (O'Donohoe, 1985). The authors conclude from their study that epilepsy in children is most likely to be the result of a pre-existing disorder, not of a history of seizures *per se* (Madge *et al.*, 1993). The data of Shinnar and his associates concerning the outcome of a first unprovoked seizure or status epilepticus in infants and children also support this conclusion (Shinnar *et al.*, 1990, 1992).

One of the shortcomings of ongoing prospective studies such as these is that the follow-up is brief relative to the term of the disease, and may not permit the identification of patients who will go on to develop epilepsy after a latent period of perhaps a decade or more. It has been proposed that kindling-like processes may take place during this latent period: for example, kindling could explain the delay between the occurrence of head trauma and the actual onset of post-traumatic epilepsy (Goddard, 1983). During the latent period, neuronal plastic changes could lead progressively to increased local excitability, repetitive firing, epileptiform discharges and eventually the emergence of clinical seizures (McNamara *et al.*, 1986). Similarly, a kindling-like mechanism has been postulated to explain the occurrence of intractable partial seizures in children who have experienced many febrile seizures in infancy (Holthausen, this volume). The argument against this is that, in both clinical situations, the typical progression of kindled seizures observed in laboratory animals, from focal to generalized, does not usually occur. Generalized seizures often precede the onset of partial seizures, which is not the case with classical kindling. The need for long-term prospective studies is obvious.

Another form of kindling in humans could consist of a progressive worsening of the severity of seizures. There is no doubt that some partial seizures are difficult to control. Although these seizures may occur frequently, however, they are not necessarily more severe. Many of these seizures are auras (Engel & Cahan, 1986). In fact, with age the incidence of secondarily generalized seizures diminishes (Gastaut *et al.*, 1975), and those that do occur are not longer in duration than before. In addition, there are well-described epileptic syndromes characterized by a period of time during which a person experiences many epileptic seizures and then suddenly the seizures spontaneously remit (Shinnar & Moshé, 1991). The existence of such syndromes contradicts the clinical relevance of kindling.

It can be argued that the transition from generalized to focal seizures may still be a form of kindling in the sense that the partial seizures are more frequent. Furthermore, it is quite possible that the expression of generalized convulsions may be suppressed by powerful inhibitory processes that become more apparent with maturation (Moshé & Albala, 1983). The development of such inhibitory mechanisms may underlie the differences in kindling observed along the phylogenetic scale (Moshé & Ludvig, 1988; Hiyoshi & Wada, 1992): rhesus monkeys seldom have generalized kindled seizures despite numerous stimulations (Wada *et al.*, 1978). This issue remains unresolved.

Shewmon and colleagues have proposed a different concept of secondary epileptogenesis based on their studies of infantile spasms (Shewmon *et al.*, 1990; Engel & Shewmon, 1991). They found some of their patients to have focal structural abnormalities, seen as altered functionality by positron emission tomography scans or more rarely by EEG. Removal of the identified focus improved patients' seizures. Accordingly, these authors suggested that, early in life, focal lesions may produce secondary epileptogenesis, altering the epileptic potential of other brain sites and leading to the development of multifocal seizures clinically expressed as infantile spasms or Lennox–Gastaut syndrome. This hypothesis suggests that secondary epileptogenesis can occur at least in the abnormal immature human brain, and argues for early intervention to prevent the development of independent foci.

The hypothesis of secondary epileptogenesis in humans, as well as the fact that kindling in animals progresses even when only subclinical epileptiform discharges occur (Goddard *et al.*, 1969), raises an important question: do we need to treat not just seizures but also subclinical epileptiform activity such as spikes (Moshé & Shinnar, 1993)? An answer is not available, although it should be noted that carbamazepine and phenytoin, used widely to prevent partial seizures, do not suppress focal spikes (Cereghino *et al.*, 1974; Rodin *et al.*, 1974; Bustamante *et al.*, 1981). In fact, none of the drugs commonly used in treating epilepsy has been shown to be antiepileptogenic in the sense of preventing the establishment of a chronic seizure disorder (Temkin *et al.*, 1990).

It has been suggested that there are other possible forms of secondary epileptogenesis that should be taken into account (Moshé & Shinnar, 1993). For example, based on his work on primate kindling, J.A. Wada (personal communication) has found it extremely difficult to elicit ADs from the area homotopic to the primary stimulation site, an observation similar to the aforementioned 'kindling antagonism' (Burchfiel, Serpa & Duffy, 1982). Wada interpreted his findings as evidence for 'inhibitory secondary epileptogenesis' and was concerned as to the functional consequences for homotopic and other brain areas bombarded by seizure discharges. These results, however, may reflect changes in plasticity of the brain; they do not address the issue of seizure generation that the term secondary epileptogenesis inherently implies. Furthermore, this mechanism may not be present in the developing brain since the evidence from kindling studies indicates that kindling antagonism does not occur in developing rats. Instead, these results suggest that in the immature brain there may be a great potential for the development of multiple seizure foci which develop simultaneously, reinforcing each other in a synergism (Haas *et al.*, 1990). It is not clear, however, if this may be the possible substrate of Shewmon's hypothesis of secondary epileptogenesis: the data do not indicate whether one site is responsible for the development of the other sites.

Conclusion

In this chapter we have described current concepts of secondary epileptogenesis and the evidence from animal and human studies for and against its involvement. It is clear from these studies that the immature brain has a greatly increased capacity for epileptogenesis. To date, however, the available clinical data do not support the hypothesis that kindling mechanisms are responsible for the creation of seizure foci in humans, although some progressive changes that occur in human epilepsy *are* reminiscent of kindling phenomena. Unfortunately, there are few clear answers: the argument as to whether secondary epileptogenesis or kindling occurs in humans is sure to continue. A major obstacle to this argument's resolution is that kindling-like processes may occur only slowly in humans, necessitating long follow-up studies.

Nevertheless, the obvious importance of secondary epileptogenesis to clinical judgements, weighing the risks of intervention against those of progression and disability, demands that continued attention be paid to this issue. It is to be hoped that the study of kindling during ontogenesis will shed additional light on these mechanisms, leading to the introduction of new treatments that are aetiologically related to the precise developmental state and pathophysiology of the human condition.

Acknowledgements

The authors thank Drs Ellen Sperber, Libor Velíšek, Shlomo Shinnar, Patric Stanton, Kurt Haas and Nandor Ludvig for their contributions. This work was supported in part by US Public Health Service Grant NS2024.

References

Ackermann, R.F., Chugani, H.T., Handforth, A. & Moshé, S.L. (1986): Autoradiographic studies of cerebral metabolism and blood flow in rat amygdala kindling. In: *Kindling 3*, ed. J.A. Wada, pp. 73–87. New York: Raven.

Aihara, H., Araki, H. & Ohzeki, M. (1982): Hippocampal kindling and effects of antiepileptic drugs. *J. Pharmacol.* **32**, 37–45.

Albala, B.J., Moshé, S.L. & Okada, R. (1984): Kainic-acid-induced seizures: a developmental study. *Dev. Brain Res.* **13**, 139–148.

Applegate, C.D. & Burchfiel, J.L. (1990): Evidence for a norepinephrine-dependent brain-stem substrate in the development of kindling antagonism. *Epilepsy Res.* **6,** 23–32.

Applegate, C.D., Burchfiel, J.L. & Konkol, R.J. (1986): Kindling antagonism: effects of norepinephrine depletion on kindled seizure suppression after concurrent alternating stimulation in rats. *Exp. Neurol.* **94,** 379–390.

Applegate, C.D., Konkol, R.J. & Burchfiel, J.L. (1987): Kindling antagonism: a role for hindbrain norepinephrine in the development of site suppression following concurrent, alternate stimulation. *Brain Res.* **407,** 212–222.

Baram, T.Z., Hirsch, E. & Schultz, L. (1993): Short-interval amygdala kindling in neonatal rats. *Dev. Brain Res.* **73,** 79–83.

Baudry, M., Arst, D., Oliver, M. & Lynch, G. (1981): Development of glutamate binding sites and their regulation by calcium in the rat hippocampus. *Dev. Brain Res.* **1,** 37–48.

Ben-Ari, Y., Tremblay, E., Riche, D., Ghilini, G. & Naquet, R. (1981): Electrographic, clinical and pathological alterations following systemic administration of kainic acid, bicuculline or pentetrazole: metabolic mapping using the deoxyglucose method with special reference to the pathology of epilepsy. *Neuroscience* **6,** 1361–1391.

Benjamin, J.A. & McKhann, G.M. (1981): Development, regeneration and aging of the brain. In: *Basic neurochemistry*, eds. G.J. Siegel, R.W. Albers, B.W. Agranoff & R. Katzman, pp. 445–469. Boston: Little Brown.

Bliss, T.V.P. & Lømo, T. (1973): Long-lasting potentiation of synaptic transmission in the dentate area of the anaesthetized rabbit following stimulation of the perforant path. *J. Physiol.* **232,** 331–356.

Bonhaus, D.W., Walters, J.R. & McNamara, J.O. (1986): Activation of substantia nigra neurons: Role in the propagation of seizures. *J. Neurosci.* **6,** 3024–3030.

Browning, R.A. (1985): Role of the brain-stem reticular formation in tonic–clonic seizures: lesion and pharmacological studies. *Fed. Proc.* **44,** 2425–2431.

Browning, R.A. & Nelson, D.K. (1986): Modification of electroshock and pentylenetetrazol seizure patterns in rats after precollicular transections. *Exp. Neurol.* **93,** 546–556.

Burchfiel, J.L., Serpa, K.A. & Duffy, F.H. (1982): Further studies of antagonism of seizure development between concurrently developing kindled limbic foci in the rat. *Exp. Neurol.* **75,** 476–489.

Bustamante, L., Luders, H., Pippenger, C. & Goldensohn, E.S. (1981): Quantitative evaluation of anticonvulsant effects on penicillin-induced spike foci in cats. *Neurology* **31,** 1163–1166.

Carey, E. (1982): The biochemistry of fetal brain development and myelination. In: *Biochemical development of the fetus and neonate*, ed. C. Jones, pp. 287–336. Amsterdam: Elsevier Biomedical Press.

Cavalheiro, E.A., Silva, D.F. & Turski, W.A. (1987): The susceptibility of rats to pilocarpine-induced seizures is age dependent. *Dev. Brain Res.* **37,** 43–58.

Cavalheiro, L.A., Riche, D.A. & Le Gal La Salle, G. (1982): Long-term effects of intrahippocampal kainic acid injection in rats: a method for inducing spontaneous recurrent seizures. *Electroencephalogr. Clin. Neurophysiol.* **53,** 581–589.

Cavazos, J.E. & Sutula, T.P. (1989): Progressive neuronal loss induced by kindling: a possible mechanism for mossy fiber synaptic reorganization and hippocampal sclerosis. *Epilepsia* **30,** 702.

Cavazos, J.E., Golarai, G. & Sutula, T.P. (1991): Mossy fiber synaptic reorganization induced by kindling: time course development, progression, and permanence. *J. Neurosci.* **11,** 2795–2803.

Cereghino, J., Brock, J., Van Meter, J., Penry, J.K., Smith, L. & White, B. (1974): Carbamazepine for epilepsy. *Neurology* **24,** 401–410.

Davison, A. & Dobbing, J. (1968): The developing brain. In: *Applied neurochemistry*, eds. A. Davison & J. Dobbing, pp. 253–268. Oxford: Blackwell Scientific Publications.

Dhuna, A., Pascual-Leone, A. & Langendorf, F. (1991): Chronic, habitual cocaine abuse and kindling: a case report. *Epilepsia* **32,** 890–894.

Engel, J.J. & Cahan, L. (1986): Potential relevance of kindling to human partial epilepsy. In: *Kindling 3*, ed. J.A. Wada, pp. 37–51. New York: Raven Press.

Engel, J. & Shewmon, D.A. (1991): The impact of the kindling phenomenon on clinical epileptology. In: *Kindling and synaptic plasticity: the legacy of Graham Goddard*, ed. F. Morrell, pp. 195–210. Boston: Birkhäuser.

Engel, J.J., Wolfson, L. & Brown, L.L. (1978): Anatomical correlates of electrical and behavioral events related to amygdaloid kindling. *Ann. Neurol.* **3,** 538–544.

Gale, K. (1988): Progression and generalization of seizure discharge: anatomical and neurochemical substrates. *Epilepsia* **29** (suppl. 2), S15–S34.

Garant, D.S., Velíšek, L., Sperber, E. & Moshé, S.L. (1992): Why do infants have seizures? *Int. Pediatr.* **7,** 199–212.

Gastaut, H., Gastaut, J.L., Gonzalez e Silva, S.E. & Fernandez-Sanchez, G.E. (1975): Relative frequency of different types of epilepsy: a study employing the classification of the International League Against Epilepsy. *Epilepsia* **16,** 457–461.

Gibbs, F.A. & Gibbs, E.L. (1963): Age factor in epilepsy. *N. Engl. J. Med.* **269,** 1230–1236.

Gilbert, M.E. & Cain, D.P. (1982): A developmental study of kindling in the rat. *Brain Res.* **2,** 321–328.

Goddard, G.V. (1983): The kindling model of epilepsy. *Trends Neurosci.* **7,** 275–279.

Goddard, G.V., McIntyre, D.C. & Leech, C.K. (1969): A permanent change in brain function resulting from daily electrical stimulation. *Exp. Neurol.* **25,** 295–330.

Goldensohn, E.S. (1984): The relevance of secondary epileptogenesis to the treatment of epilepsy: Kindling and the mirror focus. *Epilepsia* **25**(suppl. 2), S156–S168.

Gottlieb, A., Keydor, I. & Epstein, H.T. (1977): Rodent brain growth stages: an analytical review. *Biol. Neonate* **32,** 166–176.

Gowers, W.R. (1881): *Epilepsy and other chronic convulsive disorders: their causes, symptoms, and treatment.* London: Churchill.

Haas, K., Sperber, E.F. & Moshé, S.L. (1990): Kindling in developing animals: expression of severe seizures and enhanced development of bilateral foci. *Dev. Brain Res.* **56,** 275–280.

Haas, K., Sperber, E.F. & Moshé, S.L. (1992): Kindling in developing animals: interactions between ipsilateral foci. *Dev. Brain Res.* **68,** 140–143.

Hablitz, J.J. & Heinemann, U. (1987): Extracellular K^+ and Ca^{2+} changes during epileptiform discharges in the immature rat neocortex. *Brain Res.* **433,** 299–303.

Hablitz, J.J. & Heinemann, U. (1989): Alterations in the microenvironment during spreading depression associated with epileptiform activity in the immature neocortex. *Dev. Brain Res.* **46,** 243–252.

Handforth, A. (1982): Postseizure inhibition of kindled seizures by electroconvulsive shock. *Exp. Neurol.* **78,** 483–491.

Harris, K.H. & Teyler, T.J. (1984): Developmental onset of long-term potentiation in area CA1 of the rat hippocampus. *J. Physiol.* **346,** 27–48.

Hauser, W.A. & Kurland, L.T. (1975): The epidemiology of epilepsy in Rochester, Minnesota, 1935–1967. *Epilepsia* **16,** 1–66.

Hiyoshi, T. & Wada, J. (1990): Failure of nine-month phenobarbital administration to reverse amygdaloid-kindled seizure susceptibility in cats. *Ann. Neurol.* **28,** 568–573.

Hiyoshi, T. & Wada, J.A. (1992): Lasting nature of both transfer and interference in amygdaloid kindling in cats: observation upon stimulation with 11-month rest following primary. *Epilepsia* **33,** 222–227.

Holmes, G.L. & Thompson, J.L. (1987): Rapid kindling in the prepubescent rat. *Brain Res.* **433,** 281–284.

Holmes, G.L. & Thompson, J.L. (1988): Effects of kainic acid on seizure susceptibility in the developing brain. *Dev. Brain Res.* **39,** 51–59.

Holmes, G.L. & Weber, D.A. (1983): Increased susceptibility to pentylenetetrazol-induced seizures in adult rats following electrical kindling during brain development. *Dev. Brain Res.* **11,** 312–314.

Holmes, G.L. & Weber, D.A. (1986): Effects of ACTH on seizure susceptibility in the developing brain. *Ann. Neurol.* **20,** 82–88.

Kleinrok, Z., Czuczwar, S.J. & Kozicka, M. (1980): Effect of dopaminergic and GABA-ergic drugs given alone or in combination on the anticonvulsant action of phenobarbital and diphenylhydantoin in the electroshock test in mice. *Epilepsia* **21,** 519–529.

Konkol, R.J., Holmes, G.L. & Thompson, J.L. (1990): The effect of regional differences in noradrenergic growth patterns on juvenile kindling. *Dev. Brain Res.* **52,** 25–29.

Lee, S., Kawawaki, H., Matsuoka, O. & Murata, R. (1986): Effect of Ca-antagonist (flunarizine) on kindling seizures in suckling rats. *No To Hattatsu* **18,** 292–298.

Leite, J.P., Bortolotto, Z.A. & Cavalheiro, E.A. (1990): Spontaneous recurrent seizures in rats: an experimental model of partial epilepsy. *Neuroscience* **14,** 511–517.

Lerner-Natoli, M., Rondouin, G. & Baldy-Moulinier, M. (1984): Evolution of wet dog shakes during kindling in rats: comparison between hippocampal and amygdala kindling. *Exp. Neurol.* **83,** 1–12.

Lothman, E.W. & Collins, R.C. (1981): Kainic acid induced limbic seizures: metabolic, behavioral, electroencephalographic and neuropathological correlates. *Brain Res.* **218,** 299–318.

Luhmann, H.J. & Prince, D.A. (1990): Transient expression of polysynaptic NMDA receptor-mediated activity during neocortical development. *Neurosci. Lett.* **111,** 109–115.

McIntyre, D.C. (1975): Split-brain rat: transfer and interference of kindled amygdala convulsions. *Can. J. Neurol. Sci.* **2,** 429–437.

McIntyre, D.C. & Goddard, G.V. (1973): Transfer, interference and spontaneous recovery of convulsions kindled from the rat amygdala. *Electroencephalogr. Clin. Neurophysiol.* **35,** 533–543.

McIntyre, D.C. & Racine, R.J. (1986): Kindling mechanisms: current progress on an experimental epilepsy model. *Prog. Neurobiol.* **27,** 1–12.

McNamara, J.O., Bonhaus, D.W., Shin, C. *et al.* (1986): The kindling model of epilepsy: a critical review. *Crit. Rev. Clin. Neurobiol.* **1,** 341–391.

Madge, N., Diamond, J., Miller, D., Ross, E., McManus, C., Wadsworth, J. & Yule, W. (1993): The national childhood encephalopathy study: A 10-year follow-up. *Dev. Med. Child Neurol.* **35** (suppl. 68) (7), 1–118.

Mareš, P. (1973a): Ontogenetic development of bioelectrical activity of the epileptogenic focus in rat neocortex. *Neuropädiatrie* **4,** 434–445.

Mareš, P. (1973b): Symmetrical epileptogenic foci in cerebral cortex of immature rat. *Epilepsia* **14,** 427–435.

Mareš, P. & Marešová, D. (1989): Excitability cycles of epileptic after-discharges in rats. *Physiol. Bohemoslov.* **38,** 55–61.

Mareš, P. & Zouhar, A. (1988): Do we possess adequate models of childhood epilepsies? *Physiol. Bohemoslov.* **37,** 1–9.

Marešová, D. & Mareš, P. (1988): Ontogenetic development of wet dog shakes accompanying hippocampal epileptic after-discharges in rats. *Arctiv. Nerv. Sup. (Praha)* **30,** 254.

McCaughran, J.A.J., Corcoran, M.E. & Wada, J.A. (1977): Facilitation of secondary-site amygdaloid kindling following bisection of the corpus callosum and hippocampal commissure in rats. *Exp. Neurol.* **57,** 132–141.

McCaughran, J.A.J., Corcoran, M.E. & Wada, J.A. (1978): Role of the forebrain commissures in amygdaloid kindling in rats. *Epilepsia* **19,** 19–33.

Michelson, H. & Lothman, E. (1991): An ontogenetic study of kindling using rapidly recurring hippocampal seizures. *Dev. Brain. Res.* **61,** 79–85.

Michelson, H.B., Williamson, J.M. & Lothman, E.W. (1989): Ontogeny of kindling: the acquisition of kindled responses at different ages with rapidly recurring hippocampal seizures. *Epilepsia* **30,** 672.

Mody, I. & Heinemann, U. (1987): NMDA receptors of dentate gyrus granule cells participate in synaptic transmission following kindling. *Nature* **326,** 701–704.

Monroe, R.R. (1970): *Episodic behavioral disorders: a psychodynamic and neurophysiological analysis.* Cambridge, MA: Harvard University Press.

Morrell, F. (1969): Physiology and histochemistry of the mirror focus. In: *Basic mechanisms of the epilepsies*, eds. H.H. Jasper, A.A. Ward & A. Pope, pp. 357–370. Boston: Little Brown.

Morrell, F. (1985): Secondary epileptogenesis in man. *Arch. Neurol.* **42,** 318–355.

Morrell, F. (1989): Varieties of human secondary epileptogenesis. *J. Clin. Neurophysiol.* **6,** 227.

Morrell, F. (ed.) (1991a): *Kindling and synaptic plasticity: the legacy of Graham Goddard.* Boston: Birkhäuser.

Morrell, F. (1991b): The role of secondary epileptogenesis in human epilepsy. *Arch. Neurol.* **48,** 1221–1224.

Morrell, F. & de Toledo-Morrell, L. (1986): Kindling as a model of neuronal plasticity. In: *Kindling 3*, ed. J. Wada, pp. 17–33. New York: Raven Press.

Morrell, F., Rasmussen, T., Gloor, P. & de Tol-Morrell, L. (1983): Secondary epileptogenic foci in patients with verified temporal lobe tumors. *Clin. Neurophysiol.* **84,** 26.

Morrell, F., Rasmussen, T., de Toledo-Morrel, L., Quesney, L.F. & Gloor, P. (1984): Frontal lobe epilepsy neoplastic etiology: incidence of secondary epileptogenesis. *Epilepsia* **26,** 654–655.

Moshé, S.L. (1987): Epileptogenesis and the immature brain. *Epilepsia* **28** (suppl.), S3–S15.

Moshé, S.L. (1989): Ontogeny of seizures and substantia nigra modulation. In: *Problems and concepts in developmental neurophysiology*, eds. P. Kellaway & J.F. Noebels, pp. 247–262. Baltimore: Johns Hopkins Press.

Moshé, S.L. & Albala, B.J. (1982): Kindling in developing rats: persistence of seizures into adulthood. *Dev. Brain Res.* **4,** 67–71.

Moshé, S.L. & Albala, B.J. (1983): Maturational changes in postictal refractoriness and seizure susceptibility in developing rats. *Ann. Neurol.* **13,** 552–557.

Moshé, S.L. & Albala, B.J. (1984): Nigral muscimol infusions facilitate the development of seizures in immature rats. *Dev. Brain Res.* **13,** 305–308.

Moshé, S.L. & Ludvig, N. (1988): Kindling. In: *Recent advances in epilepsy*, eds. T.A. Pedley & B.S. Meldrum, pp. 21–44. Churchhill Livingstone.

Moshé, S.L. & Shinnar, S. (1993): Early intervention. In: *Surgical treatment of the epilepsies*, ed. J. Engel, Jr, pp. 123–132. New York: Raven Press.

Moshé, S.L. & Sperber, E.F. (1990): Substantia nigra-mediated control of generalized seizures. In: *Generalized epilepsy: cellular, molecular and pharmacological approaches*, eds. G. Gloor, R. Kostopoulos, M. Naquet & P. Avoli, pp. 355–367. Boston: Birkhäuser.

Moshé, S.L., Sharpless, N.S. & Kaplan, J. (1981): Kindling in developing rats: afterdischarge thresholds. *Brain Res.* **211,** 190–195.

Moshé, S.L., Albala, B.J., Ackermann, R.F. & Engel, J.J. (1983): Increased seizure susceptibility of the immature brain. *Dev. Brain Res.* **7,** 81–85.

Moshé, S.L., Holmes, G.L. & Mareš, P. (1991): Epileptogenesis and the immature brain: subcortical mechanisms. *Exp. Brain Res.* **20,** 151–153.

Muller, D., Oliver, M. & Lynch, G. (1989): Developmental changes in synaptic properties in hippocampus of neonatal rats. *Dev. Brain Res.* **49,** 105–114.

Nelson, K.B. & Ellenberg, J.H. (1976): Predictors of epilepsy in children who have experienced febrile seizures. *N. Engl. J. Med.* **295,** 1029–1033.

Nelson, K.B. & Ellenberg, J.H. (1978): Prognosis in children with febrile convulsions. *Pediatrics* **61,** 720–727.

Nobrega, J.N. & Gaito, J. (1978): Long term induction of kindled seizures in rats: interhemispheric factors. *Can. J. Neurol. Sci.* **5,** 223–230.

O'Donohoe, N.V. (1985): *Epilepsies of childhood*, 2nd edn. London: Butterworth.

Okada, R., Moshé, S.L. & Albala, B.J. (1984): Infantile status epilepticus and future seizure susceptibility in the rat. *Dev. Brain Res.* **15,** 177–183.

Olney, J.W., Rhee, V. & DeGubareff, T. (1974): Kainic acid: a powerful neurotoxic analogue of glutamate. *Brain Res.* **77,** 507–512.

Peterson, S.L., Albertson, T.E. & Stark, L.G. (1981): Intertrial intervals and kindled seizures. *Exp. Neurol.* **71,** 144–153.

Pinel, J.P.J. & Rovner, L.I. (1978): Experimental epileptogenesis: kindling induced epilepsy in rats. *Exp. Neurol.* **58,** 190–202.

Pisa, M., Sanberg, P.R., Corcoran, M.E. & Fibiger, H.C. (1980): Spontaneously recurrent seizures after intracerebral injections of kainic acid in rat: a possible method of human temporal lobe epilepsy. *Brain Res.* **200,** 481–487.

Prince, D.A. & Gutnick, M.J. (1972): Neuronal activities in epileptogenic foci of immature cortex. *Brain Res.* **45,** 455–468.

Racine, R.J., Okujava, V. & Senera, C. (1972): Modification of seizure activity by electrical stimulation: III. Mechanisms. *Electroencephalogr. Clin. Neurophysiol.* **32,** 295–299.

Racine, R.J., Rose, P.A. & Burnham, W.M. (1977): Afterdischarge thresholds and kindling rates in dorsal and ventral hippocampus and dentate gyrus. *Can. J. Neurol. Sci.* **4,** 273–278.

Racine, R.J. (1972a): Modification of seizure activity by electrical stimulation: I. After-discharge threshold. *Electroencephalogr. Clin. Neurophysiol.* **32,** 269–279.

Racine, R.J. (1972b): Modification of seizure activity by electrical stimulation: II. Motor seizures. *Electroencephal.ogr. Clin. Neurophysiol.* **32,** 281–294.

Racine, R J., Burnham, W.M., Gartner, J.G. & Levitan, D. (1973): Rates of motor seizure development of rats subjected to electrical brain stimulation: strain and interstimulation interval effects. *Electroenceph. Clin. Neurophysiol.* **35,** 553–556.

Rodin, E., Rim, C. & Rennick, P. (1974): The effects of carbamazepine on patients with psychomotor epilepsy: Results of a double-blind study. *Epilepsia* **15,** 547–561.

Seidel, W.T. & Corcoran, M.E. (1986): Relations between amygdaloid and anterior neocortical kindling. *Brain Res.* **385,** 375–378.

Shewmon, D.A., Shields, W.D., Chugani, H.T. & Peacock, W.J. (1990): Contrasts between pediatric and adult epilepsy surgery: rationale and strategy for focal resection. *J. Epilepsy* (suppl.), 1–15.

Shinnar, S. & Moshé, S.L. (1991): Age specificity of seizure expression in genetic epilepsies. In: *Genetic strategies in epilepsy research*, eds. V.E. Anderson, W.A. Hauser, I.E. Leppik, J.L. Noebels & S.S. Rich, pp. 69–85. Amsterdam: Elsevier.

Shinnar, S., Berg, A.T., Moshé, S.L., Petix, M., Maytal, J., Kang, H., Goldensohn, E.S. & Hauser, W.A. (1990): The risk of seizure recurrence following a first unprovoked seizure in childhood: a prospective study. *Pediatrics* **85,** 1076–1085.

Shinnar, S., Maytal, J., Krasnoff, L. & Moshé, S.L. (1992): Recurrent status epilepticus in children. *Ann. Neurol.* **31,** 598–604.

Shouse, M.N., King, A., Langer, J., Vreeken, T., King, K. & Richkind, M. (1990): The ontogeny of feline temporal lobe epilepsy: kindling a spontaneous seizure disorder in kittens. *Dev. Brain Res.* **52,** 215–224.

Sperber, E.F., Haas, K.Z. & Moshé, S.L. (1991a): Presence of spontaneous seizures and lack of kindling antagonism in rat pups. *Epilepsia* **32,** 32.

Sperber, E.F., Haas, K., Stanton, P.K. & Moshé, S.L. (1991b): Resistance of the immature brain to seizure-induced synaptic reorganization. *Dev. Brain Res.* **60,** 88–93.

Squillance, K., Post, R. & Pert, A. (1980): Development of wet dog shakes during amygdala kindling in the rat. *Exp. Neurol.* **70,** 487–497.

Sramka, M., Sedlak, P. & Nadvornik, P. (1977): Observation of the kindling phenomenon in treatment of pain by stimulation in thalamus. In: *Neurosurgical treatment in psychiatry, pain, and epilepsy*, ed. W.H. Sweet, pp. 651–654. Baltimore: University Park Press.

Stanton, P.K. (1991): Phasic stimulus patterns controlling long-term potentiation and depression of synaptic strengths in the hippocampus. In: *Kindling and synaptic plasticity: the legacy of Graham Goddard*, ed. F. Morrell, pp. 78–91. Boston: Birkhäuser.

Stark, L.G., Albertson, T.E. & Joy, R. M. (1986): The acquisition of a kindled response in developing rats using 24-h intertrial interval. *Dev. Brain Res.* **24,** 291–294.

Temkin, N.R., Dikmen, S.S., Wilensky, A.J., Keihm, J., Chabal, S. & Winn, H.R. (1990): A randomized, double-blind study of phenytoin for the prevention of post-traumatic seizures. *N. Engl. J. Med.* **323,** 497–502.

Thompson, J.L., Stafstrom, C.E., Chronopoulos, A., Thurber, S. & Holmes, G.L. (1990): Effect of age on seizure susceptibility following kainic acid induced status epilepticus. *Epilepsia* **31,** 634.

Torres, F. & Jacome, D. (1982): Secondary epileptogenesis in the human. In: *Secondary epileptogenesis*, eds. A. Mayersdord & R.P. Schmidt, pp. 15–26. New York: Raven Press.

Turski, L., Cavalheiro, E.A., Schwarz, M., Turski, W.A., Mello, L.E.A.M., Bartolotto, Z.A., Klockgether, T. & Sontag, K.H. (1986): Susceptibility to seizures produced by pilocarpine in rats after microinjection of isoniazid or γ-vinyl GABA into the SN. *Brain Res.* **370**, 294–309.

Velíšek, L. & Mareš, P. (1991): An increased epileptogenesis in the hippocampus of developing rats. *Exp. Brain Res.* **20,** 183–185.

Velíšek, L.S., Moshé, S.L. & Stanton, P.K. (1993): Age dependence of homosynaptic non-NMDA mediated long-term depression in field CA1 of rat hippocampal slices. *Brain Res. Dev.* **75,** 253–260.

Velíšek, L.S., Sperber, E F. & Moshé, S.L. (1993): Kindling in developing animals. In: *Epileptogenic and excitotoxic mechanisms*, eds. G. Avanzini, R. Fariello, U. Heinemann & R. Mutani, pp. 121–134. London: John Libbey.

Wada, J.A. (1986): Preface. In: *Kindling 3*, ed. J.A. Wada, pp. v–vi. New York: Raven Press.

Wada, J.A. & Sato, M. (1974): Generalized convulsive seizures induced by daily stimulation of the amygdala in cats. *Neurology* **24,** 565–574.

Wada, J.A., Sato, M. & Corcoran, M.E. (1974): Persistent seizure suceptibility and recurrent spontaneous seizures in kindled cats. *Epilepsia* **15,** 465–478.

Wada, J.A., Sato, M. & McCaughran, J.A.J. (1975): Cortical electrographic correlates on convulsive seizure development induced by daily electrical stimulation of the amygdala in rats and cats. *Folia Psychiatr. Neurol. Japan* **29,** 329–339.

Wada, J.A., Mizoguchi, T. & Osawa, T. (1978): Secondarily generalized convulsive seizures induced by daily amygdaloid stimulation in rhesus monkeys. *Neurology* **28,** 1026–1036.Ward, A. (1969): The epileptic neuron: chronic foci in animals and man. In: *Basic mechanisms of the epilepsies*, eds. H. Jasper, A. Ward & A. Pope, pp. 263–288). Boston: Little, Brown.

Woodbury, L.A. (1977): Incidence and prevalence of seizure disorders including the epilepsies in the USA. a review and analysis of the literature. In: *Plan for the nationwide action on epilepsy*, pp. 24–77. Washington, DC: DHEW Publication.

Wright, F. & Bradley, W. (1968): Maturation of epileptiform activity. *Electroencephalogr. Clin. Neurophysiol.* **25,** 259–265.

Zaide, J. (1974): Differences between Tryon Bright and Dull rats in seizure activity evoked by amygdala stimulation. *Physiol. Behav.* **12,** 527–534.

Zhao, D.Y. & Moshé, S.L. (1987): Deep prepiriform cortex and amygdala interactions. *Epilepsy Res.* **1,** 94–101.

Epileptic Seizures and Syndromes, Edited by Peter Wolf
© 1994 John Libbey & Company Ltd., pp. 505–521

Chapter 51

Secondary epileptogenesis: concepts and controversies

Eric W. Lothman

Comprehensive Epilepsy Program, Department of Neurology, Box 394, University of Virginia Health Sciences Center, Charlottesville, VA 22908, USA

Summary

The concept of secondary epileptogenesis in which a region of brain can be converted, by the proper exposure to seizures imposed from outside that region, from a normal state to a primary epileptic focus, capable itself of giving rise to spontaneous seizures, has theoretical and practical implications. The pragmatic clinical ramifications of such a process in humans would be that it provides a means by which the number of epileptic foci could proliferate and become a substrate for progressive epilepsy. Some clinical data suggest secondary epileptogenesis may occur in humans, but this is quite controversial. As an alternative to human studies, experimental animal models have been examined and found to support the idea of secondary epileptogenesis. From a historical perspective, the two most cited models are the mirror focus and kindling. These two models have produced examples of secondary epileptogenesis in the time and space domains but the data have been questioned for their relevance to humans. Much of the objection can be understood as definitional differences and what the counterparts of the phenomena in the animal models are expected to be in humans, especially with regard to experimental paradigms. In the discussion, a wider perspective for interpreting models is proposed. On this basis recent information is reviewed that supports the concept of secondary epileptogenesis in animal models, including kindling and other 'newer' models that share several features with human epilepsy. Insight into the mechanism of secondary epileptogenesis in these models promises to aid our understanding of the neurobiology of epilepsy in man and the potential for new types of therapy.

Introduction

Most patients with epilepsy can be adequately treated with antiepileptic drugs. However, in up to a third of patients (Engel, 1989; Rogowski & Porter, 1990; Wieser *et al.*, 1993) seizures remain refractory to medical therapy. For many of these individuals, seizures are partial (focal) in onset, often with secondary generalization, and accordingly they can be considered for surgical treatment for intractable epilepsy. The strategy in these cases is to seek an 'epileptic focus' in which seizures begin and from which they propagate to other regions. If an appropriate focus is found and it can be removed without unacceptable neurological consequences, then there is excellent prognosis that seizures will come under better control or even remit.

Yet the situation often does not prove this simple. One complication is that a single discrete focus may not be found. At the extreme, seizures may be found to arise in multiple regions throughout both hemispheres. In situations with less 'dissemination of epileptic foci', seizures may arise bilaterally from homotopic sites or from more than one region in a single hemisphere. In these latter instances, there are clear-cut practical implications for presurgical evaluation and for surgical treatment. More controversial are certain theoretical ramifications that offer the promise of shedding light on the neurobiology of epilepsy. One such ramification is the idea of *secondary epileptogenesis*. There has been considerable debate as to whether or not secondary epileptogenesis occurs in humans or whether it represents a phenomenon restricted to certain animal models of epilepsy, such as kindling.

In part, the controversy about secondary epileptogenesis in humans can be linked to defining what secondary epileptogenesis is and how can it be recognized. These points will be considered further below. Here I will define secondary epileptogenesis as the process by which a particular brain region, originally normal, develops an enduring functional alteration with enhanced epileptogenic properties as a consequence of being exposed to repeated seizures imposed from outside that region. The argument will be advanced below that secondary epileptogenesis, so defined, does occur, at least in animal models of epilepsy, that elucidating the basic mechanisms underlying such secondary epileptogenesis in experimental animals will advance our general understanding of the neurobiology of epilepsy, and that by properly using such information one can better understand and treat humans with epilepsy. Furthermore, it will be argued that the events of secondary epileptogenesis can be envisioned to operate in two domains. In the *spatial domain*, secondary epileptogenesis serves to multiply the number of regions critically operating in the initiation and elaboration of seizures. In the *time domain*, secondary epileptogenesis serves as a means by which epilepsy can become progressive, thereby increasing the 'severity of epilepsy'.

Secondary epileptogenesis: historical perspective

Several of the concepts addressed in this chapter have been argued about for several decades (Rodin, 1968; Wilder, 1972). The debate has been fuelled by information derived both from animal work and from clinical epileptology. All past literature will not be reviewed here; rather our considerations will begin with the extended discussion provided by Morrell (1985).

Salient features of Morrell's paper were: a definition of secondary epileptogenesis; a review of data from animal studies; and a presentation of new information from a particular group of patients that supported the hypothesis that secondary epileptogenesis does occur in humans. Morrell defined secondary epileptogenesis as the process by which an actively discharging epileptogenic region may induce similar behaviour in cellular elements of an otherwise normal network.

Morrell's discussion of secondary epileptogenesis in animals centred on two models, the mirror focus and kindling. These two models are interrelated but not identical. There are differences in the neuroanatomical systems that are best suited to each of the models. The mirror focus model involves the placement of an irritant or convulsant at one site in the brain, thereby making this site a primary 'epileptic focus'. Under appropriate circumstances, the homotopic region in the contralateral hemisphere later becomes an epileptic focus in its own right. The neocortex is well suited to the mirror focus model, in part because of its access to callosal pathways that provide the necessary anatomical substrate for the mirror focus phenomena. The kindling model involves the *repetitive* delivery of a fixed-intensity stimulus that induces an acute seizure at the site of the stimulus. Upon repetition, the seizures at the stimulus site become more elaborate and longer and the extent to which the seizures propagate from the seizure site becomes greater. While kindling has been done with chemical agents, delivered either systemically (Post *et al.*, 1984) or intracerebrally (Wasterlain & Jonec, 1980), the customary protocol is to use focal intracerebral stimuli through implanted electrodes. Although kindling has been observed when neocortical regions are selected as the kindling site (Albright & Burnham, 1980; Santori & Collins, 1988), limbic regions are particularly well suited to the kindling model. In contrast to the mirror focus model with its emphasis on callosal pathways and homotopic regions, the kindling model involves propagation amongst limbic structures on the same side of the brain and propagation to regions outside the limbic system, including subcortical sites and cortical sites. Depending on the species, a variety of commissural systems in addition to the corpus callosum are important for the spread of seizures in the kindling model.

Morrell reviewed electroencephalographic (EEG)features and clinical seizure manifestations in the kindling and mirror focus models. On the basis of this information, he postulated three stages of secondary epileptogenesis. In the first (dependent) stage, epileptiform discharges detected in the secondary focus were driven by the primary focus. In the second (intermediate) stage, epileptiform discharges were detected in the secondary focus and initially persisted after removal of the primary focus, but eventually 'ran down' and disappeared. In the third (independent) stage, epileptiform discharges in the secondary focus persisted after removal of the primary focus without run-down. Because the epileptiform discharges in the secondary focus could be full-fledged electrographic seizures and be accompanied by clinical seizures, this region was stated to have become a 'mature' epileptic focus.

Morrell also reviewed pharmacotherapy in the models of secondary epileptogenesis. He noted that a broad spectrum of drugs used in the treatment of epilepsy had the ability to suppress seizure occurrence when present in sufficient concentrations. In brief, these agents exerted an antiepileptic or anticonvulsant effect in the conventional sense and manner of use, that of suppressing seizures but not affecting the underlying cause of epilepsy. Morrell also distinguished the ability of certain, but not all, antiepileptic drugs to retard or prevent the development of secondary epileptogenesis. This distinction pointed out by Morrell was marshalled as experimental evidence that there was a process of secondary epileptogenesis because it had a distinct pharmacology. In other words, particular pharmaceutical agents exert an antiepileptogenic effect, opposing the very mechanisms that cause epileptogenesis, and this action can be theoretically distinguished from an antiepileptic/anticonvulsant effect.

The point of antiepileptogenic vs. antiepileptic/anticonvulsant actions of drugs is currently of great interest since it provides a means of treating the aetiology of epilepsy instead of its symptoms. While not the primary focus of the current discussion, some points on this topic are in order. First, a drug's having an antiepileptogenic action does not preclude its having an antiepileptic/anticonvulsant action. On the other hand, a single drug does not have to have both actions. Second, in a fashion like the expression of seizures involving a variety of pathophysiological events, there are probably a variety of mechanisms of epileptogenesis. Therefore, just as multiple types of antiepileptic/anticonvulsant drugs are currently in use, each with its own mode of action in opposing the expression of seizures (Macdonald & McLean, 1982; Stringer & Lothman, 1991), one can anticipate the potential future use of several different classes of antiepileptogenic agents. Third, should effective antiepileptogenic agents be identified, then a restructuring of the way in which drugs are used in epileptic patients may be in order. For example, for patients with an ongoing risk of seizures, an indefinite period of treatment with antiepileptic/anticonvulsant drugs is appropriate. If a time-limited period of epileptogenesis exists, then treatment with an antiepileptogenic agent can be restricted. Given the possibility of multiple means of opposing epileptogenesis and the separation of antiepileptogenic *vs.* antiepileptic/anticonvulsant drug actions, polypharmacy may become a principle for treating epileptic patients. Just as with the identification of antiepileptic/anticonvulsant drugs, the identification of antiepileptogenic agents would be facilitated by animal studies. The challenge, then, is to identify: (a) epileptogenic processes in animal models; (b) means to pharmacologically attenuate or prevent these processes; (c) which epileptogenic mechanisms are shared by animal models and patients with epilepsy; and (d) clinically useful antiepileptic agents in terms of efficacy and toxicity.

Morrell's considerations of the pathophysiology of secondary epileptogenesis in animal models brought up two factors as being important in secondary epileptogenesis. The first factor was that of spatial connections and their density. The second factor was that of temporal patterns of epileptiform discharges. Since the functional anatomy of the mirror focus and kindling models are not identical (see above) but both can be considered as appropriate means to study secondary epileptogenesis, Morrell proposed a 'loosening' of the way in which one might envision the spatial domain of secondary epileptogenesis. He mentioned the idea of a juxtahomotopic focus that in the strictest sense is not a mirror focus but does conform to a more general concept of contralateral hemisphere secondary focus. Morrell also pointed out that secondary foci may be distributed in the same hemisphere in the fashion of secondary epileptogenesis in the kindling model and also postulated that 'higher-order foci' (i.e. beyond secondary foci) may occur. Considering these ideas, one can envision a rich array of networks, encompassing several types of target areas, that provides the functional anatomy for secondary epileptogenesis, schematized in Fig. 1.

To extend his line of argument that secondary epileptogenesis takes place in humans, thereby producing phenomena like those in the kindling and mirror focus models, Morrell selected a set of patients with unilateral cerebral tumours on the basis of the following reasoning. One can take issue with human studies directed at demonstrating secondary epileptogenesis with traumatic, vascular or infectious aetiologies because the primary disease process may establish multiple primary epileptic foci. However, Morrell argued that the possibility of this occurrence was vanishingly low in the case of tumour pathology. In his personal series of 47 patients with tumours and seizures, Morrell reported

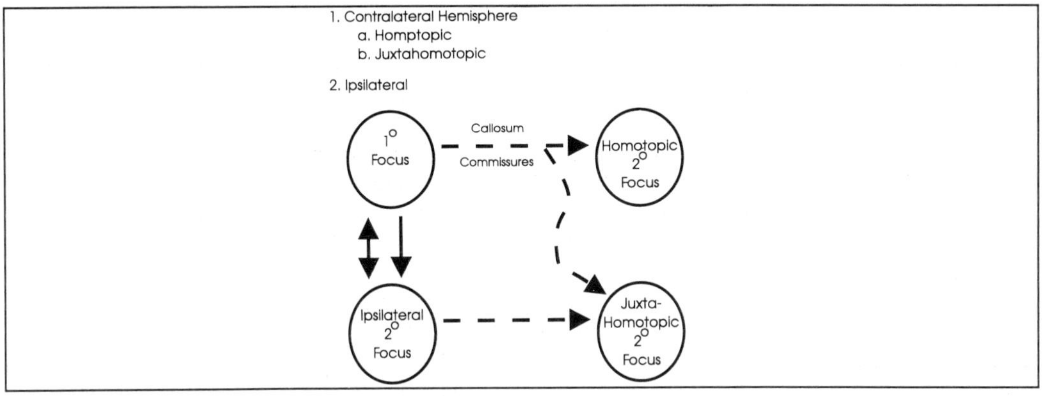

Fig. 1. Target areas in secondary epileptogenesis. Schematic representation of types of secondary epileptogenic foci, including those in the contralateral hemisphere (right side) and in the ipsilateral hemisphere (lower left), relative to the primary focus.

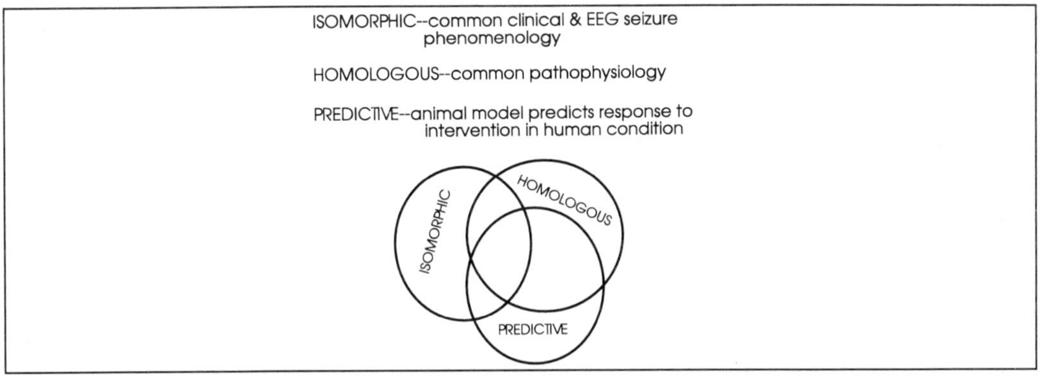

Fig. 2. Classes of animal models of epilepsy and epileptogenesis. The three 'classes' of models introduced in the text are illustrated. Note that any particular model may have one, two or three of the specified characteristics.

that 34 per cent had evidence of the later two (intermediate and independent) stages of epileptogenesis on the basis of EEG data. The thrust of this analysis was to analyse for comparisons with the mirror focus model. For details, the reader is referred to the original paper (Morrell, 1985).

Other parameters that may reflect the consequences of secondary epileptogenesis, in the clinical realm, are the frequency of seizures over time, the time between seizures and development of pharmacoresistance (decreased efficacy of antiepileptic drugs for suppressing seizures). These topics remain to be fully explored. However, Reynolds *et al.* (reviewed by Reynolds, Chapter 59) have documented a progressive decrease in the interval between successive seizures in a cohort of patients followed from the time of their first seizure. This may be viewed as an indication of the progressive nature of epilepsy. It may also be that the processes that account for successive seizures coming closer together share mechanisms with the animal models of secondary epileptogenesis that are reviewed below. This speculation remains to be studied.

Kindling as a model of secondary epileptogenesis

Since the report of Morrell in 1985, attention paid to the mirror focus model has been limited while there has been considerable work with the kindling model. In fact, today the kindling model is probably the best studied model of chronic epilepsy in experimental animals. It is therefore appropriate to consider what the kindling model can teach us about secondary epileptogenesis.

We begin by considering the broader issue of the role of animal models for epilepsy. Animal models may be envisioned in several ways, three of which are schematized in Fig. 2. An isomorphic model presents phenomena to the investigator (e.g. EEG and clinical seizures) that appear like those that occur in human epilepsy. A homologous model produces a pathophysiology in animals that shares common features with particular epileptic conditions in humans. A predictive model predicts the response to intervention in human patients on the basis of how that intervention affects the model. It is important to note that individual models may possess some or all of these features. Thus, on the one hand, a model may produce EEG and clinical seizures that are identical to those detected in human patients with epilepsy, will display functional and pathological alterations identical to those found in the brains of patients with epilepsy and will respond to an intervention (e.g. drug treatment) in the same way that the seizures in patients do. Such a model would be highly useful, being able to address a variety of experimental questions. On the other hand, a model may be linked to a particular human epileptic condition only in one or two of the ways under consideration. For example, the induction of motor convulsions in rodents with pentylenetetrazole is predictive for agents effective against absence seizures, but the two types of seizures cannot be considered to be isomorphic. The range of questions that this sort of model can answer is more limited, but with appropriate experimental design the information provided is useful. In fact, it is possible that a particular model may provide a large amount of information that is consistently of clinical relevance in one, and only one, of the identified areas, while another model may provide information in more areas, but less consistently. Thus, it is of paramount importance to know the characteristics, strengths and limitations of a particular model in order to be able to properly extrapolate the results to the clinical realm.

We may now turn to the kindling model. This model, including its name, was originally developed by Goddard and his colleagues (Goddard *et al.*, 1969). Since then hundreds of papers have been published and several reviews have appeared on this model (e.g. Racine, 1978; Goddard *et al.*, 1986; McNamara *et al.*, 1985; Löscher *et al.*, 1986). Only certain points pertinent to the present discussion will be considered here.

The most frequently used definition of the kindling model is that this represents the situation where, upon repetition of an initially subconvulsive stimulus, seizure responses intensify, culminating in the consistent expression of a generalized convulsion. Kindling has been reported in various species including rats, dogs, cats and primates (Goddard *et al.*, 1969, 1986; Wada *et al.*, 1974; Wada & Osawa, 1976; Wada, 1982; McNamara *et al.*, 1985; Löscher *et al.*, 1986). The generalized convulsion, as identified in rats, is quite distinct, consisting of forelimb clonus, rearing and falling, and has been called a kindled motor seizure (KMS). KMS, therefore, are customarily employed as the principle observation in kindling studies. Before KMS appear, a sequence of less severe seizures appear that are conventionally separated into five stages and are used as the primary index for monitoring the course of kindling. Therefore, staging in kindling is typically followed by noting the most severe behavioural seizure manifest in response to a fixed test stimulus, i.e. a form of 'end-point' marking is used. After an animal has been fully kindled, the test stimulus will consistently elicit a KMS, even if the animal is studied after several months without giving the test stimulus. Hence, the kindled state appears to be permanent for the life of the animal. Consequently, the kindling model is traditionally conceptualized as having two phases: (a) an initial dynamic progressive phase (*kindling acquisition*), in which behavioural seizures worsen until KMS appear; (b) a later enduring (permanent) stable phase (*kindled state*) with KMS to each stimulus.

Hence the kindling model is widely studied by following *behavioural* seizures that are *triggered* by an experimenter-controlled stimulus. Furthermore, the effect of experimental manipulations on the acquisition of kindling are typically assessed by the number of stimuli needed before KMS appear (or a certain number of consecutive KMS have elapsed); the effect of experimental manipulations on the stable kindled state is typically assessed by the suppression of KMS. With this approach, a hierarchy of sites has been identified predicated on the basis of number of stimuli to that site before KMS appear. While different stimulus protocols have been employed, a once daily stimulation with 50–60 Hz/1–2 s train of pulses is typically used 'to kindle'. With this approach, a variety of areas in the limbic system have been found suited to kindling, including the hippocampus, amygdala and septum. The site most often used in kindling is the amygdala; with the traditional once-daily stimulus mentioned above, kindling from the amygdala takes about 2 weeks. Kindling has also been done by delivering the stimulus to the neocortex. With neocortical kindling, the initial behavioural seizures differ from those obtained with limbic site stimulation, but eventually typical KMS occur. Consequently, it is reasonable to postulate that eventually neocortical kindling activates the same set of brain structures as limbic kindling by gaining access to limbic circuits. Studies using functional mapping have supported this idea (Albright & Burnham, 1980; Santori & Collins, 1988).

If a stable kindled state is established by stimulating one site and then another, physically separate, site is stimulated, the number of stimuli needed to elicit KMS from the second site is fewer than if no stimuli had been given to the primary site. In the case of the sequential stimulation of two sites, the increased epileptogenesis to primary site stimulation (as manifest by increased seizure response (KMS)) is said to be transferred to the secondary site. (No consideration will be given here to the interesting phenomenon that alteration of stimuli to two separate sites during the course of the initial kindling may retard kindling – Burchiel *et al.*, 1982; see also Garant, Chapter 50.)

It is important to note that the end-point-marking procedure and focusing on KMS discussed above can obscure certain aspects of the kindling model *vis-à-vis* human epilepsy. When considered on the basis of isomorphic models, kindling can be conceptualized as an experimental counterpart of complex partial seizures with secondary generalization. The involvement of limbic circuits (on the basis of their direct stimulation or by entry from neocortical site stimulation), the functional anatomy of circuits activated (Engel *et al.*, 1978; Lothman *et al.*, 1985b) and the nature of behavioural seizures all support this idea. Indeed, all KMS progress through the same sequence of behavioural seizure events that marks the acquisition phase of kindling. Moreover, it is known that the events responsible for kindling are the production of a local electrographic seizure (after-discharge) at the site of stimulation, prolongation of the after-discharge at that site, capture of sites anatomically coupled to the stimulus site into the seizure and eventual spread of the seizures into motor centres when the afterdischarge is long enough and involves enough limbic regions (Racine, 1972). On the basis of these data, it seems appropriate to concentrate on epileptogenesis in limbic networks in the kindling model. To be sure, the study of KMS may be instructive for understanding generalization of seizures from limbic areas with subsequent secondary convulsions. However, in the context of surgical treatment of patients with epilepsy, understanding epileptogenesis in limbic circuits promises to be more rewarding. From this perspective the study of electrographic seizures is as valid as the study of behavioural seizures.

The argument just presented is that seizures in the kindling model, once triggered, are isomorphic to complex partial seizures with secondary generalization. A concern with the seizures in the kindling model is that, in contrast to the situation with human epilepsy, they are not spontaneous. The occurrence of interictal spikes in limbic regions in kindled animals is well recognized (Kairiss *et al.*, 1984). The objection to this finding is that, while interictal spikes are recognized as markers of an epileptogenic brain, they are of uncertain significance for precise anatomical identification of an epileptic focus, which depends on detection of seizures. Yet some workers have shown the occurrence of recurrent, spontaneous seizures in the kindling. This was reported over 15 years ago for rats (Pinel & Rovner, 1978), cats (Wada *et al.*, 1974) and primates (Wada & Osawa, 1976).

Given the major concern about whether spontaneous seizures occur in the kindling model, one may wonder why more studies of this type have not been done. At least two sets of explanations can be offered. First, spontaneous seizures were detected only after many triggered kindling/kindled seizures. For example, the study of Pinel & Rovner (1978) needed over 300 stimuli. Thus, it seems that many seizures may need to take place before secondary epileptogenesis with spontaneous seizures occurs. If we extrapolate from the clinical side, this requirement would not be surprising. The second set of explanations relates to procedures for documenting spontaneous seizures. The detection of the spontaneous seizures is far more difficult experimentally than that of triggered seizures which occur at the whim of the investigator, up to many times per day. Furthermore, spontaneous seizure detection is complicated. Besides the issue of extended monitoring periods, there is the issue of how seizures should be detected. Behavioural observations can be used. However, if seizures arise in limbic regions, as one would expect in the kindling model, they would be expected to be more subtle than KMS unless all such spontaneous seizures generalize and are accompanied by convulsions. Accordingly, it is suggested that the proper means for detecting spontaneous seizures, with computer-assisted monitoring and seizure detection, has only recently become available and has not yet been adequately applied to the kindling model. Questions that should be addressed include the following: What type of epileptiform events occur in the kindling model–interictal spikes, spontaneous recurrent seizures, or both? What sort of epileptic history, in terms of triggered seizures, is needed for the establishment of this 'fully developed' secondary epileptogenic condition? What is the functional anatomy of such recurrent seizures if they occur? Do seizures begin only at the site used to elicit triggered seizures or from (spatially) separate secondary sites? What are the clinical accompaniments of such seizures? By answering these questions, we will have better insight into how isomorphic the kindling model is to human complex partial seizures arising in limbic regions, using the strict criteria of spontaneous recurring seizures.

For obvious reasons, data on whether kindling occurs in humans, as evidenced by responses to recurrent electrical stimuli, is sparse. While limited to a single patient, the work of Sramka *et al.* (1975) attracts attention. These investigators implanted stimulators in three thalamic sites in a patient, without previous epilepsy, for pain. After 3 weeks of stimulation, the patient began noticing limb movements coincident with the stimulation. The electrodes were removed, but the patient experienced Jacksonian seizures and exhibited electrographic paroxysms. The interpretation of Sramka and co-workers was that the seizures were a sequela of the electrode implantation and stimulation and that the patient had shown a form of kindling. Several points merit comment. This is a single case report and alternative explanations for the aetiology of the seizures, such as scar tissue from electrode implantation, can be advanced. The site of stimulation and motor manifestations were atypical for kindling as standardly examined in animals (see above). Furthermore, the occurrence of *spontaneous* seizures in this patient is at variance with the *triggered* seizures typically studied in kindling. The spontaneous seizures developed after a short period of stimulation, which seems to be different from the case in animals, at least rodents (see above). Despite these caveats, this report is provocative in suggesting that kindling, especially the occurrence of spontaneous seizures, may occur in humans.

If one accepts the idea that increased severity of *triggered* seizures (length of after-discharges and/or nature of clinical seizures) is a valid means of examining epileptogenesis, then the finding of transference in the kindling model (see above) is of interest. On this basis it can be argued that secondary epileptogenesis, in the spatial domain, occurs experimentally. One can consider the enhancement of elicited seizure responses seen during kindling acquisition as representing progressive epileptogenesis, although some might counter that this is a trivial example. Less debatable is the important issue of whether repeated provoked seizures adequately prime limbic circuits for the occurrence of spontaneous recurrent seizures, a topic considered above. Furthermore, there is evidence that, with repeated application of a constant stimulus, kindled responses show additional progression during the 'stable' fully kindled state. For example, the times to reach the various sequential behavioural events that stage the evolution of a kindled seizure become shorter. Concomitantly, the lengths of after-discharges shorten. At the same time, triggered kindled seizures appear to become more resistant to antiepileptic drugs, occasioning the opinion that under these conditions they are especially suited to serve as a model of refractory epilepsy (Löscher *et al.*, 1986).

Emerging concepts of secondary epileptogenesis

Epileptic networks

For a number of years our laboratory has been studying epileptogenesis using models derived from adaptations of the traditional kindling approach introduced above. Instead of once-daily stimulation in the amygdala, we have elicited seizures with stimulation of the ventral hippocampus with interstimulus intervals measured in minutes to hours. The discussion here will centre on our studies of secondary epileptogenesis using the two models schematized in Fig. 3. Both models utilize the same type of stimulus (50 Hz/10 s trains to the ventral CA3 region), but with different patterns. If given once every 30 min, such trains cause a lengthening of after-discharges and progression through

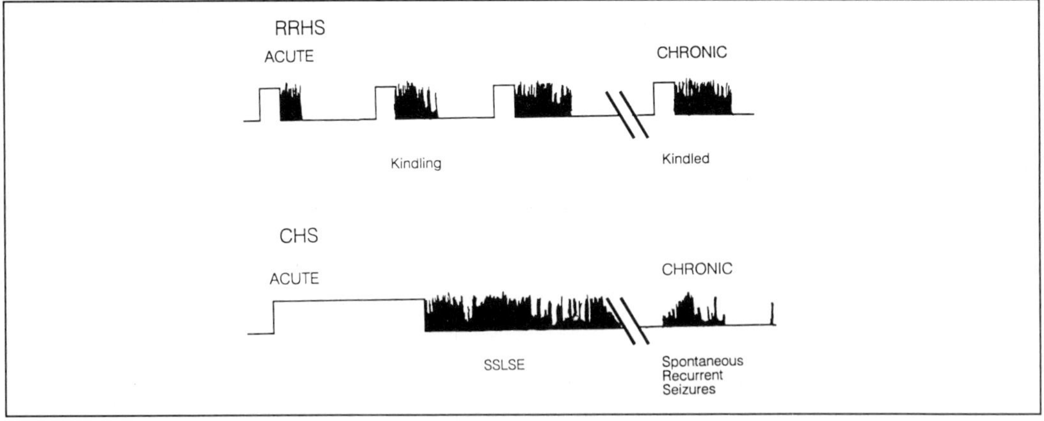

Fig. 3. Electrical stimulus-induced models of hippocampal seizures used to examine aspects of secondary epileptogenesis. Two stimulus protocols (rapidly recurring hippocampal seizures – RRHS – shown at the top and continuous hippocampal stimulation–CHS – shown at the bottom) that rely on the same fundamental stimulus, but differ with respect to the temporal patterning of that stimulus are given. For both models acute changes are shown on the left while chronic changes are on the right. The RRHS model results in kindling or triggered seizures. The CHS protocol establishes two forms of stimulus-independent seizures, self-sustaining limbic status epilepticus (SSLSE) that develops early and a chronic sequela of spontaneous recurrent

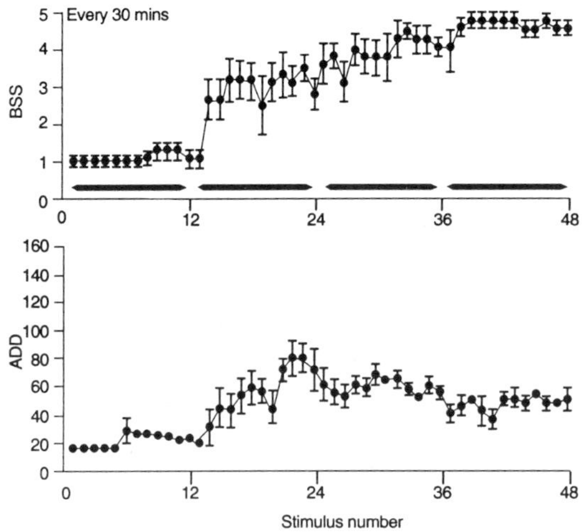

Fig. 4. Rapid kindling with RRHS protocol. Stimulus trains were given every 30 min, with 12 stimuli given per day over 4 consecutive days. Top panel presents behavioural seizure scores (BSS) on the ordinate and bottom panel presents after-discharge duration (ADD) in seconds on the ordinate for each stimulus (abscissae).

behavioural seizure stages identical to traditional kindling (Lothman *et al.*, 1985a; Lothman & Williamson, 1993), as shown in Fig. 4. If given with only a few seconds between or immediately next to each other for a period of 30–90 min, such trains establish a condition of non-convulsive self-sustaining status epilepticus marked by electrographic seizures in limbic circuits (Lothman *et al.*, 1989; VanLandingham & Lothman, 1991). The electrographic seizures progress through a sequence known to occur in humans (Treiman *et al.*, 1989). Subsequently, spontaneous recurrent seizures are detected with bipolar hippocampal electrodes. Our initial report detected such spontaneous seizures in 50 per cent of animals with intermittent monitoring (Lothman *et al.*, 1990); with extended periods of continuous computer-assisted monitoring, spontaneous seizures were detected in 90 per cent of animals (unpublished).

Thus, several epileptic phenomena have been identified with these models that can be considered secondary epileptogenesis in the time domain. In the acute time frame, the repetition of triggered seizures with the rapidly recurring hippocampal seizure protocol (Fig. 3) establishes a self-reinforcing situation wherein the seizures become longer and behavioural seizures worsen. This situation is phenomenologically similar to traditional kindling and the discussion given above applies. If one disregards stimulus-locked seizures as providing information about epileptogenesis and attends only to spontaneous seizures, the models in Fig. 3 pertain. In the acute time frame, the application of the 'continuous' hippocampal stimulation protocol produces a situation with spontaneous (*not* stimulus-locked) seizures, albeit of a special sort – status epilepticus. The chronic condition of spontaneous recurrent hippocampal seizures that develops as a sequela of the status epilepticus just discussed replicates the spontaneity of seizures in patients with epilepsy. With the strictest interpretation, this situation is isomorphic to temporal lobe epilepsy in humans with a preceding history of status epilepticus. In other words the situation can be envisioned to be a model of the human mesial temporal lobe epilepsy syndrome (Wieser *et al.*, 1993).

In our studies we have addressed the issue of secondary epileptogenesis in the spatial domain and have also addressed mechanisms. Recall that the stimulating electrodes are positioned in the ventral hippocampus of rats, which corresponds to the anterior hippocampus of humans. The intrahippocampal positioning was selected on the basis of information indicating that this structure is important for

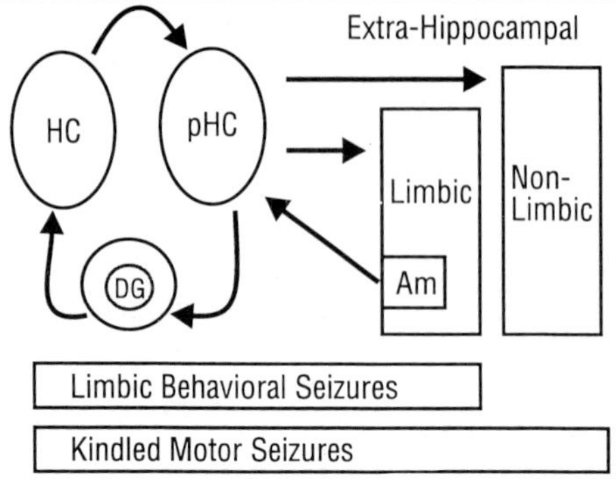

Fig. 5. Epileptic networks involved in the epileptogenic responses with the models introduced in Fig. 3. On the left the hippocampal–parahippocampal loop is shown, consisting of the hippocampus (HC), parahippocampus (pHC) and dentate gyrus (DG) linked in a serial circuit. The HC and pHC, especially the entorhinal cortex, possess a high propensity for ictal activity while the dentate gyrus normally resists developing seizures. Consequently, the potential for reverberatory activity is opposed by the DG until it develops seizure activity, like the maximal dentate activation described in the text. In this circumstance, reverberatory activity develops in the hippocampal–parahippocampal loop, leading to self-reinforcing triggered seizures (kindling) or self-sustaining, stimulus-independent seizures (limbic status epilepticus). For the models described in the text, seizures are initiated with stimuli in the hippocampus (CA3), but are associated with changes in the dentate gyrus on the sides ipsilateral and contralateral to the CA3 stimulation, examples of secondary epileptogenesis in the spatial domain. The hippocampal–parahippocampal loop can also be activated from other sides, such as the amygdala (Am), as discussed in the text.

generating many seizures in humans (Wieser, 1983). Using depth electrodes and 2-deoxyglucose autoradiography, we compared the functional anatomy of seizures before kindling with those after kindling (Lothman *et al.*, 1985a). As might be expected, a number of brain structures implicated in motor activity and seizure generalization become activated with kindled responses that were not activated with seizures before kindling. Because of our interest in epileptogenesis in limbic circuits, we carried out experiments addressing changes at the network, cellular, and molecular level that could account for heightened epileptogenesis in these models. What follows is a selected overview of the findings, combined with additional work from other laboratories.

While the after-discharges were initiated with focal stimulation in the hippocampus, we also detected electrographic seizures in structures adjacent to the hippocampus. These parahippocampal regions included the subiculum and entorhinal cortex. Pertinent details about the anatomical connections between these regions are given in Fig. 5 (the hippocampal–parahippocampal(HC–pHC) loop). The propensity of the hippocampus for generating seizures has been well known for decades. More recently, a similar tendency has been shown for the parahippocampal region, especially the entorhinal cortex (Jones, 1993). Because of the intrinsic properties of the parahippocampal region and the hippocampus and their interconnections, the opportunity for reverberatory activity in this chain of structures exists. However, an additional structure must be considered – the dentate gyrus. The granule cells of the dentate gyrus have often been shown to resist the development of seizures when studied *in vitro* under the influence of chemoconvulsants (Westbrook & Lothman, 1983; Prince, 1988). However, under the appropriate conditions *in vivo* (Stringer *et al.*, 1989) or *in vitro* (Schweitzer *et al.*, 1992; D.A. Rempe & E.W. Lothman, unpublished), dentate granule cells develop a stereotyped, robust type of paroxysmal discharge – termed maximal dentate activation. Consequently, the dentate gyrus is situated as a control point for the generation of seizures in the hippocampus and the closely connected parahippocampal regions. When the granule cells do not participate in seizures, the dentate operates as a 'brake' to retard seizures. When the granule cells do participate in seizures, the hippocampus and parahippocampal regions can participate in self-reinforcing seizures. Details of the operation of the HC–pHC loop, with the dentate gyrus as a control point, are summarized in Fig. 5.

Of interest to the present consideration is the finding that, when the dentate gyrus does not develop maximal activation, lengthening of successive hippocampal stimulus-triggered after-discharges does not take place and kindling does not occur. However, when maximal dentate activation develops, prompt lengthening of after-discharges happens (see Fig. 32 in Lothman *et al.*, 1991). In addition, maximal dentate activation can be elicited by stimulation in the *amygdala* (Stringer *et al.*, 1991). Before the elicitation of maximal dentate activation, neither lengthening of amygdala after-discharges nor kindling or behavioural seizures take place; after maximal dentate activation occurs, both lengthening of afterdischarges and behavioural kindling proceed. Furthermore, in kindled animals, chronic alterations in the dentate gyrus exist that make it easier to elicit maximal dentate activation (Stringer & Lothman, 1989).

The findings for changes in the dentate gyrus just discussed are linked to triggered seizures. Accordingly, the points raised above about the traditional model of kindling obtain. If one accepts triggered seizures as an adequate means to study epileptogenesis, then the studies just presented establish that secondary epileptogenesis in the spatial domain does occur since chronic functional changes in the dentate gyrus are established with repeated focal stimulation to the hippocampus.

The involvement of the HC–pHC loop in the induction of the acute condition of self-sustaining limbic status epilepticus, introduced above, has also been indicated by studies in our laboratory (VanLandingham & Lothman, 1991). The elucidation of permanent changes underlying increased epileptogenesis in the dentate gyrus in the post-self-sustaining limbic status epilepticus model with spontaneous recurrent seizures (right-hand side of Fig. 3) is a topic of current research in our laboratory. Studies of altered function are under way. Morphological findings of mossy fibre sprouting have been reported (Lothman & Bertram, 1993). The significance of such sprouting is discussed below.

Mechanisms of epileptogenesis

A fundamental question is how the enduring alterations of epileptogenesis discussed above come about. In recent years, several potential ways this may occur have been suggested on the basis of work with the traditional kindling model. In addition, certain investigations from the models studied in our laboratory have provided insight into this issue.

One way in which a permanent change in epileptogenesis could take place is via a rearrangement of

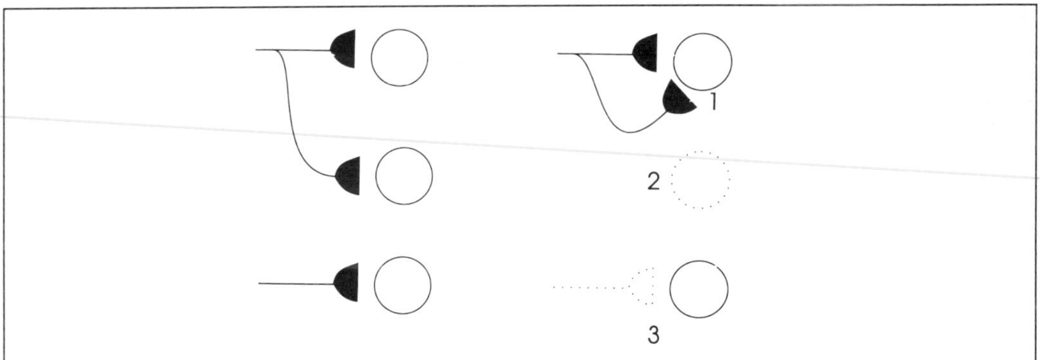

Fig. 6. Alterations in connectivity as substrates for augmented epileptogenesis. On the left side, presynaptic terminals (black knobs) are shown synapsing on postsynaptic targets (open circles). On the right-altered connectivity of the type found in models of chronic epilepsy are shown. Aberrant sprouting is illustrated at the upper right with a quantitative increase in a type of contact present in the normal brain (1); a potential signal for this sprouting is loss of the normal synaptic target for terminals (2). At the lower right, loss of connectivity is shown (3).

the connectivity between neurones. Two types of such rearrangements are schematized in Fig. 6. In the left-hand panel the normal situation is represented with a series of axon terminals (darkened knobs) shown ending on postsynaptic targets (open circles). In the upper part of the right-hand panel, the condition of aberrant sprouting is illustrated. Notice that, at the spot marked 1, axon terminals form contacts with a postsynaptic cell at a site where they normally do not form contacts. This example of aberrant sprouting arises from an increase in the number of a type of contact normally present, a quantitative change. It is also possible that qualitative changes, in which new types of synapse, not present in the normal brain, develop (not illustrated).

Attention was drawn to the class of qualitative morphological change in the kindled brain by the work of Sutula's laboratory through their studies on sprouting of the axons of dentate granule cells, so-called mossy fibres (Sutula *et al.*, 1988, 1992). Because such axons contain zinc, they are imaged with Timm's staining. In the normal brain, mossy fibres contact neurones in the dentate hilus and CA3 pyramidal cells but do not reach dentate granule cells. In brains removed from kindled animals, Timm's staining of axon terminals is detected around dentate granule cells. Since mossy fibres putatively release glutamate, such sprouting places them in a position to contact granule cells and thereby provide excess excitatory drive between granule cells, which, in turn, could establish enhanced epileptogenesis. This proposed scheme is predicated on morphological findings. To corroborate the importance of the morphological findings, physiological studies establishing altered functioning must be completed. Sutula has obtained data supporting the idea of altered function (Sutula *et al.*, 1992).

It should be noted that sprouting has been detected in other models of chronic epilepsy, including those with spontaneous seizures, such as after administration of kainic acid (Tauck & Nadler, 1985; Cronin *et al.*, 1992; Sloviter, 1992; see also Represa & Ben-Ari, chapter 53) or pilocarpine (Cavalheiro *et al.*, 1991), or that established with protracted electrical stimuli (R.S. Sloviter, pers. comm.). We have also found mossy fibre sprouting in the model of kindling achieved with rapid kindling (unpublished) and in the model of spontaneous recurrent seizures that develops as a sequela of self-sustaining limbic status epilepticus established with continuous hippocampal stimulation (Lothman & Bertram, 1993). For these models, all of which display spontaneous seizures, the density of mossy fibre sprouting is typically robust. This observation is consistent with, but certainly does not prove, mossy fibre sprouting as a factor for enhanced epileptogenesis. Moreover, it is possible that the type of mossy fibre sprouting under consideration is related to the lowered threshold for maximal dentate activation in the kindled brain, another measure of augmented epileptogenesis (see above). If these linkages are ultimately proved, then secondary epileptogenesis in the spatial domain will be established, at least in the animal models, because the change in the dentate gyrus comes about with stimuli at other sites such as the hippocampus or entorhinal cortex. The potential importance of this line of investigation is underscored by the fact that several laboratories have found mossy fibre sprouting in the dentate gyrus of patients obtained from patients with temporal lobe epilepsy (Sutula *et al.*, 1989; Babb *et al.*, 1991).

The mechanism responsible for mossy fibre sprouting is not established but one signal that has been suggested is loss of the usual targets for mossy fibres (see 2 in Fig. 6). It is reasonable to think that other types of axons than mossy fibres sprout in the epileptic brain, but work to date has focused on this finding because of the convenience of Timm's staining. Work by Sloviter (1992) and Dudek's laboratory (Cronin *et al.*, 1992) has indicated that mossy fibre sprouting can cause quantitative changes in which types of synapses normally present in the brain proliferate (cf. top right of Fig. 6). These workers found evidence of sprouting of mossy fibres on to hilar γ-aminobutyric acidergic (GABA-ergic) interneurones resulting in a hyperabundance of a kind of synapse normally present.

Another sort of change that can account for epileptogenesis is illustrated in the lower right-hand corner of Fig. 6. In this situation, instead of the formation of new synapses as was just considered, there is a *loss* of connections normally present. Evidence implicating this type of alteration has been obtained with the model of spontaneous recurring hippocampal seizures that develops as a sequela of

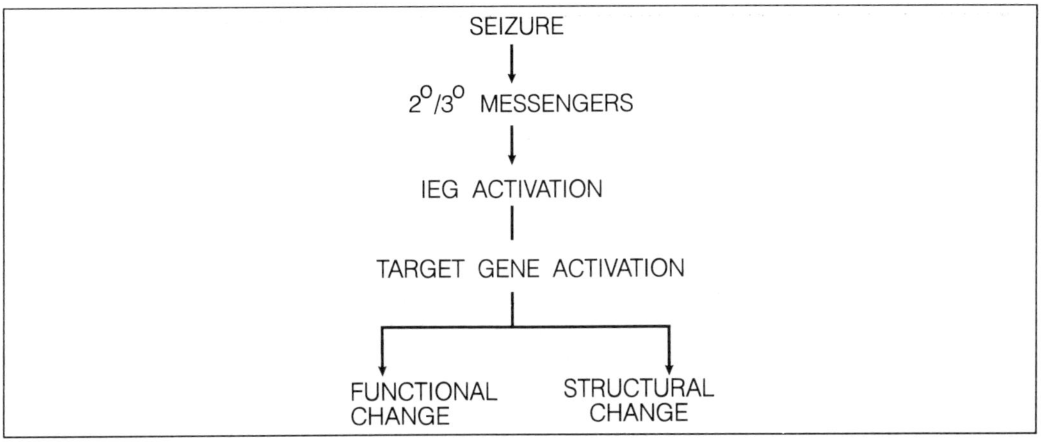

Fig. 7. Scheme for genomic activation by seizures that participates in chronic augmented epileptogenesis. For details see text.

self-sustaining limbic status epilepticus. GABA-mediated inhibition was recorded in CA1 pyramidal cells, comparing responses in the post-status epilepticus condition to those in the normal condition (Bekenstein & Lothman, 1993). 'Far-site' stimuli were used to activate GABA-ergic interneurones indirectly by first exciting the excitatory terminals that impinge on the interneurones. 'Near-site' stimuli, in the presence of antagonists to block glutamatergic excitation, were used to directly activate the GABA-ergic interneurones. With 'far-site' stimuli, GABA-mediated inhibitory postsynaptic potentials (IPSPs) were markedly attenuated in the post-status epilepticus condition compared with controls, whereas there was no difference in IPSPs between the two conditions with 'near-site' stimuli. Thus, the neuronal machinery for effecting inhibition is intact but disconnected from the usual routes of activation.

One may ask how the changes in connectivity just discussed arise. Recent work with the kindling model has begun to shed light on this question, particularly with regard to activation of gene products. Interest in this area is keen because it offers potential sites for antiepileptogenic interventions, separate from anticonvulsant/antiepileptic drugs directed at suppressing seizures once epileptogenesis has matured. Changes in connectivity could arise from morphological alterations of the kind discussed above and/or from functional changes, independent of structural pathology. Instances of this second type of pathophysiology would be alterations in receptors or enzymes responsible for synthesizing or catabolizing neurotransmitters. In this case, one would expect an enduring alteration in the expression of a particular gene or set of genes, a constitutive change. Clear-cut examples of constitutive expression of genes in the animal models of epileptogenesis discussed above remain to be established. On the other hand, a number of transient alterations in gene expression have been reported. One gene family that has received marked attention is that of immediate-early genes (IEG) shown in Fig. 7. The transcription and translation of IEG increase rapidly in response to diverse signals involving secondary and tertiary messages and subsequently up- or down-regulate the expression of later target genes. Thus, a set of events can be envisioned to occur after a seizure, involving activation of a variety of IEG and target genes. The target gene activation could be transient or longer-lasting. It seems likely that a complex intermixture of such activations comes into play and that the composite assembly of molecular processes is responsible for establishing sequelae, including enduring alterations in epileptogenesis. Furthermore, for a given region the potential for secondary epileptogenesis can be affected by the pattern of epileptic activity impinging on that region over time and the profile of where that activity comes from. From this perspective, the importance of temporal and spatial factors,

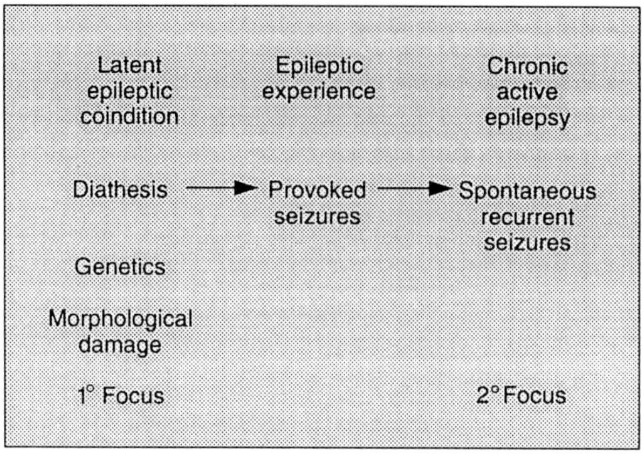

Fig. 8. Generalized scheme for epileptogenesis. The steps for secondary epileptogenesis are shown at the bottom, in which seizures from a primary focus bombard a distant site; eventually this epileptic experience converts the distant site to a secondary focus. The same overall plan can be envisioned for the development of a chronically active epileptic condition from a 'latent' epileptic condition such as that which may arise from morphological damage to the brain (acquired or developmental) or genetic diathesis for epileptogenesis.

introduced in older studies on secondary epileptogenesis, come into sharper focus. However, our understanding in this area is quite rudimentary and much work remains to be done.

Conclusions

An important clinical question is whether secondary epileptogenesis occurs in humans. If so, then a region remote from a primary epileptic focus can assume the role of a primary epileptic focus, serving as a nidus where seizures can originate independently even if the original focus is removed. If this process is repeated, several 'generations' of foci could arise. This duplication could also provide a substrate for progressive epilepsy. In both instances, spatial and temporal distributions of recurrent seizures are important factors. The nature of biological responses predicts that secondary epileptogenesis in space and time would vary among different individuals. Accordingly, detection of this process in all individuals would not be expected. Rather, the concerns become whether secondary epileptogenesis can occur, how often and under what circumstances, and whether this possibility should have an impact on the timing of surgical treatment for epilepsy.

Experimental studies in animals have shown that secondary epileptogenesis does occur under particular circumstances and with certain criteria used to detect it. With kindling protocols involving repetitive, spaced, triggered seizures, the activation of self-reinforcing mechanisms takes place, augmenting the duration and severity of these evoked seizures. There are indications that spontaneous seizures also occur in the kindling model, thereby imparting an important aspect for the isomorphism of this model to human epilepsy, but this topic merits additional study. If triggered seizures are moved close together, an acute condition of self-sustaining seizures arises that is followed later by a chronic condition of spontaneous recurrent seizures. In this situation, secondary epileptogenesis in the temporal domain is established and the isomorphic and homologous aspects of this model to human temporal lobe epilepsy are evident. Since epileptiform properties are manifest at sites remote from those used to establish the original status epilepticus (e.g. in the dentate gyrus whereas the stimulus was in the hippocampus), an argument for secondary epileptogenesis in the spatial domain can be advanced.

By examining the models in use in our laboratory and those used by others, additional insights have been provided into secondary epileptogenesis, at least in the context of the specified models. A sceptical view would be that the experimental procedures used in the animal models do not apply at all in humans, that the epileptic phenomena observed in the models are not identical to the phenomena observed in humans, and that the studying of secondary epileptogenesis in humans can only be done with studies in patients. Alternatively, one may accept the procedural or observational differences and use the information gained from the animal work to extrapolate to the clinical realm. Following this line of reasoning one step further, our understanding of epileptogenesis in general may be advanced by studies on models of secondary epileptogenesis (Fig. 8).

Acknowledgements

Supported by a grant from the National Institute of Neurological Disease and Stroke (NINDS). I thank Rose Powell for her assistance in preparation of the manuscript.

References

Albright, P.S. & Burnham, W.M. (1980): Development of a new pharmacological seizure model: effects of anticonvulsants on cortical and amygdala-kindled seizures in the rat. *Epilepsia* **21,** 681–689.

Babb, T.L., Kupfer, W.R., Pretorius, J.K., Crandall, P.H. & Levesque, M.F. (1991): Synaptic reorganization by mossy fibers in human epileptic fascia dentata. *Neuroscience* **42,** 351–363.

Bekenstein, J.W. & Lothman, E.W. (1993): Dormancy of inhibitory interneurons in a model of temporal lobe epilepsy. *Science* **259,** 97–100.

Burchiel, J.L., Serpa, K.A. & Duffy, F.H. (1982): Kindling antagonism: interactions of dorsal and ventral entorhinal cortex with the septum during concurrent kindling. *Brain Res.* **238,** 3–10.

Cavalheiro, E.T., Leito, J.P., Bortulotto, Z.A., Turski, W.A., Ikonomidou, C. & Turski, L. (1991): Long-term effects of pilocarpine in rats: structural damage of the brain triggers kindling and spontaneous recurrent seizures. *Epilepsia* **32,** 778–782.

Cronin, J., Obenans, A., Houser, C.R. & Dudek, F.E. (1992): Electrophysiology of dentate granule cells after kainate-induced synaptic reorganization of the mossy fibers. *Brain Res.* **573,** 305–310.

Engel, J., Jr (1989): *Seizures and epilepsy*, p. 536. Philadelphia: F.A. Davis.

Engel, J., J, Wolfson, L. & Brown, L. (1978): Anatomical correlates of electrical and behavioral events related to amygdaloid kindling. *Ann. Neurol.* **3,** 538–544.

Goddard, G.V., McIntyre, D.C. & Leech, C.K. (1969): A permanent change in brain function resulting from daily electrical stimulation. *Exp. Neurol.* **25,** 295–330.

Goddard, G.V., Dragunow, M., Maru, E. & Macleod, E.K. (1986): Kindling and the forces that oppose it. In: *The limbic system: functional organization and clinical disorders*, eds. B.K. Doane & K.E. Livingston, pp. 95–108. New York: Raven Press.

Jones, R.S.G. (1993): Entorhinal–hippocampal connections: a speculative view of their function. *Trends Neurosci.* **16,** 58–64.

Kairiss, E.W., Racine, R.J. & Smith, G.K. (1984): The development of the interictal spike during kindling in the rat. *Brain Res.* **322,** 101–110.

Löscher, W., Jackel, R. & Czuczwar, S.J. (1986): Is amygdala kindling in rats a model for drug-resistant partial epilepsy? *Exp. Neurol.* **93,** 211–226.

Lothman, E.W. & Bertram, E.H. (1993): Epileptogenic effects of status epilepticus. *Epilepsia* **34** (suppl 1), S59–S70.

Lothman, E.W. & Williamson, J.M. (1993): Rapid kindling with recurrent hippocampal seizures: effect of stimulus frequency and train duration. *Epilepsy Res.* **14,** 209–220.

Lothman, E.W., Hatlelid, J.M., Zorumski, C.F., Conry, J.A., Moon, P.F. & Perlin, J.B. (1985ba): Kindling with rapidly recurring hippocampal seizures. *Brain Res.* **360,** 83–91.

Lothman, E.W., Hatlelid, J.M. & Zorumski, C.F. (1985b): Functional mapping of limbic seizures originating in the hippocampus: a combined 2-deoxyglucose and electrophysiologic study. *Brain Res.* **360,** 92–100.

Epileptic Seizures and Syndromes, Edited by Peter Wolf
© 1994 John Libbey & Company Ltd., pp. 523–532

Chapter 52

Status epilepticus and secondary epileptogenesis in the pilocarpine model of epilepsy

Esper A. Cavalheiro

Neurologia Experimental, Escola Paulista de Medicina, Rua Botucatu, 862, 04023–900 Sao Paulo, Brazil

Summary

Pilocarpine induces in rats limbic seizures that become secondarily generalized and evolve to status epilepticus. Spontaneous recurrent seizures (SRSs) are registered during the long-term period following the systemic administration of pilocarpine in rats. Electroencephalographic, behavioural and pathological features resemble those of human complex partial seizures. In this chapter we review some characteristics of the pilocarpine model of epilepsy considering (a) the evolution of SRSs, which proceeds through kindling-like phenomena, (b) the effect of antiepileptic drugs against SRSs, (c) the neurochemical changes in the hippocampus of rats during the periods that lead to SRSs, (d) the supragranular dentate sprouting observed in the hippocampal formation of rats displaying SRSs, and (e) the relationship between the duration of status epilepticus and the late development of spontaneous seizures.

Introduction

Status epilepticus (SE) has been implicated in the production of brain damage in several neuropathological studies (Oxbury & Whitty, 1971; Maytal *et al.*, 1989). In close association with these findings is the strong evidence that links SE in infancy with the later development of epilepsy (Aicardi & Chevrie, 1983; Brown & Hussain, 1991), although the nature of this relationship cannot be inferred from retrospective studies. Furthermore, we can hypothesize that secondary epileptogenesis following SE implies that the massive epileptic activation during SE and the subsequent neuronal damage may induce plastic changes which will underlie the ensuing epileptogenesis.

We have recently shown (Cavalheiro *et al.*, 1991) that rats with brain damage secondary to SE induced by systemic administration of a cholinergic muscarinic agonist, pilocarpine, develop spontaneous recurrent seizures (SRSs) in the long run. First SRSs are usually observed 4–44 days after pilocarpine-induced SE. The mean 'seizure-silent period' lasts for 14.8 ± 3 days (mean ± SEM; n = 19). During the 'chronic period' SRSs are observed with a frequency of 2–4 per animal/week. No spontaneous remission of SRSs has been observed for periods as long as 6 months. Due to its characteristics, SRSs monitored during the 'chronic period' has been considered a good model for human temporal epilepsy (Leite *et al.*, 1990; Cavalheiro *et al.*, 1991) and useful for studying the development of an 'epileptic brain' after SE.

Kindling-like mechanisms underlie the development of epileptic foci

The evolution of SRSs that appear some days after pilocarpine-induced SE follows the behavioural and electrographic stages of kindling. In these animals the first seizure is normally characterized by paroxysmal discharges localized in the hippocampal leads without changes in cortical records. Behavioural correlates of such seizures comprise an arrest reaction followed by eye-blinking, chewing and head-nodding, as in kindling stage 1 or 2 (Racine, 1972). The following SRSs show electrographically gradual synchronization of cortical and hippocampal records and longer duration of ictal events. Clonus of the forelimbs and rearing with falling (kindling stage 4 or 5) are the hallmarks of such seizures. However, the evolution of spontaneous kindling is variable in terms of both duration of paroxysmal discharges and sequence of behavioural stages in every individual animal. Several seizure stages of similar or less intensity than the subsequent convulsion can be observed before final kindling stage 5 is reached. Once stage 5 kindled seizures are reached, then the vast majority of the following seizures are also generalized. These observations demonstrate that in the majority of rats the evolution of SRSs resulting from pilocarpine treatment follows stages of kindling (Leite *et al.*, 1990; Cavalheiro *et al.*, 1991). The common characteristics of such seizures are (1) primary activation of the hippocampus (before the cortex), (2) variable duration of discharges from one seizure to another which interferes with stereotyped progression until secondary generalization, and (3) random duration of discharges after secondary generalization (Turski & Cavalheiro, 1992).

Effect of antiepileptic drugs on SRSs

The validity of an experimental model of epilepsy is usually challenged by the profile of action of antiepileptic drugs (Meldrum, 1986). Accordingly, studies on the efficacy of antiepileptic drugs against SRSs registered during the long-term period following pilocarpine-induced SE in rats would provide the necessary information about the validity of this experimental model. To reach this goal, five clinically utilized antiepileptic drugs, phenobarbital (PHB), carbamazepine (CBZ), phenytoin (PHT), valproic acid (VPA) and ethosuximide (ESM), were administered after the establishment of the baseline seizure frequency for each rat. Seizure frequency during the 2 weeks of treatment was compared with equivalent periods before and after treatment.

PHB (40 mg/kg), PHT (100 mg/kg) and CBZ (120 mg/kg) given daily were effective against SRS (Fig. 1). VPA (450 mg/kg) was only weakly active and ESM (400 mg/kg) was completely ineffective against SRSs during the 2 weeks of treatment (Fig. 2) (Leite & Cavalheiro, 1991). The results obtained in this study indicated an excellent parallelism between antiepileptic drugs which are more effective against SRSs and their ability to protect against human complex partial seizures (Eadie, 1981). Among these drugs, CBZ and PHT are clearly drugs of first choice for complex partial seizures. PHB is probably virtually equipotent, but its use is avoided because of undesirable side-effects (Porter, 1986). Although VPA is effective in control of human partial-onset seizures (Bourgeois, 1989), its weak activity against SRSs may be due to its rapid metabolization in rats. ESM, which did not protect against SRSs, has no effect upon human partial seizures (Eadie, 1985). The similar profile of drug action, together with the evidence that electrographic, behavioural and neuropathological features reproduce clinical phenomenology, validates SRSs as a useful model of temporal lobe epilepsy.

Neurochemical changes in the hippocampus during the development of SRSs

Seizure activity is associated with a wide range of local biochemical alterations. Among them are changes in the turnover of various neurotransmitters, glucose metabolism, several second messengers and gene expression, leading to pathophysiological processes responsible for the long-term changes

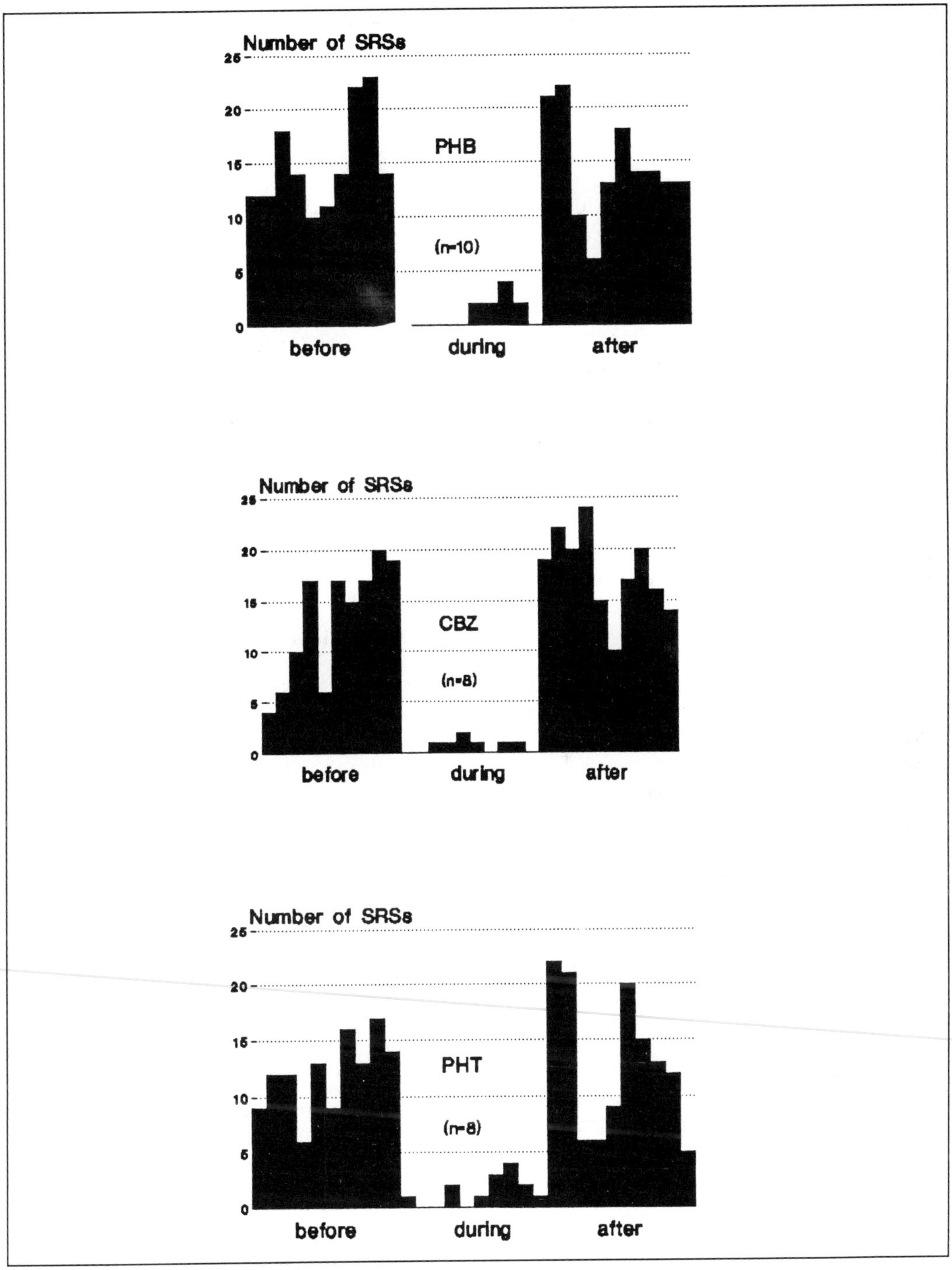

Fig. 1. Effect of phenobarbital (PHB), carbamazepine (CBZ) and phenytoin (PHT) on spontaneous recurrent seizures (SRSs) in rats. The histogram represents the cumulative frequency of SRSs in animals (number in brackets) before, during and after drug treatment. The total number of SRSs was calculated for a 1-day period.

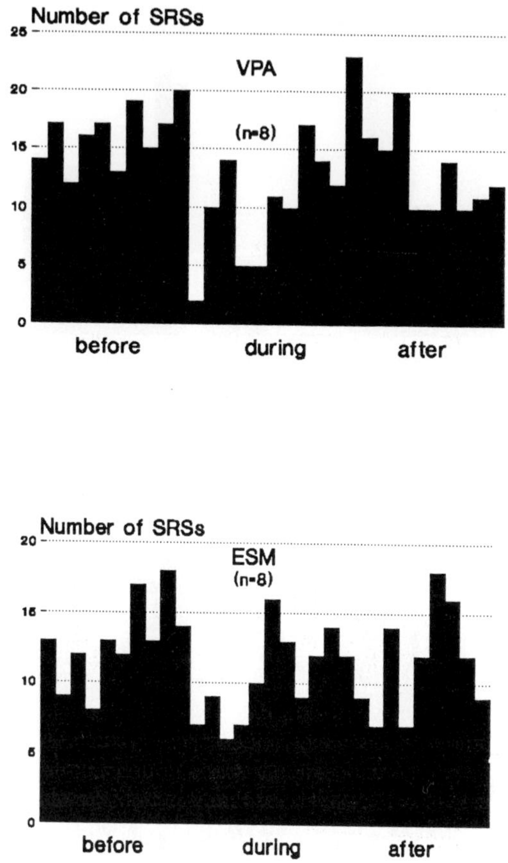

Fig. 2. Effect of valproate (VPA) and ethosuximide (ESM) on spontaneous recurrent seizures (SRSs) in rats. The histogram represents the cumulative frequency of SRSs in animals (number in brackets) before, during

in neuronal behaviour (Meldrum, 1991). In spite of numerous studies that clearly indicate the importance of monoamines and amino acids in epilepsy, the mechanisms by which these neurotransmitters influence seizures are not completely understood. As already reported (Cavalheiro *et al.*, 1991), the development of SRSs is characterized by paroxysmal activity initially localized in the hippocampal formation. Spreading of paroxysmal activity from hippocampal to cortical recordings was demonstrated characterizing the hippocampal formation as an important structure in the organization of the epileptic activity in this model. With the purpose of following the changes that occur during the establishment of an epileptic focus, the levels of monoamines and their metabolites as well as those of amino acid neurotransmitters were determined in the rat hippocampus during (a) the pilocarpine-induced SE, (b) the seizure-silent period and (c) the chronic period when SRSs occur.

Hippocampal noradrenaline (NA) level was decreased while that of dopamine (DA) was increased in all periods mentioned above. Serotonin (5-hydroxytryptamine (5HT)) content was increased only in the hippocampus of rats killed during pilocarpine-induced SE. In accordance with these results, the utilization rate of NA was increased and that of DA was decreased during the three periods. The turnover of 5HT was increased only in the SE period (Fig. 3, top) (Cavalheiro *et al.*, 1992, 1993).

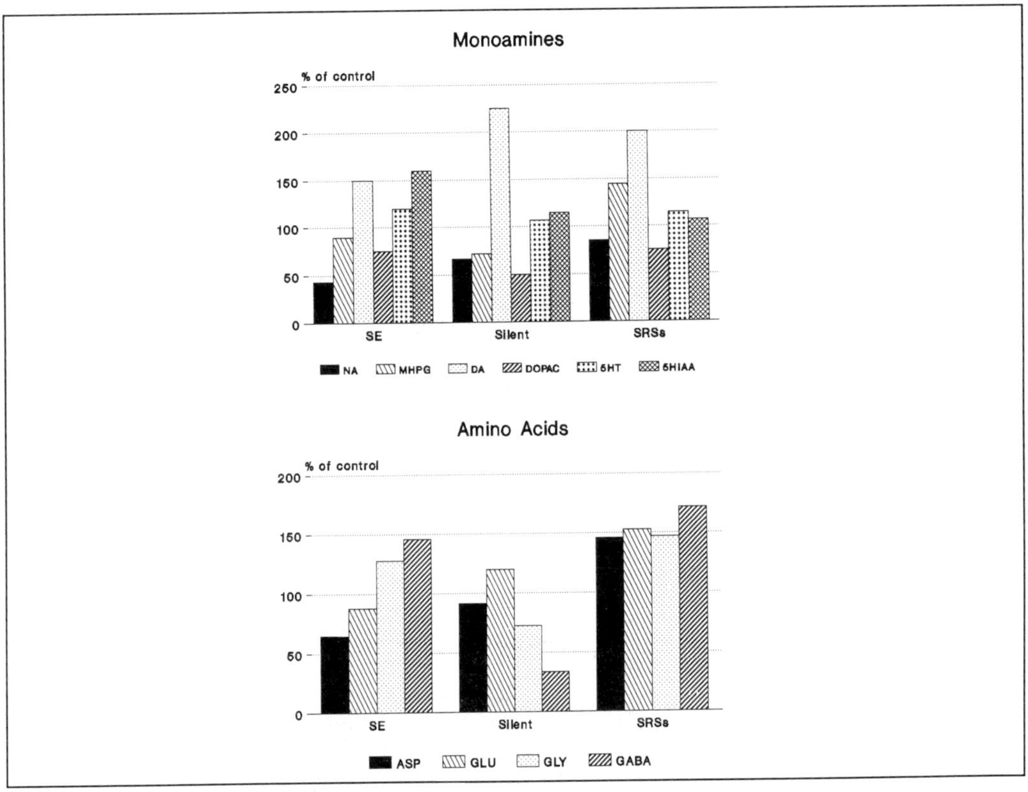

Fig. 3. Hippocampal level of monoamines, their metabolites (top) and amino acids (bottom), expressed as percentage of control values, during the development of spontaneous recurrent seizures in rats. SE = period of pilocarpine-induced status epilepticus; Silent = seizure-free silent period; SRSs = period of spontaneous recurrent seizures; NA = noradrenaline; MHPG = 4-hydroxy-3-methoxyphenylglycol; DA = dopamine; DOPAC = dihydroxyphenylacetic acid; 5HT = serotonin; 5HIAA = 5-hydroxyindoleacetic acid; ASP = aspartate; GLU = glutamate; GLY = glycine; GABA = γ-aminobutyric acid.

During the period of SE, hippocampal concentrations of aspartate (Asp) and glutamate (Glu) were decreased while that of γ-aminobutyric acid (GABA) was increased. The seizure silent period was characterized by decreases in GABA and glycine (Gly) levels and an increase in Glu concentration. During the chronic period, when SRSs occur, the concentration of all four amino acids was increased (Fig. 3 bottom).

These results show that, although cholinergic routes were activated by pilocarpine, several neurotransmitter systems were involved which could be implicated in the initiation, maintenance or both of seizures during the establishment of this model of epilepsy. Due to dependence existing between all neurotransmitter systems, it is difficult to determine which one triggers the neurochemical changes observed in this study. The time elapsing from brain injury to the appearance of the epileptic focus in humans may be the analogue of the seizure-silent period of the pilocarpine model and some neurochemical intervention during this period may modify the focus development (Cavalheiro *et al.*, 1993).

Synaptic reorganization in the hippocampus of rats with SRSs

As mentioned before, pilocarpine-induced SE invariably led to cell loss in the hippocampal subfields

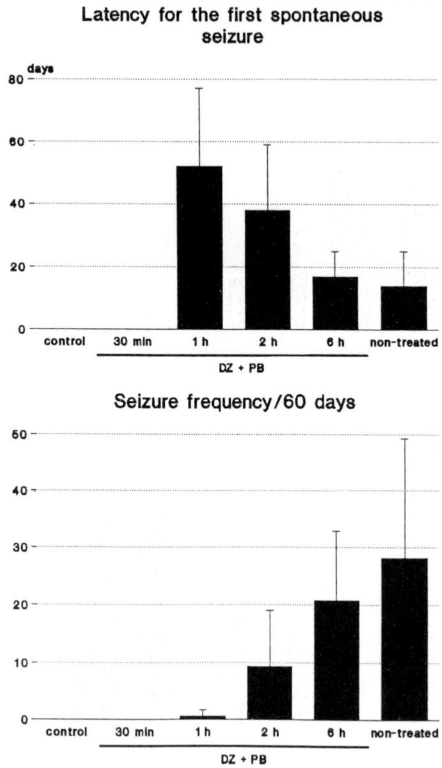

Fig. 4. Latency for the appearance of the first spontaneous seizure (top) and seizure frequency for 60 days (bottom) in rats submitted to 30 min, 1, 2 and 6 h of pilocarpine-induced status epilepticus (SE). Control = animals that were not submitted to SE; Non-treated = animals with spontaneous remission of SE; DZ = diazepam; PB = pentobarbital.

CA1 and CA3 and in the hilus of the dentate gyrus. Cell loss is also often seen in the septum, olfactory tubercle, amygdala, piriform cortex, neocortex and thalamic nuclei (Turski *et al.*, 1983, 1986). Timm staining of the hippocampal formation has shown supragranular sprouting of the mossy fibres, which increases with time after the epileptogenic insult (see Fig. 6f). The sprouting starts as early as 4 days after SE and reaches a plateau by 100 days after SE induction (Mello *et al.*, 1993). The time course for the development of supragranular mossy fibre sprouting in the pilocarpine model is similar to that seen after epileptogenic or non-epileptogenic lesions of the hippocampal complex (Steward *et al.*, 1974, 1988; Nadler *et al.*, 1980; Cavazos *et al.*, 1991). These results suggest that cell loss within the dentate hilus is a critical step that activates a cascade of events, leading to mossy fibre sprouting and *de novo* recurrent excitation of granule cells, culminating in SRSs. In the pilocarpine model, as in clinical epilepsy, the silent period presumably represents an interval of active synaptic reorganization and sprouting, during which an initial insult produces a permanently diseased brain. Accordingly, it is during this interval that therapeutic intervention could halt or redirect synaptic reorganization so as to prevent epileptogenesis.

The development of SRSs is related with the duration of status epilepticus

One interesting question linking SE with secondary epileptogenesis regards how much of SE is needed

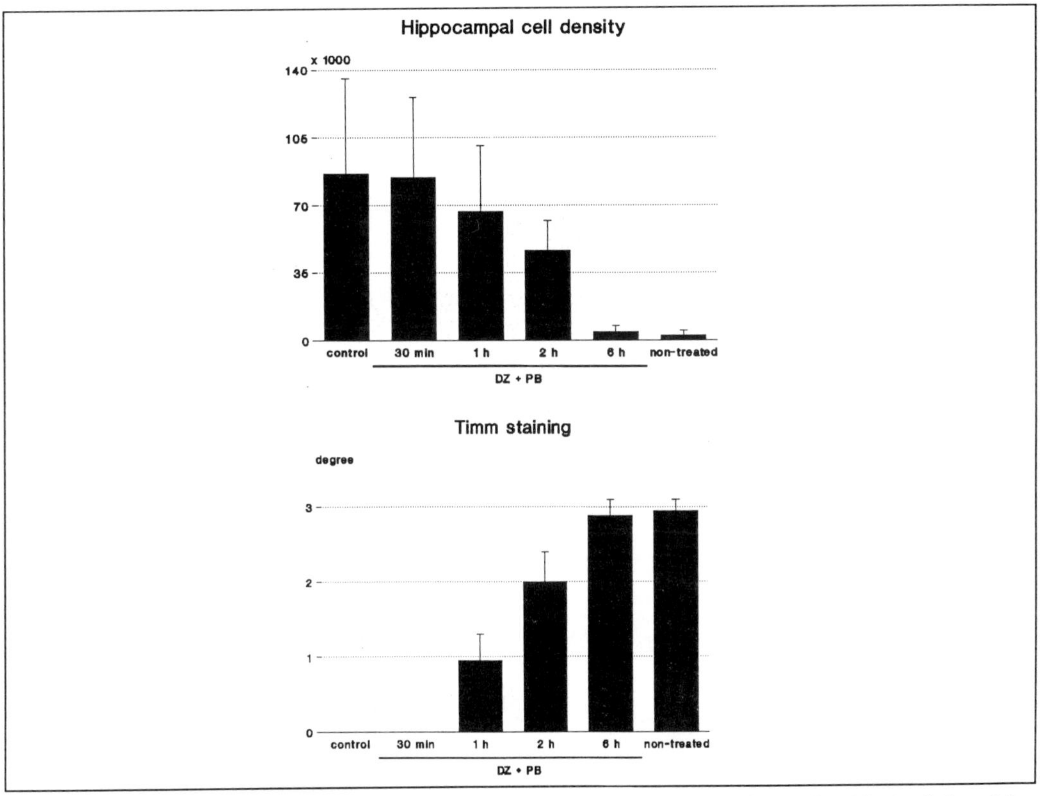

Fig. 5. Hippocampal cell density (top) and Timm staining (bottom) in rats submitted to 30 min, 1, 2 and 6 hours of pilocarpine-induced status epilepticus (SE). Control = animals that were not submitted to SE; Non-treated = animals with spontaneous remission of SE; DZ = diazepam; PB = pentobarbital. See text for explanation on cell counting and Timm staining scores.

for the establishment of an epileptic focus. To approach this problem we investigated the relationship between the duration of pilocarpine-induced SE, the latency for the appearance of the first SRSs, the frequency of such seizures, the cell density in the hippocampal formation (according to Mouritzen-Dam, 1982) and the intensity of the reactive synaptogenesis observed through the Timm's method. The subjective scores used for assessing supragranular Timm staining were: 0 = no stain; 1 = mild patch stain; 2 = moderate continuous stain; 3 = very intense staining along the septotemporal axis of the hippocampus. Following SE induction through the systemic administration of pilocarpine, an association of diazepam plus pentobarbital was used to interrupt SE 30 min, 1, 2 or 6 h after its beginning. SE remitted spontaneously in some non-treated rats.

Animals submitted to 30 min of SE did not evolve to the chronic period of the pilocarpine model and did not show any seizure in the long-term period of observation, which lasted up to 120 days after SE induction. A significant increase in the mean latency for the first spontaneous seizure (Fig. 4, top) and a significant decrease in seizure frequency (Fig. 4, bottom) were observed in animals with SE of shorter duration, i.e. 1 and 2 h. The behavioural and electrographic evolution of animals submitted to 6 h of SE was indistinguishable from that observed in non-treated rats, with spontaneous remission of SE. Cell loss in the hippocampal formation (Fig. 5, top) as well as the intensity of neo-Timm staining (Fig. 5, bottom) varied proportionally with the duration of SE induced by pilocarpine (Lemos & Cavalheiro, 1991).

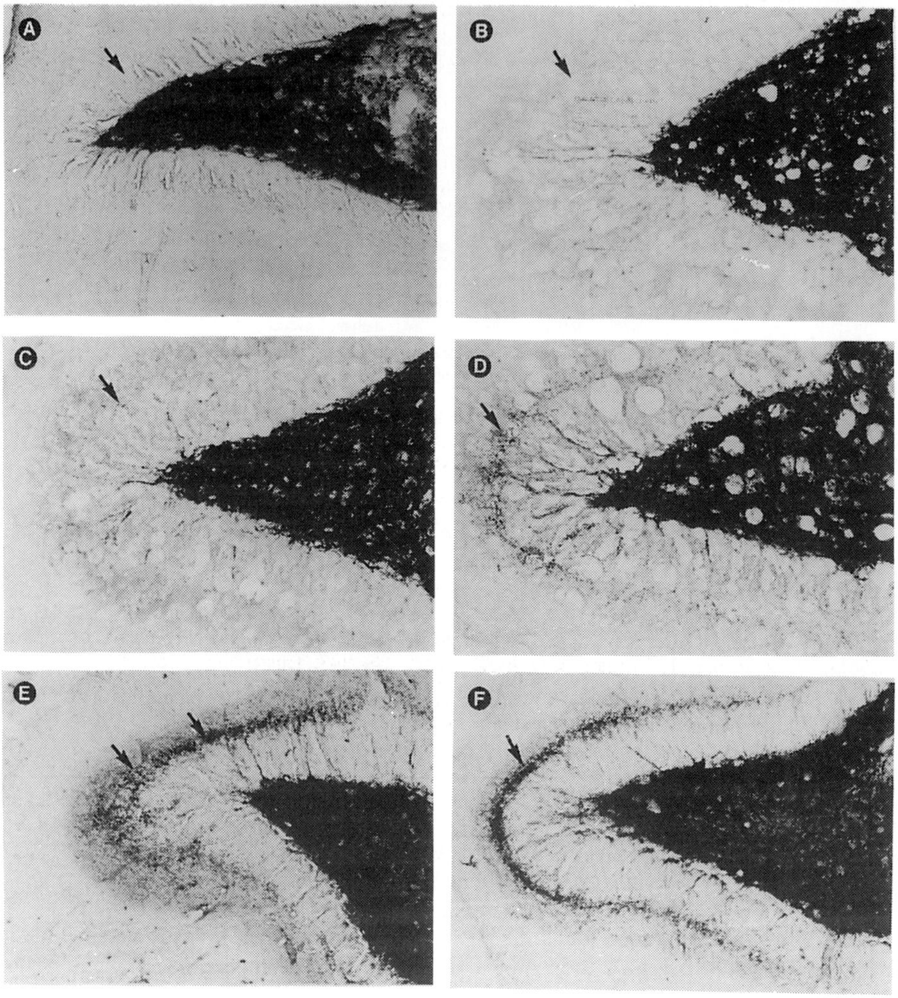

Fig. 6. Histological evidence for synaptic reorganization associated with SRSs. The pattern of Timm staining in the inner dentate molecular layer of a control animal is shown in (A). (B), (C), (D) and (E) show, respectively, Timm staining in the same region of animals submitted to 30 min, 1, 2 and 6 h of pilocarpine-induced status epilepticus (SE). Timm staining in a non-treated rat with spontaneous remission of SE is shown in (F).

These results show that the development of late epilepsy is closely related to the duration of SE. This relationship seems to be dependent on neuronal cell loss in the hippocampal formation and the subsequent synaptic reorganization in this structure.

Conclusion

The series of experiments reported here show that behavioural, electrographic, neuropathological and pharmacological profiles of SRSs resemble some of the characteristic hallmarks of human focal epilepsy (Cavalheiro *et al.*, 1991, 1994; Leite & Cavalheiro, 1991; Lemos & Cavalheiro, 1991; Mello *et al.*, 1993). Therefore, this novel and unique experimental approach may serve as a model of epilepsy resembling the human condition. Furthermore, the evolution of SRSs following pilocarpine-induced SE indicates that several biochemical changes induced by the massive activation of hippocampal circuitry during SE leads to cell death and synaptic reorganization, which seems to underlie the development of the epileptic focus. Therapeutic intervention controlling the duration of SE or during the seizure-silent period can modify the formation of such a focus and thus avoid the later occurrence of SRSs.

Acknowledgements

The author thanks L. Calderazzo, M.J. Fernandes, J.P. Leite, T. Lemos, L.E.A.M. Mello and M.G. Naffah-Mazzacoratti for their participation in the experiments reported here. This research was supported by FAPESP, CNPq and FINEP from Brazil.

References

Aicardi, J. & Chevrie, J.J. (1983): Consequences of status epilepticus in infants and children. In: *Status epilepticus: mechanisms of brain damage and treatment*, eds. A.V. Delgado-Escueta, C.G. Wasterlain, D.M. Treiman & R.J. Porter, pp. 115–125. New York: Raven Press.

Bourgeois, B.F.D. (1989): Valproate: clinical use. In: *Antiepileptic drugs*, eds. R. Levy, R. Mattson, B. Meldrum, J.K. Penry & F.E. Dreifuss, pp. 633–642. New York: Raven Press.

Brown, J.K. & Hussain, I.H.M. (1991): Status epilepticus: pathogenesis. *Dev. Med. Child Neurol.* **33,** 3–17.

Cavalheiro, E.A., Leite, J.P., Bortolotto, Z.A., Turski, W.A., Ikonomidou, C. & Turski, L. (1991): Long-term effects of pilocarpine in rats: structural damage of the brain triggers kindling and spontaneous recurrent seizures. *Epilepsia* **32,** 778–782.

Cavalheiro, E.A., Fernandes, M.J., Turski, L. & Mazzacoratti, M.G.N. (1992): Neurochemical changes in the hippocampus of rats with spontaneous recurrent seizures. In: *Molecular neurobiology of epilepsy*, eds. J. Engel, Jr, C. Wasterlain, E.A. Cavalheiro, U. Heinemann & G. Avanzini, pp. 239–248. Amsterdam: Elsevier.

Cavalheiro, E.A., Fernandes, M.J., Turski, L. & Naffah-Mazzacoratti, M.G. (1994): Spontaneous recurrent seizures in rats: amino acid and monoamine determination in the hippocampus. *Epilepsia* **35,** 1–11.

Cavazos, J.E., Golarai, G. & Sutula, T.P. (1991): Mossy fiber synaptic reorganization induced by kindling: time course of development, progression and permanence. *J. Neurosci.* **11,** 2795–2803.

Eadie, M.J. (1981): Anticonvulsant therapy: present and future. *Trends Pharmacol. Sci.* **2,** 37–39.

Eadie, M.J. (1985): Clinical use of antiepileptic drugs. In: *Antiepileptic drugs*, eds. H.H. Frey & D. Janz, pp. 765–790. Berlin: Springer.

Leite, J.P. & Cavalheiro, E.A. (1991): Antiepileptic drugs and their antagonism of spontaneous seizures in rats. *Epilepsia* **32** (suppl. 1), 35.

Leite, J.P., Bortolotto, Z.A. & Cavalheiro, E.A. (1990): Spontaneous recurrent seizures in rats: an experimental model of partial epilepsy. *Neurosci. Biobehav. Rev.* **14,** 511–517.

Lemos, T. & Cavalheiro, E.A. (1991): Reorganização sináptica e ocorrência de crises espontâneas em ratos. *J. Liga Bras. Epil.* **5,** 135–138.

Maytal, J., Shinnar, S., Moshé, S.L. & Alvarez, L.A. (1989): Low morbidity and mortality of status epilepticus in children. *Pediatrics* **83,** 323–331.

Meldrum, B.S. (1991): Neurochemical substrates of ictal behavior. In: *Neurobehavioral problems in epilepsy,* eds. D. Smith, D. Treiman & M. Trimble, pp. 35–45. New York, Raven Press.

Meldrum, B.S. (1986): Preclinical test systems for evaluation of novel compounds. In: *New anticonvulsant drugs*, eds. B.S. Meldrum, & R.J. Porter, pp. 31–48. London: John Libbey.

Mello, L.E.A.M., Cavalheiro, E.A., Tan, A.M., Kupfer, W.R., Pretorius, J.K., Babb, T.L. & Finch, D.M. (1993): Circuit mechanisms of seizures in the pilocarpine model of chronic epilepsy: cell loss and mossy fiber sprouting. *Epilepsia* 34, 985–995.

Mouritzen-Dam, A. (1982): Hippocampal neuron loss in epilepsy and after experimental seizures. *Acta Neurol. Scand.* **66,** 601–642.

Nadler, J.V., Perry, B.W. & Cotman, C.W. (1980): Selective reinnervation of hippocampal area CA1 and the fascia dentata after destruction of CA3–CA4 afferents with kainic acid. *Brain Res.* **182,** 1–9.

Oxbury, J.M. & Whitty, W.M. (1971): Causes and consequences of status epilepticus in adults. *Brain* **94,** 733–744.

Porter, R.J. (1986): Antiepileptic drugs: efficacy and inadequacy. In: *New anticonvulsant drugs*, eds. B.S. Meldrum & R.J. Porter, pp. 3–15. London: John Libbey.

Racine, R.J. (1972): Modification of seizure activity by electrical stimulation. II. Motor seizure. *Electroencephalogr. Clin. Neurophysiol.* **32,** 281–284.

Steward, O., Cotman, C.W. & Linch, G.S. (1974): Growth of a new fiber projection in the brain of adult rats: reinnervation of the dentate gyrus by the contralateral entorhinal cortex following ipsilateral entorhinal lesions. *Exp. Brain Res.* **20,** 45–66.

Steward, O., Vinsant, S.L. & Davis, L. (1988): The process of reinnervation in the dentate gyrus of adult rats: an ultrastructural study of changes in presynaptic terminals as a result of sprouting. *J. Comp. Neurol.* **267,** 24–33.

Turski, L. & Cavalheiro, E.A. (1992): Seizures induced by pilocarpine: relevance in epilepsy. In: *Current aspects of the neurosciences*, ed. N.N. Osborne, pp. 127–158. New York: Macmillan.

Turski, W.A., Cavalheiro, E.A., Schwarz, M., Czuczwar, S.J., Kleinrok, Z. & Turski, L. (1983): Limbic seizures produced by pilocarpine in rats: behavioural, electroencephalographic and neuropathological study. *Behav. Brain Res.* **9,** 315–335.

Turski, L., Cavalheiro, E.A., Sieklucka-Dziuba, M., Ikonomidou-Turski, C., Czuczwar, S.J. & Turski, W.A. (1986): Seizures produced by pilocarpine: neuropathological sequelae and activity of glutamate decarboxylase in the rat forebrain. *Brain Res.* **398,** 37–48.

Epileptic Seizures and Syndromes, Edited by Peter Wolf
© 1994 John Libbey & Company Ltd., pp. 533–539

Chapter 53

Sprouting and synaptogenesis of hippocampal mossy fibres in epileptic rats

Alfonso Represa and Yehezkel Ben-Ari

INSERM U29, 123 Bd. Port Royal, 75674 Paris Cedex 14, France

Summary

Experimentally induced epilepsy (kindling and kainate treatment) elicits collateral sprouting of mossy fibres in rat hippocampus. Collateral branches invade the hilus, cross the granule cell layer and distribute throughout the inner third of the molecular layer. These newly developed collaterals may acquire the typical features of mossy fibres including giant synapses. Granule cell dendrites may develop giant thorny excrescences, suggesting that the target of these collaterals are granule cells. In kindled rats we also observed a terminal sprouting and synaptogenesis of mossy fibres in the infrapyramidal layer of CA3. Targets for mossy fibres were the basilar dendrites of CA3 pyramidal neurones, which developed the characteristic thorny excrescences at the contact with the newly developed mossy fibre terminals. The mechanisms and the consequences of this seizure-related sprouting are discussed.

Epilepsy may be considered as the result of a permanent enhancement of synaptic activity (Douglas & Goddard, 1975). In fact, persistent increase in synaptic efficacy has now been observed *in vitro*, following short application of various convulsants (see refs. in Ben Ari & Gho, 1988). Different studies support the hypothesis that such functional changes may be sustained by a synaptic remodelling. This has been mainly analysed in two different models of temporal lobe epilepsy: the kindling of limbic structures (Goddard *et al.*, 1969) and the administration of kainic acid (KA) (Nadler, 1981; Ben-Ari, 1985). In the present report we review recent data from our laboratory showing that in both models of epilepsy hippocampal mossy fibres (MF) sprout and made aberrant synaptic contacts with granule cell dendrites and, in some conditions, with basilar dendrites of CA3 pyramidal neurones. Although the mechanisms responsible for this sprouting are at present unclear, different reports have shown that a brief seizure episode can evoke sequential changes on the expression of different molecules, including transcription factors, trophic factors and cytoskeleton proteins. These changes may constitute different steps in the process from an episode of abnormal hyperactivity to sprouting and synaptogenesis and are therefore discussed in this chapter. Finally, the consequences of this MF sprouting and synaptogenesis are discussed.

The inferior region of the hippocampus: organization and unique features

The granule cells of the dentate gyrus constitute a major gateway to the hippocampus since they are the target of the perforant pathway, i.e. the principal cortical input to the hippocampus which originates in the entorhinal cortex.

The axons of granular cells, the MF, establish synaptic contacts with the ipsilateral giant pyramidal CA3 neurones and with various interneurones in the inferior region. Each MF makes synaptic contacts with several different target cells. The MF synaptic complex is the largest in the brain; in our study they had a mean size of $7.32 \pm 2.7\ \mu m^2$ (Represa & Ben-Ari, 1992). This synapse appears as a giant multi-invaginated bouton which establishes multiple synaptic contacts with the giant spines of the proximal part of the apical dendrite of CA3 pyramidal neurones (Blackstad & Kjaerheim, 1961; Hamlyn, 1962). CA3 pyramidal cells are well interconnected by the recurrent collaterals, which make synaptic contacts with the distal part of the apical dendrites, in the stratum radiatum (see refs. in Miles & Wong, 1986). MF and recurrent collaterals may therefore contribute to the synchronization of CA3 pyramidal cells and explain the particular vulnerability of this structure to the epileptic procedures.

Synchronized burst generated in CA3 neurones

In keeping with earlier *in vivo* data, several experiments performed on hippocampal slices illustrate the unique ability of the CA3 region to generate a synchronized burst following certain electrical procedures or the application of various convulsive agents. Thus, brief applications of any of the following solutions – high K^+ solution, mast cell-degranulating peptide, reduced Mg^{2+} concentrations, α-tubocurarine, γ-aminobutyric acid A (GABA-A) receptor channel-blockers, excitatory amino acids – or repetitive electrical stimulation (kindling) generate repetitive synchronized bursts, which persist for the duration of the application and often for several minutes after washing (Miles & Wong, 1986; Ben-Ari & Gho, 1988; Neuman *et al.*, 1988). These bursts are giant excitatory postsynaptic potentials (EPSP) and not endogenous pacemaker events. They are generated by the excitatory recurrent collaterals of the axons of CA3 neurones (Ben-Ari & Gho, 1988). Electrophysiological and 'modelling' studies have shown that this recurrent system underlies the susceptibility of the CA3 region to paroxysmal activity, since it amplifies the excitatory signals which impinge on CA3 neurones from various extrinsic and intrinsic afferents, mainly MF (Traub & Wong, 1982). Furthermore, once excitability has been enhanced, for example by blocking GABA-ergic inhibition or activating KA receptors (Gho *et al.*, 1986; Miles & Wong, 1987; Neuman *et al.*, 1988), further intracellular stimulations of a CA3 pyramidal neurone will evoke a synchronized burst. Using dual intracellular stimulation of CA3 pyramidal neurones, Miles and Wong (1986) have also shown that, during paroxysmal activity, polysynaptic excitatory responses can be recorded between two previously non-interacting cells. This type of plasticity can lead to the emergence of a synchronous discharge in a group of closely interacting CA3 neurones. Although there is no compelling evidence, glutamate is probably the neurotransmitter used by the recurrent excitatory collateral synapses (like the CA3 collateral axons innervating CA1 pyramidal neurones), acting on non-*N*-methyl-D-aspartate (NMDA) receptors. In fact, blockade of non-NMDA receptors by selective antagonists such as, 6-cyano-7-nitroquinoxaline-2,3-dione (CNQX), completely blocked the synchronized bursts (see refs. in Neuman *et al.*, 1988). In keeping with this observation, laminar profile analysis confirmed that these bursts, which have a reversal potential of 0 mV, were generated in the apical dendrites of CA3 neurones, where the recurrent collateral synapses are present (Ben-Ari & Gho, 1988).

Summing up, the recurrent excitatory collateral system therefore provides a unique system to amplify CA3 excitatory responses (mainly produced by MF stimulation) and to generate synchronized network-driven events in a population of CA3 neurones, once the GABA-ergic and voltage-dependent K^+ channels have been inhibited. These neurones will in turn generate paroxysmal activity in the entire hippocampal circuit.

Paroxysmal activity induces collateral and terminal sprouting and synaptogenesis of MF

As previously reported (Nadler, 1981; Ben-Ari, 1985) the hippocampus of KA-treated rats develops a sclerosis characterized in the CA3 field by the disappearance of all CA3 pyramidal cells and a glial proliferation (Represa *et al.,* 1993). The fascia dentata of these animals also presents a lack of hilar cells (from 47 ± 5 in slices of controls to 7 ± 13 in KA-treated rats; $P < 0.001$ (Represa *et al.*, 1993a). In kindled rats, in keeping with Goddard *et al.* (1969), we do not find signs of lesion, glial proliferation or neuronal degeneration (Represa & Ben-Ari, 1992; Represa *et al.*, 1993a). Thus, the mean surface of both hilus and molecular layer of fascia dentata remains similar to that of controls. In the hilus of our kindled animals the number of neuronal cells (polymorph cells) is not significantly reduced (40 ± 9 hilar cells/slice).

In the fascia dentata of both kindled and KA-treated rats we have observed collateral sprouting of MF (Represa *et al.*, 1993a). In fact, numerous branches originating from MF in the hilus distribute within the plexiform layer or pass through the granule cell layer and form a complex plexus in the inner third of the molecular layer (Fig. 1). Whereas in the hilus MF present numerous conventional MF varicosities (about 5.2 ± 1.4 µm diameter), in the molecular layer collateral sprouted branches only have a few varicosities. Although some of these varicosities are of great size, their mean diameter is thinner than the characteristic mousses (1.53 ± 0.2 µm and 1.85 ± 0.1 µm in kindled and KA-treated rats respectively (Represa *et al.*, 1993a).

The granule cells of epileptic rats show a normal dendritic arborization. Some impregnated neurones (about 10 per cent of impregnated cells) display clusters of giant excrescences in their primary or secondary dendrites or both. In some impregnated granule cells from KA-treated rats, but not from kindled rats, clear giant thorny excrescences have been observed (Represa *et al.*, 1993a).

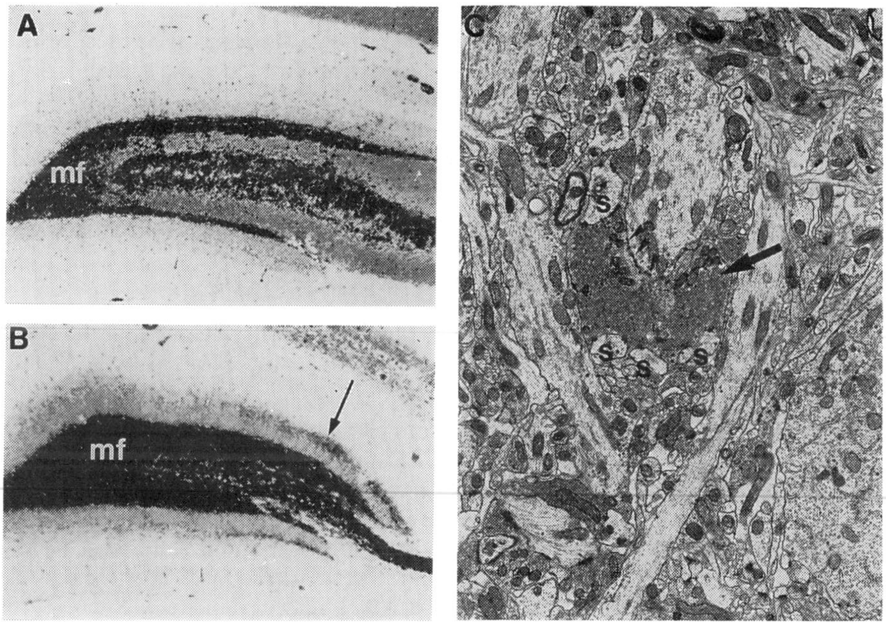

Fig. 1. Collateral sprouting and synaptogenesis of mossy fibres after KA treatment.
(A, B) Timm staining of mossy fibres (dark silver deposits) depicting the distribution of mossy fibres (mf) in control rat (A) and an epileptic rat (B) sacrificed 30 days after KA administration. Note that, after KA, Timm deposits invade the hilus and form an ectopic band in the inner third of the molecular layer.
(C) Electron micrograph depicting the presence of ectopic mossy fibre boutons (arrow) in the zones of sprouting. This bouton has a complex shape, desmosome-like contacts with dendritic shafts (arrow heads), multiple asymmetric contacts with giant complex spines (s) and a high density of synaptic vesicles.

In the fascia dentata of epileptic animals (kindled and KA-treated rats), giant synaptic boutons develop in the inner third of the molecular layer (Fig. 1c). These boutons have all the characteristic features of mossy boutons: relative giant size (mean cross-sectional area of 5.9 ± 3.2 μm^2), complex shape, multiple synaptic contacts (2.7 ± 1.7 per bouton) with complex dendritic spines (2.5 ± 0.9 spines per bouton), high density of synaptic vesicles, desmosome-like contacts with dendritic spines or other MF boutons and postsynaptic spines embedded in the bouton (Represa *et al.*, 1993a). Interestingly, the analysis of the synaptic profiles revealed that the number of synaptic boutons measuring 2–2.5 μm (diameter) was increased in kindled rats. These boutons have not been considered as MF boutons. The mean number of characteristic MF ectopic boutons/mm^2 in kindled rats was 285 ± 106 (with a maximum of 370 and a minimum of 156 boutons/mm^2) These characteristic MF boutons represent 0.40 ± 0.15 MF boutons per granule cell (the number of total synapses per granule cells was estimated to be about 2706 in this field).

We now have evidence that experimental epilepsy is associated with sprouting of MF, not only in the fascia dentata (see refs. in Ben-Ari & Represa, 1990) but also in the infrapyramidal band of CA3 (Represa & Ben-Ari, 1992). This terminal sprouting only develops in epileptic rats which have no CA3 degeneration (kindled rats). This sprouting is also associated with the formation of ectopic, axospinous MF synapses with basilar dendrites of CA3 pyramidal neurones. In the stratum oriens of the midseptal pole of the hippocampus we counted 0.1 ± 0.1 MF boutons/neurone and 1.9 ± 0.4 MF boutons/neurone in control and kindled rats respectively. The difference between control and kindled is significant ($P < 0.01$) and may represent for each neurone 7.2 additional asymmetric synaptic contacts since each MF bouton made 3.82 ± 2.7 synaptic contacts with 3.4 ± 1.7 spines (Represa & Ben-Ari, 1992).

When comparing these results, it is quite clear that collateral synaptogenesis is more restricted than terminal synaptogenesis. Although the new MF collaterals may develop without establishing synaptic contacts, our results rather suggest that collateral MF make additional synapses without the characteristic features of MF boutons: they may be of smaller size and have a less classical MF configuration. This supports the hypothesis that collateral (but not terminal) MF sprouting was associated with the development of 'hypotrophic' MF boutons. If this is the case, the density of newly developed MF synapses would be greater than our estimation.

Molecular changes induced by seizures

In the hippocampus of epileptic rats, particularly in the granule cells, a cascade of molecular events develops after seizures and precedes the sprouting and synaptogenesis of mossy fibers. These changes may be summarized as follows:

(1) A rapid activation (within the first hours following the seizure onset), the proto-oncogenes c-*fos* (Dragunow & Roberstson, 1987; Morgan *et al.*, 1987; Popovici *et al.*, 1990), ZIF/268, c-*jun* and *jun*-B (Saffen *et al.*, 1988). These factors are known to be implicated in the regulation of gene transcription, as either a negative or a positive regulatory element (i.e. inducing the activation of trophic factors or different effector genes) and probably have an important role in coupling short-term events, elicited by cellular stimuli, with long-term alterations in target gene expression. These factors may play a crucial role in the cascade of molecular events induced by seizures (Ben-Ari & Represa, 1990).

(2) Concomitantly with this activation, the levels of messenger ribonucleic acid (mRNA) for trophic factors, such as nerve growth factor (NGF) (Gall & Isackson, 1989; Zafra *et al.*, 1990) and brain-derived growth factor (Zafra *et al.*, 1990), increase first in dentate granule cells and then in other limbic regions, including CA3. In contrast, the levels of neurotrophin-3 (NT-3) mRNA transiently decrease in the hippocampus after KA treatment (Rocamora *et al.*, 1992) or have no change at all after kindling (Ernfors *et al.*, 1991). These changes are concomitant with a transient alteration of high-affinity receptors of neurotrophic factors: the tyrosine kinase receptors (trk) (Bengzon *et al.*, 1993). Thus, whereas the hippocampal levels of mRNAs encoding for trkA and trkB receptors, which

mainly mediate the effects of NGF and brain derived neutrotrophic factor (BDNF), are increased in the granule cells of kindled rats, the levels of trkC mRNA, which rather mediate the effects of NT-3, do not change (Bengzon *et al.*, 1993). There is now evidence that these changes in mRNA are associated with alterations of the levels of neurotrophin and receptor proteins (see refs. in Bengzon *et al.*, 1993). The precise role of neurotrophins in adult brain is at present unknown but it is assumed that neurotrophins may be involved in some plastic changes, like those observed in epileptic animals, and in the protection of neurones from different insults (i.e. granule cells do not degenerate after seizures).

(3) Finally, we studied the changes induced by the administration of KA in the expression of the most prominent cytoskeleton element within developing and mature neurones, the microtubules, by combining *in situ* hybridization and immunocytochemistry (Represa *et al.*, 1993a). In our study the levels of mRNAs encoding for α-tubulin increased in the dentate granule cell bodies after 3 days of KA treatment; peak levels were found on day 12. These changes correlated with an enhancement of α-tubulin immunoreactivity in both granule cell dendrites and MF, already noticeable 4 days after KA (Represa *et al.*, 1993a).

From a transient abnormal activity to fibre sprouting

Although the links between these steps (gene activation, increased expression of cytoskeleton proteins and fibre sprouting) have not been fully clarified and the precise role of these trophic factors has not yet been well elucidated, *in vitro* studies suggest they are all components of the same process. In fact, seizure episodes trigger a large calcium influx in hippocampal neurones (see refs. in Ben-Ari & Represa, 1990). Calcium influx has been found to regulate c-*fos* expression (Morgan & Curran, 1991), while c-*fos* and c-*jun* regulate NGF expression in cultures of fibroblasts of transgenic mice (Hengerer *et al.*, 1990).

Consequences of MF sprouting and synaptogenesis

Several lines of evidence strongly support a major role for MF in the induction and propagation of epileptic discharges and underlying pathological changes (Ben-Ari, 1985; Okazaki & Nadler, 1988). In fact, limbic motor seizures and the subsequent sclerosis of Ammon's horn did not develop before the maturation of MF had taken place (Nitecka *et al.*, 1984). The destruction of MF (by γ-ray irradiation or colchicine injection) also had a protective effect on adult animals, since epileptic status failed to be produced and pyramidal cells did not degenerate in such animals (Okazaki & Nadler, 1988).

It is therefore likely that an aberrant and enhanced MF synaptogenesis may impair hippocampal function and contribute to the maintenance of the epilepsy (Tauck & Nadler, 1985). The increased number of MF synapses represent at last an amplification of the excitatory signal impinging on CA3 neurones or in granule cells. Since each MF will innervate a greater number of target cells in epileptics, MF sprouting will facilitate their synchronization.

In regard to the repercussions of MF sprouting, it is interesting to note that in epileptic rats MF sprouting was associated with a selective increase in binding for ^{3}H-kainate. In fact, KA binding sites were significantly increased in the molecular layer of both kindled and KA-treated rats (up to 30 per cent as compared with control rats (Represa *et al.*, 1987, 1989). Furthermore, in the stratum oriens of the CA3 field, KA binding dramatically increased after kindling and formed an ectopic band of labelling (Represa *et al.*, 1989). These changes in binding were without effect on the affinity constant and probably reflect an increase in the mean number of KA receptors. The increased density of KA receptors will promote further excitability of the hippocampal circuitry.

The stoichiometry of glutamate receptors is not yet well understood but it seems clear that different subunits so far cloned may confer on the receptors different functional properties, mainly in calcium permeability. It should be of interest to determine whether permanent or transient changes in the molecular composition of glutamatergic receptors develop during seizures. Recent publications have already suggested that in kindled rats the sensitivity of the d-amino-3-hydroxy-5-methyl-4-isoxazole-propionate (AMPA) subtype of glutamate receptors is increased in granule cells as a result of alternative splicing (Kamphuis *et al.*, 1992). These changes may be related to the collateral sprouting and synaptogenesis of MF, but may also develop in the absence of other histopathological alterations. They may be induced by paroxysmal activity. This point deserves emphasis, since many epileptic processes which develop in the absence of major signs of histopathological changes would be sustained by a remodelling of glutamate receptors. A better understanding of such changes would help the research on antiepileptic drugs.

References

Ben-Ari, Y. (1985): Limbic seizures and brain damage produced by kainic acid: mechanisms and relevance to human temporal lobe epilepsy. *Neuroscience* **14,** 375–403.

Ben-Ari, Y. & Gho, M. (1988): Long-lasting modification of the synaptic properties of rat CA3 hippocampal neurones induced by kainic acid. *J. Physiol.* **404,** 365–384.

Ben-Ari, Y. & Represa, A. (1990): Brief seizure episodes induce long-term potentiation and mossy fibre sprouting in the hippocampus. *Trends Neurosci.* **13,** 312–318.

Bengzon, J., Kokaia, Z., Ernfors, P., Kokaia, M., Leanza, G., Nilsson, O.G., Persson, H. & Lindvall, O. (1993): Regulation of neurotrophin and trkA, trkB and trkC tyrosine kinase receptor messenger RNA expression in kindling. *Neuroscience* **53,** 433–446.

Blackstad, T.W. & Kjaerheim, Å. (1961): Special axo-dendritic synapses in the hippocampal cortex: electron and light microscopic studies on the layer of the mossy fibers. *J. Comp. Neurol.* **117,** 113–159.

Douglas, R.M. & Goddard, G.V. (1975): Long-term potentiation of the perforant path–granule cell synapse in the rat hippocampus. *Brain Res.* **86,** 205–215.

Dragunow, M. & Robertson, H.A. (1987): Kindling stimulation induces c-*fos* protein(s) in granule cells of the rat dentate gyrus. *Nature* (London) **329,** 441–442.

Ernfors, P., Bengzon, J., Kokaia, Z., Persson, H. & Lindvall, O. (1991): Increased levels of messenger RNAs for neurotrophic factors in the brain during kindling epileptogenesis. *Neuron* **7,** 165–176.

Gall, C.M. & Isackson, P.J. (1989): Limbic seizures increase neuronal production of messenger RNA for nerve growth factor. *Science* **245,** 758–761.

Gho, M., King, A.E., Ben-Ari, Y. & Cherubini, E. (1986): Kainate reduces two voltage-dependent potassium conductances in rat hippocampal neurons *in vitro*. *Brain Res.* **385,** 411–414.

Goddard, G.V., McIntyre, D.C. & Leech, C.K. (1969): A permanent change in brain function resulting from daily electric stimulation. *Exp. Neurol.* **25,** 295–330.

Hamlyn, L.H. (1962) The fine structure of the mossy fiber endings in the hippocampus of the rabbit. *J. Anat.* (London)**96,** 112–120.

Hengerer, B., Lindholm, D., Heumann, R., Rüther, U., Wagner, E.F. & Thoenen H. (1990): Lesion-induced increase in nerve growth factor mRNA is mediated by c-*fos*. *Proc. Nat. Acad. Sci. USA* **87,** 3899–3903.

Kamphuis, W., Monyer, H., De Rijk, T.C. & Lopes da Silva, F.H. (1992): Hippocampal kindling increases the expression of glutamate receptor-A Flip and B Flip mRNA in dentate granule cells. *Neurosci. Lett.* **148,** 51–54.

Miles, R. & Wong, R.K.S. (1986): Excitatory synaptic interactions between CA3 neurons in the guinea-pig hippocampus. *J. Physiol.* **373,** 371–373.

Miles, R. & Wong, R.K.S. (1987): Latent synaptic pathways revealed after tetanic stimulation in the hippocampus. *Nature* **329,** 724–726.

Morgan, J.I. & Curran, T. (1991): Proto-oncogene transcription factors and epilepsy. *Trends Pharmacol. Sci.* **12,** 343–349.

Morgan, J.I., Cohen, D.R., Hempstead, J.L. & Curran, T. (1987): Mapping patterns of c-Fos expression in the central nervous system after seizure. *Science* **237,** 192–197.

Nadler, J.V. (1981): Kainic acid as a tool for the study of temporal lobe epilepsy. *Life Sci.* **29,** 2031–2042.

Neuman, R.S., Ben-Ari, Y. & Cherubini, E. (1988): Antagonism of spontaneous and evoked burst by 6-cyano-7-nitroquinoxaline-2,3-dione (CNQX) in the CA3 region of the *in vitro* hippocampus. *Brain Res.* **474,** 201–203.

Nitecka, L., Tremblay, E., Charton, G., Bouillot, J.P., Berger, M.L. & Ben-Ari, Y. (1984): Maturation of kainic acid seizure–brain damage syndrome in the rat. II Histopathological sequelae. *Neuroscience* **13,** 1073–1094.

Okazaki, M.M. & Nadler, J.V. (1988): Protective effects of mossy fiber lesions against kainic acid-induced seizures and neuronal degeneration. *Neurosci.ence* **26,** 763–781.

Popovici, T., Represa, A., Crépel, V., Barbin, G., Beaudoin, M. & Ben-Ari, Y. (1990): Effects of kainic acid-induced seizures and ischemia on c-*fos*-like proteins in rat brain. *Brain Res.* **536,** 183–194.

Represa, A. & Ben-Ari, Y. (1992): Kindling is associated with the formation of novel mossy fiber synapses in the CA3 region. *Exp. Brain Res.* **92,** 69–78.

Represa, A., Tremblay, E. & Ben-Ari, Y. (1987): Kainate binding sites in the hippocampal mossy fibers: localization and plasticity. *Neuroscience* **20,** 739–748.

Represa, A., Le Gal La Salle, G. & Ben-Ari, Y. (1989): Hippocampal plasticity in the kindling model of epilepsy in rats. *Neurosci. Lett.* **99,** 345–350.

Represa, A., Jorquera, I., Le Gal La Salle, G. & Ben-Ari, Y. (1993a): Epilepsy induced collateral sprouting of hippocampal mossy fibers: does it induce the development of ectopic synapses with granule cell dendrites? *Hippocampus* **3,** 257–268.

Represa, A., Niquet, J., Charriaut-Marlangue, C. & Ben-Ari, Y. (1993b): Reactive astrocytes in the KA-damaged hippocampus have the phenotypic features of type-2 astrocytes. *J. Neurocytol.* **22,** 299–310.

Represa, A., Pollard, H., Moreau, J., Ghilini, G., Krestchatisky, M. & Ben-Ari, Y. (1993c): Mossy fiber sprouting in epileptic rats is associated with a transient increased expression of α-tubulin. *Neurosci. Lett.* **153,** 149–152.

Rocamora, N., Palacios, J.M. & Mengod, G. (1992): Limbic seizures induce a differential regulation of the expression of nerve growth factor, brain-derived neurotrophic factor and neurotrophin-3, in the rat hippocampus. *Mol. Brain Res.* **13,** 27–33.

Saffen, D.W., Cole, A.J., Worley, P.F., Christy, B.A., Ryder, K. & Baraban, J.M. (1988): Convulsant-induced increase in transcription factor messenger RNAs in rat brain. *Proc. Nat. Acad. Sci. USA* **85,** 7795–7799.

Tauck, D.L. & Nadler, J.V. (1985): Evidence for functional mossy fiber sprouting in hippocampal formation of kainic acid treated rats. *J. Neurosci.* **5,** 1016–1022.

Traub, R.D. & Wong, R.K.S. (1982): Cellular mechanism of neuronal synchronization in epilepsy. *Science* **216,** 745–747.

Zafra, F., Hengerer, B., Leibrock, J., Thoenen, H. & Lindholm, D. (1990): Activity dependent regulation of BDNF and NGF mRNAs in the rat hippocampus is mediated by non-NMDA glutamate receptors. *EMBO J.* **9,** 3545–3550.

Epileptic Seizures and Syndromes, Edited by Peter Wolf
© 1994 John Libbey & Company Ltd., pp. 541–546

Chapter 54

Ictogenesis and chaos

Christian E. Elger and Klaus Lehnertz

Univ. Nervenklinik Epileptologie, Sigmund Freud Strasse 25, 53127 Bonn, Germany

Introduction

Since the early observations of Goldensohn and Pupura (1963) and Matsumoto and Ajmone-Marsan (1964a, b) it has been known that the most prominent behaviour of neurons within the epileptic focus is the so-called paroxysmal depolarization shift (PDS). The PDS is characterized by a slow membrane depolarization which elicits a high-frequency burst of action potentials. Although the epileptic focus is surrounded by a zone of strong inhibition (Prince & Wilder, 1967; Elger & Speckmann, 1983), epileptiform activity can spread to adjacent neurons so that a larger neuronal population is recruited into the epileptic process. Furthermore, single-unit recordings in animals with experimental epilepsy (Wyler, 1983) have shown that, in contrast to physiological behaviour, epileptic neurons do not show a correlated response during a specific operant task. Instead, they exhibit high-frequency bursts of action potentials that occur more or less randomly (Fig. 1).

The result might be that during the development and manifestation of the epileptic process the activity of involved neurons undergoes a reduction or even a complete loss of complexity features, leading to a decreased responsiveness. If this explanation holds true, it can be assumed that the estimation of a reduced neuronal complexity might help to establish the spatiotemporal extent of the epileptogenic zone, which is the main aim of presurgical evaluation in patients with pharmacoresistant epilepsies (Lüders & Awad, 1992).

A mathematical approach to quantify the complexity of a neuronal system can be based on complexity-related concepts such as non-stationarity and non-predictability (Barlow, 1985; Jansen, 1991), reflected in the electromagnetic signals recorded by the electroencephalogram (EEG), electrocorticogram (ECoG), magnetoencephalogram (MEG) that originate from neuronal processes (Fig. 2).

A first concept is to regard the underlying neuronal system as highly complex but linear. Quantifying methods, such as estimation of spectra or autoregressive modelling, have proven to be successful in only a limited number of cases.

An alternative concept is characterized by modelling the neuronal system as relatively simple (in terms of number of parameters required for a mathematical description) but highly non-linear. From the theory of non-linear dynamics (Schuster, 1984), it is known that special non-linear systems with only a few degrees of freedom may exhibit chaotic behaviour that is characterized by broad-band spectra or rapid decaying autocorrelation functions; this type can often be observed in the analysis of neuronal behaviour.

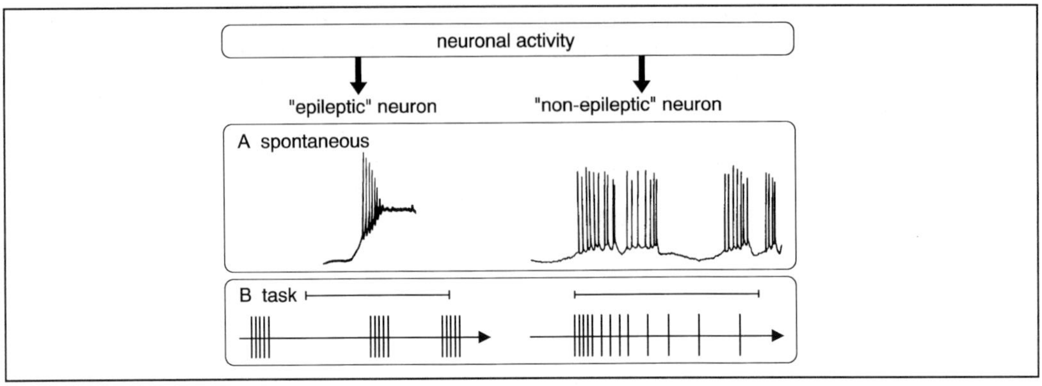

Fig. 1. Schematic drawings of membrane potential changes occurring spontaneously (A) and discharge rates related to a specific operant task (B) of 'epileptic' and 'non-epileptic' neurons.

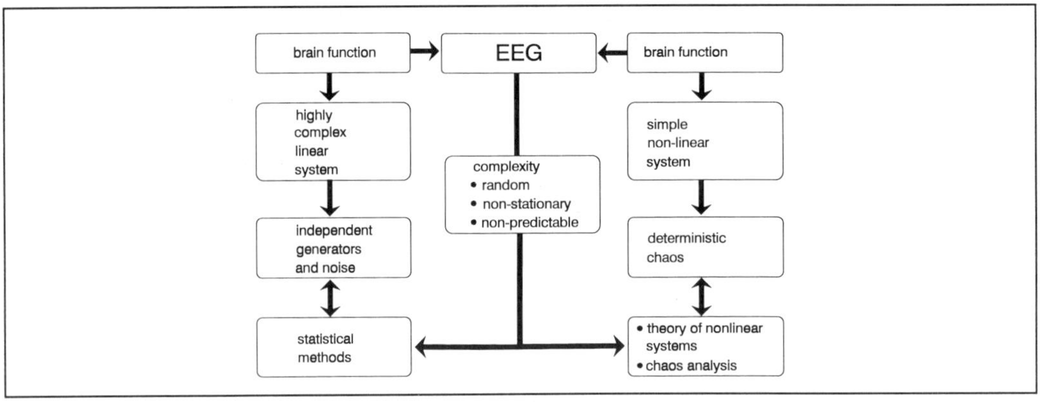

Fig. 2. Linear vs. non-linear modelling of brain function derived from complexity features of the accompanying electromagnetic signals.

This second approach offers different measures to parameterize chaotic behaviour either statically or dynamically. In particular, the dimension is a measure to quantify the complexity in terms of number of degrees of freedom. Several authors have shown that different dimensions reflect different brain states, where synchronized states are characterized by low dimension values and vice versa (Babloyantz *et al.*, 1985; Babloyantz & Destexhe, 1986; Mayer-Kress & Layne, 1987; Röschke & Basar, 1989; Frank *et al.*, 1990; Pijn *et al.*, 1991).

Methods

In order to quantify the spatiotemporal extent of complexity changes related to epilepsy, we examined the ECoG of patients with pharmacoresistant temporal lobe epilepsy by means of a moving-window dimension analysis. The ECoG was recorded during the presurgical work-up, using subdural strip electrodes and intrahippocampal depth electrodes. The data sets consisted of ictal activity (including pre- and postictal phase) as well as interictal activity (regardless of whether or not pathological activity was present) and were taken from selected electrodes located in the hypothesized focal area, adjacent areas and from homologous electrodes on the contralateral side, using a priori information gained from a visual inspection of the localization of seizure onset and propagation. The data sets were segmented into 30 s epochs with a 50 per cent overlap and for each segment the dimension (D_2 correlation dimension) was calculated, using a method proposed by Grassberger and Procaccia (1983). Since the absolute value of the dimension depends on calculational as well as on recording parameters (Albano *et al.*, 1987; Smith, 1988; Möller *et al.*, 1989; Lehnertz, 1992), only changes of the dimension (for a fixed setting of calculation and recording parameters) were taken into account by compiling a time-dependent 'dimension profile' for all recording locations. For reasons of simplicity, unresolved estimates and dimension values greater than a predefined upper limit were regarded equal to a selected cut-off value D*.

Results

A typical set of dimension profiles obtained from different recording locations during the ictal (including pre- and postictal) phase is shown in Fig. 3.

In the ictal phase there is a low dimension state reflecting highly synchronized activity. Preictally, pronounced transitions from high- to low-dimensional system states are found, especially in the focal area (temporobasal and hippocampal locations) and – less pronounced – in adjacent areas. Here the degree of dimension changes seems to depend on whether or not these brain areas are recruited during seizure spread. At remote locations (e.g. the contralateral side, excluding the contralateral hippocampus), only minor or no dimension changes can be found during the whole observation time. Furthermore, in the focal area a dropping to a more or less stable low-dimensional state is observed approximately 10 min before seizure onset. One might speculate if such a long-lasting synchronization

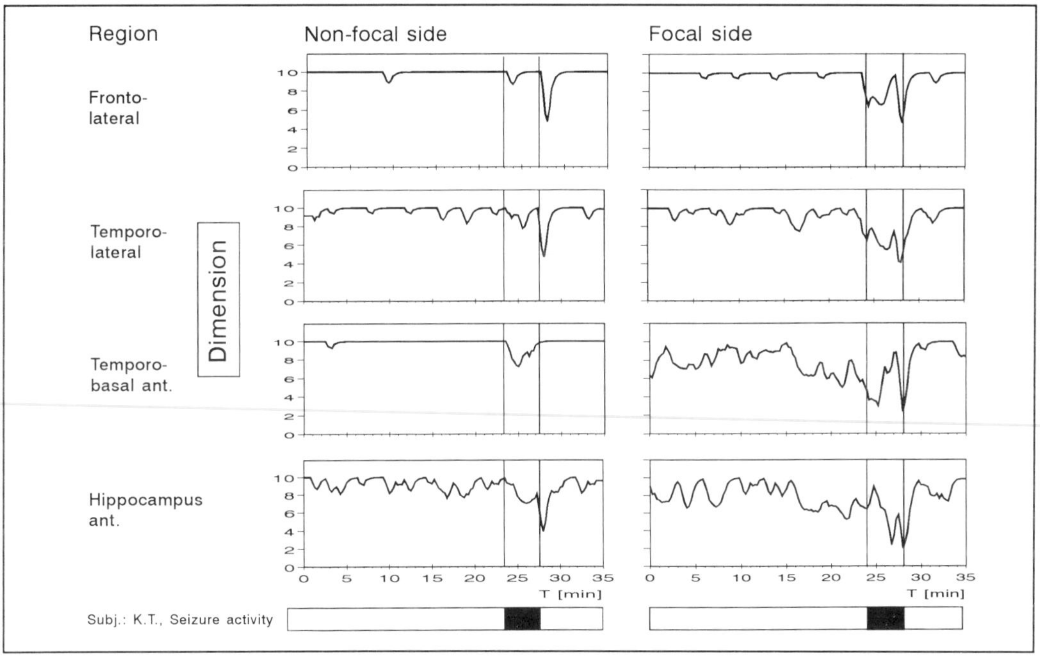

Fig. 3. Dimension profiles obtained from an ictal ECoG segment (including pre- and postictal phase) at different recording locations (focal and homologous non-focal side). Unresolved dimension estimates are regarded as equal to an upper limit of 10. The two vertical lines denote the beginning and end of the clinical seizure (complex partial seizure of temporal lobe origin; histology: Ammon's horn sclerosis).

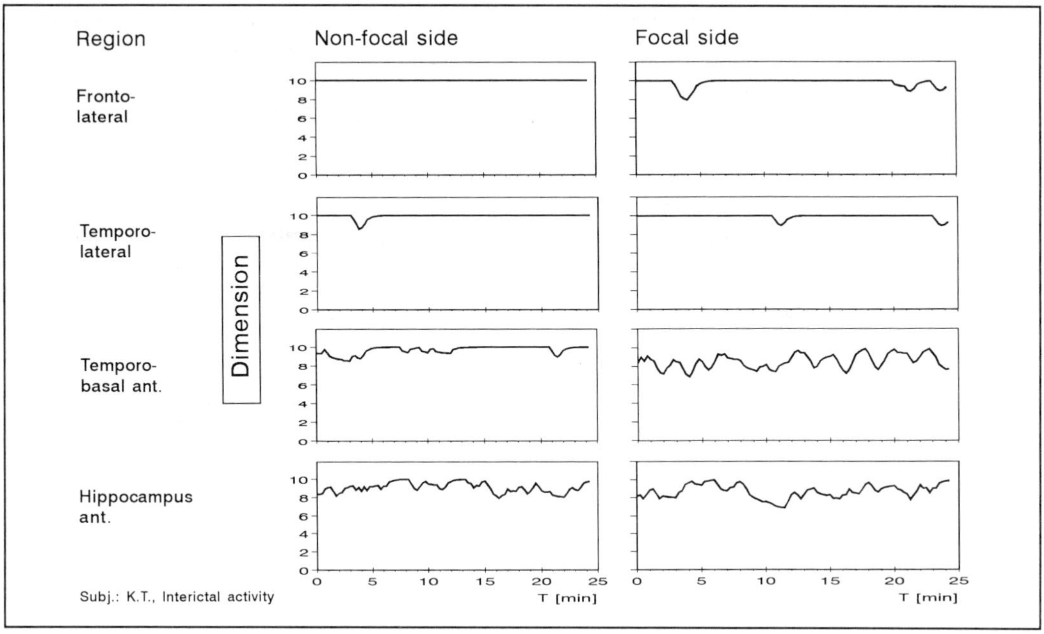

Fig. 4. Same patient as in Fig. 3; interictal ECoG segment.

phenomenon of neuronal activity in the focal area can be regarded as an indicator of an imminent seizure.

Interictally, similar but less pronounced transitions that compare to those found in the preictal phase can be found only in the focal area, while at adjacent and remote locations the dimension remains nearly constantly high (Fig. 4).

A further reduction of information is gained by condensing the information of the dimension profile into a single number, namely by calculating the area between the profile and the cut-off line representing unresolved estimates. If this value is normalized with respect to the observation length, one obtains a time-independent measure (which we call 'complexity loss measure') that quantifies neuronal complexity reduction as a single number for each recording location. Maximum values of this measure were found in those brain areas that correspond to the epileptogenic zone as it was established during the presurgical evaluation by other methods (Fig. 5).

A comparison of complexity loss measures obtained from interictal ECoG data sets recorded on different days yielded only minor variations in time for the non-focal recording locations. In the focal area, however, a high variablility was observed. Relating these findings to the initially formulated hypothesis (for instance, the relation between the neuronal complexity loss and the degree of epileptogenic disturbance), it seems natural to take into consideration a variable which is commonly accepted to influence the epileptic process: the anticonvulsant medication. As depicted in Fig. 6, the complexity loss measure shows an inverse correlation with the serum level of e.g. carbamazepine in the focal area only, while no correlation could be observed in non-focal recording locations.

Discussion

The results obtained so far indicate a graded complexity loss which fits the following spatial versus temporal distribution scheme:

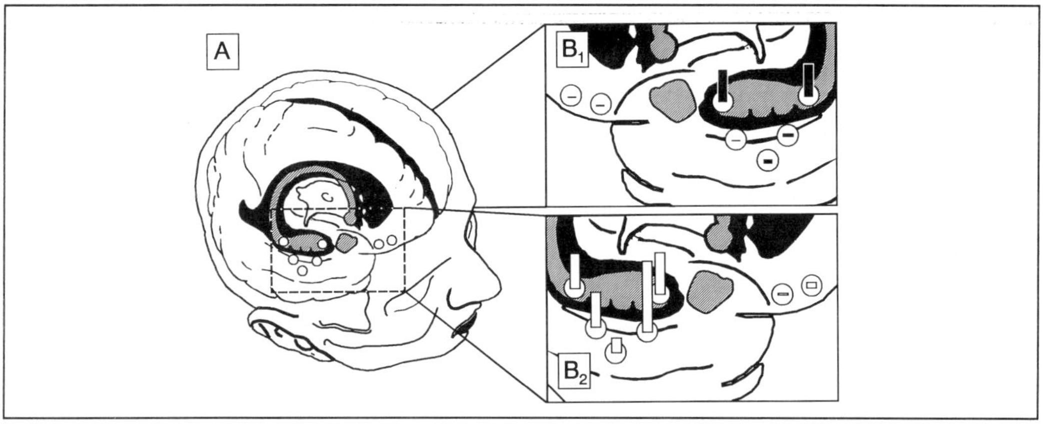

Fig. 5. Spatial distribution of the complexity loss measure schematically plotted according to the anatomical recording locations (total view A; close-up view of contralateral B1 and ipsilateral side B2).

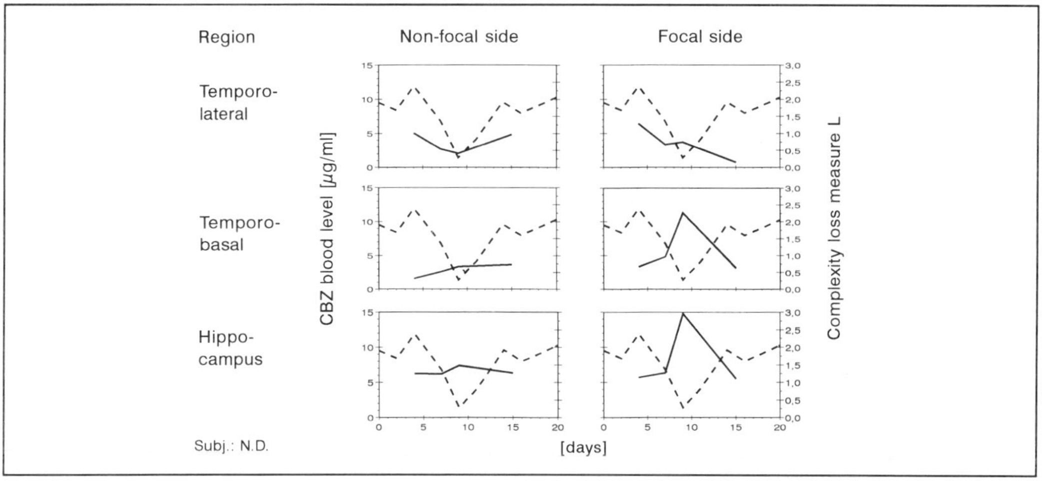

Fig. 6. Spatiotemporal dependence of the complexity loss measure in relation to anticonvulsant medication carbamazepine (CBZ). The time profile of the serum blood level during the phase of presurgical evaluation is shown as dashed lines; the solid lines represent the time profiles of the complexity loss measure from different recording (focal and homologous non-focal) locations (complex partial seizures of temporomesial origin; histology: loss of hippocampal ganglion cells in the pyramidal layer with reactive gliosis).

(a) In the focal area there is a marked loss during interictal states. Approximately 10–15 min before seizure onset a pronounced increase of the complexity loss can be observed, which reaches its maximum during the ictal state.
(b) In adjacent areas the complexity loss is less pronounced during interictal states as compared with the focal area; it might increase during preictal and ictal states dependent on the degree of the involvement during seizure spread.
(c) In remote non-focal areas there are interictally no hints of a reduced complexity. However, during ictal states, a tendency to a slightly increased temporary reduction exists in those areas that are recruited during seizure development.

Up to now these findings are based on the analysis of 30 ictal and interictal ECoG data sets with a mean duration of 20 min in seven patients. The results obtained confirm the findings of the presurgical work-up. However, the conclusion, particularly concerning the localization and delineation of the epileptogenic zone, has to be confirmed in a larger number of cases.

References

Albano, A.M., Mees, A.F., de Guzman, G.C. & Rapp, P.E. (1987): Data requirements for reliable estimation of correlation dimensions. In: *Chaos in biological systems*, eds. H. Degn, A.V. Holden & L.F. Olsen, pp. 207–219. New York: Plenum Press.

Babloyantz, A. & Destexhe, A. (1986): Low-dimensional chaos in an instance of epilepsy. *Proc. Nat. Acad. Sci. USA* **83,** 3513–3517.

Babloyantz, A., Nicolis, C. & Salazar, M. (1985): Evidence of chaotic dynamics of brain activity during the sleep cycle. *Phys. Lett. A.,* **111,** 152–156.

Barlow, J.S. (1985): Methods of analysis of nonstationary EEGs with emphasis on segmentation techniques: a comparative review. *J. Clin. Neurophysiol.* **2(3),** 267–304.

Elger, C.E. & Speckmann, E.-J. (1983): Penicillin induced epileptic foci in the motor cortex: vertical inhibition. *Electroencephalogr. Clin. Neurophysiol.* **56,** 604–622.

Frank, G.W., Lookman, T., Nerenberg, M.A.H. & Essex, C. (1990): Chaotic time series analysis of epileptic seizures. *Physica D* **46,** 427–438.

Goldensohn, E.S. & Pupura, D.P. (1963): Intracellular potentials of cortical neurons during focal epileptogenic discharges. *Science* **139,** 840–842.

Grassberger, P. & Procaccia, I. (1983): Characterization of strange attractors. *Phys. Rev. Lett.* **50,** 346–349.

Jansen, B.H. (1991): Quantitative analysis of electroencephalograms: is there chaos in the future? *Int. J. Biomed. Comput.* **27,** 95–123

Lehnertz, K. (1992): Influence of sampling rate and filtering on the correlation dimension of the human alpha EEG and MEG. In: *Biomagnetism: clinical aspects*, eds. M. Hoke, S.N. Erne, Y.C. Okada & G.L. Romani. Elsevier: Amsterdam.

Lüders, H.O. & Awad, I. (1992): Conceptual considerations. In: *Epilepsy surgery*, ed. H.O. Lüders, pp. 51–62. New York: Raven Press.

Matsumoto, H. & Ajmone-Marsan, C. (1964a): Cortical cellular phenomena in experimental epilepsy: interictal manifestations. *Exp. Neurol.* **9,** 286–304.

Matsumoto, H. & Ajmone-Marsan, C. (1964b): Cortical cellular phenomena in experimental epilepsy: ictal manifestations. *Exp. Neurol.* **9,** 305–326.

Mayer-Kress, G. & Layne, S.P. (1987): Dimensionality of the human electroencephalogram. In: *Perspectives in biological dynamics and theoretical medicine*, eds. S.H. Koslow, A.J. Mandell & M.F. Shlesinger. *Ann. NY Acad. Sci.* **504,** 62–87.

Möller, M., Lange, W., Mitschke, F., Abraham, N.B. & Hübner, U. (1989): Errors from digitizing and noise in estimating attractor dimensions. *Phys. Lett. A* **138,** 176–182.

Pijn, J.P., van Neerven, J., Noest, A. & Lopes da Silva, F.H. (1991): Chaos or noise in EEG signals: dependence on state and brain site. *Electroencephalogr. Clin. Neurophysiol.* **79,** 371–381.

Prince, D.A. & Wilder, B.J. (1967): Control mechanisms in cortical epileptogenic foci: 'surround' inhibition. *Arch. Neurol.* **16,** 194–202.

Röschke, J. & Basar, E. (1989): Correlation dimensions in various parts of cat and human brain in different states. In: *Springer series in brain dynamics* 2, eds. E. Basar & T.H. Bullock, pp. 131–148. Berlin, Heidelberg: Springer.

Schuster, H.G. (1984): *Deterministic chaos.* Weinheim: Physik-Verlag.

Smith, L.A. (1988): Intrinsic limits on dimension calculations. *Phys. Lett. A.* **133(6),** 283–288.

Wyler, A.R. (1983): Firing patterns of epileptic neurons from motor cortex of awake, behaving monkeys. In: *Epilepsy and motor system*, eds. E.-J. Speckmann & C.E. Elger, pp. 179–200. Munich, Vienna, Baltimore: Urban and Schwarzenberg,

Epileptic Seizures and Syndromes, Edited by Peter Wolf
© 1994 John Libbey & Company Ltd., pp. 547–561

Chapter 55

Pathophysiology of focal and generalized convulsive versus that of generalized non-convulsive seizures

Massimo Avoli and Pierre Gloor

Montreal Neurological Institute and Department of Neurology and Neurosurgery, McGill University, 3801 University Street, Montreal, Quebec, Canada H3A 2B4

Introduction

In the light of their underlying pathophysiological mechanisms and their electrographic and clinical manifestations, two types of seizures can be distinguished. The first is the prototype of non-convulsive generalized epilepsy as epitomized by pure absence seizures. It is characterized by a stable, generalized non-evolving electroencephalographic (EEG) pattern consisting of a 3 Hz spike-and-wave rhythm which is not followed by postictal depression. The second type is focal or generalized, but in the latter case it is convulsive (tonic, clonic or both). It differs from the first type by an evolving EEG pattern and the presence of postictal depression. Such a seizure starts with fast, low-voltage activity, which gradually changes into a repetitive rhythmic pattern of progressively increasing amplitude and decreasing frequency (the tonic phase), followed by interrupted bursts of discharges separated by brief periods of silence (the clonic phase). One characteristic of the evolving nature of these seizures is their tendency, if focal in onset, to spread, which may lead to generalization of the seizure discharge. The end of the seizure is followed by postictal depression. The clinical manifestations depend on the area of cortex involved, but, if the discharges involve motor regions, they are convulsive and there are postictal signs of depression, such as Todd's paralysis. If they involve the temporal lobe, the manifestations are often non-convulsive (unresponsiveness, automatism), the postictal signs being confusion and amnesia.

What distinguishes these two types of seizures is not that one is non-convulsive and the other convulsive, but two other features: non-evolution of the EEG pattern and lack of postictal changes in the first, and an evolving pattern followed by postictal depression in the second. In 1979 one of us proposed the term first and second degree of epileptogenesis to characterize these two types of seizures (Gloor, 1979). For simplicity's sake we shall hereafter call the first type grade 1 and the second grade 2 type of seizure. The goal of this chapter is to offer an explanation for some of the differences that exist at the cellular level between these two epileptic conditions in humans. Although there are several ways of inducing experimentally focal and generalized epileptiform discharges, we shall focus on models which are induced by convulsants such as penicillin, bicuculline or picrotoxin. These drugs share the ability to interact with the γ-amino-butyric acid ($GABA_A$) receptor–ionophore complex (for review, see Avoli, 1988).

Within these experimental limits, three examples of epileptiform EEG patterns similar to those encountered in humans can be defined. First, there is the focal interictal discharge evoked by topical application of penicillin to the neocortex or hippocampus (Kooi & Beck, 1956; Gloor *et al.*, 1966; Ajmone-Marsan, 1969; Ayala *et al.*, 1973). This type of discharge is commonly found interictally in the EEG of patients suffering from focal (partial) seizures. It consists of a large-amplitude, sharp transient which, in the experimental situation, is localized to the region exposed to the epileptogenic agent (Fig. 1A). Second, there are the generalized epileptiform discharges of feline generalized penicillin epilepsy induced by intramuscular (IM) injection of large doses of penicillin in the cat (Prince & Farrell, 1969; Gloor, 1988; Gloor & Fariello, 1988). The EEG pattern resulting from such an injection consists of generalized, bilaterally synchronous spike-and-wave discharges. The EEG pattern and the behavioural manifestations in the cat closely approximate those of human absence attacks (Fig. 1B). This type of epileptic activity is ictal but non-convulsive, as in human absence attacks. Both in humans and in the cat the clinical manifestations of generalized spike-and-wave discharges are mild and the discharges are not followed by postictal depression. Third, there are seizures caused by the topical application of a convulsant drug (Fig. 2A), which can secondarily evolve into a generalized seizure. Moreover, this type includes convulsive seizures which occasionally evolve from the just-described non-convulsive spike-and-wave pattern of feline generalized

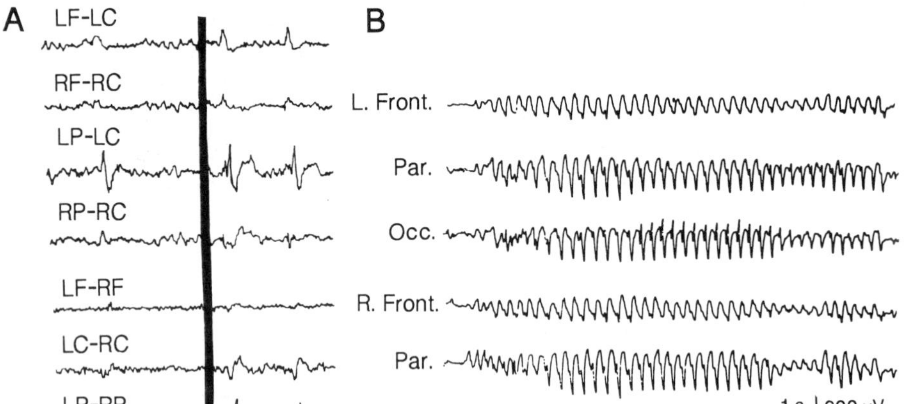

Fig. 1A. Interictal focal epileptiform activity induced in the cat cerebral cortex by local injection of penicillin in the left visual cortex of the cat. Focal spike discharges occurring spontaneously (A) and activated by light flashes (B) are maximal in the area of penicillin application. Abbreviations: L: left; R: right; F: frontal; C: central; P: posterior. Reproduced with permission from Kooi & Beck (1956). In Fig. 1B the EEG pattern of feline generalized penicillin epilepsy recorded with electrodes inserted chronically in the skull displays features similar to those observed in human generalized spike-and-wave discharges associated with absence attacks. Abbreviations are: L, left; R, right; Front., frontal; Par., parietal; Occ., occipital. Reproduced with permission from Guberman et al. (1975).

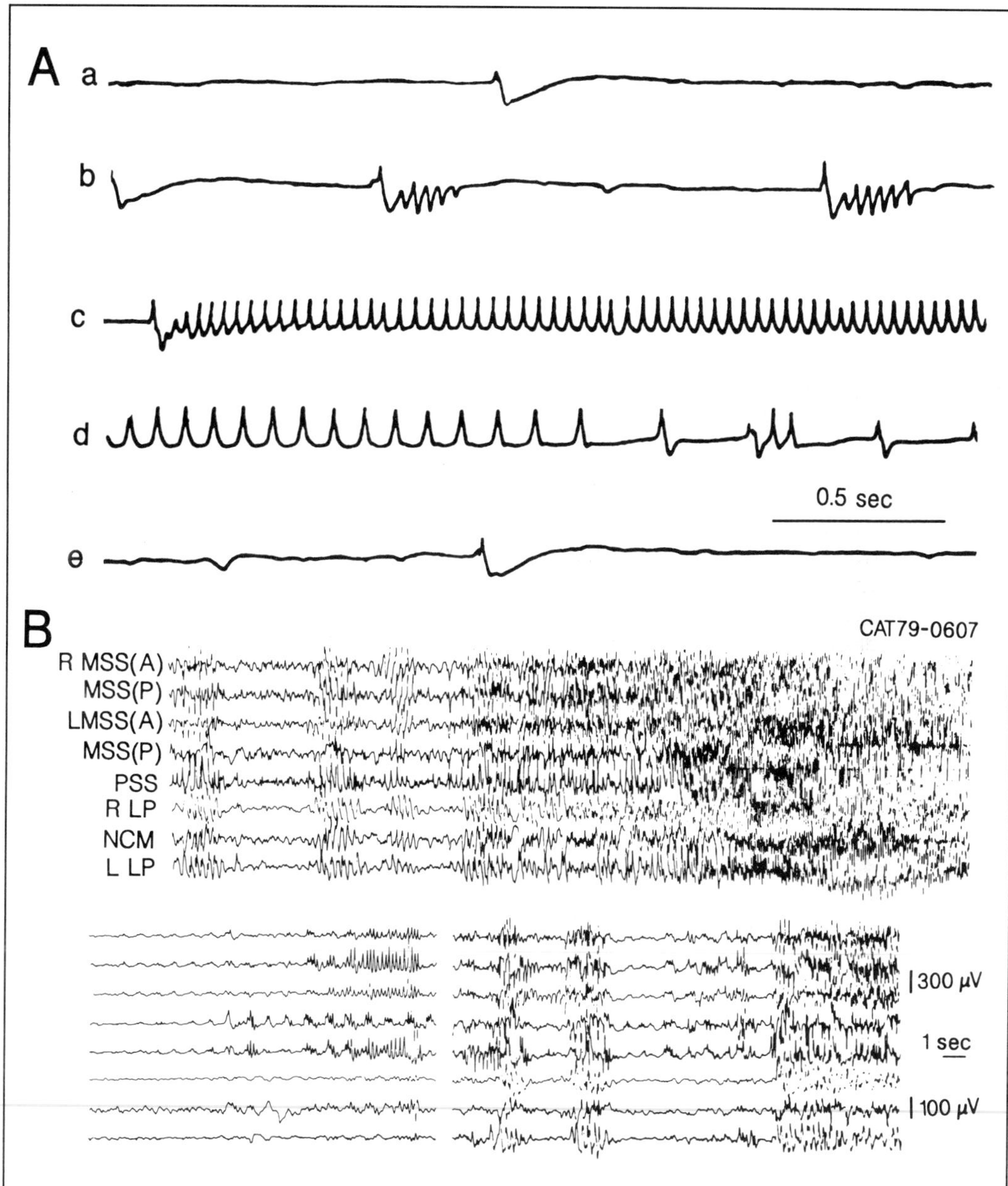

Fig. 2A. Transition from interictal focal epileptiform activity (a and b) to convulsive tonic (c) and clonic (d) EEG pattern in the penicillin-induced focus in the cat cortex in situ. The recovery of interictal activity following postictal depression (not shown) is illustrated in e. Reproduced with permission from Ajmone–Marsan (1969). Fig. 2B. Transition from generalized spike-and-wave discharges (grade 1) to generalized convulsive (grade 2) EEG pattern. Postictal depression (lower left panel), recorded 2 min after the end of the seizure, characterized by low-voltage pattern with slow waves followed by the appearance of spindles. Another generalized convulsive seizure occurs 13 min later (lower right panel). Abbreviations are: MSS, middle suprasylvian gyrus; PSS, posterior suprasylvian gyrus; LP, nucleus lateralis posterior; NCM, nucleus centralis medialis; R, right; L, left; A, anterior; P, posterior. Reproduced with permission from Avoli et al. (1981).

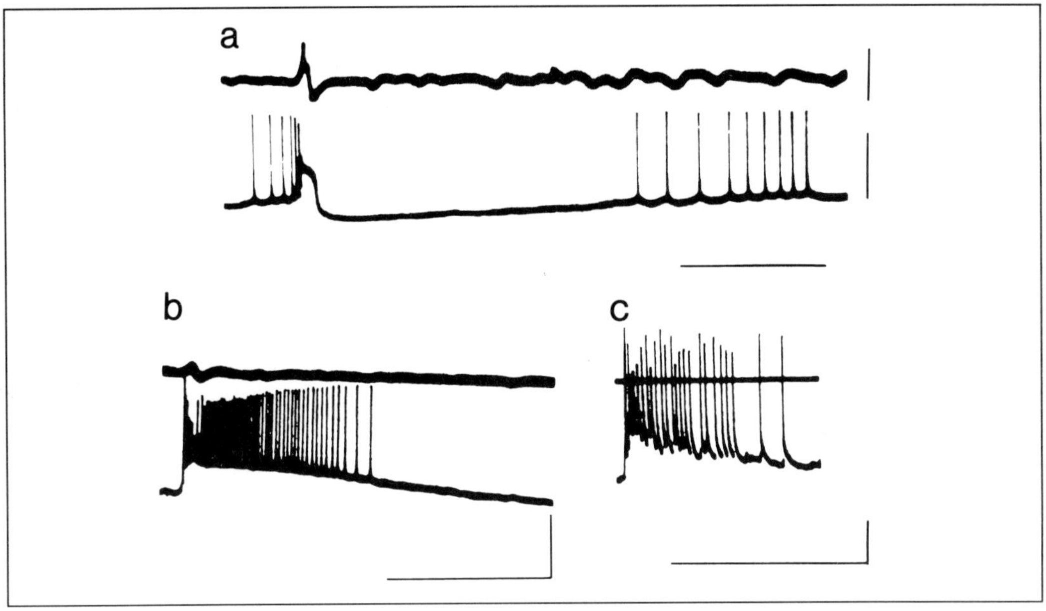

Fig. 3. Similarities between PDSs recorded in vivo (a, b) and in vitro (c). a. EEG (top trace) and intracellular (bottom trace) recordings from the cortex of an intact, anaesthetized cat show a typical spontaneously occurring interictal discharge, the PDS being followed by a long-lasting hyperpolarization (calibrations: 1 mV for the EEG, 40 mV for the intracellular trace and 400 ms); b. same experimental conditions as in a showing a spontaneously occurring PDS followed by a long-lasting depolarization associated with discharge of action potentials (calibrations: 25 mV for the intracellular signal and 500 ms); c. spontaneous PDS generated by a CA1 pyramidal cell of a guinea pig hippocampal slice bathed in medium containing 2 mM penicillin. Reproduced with permission from Schwartzkroin & Pedley (1979).

penicillin epilepsy (Fig. 2B). Although the onset of the convulsive seizure markedly differs in these two situations, the evolution of the EEG pattern of the seizure is similar in the two instances and the end of the discharge is followed in both cases by postictal depression.

The first and third patterns are hallmarks of grade 2 seizures, the second of grade 1 seizures.

Cellular patterns associated with grade 1 and with grade 2 epileptiform discharges

The cellular counterpart of the focal interictal discharge induced by convulsant drugs such as penicillin, bicuculline or picrotoxin is a large-amplitude depolarization associated with a prolonged burst of action potentials, sometimes followed by a long-lasting hyperpolarization (Fig. 3). This phenomenon is known under the term of paroxysmal depolarizing shift (PDS; see Matsumoto & Ajmone-Marsan, 1964b) and can be reproduced both *in vivo* and *in vitro* (for review see Ayala *et al.*, 1973; Prince & Connors, 1986). The similarities which exist between *in vivo* and *in vitro* PDSs are illustrated in Fig. 3.

The PDS is a network event with an underlying giant excitatory postsynaptic potential (EPSP) presumably resulting from the synchronous activation of recurrent excitatory pathways (Ayala *et al.*, 1973; Johnston & Brown, 1981, 1984; Traub & Wong, 1983). However, non-synaptic processes contribute to the PDS's depolarizing envelope and to the associated firing of action potentials. This is shown in Fig. 4A, where a PDS was recorded from a human cell in a neocortical slice that was bathed in a medium containing bicuculline. In this experiment the epileptiform response was elicited

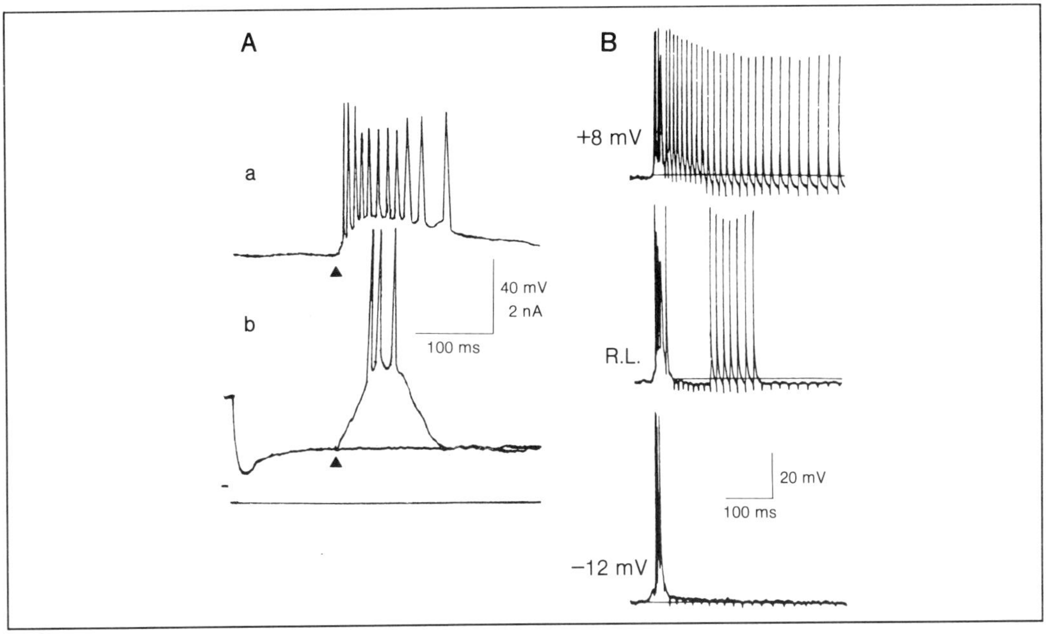

Fig.4A. Current-clamp recording from a human neocortical neurone bathed in bicuculline methiodide shows the contribution of voltage-dependent conductances to the PDS induced by extracelluar stimuli of same intensity in both a and b. B. Evidence for field (ephaptic) effects during PDS generated by a rat CA1 hippocampal neurone bathed in penicillin (3.2 mM) and high K^+ (7.25 mM). Note that action potentials of ephaptic origin are generated during the hyperpolarization that follows the burst (+ 8 mV and RC traces). Reproduced with permission from Tancredi & Avoli (1987).

by extracellular focal stimuli of identical intensity at resting membrane potential (sample a) and at a hyperpolarized membrane potential approximately 30 mV more negative than rest (sample b). Hyperpolarizing the membrane potential increases the amplitude of the depolarizing envelope of the PDS, but shortens its duration. Furthermore, ephaptic field effects (see Fig. 4B), action potentials of ectopic origin and long duration, low-amplitude action potentials (suggesting the presence of Ca^{2+}-mediated regenerative processes of dendritic origin) can occur during the PDS (Prince, 1978). Therefore the cellular correlates of the experimental focal interictal discharge are quite different from normal EPSPs recorded in hippocampal or neocortical cells following orthodromic stimuli, even when these are delivered at high strength or during low-frequency repetitive stimulation.

The characteristics of the PDS contrast with the intracellular correlate of generalized spike-and-wave discharges induced by IM injection of penicillin in cats (Fig. 5). As shown initially in Prince's laboratory (Fisher & Prince, 1977) and later confirmed by us (Giaretta *et al.*, 1987), the cellular counterpart of generalized spike-and-wave discharges is an alternating sequence of depolarizing and hyperpolarizing potentials. The depolarizing component, which is synchronous with the 'spike' of the spike-and-wave complex, is similar to a normal EPSP and rarely elicits more than two or three action potentials. Intracellular recordings do not reveal any sign of 'atypical' generation of action potentials, such as fractionated or partial spikes or any good evidence of Ca^{2+} spike generation (Fisher & Prince, 1977; Giaretta *et al.*, 1987). The synaptic nature of the depolarizing potential coinciding with the spike of the spike-and-wave complex is indicated by its behaviour during injection of steady hyperpolarizing current, since it increases in amplitude (Fig. 5B). These experiments also indicate that the hyperpolarization which follows the depolarizing component and correlates in time with the

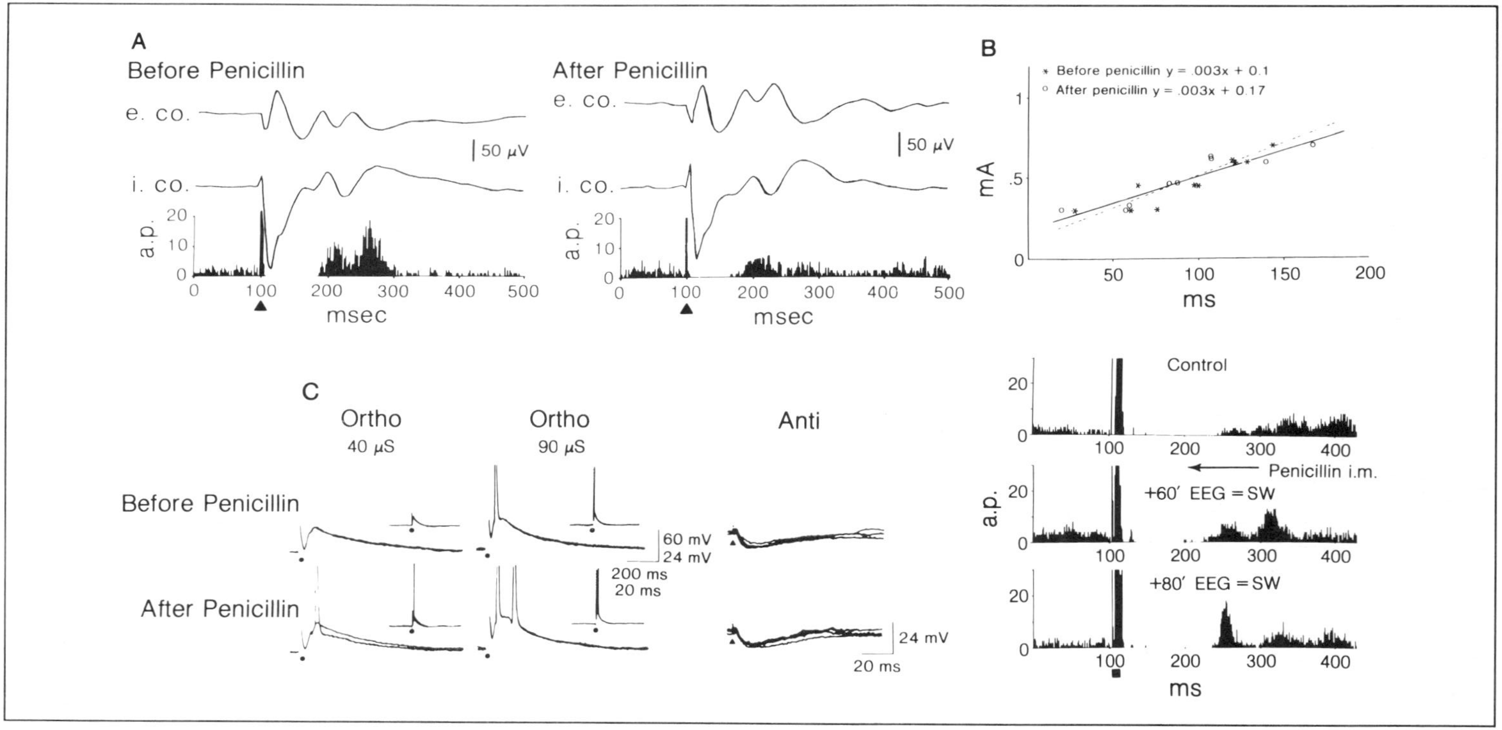

Fig. 6A. Lack of changes in recurrent inhibition induced by electrical stimulation of the cerebral peduncle (triangle) before and after IM injection of penicillin, sufficient to induce generalized spike-and-wave discharge. Averages of the field potentials recorded from the cortical surface (e.co.) and the intracortical (i.co.) layers of the pericruciate gyrus. Single-unit peristimulus time histograms of the activity of a cortical cell antidromically activated from the cerebral peduncle. The duration of the inhibitory pause is unchanged after IM penicillin. Reproduced with permission from Kostopoulos et al. (1983). B. Upper part: relationship between intensity of the direct cortical shock (mA) and duration of the inhibitory period (ms) before (solid line) and after IM penicillin; lower part: peristimulus time histograms of a neurone of the middle suprasylvian gyrus in response to direct cortical shock at the indicated time after IM penicillin. Length of inhibitory pause unchanged. Reproduced with permission from Giaretta et al. (1985). C. Low concentrations of penicillin (0.34 mM) induce in a CA1 pyramidal cell of the rat hippocampal slice an increase in the amplitude and half-width of the EPSP as well as the discharge of two action potentials following orthodromic stimuli without changing the amplitude or the duration of the recurrent IPSP. Reproduced with permission from Avoli (1984).

(Fig. 6A, B) (Kostopoulos *et al.*, 1983; Giaretta *et al.*, 1985). Therefore, in contrast to penicillin-induced focal, interictal epileptogenesis, generalized spike-and-wave activity induced by parenteral penicillin is associated with the preservation of Cl^--mediated, hyperpolarizing potentials caused by the activation of $GABA_A$ receptors and presumably the operation of $GABA_B$-mediated K^+ hyperpolarizations. This conclusion is further supported by the preserved sensitivity of cortical neurones to iontophoretically applied GABA following IM penicillin injection up to and beyond the period of spike-and-wave activity in feline generalized penicillin epilepsy (Kostopoulos, 1986). To sum up: epileptic discharges representative of grade 1 type epileptogenesis are characterized by the preservation of $GABA_A$ receptor-mediated inhibition, while in those that are representative of grade 2 type epileptogenesis $GABA_A$ receptor-mediated inhibition is impaired or abolished.

A possible explanation for the penicillin-induced increase in excitability in feline generalized epilepsy is that this drug causes an impairment of the dendritic depolarizing GABA-ergic potentials without decreasing noticeably the somatic hyperpolarizing $GABA_A$ mechanism, although another hypothesis involving glutamate leakage has also been proposed (van Gelder *et al.*, 1984). The first of these hypotheses is supported by the following findings: (i) the concentration of penicillin in the cortex following IM injection in amounts producing generalized spike-and-wave discharges is at least 10-fold less than that used to induce a cortical epileptogenic focus (Quesney & Gloor, 1978; Davenport *et al.*, 1979); (ii) the depolarizing potential caused by $GABA_A$ receptors located mainly on the dendrites appears to be sensitive to very low concentrations of penicillin (Alger & Nicoll, 1982a). Accordingly, doses of penicillin similar to those present in the cat brain following IM injection, when applied in the medium which perfuses the hippocampal slice, are capable of inducing an increase of the orthodromic EPSP without any measurable decrease of the amplitude of the recurrent IPSP induced by stimulation of the alveus (Fig. 6C) (Avoli, 1984).

Some observations on feline generalized penicillin epilepsy are also pertinent with regard to the mechanism of grade 2 seizures. Occasionally in this condition the EEG pattern will change from one typical for grade 1 seizures (generalized spike-and-wave discharges) to one that characterizes generalized convulsions (repetitive evolving type of discharge followed by postictal depression) as shown in Fig. 2B. When this occurs the depression of firing (corresponding to the $GABA_A$ receptor-mediated inhibitory pause) which follows upon stimuli delivered in the thalamus, in the cortex or to the cerebral peduncle disappears shortly before the onset as well as during the type 2 seizure discharge (Figs. 2B and 7) (Kostopoulos *et al.*, 1983; Giaretta *et al.*, 1985). Thus the transition from the pattern of generalized spike-and-wave discharge to that characteristic of convulsive seizures is accompanied and possibly caused by the breakdown of one or more than one hyperpolarizing inhibitory potentials in the brain. This view is in keeping with the observation that, in the neocortex of a cat which had received a topical application of penicillin, post-PDS hyperpolarizations disappear before the onset of focal ictal discharge and are barely observed during such discharge (Matsumoto & Ajmone-Marsan, 1964a, b). A breakdown of GABA-ergic potentials has also been reported for epileptiform responses evoked in the rat hippocampus by repetitive electrical stimulation (Ben Ari *et al.*, 1981) and in the *in vitro* olfactory cortex during seizure-like activity induced by application of 4-aminopyridine (Galvan *et al.*, 1982).

Several mechanisms might be responsible for the decreased efficacy and eventual disappearance of GABA-mediated potentials observed immediately before the onset of and during the grade 2 type of ictal discharge. There is much evidence for a failure of inhibition during conditions that are conducive to focal or generalized grade 2 type discharges. These include a use-dependent depression of inhibitory potentials, which can occur both pre- and postsynaptically (McCarren & Alger, 1985), and a decreased efficacy of GABA-ergic potentials resulting from the changes in the ionic composition of the extracellular environment which accompany epileptiform discharges. For instance, as has been documented in several models of epilepsy, $[K^+]_o$ increases from a baseline of 3 mM up to 15–20 mM during seizure activity (Lux *et al.*, 1986). This change in $[K^+]_o$ can influence the efficacy of GABA-ergic conductances by causing a shift of the Cl^- equilibrium potential in the positive direction

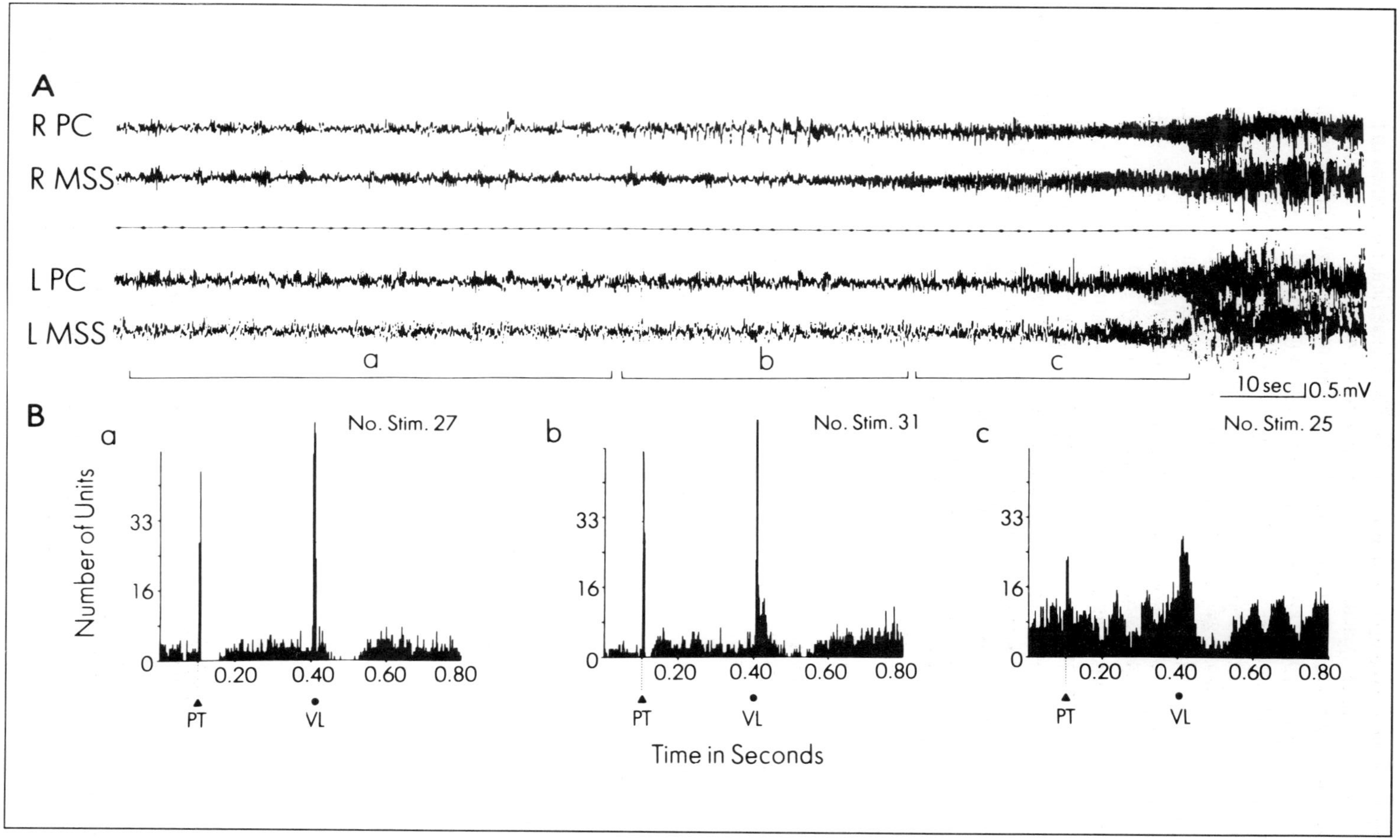

Fig. 7. Peristimulus time histograms (panel B) of an identified pyramidal tract cell recorded at a stage when spike-and-wave discharges were cyclically turning into convulsive seizure activity (panel A). Computation of each histogram was limited to the period associated with one of the three different patterns of EEG activity shown in A. Note the gradual disappearance of the inhibitory pause following antidromic pyramidal tract (PT) or orthodromic thalamic (VL) stimulation as the convulsive seizure activity approaches. Abbreviations in A as in Fig. 2b. Reproduced with permission from Avoli (1988).

and thus a decrease in the drive of the hyperpolarizing IPSPs mediated through $GABA_A$ receptors. Furthermore, an increase in $[K^+]_o$ will diminish the chemical gradient for this cation and thus it will decrease the amount of K^+ outward current caused by the activation of the $GABA_B$ receptor.

$[K^+]_o$ increases only by 1.2–1.8 mM during spike-and-wave discharges (grade 1 type activity) (Fig. 8A and B, left sample), while it can reach values as high as 16 mM during the 'tonic–clonic' (grade 2 type) activity (Fig. 8B, right sample). Concomitant analysis of $[Ca^{2+}]_o$ during the two types of discharges induced in the cat by penicillin IM has also shown that Ca^{2+} only decreases by 0.2–0.4 mM during spike-and-wave discharge but can drop by 1 mM during 'tonic–clonic' seizure activity. This is in agreement with the observation made by Pumain *et al.* (1985) in the photosensitive baboon where the drop in $[Ca^{2+}]_o$ was minimal during photically evoked spike-and-wave discharge, but became large when the convulsive seizure appeared.

A depressant effect on the IPSP can also be caused by the decrease in extracellular $[Ca^{2+}]_o$ which accompanies and at times precedes the onset of seizure activity (Heinemann *et al.*, 1977; Pumain *et al.*, 1985). A deficiency of Ca^{2+} would affect particularly the release of GABA and thus the efficacy of the IPSP. Furthermore, Connor *et al.* (1988) have shown that in response to glutamate-induced depolarization Ca^{2+} enters the cell, and especially in response to repeated glutamate pulses its intracellular concentration may continue to rise. This may be an additional factor in decreasing the GABA response (Stelzer *et al.*, 1988).

Possible relevance for human epilepsy

The differences in the cellular mechanisms underlying grade 1 and grade 2 types of epileptiform discharges discussed in this review might explain some differences in the clinical consequences of

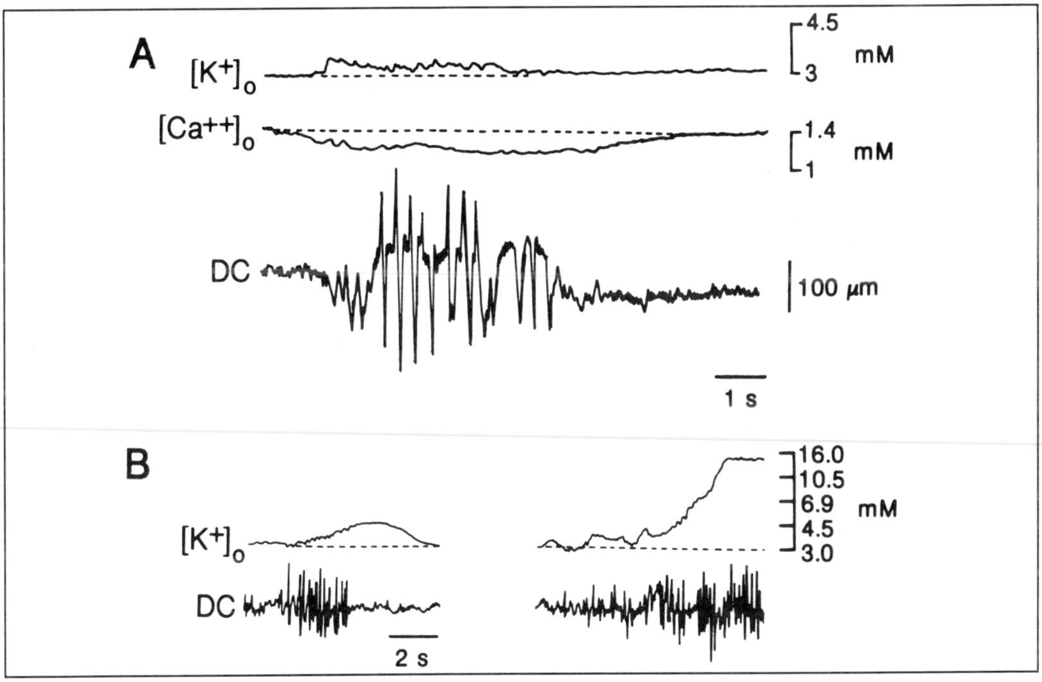

Fig. 8A. Measurement of $[K^+]_o$ and $[Ca^{2+}]_o$ during a spike-and-wave discharge (DC) recorded in the middle suprasylvian gyrus of a cat injected with IM penicillin. B. Changes in $[K^+]_o$ during spike-and-wave discharge (left panel) and 'tonic–clonic' activity (right panel) (unpublished data from G. Kostopoulos, C. Drapeau & M. Avoli).

pure absence epilepsy with spike-and-wave discharge as compared with seizure disorders associated with generalized convulsive or partial seizures (Gloor, 1989). Absence epilepsy uncomplicated by generalized convulsions is probably the most benign form of epilepsy (Lennox & Lennox, 1960; Dalby, 1969; Berkovic *et al.*, 1987) and is the prototype of a grade 1 type of seizure disorder. Its EEG manifestation, the generalized spike-and-wave discharge, is a non-evolving seizure pattern that is not followed by any postictal depression either electrographically or clinically, indicating the likely lack of any deleterious after-effects of the discharge. Pure absence epilepsy uncomplicated by convulsive seizures tends to have a benign course, since it often remits either spontaneously or under treatment (Gloor, 1989). In contrast, the EEG pattern of grade 2 type seizures, whether partial or generalized, is followed by both EEG and clinical signs of postictal depression. These seizures are more resistant to therapy and may have short or more enduring deleterious consequences.

The experiments reviewed here indicate that, during generalized spike-and-wave discharges induced in the cat by the IM injection of penicillin, hyperpolarizing mechanisms mediated through GABA receptors are fully preserved, at least at the level of the neuronal soma. One important implication deriving from the preserved efficacy of hyperpolarizing GABA-ergic mechanisms is that in the experimental model of generalized spike-and-wave discharge the ionic conductance changes caused by activation of the *N*-methyl-D-aspartate (NMDA) receptor through the action of the excitatory aminoacids glutamate and aspartate are probably very limited. The NMDA receptor is coupled with an ionophore which displays a voltage-dependent block exerted by Mg^{2+} present in the extracellular space (Novak *et al.*, 1984). Such NMDA-induced, depolarizing events are associated with the entry of Ca^{2+} into the neuronal compartment.

This condition is bound to change when inhibition breaks down, as in the case of the transition from interictal to ictal epileptiform activity in partial (focal) epilepsy or from generalized spike-and-wave discharge to generalized convulsive seizure activity. Thus, during the transition from one state to the other in these two types of seizures, a breakdown of inhibitory hyperpolarizing mechanisms occurs. Through prolonged depolarization of the membrane, this will relieve the blockade of the NMDA channel exerted by Mg^{2+}. Hence, the NMDA–ionophore will become fully permeant to cations and in particular to Ca^{2+}. Consequently, during seizures in which a breakdown of GABA-mediated inhibitory mechanisms occurs, a large amount of Ca^{2+} will enter the intracellular compartment as shown by extracellular measurements of the Ca^{2+} activity.

This Ca^{2+} influx into the cells, which is likely to occur during any form of grade 2 type epileptic seizures, but not in absence attacks, will undoubtedly cause a number of intracellular responses, some of which are mediated directly by Ca^{2+}, others indirectly through the activation of one or several second-messenger systems. In most instances, these effects are probably only temporary and relatively benign, expressing themselves in the well-known postictal depression evident in the EEG in the form of slow waves or clinically in the form of Todd's paralysis, mental confusion or postictal amnesia. Postictal depression (evident both clinically and in the EEG) and the risk of prolonged memory disturbances after seizures are most pronounced in grade 1 type seizures with a temporal lobe origin. This may reflect the fact that the hippocampus is that part of the brain, especially its sector CA1, which shows the highest concentration of NMDA receptors anywhere in the brain (Cotman & Monaghan, 1987). The integrity of the brain is thus not only at risk in prolonged convulsive seizures, but also in prolonged or frequently repeated non-convulsive temporal lobe seizures. Plastic neuronal changes analogous to those underlying kindling may also occur and could cause the seizure tendency to become more firmly entrenched in the brain. This may explain the relative therapy resistance of long-standing seizure disorders (Reynolds *et al.*, 1983). Prolonged and massive entry of Ca^{2+} as it occurs during grade 2 seizures may exert deleterious consequences, which may include reversible or irreversible cell damage and even cell death. None of these deleterious consequences are known to occur in pure absence epilepsy characterized by generalized spike-and-wave discharge (Gloor, 1989).

Acknowledgements

This work was supported by Medical Research Council (MRC) grant MT-8109 to MA.

References

Ajmone-Marsan, C. (1969): Acute effects of topical epileptogenic agents. In: *Basic mechanisms of the epilepsies*, eds. H.H. Jasper, A.A.J. Ward & A. Pope, pp. 299–319. Boston: Little, Brown.

Alger, B.E. & Nicoll, R.A. (1982a): Feed-forward dendritic inhibition in rat hippocampal pyramidal cells studied *in vitro*. *J. Physiol. (Lond.)* **328,** 105–123.

Alger, B.E. & Nicoll, R.A. (1982b): Pharmacological evidence for two kinds of GABA receptors on rat hippocampal pyramidal cells studied *in vitro*. *J. Physiol.* (Lond.) **328,** 125–141.

Andersen, P., Eccles, J.C. & Loyning, Y. (1964a): Location of postsynaptic inhibitory synapses on hippocampal pyramids. *J. Neurophysiol.* **27,** 592–607.

Andersen, P., Eccles, J.C. & Loyning, Y. (1964b): Pathway of postsynaptic inhibition in the hippocampus. *J. Neurophysiol.* **27,** 608–619.

Andersen, P., Dingledine, R., Gjerstad, L., Langmoen, I.A. & Mosfeldt-Laursen, A. (1980): Two different responses of hippocampal pyramidal cells to application of γ-amino butyric acid. *J. Physiol.* (Lond.) **305,** 279–296.

Avoli, M. & Gloor, P. (1981): The effects of transient functional depression of the thalamus on spindles and on bilateral synchronous discharges of feline generalized penicillin epilepsy. *Epilepsia* **22,** 443–452.

Avoli, M. (1984): Penicillin-induced hyperexcitability in the *in vitro* hippocampal slice can be unrelated to impairment of somatic inhibition. *Brain Res.* **323,** 154–158.

Avoli, M. (1988): GABAergic mechanisms and epileptic discharges. In: *Neurotransmitters and cortical functions: from molecules to mind*, eds. M. Avoli, T.A. Reader, R.W. Dykes & P. Gloor, pp. 187–205. New York, London: Plenum Press.

Avoli, M. (1992): Synaptic activation of $GABA_A$ receptors causes a depolarizing potential under physiological conditions in rat hippocampal pyramidal cells. *Eur. J. Neurosci.* **4,** 16–26.

Ayala, G.F., Dichter, M., Gumnit, R.J., Matsumoto, H. & Spencer, W.E. (1973): Genesis of epileptic interictal spikes: new knowledge of cortical feedback systems suggests a neurophysiological explanation of brief paroxysms. *Brain Res.* **51,** 1–17.

Ben Ari, Y., Krnjevic, K., Reiffenstein, R.J. & Reinhardt, W. (1981): Inhibitory conductance changes and action of GABA in rat hippocampus. *Neuroscience* **6,** 2445–2463.

Berkovic, S.F., Andermann, F., Andermann, E. & Gloor, P. (1987): Concepts of absence epilepsies: discrete syndromes or biological continuum. *Neurology* **37,** 993–1000.

Connor, J.A., Wadman, W.J., Hodeberger, P.E. & Wong, R.K.S. (1988): Sustained dendritic gradients of Ca^{2+} induced by excitatory amino acids in CA1 hippocampal neurons. *Science* **240,** 649–653.

Cotman, C.W. & Monaghan, D.T. (1987): Organization of amino acid receptors: functional implications. In: *Excitatory amino acid transmission*, eds. T.P. Hicks, D. Lodge & H. McLennan, pp. 325–332. New York: Alan R. Liss.

Dalby, M.A. (1969): Epilepsy and 3 per second spike and wave rhythms: a clinical, electroencephalographic and prognostic analysis of 346 patients. *Acta Neurol. Scand.* **45** (Suppl. 40), 183.

Davenport, J., Schwindt, P.C. & Crill, W.E. (1979): Epileptic doses of penicillin do not reduce a monosynaptic GABA-mediated post-synaptic inhibition in the intact anesthetized cat. *Exp. Neurol.* **65,** 552–572.

Dingledine, R. & Gjerstad, L. (1980): Reduced inhibition during epileptiform activity in the *in vitro* hippocampal slice. *J. Physiol.* (Lond.) **305,** 297–313.

Dreifuss, J.J., Kelly, J.S. & Krnjevic, K. (1969): Cortical inhibition and gamma-aminobutyric acid. *Exp. Brain Res.* **9,** 137–154.

Fisher, R.S. & Prince, D.A. (1977): Spike-wave rhythms in cat cortex induced by parenteral penicillin. II. Cellular features. *Electroencephalogr. Clin. Neurophysiol.* **42,** 625–639.

Galvan, M., Grafe, P. & ten Bruggencate, G. (1982): Convulsant actions of 4-aminopyridine on the guinea pig olfactory cortex slice. *Brain Res.* **241,** 75–86.

Giaretta, D., Kostopoulos, G., Gloor, P. & Avoli, M. (1985): Intracortical inhibitory mechanisms are preserved in feline generalized penicillin epilepsy. *Neurosci. Lett.* **59,** 203–208.

Giaretta, D., Avoli, M. & Gloor, P. (1987): Intracellular recordings in pericruciate neurons during spike and wave discharges of feline generalized penicillin epilepsy. *Brain Res.* **405,** 68–79.

Gloor, P. (1979): Generalized epilepsy with spike and wave discharge: a reinterpretation of its electrographic and clinical manifestations. *Epilepsia* **20,** 571–588.

Gloor, P. (1988): Neurophysiological mechanism of generalized spike-and-wave discharge and its implications for understanding absence seizures. In: *Elements of petit mal epilepsy,* eds. M.S. Myslobodsky & A.F. Mirsky, pp. 159–209). New York, Berne, Frankfurt, Paris: Peter Lang.

Gloor, P. (1989): Epilepsy: relationships between electrophysiology and intracellular mechanisms involving second messengers and gene expression. *Can. J. Neurol. Sci.* **16,** 8–21.

Gloor, P. & Fariello, R.G. (1988): Generalized epilepsy: some of its cellular mechanisms differ from those of focal epilepsy. *Trends Neurosci.* **11,** 63–68.

Gloor, P., Hall, G. & Coceani, F. (1966): Differential sensitivity of various brain structures to the epileptogenic action of penicillin. *Exp. Neurol.* **16,** 333–348.

Heinemann, U., Lux, H.D. & Gutnick, M.J. (1977): Extracellular free calcium and potassium during paroxysmal activity in the cerebral cortex of the cat. *Exp. Brain Res.* **27,** 237–243.

Hotson, J.R. & Prince, D.A. (1980): A calcium-activated hyperpolarization follows repetitive firing in hippocampal neurons. *J. Neurophysiol.* **43,** 409–419.

Johnston, D. & Brown, T.H. (1981): Giant synaptic potential hypothesis for epileptiform activity. *Science* **211,** 294–297.

Johnston, D. & Brown, T.H. (1984): Mechanisms of neuronal burst generation. In: *Electrophysiology of epilepsy,* eds. P.A. Schwartzkroin & H.V. Wheal, pp. 277–301. London: Academic Press.

Kooi, K.A. & Beck, E.C. (1956): Frequency of photic stimulation as a variable in the activation of experimental convulsions. *Electroencephalogr. Clin. Neurophysiol.* **8,** 653–663.

Kostopoulos, G. (1986): Neuronal sensitivity to GABA and glutamate in generalized epilepsy with spike and wave discharges. *Exp. Neurol.* **9,** 20–36.

Kostopoulos, G., Avoli, M. & Gloor, P. (1983): Participation of cortical recurrent inhibition in the genesis of the spike and wave discharges in feline generalized penicillin epilepsy. *Brain Res.* **267,** 101–112.

Krnjevic, K. & Schwartz, S. (1967): The action of γ- aminobutyric acid on cortical neurons. *Exp. Brain Res.* **3,** 320–336.

Lennox, W.G. & Lennox, M.A. (1960): *Epilepsy and related disorders.* Boston: Little, Brown.

Lux, H.D., Heinemann, U. & Dietzel, I. (1986): Ionic changes and alterations in the size of the extracellular space during epileptic activity. In: *Advances in neurology,* eds. A.V. Delgado-Escueta, A.A.J. Ward, D.M. Woodbury & R.J. Porter, pp. 619–639. New York: Raven Press.

McCarren, M. & Alger, B.E. (1985): Use-dependent depression of IPSPs in rat hippocampal pyramidal cells *in vitro. J. Neurophysiol.* **53,** 557–571.

Matsumoto, H. & Ajmone-Marsan, C. (1964a): Cortical cellular phenomena in experimental epilepsy: interictal manifestations. *Exp. Neurol.* **9,** 286–304.

Matsumoto, H. & Ajmone-Marsan, C. (1964b): Cortical cellular phenomena in experimental epilepsy: ictal manifestations. *Exp. Neurol.* **9,** 305–326.

Newberry, N.R. & Nicoll, R.A. (1984): A bicuculline-resistant inhibitory post-synaptic potential in rat hippocampal pyramidal cells *in vitro. J. Physiol.* (Lond.) **348,** 239–254.

Newberry, N.R. & Nicoll, R.A. (1985): Comparison of the action of baclofen with #y-aminobutyric acid on rat hippocampal pyramidal cells *in vitro. J. Physiol.* (Lond.) **360,** 161–185.

Novak, L., Bregestovski, P., Ascher, P., Herbert, A. & Prochiantz, A. (1984): Magnesium gates glutamate-activated channels in mouse central neurons. *Nature* **307,** 462–465.

Prince, D.A. & Connors, B.W. (1986): Mechanisms of interictal epileptogenesis. In: *Advances in neurology,* eds. A.V. Delgado-Escueta, A.A.J. Ward, D.M. Woodbury & R.J. Porter, pp. 275–299. New York: Raven Press.

Prince, D.A. & Farrell, D. (1969): 'Centrencephalic' spike-wave discharges following parenteral penicillin injection in the cat. *Neurology* **19,** 309–310.

Pumain, R., Menini, C., Heinemann, U., Louvel, J. & Siva-Barrat, C. (1985): Chemical synaptic transmission is not necessary for epileptic seizures to persist in the baboon *Papio papio. Exp. Neurol.* **89,** 250–258.

Quesney, L.F. & Gloor, P. (1978): Generalized penicillin epilepsy in the cat: correlation between electrophysiological data and distribution of ^{14}C-penicillin in the brain. *Epilepsia* **19,** 34–45.

Reynolds, E.H., Elwes, R.D.C. & Shorvon, S.D. (1983): Why does epilepsy become intractable? *Lancet* **ii,** 952–954.

Schwartzkroin, P.A. & Pedley, D. (1979): Slow depolarizing potentials in 'epileptic' neurons. *Epilepsia* **20,** 267–277.

Schwartzkroin, P.A. & Prince, D.A. (1980): Changes in excitatory and inhibitory synaptic potentials leading to epileptogenic activity. *Brain Res.* **183,** 61–76.

Stelzer, A., Kay, A.R. & Wong, R.K.S. (1988): GABA$_A$-receptor function in hippocampal cell is maintained by phosphorylation factors. *Science* **241,** 339–341.

Tancredi, V. & Avoli, M. (1987): Control of spontaneous epileptiform discharges by extracellular potassium: an '*in vitro*' study in the CA1 subfield of the hippocampal slice. *Exp. Brain Res.* **67,** 363–372.

Thallman, R.H. & Ayala, G.F. (1983): A late increase in K conductance follows synaptic stimulation of granule neurons of the dentate gyrus. *Neurosci. Lett.* **23,** 243–248.

Traub, R.D. & Wong, R.K.S. (1983): Synchronized burst discharge in disinhibited hippocampal slice. II. Model of cellular mechanism. *J. Neurophysiol.* **49,** 459–471.

van Gelder, N.M., Siatitsas, I., Menini, C. & Gloor, P. (1984): Feline generalized penicillin epilepsy: changes in glutamic acid and taurine parallel the progressive increase in excitability of the cortex. *Epilepsia* **24,** 200–213.

Epileptic Seizures and Syndromes, Edited by Peter Wolf
© 1994 John Libbey & Company Ltd., pp. 563–578

Chapter 56

Interplay of interictal discharges and seizures: some clinical and EEG findings

Heinz-Gregor Wieser, Mima Bjeljac, Nadja Khan, Suzanne Müller, Adrian M. Siegel and Yasuhiro Yonekawa

EEG-Abteilung und Epileptologie, Neurologische Klinik, Universitätsspital Zürich, 8091 Zürich, Switzerland

Summary

Interictal epileptiform EEG potentials ('spikes') are considered the hallmark of many – although not all – epilepsies. The epilepsies are characterized by recurrent unprovoked seizures.

The relationship between interictal spikes and ictal seizure discharges is, however, not always that of a simple and steady increase of the interictal spikes culminating in a seizure. On the contrary the interplay and transition between interictal and ictal states more often resemble a fundamental qualitative change rather than a pure quantitative increase. Clinically a theory postulating some kind of categorically different flip-flop behaviour would be a more appropriate description than a more gradual difference bertween the interictal and ictal state. Never the less, preictal changes lasting from several seconds to hours can be observed under certain circumstances. These preictal changes are phenomenologically described and discussed reviewing the most important clinical, electroencephalographic and experimental data observed mainly in candidates of surgical therapy for epilepsy.

Modern understanding of the epilepsies is that of an epileptogenic process and therefore includes the dimensions of space and time. Whereas understanding in space, i.e. localization, has witnessed a remarkable progress during the last decades, little is known about the epileptic process in the dimension of time. Its characterization with respect to interictal vs. ictal is useful, because self-evident, but the *transition* and the *interplay* between these conditions are poorly understood. Even in a pragmatic clinical sense it is necessary to expand this categorization in time by introducing terms such as 'preictal and postictal', 'semi-ictal', 'infraclinical discharges' and various forms of 'electrical and/or clinical, continuous or intermittent status epilepticus'.

Advanced concepts include under the term epileptogenesis not only the propensity for the occurrence of spontaneous seizures, i.e. ictal events, but also interictal perturbations, which are frequently allied with seizures. Seizures, without doubt, implicate the phenomena of recruiting and spread of seizure discharges. In this context it is interesting that recent experimental research distinguishes more sharply between *anticonvulsant, antiepileptic and antiepileptogenic properties of drugs*. Whereas anticonvulsants mainly prevent the spread of seizures, antiepileptic drugs mainly interfere with the recruitment mechanism at the primary epileptogenic area. Antiepileptogenic drugs, such as

N-methyl-D-aspartate (NMDA)-receptor antagonists, however, might function irrespectively of their anticonvulsant and antiepileptic effectiveness (Lothman, 1991). Indeed, it has been shown that NMDA-receptor antagonists, such as MK-801, can prevent motor kindling (Hosford & McNamara, 1990), abolish electrographic kindling and associated electrophysiological alterations (Stringer & Lothman, 1990) and prevent neuronal degeneration (Clifford *et al.*, 1989).

The search for better understanding of the *interplay and transition between interictal and ictal conditions* is motivated by the urgent need for therapeutically applicable *seizure-preventing strategies* including *warning devices*. In this respect the ultimate goal is a time- and location-specific therapy (Efron, 1956; Aird, 1983), i.e. the application of a specific drug or a stimulus (Dahl, 1992; Düchting-Röth *et al.*, 1992; Reker *et al.*, 1993), e.g. electrical stimulation of the vagal nerve (Hufnagel *et al.*, 1993; Bongartz *et al.*, 1993; Helmstaedter *et al.*, 1993), at – or acting at – a certain, well-defined brain region in a time-limited fashion.

In this chapter we will discuss some clinical and electrophysiological preictal changes lasting from several seconds to hours, which include subtle clinical manifestations such as non-specific and specific prodromes; electrophysiological phenomena, such as preictal spike-rate changes, loss of variability of spikes, changes of electroencephalographic (EEG) background activity ('rigidity phenomenon', Wang & Wieser, 1994), including changes of dimensionality (as evidenced by chaos analysis, Basar, 1990; Babloyantz & Destexhe, 1986, 1987), attenuation and 'forced normalization' (Landolt, 1960, 1963). Furthermore, we will review possible changes of the functional connectivity of the brain as evidenced by altered evoked potentials after electrical brain stimulations. In addition, electrical and magnetic direct current (DC) stimulation is mentioned. Finally, we shall mention some biochemical data, i.e. changes of transmitters measured by microdialysis and push–pull techniques in the extracellular fluid of the human epileptogenic focus during various interictal and ictal states.

Clinical preictal changes

Preictally many patients suffer from distinct signs and symptoms which manifest themselves up to several hours prior to the seizure. These *prodromes* may be ill-defined, i.e. are difficult to describe, and commonly consist of non-specific symptoms, such as so-called 'nervousness', increase of irritability, attention difficulties, sleep and vigilance disturbances, headache and vegetative signs, including diarrhoea, increased sweating, etc (Ginccioli *et al.*, 1988, 1990; Hughes *et al.*, 1993). It is not uncommon that patients report these symptoms occurring with a slowly increasing intensity until they ultimately culminate in the ictus. Many patients have learned that these prodromes herald their impending seizures and therefore respond to them with self-protective behavioural reactions, such as going to bed, discontinuing potentially dangerous work, etc.

These non-specific prodromes must be clearly distinguished from the *aura* which, by definition, represents already a simple partial seizure or the initial part of a more severe and prolonged complex partial seizure with or without secondary generalization. Whereas the patients with prodromes usually behave expectantly and try to protect themselves in a non-specific manner, many patients with characteristic habitual auras have developed rather specific *seizure-preventing/suppressing strategies.*

These strategies of aura interruption (see Wolf, Chapter 66) sometimes appear extremely sophisticated. In addition, they are meaningful in that they obviously interfere with the recruitment of the neuronal population within the epileptogenic area. In a few patients, we had the opportunity to study the efficacy of seizure-preventing/suppressing strategies in the epileptogenic area by stereotactically placed depth electrodes. The nature of the observed seizure-preventing/suppressing manoeuvre was usually such that it influenced the neuronal population in danger of being recruited by appropriate internal or external sensory stimuli. Neurones at risk for recruitment ('group II neurones', Wyler, 1980) can be synaptically influenced and it seems logical to assume that appropriate stimuli, under certain circumstances, may 'occupy them physiologically' and in this way prevent their recruitment into the burst activity of the intrinsically abnormal 'epileptic pacemaker' or 'group I neurones' (Wyler & Fetz, 1974; Wyler, 1980; Wyler & Ward, 1980; Wieser, 1989a).

It is obvious that seizure-preventing strategies are closely linked to seizure-inducing mechanisms on the one hand, and to the sensory evoked and reflex epilepsies on the other (Wieser, 1989a). Based on experimental studies in monkeys on mechanisms of operant control of brain activity in general, and the behavioural control of firing patterns of normal and abnormal neurones in chronic epileptic cortical foci in particular (Wyler & Fetz, 1974; Wyler, 1980; Wyler & Ward, 1980), behavioural therapy in human epileptics has aroused considerable interest during recent years, and some promising results have been reported (Efron, 1956; Aird, 1983; Dahl, 1992; Düchting-Röth *et al.*, 1992; Reker *et al.*, 1993).

Electrophysiological preictal changes

Even in the older literature, extensive work has been devoted to this topic (Ralston, 1958). It might be useful to differentiate between experimental findings mainly derived from acute penicillin foci, and clinical examinations. Walker *et al.* (1945) described a steady increase of the *interictal spike rate prior to a seizure*. King *et al.* (1953) reported on a decrease of the EEG amplitude and Gastaut (1954) on an increase of the interictal spike during the preictal phase. In cats, in the penicillin focus, Angeleri *et al.* (1972) observed an abrupt increase of the spike rate 5 s prior to the seizures. When studying this phenomenon, however, in 40 patients with temporal lobe epilepsy (TLE) the same authors (Angeleri *et al.*, 1970) had arrived at much more divergent results: in 70 per cent of patients there were no significant changes, in 20 per cent there was an increase and in 10 per cent a decrease of the preictal spike rate. In 1989 we quantitatively studied 21 spontaneous seizures in nine patients suffering from TLE with drug-resistant complex partial seizures. With the exception of two patients with stereotactic depth electrodes (Wieser, 1987), all others had bilaterally implanted four contact foramen ovale electrodes (Wieser, 1991a). Spike rate and vigilance were simultaneously studied, using the

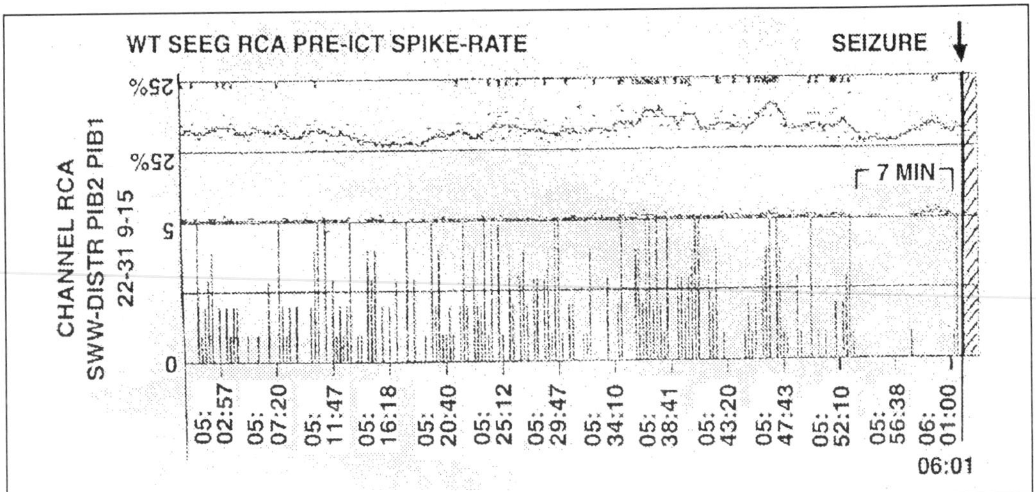

Fig. 1. Automatic spike analysis of right hippocampal EEG before a habitual seizure, which occurred at 06.01 (arrow). The preictal phase has been analysed using SPECTRAMED program EPI-4, plotting vigilance (power in band 9–15 Hz (PIB1) and power in band 22–31 Hz (PIB2)). Full vertical bars at bottom (SSW-DISTR) represent a spike incidence of five spikes per analysis interval. Note the cessation of spikes 7 min before the occurrence of the seizure.

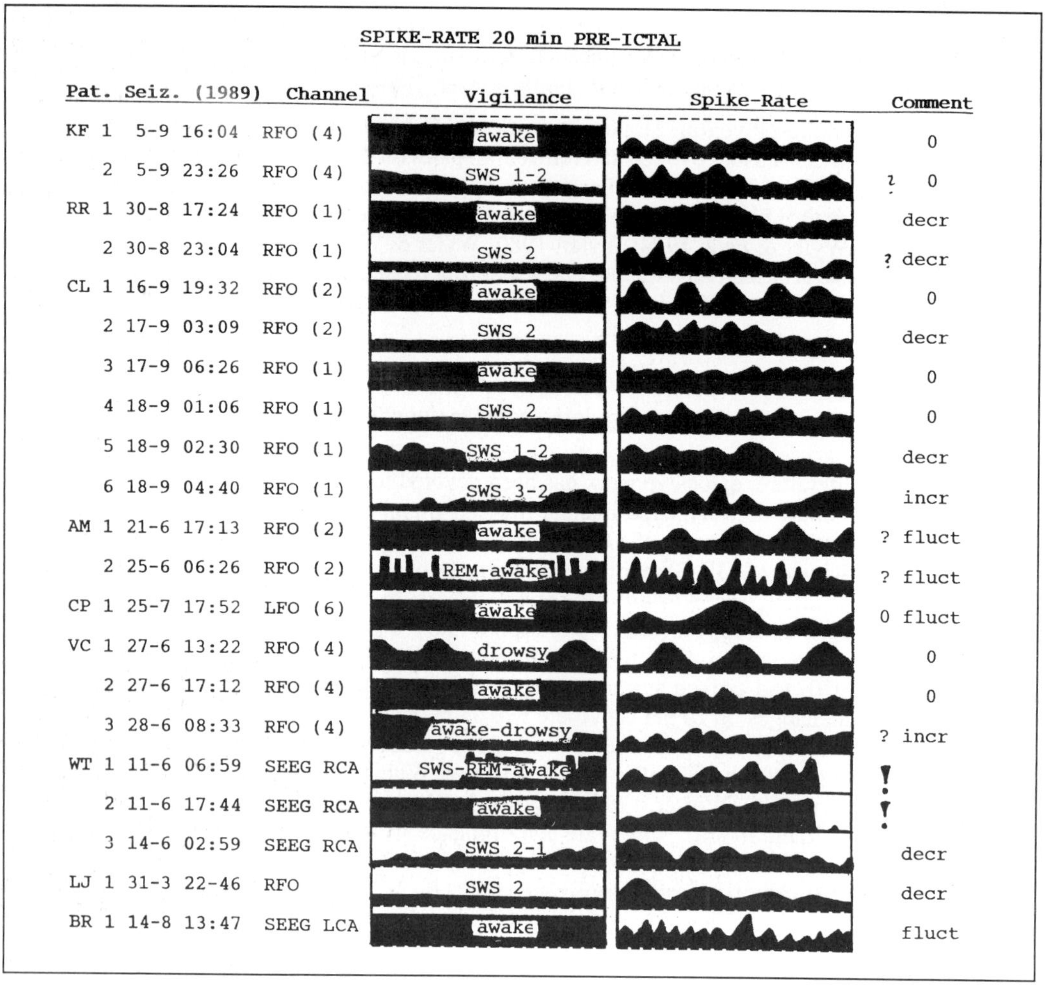

Fig. 2. Synopsis of preictal vigilance and spike rate changes of mesiobasal limbic EEG in 21 seizures of nine patients with temporal lobe epilepsy. Vigilance is visualized following the usual somnographic presentation: awake is at top, slow-wave sleep (SWS) is at bottom. Sleep staging is according to Rechtschaffen and Kales. Spike rate is depicted as shown in Fig. 1. Note that only patient WT (also illustrated in Fig. 1) exhibits a significant preictal decrease of the spike rate.

computer programme Epiplot 4 (Spectralab Fricker), i.e. automatic spike detection and vigilance description (see Fig. 1), and Gotman's Stellate® system algorithms.

The simple counting of the spike rate prior to seizure was, however, not very enlightening (Wieser, 1989b; Fig. 2). Likewise, Katz *et al.* (1991) and Gotman *et al.* (1982) did not find consistent changes in preictal spike rates.

In chronically isolated cortex, Prince (1965a) found cyclical spike driving, and in the penicillin spike focus long-duration periodic changes in its excitability (Prince, 1965b). Using the penicillin focus in cats, Sherwin (1978), however, described a steadily increasing preference of pairwise penicillin spike intervals prior to a seizure. In accordance with this finding are results on interictal excitability fluctuations, studied by electrical double-pulse stimulation (Scobey & Gabor, 1977), leading to the idea of a *preferred interictal spike frequency*. Indeed, many observations of clinical electroencephalographers, such as the periodic paroxysmal complexes seen in herpes encephalitis, in Creutzfeld–Jakob disease, and sometimes in limbic mesial temporal discharges ('Uhrwerk Fokus') and periodic lateralized epileptiform discharges (PLEDS), are in accordance with the notion of a preferred interictal spike frequency depending on the neuronal circuits involved.

Summarizing this and other work on the relation between interictal spike rate and seizures, one can formulate two models. *Model I* assumes that there is a continuum between interictal and ictal events, i.e. according to this notion the differences between the interictal spike and the seizure are viewed as having a quantitative but not a qualitative nature. This model has been supported by Ajmone-Marsan (1961) and Dichter and Spencer (1969). In contrast, *model II* assumes a qualitative difference between the interictal and ictal states. Some authors even suggest a reciprocal relationship. Model II is mainly supported by clinical observations, e.g. the findings on human 3/s spike-wave petit mal epilepsy of Stevens *et al.* (1972). It is also supported by Elazar and Blum (1974), who showed that certain interictal spike rates might prevent seizures.

During the last two decades some authors have tackled this problem using more sophisticated approaches. Rossi *et al.* (1980) and Lieb *et al.* (1978), for instance, described the *independence of spike rate from vigilance* ('rigidity of spikes') as a useful indicator for the primary epileptogenic zone. Recently, Wang and Wieser (1994) showed that the independence of EEG background activity from vigilance is a similar good descriptor for the epileptogenic zone.

Studies on the regional coherence of EEG activity have been instrumental in the understanding of ictal seizure spread (Duckrow & Spencer, 1992). The interhemispheric *coupling of epileptiform potentials* was studied by Lange *et al.* (1983). Most interestingly, these authors found an increased coupling starting already 60 min prior to the seizure in some patients.

Using *chaos theory*, Babloyantz and Destexhe (1986, 1987), Sackellares *et al.* (1989) and Basar (1990) arrived at similar results. For instance, Sackellares *et al.* (1989) found 30 s prior to a seizure a decrease of the Lyapunov exponent, a measure of the degree of dimensionality (see also Elger & Lehnertz, Chapter 54). Of course, these EEG studies do not answer the question as to the nature of this stronger coupling of various scalp or brain sites prior to the seizure. Experimental (Caspers, 1959; Caspers & Speckmann, 1969) and some clinical DC-EEG recordings (Stodieck & Wieser, 1983, 1984, 1987) showed that seizures are accompanied by a stepwise negative DC shift. Therefore, it is tempting to assume that the stronger coupling of various brain regions is linked to a DC change.

Attenuation and 'forced normalization'

Landolt (1960, 1963) has popularized the concept of a reciprocal relationship between the degree of epileptiform EEG abnormalities and behavioural peculiarities in the sense of accentuation of psychiatric disturbances. He and others (Tellenbach, 1965) observed that forced normalization of the EEG could be associated with the appearance of psychiatric signs and symptoms to the degree of psychosis. Besides the disappearance of interictal spikes, an attenuation of the background EEG rhythms was observed. Specific drugs were believed to play an important role in this phenomenon (Wolf & Köhler, 1980). More recent experiences with γ-aminobutyric acidergic (GABA-ergic) antiepileptic drugs, such as vigabatrin, seem to support this notion (Sälke-Kellermann *et al.*, 1993; Wolf, 1994).

Attenuation, i.e. flattening of background EEG activity, is sometimes associated with spike suspension. If regional, it can represent the characteristic manifestation of seizures, in particular of mesial temporal lobe seizures (Fig. 3). If prolonged, it is difficult to decide, without depth recordings, whether this attenuation reflects an already present, localized mediobasal seizure discharge or whether this phenomenon should be viewed as preictal. Our experience speaks in favour of the first assumption. Elsewhere (Wieser *et al.*, 1981; Wieser, 1983a, b) we have discussed the reciprocal relationship between temporal archi- and neocortex and possible relationships with negative DC shifts. If attenuation is viewed as a preictal phenomenon, it would be tempting to relate these EEG phenomenon

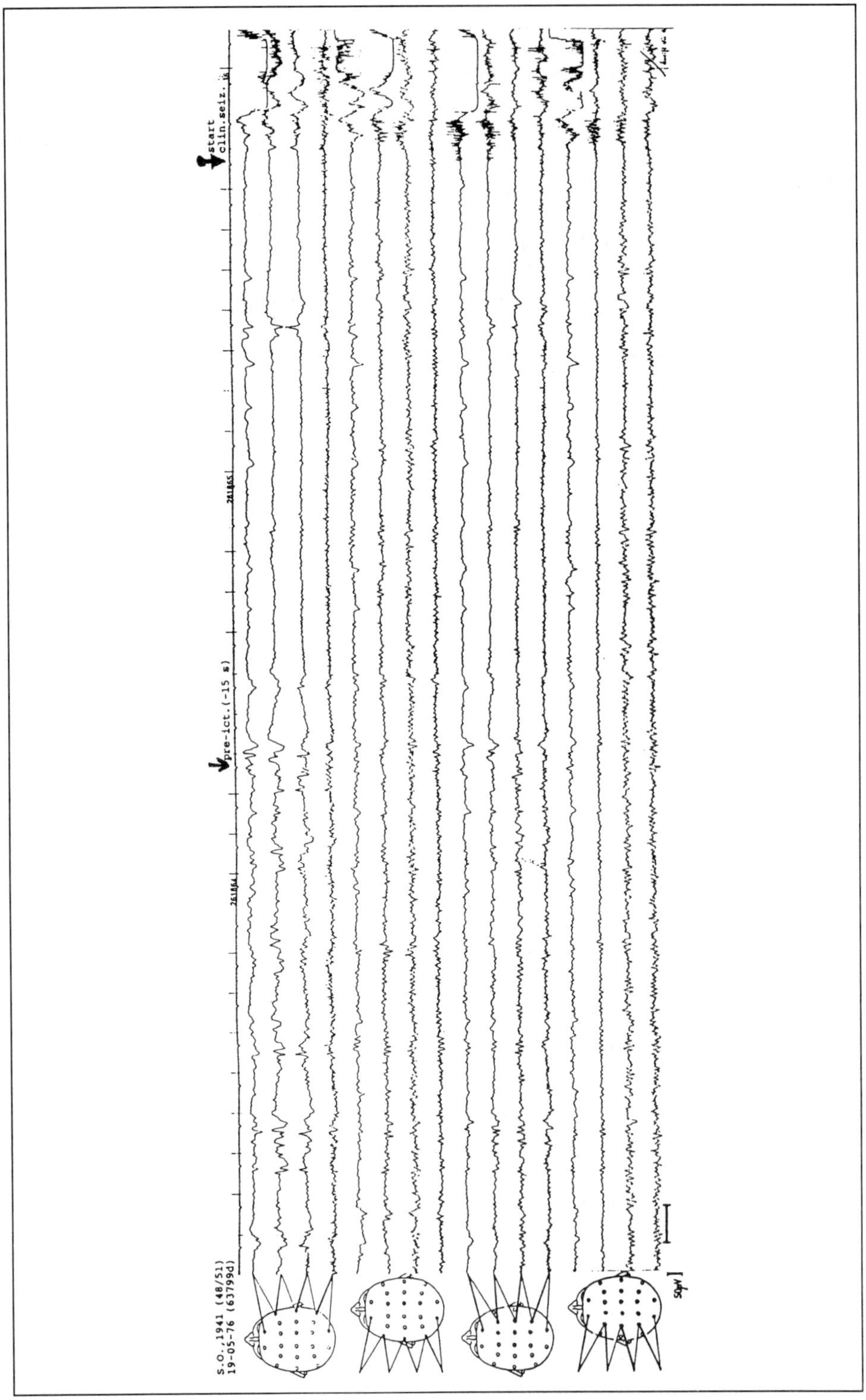

Fig. 3. Regional attenuation of background scalp EEG activity associated with preictal cessation of spikes (arrow) in a patient with a medically refractory right temporal lobe epilepsy with proved seizure origin in right amygdala (at clinical seizure onset). Following stereo-EEG, this patient underwent a stereotactic electrocoagulation of the right amygdala, which rendered him seizure-free for more than 10 years.

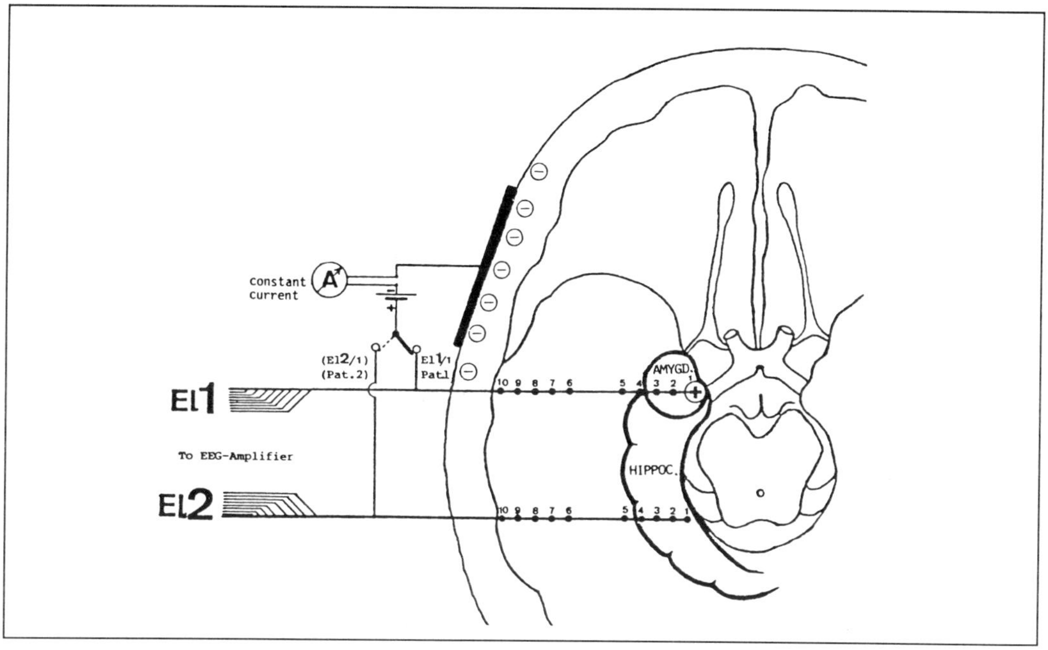

Fig. 4. Schematic view of two multiple-contact hollow-core depth electrodes located with their tips in the amygdala (El-1) and hippocampus (El-2). Polarizing current was injected by a constant-current device through the innermost amgdalar or hippocampal contact. Current return was provided by a large (25 cm^2) ipsilateral frontotemporal scalp electrode.

to possible biochemical changes (see below) facilitating the occurrence of the seizure. A third interpretation of the attenuation phenomenon is that of a general or regional arousal reaction, which either accompanies an aura produced by localized seizure discharges or, conversely, occurs with an arousing stimulus and thereby leads through seizure-facilitating vigilance fluctuations to the overt seizure (Niedermeyer, 1991).

Possible changes of the functional connectivity of the brain as evidenced by altered evoked potentials

Since the pioneering work of Buser *et al.* (1968) describing 'réponses paroxystiques' as landmarks of the epileptogenic zone, several groups, including ourselves, have sought ways of examining whether evoked potentials after intracerebral electrical stimulation show preictal and ictal changes compared with the interictal state. Distribution, latencies and the overall localization-specific configuration of the intracranially recorded evoked potentials have been been studied in different vigilance states with the expectation of finding characteristic alterations in relation to seizure-prone vigilance stages. Indeed, it was possible to demonstrate facilitated propagation of evoked potentials along those functional pathways used by the seizure spread (Wieser, 1983b, 1991b; Spencer *et al.*, 1992a, b). Wilson *et al.* (1990, 1991) found it easy to obtain functional verification of significant ipsilateral pathways in the human limbic system but no, or only very weak, evidence was evident for contralateral functional connections in the interictal state.

In one epileptic patient we had the opportunity to record visual evoked potentials (VEP) interictally, preictally and ictally. There were marked alterations of the VEP following chequer-board stimulation

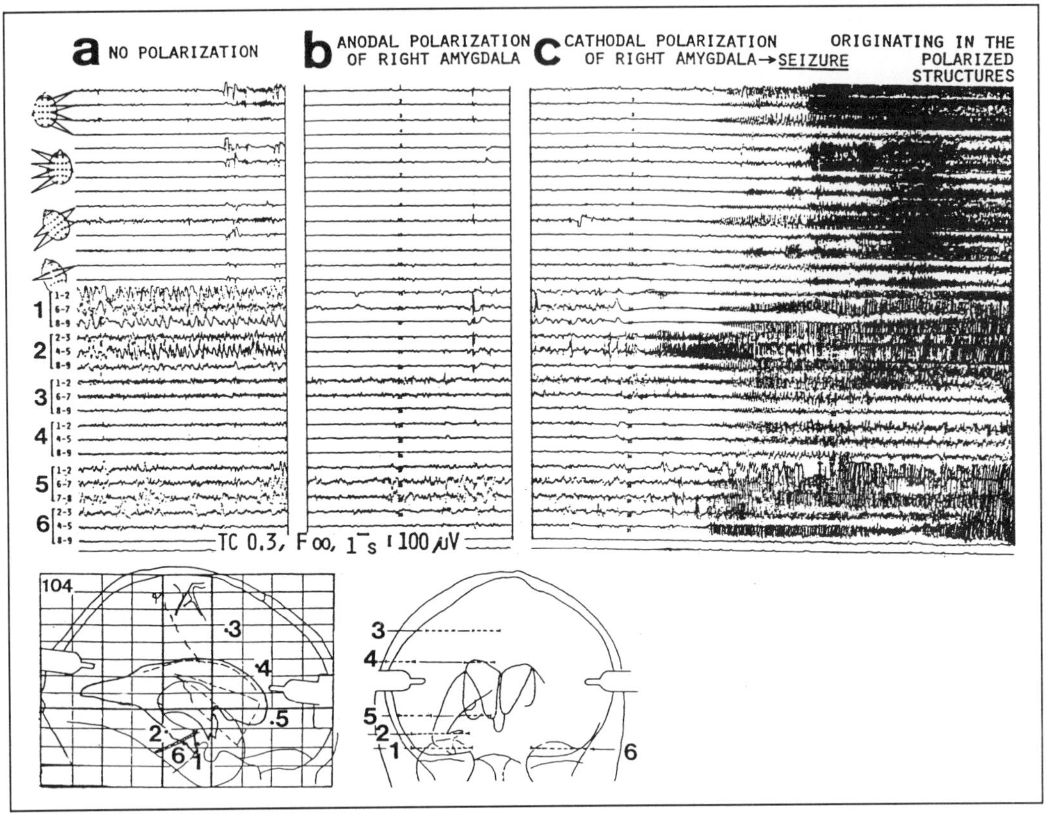

Fig. 5. Baseline EEG (a) and effects of anodal (b) as well as cathodal polarization (c) of right amygdala. Whereas anodal polarization (b, middle part) led to a suspension of spontaneously present spikes in the primary epileptogenic zone, cathodal polarization (c, right part) provoked a seizure.

during a complex partial seizure of right temporal-occipital origin. The latencies of N100 were prolonged and the formal configuration of the evoked potential was completely changed.

Electrical and magnetic DC stimulation

It has been shown that the excitability of neural tissue can be influenced by a polarizing continuous DC. Naturally occurring local DC shifts are though to modulate repetitive actions of single neurones. Therefore it can be expected that adequate polarization might inhibit generation and spread of epileptic activity. To test this hypothesis we polarized mesiobasal limbic epileptic foci in three medically refractory patients before surgical removal of these structures. The patients underwent presurgical evaluation with prolonged seizure monitoring, using stereo-EEG. With the depth electrodes still *in situ*, we applied weak constant DC (1–200 µA) to the amygdala or hippocampus and simultaneously recorded scalp and depth EEG (Fig. 4). Anodal (positive) polarization of the mesiobasal structures tended to decrease spike-incidence, whereas cathodal current had the opposite effect and even induced seizures (Fig. 5). Intracerebrally evoked responses were altered in shape. The phase with opposite polarity to the applied DC field was increased in amplitude and duration (Fig. 6). In one patient polarization was followed by a transient psychotic state and two months of complete seizure relief.

Recently we have discovered a hitherto unknown effect of electromagnetic field exposure on human

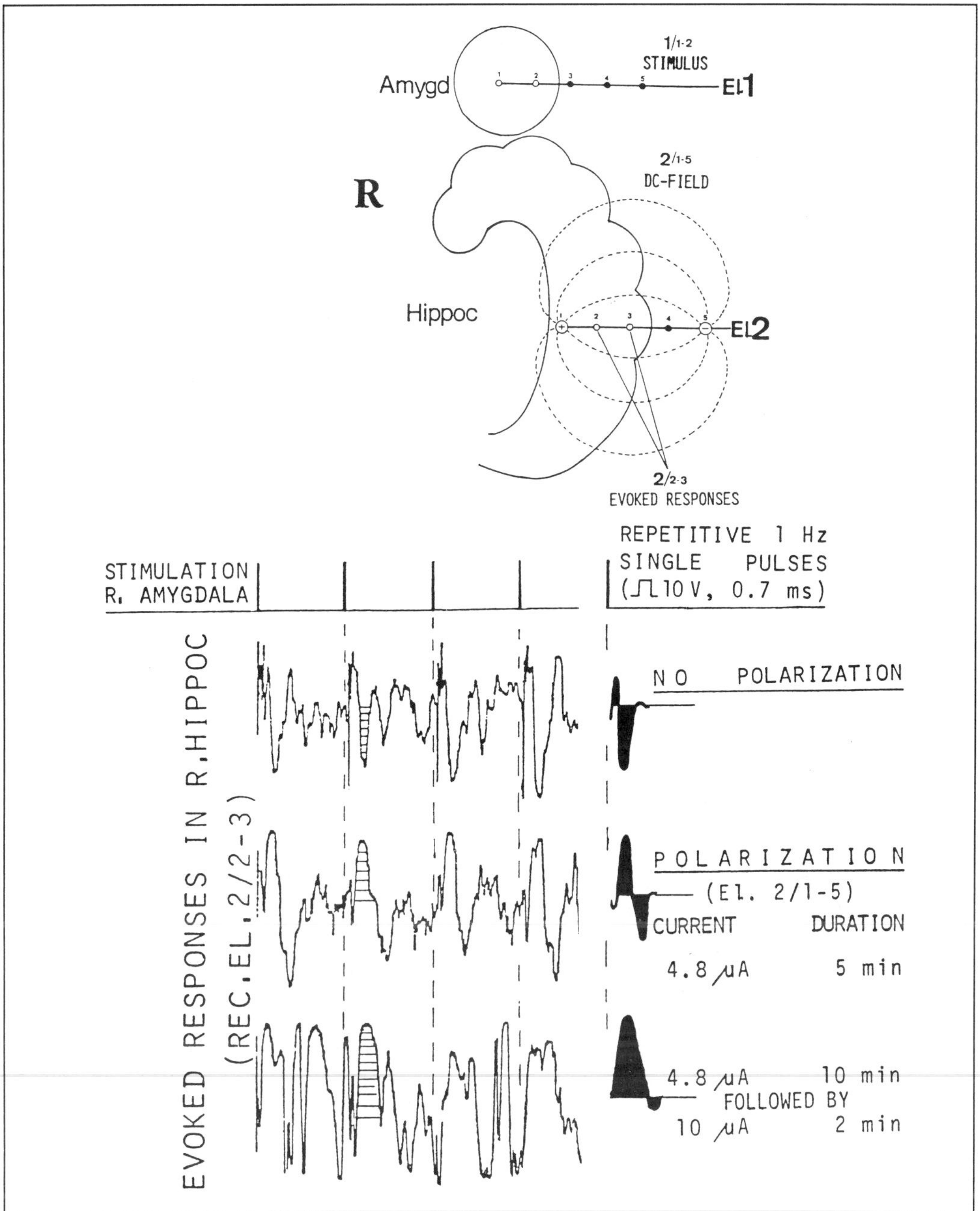

Fig. 6. Effects of polarization of right hippocampus on responses evoked by electrical stimulation of right amygdala (stimulation parameters: 1 Hz/10 V/0.7 ms duration). DC (4, 8 and 10 µA) was applied across the right hippocampus (El 2/1–5) using a 9V battery-powered constant-current device with an additional continuous monitoring of current flow by an amperemeter. Responses were recorded within the right hippocampus (El 2/2–3). Note the changes of the hippocampal responses: the phase with opposite polarity to the applied DC field increase in amplitude and duration. Left: individual responses; right: averaged responses (in black).

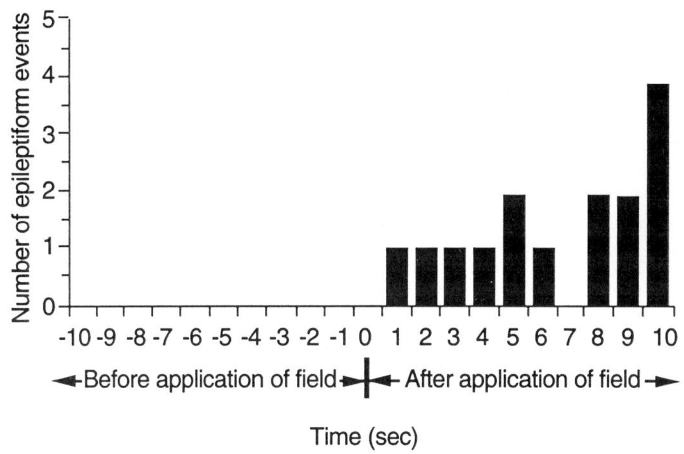

Fig. 7. Anomalous epileptiform events recorded by the use of foramen ovale electrodes and evoked by weak magnetic field changes in patient SA, suffering from the syndrome of mesial temporal lobe epilepsy. Random activity is represented by the incidence of epileptiform events in the 10 s intervals prior to field application. DC magnetic fields were in the order of 1–4 mT. (From Fuller et al., in press, with permission.)

epileptic foci (Dobson *et al.*, in press; Fuller *et al.*, in press; Kerr, 1993). As part of our preoperative evaluation protocol of medically refractory patients, we recorded the EEG directly from the mesio-basal temporal lobe, using electrodes inserted through the foramen ovale (Wieser, 1991a). A constant, uniform magnetic field of intensity 1–2 mT was applied to the heads of epilepsy patients and the effects of electromagnetic field exposure were studied in the foramen ovale electrode EEG of these patients. Application of the magnetic field caused a significant increase in epileptiform activity detected at the electrodes sites.

Human sensitivity to magnetic fields is not an entirely unexpected finding. There are precedents that indicate that this sensitivity is an entirely reasonable phenomenon. For example, some animal species are very sensitive to magnetic fields. Ethologists studying migratory birds (Wiltschko & Wiltschko, 1991) and bees (Walker & Bittermann, 1989) have demonstrated that many species can detect the geomagnetic field with sufficient sensitivity to obtain navigational cues. Moreover, Semm and Beason (1990) showed that magnetic fields can induce significant electrical activity in the trigeminal nucleus of the bobolink, *Dolichonyx oryzivorous*. There is a growing body of evidence that circadian rhythms are influenced by electromagnetic fields (Moore-Ede *et al.*, 1992). In particular, Wever (1974) demonstrated that entrainment of several circadian processes in human subjects was dependent on the naturally occurring low-frequency electromagnetic fields present in the environment. The implications of the discovery of magnetic field effects are manifold and exciting: it may be that they are very important for the healthy functioning of the human organism. Also, these effects could explain why many epileptic patients report a hitherto unexplained clustering of their seizures in relation to changes of the geomagnetic field, such as those associated with lunar cycles. In addition, if it holds true that these weak magnetic fields, which are not consciously sensed by humans, can be used to generate the required neural activation of the epileptogenic area on demand, it may become feasible to provide more immediate diagnosis in a much easier fashion for a greater number of patients suffering from epilepsy.

Further studies are, however, necessary to answer the question as to the importance of these findings in explaining the transition from the interictal to the ictal state.

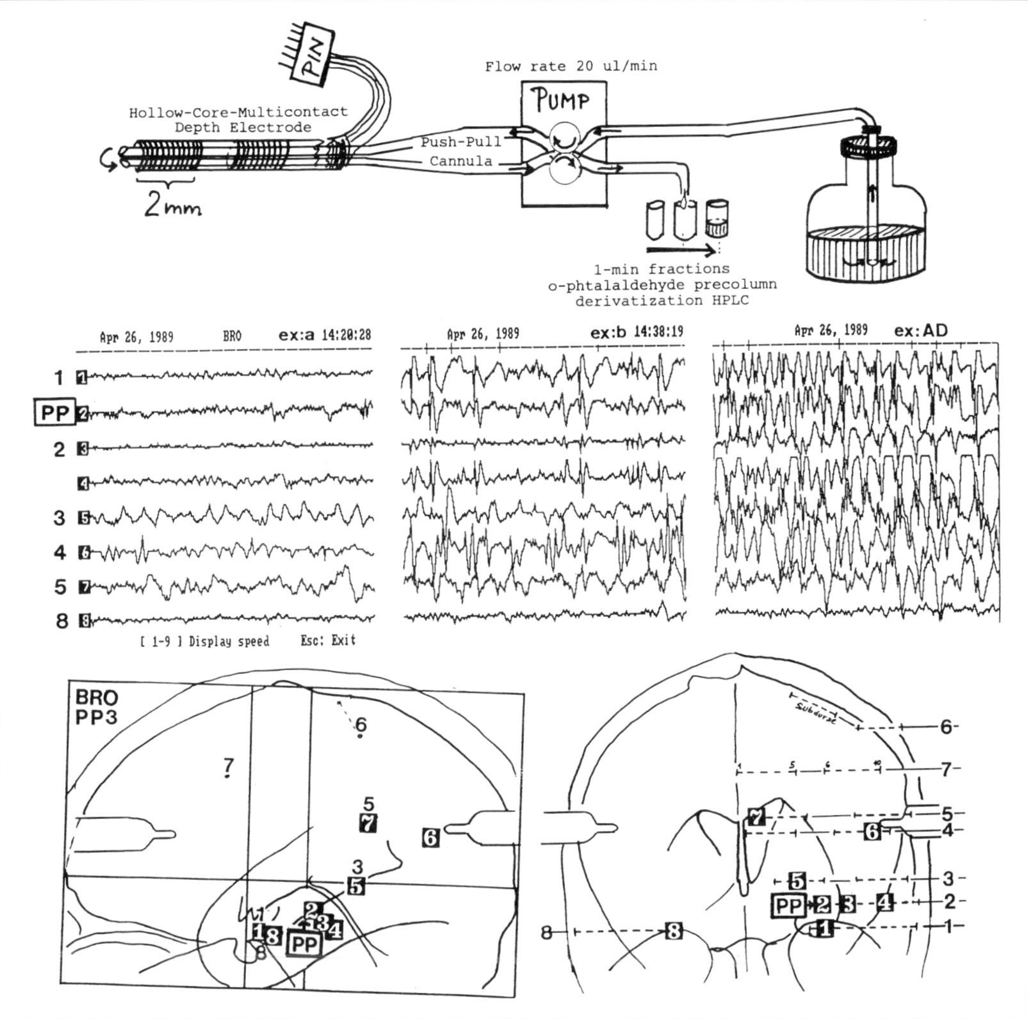

Fig. 8. Schematic design of the push–pull cannula device (top) showing the push–pull cannula inserted into a standard hollow-core electrode with the target in the hippocampus (bottom, PP, electrode 2). The push–pull cannula is connected to a pump, allowing for continuous collection and analysis of 1-min fractions of perfusates. The middle part of the figure shows three examples of depth-recorded EEG. Black numbers on white identify the depth electrodes, and white numbers on black squares the depicted channels and the anatomical recording sites. The left EEG section shows a period without spikes (example a, ex:a), the middle section with moderate spiking (ex:b) and the right section an electrically induced after-discharge (ex: AD).

Changes of transmitters measured by the use of microdialysis and push–pull in the extracellular fluid of the human epileptogenic focus during various interictal and ictal states

In the course or presurgical stereo-EEG evaluation of candidates for epilepsy surgery, dialytrodes (During *et al.*, 1989) or the push–pull technique can be used to collect extracellular fluid from the primary epileptogenic area. Our study, using the push–pull technique, was approved by our Ethical Commission. Informed consent was obtained from the patients. A push–pull cannula device was introduced into the lumen of a standard hollow-core multicontact depth probe (Comte *et al.*, 1983).

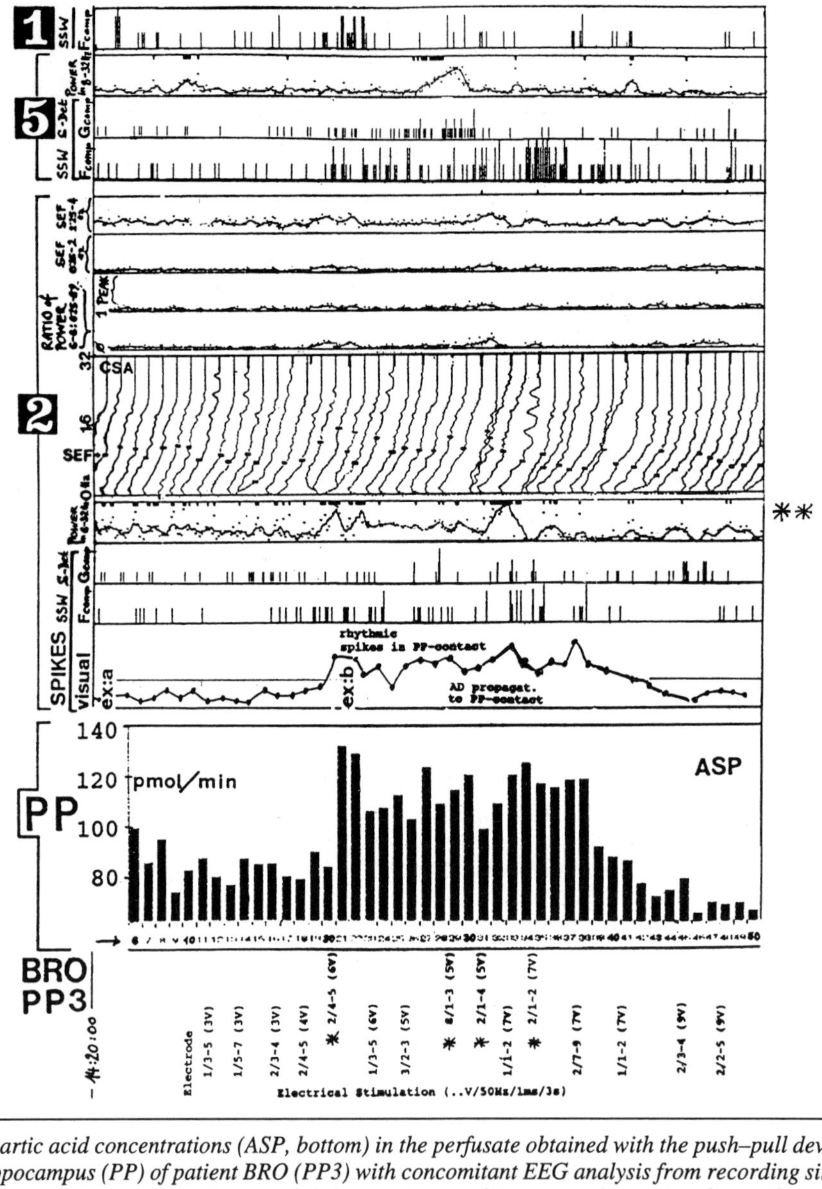

*Fig. 9. Aspartic acid concentrations (ASP, bottom) in the perfusate obtained with the push–pull device from the left hippocampus (PP) of patient BRO (PP3) with concomitant EEG analysis from recording site 2 (left hippocampus, close to PP), recording site 5 (left posterior parahippocampal gyrus) and recording site 1 (left amygdala). Automatic spike detection (SSW S-Det) was performed with two algorithms (Fcomp and Gcomp, i.e. Spectramed® and Stellate® software), in addition to visual spike counting (visual). Where indicated, the spectral power for a given frequency range (Power) and ratios of power, as well as compressed spectral arrays (CSA) with appropriate sensitive spectral edge frequencies (SEF), have been plotted too. At the very bottom electrical stimulations are indicated in terms of stimulated sites (electrode/contacts – see Fig. 8) and strength (voltage, in brackets). Those four stimulations which led to an after-discharge are indicated by *. The EEG examples depicted in Fig. 8 are indicated as ex:a, ex:b and AD (with propagation to PP-close contacts). Note the good correspondence between fluctuations of the aspartic acid concentration (in pmol/min) and the spike rate at limbic recording sites 2 and 5, but also with power in band 8–32 Hz of the EEG at recording site 2 (**; left hippocampus).*

A very sensitive and highly specific high-performance liquid chromatography (HPLC) method was used (Do *et al.*, 1986). Extracellular fluid collection was at the rate of 1 min over a period of 1 h. The content of various neurotransmitters (GABA, glycine, β-alanine, glutamate, aspartate, homocysteate, glutamine, taurine) was measured in the perfusates. In all patients of this study the target was the hippocampus. A computer-assisted analysis of the background depth EEG (using fast Fourier transform with compressed spectral array and spectral vigilance programs) and of spontaneous and electrically provoked epileptiform events (using automatic seizure and spike detection algorithms) was performed and these results were correlated with the biochemical measurements. To date, this work in progress has revealed that the amount of some – but not all – measured neurotransmitters, in particular aspartic acid, shows fluctuations in the extracellular perfusates. Moreover, a positive correlation was obtained between changes of some neurotransmitters, in particular aspartate, and spontaneous and electrically provoked epileptiform depth-EEG changes (Wieser *et al.*, 1989; Cuénod *et al.*, 1990; Do *et al.*, 1991).

References

Aird, R.B. (1983): The importance of seizure-inducing factors in the control of refractory forms of epilepsy. *Epilepsia* **24,** 567–583.

Ajmone-Marsan, C. (1961): Electrographic aspects of 'epileptic' neuronal aggregates. *Epilepsia* **2,** 22–38.

Angeleri, F., Giaquinto, S. & Marchesi, G.F. (1970): Registrazione elettro-clinica delle crisi temporali e scariche intercritiche nell sonno notturno. *Rev. Neurol.* **40,** 321–327.

Angeleri, F., Giaquinto, S. & Marchesi, G.F. (1972): Temporal distribution of interictal and ictal discharges from penicillin foci in cats. In: *Synchronization of EEG activity in epilepsies,* eds. H. Petsche & M.A.B. Brazier, pp. 221–234. New York: Springer.

Babloyantz, A. & Destexhe, A. (1986): Low-dimensional chaos in an instance of epilepsy. *Proc. Nat. Acad. Sci.* USA **83,** 3513–3517.

Babloyantz, A. & Destexhe, A. (1987): Chaos in neuronal networks. In: *Proceedings of the IEEE First International Conference on Neural Networks*, eds. M. Caudill & C. Butler, pp. 31–40.

Basar, E. (ed.) (1990): *Chaos in brain function.* Berlin: Springer.

Bongartz, U., Burr, W., Dümpelmann, M., Hufnagel, A., Hefner, G. & Elger, C.E. (1993): Die chronische Elektrostimulation des N. vagus zur Prophylaxe epileptischer Anfälle. II. Kein Hinweis auf stimulationbedingte EEG-Veränderungen. In: *Epilepsie 92*, ed. H. Stefan, pp. 383–387. Berlin: Deutsche Sektion ILAE.

Buser, P., Talairach, J. & Bancaud, J. (1968): Potentiels évoqués, réponses paroxystique aux stimulations périphériques et zone épileptogène. *Rev. Neurol.* **118,** 514.

Caspers, H. (1959): Über die Beziehungen zwischen Dendritenpotential und Gleichspannung an der Hirnrinde. *Pflügers Arch. Ges. Physiol.* **269,** 157.

Caspers, H. & Speckmann, E.-J. (1969): DC potential shifts in paroxysmal states. In: *Basic mechanisms of the epilepsies*, eds. H.H. Jasper, A.A. Ward & A. Pope, pp. 375–388. Boston: Little, Brown.

Clifford, D.B., Zorumski, C.F. & Olney, J.W. (1989): Ketamine and MK-801 prevent degeneration of thalamic neurons induced by focal cortical seizures. *Exp. Neurol.* **105,** 272–279.

Comte, P., Siegfried, J. & Wieser, H.G. (1983): Multipolar hollow-core electrode for brain recordings. *Appl. Neurophysiol.* **46,** 41–46.

Cuénod, M., Audinat, E., Do, K.Q., Gähwiler, B.H., Grandes, P., Herrling, P., Knöpfel, T., Perschak, H., Streit, P., Vollenweider, F. & Wieser, H.G. (1990): Homocysteic acid as transmitter candidate in the mammalian brain and excitatory amino acids in epilepsy. In: *Excitatory amino acids and neuronal plasticity*, ed. Y. Ben-Ari, pp. 57–63. New York: Plenum Press.

Dahl, J. (1992): Ein verhaltensmedizinischer Ansatz zur Diagnostik und Behandlung bei Epilepsien. In: *Epilepsie 91*, ed. D. Scheffner, pp. 303–316. Reinbek: Einhorn Presse Verlag.

Dichter, M. & Spencer, W.A. (1969): Penicillin-induced interictal discharges from the cat hippocampus. II. Mechanisms underlying origin and restriction. *J. Neurophysiol.* **32,** 663–687.

Do, K.Q., Mattenberger, M., Streit, P. & Cuénod, M. (1986): *In vitro* release of endogenous excitatory sulfur- containing amino acids from various rat brain regions. *J. Neurochem.* **46,** 779–786.

Do, K.Q., Klancnik, J., Gähwiler, B., Perschak, H., Wieser, H.G. & Cuénod, M. (1991): Release of EEA: animal studies and epileptic foci studies in human. In: *Excitatory amino acids*, eds. B.S. Meldrum, F. Moroni, R.P. Simon & J.H. Woods, pp. 677–685. New York: Raven Press.

Dobson, J.P., Fuller, M., Moser, S., Wieser, H.G., Dunn, J.R. & Zoeger, J. (1993): Evocation of epileptiform activity by weak DC magnetic fields and iron biomineralization in the human brain. In: *Advances in biomagnetism*, ed. L. Deecke, C. Baumgartner, G. Stronik & S.J. Williams. New York: Plenum Press (in press).

Düchting-Röth, A., Reker, M. & Wolf, P. (1992): Unterbrechung auraeingeleiteter epileptischer Anfälle (unter Verwendung einer biofeedback-unterstützten Kontrolltechnik). In: *Epilepsie 91*, ed. D. Scheffner, pp. 317–321. Reinbek: Einhorn Presse Verlag.

Duckrow, R.B. & Spencer, S.S. (1992): Regional coherence and the transfer of ictal activity during seizure onset in the medial temporal lobe. *Electroencephalogr. Clin. Neurophysiol* **82,** 415–422.

During, M.J., Anderson, G.M., Roth, R.H. & Spencer, D.D. (1989): A human dialytrode: *in vivo* measurements of neuroactive substances in the human hippocampus with simultaneous depth EEG recordings. *Soc. Neurosci. Abstr.* **15,** 340.

Efron, R. (1956): The effect of olfactory stimuli in arresting uncinate fits. *Brain* **79,** 267–281.

Elazar, Z. & Blum, B. (1974): Interictal discharges in tungsten foci and EEG seizure activity. *Epilepsia* **15,** 599–610.

Fuller, M., Dobson, J.P., Wieser, H.G. & Moser, S. (1993): On the sensitivity of the human brain to magnetic fields – evocation of epileptiform activity. *Brain Res. Bull.* (in press).

Gastaut, H. (1954): *The epilepsies: electroclinical correlations* (English translation by M.A.B. Brazier), Springfield, Ill.: Thomas.

Ginccioli, D., Erdmann, H.Z. & Wolf, P. (1988): Epilepsie und Prodromi. In: *Epilepsie 87*, ed. E.J. Speckmann & B.J. Palm, pp. 513–516. Reinbek: Einhorn Presse Verlag.

Ginccioli, D., Czuczwana, H., Finkler, J., Leitenberger, J., May, Th., Nothbaum, N. & Wolf, P. (1990): Epilepsie und Prodromi: Eine prospektive Untersuchung. In: *Epilepsie 89*, ed. P. Wolf, pp. 312–321. Reinbek: Einhorn Presse Verlag.

Gotman, J., Ives, J., Gloor, P., Olvier, A. & Quesney, L.F. (1982): Changes in interictal EEG spiking and seizure occurrence in humans. *Epilepsia* **23,** 432–433.

Helmstaedter, C., Hefner, G., Bongartz, U., Hufnagel, A. & Elger, C.E. (1993): Die chronische Elektrostimulation des N. vagus zur Prophylaxe epileptischer Anfälle: Kognitive Leistungsänderungen. In: *Epilepsie 92*, ed. H. Stefan, pp. 433–436. Berlin: Deutsche Sektion ILAE.

Hosford, D.A. & McNamara, J.O. (1990): Basic mechanism of the epilepsies. *Curr. Opin. Neurol. Neurosurg.* **3,** 262–265.

Hufnagel, A., Zentner, J., Hefner, G., Bongartz, U., Helmstaedter, C., Peter, B. & Elger, C.E. (1993): Die chronische Elektrostimulation des N. vagus. I. Methode und Auswirkungen auf die Anfallssituation. In: *Epilepsie 92*, ed. H. Stefan, pp. 51–56. Berlin: Deutsche Sektion ILAE.

Hughes, J., Devinsky, O., Feldmann, E. & Bromfield, E. (1993): Premonitory symptoms in epilepsy. *Seizure* **2,** 201–203.

Katz, A., Marks, D.A., McCarthy, G. & Spencer, S.S. (1991): Does interictal spiking change prior to seizures? *Electroencephalogr. Clin. Neurophysiol.* **79,** 153–156.

Kerr, R.A. (1993): Magnetism triggers a brain response (research news article). *Science* **260,** 1590.

King, R.B., Schricker, J. & O'Leary, J.L. (1953): An experimental study of the transition from normal to convulsoid cortical activity. *J. Neurophysiol.* **16,** 286–298.

Landolt, H. (1960): *Die Temporallappen-Epilepsie und ihre Psychopathologie.* Basle, New York: Karger.

Landolt, H. (1963): Die Dämmer- und Verstimmungszustände bei Epilepsie und ihre Elektroencephalographie. *Dtsch. Z. Nervenheilk.* **185,** 411–430.

Lange, H.H., Lieb, J.P., Engel, J., Jr & Crandall, P.H. (1983): Temporo-spatial patterns of pre-ictal spike activity in human temporal lobe epilepsy. *Electroencephalogr. Clin. Neurophysiol.* **56,** 543–555.

Lieb, G.P., Woods, S.C., Siccardi, A., Crandall, P.H., Walter, D.O. & Leake, B. (1978): Quantitative analysis of depth spiking in relation to seizure foci in patients with temporal lobe epilepsy. *Electroencephalogr. Clin. Neurophysiol.* **44,** 641–663.

Lothman, E.W. (1991): Basic mechanism of the epilepsies. *Curr. Opin. Neurol. Neurosurg.* **4,** 253–258.

Moore-Ede, M.C., Campbell, S.S. & Reiter, R.J. (1992): *Electromagnetic fields and circadian rhythmicity,* 210pp. Boston: Birkhäuser.

Niedermeyer, E. (1991): Awakening epilepsy ('Aufwach-Epilepsie') revisited. In: *Epilepsy, sleep and sleep deprivation*, 2nd edn, (*Epilepsy Res.* Suppl. 2), eds. R. Degen & E.A. Rodin, pp. 37–42. Amsterdam: Elsevier.

Prince, D.A. (1965a): Cyclical spike driving in chronically isolated cortex. *Epilepsia* **6,** 226–242.

Prince, D.A. (1965b): Long duration periodic changes in excitability of penicillin spike foci: cyclical spike driving. *Electroencophalogr. Clin. Neurophysiol.* **19,** 139–151.

Ralston, B.L. (1958): The mechanism of transition of interictal spiking foci into ictal seizure discharges. *Electroencephalogr. Clin. Neurophysiol.* **10,** 217–232.

Reker, M., Düchting-Röth, A. & Wolf, P. (1993): Das Anfallsunterbrechungsprojekt in Bethel: Bewertung erster Ergebnisse von fünf Therapieverläufen. In: *Epilepsie 92*, ed. H. Stefan, pp. 40–45. Berlin: Deutsche Sektion ILAE.

Rossi, G.F., Colicchio, G., Gentilomo, A., Pola, P. & Scerrati, M. (1980): The stereoelectroencephalogram as a means to locate epileptogenic lesions. In: *Advances in epileptology: XIth Epilepsy International Symposium*, ed. R. Canger, F. Angeleri & J.R. Penry, pp. 91–101. New York: Raven Press.

Sackellares, J.C., Iasemidis, L.D., Zaveri, H.P. & Williams, W.J. (1989): Measurement of chaos to localize seizure onset. *Epilepsia* **30,** 5.

Sälke-Kellermann, A., Baier, H., Rambeck, B., Boenigk, H.E. & Wolf, P. (1993): Acute encephalopathy with vigabatrine. *Lancet* **342,** 185.

Scobey, R.P. & Gabor, A.J. (1977): Properties of epileptogenic focus: activation field. *J. Neurophysiol.* **40,** 1199–1213.

Semm, P. & Beason, R.C. (1990): Responses to small magnetic variations by the trigeminal system of the bobolink. *Brain Res. Bull.* **25,** 735–740.

Sherwin, I. (1978): Interictal–ictal transition in the feline penicillin epileptogenic focus. *Electroencephalogr. Clin. Neurophysiol.* **45,** 525–534.

Spencer, S.S., Guimaraes, P., Katz, A., Kim, J. & Spencer, D.D. (1992a): Morphological patterns of seizures recorded intracranially. *Epilepsia* **33,** 537–545.

Spencer, S.S., Marks, D., Katz, A., Kim, J. & Spencer, D.D. (1992b): Anatomic correlates of interhippocampal seizure propagation time. *Epilepsia* **33,** 862–873.

Stevens, J.R., Lonsbury, B.L. & Goel, S.L. (1972): Seizure occurrence and interspike interval: telemetered electroencephalogram studies. *Arch. Neurol.* (Chic.) **26,** 409–419.

Stodieck, S.R.G., & Wieser, H.G. (1983): The effects of polarization on human epileptic foci. In: *Proceedings of First* Vienna International Workshop on Functional Electrostimulation, ed. H. Thoma. Vienna: University Press.

Stodieck, S.R.G. & Wieser, H.G. (1984): Effects of polarization on human epileptic foci. *Artif. Organs* **8** (3), 392.

Stodieck, S.R.G. & Wieser, H.G. (1987): Epicortical DC changes in epileptic patients. In: *Advances in epileptology*, Vol. 16, eds. P. Wolf, M. Dam, D. Janz & F.E. Dreifuss, pp. 123–127. New York: Raven Press.

Stringer, J.L. & Lothman, E.W. (1990): Use of maximal dentate activation to study the effects of drugs on kindling and kindled responses. *Epilepsy Res.* **6,** 180–186.

Tellenbach, H. (1965): Epilepsie als Anfallsleiden und als Psychose. *Nervenarzt* **36,** 190–202.

Walker, A.E., Johnson. H.C. & Kollros, J.J. (1945): Penicillin convulsions: the effect of penicillin applied to the cortex of monkey and man. *Surg. Gynecol. Obstetr.* **81,** 692–701.

Walker, M.M. & Bitterman, M.E. (1989): Honeybees can be trained to respond to very small changes in the geomagnetic field intensity. *J. Exp. Biol.* **145,** 489–494.

Wang, J. & Wieser, H.G. (1994): The regional 'rigidity' of background EEG activity in the epileptogenic zone. *Epilepsia* **35,** 495–504.

Wever, R. (1974): ELF effects on human circadian rhythms. In: *ELF and VLF electromagnetic field effects*, ed. M. Persinger, pp. 101–104. New York: Raven Press.

Wieser, H.G. (1983a): Depth recorded limbic seizures and psychopathology. *Neurosci. Biobehav. Rev.* **7,** 427–440.

Wieser, H.G. (1983b): *Electroclinical features of the psychomotor seizure.* Stuttgart, London: Fischer, Butterworths.

Wieser, H.G. (1987): Stereo-electroencephalography. In: *Presurgical evaluation of epileptics*, eds. H.G. Wieser & C.E. Elger, pp. 192–204. Berlin: Springer.

Wieser, H.G. (1989a): Seizure-inducing and -preventing mechanisms. In: *Reflex seizures and reflex epilepsies*, ed. A. Beaumanoir, H. Gastaut & R. Naquet, pp. 49–55. Geneva: Editions Médecine & Hygiène.

Wieser, H.G. (1989b): Preictal EEG findings. *Epilepsia* **30,** 669.

Wieser, H.G. (1991a): Semi-invasive EEG: foramen ovale electrodes. In: *Epilepsy surgery*, ed. H. Lüders, pp. 361–370. New York: Raven Press.

Wieser, H.G. (1991b): Temporal lobe epilepsy, sleep and arousal: stereo-EEG findings. In: *Epilepsy, sleep and sleep deprivation*, 2nd edn (*Epilepsy Res.* suppl. 2), eds. R. Degen & E.A. Rodin, pp. 97–119. Amsterdam: Elsevier.

Wieser, H.G., Siegfried, J. & Bernoulli, C. (1981): Corrélations stéréo- electroencéphalographiques des manifestations psychiatriques dans l'épilepsie. *Méd. Hyg.* **39,** 1920–1928.

Wieser, H.G., Do, K.Q., Perschak, H. & Cuénod, M. (1989): Modulation of extracellular aspartate level during epileptiform events in primary epileptogenic area of patients. Abstracts: Satellite Symposium of the XXXI International Congress of Physiological Sciences, p. 68. Frankfurt.

Wilson, C.L., Isokawa, M., Babb, T.L. & Crandall, P.H. (1990): Functional connections in the human temporal lobe. I. Analysis of limbic system pathways using neuronal responses evoked by electrical stimulation. *Exp. Brain Res.* **82,** 279–292.

Wilson, C.L., Isokawa, M., Babb, T.L., Crandall, P.H., Levesque, M.F. & Engel, J., Jr (1991): Functional connections in the human temporal lobe. II. Evidence for a loss of functional linkage between contralateral structures. *Exp. Brain Res.* **85,** 174–187.

Wiltschko, W. & Wiltschko, R. (1991): Orientation in birds: magnetic orientation and celestial cues in migratory orientation. *EXS* **60,** 16–37.

Wolf, P. (1994): New antiepileptic drugs already registered. In: *Proceedings of the Zurich Consensus Conference on New Antiepileptic Drugs*, ed. H.G. Wieser, F. Dreifuss & U. Heinemann. *Epilepsia* 35 (suppl. 5), S22–S24.

Wolf, P. & Köhler, C.K. (eds.) (1980): Psychopathologische und pathogenetische Probleme psychotischer Syndrome bei Epilepsie. Bern: Huber.

Wyler, A.R. (1980): Operant control of CNS activity. In: *Epilepsy, a window to the brain mechanisms*, eds. J.S. Lockard & A.A. Ward, Jr, pp. 69–82. New York: Raven Press.

Wyler, A.R. & Fetz, E.F. (1974): Behavioral control of firing patterns of normal and abnormal neurons in chronic epileptic cortex. *Exp. Neurol.* **42,** 448–464.

Wyler, A.R. & Ward, A.A. Jr (1980): Epileptic neurons. In: *Epilepsy, a window to the brain mechanisms*, eds. J.S. Lockard, & A.A. Ward, Jr, pp. 51–68. New York: Raven Press.

Epileptic Seizures and Syndromes, Edited by Peter Wolf
© 1994 John Libbey & Company Ltd., pp. 579–588

Chapter 57

Interplay between interictal and ictal foci in the electrogenesis of hippocampal seizures

Yoel Yaari, Rony Azouz and Morten S. Jensen*

Department of Physiology, Hebrew University–Hadassah School of Medicine, Jerusalem 91010, Israel;
**PharmaBiotech, Institute of Physiology, Aarhus University, 8000 Aarhus, Denmark*

Summary

Rat hippocampal slices perfused with artificial cerebrospinal fluid containing a moderately elevated concentration of potassium ($[K^+]_o$) manifest epileptiform activity that arises in two separate and functionally different epileptogenic foci. An interictal focus in the CA3 field intermittently generates brief bursts of synchronous discharges which normally propagate into CA1. The interictal bursts evolve through enhanced excitatory (glutamatergic) synaptic interactions and therefore are blocked by glutamatergic antagonists. In the CA1 field an ictal focus repeatedly generates sustained paroxysms that spread within, but are spatially limited to, this area. These episodes are presumably produced by the regenerative accumulation of $[K^+]_o$, which produces marked neuronal excitation within and around the primary focus. Direct electrical interactions between juxtaposed neurones contribute to the marked synchronization of neuronal firing that develops during these events. Since these excitatory interactions are non-synaptic in nature, they resist blockage by glutamatergic antagonists.

Interictal activity generated in CA3 interacts with the ictal focus in CA1. When arriving immediately after an episode of sustained population discharge, that is, when $[K^+]_o$ is still elevated, interictal inputs trigger giant bursts in CA1. Consequently, ictal episodes in CA1 appear biphasic, consisting of a tonic phase of sustained discharge lasting several seconds followed by a clonic phase of intermittent giant bursts, which lasts a minute or more.

Thus, the analyses of this *in vitro* model of focal hippocampal epilepsy demonstrate an interplay between interictal and ictal foci that can produce tonic–clonic sequences of seizure discharge resembling those seen in animal experiments and in the clinical situation.

Introduction

In the description and analysis of electrical phenomena characteristic of the epileptic condition, a useful distinction is made between the *ictal* state, or seizure proper, which is associated with peripheral epileptic manifestations, and the *interictal* state, which clinically is relatively silent. Throughout the ictal state, large neuronal aggregates in many brain regions discharge synchronously and excessively, thereby interrupting normal brain function for a minute or more. In contrast, only brief (*c.* 100 ms) and spatially restricted bursts of synchronous electrical activity (reflected as electroencephalographic (EEG) 'spikes') are generated by the epileptic neuronal aggregate during the interictal state (Ajmone Marsan, 1961; Dichter & Ayala, 1987).

Focal application of convulsant agents to the neocortex or hippocampus of experimental animals produces recurring ictal episodes intersperesed by interictal bursts (Ajmone Marsan, 1961). Intracellular recordings from pyramidal cells have disclosed that neurones in the epileptogenic focus depolarize simultaneously during each interictal event (Matsumoto & Ajmone Marsan, 1964a). This interictal depolarization shift (DS) is attributed primarily to recurrent excitatory postsynaptic potentials (EPSPs), which are enhanced following convulsant-induced disinhibition (Ayala *et al.*, 1973; Johnston & Brown, 1981). The interictal DS is curtailed by a long-lasting hyperpolarization that consists of a mixture of intrinsic spike after-potentials and inhibitory postsynaptic potentials underlain by increased conductances to potassium and chloride (Matsumoto & Ajmone Marsan, 1964a; Dichter & Ayala, 1987).

A typical ictal episode appears to develop progressively from, and in suggestively close relationship with, the interictal events. At the single-cell level, the earliest detectable sign of an impending ictal episode is the progressive decrease and disappearance of hyperpolarization that follows each interictal DS (Matsumoto & Ajmone Marsan, 1964b). The DSs increase in amplitude and duration, causing the neurone to generate increasingly longer spike trains (*after-discharges*; Ralston, 1958). Eventually the membrane potential reaches and maintains a very low level of polarization, on top of which individual DSs can no longer be discerned. The sustained (or tonic) depolarization drives the neurone to fire repetitively until its spike mechanism inactivates. These changes occurring simultaneously in many neurones are reflected in repetitive synchronous firing of the epileptic population and in marked elevation of the extracellular concentration of $[K^+]$ ($[K^+]_o$; Fisher *et al.*, 1976; Heinemann *et al.*, 1977). Consequent to the loss of inhibitory responses the epileptic discharges can also spread into normal neuronal aggregates and in some situations even generalize throughout the brain. This cellular behaviour, which lasts 5–10 s, comprises the tonic phase of seizure.

The first phase is followed by the *clonic* phase of seizure, during which neurones slowly repolarize and large DSs reappear intermittently, causing the neuronal population to generate a series of synchronous giant bursts for a minute or more (Matsumoto & Ajmone Marsan, 1964b). Eventually the membrane potential reaches, and occasionally exceeds, the resting potential at which point the ictal episode ends. It is followed by a period of neuronal inactivity of variable duration (*postictal depression*).

Whereas the cellular mechanisms underlying the transition from the interictal to the ictal state have been investigated thoroughly (Dichter, 1988; Jensen & Yaari, 1988, 1992; Prince, 1988; Yaari & Jensen, 1988), much less is known about the processes mediating the transformation of tonic to clonic discharge. We have employed an *in vitro* model of focal hippocampal epilepsy, namely the high-K^+ model (Jensen & Yaari, 1988; Traynelis & Dingledine, 1988), to study this phenomenon. Our results suggest that tonic and clonic discharges are not just morphological variations of the same epileptogenic process. Rather, they are triggered by fundamentally different mechanisms and reflect a dynamic interplay between two types of epileptogenic foci.

Interictal and ictal epileptogenesis in rat hippocampal slices

Rat hippocampal slices perfused with artificial cerebrospinal fluid containing a moderately elevated concentration of potassium (e.g. 7.5 mM instead of the normal 3.5 mM $[K^+]$) generate two forms of epileptiform activity that may be categorized electrographically as either interictal or ictal events (Fig. 1a). Interestingly, the two types of epileptiform events are generated in separate foci (Yaari & Jensen, 1988). The focus of interictal events is localized to the CA3 field (Rutecki *et al.*, 1985; Korn *et al.*, 1987). Brief (*c.* 50–100 ms) synchronous bursts arise in this focus every 1 or 2 s through a regenerative process that is largely mediated by recurrent synaptic excitation (Chamberlin *et al.*, 1990). These bursts propagate into the adjacent CA1 field via the Schaffer collaterals of CA3 pyramidal cells, which

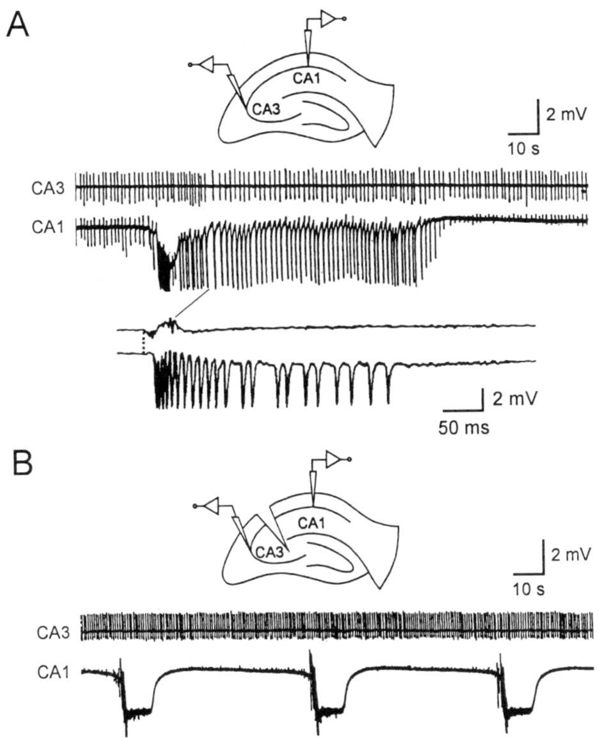

Fig. 1. Elevating the concentration of K^+ in the perfusing artificial cerebrospinal fluid ($[K^+]_o$) to 7.5 mM induces an interictal focus in CA3 and an ictal focus in CA1. Simultaneous extracellular recordings with NaCl-filled (1 M) microelectrodes were made in the pyramidal layers of CA3 and CA1, as depicted in the schemes. A. Intact slice. Upper traces show, on a slow time-scale, the interictal bursts generated in CA3 and propagated to CA1, and a single ictal episode in CA1 consisting of tonic and clonic phases. Note the high-frequency repetitive discharge characteristic of the tonic phase that lasts almost 10 s, and the giant clonic bursts that recur for more than a minute and are followed by postictal depression. A single clonic event is shown on an expanded time scale in the lower traces. The clonic burst in CA1 is preceded by an interictal burst in CA3. B. Cut slice. If the connections between CA3 and CA1 are severed, elevating $[K^+]_o$ induces independent foci in CA3 and in CA1. In this preparation the activity of the ictal focus can be isolated from the modulatory effects of the interictal focus. Note that ictal episodes lack a clonic phase, suggesting that it requires an extraneous trigger (normally furnished by the CA3 interictal focus).

make excitatory synaptic contacts with CA1 pyramidal cells. Since EPSPs in these hippocampal fields are mediated by the amino acid neurotransmitter glutamate, the generation and spread of interictal bursts is readily suppressed by application of glutamate receptor antagonists (Chamberlin *et al.*, 1990; Yaari & Jensen, 1992; Jensen & Yaari, 1991; see below, Fig. 3).

In addition to interictal events that develop in all slices exposed to an elevated extracellular concentration of [K+] ($[K^+]_o$), ictal episodes appear in the CA1 field of some slices. Once established, these events recur quite regularly once every few minutes (Traynelis & Dingledine, 1988). In many cases the transition from interictal bursts to ictal discharge involves the loss of post-DS hyperpolarizations, the progressive growth of interictal DSs and the appearance of after-discharges (Jensen & Yaari, 1988, 1992). Each ictal episode consists of a sequence of tonic and clonic discharges, which closely resemble the sequence of seizure discharges recorded in animal models of focal epileptogenesis (Fig. 1a). During the tonic phase pyramidal neurones depolarize 10–20 mV for several seconds

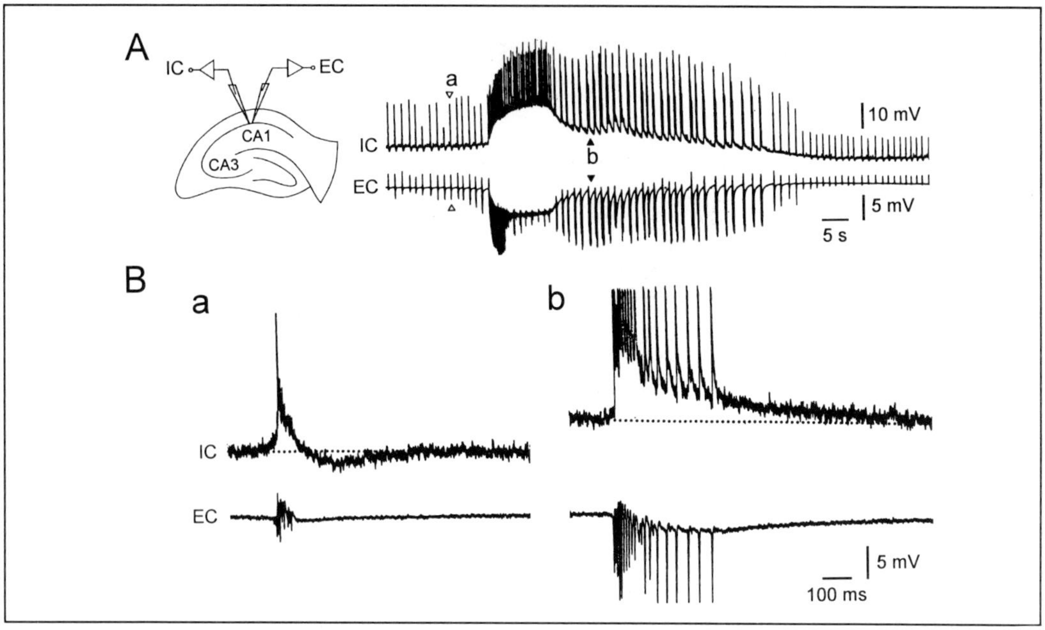

Fig. 2. Intracellular and extracellular manifestations of a tonic–clonic episode in an intact hippocampal slice perfused with high $[K^+]_o$ artificial cerebrospinal fluid. A pyramidal neurone was impaled with a K-acetate- (4 M) filled microelectrode. A. Simultaneous intra- (IC) and extracellular (EC) recordings were obtained in CA1, as illustrated in the scheme (left). A tonic–clonic ictal episode preceded and followed by interictal bursts is depicted on a slow time-scale. Note the sustained depolarization during the tonic phase that underlies high-frequency repetitive discharge. B. Comparison of interictal (a) and clonic (b) bursts. The arrows in A indicate the events that are expanded in B. Note that the interictal burst consists of a depolarizing shift (DS) followed by a hyperpolarization. In contrast, the clonic burst is a prolonged, giant DS that evokes intense burst firing and after-discharges.

and fire repetitively at a high frequency (Fig. 2a). In the following clonic phase, which lasts from 10 s to a minute or more, the neurones repolarize slowly and then hyperpolarize, while intermittent DSs reappear and assume a gigantic size (Fig. 2a, b). Throughout the course of a tonic–clonic episode, the firing of individual neurones coincides with the firing of their neighbouring cells. The marked neuronal synchrony is reflected in the appearance of large population spikes in the zone of intense firing (Fig. 2).

Electrogenesis of tonic discharge

If the connections between the CA3 and CA1 fields are severed, interictal bursts arising in CA3 can no longer propagate into CA1. In such cut slices ictal episodes can still be induced in CA1 by moderately raising $[K^+]_o$, but they lack the clonic component (Fig. 1b). Likewise, blockage of glutamatergic EPSPs by glutamate receptor antagonists or by addition of cadmium (which blocks evoked neurotransmitter release) suppresses interictal bursts in both CA3 and CA1 and also abolishes the clonic component of ictal episodes (Fig. 3; Jensen & Yaari, 1988, 1991). These findings reinforce the view that the ictal focus is localized to CA1 and can trigger tonic ictal episodes independent of the interictal drive from CA3. Furthermore, they indicate that these episodes evolve through non-synaptic excitatory neuronal interactions (Yaari *et al.*, 1986; Yaari & Jensen, 1988, 1990).

Previous work has suggested that, since CA1 pyramidal cells are tightly packed (Green & Maxwell, 1961), K^+ released into the interstitium by intensely firing neurones may accumulate to levels that

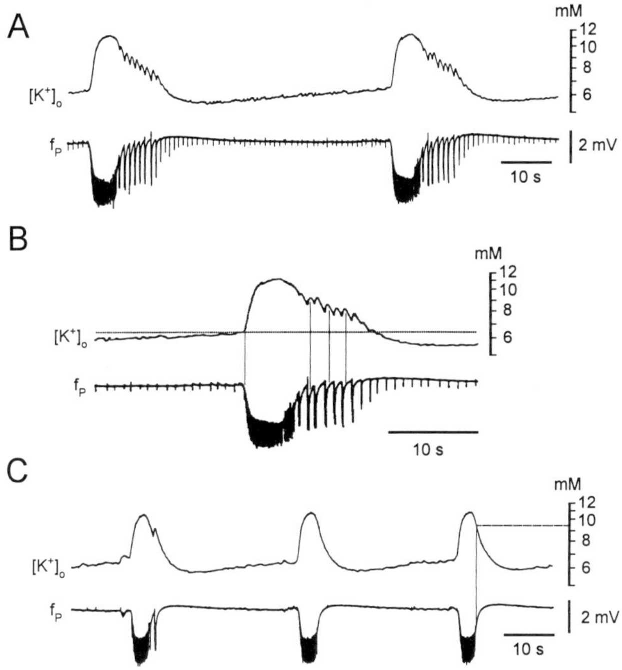

Fig. 3. Seizure-related changes in $[K^+]_o$ in an intact hippocampal slice. A double-barrelled K^+-selective microelectrode (Yaari et al., 1986) was used to simultaneously record $[K^+]_o$ (upper traces) and the extracellular potential (f_P, lower traces) from the CA1 pyramidal layer. Ictal episodes were induced by raising $[K^+]$ in the artificial cerebrospinal fluid to 7.5 mM. A. Changes in $[K^+]_o$ associated with two consecutive ictal episodes. Note the gradual build-up of $[K^+]_o$ before, and the rapid increase in $[K^+]_o$ during, the onset of tonic discharge. B. A single ictal episode shown on an expanded time-scale. Note that at seizure threshold $[K^+]_o$ is about 6.5 mM and it rapidly reaches a ceiling level of about 11 mM. During the clonic phase $[K^+]_o$ remains elevated and each clonic burst is associated with a transient increase in $[K^+]_o$ C. Following suppression of glutamatergic EPSPs with the glutamate receptor antagonist 1-(p-chlorobenzoyl)-piperazine-2, 3-dicarboxylic acid (pCB-PzDA; 0.5 mM), the interictal and clonic bursts disappear, and ictal episodes consist of a tonic component only. Note that $[K^+]_o$ remains elevated for several seconds after cessation of tonic discharge.

will excite the neuronal population even further, thereby triggering a regenerative process of neuronal recruitment and K^+_o increase (Fertziger & Ranck, 1970). Such a process may contribute to the development of seizure discharge within an ictal focus. Furthermore, the dispersion of $[K^+]_o$ from the focus into adjacent regions (e.g. by the glial spatial buffer; Walz, 1989) would excite surrounding neuronal aggregates and may mediate the spatial spread of ictal discharge even if EPSPs are blocked (Konnerth *et al.*, 1984; Yaari *et al.*, 1986). This *K^+ accumulation hypothesis* is compatible with direct measurements of $[K^+]_o$ in ictal foci using ion-selective microelectrodes. As illustrated in Fig. 3, each ictal episode is precipitated by a slow rise in $[K^+]_o$. At the onset of ictal discharge, the rise in $[K^+]_o$ is also markedly accelerated. Consequently $[K^+]_o$ rapidly rises until it reaches a ceiling level of 11–12 mM during the tonic phase of seizure. The $[K^+]_o$ also remains elevated during the clonic phase and then decays slowly to a postictal low level (Fig. 3b).

High $[K^+]_o$ exerts several excitatory effects on hippocampal neurones, which may account for its suggested role in neuronal recruitment during seizure, (see below). However, the K^+_o accumulation hypothesis cannot readily explain the marked neuronal synchronization that develops during the course of an ictal episode. Several lines of evidence suggest that neuronal synchronization within the time frame of a population spike (*c.* 5 ms) results from direct electrical (*ephaptic*) interactions between the tightly packed pyramidal neurones (Dudek *et al.*, 1986).

The excitatory interactions mediated by $[K^+]_o$ and by the electric field may be enhanced further by shrinkage of the extracellular space due to the activity-induced reduction in extracellular osmolality (Lux *et al.*, 1986). Indeed, perfusing the slices with hyperosmolar artificial cerebrospinal fluid, which increases the volume fraction of the extracellular space, can suppress ictal electrogenesis (Traynelis & Dingledine, 1989).

Electrogenesis of clonic discharge

The dependence of clonic bursts on the integrity of the pathways connecting CA3 to CA1 and on functional EPSPs suggests that they are evoked synaptically by the interictal bursts propagating from CA3. Indeed, each clonic burst in CA1 appears time-locked to an interictal burst in CA3 with a delay (~10 ms) consistent with feed-forward synaptic excitation (Fig. 1a). Furthermore, the generation of clonic bursts can be mimicked by delivering just-suprathreshold stimuli at 0.5–1 Hz to afferent fibres in the stratum radiatum of isolated CA1 slices (Fig. 4). When delivered *before* a tonic episode, these stimuli evoke only small interictal-like bursts. In contrast, when applied immediately *after* the tonic episode, each stimulus triggers a giant clonic-like burst (Fig. 4). If stimulation is delayed more than 1 or 2 s after the cessation of tonic discharge, clonic-like bursts can no longer be induced.

These observations indicate that clonic bursts arise in CA1 if a critical mass of neurones is activated within a narrow time window after the tonic episode. In an intact slice the interictal focus in CA3 thus provides an appropriate trigger for clonic bursts. That is to say, by generating propagating bursts every 1–2 s, it can reliably activate CA1 at the appropriate time for evoking clonic activity. Although an external trigger is required, the actual process of neuronal recruitment and synchronization during clonic discharge is mediated by recurrent excitation within the CA1 network. This is indicated by the finding that prolonged clonic bursts (consisting of 10–20 population spikes) can be evoked in isolated

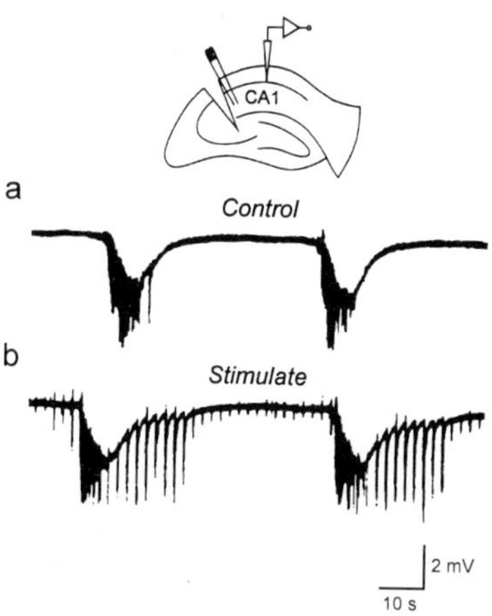

Fig. 4. Induction of clonic-like bursts in isolated CA1 by afferent fibre stimulation. The slice was cut as depicted in the scheme. A bipolar stimulation electrode was positioned in the apical dendritic layer (stratum radiatum), which contains afferent fibres to CA1 neurones. Extracellular recordings were made in the pyramidal layer. a. Elevating $[K^+]_o$ to 7.5 mM induced recurring ictal episodes consisting of only tonic components. b. Single-shock stimuli (3 V; 0.5 Hz) evoked interictal-like bursts when delivered before each tonic episode. The same stimuli delivered immediately after tonic discharge evoked giant clonic-like bursts.

CA1 slices even by just-suprathreshold, single-shock stimuli (Fig. 4). Thus, despite cessation of spontaneous firing, the CA1 neuronal aggregate continues to possess a high epileptogenic potential a few seconds after the tonic phase of seizure. This potential can easily be transformed into synchronous burst firing by an appropriately timed synaptic input to CA1.

Cellular basis of clonic bursts

Intracellular recordings in conditions of blocked EPSPs (and blocked clonic bursts) have shown that following tonic discharge pyramidal neurones hyperpolarize beyond their resting membrane potential for several seconds. This hyperpolarization is presumably is mediated by electrogenic Na^+/K^+ pumping activated by the perturbed concentrations of Na^+ and K^+ (Konnerth *et al.*, 1986). Neuronal hyperpolarization is normally associated with decreased excitability and would be expected to reduce the epileptogenic potential of the CA1 network. What mechanism, then, accounts for the enhanced responsiveness of these neurones just after a tonic episode?

We believe that a clue to this paradox is provided by Fig. 3c, which describes the $[K^+]_o$ changes associated with pure tonic events (isolated by blocking glutamatergic EPSPs). It can be seen that the changes in $[K^+]_o$ do not mirror exactly the time course of tonic discharge. Rather, at the point at which tonic discharge ceases, $[K^+]_o$ is still markedly elevated (*c.* 9.5 mM), and it decays to preictal levels only 3–5 s thereafter. We suggest that this tail of elevated $[K^+]_o$ confers on the CA1 network the enhanced responsiveness that follows a tonic event.

There are several mechanisms by which elevated $[K^+]_o$ can promote a synchronous burst response to a just-suprathreshold stimulus. As noted above, recurrent synaptic excitation is markedly enhanced in high $[K^+]_o$ (Chamberlin *et al.*, 1990). This may reflect a direct facilitatory effect of high $[K^+]_o$ on glutamate release and/or an indirect effect mediated by attenuation of γ-aminobutyric acidergic (GABA-ergic) inhibition (Korn *et al.*, 1987; however, see Jensen *et al.*, 1993b). Furthermore, as illustrated in Fig. 5, raising $[K^+]_o$ from 3.5 to 7.5 mM markedly affects the intrinsic firing properties of CA1 pyramidal cells, transforming many regular firing neurones into intrinsic burst firing cells (Jensen *et al.*, 1993a). The presence of a large fraction of burst-firing cells in a network of neurons that are reciprocally connected by excitatory synapses would greatly amplify the response to a given synaptic input (Traub & Wong, 1982). Taken together, these cellular effects of elevated $[K^+]_o$ may

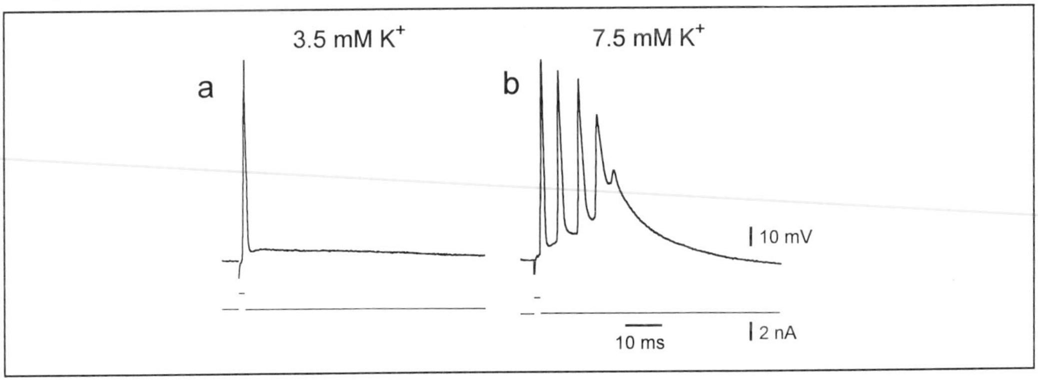

Fig. 5. Effects of raising $[K^+]_o$ on the firing pattern of a CA1 pyramidal neurone. The neurone was impaled with a K-acetate-filled microelectrode and was activated by brief (2 ms) depolarizing current pulses delivered through the intracellular microelectrode. a. In normal $[K^+]_o$ (3.5 mM; resting potential –68 mV), the stimulus evoked a single action potential that was followed by a prominent after-depolarization. b. In high $[K^+]_o$ (7.5 mM) the same stimulus evoked a burst of five spikes capping a huge depolarizing shift. High $[K^+]_o$ also depolarized the neurone by 5 mV. However, the burst response was seen both in the depolarized condition and after repolarizing the cell with constant negative current.

provide a sufficient positive feedback for the generation of a giant clonic burst immediately after the termination of tonic discharge.

Since each clonic burst induces a transient elevation in $[K^+]_o$ (Fig. 3b), the decay of $[K^+]_o$ to preictal levels would be delayed by clonic activity. Consequently, an external stimulus arriving in CA1 immediately after the first clonic burst would also encounter a high epileptogenic potential and thus would trigger a second clonic burst, which in turn would sustain the elevated $[K^+]_o$ for another short while. In this way, a series of clonic bursts can be triggered consecutively in CA1 by an external pacemaker, such as the interictal focus in CA3. This process would continue until $[K^+]_o$ is reduced sufficiently by Na^+/K^+ pumping and other K^+_o buffering mechanisms.

Discussion

The data summarized in this chapter show that moderately elevating baseline $[K^+]_o$ can induce two types of epileptogenic foci in rat hippocampal slices: an interictal focus in CA3 and an ictal focus in CA1. The mechanisms underlying the generation of epileptiform activity in the two foci appear to be entirely different. Previous work has shown that interictal bursts in CA3 are generated by excitatory synaptic interactions, which are presumably enhanced directly and/or via the disinhibitory effects of elevated $[K^+]_o$ (Korn *et al.*, 1987; Chamberlin *et al.*, 1990). By contrast, tonic paroxysms evolve in CA1 through surrounding excitation, presumably mediated by the regenerative accumulation of $[K^+]_o$ (Yaari *et al.*, 1986) and reinforced by ephaptic interactions (Dudek *et al.*, 1986) and shrinkage of the extracellular space (Lux *et al.*, 1986).

Since CA3 is normally connected to CA1 via the Schaffer collaterals, the interictal focus provides a regular excitatory input to CA1. The intensity of the epileptiform responses evoked in CA1 by this input largely depends on the properties of the CA1 network, which vary according to activity of the ictal focus in CA1. An important determinant of these properties is K^+_o, whose accumulation in the extracellular space markedly enhances the epileptogenic potential of the CA1 network by a variety of excitatory effects. Because $[K^+]_o$ in CA1 rises slowly before the onset of an ictal episode, interictal bursts evoked in CA1 during the preictal period gradually build up in size and duration. This may produce the apparently smooth transition from interictal to ictal discharge that is often observed in this model (Jensen & Yaari, 1988). Likewise, since $[K^+]_o$ is markedly elevated during and immediately after a tonic episode, bursts evoked in CA1 shortly after cessation of tonic discharge are gigantic in size and appear as a distinct clonic phase in the ictal episode. Thus, interictal–ictal and tonic–clonic transitions are, respectively, reflections of $[K^+]_o$ build-up before and clearance after a tonic ictal episode.

Taken together, the analyses of this *in vitro* model of hippocampal epilepsy suggests that the interplay between interictal and ictal foci can produce tonic–clonic sequences of seizure discharge that resemble those seen *in vivo*. Although the evidence relating these sequences to dynamic changes in $[K^+]_o$ is still circumstantial, the K^+_o accumulation hypothesis provides a testable framework for future studies of ictal electrogenesis.

Acknowledgements

Supported by the Wolfson Foundation administered by the Israel Academy of Sciences and Humanities and the Danish Medical Research Council.

References

Ajmone Marsan, C. (1961): Electrographic aspects of 'epileptic' neuronal aggregates. *Epilepsia* **2,** 22–38.

Ayala, G.F., Dichter, M.A., Gumnit, R.J., Matsumoto, H. & Spencer, W.A. (1973): Genesis of epileptic interictal spikes: new knowledge of cortical feedback systems suggests a neurophysiological explanation of brief paroxysms. *Brain Res.* **52,** 1–17.

Chamberlin, N.L., Traub, R.D. & Dingledine, R. (1990): Role of EPSPs in initiation of spontaneous synchronized burst firing in rat hippocampal neurons bathed in high potassium. *J. Neurophysiol.* **64**, 1000–1008.

Dichter, M.A. (1988): Modulation of inhibition and the transition to seizure. In: *Mechanisms of epileptogenesis: the transition to seizure*, ed. M.A. Dichter, pp. 169–182. New York: Plenum Press.

Dichter, M.A. & Ayala, G.F. (1987): Cellular mechanisms of epilepsy: a status report. *Science* **237**, 157–164.

Dudek, F., Snow, R. & Taylor, C. (1986): Role of electrical interactions in synchronization of epileptiform bursts. *Adv. Neurol.* **44**, 593–617.

Fertziger, A. & Ranck, J., Jr (1970): Potassium accumulation in interstitial space during epileptiform seizures. *Exp. Neurol.* **26**, 571–585.

Fisher, R.F., Pedely, T.A., Moody, W.J., Jr & Prince, D.A. (1976): The role of extracellular potassium in hippocampal epilepsy. *Arch. Neurol.* **33**, 76–83.

Green, J. & Maxwell, D. (1961): Hippocampal electrical activity. I. Morphological aspects. *Electroencephalogr. Clin. Neurophysiol.* **13**, 854–867.

Heinemann, U., Lux, H.D. & Gutnick, M.J. (1977): Extracellular free calcium and potassium during paroxysmal activity in the cerebral cortex of the cat. *Exp. Brain. Res.* **27**, 237–243.

Jensen, M.S. & Yaari, Y. (1988): The relationship between interictal and ictal paroxysms in an *in vitro* model of focal hippocampal epilepsy. *Ann. Neurol.* **24**, 591–598.

Jensen, M.S. & Yaari, Y. (1991): Role of glutamate receptors in potassium-induced paroxysms in rat hippocampal slices. *Exp. Brain Res.* **S20**, 85–88.

Jensen, M.S. & Yaari, Y. (1992): Potassium-induced endogenous bursting and disinhibition: role in interictal–ictal transitions in rat hippocampal slices. In: *Epilepsy and inhibition*, eds. E.-J. Speckmann & M.J. Gutnick, pp. 229–240. Munich: Urban & Schwartzenberg.

Jensen, M.S., Cherubini, E. & Yaari, Y. (1993a): Opponent effects of potassium on $GABA_A$-mediated postsynaptic inhibition in the rat hippocampus. *J. Neurophysiol.* **69**, 764–771.

Jensen, M.S., Azouz, R. & Yaari, Y. (1993b): Varient firing patterns in rat hippocampal pyramidal cells modulated by extracellular potassium. *J. Neurophysiol.* **71**, 831–839.

Johnston, D. & Brown, T.H. (1981): Giant synaptic potential hypothesis for epileptiform activity. *Science* **211**, 294–297.

Konnerth, A., Heinemann, U. & Yaari, Y. (1984): Slow transmission of neural activity in hippocampal area CA1 in the absence of active chemical synapses. *Nature* **307**, 69–71.

Konnerth, A., Heinemann, U. & Yaari, Y. (1986): Nonsynaptic epileptogenesis in the mammalian hippocampus *in vitro*. I. Development of seizure-like activity in low extracellular calcium. *J. Neurophysiol.* **56**, 409–423.

Korn, S.J., Giacchino, J.L., Chamberlin, N.L. & Dingledine, R. (1987): Epileptiform burst activity induced by potassium in the hippocampus and its regulation by GABA-mediated inhibition. *J. Neurophysiol.* **57**, 325–340.

Lux, H.D., Heinemann, U. & Dietzel, I. (1986): Ionic changes and alterations in the size of the extracellular space during epileptic activity. *Adv. Neurol.* **44**, 619–640.

Matsumoto, H. & Ajmone Marsan, C. (1964a). Cortical cellular phenomena in experimental epilepsy: interictal manifestations. *Exp. Neurol.* **9**, 286–304.

Matsumoto, H. & Ajmone Marsan, C. (1964b): Cortical cellular phenomena in experimental epilepsy: ictal manifestations. *Exp. Neurol.* **9**, 305–326.

Prince, D.A. (1988): Cellular mechanisms of interictal-ictal transitions. In: *Mechanisms of epileptogenesis: the transition to seizure*, ed. M.A. Dichter, pp. 57–72. New York: Plenum Press.

Ralston, B.L. (1958): The mechanism of transition of interictal spiking foci into ictal seizure discharges. *Electroencephalogr. Clin. Neurophysiol.* **10**, 217–232.

Rutecki, P.A., Lebeda, F.J. & Johnston, D. (1985): Epileptiform activity induced by changes in extracellular potassium in hippocampus. *J. Neurophysiol.* **54**, 1363–1374.

Traub, R.D. & Wong, R.K.S. (1982): Cellular mechanisms of neuronal synchronization in epilepsy. *Science* **216**, 745–747.

Traynelis, S.F. & Dingledine, R. (1988): Potassium-induced spontaneous electrographic seizures in the rat hippocampal slice. *J. Neurophysiol.* **59**, 259–276.

Traynelis, S.F. & Dingledine, R. (1989): Role of extracellular space in hyperosmotic suppression of potassium-induced electrographic seizures *J. Neurophysiol.* **61**, 927–938.

Walz, W. (1989): Role of glial cells in the regulation of the brain microenvironment. *Prog. Neurobiol.* **33,** 309–333.

Yaari, Y. & Jensen, M.S. (1988): Nonsynaptic mechanisms and interictal–ictal transitions in the mammalian hippocampus. In: *Mechanisms of epileptogenesis: the transition to seizure*, ed. M.A. Dichter, pp. 183–198. New York: Plenum Press.

Yaari, Y. & Jensen, M.S. (1992): Two types of epileptic foci generating brief and sustained paroxysms in the *in vitro* rat hippocampus. In: *Neurotransmitters in epilepsy*, Vol. 4, ed. G. Avanzini, R.G. Fariello & U. Heinemann, pp. 359–368. New York: Demos Publications.

Yaari, Y., Konnerth. A. & Heinemann, U. (1986): Nonsynaptic epileptogenesis in the mammalian hippocampus *in vitro*. II. Role of extracellular potassium. *J. Neurophysiol.* **56,** 424–438.

Section VI

Therapy resistance

The ultimate goal of all research in epileptology, clinical as well as theoretical, is the improvement of therapy, and the great challenge here is therapy resistance.

This section deals both with the definition and establishment of pharmacoresistance and with an analysis of its possible causative factors. Both clinical and theoretical views are presented concerning the question whether therapy resistance develops in the course of clinical epilepsy or intractable epilepsies are primarily different.

Morphological findings with specific pharmacoresistant epilepsies have been reported above (Chapters 43 and 46), whereas the problem of resistance to surgical treatment, which was touched upon in Chapter 37, is not further explored.

As for the West syndrome, a condition which is considered to be especially inaccessible to treatment, the therapeutic approaches currently prevailing in Germany are discussed along with new and more promising strategies.

Epileptic Seizures and Syndromes, Edited by Peter Wolf
© 1994 John Libbey & Company Ltd., pp. 591–597

Chapter 58

Establishment of pharmacoresistance

Blaise F.D. Bourgeois

Department of Neurology, Washington University, 660 S. Euclid Avenue, St. Louis, Mo 63110, USA

Summary

The initial goal of therapy in any patient with epilepsy is obviously not to establish that she or he is medically intractable, but to use drugs systematically, assuming that the patient's seizures will come under control. However, the possibility of pharmacoresistance should be accepted and tested, in order not to delay unnecessarily the option of epilepsy surgery. There is no single step in the drug management that separates a potentially treatable from an intractable epilepsy. In a patient who is being considered for epilepsy surgery, the criteria for medical intractability are probably met if the degree of seizure control is not satisfactory to the patient despite adequate trials with the major antiepileptic drugs at the maximal tolerated doses. Unfortunately, these criteria are not universal and need to be redefined for every patient. An adequate drug trial in a refractory epilepsy is determined not only by the maximal tolerated dose, but also by the optimal choice of drugs and by the appropriate duration of the treatment at that dose. Finally, there are several reasons why the process of establishing of pharmacoresistance should be as short as possible. Firstly, if the patient is not truly medically intractable, the successful therapeutic step will occur sooner. Secondly, in a patient who becomes seizure-free after surgery, the long-term psychosocial outcome is likely to be better if the surgery is performed earlier. Thirdly, it is suspected that the seizure reduction following epilepsy surgery is enhanced by early intervention. Finally, there are data suggesting that a cognitive improvement following surgery is more likely if the interval between onset of the epilepsy and surgery is shorter.

Introduction

The pharmacoresistance of epilepsy is probably the main challenge for the physician taking care of patients with epilepsy. Patients who are pharmacoresistant represent a disproportionately large group in any epileptological practice. Even after optimal use of the available antiepileptic drugs, approximately one-third of patients diagnosed with epilepsy do not become seizure-free. The terms 'pharmacoresistance' and 'medical intractability' are used synonymously by some, whereas others may define intractability as absence of seizure freedom and pharmacoresistance as absence of any response to antiepileptic drug therapy. The two terms will be used synonymously here to refer to the inability to achieve complete or almost complete seizure control with medications.

Medical intractability of epilepsy can be considered from two apparently diametrically opposed viewpoints. The initial goal of therapy in any patient with epilepsy is obviously not to establish that she or he is medically intractable, but to use drugs systematically, assuming that the patient's seizures will come under control unless proved otherwise. On the other hand, in any patient who appears to be difficult to control, the possibility of pharmacoresistance should be accepted and tested, in order not to delay unnecessarily the option of epilepsy surgery. Fortunately, trying to overcome drug failure and documenting intractability constitute only one and the same therapeutic approach, since intractability can be defined in broad terms as the failure of optimal therapy. However, the fact that epilepsy surgery is now widely available creates a pressure to decide after how much optimal therapy a patient is unlikely to become completely controlled at any time in the future.

The establishment of pharmacoresistance remains one of the absolute prerequisites for epilepsy surgery. Yet there is no unequivocal definition of pharmacoresistance. There is no single step in the drug management that separates a potentially treatable from an intractable epilepsy. Accordingly, there are no universally accepted criteria regarding the establishment of pharmacoresistance and, in publications on epilepsy surgery, diverse or vague statements are made. Epilepsy surgery is not the only therapeutic procedure requiring the establishment of medical intractability. To some extent, resistance to conventional drugs is also a prerequisite for trials with experimental antiepileptic drugs or for alternative measures, such as vagal stimulation. The definition of intractability in these two situations may be different from that in the case of surgery, which is a definitive and irreversible intervention.

Definition of the concept of intractability

Theoretically, and ideally, absolute intractability can be defined as persistence of seizures despite treatment with the maximal tolerated doses of *all* available antiepileptic drugs in monotherapy and with *all possible combinations*. This definition appears quite simple, but its practical application is virtually impossible. There is a relatively large number of antiepileptic drugs on the market and the number of possible combinations is an exponential function of that number. Even with the shortest possible observation time on each drug or on each combination of drugs, it might well take a decade or more to satisfy the above definition. This is clearly too long in a patient in whom the probability of complete seizure control by epilepsy surgery is above 50 per cent. Thus, pharmacoresistance will remain a relative concept. Also, the certainty that a patient's seizures cannot be fully controlled with medication will only be approached progressively and in an asymptotic fashion. Intractability will have to be defined in every patient in light of the specific alternative measure under consideration. In dealing with the question of possible evaluation for an experimental antiepileptic drug trial or for epilepsy surgery, the physician is confronted with two questions: first, how to establish intractability for these purposes, and secondly, how and how rapidly intractability can be documented in a patient who could not be controlled so far. These questions should not only preoccupy those working centres performing trials with experimental antiepileptic drugs or epilepsy surgery, but also those who refer patients to such centres.

In a patient who is being considered for epilepsy surgery, the criteria for medical intractability are probably met if the degree of seizure control is not satisfactory to the patient despite adequate trials with the major antiepileptic drugs at the maximal tolerated doses, i.e. with acceptable side-effects. Unfortunately, these criteria are not universal and need to be redefined for every patient, because satisfactory seizure control, adequate trial and maximal tolerated dose may vary from patient to patient. With resective epilepsy surgery as the only alternative, satisfactory seizure control may not necessarily mean complete seizure control. Depending on their level of functioning and on the severity of the seizures, some patients may consider that an occasional seizure is preferable to the prospect of brain surgery. Others may come to the conclusion that even a rare seizure affects their quality of life sufficiently to justify the prolonged evaluation and the risk associated with epilepsy surgery. For these patients, usually high-functioning individuals, two major factors often affect their decision: the inability to drive and the fear of a seizure. It is fair to say that complete seizure control is actually only achieved when the patient loses her or his fear of a seizure, because a fully normal life is only possible when the patient feels confident that there will most probably be no further seizure. Finally, whether the persisting seizure frequency justifies a surgical intervention also depends on the expected postoperative results. The higher the probability of complete seizure control after a given resection, the lower the threshold below which the seizure frequency will be considered satisfactory. In conclusion, the criteria for unsatisfactory seizure control for the purpose of epilepsy surgery are met when a patient is willing to undergo presurgical monitoring and to take the risks involved in the surgery. There is one limit to this rule: surgery is not offered to patients who are seizure-free and want the surgery in order to possibly be off medications in the future.

What represents acceptable or unacceptable side-effects is also subject to individual variation, whether these side-effects are dose-related or not. Sedation or cognitive impairment does not have the same impact on every patient's quality of life. Similarly, weight gain, tremor, increased body hair and teratogenicity may represent a serious problem for some and be an irrelevant issue for others. The concept of the maximal tolerated dose is somewhat easier to define than unsatisfactory seizure control, but it is often misunderstood or not applied. The maximal tolerated dose is not the highest daily dose that the patient ever took . . . and tolerated. It is the highest dose that a patient can tolerate without experiencing recurrent dose-related toxicity. The maximal tolerated dose can only be determined by progressively increasing the daily dose until the patient actually experiences recurrent dose-related toxicity, even if only for a day or two, and then decreasing the dose to the highest level the patient had tolerated without evidence of toxicity. In publications reporting series of epilepsy surgeries, this issue is often not clearly addressed. In the methods section, the following definitions of intractability can be found: . . . 'intensive and methodological treatment with anticonvulsant agents must be ineffective in controlling seizures despite adequate serum anticonvulsant levels' (Meyer *et al.*, 1986); or 'seizures uncontrolled despite an adequate trial of phenytoin, carbamazepine and phenobarbital or primidone. 'Adequate trial' refers to antiepileptic drug concentration within the accepted "therapeutic range" or intolerance to the medication' (King *et al.*, 1986). All too often, drug levels within the so called therapeutic range are used as the criterion for an adequate dose. The general trend, however, is to consider an antiepileptic drug ineffective in a patient only when seizures persist at the maximal tolerated dose, regardless of the blood levels or their therapeutic range (Cramer *et al.*, 1983; Lesser *et al.*, 1984; Dasheiff *et al.*, 1986). For instance, 17 of 30 patients who had seizures at least weekly at phenytoin levels below 20 mg/l became seizure-free at levels above 20 mg/l, with no clinical evidence of toxicity (Cobos, 1987). On the basis of the concept of the maximal tolerated dose, Schmidt (1986) proposed an intractability scale of 1 to 5. A score of 5 is defined as the failure of more than one major drug of first choice in monotherapy at the maximal tolerated dose.

An adequate drug trial in a refractory epilepsy is determined not only by the maximal tolerated dose but also by the optimal choice of the drugs and by the appropriate duration of the treatment at that dose. Diagnostic aspects need to be taken into account. One needs to be certain that the seizure diagnosis is correct, and thus the appropriate drug is used. Also, among patients who are evaluated for intractable seizures, there is always a relatively high percentage of patients with psychogenic seizures (Janz, 1978; Rodin *et al.*, 1982). How long does one need to wait before coming to the conclusion that the drug being tried is unlikely to provide satisfactory seizure protection? Here again, there is no universal answer and the main individual parameter that will determine the duration of a trial is the seizure frequency. In a patient who has had an average of three seizures per week and continues to have three seizures per week, it will not take as long to be convinced of a failure than in a patient who has had about one seizure per month and continues to have an average of one seizure per month. This effect of the pre-existing seizure frequency on the necessary time of observation at the maximal tolerated dose of a drug can be used to establish guidelines. One can determine the average seizure interval before a given trial with a drug and calculate the subsequent period of observation as five to 10 times this seizure interval. For instance, let us assume that a patient has an average seizure frequency of one per week and then has the drug dose increased to the maximal tolerated dose. If this patient continues to present seizures 5–10 weeks later, the drug is likely to fail even if given beyond that time. Of course, one will wait until the patient has more than one or two seizures before deciding that a given trial has failed, no matter what the original seizure frequency was. Also, the time of observation may be prolonged by an initial but transient decrease of the seizure frequency after a drug change or a dosage increase.

Although medical intractability to conventional drugs is a prerequisite for both epilepsy surgery and experimental antiepileptic drug trials, the definition of intractability may differ slightly between these two situations. In general, more rigorous criteria should be used in surgical candidates because of the greater risk and the potentially irreversible deficits associated with surgery. On the other hand, intractability criteria should also be applied to patients who are being screened for experimental antiepileptic drug trials. There are at least three reasons for this: (1) a trial with an experimental antiepileptic drug is associated with a somewhat higher risk of unexpected problems than with a conventional drug; (2) if experimental antiepileptic drugs are tested only in patients having met certain intractability criteria, the study groups will be more homogeneous; and (3) drug trials should select out new drugs that are more effective than the existing drugs and that will achieve what the available drugs have not achieved.

Practical application of intractability criteria

If one accepts the above guidelines as criteria for establishing pharmacoresistance, the next step is to implement these guidelines in a particular patient in whom the option of using an experimental antiepileptic drug or of epilepsy surgery is considered. Patients are referred or first seen at various stages in the course of the medical management of their epilepsy. The very first step will be to verify the diagnosis. Then, one should attempt to compile a list of all antiepileptic drugs that have been used, whether alone or in combination, with the maximal dose and level that was attained, the duration of trials, idiosyncratic or dose-related side-effects and changes in seizure frequency. Based on this list, it should be possible to determine which drugs have failed despite an adequate trial and which drugs should not be used again because of an idiosyncratic reaction. Patient reports of ‘allergic reaction’ or ‘toxicity’ should be evaluated very carefully. An ‘allergic reaction’ may represent early toxicity after rapid introduction, and ‘toxicity’ may have represented a level above the individual therapeutic range. Whether the patient should undergo further trials with other drugs or drug combinations or whether a drug should be used again because it had not been used adequately in the past will depend on an additional element in the definition of medical intractability: which drugs and which drug combinations need to be tried against a given seizure type in order to demonstrate pharmacoresistance. This is a point on which there seems to be the widest divergence of opinion. The spectrum of opinion goes from using two major drugs at the maximal tolerated dose (Schmidt, 1986) to using four major drugs and six combinations of these four drugs, which amounts to a total of 10 trial periods (D.M. Treiman, pers. comm.). In the case of partial-onset seizures, which are the ones most likely to be considered for surgery, there are now five major drugs that are considered equally effective.

In the first Veterans Administration collaborative study (Mattson *et al.*, 1985), carbamazepine, phenytoin, phenobarbital and primidone were found to be equally effective in terms of seizure control. Valproate was shown to be as effective in untreated patients when it was compared with phenytoin (Turnbull *et al.*, 1982) or with carbamazepine and phenytoin (Callaghan *et al.*, 1985). In the second Veterans Administration collaborative study (Mattson *et al.*, 1992), valproate and carbamazepine were shown to be about equally effective. When scores of efficacy and toxicity were considered, carbamazepine and phenytoin fared better than the other three drugs. Thus, the absolute minimal requirement for demonstrating intractability would be failure of carbamazepine and phenytoin in monotherapy at the maximal tolerated dose. Beyond that, the next step would be a trial with valproate, preferably in monotherapy because of both the cumulative toxicity that is seen with drug combinations and the fact that high levels of valproate are difficult to achieve in the presence of carbamazepine and phenytoin. However, in a group of patients in whom carbamazepine, phenytoin, phenobarbital and primidone had failed, only one patient became seizure-free with valproate therapy (Dasheiff *et al.*, 1986). Many physicians will still want to try phenobarbital before labelling a patient as pharmacoresistant. In that case, primidone should be considered instead of phenobarbital. The reason is that primidone is converted to phenobarbital. A failure of primidone at the maximal tolerated dose most probably implies that phenobarbital would also have failed. The opposite is less certain. It has been demonstrated repeatedly in animal experiments that primidone provides seizure protection in the absence of phenobarbital and that primidone probably also has a different mechanism of action (Bourgeois *et al.*, 1983). A difference between phenobarbital treatment and primidone treatment could never be demonstrated clearly in patients with epilepsy. Of two studies comparing the efficacy of primidone and phenobarbital therapy at similar phenobarbital levels, one suggested equal efficacy (Oleson & Dam, 1967), whereas the other suggested that therapy with primidone was slightly more effective (Oxley *et al.*, 1980). Giving primidone the benefit of the doubt, one could consider that using primidone instead of phenobarbital could save one therapeutic step in the establishment of pharmacoresistance of partial onset seizures. Beyond the major drugs, so far there is no evidence to suggest that the use of secondary drugs will bring a success that could not be achieved (Dasheiff *et al.*, 1986). However, the concept of the number of drugs to be included will soon have to be re-evaluated when new antiepileptic drugs are introduced. The exact role of such drugs as felbamate, vigabatrin, gabapentin and lamotrigine remains to be established.

A question that may arise is whether a major drug should be tried again in monotherapy, if it has been tried previously only in combination with another drug. It may be advisable to do so for two reasons. First, the neurotoxicity of two antiepileptic drugs is most probably additive (Bourgeois & Dodson, 1988). Secondly, the efficacy of a drug can be impaired by pharmacokinetic interactions. For instance, the maximal tolerated level of carbamazepine might be lower in the presence of phenobarbital or phenytoin. Also, the elimination half-life of carbamazepine is shortened by phenobarbital and by phenytoin, resulting in wider fluctuations of the levels from dose to dose, with higher peak levels and lower trough levels in relation to the average concentrations. If the peak levels are to be kept below values that cause side-effects, the highest tolerated average concentration will be lower during combination therapy than during carbamazepine monotherapy.

Is it necessary to use combinations of antiepileptic drugs in order to demonstrate intractability for the purpose of experimental antiepileptic drug trials or epilepsy surgery? There is probably no scientific answer to this question. In order to justify the inclusion of drug combinations, one would have to clearly demonstrate that certain combinations, at the maximal tolerated dose of both medications, can provide complete seizure control that could not be achieved with either drug alone, also at the maximal tolerated dose. In other words, the pharmacodynamic interaction should provide a better therapeutic index than either drug alone. Experimental studies on pharmacodynamic interactions between drugs suggest that most antiepileptic interactions are additive and not supra-additive (Bourgeois & Dodson, 1988). Neurotoxic interactions may be either additive or infra-additive. Among the major drugs against partial-onset seizures, only the association of valproate with carbamazepine or with phenytoin appears to be beneficial according to this animal model. Against absence seizures, the combination of valproate with ethosuximide is potentially advantageous (Bourgeois, 1988). Clinical studies in patients with partial-onset seizures all suggest only limited success for combinations when appropriate monotherapy has failed, with significant improvement seen only in 10–15 per cent of patients (Schmidt, 1982; Mattson *et al.*, 1985; Reynolds, 1987). Unfortunately, the figures are not very different for a second drug in monotherapy after a first adequate monotherapy trial has failed (Schmidt & Richter, 1986).

Finally, there are several reasons why the process of establishing pharmacoresistance should be as short as possible. Firstly, if the patient is not truly medically intractable, the successful therapeutic step will occur sooner or experimental antiepileptic drugs can be tried earlier. Secondly, in a patient who becomes seizure-free after surgery, the long-term psychosocial outcome is likely to be better if the surgery is performed earlier. This is particularly true for the crucial formative years of adolescence and early adulthood. Thirdly, it is suspected that the seizure reduction following epilepsy surgery is enhanced by early intervention. Finally, there are data suggesting that a cognitive improvement following surgery is more likely if the interval between onset of the epilepsy and surgery is shorter (Meyer *et al.*, 1986).

A time span of about 2 years between the onset of the epilepsy and the establishment of pharmacoresistance is a desirable and realistic goal in a persistently refractory patient. Experience has shown that seizure control is seldom achieved in a patient who continues to have seizures after 2 years of adequate therapy. In a group of 21 refractory patients, Reynolds (1987) was able to demonstrate that pharmacoresistance was established within 2 years in 19 patients. In current practice, however, most patients who are operated have had epilepsy for over 10 years. Of course, the time required to establish pharmacoresistance varies substantially from one patient to the next. It will be relatively short in patients with frequent seizures who show little or no response to any drug. Inversely, it will be relatively long in patients with a low seizure frequency and prolonged remissions after drug changes. In any case, drug changes and dosage increases should never be delayed whenever it becomes apparent that the present drug regimen is not successful.

References

Bourgeois, B.F.D. (1988): Combination of valproate and ethosuximide: antiepileptic and neurotoxic interaction. *J. Pharmacol. Exp. Ther.* **247,** 1128–1132.

Bourgeois, B.F.D. & Dodson, W.E. (1988): Antiepileptic and neurotoxic interactions between antiepileptic drugs. In: *Antiepileptic drug interactions*, ed. W.H. Pitlick, pp. 209–218. New York: Demos.

Bourgeois, B.F.D., Dodson, W.E. & Ferrendelli, J.A. (1983): Primidone, phenobarbital and PEMA: seizure protection, neurotoxicity and therapeutic index of individual compounds in mice. *Neurology* **33,** 283–290.

Callaghan, N., Kenny, R.A., O'Neill, B., Crowley, M. & Goggin, T. (1985): A prospective study between carbamazepine, phenytoin and sodium valproate as monotherapy in previously untreated and recently diagnosed patients with epilepsy. *J. Neurol. Neurosurg. Psychiatry* **48,** 639–644.

Cobos, J.E. (1987): High-dose phenytoin in the treatment of refractory epilepsy. *Epilepsia* **28,** 111–114.

Cramer, J.A., Smith, D.B., Mattson, R.H., Delgado-Escueta, A.V. & Collins, J.F. (1983): A method of quantification for the evaluation of antiepileptic drug therapy. *Neurology* **33** (suppl. 1), 26–37.

Dasheiff, R.M., McNamara, D. & Dickinson, L.V. (1986): Efficacy of second line antiepileptic drugs in the treatment of patients with medically refractive complex partial seizures. *Epilepsia* **27,** 124–127.

Janz, D. (1978): Über Pharmakoresistenz in der Epilepsiebehandlung. *Dtsch. Med. Wochenschr.* **41,** 1612–1619.

King, D.W., Flanigin, H.F., Gallagher, B.B., So, E.L., Murvin, A.J., Smith, D.B., Oommen, K.J., Feldman, D.S. & Power, J. (1986): Temporal lobectomy for partial complex seizures: evaluation, results, and 1-year follow-up. *Neurology* **36,** 334–339.

Lesser, R.P., Pippenger, C.E., Lüders, H. & Dinner, D.S. (1984): High-dose monotherapy in the treatment of intractable seizures. *Neurology* **34,** 707–711.

Mattson, R.H., Cramer, J.A., Collins, J.F., Smith, D.B., Delgado-Escueta, A.V., Browne, T.R., Williamson, P.D., Treiman, D.M., McNamara, J.O., McCutchen, C.B., Homan, R.W., Crill, W.E., Lubozynski, M.F., Rosenthal, N.P. & Mayersdorf, A.s (1985): Comparison of carbamazepine, phenobarbital, phenytoin and primidone in partial and secondarily generalized tonic–clonic seizures. *N. Engl. J. Med.* **313,** 145–151.

Mattson, R.H., Cramer, J.A., Collins, J.F. and the Department of Veterans Affairs Epilepsy Cooperative Study No. 264 Group (1992): A comparison of valproate with carbamazepine for the treatment of complex partial seizures and secondarily generalized tonic–clonic seizures in adults. *N. Engl. J. Med.* **327,** 765–771.

Meyer, F.B., Marsh, W.R., Laws, E.R. & Sharbrough, F.W. (1986): Temporal lobectomy in children with epilepsy. *J. Neurosurg.* **64,** 371–376.

Oleson, O.V. & Dam, M. (1967): The metabolic conversion of primidone to phenobarbitone in patients under long-term treatment. *Acta Neurol. Scand.* **43,** 348–356.

Oxley, J., Hebdige, S., Laidlaw, J., Wadsworth, J. & Richens, A. (1980): A comparative study of phenobarbitone and primidone in the treatment of epilepsy. In: *Antiepileptic therapy: advances in drug monitoring*, eds. S.I. Johannessen, P.L. Morselli, C.E. Pippenger, A. Richens, D. Schmidt & H. Meinardi, pp. 237–245. New York: Raven Press.

Reynolds, E.H. (1987): Early treatment and prognosis of epilepsy. *Epilepsia* **28,** 97–106.

Rodin, E., Klutke, G. & Chayasirisobohn, S. (1982): Epileptic patients who are refractory to anticonvulsant medications. *Neurology* **32,** 1382–1384.

Schmidt, D. (1982): Two antiepileptic drugs for intractable epilepsy with complex-partial seizures. *J. Neurol. Neurosurg. Psychiatry* **45,** 1119–1124.

Schmidt, D. (1986): Diagnostic and therapeutic management of intractable epilepsy. In: *Intractable epilepsy*, eds. D. Schmidt & P.L. Morselli, pp. 237–257. New York: Raven Press.

Schmidt, D. & Richter, K. (1986): Alternative single anticonvulsant drug therapy for refractory epilepsy. *Ann. Neurol.* **19,** 85–87.

Turnbull, D.M., Rawlings, M.D. Weightman, D. & Chadwick, D.W. (1982): A comparison of phenytoin and valproate in previously untreated adult epileptic patients. *J. Neurol. Neurosurg. Psychiat.* **45,** 55–59.

Epileptic Seizures and Syndromes, Edited by Peter Wolf
© 1994 John Libbey & Company Ltd., pp. 599–603

Chapter 59

Mechanisms of intractability

Edward H. Reynolds

Institute of Epileptology, Maudsley and King's College Hospitals, Denmark Hill, London SE5 8AZ, UK

Changing view of epilepsy prognosis

When I was training in neurology during the 1960s the question of how epilepsy became intractable was, to my knowledge, never asked either clinically or experimentally. This may be because at that time epilepsy was widely perceived to be chronic in most patients. In 1968 Rodin published his authoritative monograph which reviewed the literature on prognosis over nearly a century, from Gowers (1881) to his own studies. Rodin concluded that only about a third of epileptic patients were likely to achieve a terminal remission of at least 2 years; that the longer patients were followed up the more likely they were to have a relapse; and that four-fifths of all patients with epilepsy were likely to have a chronic seizure disorder. He regarded epilepsy as a chronic condition with remissions and exacerbations. The view at that time was that the drugs available, which included phenobarbitone and phenytoin, were not powerful enough to suppress what was regarded as severe and chronic epilepsy in most patients.

In the last two decades there has been a considerable change in our perspective of the prognosis of epilepsy. Elsewhere I have reviewed the new community- and hospital-based studies, which suggest that no more than one-quarter to one-third of newly diagnosed patients go on to develop chronic epilepsy (Elwes & Reynolds, 1990; Reynolds, 1990). Has there been a revolution in the treatment of epilepsy in these two decades which could explain such a remarkably better prognosis? I rather doubt it, even though there have been improvements in management, for example, some new drugs, the application of drug monitoring and a more rational approach to treatment, e.g. less polytherapy. Our own and other studies have recently shown that some of the newer drugs are no more efficacious in controlling seizures than phenobarbitone and phenytoin (Mattson *et al.*, 1985; Heller *et al.*, 1989; De Silva *et al.,* 1989).

Why does epilepsy become intractable?

As a result of our own hospital-based prospective studies of the treatment of newly diagnosed epileptic patients in the 1970s, which showed a surprisingly good prognosis (Reynolds *et al.*, 1976; Shorvon *et al.*, 1978; Elwes *et al.*, 1984), my colleagues and I first began to consider the question: why do the minority of patients go on to develop chronic intractable epilepsy (Reynolds *et al.*, 1983; Shorvon 1984)? The standard and traditional view then and now is the notion that this subgroup has more 'severe' epilepsy, too severe for currently available drugs to suppress the seizures. However, we considered an alternative or additional possibility that chronicity was not inevitable, that epilepsy should be viewed as a process and that to some extent intractable epilepsy might be prevented by earlier more effective treatment (Shorvon & Reynolds, 1982; Reynolds, 1987, 1989). This idea owed something to Gowers (1881), who showed that the longer the history of epilepsy the worse the prognosis, and who proposed that seizures might beget further seizures. Gowers' tentative views, long since forgotten and for which admittedly he had little evidence, were totally overshadowed by the views of his colleague Jackson, which were later reinforced by Berger's discovery of electroencephalography (EEG), that seizures represented neuronal discharges which needed suppressing.

Factors contributing to intractability

Both the older studies of patients with chronic epilepsy (Rodin, 1968) and more recent studies of newly diagnosed patients (Okuma & Kumashiro, 1981; Elwes *et al.*, 1984; Beghi & Tognoni, 1988) show that certain factors have an adverse influence on long-term prognosis. These include partial or mixed seizure types (as compared with tonic–clonic seizures); symptomatic epilepsy; clinical or computed tomographic evidence of cerebral disease; and intellectual handicap, psychiatric illness, personality change or social problems. Older age, a family history of epilepsy and severe background or 'epileptiform' abnormalities on EEG are less certain indicators of a poorer prognosis. In this chapter I am concerned with additional factors related to the concept of a process of epilepsy leading to intractability and sometimes to remission.

The process of epilepsy

Our own prospective studies of newly diagnosed epilepsy confirmed that the longer seizures continued after the start of treatment, the worse the subsequent prognosis (Elwes *et al.*, 1984), as had also been noted by Rodin (1968) in studies of chronic patients. In examining the possible reasons why 21 of the first 106 newly diagnosed patients we studied developed chronic epilepsy, poor compliance with treatment and the presence of brain pathology stood out as the most significant factors (Chesterman *et al.*, 1987).

One of the difficulties in examining the question of the influence of antiepileptic drugs on the prognosis of epilepsy is that we know so little about the natural history of *untreated* epilepsy. For ethical reasons there have been no placebo-controlled studies of treatment in newly diagnosed patients. Because prospective studies of untreated patients are questionable, Elwes *et al.* (1988) attempted a limited retrospective study in patients presenting to the neurology department at King's College Hospital with between two and five untreated tonic–clonic seizures. They examined the time intervals between each seizure in 183 patients in whom it was possible to accurately date the attacks. This was possible in many patients presenting with the more dramatic tonic–clonic seizures but is rarely possible in patients presenting with partial seizures, many of which are uncountable or even unknown to the patient. Overall, they found a steadily declining time interval between attacks, whether patients presented with three, four or five seizures. In only 20 per cent of patients were there examples of increased intervals between two successive time periods. Such a study has several methodological weaknesses related to its retrospective hospital-based nature, dictated by ethical considerations. Nevertheless, the findings are in keeping with the concept of an escalating process of epilepsy, at least in its early stages, and again emphasize the need to find some way of examining the issues prospectively.

In the last decade my colleagues and I have undertaken two separate prospective studies of the comparative efficacy and toxicity of four major antiepileptic drugs (phenobarbitone, phenytoin, carbamazepine and sodium valproate) in 243 adults and 167 children with newly diagnosed previously untreated epilepsy (at least two tonic–clonic ± partial seizures) (De Silva *et al.*, 1989; Heller *et al.*, 1989). In both studies we found no significant differences in efficacy between the four drugs and, as previously noted, the overall prognosis with each of the drugs was very good in both adults and children. By combining the data from each of the four drug groups we were able to examine those factors other than drug therapy which influence long-term prognosis (Reynolds *et al.*, 1989). Remarkably, in both adults and children, the most significant prognostic factor was the number of seizures prior to treatment; the more untreated seizures the worse the prognosis, as measured either by time to first seizure recurrence after treatment, or by number of patients entering 1 year remission (see Reynolds, 1991). We were also able to show that the phenomenon can be demonstrated for tonic–clonic or partial seizures alone respectively. As might be expected, we also found that the *frequency* of seizures prior to the start of treatment was an important influence on prognosis. The more frequent the attacks the worse the prognosis, but this factor was less important than the *number* of seizures.

In contrast to Gowers (1881), Rodin (1968) and Elwes *et al.* (1984), Feksi *et al.* (1991) suggest that the duration of epilepsy does not influence the outcome of treatment. This conclusion, in the context of a comparative trial of phenobarbitone and carbamazepine for 12 months, in a previously largely untreated population of patients in a primary health-care setting in East Africa, is based simply on dividing their patients into two groups, with more than or less than 5 years of epilepsy. This should be interpreted with some caution, all the more so as the data were collected retrospectively by many health-care workers from poorly educated patients with a mean duration of epilepsy of 7 years.

Two recent prospective controlled trials of treatment against no treatment of a first unprovoked seizure suggest that treatment significantly reduces the risk of recurrence. Chandra (1992) randomized 228 patients either to sodium valproate or placebo. The code was broken after a second seizure and placebo patients were then given sodium valproate. After 12 months the recurrence rate was 4.3 per cent in the treatment group and 55.7 per cent in the placebo group. In an Italian multicentre study Musicco *et al.* (1993) randomised 397 patients to either treatment or no treatment. Again, treatment was instituted in the no-treatment group after a recurrence. After 24 months the cumulative time-dependent risk of relapse was 25 per cent in the treated group and 51 per cent in the untreated subjects. The risk of relapse was 2.8 times higher for untreated subjects. The possibility that drug treatment influences the natural history of epilepsy as well as suppressing seizures is supported by the observation of the MRC Antiepileptic Drug Withdrawal Study Group (1991) that the most important factor determining outcome was the duration of seizure freedom: the longer the control of epilepsy, the lower the risk of recurrence on drug withdrawal. The possible mechanisms of the process of remission in epilepsy (Reynolds, 1991) are not the subject of this review.

Relevance of kindling

Is the process of evolving epilepsy which I have discussed related in any way to the phenomenon of kindling (Reynolds, 1989)? There must be some doubt about this if kindling is defined strictly in terms of the experimental (and possible clinical) effects of repeated subclinical stimuli which culminate in the occurrence of the first seizure. The events I have been concerned with occur after the first seizure. Is this an extension of kindling or a completely different phenomenon? Although recurrent spontaneous seizures have been described in the kindling model in some species, this aspect seems to have received less attention. Furthermore, for the most part kindling studies are undertaken in animals which are not genetically predisposed to spontaneous seizures, whereas a genetic background of varying degree is widely suspected in clinical epilepsy.

For the time being it seems appropriate to consider the process of epilepsy as separate and distinct from kindling, even though the analogies between the two are readily apparent and probably would have fascinated Gowers. Both take a longitudinal view of seizure processes over time. In the case of kindling it is the impact of suitably spaced successive subclinical stimuli (SSSSS) that is the key. In the Gowers process we are concerned with the effect of suitably spaced successive seizures (SSSS). Exactly how each stimulus leaves its mark on the nervous system in kindling is unknown, but if a subclinical stimulus can leave its unidentified but undoubted imprint is it not reasonable to suppose that a seizure itself can do something similar (Reynolds, 1988, 1989)? Perhaps both phenomena have more in common with memory and learning. In the former the brain is 'learning' to develop a seizure, in the latter 'learning' to have more seizures. In both processes 'inhibitory' phenomena come into play, which is why the spacing of the stimuli or the seizures is important.

Conclusion

The traditional view of intractability, which can be traced to Jackson and Berger, suggests that drug treatment is not powerful enough to suppress the seizure discharges in patients with more 'severe' forms of epilepsy, e.g. due to brain lesions. An alternative or additional view, which I have outlined here, is that epilepsy should be viewed as a process with the potential in some patients to evolve into intractability. According to this view, chronicity is not inevitable and the potential exists to some degree to influence the natural history and to prevent intractability by early effective treatment to 'arrest' (Gowers) the process.

References

Beghi, E. & Tognoni, G. (1988): Prognosis of epilepsy in newly referred patients: a multi-center prospective study. *Epilepsia* **29,** 236–243.

Chandra, B. (1992): First seizure in adults: to treat or not to treat. *Clin. Neurol. Neurosurg.* **94**(suppl.), S61–S63.

Chesterman, P., Elwes, R.D.C. & Reynolds. E.H. (1987): Failure of monotherapy in newly diagnosed epilepsy. In: *The XVIth Epilepsy International Symposium: Advances in Epileptology,* Vol. 16, eds. P. Wolf, M. Dam, D. Janz & F.E. Dreifuss, pp. 461–464. New York: Raven Press.

De Silva, M., McArdle, B., McGowan, M., Neville, B.G.R., Johnson, A.L. & Reynolds, E.H. (1989): Monotherapy for newly diagnosed childhood epilepsy: a comparative trial and prognostic evaluation. *Epilepsia* **30,** 662.

Elwes, R.D.C. & Reynolds E.H. (1990): The early prognosis of epilepsy. In: *Comprehensive epileptology,* eds. M. Dam & L. Gram, pp. 715–727. New York: Raven Press.

Elwes, R.D.C., Johnson, A.L., Shorvon, S.D. & Reynolds, E.H. (1984): The prognosis for seizure control in newly diagnosed epilepsy. *N. Engl. J. Med.* **311,** 944–947.

Elwes, R.D.C., Johnson, A.L. & Reynolds, E.H. (1988): The course of untreated epilepsy. *Brit. Med. J.* **297,** 948–950.

Feksi, A.T., Kaamugisha, J., Sander, J.W.A.S., Gatiti, S. & Shorvon, S.D. (1991): A prospective study of antiepileptic drug treatment in a primary health setting in East Africa, in a previously largely untreated population. *Lancet* **337,** 406–409.

Gowers, W.R. (1881): *Epilepsy and other chronic convulsive disorders.* London: Churchill.

Heller, A.J., Chesterman, P., Elwes, R.D.C., Crawford, P., Chadwick, D., Johnson, A.L. & Reynolds, E.H. (1989): Monotherapy for newly diagnosed adult epilepsy: a comparative trial and prognostic evaluation. *Epilepsia* **30,** 648.

Mattson, R.H., Cramer, J.A., Collins, J.F. *et al.* (1985): Comparison of carbamazepine, phenobarbital, phenytoin and primidone in partial and secondarily generalised tonic–clonic seizures. *N. Engl. J. Med.* **313,** 145–151.

MRC Antiepileptic Drug Withdrawal Study Group (1991): Randomised study of antiepileptic drug withdrawal in patients in remission. *Lancet* **337,** 1175–1180.

Okuma, T. & Kumashiro, H. (1981): Natural history and prognosis of epilepsy: report of a multi-institutional study in Japan. *Epilepsia* **22,** 35–53.

Musicco, M., Beghi, E., Bordo, B. & Viani, F. (1993): A randomized clinical trial on the efficacy of antiepileptic drugs in reducing the risk of relapse after a first unprovoked tonic–clonic seizure. *Neurology* **43,** 478–483.

Reynolds, E.H. (1987): Early treatment and prognosis of epilepsy. *Epilepsia* **28,** 97–106.

Reynolds, E.H. (1988): The prevention of chronic epilepsy. *Epilepsia* **29** (Suppl. 1), S25–28.

Reynolds, E.H. (1989): The process of epilepsy. In: *The clinical relevance of kindling,* eds. T. Bolwig & M.R. Trimble, pp. 149–160. Chichester: John Wiley.

Reynolds, E.H. (1990): Changing view of epilepsy prognosis. *Br. Med. J.* **301,** 1112–1114.

Reynolds, E.H. (1991): The influence of antiepileptic drugs on the natural history of epilepsy. In: *New antiepileptic drugs,* eds. F. Pisani, E. Perucca, G. Avanzini & A. Richens, pp. 15–19. Amsterdam: Elsevier.

Reynolds, E.H., Chadwick, D. & Galbraith, A.W. (1976): One drug (phenytoin) in the treatment of epilepsy. *Lancet* **i,** 923–926.

Reynolds, E.H., Elwes, R.D.C. & Shorvon, S.D. (1983): Why does epilepsy become intractable? Prevention of chronic epilepsy. *Lancet* **ii,** 952–954.

Reynolds, E.H., Heller, A.J., Elwes, R.D.C. *et al.* (1989): Factors influencing prognosis of newly diagnosed epilepsy. *Epilepsia* **30,** 648.

Rodin, E.A. (1968): *The prognosis of patients with epilepsy.* Springfield, Illinois: Charles C. Thomas.

Shorvon, S.D. (1984): The temporal aspects of prognosis in epilepsy. *J. Neurol. Neurosurg. Psychiatry* **47,** 1157–1165.

Shorvon, S.D. & Reynolds, E.H. (1982): Early prognosis of epilepsy. *Br. Med. J.* **285,** 1699–1701.

Shorvon, S.D., Chadwick, D., Galbraith, A.W. & Reynolds, E.H. (1978): One drug for epilepsy. *Br. Med. J.* **i,** 474–476.

Epileptic Seizures and Syndromes, Edited by Peter Wolf
© 1994 John Libbey & Company Ltd., pp. 605–617

Chapter 60

Strategies for analysing the generation and causes of drug-resistant seizures in temporal lobe epilepsy

Uwe Heinemann

Inst. Neurophysiology, Ctr. Physiology and Pathophysiology, University of Cologne, Robert Kochstr. 39, 50931 Köln, Germany

During the course of their disease about 10–20 per cent of epileptic patients turn out to be resistant against currently available antiepileptic drugs even when excellent patient compliance is provided. As a result many centres in the United States, and now increasingly also in Europe, have developed epilepsy surgery programmes. However, not all patients are suitable for such treatment. Surgery is, in addition, not without risks for the patients. Therefore strategies have to be developed which not only increase the likelihood that new anticonvulsants improve quality of life by improving seizure control with fewer side-effects but also prevent progression of epilepsies into a pharmacoresistant state. Drugs are also required which provide seizure control for such patients.

In order to understand the processes underlying development of drug-resistant epilepsies, it must be remembered that many of these epilepsies start in childhood, that they are often treated with concepts derived from the treatment of epilepsies in adulthood and that currently available drugs prevent neither generation of epilepsies after lesions nor progression of epilepsy. In discussing possible approaches to the understanding of the generation of drug-resistant seizures, I will concentrate on temporal lobe seizures (TLE). These are among the most frequent seizure types and presumably they contribute most to drug-resistant seizures.

The fact that some seizures are resistant to currently available drugs could indicate that the mode of ictogenesis in drug-resistant epilepsies differs from that in treatable forms of epilepsies. This implies that there is more than one mode of ictogenesis. Indeed, we had recently to accept that seizures have in common only that neuronal activity is strongly synchronized during ictal episodes. However, the mode and mechanisms of this synchronization differ among seizure types. Based on physiological and pharmacological characteristics, one can suggest at least two different modes of generation of fits: primarily generalized non-convulsive seizures, predominantly of thalamocortical origin, and focal or primarily and secondarily generalized convulsive seizures, which depend on the generation of high-frequency discharges in a large population of neurones.

Primarily generalized non-convulsive seizures

These respond pharmacologically to dimethadione (DMO), ethosuximide (ESM) and valproic acid (VPA). All these agents have in common that they reduce T-type Ca^{2+} currents (Coulter *et al.*, 1989; Rogawski & Porter, 1990). These channels are strongly expressed in the thalamus, in the inferior olive and, to some extent, also in the neocortex (Llinás & Yarom, 1981; Jahnsen & Llinás, 1984). In the thalamus they are strongly involved in physiological mechanisms of rhythmogenesis. The T-type Ca^{2+} channels have three states. They are inactivated at membrane potentials above –50 mV. The inactivation can be removed by hyperpolarization. Upon return to resting membrane potential, they become activated and generate a low-threshold Ca^{2+} spike. This provides the excitatory drive for generation of Na^+-dependent propagating action potentials (Deschenes *et al.*, 1984). These drive not only neocortical neurones but also γ-aminobutyric acidergic (GABA-ergic) cells in the nucleus reticularis thalami (Huguenard & Prince, 1992). The cells in this nucleus are all GABA-ergic and provide recurrent GABA- A- and GABA-B-mediated synaptic inhibition in a relatively large number of thalamocortical projection cells. A burst of action potentials in thalamocortical relay cells is therefore followed by a prolonged GABA-A- and GABA-B-mediated inhibitory postsynaptic potential (IPSP) (Avanzini *et al.*, 1989; Huguenard & Prince, 1992). During the inhibition, an inward rectifying current is activated with slow deactivation properties (McCormick & Pape, 1990). It drives the membrane potential to levels where the T-type Ca^{2+} channels open. In this type of network a hyperpolarizing event can therefore produce a series of spontaneous Ca^{2+} spike–IPSP sequences, which are readily synchronized throughout the thalamus due to the fact that the IPSP is generated in more cells than the one which initially produced a burst discharge (Andersen & Anderson, 1968).

There are various principal mechanisms by which these primarily generalized seizures can be prevented.

– Blockade of the T-type Ca^{2+} currents, as is currently done in the treatment of such seizures.
– Blockade of the slow IPSPs. This can be accomplished most effectively by agents which reduce the generation of slow IPSPs (Snead *et al.*, 1990). There are now drugs available which block GABA-B-mediated slow IPSPs and these seem to be effective in blocking experimental forms of primarily generalized absence seizures. Agents which block the activation of thalamocortical relay cells might also be effective. These could involve GABA receptor agonists which often inhibit inhibitory neurones effectively.
– Blockade of the inward rectifying current, which is sensitive to Cs^+ and to a number of catecholamines (Pape & McCormick, 1989).

– Finally the membrane potential of thalamocortical relay cells might be a target itself. The activation of T-type Ca^{2+} currents is dependent on the membrane potential of thalamocortical relay cells and such an activation does not occur when the membrane potential is held above –50 mV. It is likely that increases in vigilance shift the membrane potential of thalamocortical relay cells in a depolarizing direction. Such increases in vigilance are well known to interfere with the generation of absence seizures.

Modulation of GABA-B-receptor-mediated actions and of inward rectifying currents has some potential which might lead to drugs with fewer side-effects than those currently employed in the treatment of primarily generalized non-convulsive seizures.

Occasionally the non-convulsive primarily generalized seizures develop, especially during adolescence, into forms where convulsive seizures emerge as a result of the rhythmic activity and where, therefore, convulsive and non-convulsive seizures coexist. This suggests that absence or petit mal seizures can be progressive in themselves. The general assumption is that neurodegenerative and kindling-like effects are only brought about by intense stimulation. However, long-term potentiation, such as augmentation of synaptic transmission can also be induced by patterned stimulation (Engstrom *et al.*, 1990). Chemical kindling with pentylenetetrazole (PTZ) is produced with subconvulsive concentrations (Barkai *et al.*, 1990). Such concentrations can nevertheless produce absence-like seizures (Snead *et al.*, 1992).

For the transition of non-convulsive into convulsive seizures it has to be remembered that the thalamus in spite of its large rhythmogenic potential, is readily recruited into cortical seizures. Studies with penicillin foci and cortical electrical stimulation show that such driving is dependent on feedback from the neocortex into the thalamus (Gutnick *et al.*, 1979; Heinemann & Gutnick, 1979; Snead *et al.*, 1992). While afferent stimulation to the thalamus evokes only small rises in $[K^+]_o$, large rises accompany seizures in the neocortex. These easily corrupt GABA-B-mediated IPSPs. The latter depend on a long-lasting activation of K^+ currents. Upon extracellular potassium accumulation these GABA-B-mediated IPSPs provide, in the presence of increased extracellular potassium, a depolarizing drive which might well contribute to the ictogenesis (Rausche *et al.*, 1989) and explain some of the proconvulsant effects of GABA-B receptor agonists such as baclofen.

The fact that GABA-A receptors are the target sites for steroid hormones raises the possibility that stress conditions and circadian variations in such hormone levels and the increase in sexual hormone concentrations accompanying puberty promote transition from absence seizures to convulsive fits (Smith *et al.*, 1987).

Convulsive seizures of focal origin

Circumscribed alterations in the balance between excitation and inhibition will eventually lead to generation of focal seizures (Prince, 1978; Heinemann & Jones, 1989). Experimentally this can be achieved by blockade of GABA-A-mediated inhibition (Curtis *et al.*, 1970), by augmentation of excitatory synaptic transmission (Walther *et al.*, 1986) or by blockade of potassium currents (Baranyi & Feher, 1979). Between seizures, such foci are characterized by interictal spikes which are due to synchronized generation of unitary depolarizations (paroxysmal depolarization shifts, PDS) to –30 mV, lasting between 50 and 300 ms in a given neuronal aggregate (Matsumoto & Ajmone-Marsan, 1964). The generation of such PDS seems to depend on the release of intrinsic pacemaker cells from synaptic control (Traub *et al.*, 1987). Pacemaker cells are located in area CA3 (Wong & Prince, 1978) and layer 4/5 of the neocortex (Gutnick *et al.*, 1982). These cells produce intrinsic burst discharges upon activation and recruit synaptically neighbouring and follower cells. The recruitment and synchronization of follower cells vary with the underlying cause of the seizures. In the neocortex, superficial cells are less likely to participate in PDS when the underlying disturbance preserves synaptic inhibition (E. Barkai & M.J. Gutnick, in prep.). However, repetitive stimulation also causes in these conditions earlier or later reduction in the efficacy of synaptic inhibition and recruitment into paroxysmal activity (Thompson & Gähwiler, 1989a, b, c).

Seizures emerge from such activity only when additional excitatory feed-back develops. This may depend on independent electrogenesis in the dendrites (Traub *et al.*, 1993), in presynaptic terminals (Gutnick & Prince, 1972) or on backfiring from a follower aggregate into the focus. The seizures in such conditions are characterized by sustained depolarizations of the neuronal membranes, by high-frequency firing and, due to the increased neuronal activity, also changes of the neuronal microenvironment (Heinemann & Jones, 1989). $[K^+]_o$ can rise to levels near 10 mM in the neocortex and near 12 mM in the hippocampus and entorhinal cortex (EC). The seizures are associated with marked decreases in $[Ca^{2+}]_o$ and $[Na^+]_o$ as well as in the size of the extracellular space. Smaller decreases in the order of up to 0.3 mM can also be observed in the $[Mg^{2+}]_o$ (Lux *et al.*, 1986). Mimicking such changes precipitates seizure activity in hippocampal area CA1, suggesting that changes in the extracellular microenvironment contribute to ictogenesis (Traynelis & Dingledine, 1988). Also the slow negative field potentials due to sustained inward currents into neurones and spatial glial buffering can contribute to ictogenesis (Jefferys, 1981). Convulsant activity of this type responds either to agents which reduce repetitive firing by interfering with Na^+ channels (phenytoin

epileptiform activity in superficial layers of the EC and in the dentate gyrus (Walther *et al.*, 1986). If this filter function fails there is a great risk that epileptiform activity will build up to intense levels of activity. This is further supported by the fact that discharges generated in area CA3 find an augmenting potential already in area CA1. The subiculum and the EC are multiply interconnected, which might help to build up very intense seizures, particularly if this recurrent synaptic excitatory loop is strengthened. A strong recurrent excitation in the deep layers of medial and lateral EC could further amplify the seizure activity. Thus, once seizure activity passes though the dentate gyrus with little attenuation, the risk of reverberating activity through the EC–dentate gyrus–hippocampus and subiculum circuitry is very strong and it may build up to levels no longer controllable by the currently available drugs. The limit may not necessarily be caused by a qualitative failure of these anticonvulsants. Instead, concentrations of anticonvulsants sufficient to control such intense discharges may not be achieved, due to problems with drug toleration by the patients because of heavy systemic side-effects. Other drugs with a similar therapeutic profile but fewer side-effects could, thus, very well be effective in the treatment of currently pharmacoresistent epilepsies. There is hope that some of the new agents now becoming available will meet these requirements.

The fact that the interconnectivity in the hippocampal formation favours build-up of epileptiform activity has led to the search for abnormal connectivity. Particularly in the dentate gyrus, it has been shown that human TLE is associated with sprouting of mossy fibres (Babb *et al.*, 1991). If these were to innervate granule cells, a considerable increase in excitatory connectivity might develop (Sutula *et al.*, 1988; Represa *et al.*, 1990). Moreover, reductions in the number of mossy cells, which are part of the inhibitory control over activity propagated through the dentate gyrus, may be involved in a failure of gate control in the dentate gyrus (Sloviter, 1983, 1987). Changes in input resistance, alterations in NMDA receptor-mediated synaptic transmission and changes in the long-term efficacy of GABA-ergic synaptic transmission might also contribute (Mody & Heinemann, 1987; Mody *et al.*, 1988). A failure of feedforward inhibition might also occur in the hippocampal area CA1 (Bekenstein & Lothman, 1991). Indeed, a number of such alterations are also observed in tissue from patients with TLE (Babb *et al.*, 1991, 1992).

More recently we were able to show that SLEs propagate readily from the EC into the hippocampus proper if slices are prepared from juvenile animals (T. Gloveli, D. Albrecht & C.L. Zhang, in prep.). It might well be that the excitatory connections from the EC to area CA1 and CA3 are over-expressed in juvenile animals. During ontogenesis the precise patterns of innervation are not fully mature. Therefore one could imagine that abnormal connectivity between the EC and the hippocampus proper present during ontogenesis might stabilize when epileptiform activity is propagated along such fibres. An example for such a stabilization of abnormal circuit properties is found in sound-induced seizures. These can be induced if a rat or a seizure-prone mouse is exposed to very intense noise during the critical period for the fine tuning of the acoustic system (Greuel *et al.*, 1988; Pierson *et al.*, 1989). That the projection from the EC to hippocampal areas CA1 and CA3 is stronger during adolescence than during adulthood is indeed likely, since the dentate gyrus is the structure in the EC–hippocampal formation which develops last and largely postnatally, while the projections from the EC have already reached the hippocampus. Stabilization of such connections by abnormal activity and preservation of more abundant recurrent connectivity in area CA1 and CA3 by early-childhood seizures could be a principle involved in the formation of more seizure-prone networks in the EC–hippocampal complex. This would show in abnormal interconnectivity in the brains of patients with TLE. Surprisingly, the possibility that recurrent collaterals in the hippocampus and projections from the EC directly to area CA1 and CA3 are augmented has so far been little investigated. Such studies should be easy in *en bloc* resected temporal lobe specimens with tracers such as DiI and DiO. If such an augmented projection existed, the propagation of epileptiform activity from the EC to the hippocampus would be altered.

A final possibility to account for an abnormal and facilitated synchronization of seizures in TLE lies in the fact that during ontogenesis horizontal cells appear transiently in the outer third of the dentate gyrus. Such cells usually decrease in numbers with adolescence but seem to be quite frequent in the post-mortem specimens of TLE patients (Meencke, 1987). During adolescence such cells do not build up effective synapses (von Haebler *et al.*, 1993). However, if these cells formed active synapses, they would also provide for a feed-forward excitatory loop in the hippocampus. Infrared videomicroscopy would help to record from such cells and see whether they are synaptically interacting with granule cells in TLE.

Abnormal GABA and glutamate receptors and abnormal ionic channels in human temporal lobe epilepsy

GABA and glutamate receptors occur in a wide variety of forms which we are now beginning to understand (Draguhn *et al.*, 1990; Keinänen *et al.*, 1990; Seeburg *et al.*, 1990; Sommer *et al.*, 1990, 1991; Verdoorn *et al.*, 1990; Herb *et al.* 1992; Monyer *et al.*, 1992; Wisden *et al.*, 1992). The same applies to ionic channels (Stühmer *et al.*, 1989; Ruppersberg *et al.*, 1990). Biophysical studies show that each of these subvarieties has distinct properties with respect to ion permeability, desensitization behaviour and pharmacological properties. Changes in the subunit combination would also affect the behaviour of the respective receptors and ionic channels. *In situ* hybridization, marking with subunit-specific antibodies, localization studies with confocal microscopy and specific pharmacological tools, such as local release of agonists by light from a caged form, would all help to understand such changes. If an abnormal receptor is formed, this would be the ideal target for a drug which would not interfere with normal neuronal function but selectively influence the behaviour of the diseased part of the tissue. An example of such an alteration would be an over-expression of GABA receptors sensitive to zinc (Stühmer *et al.*, 1989; Draguhn *et al.*, 1990; Ruppersberg *et al.*, 1990). Since the zinc content increases in the tissue of TLE patients, this might cause a failure of synaptic inhibition due to activity-dependent blockade of GABA receptors. We are at present testing this hypothesis for different GABA currents in rat hippocampal slices from normal and kindled rats.

Mechanisms involved in the generation of drug-resistant epilepsies

At present four hypotheses can be formulated which could account for the generation of pharmacoresistant epilepsy. The first would suggest that developmental abnormalities cause generation of epileptiform activity in the temporal lobe. This might stabilize abnormal connections. Indeed, during ontogenesis there is a widespread over-expression of fibres propagating from one part of the brain to the other. Such interactions are seen between the primary auditory and visual cortex, a projection absent in the brains of adult animals. Similarly, the projections from parts of the visual cortex reach more extended portions of the contralateral visual cortex in young as compared with adult animals. The tuning of the preserved fibres is usually believed to depend on successful synaptic interaction. There are many examples in the literature showing that interventions with this process may lead to abnormal stabilization of such circuitry. It may well be possible but has not yet been proved that such stabilization is an important aspect in the generation of drug-resistant epilepsies. This is comparable to the ontogenetic stabilization and fine tuning of receptive field properties for cortical neurones (Greuel *et al.*, 1988). Also the recurrent collaterals seem to decrease with adolescence. An example of such a process might be found in sound-induced seizures. Often these develop in genetically suitable animals only when exposure to abnormal sound occurs during the critical period in which the properties of the acoustic system are being fine-tuned (Pierson *et al.*, 1989). Studies in the visual system of kittens have provided evidence that such processes can be treated under favourable conditions. Thus it was documented that abnormal stabilization of neural networks in the visual system can be reversed under the influence of noradrenaline perfusion (for review see e.g. Singer, 1990).

The second hypothesis is based on the kindling hypothesis. It was shown that repetitive stimulation of limbic structures will first lead to local seizures, which recruit more and more parts of the brain until after some repetitions full-blown seizures emerge (Goddard *et al.*, 1969). This process is difficult to stop by treatments with anticonvulsant drugs and therefore provides a model of generation of drug-resistant epilepsy. Kindling is less likely to occur the higher the species under study. However, since kindling epilepsy is more readily produced during adolescence (Haas *et al.*, 1990) and in epilepsy-prone animals conditions may exist which also favour the occurrence of similar phenomena in humans.

With each stimulation a number of second-messenger systems are stimulated within the activated cells and epileptogenic stimuli also cause formation of proto-oncogenes, which in turn can activate genes inside the nucleus. With some delay, after a kindling stimulation gene products regulating cell survival and formation of axon collaterals appear (Morris *et al.*, 1988; Gall & Isackson, 1989; Isackson *et al.*, 1991). Effects have also been noted on the production of opiate peptides and on receptors for such agents. Similarly, changes in glutamate receptors have been recently reported (Gall *et al.*, 1990; Kamphuis *et al.*, 1992). As a consequence of epileptogenesis, there are also changes in the calmodulin-dependent kinase (Bronstein *et al.*, 1988, 1990) and down-regulation of calcium-binding proteins (Baimbridge & Miller, 1984). These might affect the extent to which Ca^{2+} accumulates within the cell. Increases in intracellular Ca^{2+} concentration may affect the behaviour of NMDA and GABA receptors as well as the behaviour of some ionic channels. In animal models but principally also in human brain, it is possible to determine which genes are activated and which are down-regulated during the process of epileptogenesis. This can be done by modern molecular biological techniques and would provide us with a more complete catalogue of epilepsy related genomic alterations.

Moreover, during the process of epileptogenesis, microglia and astroglia may be activated. These release, among other things, interleukins, which affect glial cell (Köller *et al.*, 1993) and neuronal behaviour. Recently evidence has been presented which suggests that type II astrocytes appear following some epileptogenic processes in the hippocampus (Represa *et al.*, 1993). These cells have distinctly different properties from those of type I astroglia and may therefore contribute to epileptogenesis.

Which of these and other changes are involved in the formation of pharmacoresistant epilepsy can now be decided by comparative studies in different TLE models. Moreover transgenic mice and knock-out mice offer the possibility of affecting the expression of some of these molecules and thereby permit an analysis of processes critical for the development of drug-resistant epilepsy. In addition, slice culture perhaps offers the possibility of establishing a juvenile kindling model *in vitro*. In such a model, the above-described sequence of expression of regulatory peptides may be influenced by treatment with antisense probes which prevent the expression of defined peptides.

The third hypothesis of generation of drug-resistant epilepsy is based on the observation that many patients with TLE possess a hippocampus with a reduced cell number in the hilus, the area CA1 and CA3 and the subiculum as well as the EC. These alterations can be mimicked experimentally by inducing a prolonged period of status epilepticus. This is the case in the kainate acid lesion model, in the pilocarpine model and in a model of status epilepticus induced by prolonged stimulation of afferents to the dentate gyrus (Sloviter, 1983; Ben-Ari *et al.*, 1986; Cavalheiro *et al.*, 1991; Bertram & Lothman, 1993). Following survival from such an episode, there is usually a seizure-free period before limbic seizures become apparent. These are, at least in the electrically induced status epilepticus model, progressive in nature and mimic many of the alterations observed in human TLE (E.W.H. Lothman, in prep.). However, as far as these models have been tested, they do not reach a state of pharmacoresistance. However, this might change when the models are induced in juvenile animals.

Finally, it has been proposed that general disturbances in oxygen supply produce alterations in the cortex and hippocampus, resulting in cell death and a subsequent reorganization of cortical tissue. We have tested the possibility that such alterations affect the epileptogenicity in the hippocampus. In studies on a two-vessel occlusion model, we found, as late as 1 year after the hypoxic insult, no alterations of the epileptogenicity of the hippocampus when exposed to penicillin or low magnesium medium (L. Mudrick & U. Heinemann, in prep.). However, in the neocortex from these animals synaptic inhibition is reduced and NMDA-mediated synaptic repetitive discharges appear (H. Luhmann, T. Mittmann, L. Mudrick & U. Heinemann, in prep.). Thus, it is very possible that small lesions in the central nervous system (CNS) due to transient hypoxic episodes during seizures result in mini-lesions with subsequent rearrangement of neuronal circuitry. This would imply that neuroprotective treatments will help to prevent progression of pharmacosensitive to pharmacoresistant seizures.

In conclusion, it seems that the EC and hippocampus do not a priori possess properties which render seizures generated in this structure resistant to currently available drugs. In most cases the drug resistance appears to be an acquired phenomenon which may well have to do with effects of seizures on the developing brain. Detailed studies on the above-described hypotheses offer the possibility for the understanding of formation of drug-resistant epilepsies and may offer the possibility to prevent progression of epilepsies.

Acknowledgements

This research was supported by Deutsche Forschungsgemeinschaft grant He 1128/6–2, the Sonderforschungsbereich 194 and a grant from the Human Frontier Science Program. We are grateful for expert technical assistance to M. Bullmann and G. Heske for preparation of the manuscript. We thank A. Draguhn and H. Luhmann for reading early versions of this manuscript and for helpful discussions.

References

Albrecht, D. & Heinemann, U. (1989): Low calcium-induced epileptiform activity in hippocampal slices from infant rats. *Dev. Brain Res.* **48,** 316–320.

Alonso, A. & Garcia-Ausst, E. (1987): Neuronal sources of theta rhythm in the entorhinal cortex of the rat. I. Laminar distribution of theta field potentials. *Exp. Brain Res.* **67** (3), 493–501.

Alonso, A. & Llinás, R.R. (1989): Subthreshold Na^+-dependent theta-like rhythmicity in stellate cells of entorhinal cortex layer II. *Nature* **342,** 175–177.

Andersen, P. & Anderson, S. A. (1968): *Physiological basis of alpha rhythm.* New York: Apple-Century-Crofts.

Anderson, W.W., Lewis, D.V., Swartzwelder, H.S. & Wilson, W.A. (1986): Magnesium-free medium activates seizure-like events in the rat hippocampal slice. *Brain Res.* **398,** 215–219.

Avanzini, G., de Curtis, M., Panzica, F. & Spreafico, R. (1989): Intrinsic properties of nucleus reticularis thalami neurones of the rat studied *in vitro. J. Physiol. (Lond.)* **416,** 111–122.

Babb, T.L., Kupfer, W.R., Pretorius, J.K., Crandall, P.H. & Levesque, M.F. (1991): Synaptic reorganization by mossy fibers in human epileptic fascia dentata. *Neuroscience* **42,** 351–363.

Babb, T.L., Pretorius, J.K., Kupfer, W.R., Mathern, G.W., Crandall, P.H. & Levesque, M.F. (1992): Aberrant synaptic reorganization in human epileptic hippocampus: evidence for feedforward excitation. *Dendron* **1,** 7–25.

Baimbridge, K.G. & Miller, J.J. (1984): Hippocampal calcium binding protein during kindling-induced epileptogenesis: progressive decline and effects of anticonvulsants. *Brain Res.* **324,** 85–90.

Baranyi, A. & Feher, O. (1979): Convulsive effects of 3-aminopyridine on cortical neurones. *Electroencephalogr. Clin. Neurophysiol.,* **47,** 745–751.

Barkai, E., Golan, H., Grossman, Y. & Gutnick, M.J. (1990): Pentylenetetrazole-induced kindling is prevented by prior treatment with cysteamine. *Eur. J. Pharmacol.* **182,** 167–169.

Bekenstein, J.W. & Lothman, E.W. (1991): A comparison of the ontogeny of excitatory and inhibitory neurotransmission in the CA1 region and dentate gyrus of the rat hippocampal formation. *Dev. Brain Res.* **63,** 237–243.

Ben-Ari, Y., Represa, A., Tremblay, E. & Nitecka, L. (1986): Selective and non-selective seizure related brain damage produced by kainic acid. In: *Excitatory amino acids and epilepsy*, eds. R. Schwarcz & Y. Ben-Ari, pp. 647–657. New York, London: Plenum Press.

Bertram, E.H., III & Lothman, E.W. (1993): Morphometric effects of intermittent kindled seizures and limbic status epilepticus in the dentate gyrus of the rat. *Brain Res.* **603,** 25–31.

Bloom, F.E. & Siggins, G.R. (1987): Electrophysiological action of ethanol at the cellular level. *Alcohol* **4,** 331–337.

Bronstein, J., Farber, D. & Wasterlain, C. (1988): Decreased calmodulin kinase activity after status epilepticus. *Neurochem. Res.* **13,** 83–86.

Bronstein, J.M., Farber, D.B., Micevych, P.E., Lasher, R. & Wasterlain, C.G. (1990): Kindling induced changes in calmodulin kinase II immunoreactivity. *Brain Res.* **524,** 49–53.

Cavalheiro, E.A., Leite, J.P., Bortolotto, Z.A., Turski, W.A., Ikonomidou, C. & Turski, L. (1991): Long-term effects of pilocarpine in rats: structural damage of the brain triggers kindling and spontaneous recurrent seizures. *Epilepsia* **32,** 778–782.

Coulter, D.A., Huguenard, J.R. & Prince, D.A. (1989): Specific petit mal anticonvulsants reduce calcium currents in thalamic neurons. *Neurosci. Lett.* **98,** 74–78.

Curtis, D.R., Duggan, A.W., Felix, D. & Johnston, G.A.R. (1970): GABA, bicuculline and central inhibition. *Nature* **226** (2), 1222–1224.

Deschenes, M., Paradis, M., Roy, J.P. & Steriade, M. (1984): Electrophysiology of neurons of lateral thalamic nuclei in cat: resting properties and burst discharges. *J. Neurophysiol.* **51,** 1196–1219.

Draguhn, A., Verdorn, T.A., Ewert, M., Seeburg, P.H. & Sakmann, B. (1990): Functional and molecular distinction between recombinant rat $GABA_A$ receptor subtypes by Zn^{2+}. *Neuron* **5,** 781–788.

Dreier, J.P. & Heinemann, U. (1990): Late low magnesium-induced epileptiform activity in rat entorhinal cortex slices becomes insensitive to the anticonvulsant valproic acid. *Neurosci. Lett.* **119,** 68–70.

Engstrom, D.A., Bennett, M.C., Stevens, K.E., Wilson, R.L., Diamond, D.M., Fleshner, M. & Rose, G.M. (1990): Modulation of hippocampal primed burst potentiation by anesthesia. *Brain Res.* **521,** 148–152.

Gall, C.M. & Isackson, P.J. (1989): Limbic seizures increase neuronal production of messenger RNA for nerve growth factor. *Science* **245,** 758–761.

Gall, C., Sumikawa, K. & Lynch, G. (1990): Levels of mRNA for a putative kainate receptor are affected by seizures. *Proc. Nat. Acad. Sci. USA* **87,** 7643–7647.

Geddes, J.W., Cahan, L.D., Cooper, S.M., Kim, R.C., Choi, B.H. & Cotman, C.W. (1990): Altered distribution of excitatory amino acid receptors in temporal lobe epilepsy. *Exp. Neurol.* **108,** 214–220.

Goddard, G.V., McIntyre, D.C. & Leech, C.K. (1969): A permanent change in brain function resulting from daily electrical stimulation. *Exp. Neurol.* **25,** 295–330.

Greuel, J.M., Luhmann, H.J. & Singer, W. (1988): Pharmacological induction of use-dependent receptive field modifications in the visual cortex. *Science* **242,** 74–77.

Gutnick, M.J. & Prince, D.A. (1972): Thalamocortical relay neurons: antidromic invasion of spikes from a cortical epileptogenic focus. *Science* **176,** 406–437.

Gutnick, M.J., Heinemann, U. & Lux, H.D. (1979): Stimulus induced and seizure related changes in extracellular potassium concentration in cat thalamus (VPL). *Electroencephalogr. Clin. Neurophysiol.* **47,** 329–344.

Gutnick, M.J., Connors, B.W. & Prince, D.A. (1982): Mechanisms of neocortical epileptogenesis *in vitro. J. Neurophysiol.* **48,** 1321–1335.

Haas, K.Z., Sperber, E.F. & Moshé, S.L. (1990): Kindling in developing animals: Expression of severe seizures and enhanced development of bilateral foci. *Dev. Brain Res.* **56,** 275–280.

Hablitz, J.J. (1984): Picrotoxin-induced epileptiform activity in hippocampus: role of endogenous versus synaptic factors. *J. Neurophysiol.* **51,** 1011–1027.

Heinemann, U. & Gutnick, M.J. (1979): Relation between extracellular potassium concentration and neuronal activities in cat thalamus (VPL) during projection of cortical epileptiform discharge. *Electroencephalogr. Clin. Neurophysiol.* **47,** 345–357.

Heinemann, U. & Jones, R.S.G. (1989): Neurophysiology of epilepsy. In: *Perspectives of epilepsy*, eds. L. Gram & M. Dam, pp. 17–42. New York: Raven Press.

Heinemann, U., Franceschetti, S., Hamon, B., Konnerth, A. & Yaari, Y. (1985): Effects of anticonvulsants on spontaneous epileptiform activity which develops in the absence of chemical synaptic transmission in hippocampal slices. *Brain Res.* **325,** 349–352.

Heinemann, U., Arens, J., Dreier, J.P., Stabel, J. & Zhang, C.L. (1991): *In vitro* epileptiform activity: role of excitatory amino acids. *Epilepsy Res.* **10,** 18–23.

Herb, A., Burnashev, N., Werner, P., Sakmann, B., Wisden, W. & Seeburg, P.H. (1992): The KA-2 subunit of excitatory amino acid receptors shows widespread expression in brain and forms ion channels with distantly related subunits. *Neuron* **8,** 775–785.

Huguenard, J.R. & Prince, D.A. (1992): A novel T-type current underlies prolonged Ca^{2+}-dependent burst firing in GABAergic neurons of rat thalamic reticular nucleus. *J. Neurosci.* **12,** 3804–3817.

Isackson, P.J., Huntsman, M.M., Murray, K.D. & Gall, C.M. (1991): BDNF mRNA expression is increased in adult rat forebrain after limbic seizures: temporal patterns of induction distinct from NGF. *Neuron* **6,** 937–948.

Jahnsen, H. & Llinás, R.R. (1984): Ionic basis for the electroresponsiveness and oscillatory properties of guinea-pig thalamic neurones *in vitro. J. Physiol. (Lond.)* **349,** 227–247.

Jefferys, J.G.R. (1981): Influence of electric fields on the excitability of granule cells in guinea-pig hippocampal slices. *J. Physiol. (Lond.)* **319,** 143–152.

Jefferys, J.G.R. & Haas, H.L. (1982): Synchronized bursting of CA1 hippocampal pyramidal cells in the absence of synaptic transmission. *Nature* **300,** 448–450.

Kamphuis, W., Monyer, H., De Rijk, T.C. & Lopes da Silva, F.H. (1992): Hippocampal kindling increases the expression of glutamate receptor-A Flip and -B Flip mRNA in dentate granule cells. *Neurosci. Lett.* **148,** 51–54.

Keinänen, K., Wisden, W., Sommer, B., Werner, P., Herb, A., Verdoorn, T.A., Sakmann, B. & Seeburg, P.H. (1990): A family of AMPA-selective glutamate receptors. *Science* **249,** 556–560.

Köller, H., Siebler, M., Pekel, M. & Müller, H.W. (1993): Depolarization of cultured astrocytes by leukotriene B_4: evidence for the induction of a K^+ conductance inhibitor. *Brain Res.* **612,** 28–34.

Konnerth, A., Lux, H.D. & Heinemann, U. (1986): Ionic properties of burst generation in hippocampal pyramidal cell somata '*in vitro*'. In: *Calcium electrogenesis and neuronal functioning*, eds. U. Heinemann, M. Klee, E. Neher & W. Singer, pp. 368–374. Berlin, Heidelberg, New York, London, Paris, Tokyo: Springer Verlag.

Leschinger, A., Stabel, J., Igelmund, P. & Heinemann, U. (1993): Pharmacological and electrographic properties of epileptiform activity induced by elevated K^+ and lowered Ca^{2+} and Mg^{2+} concentration in rat hippocamal slices. *Exp. Brain Res.* **96,** 230–240.

Leweke, F.M., Louvel, J., Rausche, G. & Heinemann, U. (1990): Effects of pentetrazol on neuronal activity and on extracellular calcium concentration in rat hippocampal slices. *Epilepsy Res.* **6,** 187–198.

Llinás, R.R. & Yarom, Y. (1981): Properties and distribution of ionic conductances generating electroresponsiveness of mammalian inferior olivary neurones *in vitro. J. Physiol. (Lond.)* **315,** 569–584.

Lux, H.D., Heinemann, U. & Dietzel, I. (1986): Ionic changes and alterations in the size of the extracellular space during epileptic activity. In: *Advances in neurology,* Vol. 44: *Basic mechanisms of the epilepsies: molecular and cellular approaches,* eds. A.V. Delgado-Escueta, A.A. Ward, D.M. Woodbury & R.J. Porter, pp. 619–639. New York: Raven Press.

McCormick, D.A. & Pape, H.-C. (1990): Properties of a hyperpolarization-activated cation current and its role in rhythmic oscillation in thalamic relay neurones. *J. Physiol. (Lond.)* **431,** 291–318.

Macdonald, R.L. & McLean, M.J. (1986): Anticonvulsant drugs: mechanisms of action. In: *Advances in neurology,* Vol. 44: *Basic mechanisms of the epilepsies*, eds. A.V. Delgado-Escueta, A.A. Ward, D.M. Woodbury & R.J. Porter, pp. 713–736. New York: Raven Press.

Matsumoto, H. & Ajmone-Marsan, C. (1964): Cortical cellular phenomena in experimental epilepsy: Interictal manifestations. *Exp. Neurol.* **9,** 286–304.

Meencke, H.-J. (1987): Neuropathology of generalized primary epilepsy. *Adv. Epileptology* **16,** 1–8.

Mody, I. & Heinemann, U. (1987): NMDA receptors of dentate gyrus granule cells participate in synaptic transmission following kindling. *Nature* **326,** 701–704.

Mody, I., Stanton, P.K. & Heinemann, U. (1988): Activation of *N*-methyl-D-aspartate receptors parallels changes in cellular and synaptic properties of dentate gyrus granule cells after kindling. *J. Neurophysiol.* **59,** 1033–1054.

Monyer, H., Sprengel, R., Schoepfer, R., Herb, A., Higuchi, M., Lomeli, H., Burnashev, N., Sakmann, B. & Seeburg, P.H. (1992): Heteromeric NMDA receptors: molecular and functional distinction of subtypes. *Science* **256,** 1217–1221.

Morris, B.J., Feasey, K.J., ten Bruggencate, G., Herz, A. & Höllt, V. (1988): Electrical stimulation *in vivo* increases the expression of proenkephalin mRNA and decreases the expression of prodynorphin mRNA in rat hippocampal granule cells. *Proc. Nat. Acad. Sci. USA* **85,** 3226–3230.

Müller, W., Misgeld, U. and Heinemann, U. (1988) Carbachol effects on hippocampal neurons *in vitro* dependence on the rate of rise of carbachol tissue concentration. *Exp. Brain Res.* **72,** 287–298.

Niesen, C.E., Baskys, A. & Carlen, P.L. (1988): Reversed ethanol effects on potassium conductances in aged hippocampal dentate granule neurons. *Brain Res.* **445,** 137–141.

Pape, H.-C. & McCormick, D.A. (1989): Noradrenaline and serotonin selectively modulate thalamic burst firing by enhancing a hyperpolarization-activated cation current. *Nature* **340,** 715–718.

Perreault, P. & Avoli, M. (1989): Effects of low concentrations of 4-aminopyridine on CAl pyramidal cells of the hippocampus. *J. Neurophysiol.* **61,** 953–970.

Pierson, M.G., Smith, K.L. & Swann, J.W. (1989): A slow NMDA-mediated synaptic potential underlies seizures originating from midbrain. *Brain Res.* **486,** 381–386.

Prince, D.A. (1978): Neurophysiology of epilepsy. *Ann. Rev. Neurosci.* **1,** 395–415.

Psarropoulou, C. & Avoli, M. (1993): 4-Aminopyridine-induced spreading depression episodes in immature hippocampus: Developmental and pharmacological characteristics. *Neuroscience* **55,** 57–68.

Ramon y Cajal, S. (1993): *The structure of Ammon's horn.* London: C.C. Thomas.

Rausche, G., Sarvey, J.M. & Heinemann, U. (1989): Slow synaptic inhibition in relation to frequency habituation in dentate granule cells of rat hippocampal slices. *Exp. Brain Res.* **78,** 233–242.

Represa, A., Tremblay, E. & Ben-Ari, Y. (1990): Sprouting of mossy fibers in the hippocampus of epileptic human and rat. *Adv. Exp. Med. Biol.* **268,** 419–424.

Represa, A., Niquet, J., Charriaut-Marlangue, C. & Ben-Ari, Y. (1993): Reactive astrocytes in the kainic acid-damaged hippocampus have the phenotypic features of type-2 astrocytes. *J. Neurocytol.* **22,** 299–310.

Ribak, C.E. (1991): Epilepsy hypothesis. *Science* **238,** 1292–1293.

Rogawski, M.A. & Porter, R.J. (1990): Antiepileptic drugs: pharmacological mechanisms and clinical efficacy with consideration of promising developmental stage compounds. *Pharmacol. Rev.* **42,** 223–270.

Ruppersberg, J.P., Schröter, K.H., Sakmann, B., Stocker, M., Sewing, S. & Pongs, O. (1990): Heteromultimeric channels formed by rat brain potassium-channel proteins. *Nature* **345,** 535–537.

Schwartzkroin, P.A. & Prince, D.A. (1978): Cellular and field potential properties of epileptogenic hippocampal slices. *Brain Res.* **147,** 117–130.

Schwindt, P.C. & Crill, W.E. (1980): Properties of a persistent inward current in normal and TEA-injected motoneurons. *J. Neurophysiol.* **43,** 1700–1724.

Seeburg, P.H., Wisden, W., Verdoorn, T.A., Pritchett, D.B., Werner, P., Herb, A., Luddens, H., Sprengel, R. & Sakmann, B. (1990): The $GABA_A$ receptor family: molecular and functional diversity. *Cold Spring Harbor Symp. Quant. Biol.* **55,** 29–40.

Singer, W. (1990): The formation of cooperative cell assemblies in the visual cortex. *J. Exp. Biol.* **153,** 177–197.

Sloviter, R.S. (1983): 'Epileptic' brain damage in rats induced by sustained electrical stimulation of the perforant path. I. Acute electrophysiological and light microscopic studies. *Brain Res. Bull.* **10,** 675–697.

Sloviter, R.S. (1987): Decreased hippocampal inhibition and a selective loss of interneurons in experimental epilepsy. *Science* **235,** 73–76.

Smith, S.S., Waterhouse, B.D., Chapin, J.K. & Woodward, D.J. (1987): Progesterone alters GABA and glutamate responsiveness: a possible mechanism for its anxiolytic action. *Brain Res.* **400,** 353–359.

Snead, O.C., III, Hechler, V., Vergnes, M., Marescaux, C. & Maitre, M. (1990): Increased gamma-hydroxybutyric acid receptors in thalamus of a genetic animal model of petit mal epilepsy. *Epilepsy Res.* **7,** 121–128.

Snead, O.C., III, Depaulis, A., Banerjee, P.K., Hechler, V. & Vergnes, M. (1992): The $GABA_A$ receptor complex in experimental absence seizures in rat: an autoradiographic study. *Neurosci. Lett.* **140,** 9–12.

Sommer, B., Keinänen, K., Verdoorn, T.A., Wisden, W., Burnashev, N., Herb, A., Köhler, M., Takagi, T., Sakmann, B. and Seeburg, P.H. (1990): Flip and flop: a cell-specific functional switch in glutamate-operated channels of the CNS. *Science* **249,** 1580–1585.

Sommer, B., Köhler, M., Sprengel, R. & Seeburg, P.H. (1991): RNA editing in brain controls a determinant of ion flow in glutamate-gated channels. *Cell* **67,** 11–19.

Stühmer, W., Ruppersberg, J.P., Schröter, K.H., Sakmann, B., Stocker, M., Giese, K.P., Perschke, A., Baumann, A. & Pongs, O. (1989): Molecular basis of functional diversity of voltage-gated potassium channels in mammalian brain. *EMBO J.* **8,** 3235–3244.

Sutula, T., Xiao-Xian, H., Cavazos, J. & Scott, G. (1988): Synaptic reorganization in the hippocampus induced by abnormal functional activity. *Science* **239,** 1147–1150.

Swann, J.W. & Brady, R.J. (1984): Penicillin-induced epileptogenesis in immature rat CA3 hippocampal pyramidal cells. *Dev. Brain Res.* **12,** 243–254.

Thompson, S.M. & Gähwiler, B.H. (1989a): Activity-dependent disinhibition. I. Repetitive stimulation reduces IPSP driving force and conductance in the hippocampus *in vitro*. *J. Neurophysiol.* **61,** 501–511.

Thompson, S.M. & Gahwiler, B.H. (1989b): Activity-dependent disinhibition. II. Effects of extracellular potassium, furosemide, and membrane potential on E_{Cl^-} in hippocampal CA3 neurons. *J. Neurophysiol.* **61,** 512–523.

Thompson, S.M. & Gähwiler, B.H. (1989c): Activity-dependent disinhibition. III. Desensitization and $GABA_B$ receptor-mediated presynaptic inhibition in the hippocampus *in vitro*. *J. Neurophysiol.* **61,** 524–533.

Traub, R.D., Miles, R. & Wong, R.K.S. (1987): Models of synchronized hippocampal bursts in the presence of inhibition. I. Single population events. *J. Neurophysiol.* **58,** 739–748.

Traub, R.D., Miles, R. & Jefferys, J.G.R. (1993): Synaptic and intrinsic conductances shape picrotoxin-induced synchronized after-discharges in the guinea-pig hippocampal slice. *J. Physiol. (Lond.)* **461,** 525–547.

Traynelis, S.F. & Dingledine, R. (1988): Potassium-induced spontaneous electrographic seizures in the rat hippocampal slice. *J. Neurophysiol.* **59,** 259–276.

Verdoorn, T.A., Draguhn, A., Ymer, S., Seeburg, P.H. & Sakmann, B. (1990): Functional properties of recombinant rat $GABA_A$ receptors depend upon subunit composition. *Neuron* **4,** 919–928.

von Haebler, D., Stabel, J., Draguhn, A. & Heinemann, U. (1993): Properties of horizontal cells transiently appearing in the rat dentate gyrus during ontogenesis. *Exp. Brain Res.* **94,** 33–42.

Walther, H., Lambert, J.D.C., Jones, R.S.G., Heinemann, U. & Hamon, B. (1986): Epileptiform activity in combined slices of the hippocampus, subiculum and entorhinal cortex during perfusion with low magnesium medium. *Neurosci. Lett.* **69,** 156–161.

Wisden, W., Laurie, D.J., Monyer, H. & Seeburg, P.H. (1992): The distribution of 13 $GABA_A$ receptor subunit mRNAs in the rat brain. I. Telencephalon, diencephalon, mesencephalon. *J. Neurosci.* **12,** 1040–1062.

Wong, R.K.S. & Prince, D.A. (1978): Participation of calcium spikes during intrinsic burst firing in hippocampal neurons. *Brain Res.* **159,** 385–390.

Yaari, Y., Konnerth, A. & Heinemann, U. (1983): Spontaneous epileptiform activity of CAl hippocampal neurons in low extracellular calcium solutions. *Exp. Brain Res.* **51,** 153–156.

Epileptic Seizures and Syndromes, Edited by Peter Wolf
© 1994 John Libbey & Company Ltd., pp. 619–629

Chapter 61

West syndrome: new therapeutic strategies

Hartmut Siemes

Kinderklinik, Rittberg-Krankenhaus, Carstennstr. 58, D-1000 Berlin 45, Germany

Summary

More than 150 years since the original description of the West syndrome, still no consensus of standard care has been established. Treatment with ACTH or corticosteroids is the most effective therapy. However, hormonal therapy is burdened with frequent side-effects, some of which are very serious. The benzodiazepines (clonazepam, nitrazepam) have been used with some success: up to about 30 per cent of patients may become seizure-free. However, toxicity and tolerance may occur in a high percentage of children. High-dose pyridoxine and high-dose intravenous γ-globulins have also been reported to be beneficial in treating children with infantile spasms. However, the small number of patients treated and the heterogeneity of studies published make it difficult to assess the efficacy of these drugs. High-dose valproate seems to be the most promising alternative therapy to ACTH. The results of several studies indicate a high percentage of seizure-free patients and a favourable long-term outcome. According to a recent enquiry in German paediatric centres, a therapy-related mortality rate of 2.0 per cent can be expected with ACTH therapy, whereas the comparable figure with valproate is 0.2 per cent. Vigabatrin has been shown to be an effective and safe drug in treatment of children with refractory infantile spasms.

Introduction

In 1841 the British physician Dr West first described infantile spasms in a letter to the editor of the *Lancet* entitled 'On a peculiar form of infantile convulsions'. Being a witness to these seizures in his own child, he asked for therapeutic advice. What therapy could we recommend him today?

The West syndrome is an age-related generalized epilepsy; it nearly always starts before the age of 1 year. It is characterized by a triad of infantile spasms as a peculiar type of seizures (flexor, extensor and mixed flexor–extensor), psychomotor retardation or deterioration and a characteristic electroencephalographic (EEG) pattern of hypsarrhythmia. Infantile spasms have multiple aetiologies. The basic mechanisms of these seizures are largely unknown.

Classification of patients and long-term outcome of children with infantile spasms

The aetiological classification of patients is crucial to the evaluation of therapies and the prediction of long-term outcome. On the basis of medical and developmental history, the neurological findings and the results of neuroradiological investigations, patients can be divided into two groups, cryptogenic and symptomatic. A patient is classified as cryptogenic if he/she meets the following criteria: no known associated aetiological factor, normal development prior to the onset of the spasms, a normal neurological examination and no abnormal neuroradiological findings prior to therapy. The remainder are classified as symptomatic.

The prognosis for children with infantile spasms is grave, as has been confirmed in virtually all follow-up studies. Past studies of long-term outcome have reported a significant mortality rate (11–23 per cent) associated with hormonal treatment (Gibbs *et al.*, 1954; Trojaborg & Plum, 1960; Mizutani, 1969; Friedman & Pampiglione, 1971; Jeavons *et al.*, 1973), whereas in a more recent study a lower mortality rate (5 per cent) was documented (Glaze *et al.*, 1988).

According to many studies, 76–89 per cent of children with infantile spasms will be permanently retarded. The probability of normal mental outcome for symptomatic seizures is very low (mean about 4 per cent with a range of 0–14 per cent calculated from 690 patients of 10 therapy studies), whereas it is much higher in those with cryptogenic spasms (mean about 42 per cent with a range of 21–58 per cent calculated from 590 patients of 12 therapy studies) (Cavazzuti, 1973; Jeavons *et al.*, 1973; Gibbs & Gibbs, 1976; Fejerman & Medina, 1977; Kurokowa *et al.*, 1980; Ohtahara *et al.*, 1980; Pinsard, 1980; Singer *et al.*, 1980; Matsumoto *et al.*, 1981; Lerman & Kivity, 1982; Riikonen, 1982; Lombroso, 1983; Fois *et al.*, 1984; Glaze *et al.*, 1988; Hrachovy *et al.*, 1991). In either group, inability to control the seizures seems to indicate a poorer prognosis for normal development (Riikonen, 1982; Fois *et al.*, 1984).

The patients with infantile spasms exhibited a high percentage of further permanent deficits of the central nervous system (CNS): cerebral palsy in about 35–50 per cent of children (Seki *et al.*, 1976; Aicardi & Chevrie, 1978; Pollack *et al.*, 1979; Riikonen, 1982; Fois *et al.*, 1984), secondary epilepsies in about 35–80 per cent of patients (Dravet *et al.*, 1973; Ohtahara *et al.*, 1980; Riikonen *et al.*, 1982; Glaze *et al.*, 1988; Prats *et al.*, 1991) and psychiatric abnormalities in up to 30 per cent of patients, a substantial part of them developing autism (Taft & Cohen, 1971; Riikonen & Amnell, 1981).

Table 1. Treatment of infantile spasms – past and new strategies

Past and recent strategies
High-dosage/long-duration ACTH (40 to 160 units/day; 3 to 12 months)
Low-dosage/short-duration ACTH (5 to 40 units/day; 1 to 6 weeks)
Benzodiazepines (nitrazepam, clonazepam)
Valproate
New strategies
Low-dosage/short- to long-duration ACTH (5 to 30 units/day; 2 weeks to 6 months)
High-dose valproate (up to 300 mg/kg/day)
High-dose pyridoxine (up to 300 mg/kg/day)
High-dose gammaglobulin (1 g/kg/day for 2 days every 3 weeks for 6 months)
Vigabatrin

Past and new treatment strategies in infantile spasms

Several methodological problems make it difficult to assess the efficacy of clinical therapeutic studies (Hrachovy & Frost, 1988, 1989).

1. The natural history of infantile spasms has to be considered. It may be difficult to determine the medication effect, since after 12 months since onset of the seizures a spontaneous remission rate of 25 per cent has been described (Hrachovy *et al.*, 1991).
2. There is a multiplicity of associated aetiological factors.

Rather large groups of patients are a prerequisite for comparable results, since all investigators agree that the most important predictor of treatment efficacy and long-term outcome is the underlying cause

of the infantile spasms.
3. Few well-controlled prospective single- or double-blind studies have been performed; most studies have been retrospective.
4. Dosages of medication and duration of treatment have varied considerably.
5. Determining the acute effects of therapies requires monitoring seizure frequency by objective means (serial 24-hour EEG/video monitoring).

Table 1 gives a summary of past and new treatment strategies.

Treatment of infantile spasms with ACTH and corticosteroids

Past modalities

Since 1958 adrenocorticotrophic hormone (ACTH) and corticosteroids have been reported to be the most effective drugs for treatment of infantile spasms (Sorel & Dusaucy-Bauloye, 1958). According to numerous therapeutic, trials about 50–80 per cent of cases have shown cessation of seizures and disappearance of the hypsarrhythmic EEG pattern (Aicardi, 1986). The hormonal drugs and dosages employed and the duration of treatment have varied considerably. In the past either high dosages of ACTH and long duration of therapy (40–160 units/day for 3 to > 12 months) (Chevrie & Aicardi, 1971; Lagenstein *et al.*, 1978; Singer *et al.*, 1980; Lerman & Kivity, 1982; Lombroso, 1983; Snead *et al.*, 1983) or low-dosage ACTH therapy for relatively brief periods (5–40 units/day for 1 to 6 weeks) were utilized (Trojaberg & Plum, 1960, Jeavons & Bower, 1961, Willoughby *et al.*, 1966, Riikonen, 1982).

A high relapse rate after discontinuation of hormonal treatment has been reported; it may range between 30 and 65 per cent (Aicardi, 1986).

New strategy: low-dose ACTH

In the past there was no clear answer to the question whether high-dose or low-dose ACTH therapy produces better results. In the retrospective analysis of the results of high-dose ACTH therapy versus low-dose ACTH therapy some researchers report better control of seizures and greater EEG improvement with the higher ACTH dosage (Lombroso, 1983; Snead *et al.*, 1983). However, Riikonen (1982) and Fois and colleagues (1987) showed that higher doses produced no better results than smaller doses. Meanwhile, results of a recently published single-blind controlled study of high-dose ACTH versus low-dose ACTH indicated no major difference between the two groups (Hrachovy *et al.*, 1992). In conclusion, low-dose ACTH therapy (5–30 units/day) seems to be most reasonable, with duration of therapy varying between 2 weeks and 6 months depending on the aetiology of the spasms and the patients' response. It has already been utilized and recommended by some researchers (Fois *et al.*, 1987; Nolte *et al.*, 1988; Hrachovy & Frost, 1989; Nolte *et al.*, 1990; Kuriyama *et al.*, 1992; Nolte, 1992). In fact, patients with lower ACTH doses seem to have a better outcome and fewer side-effects (Riikonen & Donner, 1980).

Some authors consider ACTH and prednisone to be equipotential, whereas others consider ACTH to be superior (Low, 1958; Willoughby *et al.*, 1966; Snyder, 1967; Lacy & Penry, 1976; Kurokowa *et al.*, 1980; Lombroso, 1983; Snead *et al.*, 1983). Hrachovy and colleagues (1983) in a controlled study of the relative efficacies of low-dose ACTH and prednisone revealed no major difference between these two drugs in stopping the seizures and improving the EEG. Therefore it is difficult to understand why prednisone is not used more often as a first-line drug. This drug would allow easier management of therapy.

The hormonal therapy of infantile spasms is burdened with frequent side-effects, some of which are quite serious. The most common complications are listed in Table 2. Riikonen & Donner (1980) reported pronounced side-effects with the use of ACTH in 37 per cent of 162 children. The authors attributed six of eight deaths in their patients to an ACTH-facilitated infection.

Table 2. Side-effects of ACTH

Infections (immunosuppression): sepsis, meningitis
Hypertension
Cardiomyopathy
Electrolyte imbalance, retention of fluid
Osteoporosis (fractures of vertebrae)
Delayed growth
Nephrocalcinosis, renal failure
Ocular opacities
Gastrointestinal disturbances
Disturbances of behaviour: irritability, lethargy
Transient (reversible?) brain shrinkage

The pronounced side-effects of hormonal therapy have led to a permanent search for alternative medications. Various other drugs have been successfully utilized to treat infantile spasms.

Past therapies alternative to hormonal treatment

Benzodiazepines

The benzodiazepines (clonazepam and nitrazepam) have been used with some success during the last 20 years; up to about 30 per cent of patients may become seizure-free (Völzke *et al.*, 1967; Jan *et al.*, 1971; Dumermuth & Kovacs, 1973; Vasella *et al.*, 1973; Lacy & Penry, 1976; Nolte *et al.*, 1988). However, toxicity and tolerance may occur in a high percentage of children.

New therapeutic strategies alternative to hormones

High-dose pyridoxine and high-dose intravenous γ-globulins

High-dose pyridoxine (Blennow & Starck, 1986; Ohtsuka *et al.*, 1987; Ito *et al.*, 1991; Pietz *et al.*, 1991) and high-dose intravenous γ-globulins (Ariizumi *et al.*, 1987; Echenne *et al.*, 1991) have also been reported to be beneficial in treating children with infantile spasms. However, the small number of patients treated and the heterogeneity of studies published make it difficult to assess the efficacy of these drugs.

High-dose valproate

Valproate (VPA) seems to be most promising as an alternative therapy to ACTH. The results of the various studies are listed in Table 3 according to the increasing VPA dosage that has been used (Pavone *et al.*, 1981; Bachmann, 1982; Dulac *et al.*, 1982; Siemes *et al.*, 1988; Prats *et al.*, 1991; Kotlarek *et al.*, 1992). With the low dose of 20 mg/kg/d about 20 per cent of the patients became seizure-free, with dosages up to 100 mg/kg/day about 40–65 per cent of patients and with the extremely high dosage of 100–300 mg/kg/day the remarkable percentage of 78 per cent of the children became controlled. This table gives the impression that there is a positive relation between VPA dosage and efficacy of this drug demonstrated by the percentage of seizure-free patients.

The rate of relapses varied between 12 per cent and 32 per cent. No case of severe VPA-associated hepatotoxicity has been reported in these patients. The conclusion is that one should administer a high dose if one decides to use this drug.

Table 3. Valproate monotherapy of West syndrome: initial response

			Seizure-free		Rate of relapses	
Authors [a]	Patients n	Dose of valproate (mg/kg/day)	*n*	%	*n*	%
Pavone *et al.*, 1981	18	20 (–30)	4/18	(22%)	?	
Bachmann, 1982	19	(20) 40–60	8/19	(42%)	?	
Dulac *et al.*, 1982	9	15–75	4/9	(44%)	?	
Siemes *et al.*, 1988	22	40–100	14/22	(64%)	7/22	32%
Kotlarek *et al.*, 1992	74	50–100	33/70	(47%)	4/33	12%
Prats *et al.*, 1991	42	100–300[b]	33/42	(78%)	8/42	19%

n = number of patients; [a]authors listed according to increasing dosage of VPA; [b]for a maximum of 3 weeks, thereafter 30–50 mg/kg/day.

The long-term outcome in patients treated with VPA is demonstrated in Table 4. To compare VPA with ACTH, two more recently published hormone studies of Riikonen (1982) and Glaze and colleagues (1988) were chosen, since they contain detailed informations with respect to mortality, psychomotor development and secondary epilepsies. Prats and colleagues (1991) reported the long-term results of their recent VPA therapy study administering 100–300 mg/kg/day. They additionally presented comparable results of the low-dose ACTH therapy regimen that had been utilized by them in the past. Further, the data of two prospective VPA studies published by Kotlarek and colleagues (1992) and our group (Siemes *et al.*, 1993) are included.

The rather high mortality rate reported by Riikonen and colleagues may be partially explained by the long follow-up time (up to 19 years).

With administration of ACTH the percentage of normal mental outcome varies between 5 per cent and 12 per cent of patients. With VPA a much higher value of 28 per cent has been documented in two series. Accordingly the percentage of moderately to severely retarded children is lowered in these patients by about 20 per cent. Seven of the 21 living children of our own study (including all four patients with cryptogenic spasms) are now attending a regular school (some of them receiving additional educational support).

With the use of ACTH 53 per cent to 80 per cent of patients developed secondary epilepsies whereas with VPA a percentage ranging between 28 per cent and 51 per cent was found. In the study of Kotlarek and colleagues 47 out of the 74 children were VPA-resistant; these patients also received ACTH. The authors stated that only four out of the 27 VPA-responsive children later developed epilepsies; this represents the extremely low value of 15 per cent.

Regarding VPA therapy it has been objected that, compared with hormonal therapy, there is a delayed cessation of seizures and disappearance of hypsarrhythmia, which could influence the outcome negatively. This objection has been raised because a short period of spasms has been associated with a more favourable outcome (Jeavons *et al.*, 1973; Seki *et al.*, 1976; Riikonen, 1982) and hormonal therapy is more likely than any other treatment to shorten the period of seizure activity. However, the presented results indicate that the incidence of normal mental outcome and of secondary epilepsies seems to be more favourable with VPA than with ACTH.

Vigabatrin

The first indication that vigabatrin might be effective in the treatment of infantile spasms was presented by Livingston *et al.* (1989) and Luna *et al.* (1989) who used vigabatrin as add-on therapy in children with refractory epilepsy. No study using vigabatrin as primary drug for treatment of infantile spasms has been published so far. Two add-on trials in children with refractory infantile spasms suggest that vigabatrin is an effective drug in these children (Auerswald, 1992; Chiron *et al.*, 1992). There was a seizure reduction of more than 50 per cent in 71 per cent or 78 per cent of children,

Table 4. Primary treatment of infantile spasms with valproate in comparison with hormonal therapy: long-term outcome

Patients		Mortality rate		Psychomotor development								Epilepsy		Follow-up time[a]	
				Normal		Retardation									
						Slight		Moderate		Severe					
n	Treatment	*n*	%	*n*	%	*n*	%	*n*	%	*n*	%	*n*	%	(years)	Authors
214	ACTH, dexamethasone	42/214	19	23/192	12	10/192	5	20/192	10	85/192	72	136/192	71	10.4 (3–19)	Riikonen, 1982
64	ACTH, prednisone	3/64	5	3/64	5	3/64	5	14/64	21	41/64	64	34/64	53	4 (0.75–10.25)	Glaze *et al.*, 1988
45	ACTH[b]	4/45	9	6/45	9	6/45	13	35/45 (78%				32/45	80	3.4 (± 0.22)	Prats *et al.*, 1991
42	Valproate[b]	4/42	10	6/42	28	4/42	9	20/42 (62%)				20/42	51	3.4 (± 0.22)	Prats *et al.*, 1991
74	Valproate[c]	2/74	3	––	–	––	––	–	–	–	–	53/74[d]	47	4.5 (1.5–7)	Kotlarek *et al.*, 1992
21	Valproate[e]	1/22	5	6/22	27	2/22	9	3/22	14	10/22	45	6/22	27	8.5 (7–10)	Siemes *et al.*, 1993

[a]Mean ± SD or range, respectively.
[b]Study comparing ACTH and VPA, moderate and severe retardation compiled together, 7 VPA-resistant patients received ACTH.
[c]Valproate monotherapy initially, 47 VPA-resistant patients also received ACTH.
[d]Only four out of the 27 children with sole valproate monotherapy later developed epilepsy (15%).
[e] Three VPA-resistant children received dexamethasone, one patient ACTH additionally, respectively.

and 28 per cent or 38 per cent became seizure-free, respectively. In contrast to the symptomatic cases, Chiron and colleagues (1992) reported a high relapse rate in cryptogenic spasms.

The initial results of our own open, uncontrolled two-centre trial in children with refractory infantile spasms are presented in Table 5. Evaluation at a mean follow-up time of about 1 year yielded the following results: about 70 per cent of patients were still receiving vigabatrin and about 60 per cent of children were free of seizures, two-thirds of them receiving vigabatrin monotherapy. The only serious side-effect was agitation in one of these children which disappeared after decrease in the dose of vigabatrin. Thus, our study confirms the results of the earlier trials, that vigabatrin is an effective and safe drug.

Table 5. Efficacy of vigabatrin in refractory infantile spasms – results of an open study (Siemes, Brandl and Spohr, 1994)

Study design: add-on, two-centre trial of patients with previously uncontrolled infantile spasms
Patients' characteristics: $n = 23$; male = 12, female = 11
Associated aetiological factors: cryptogenic: 4/23; symptomatic: 19/23
Previous antiepileptic medication: valproate, dexamethasone, vitamin B_6, ACTH, clonazepam, clobazam, phenobarbital
Age at start of vigabatrin therapy: mean 9.5 months (range: 2.5 to 22 months)
Evaluation time since start of vigabatrin therapy: mean 11 months (range: 4–33 months)
Deaths: 2/23 (9%)
Patients still receiving vigabatrin: 15/21 (71%)
  Seizure-free*: 12/21 (57%)
    Monotherapy: 8/21 (38%)
    Polytherapy**: 4/21 (29%)
  Seizure reduction 50 %: 3/21 (14%)
  Relapses: 3/21 (14 %)
  Vigabatrin dosage: mean 83,5 mg/kg/d (range: 50–125)
Patients without medication, seizure-free: 1/21 (5%)
EEG findings:
  Hypsarrhythmia: 2/21 (10%)
  Localized epileptogenic discharges: 11/21 (52%)
  No epileptogenic discharges: 8/21 (38%)
Secondary epilepsies: 3/21 (14%)
Developmental retardation:
  Normal or slight*: 5/21 (24%)
  Moderate: 6/21 (29%)
  Severe, very severe: 10/21 (48%)

*Including four children with cryptogenic seizures; **co-medication: valproate, carbamazepine, dexamethasone.

Therapy of West syndrome: present state in Germany

Information on the therapeutic regimens applied for infantile spasms in Germany was gathered by a questionnaire completed by the physicians of various paediatric centres who are responsible for therapy. The questionnaire included data on the number of treated patients per year, on the drugs of first and second choice and their effectiveness, and on noted severe side-effects. The questionnaire was returned from 58 of 122 German paediatric hospitals, including 12 university departments. The number of treated patients per year was 231, and the average number of patients per clinic was four with a range from one to 15 patients. The German questionnaire data were used to compile Tables 6 and 7.

The drug of first choice is ACTH in the majority of the hospitals (60 per cent), either alone or together with other drugs (Table 6). Clonazepam is a first-line drug in 18 per cent of the centres and valproate in about 20 per cent, a few of them using it in combination with hormones. Only a minority use pyridoxine. The percentages of controlled patients vary considerably according to the drug administered drug but are in accordance with the data reported in the literature. The estimated therapy-related mortality was 2.0 per cent for ACTH is 0.2 per cent for VPA (Table 7). The results reflect the controversies and confusion concerning the treatment of infantile spasms. Still, no consensus of standard care has been established.

Table 6. German questionnaire data about the treatment of infantile spasms (1992): drugs of first choice in 56 paediatric hospitals (231 patients/year) and treatment response (percentage of controlled patients)

	Hospitals		Controlled
Drugs of first choice	n	%	%
ACTH	25	45	~65
ACTH or valproate	5	9	~47
ACTH or valproate or vitamin B6	1	2	~30
ACTH or vigabatrin	1	2	~45
Clonazepam	10	18	~20
Valproate	8	14	~35
Valproate plus ACTH or dexamethasone	2	3	~70
Valproate or vigabatrin	1	2	~35
Vitamin B6	3	5	~20

Table 7. German questionnaire data about the treatment of infantile spasms (1992)

Estimated therapy-related mortality during the last 6 years

	Patients/year	Mortality rate
ACTH	164	20/984 (2%)*
Valproate	89	1/534 (0.2%)*
Clonazpam	46	0/276
Dexamethasone	18	0/106

Reported non-fatal complications of therapy

ACTH: infections, hypertonus, cardiomyopathy, encephalopathy, nephrocalcinosis
Valproate: reversible increase of liver enzymes, transient thrombocytopenia
Clonazepam: upper respiratory tract infections

* Infections (sepsis or pneumonia), gastric bleeding, cardiomyopathy.
** Fatal VPA-associated hepatotoxicity.

Recommended clinical research studies

Since even low-dose ACTH therapy is burdened with severe side-effects, it appears to be reasonable and ethically justifiable to perform the following prospective studies:

1. high-dose VPA *vs.* low-dose ACTH;
2. vigabatrin *vs.* low-dose ACTH;
3. vigabatrin *vs.* high-dose valproate.

Conclusion

What therapeutic advice could we give Dr West taking into account the results of the most recent therapeutic trials?

Since his son seemed to have cryptogenic infantile spasms we would suggest low-dose/short-duration ACTH. An alternative would be high-dose VPA. In the case of symptomatic spasms most investigators would also use low-dose ACTH. One might prefer to start with high-dose valproate, and to try a corticosteroid or vigabatrin if VPA fails to control the seizures.

References

Aicardi, J. (1986): Infantile spasms. In: *Epilepsy in children. International review of child neurology series*, ed. J. Aicardi, pp. 17–38. New York: Raven Press.

Aicardi, J. & Chevrie, J. J. (1978): Les spasmes infantiles. *Arch. Fr. Pediatr.* **35,** 1015–1021.

Ariizumi, M., Baba, K., Hibio, S., Shiihara, H., Michihiro, N., Ogawa, K. & Okubo, O. (1987): Immunoglobulin therapy in the West syndrome. *Brain Dev.* **9,** 422–425.

Auerswald, G. (1992): Vigabatrin bei pharmakoresistenten Epilepsien im Kindesalter. *Akt. Neurol.* **19** (1), 26–27.

Bachmann, D.S. (1982): Use of valproic acid in treatment of infantile spasms. *Arch. Neurol.* **39,** 49–52.

Blennow, G. & Starck, L. (1986): High dose B6 treatment in infantile spasms. *Neuropediatrics* **17,** 7–10.

Cavazzuti, G.B. (1973): Infantile spasms with hypsarrhythmia. In: *Evolution and prognosis of epilepsies*, eds. E. Lugaresi, P. Pazzaglia & C.A. Tassinari, pp. 109–117. Bologna: Aulo Gaggi.

Chevrie, J.J. & Aicardi, J. (1971): Le prognostic psychique des spasmes infantiles traités par l'ACTH ou les corticoides. Analyse statisque de 78 cas suivis plus d'un . *J. Neurol. Sci.* **12,** 351–357.

Chiron, C., Dulac, O., Beaumont, D., Mondragon, S., Palacios, L. & Luna, D. (1992): Clinical trial of vigabatrin (gamma-vinyl-GABA) in infantile spasms. *Epilepsia* **33** (suppl. 3), 723 (abstract).

Dravet, C., Munari, C. & Roger, J. (1973): Evolution de 39 cas de syndrome de West en relation avec l'épilepsie ultérieure. In: *Evolution and prognosis of epilepsies*, eds. E. Lugaresi, P. Pazzaglia & C. A. Tassinari, pp. 119–131. Bologna: Aulo Gaggi.

Dulac, O., Steru, D., Rey, E. & Arthius, M. (1982): Monothérapie par le valproate de sodium dans les épilepsies de l'enfant. *Arch. Fr. Pediatr.* **39,** 347–353.

Dumermuth, G. & Kovacs, E. (1973): The effects of clonazepam (Ro5-4023) in the syndrome of infantile spasms with hypsarrhythmia and in petit mal variant or Lennox syndrome. *Acta Neurol. Scand.* **49**, (suppl. 53), 26–28.

Echenne. B., Dulac, O., Parayre-Chanez, M.J., Chiron, C., Taillebois, L., Cognot, C., Andary, M., Clot, J. & Baldy-Moulinier, M.B. (1991): Treatment of infantile spasms with intravenenous gamma-globulins: *Brain Dev.* **13,** 313–319.

Fejerman, N. & Medina, C.S. (1977): *Convulsiones en la infancia.* Buenos Aires: Editorial Ergon.

Fois, A., Malandrini, F., Balestri, P. & Giorgi, D. (1984): Infantile spasms – long term results of ACTH treatment. *Eur. J. Pediatr.* **142,** 51–55.

Fois, A., Malandrini, F. & Mostardini, R. (1987): Further observations on the treatment of infantile spasms with corticotropin. *Brain Dev.* **9,** 82–84.

Friedman, I.E. & Pampiglione, G. (1971): Prognostic implications of electroencephalographic findings of hypsarrhythmia in first year of life. *Br. Med. J.* **4,** 323–325.

Gibbs, F.A. & Gibbs, E.L. (1976): Follow-up of ACTH-treated and untreated cases of hypsarrhythmia. *Clin. Electrencephalogr.* **7,** 149–157.

Gibbs, E.L., Fleming M.M. & Gibbs, F.A. (1954): Diagnosis and prognosis of hypsarrhythmia and infantile spasms. *Pediatrics* **33,** 66–72.

Glaze, D.G., Hrachovy, R.A., Frost, J.D., Kellaway, P. & Zion, T.E. (1988): Prospective study of outcome of infants with infantile spasms treated during controlled studies of ACTH and prednisone. *J. Pediatr.* **112,** 389–396.

Hrachovy, R.A. & Frost, J.D. (1988): Infantile spasms. *Cleveland Clin. J. Med.* **56** (suppl.), 10–16.

Hrachovy, R.A. & Frost, J.D. (1989): Infantile spasms. *Pediatr. Clin. North Am.* **36,** 311–329.

Hrachovy, R.A., Frost, J.D., Kellaway, P. & Zion, T. (1983): Double-blind study of ACTH vs prednisone therapy in infantile spasms. *J. Pediatr.* **103,** 641–645.

Hrachovy, R.A., Glaze, D.G. & Frost, J.D. (1991): A retrospective study of spontaneous remission and long-term outcome in patients with infantile spasms. *Epilepsia* **32,** 212–214.

Hrachovy, R.A, Frost, J.D. & Glaze, D.G. (1992): Single-blind study of high-dose versus low-dose ACTH therapy in infantile spasms. *Epilepsia* **33** (suppl. 3), 113 (abstract).

Ito, M., Okuno, T., Hattori, H., Fujii, T. & Mikawa, H. (1991): Vitamin B6 and valproic acid in treatment of infantile spasms. *Pediatr. Neurol.* **7,** 91–96.

Jan, J.E., Riegl, J.A., Crichton, J.U. & Dunn, H.G. (1971): Nitrazepam in the treatment of epilepsy in childhood. *Can. Med. Assoc. J.* **104,** 571–575.

Jeavons, P.M. & Bower, B.D. (1961): The natural history of infantile spasms. *Arch. Dis. Child.* **36,** 17–21.

Jeavons, P.M., Bower, B.D. & Dimitrakoudi, M. (1973): Long-term prognosis of 150 cases of 'West syndrome'. *Epilepsia* **14,** 153–164.

Kotlarek, F., Groβ-Selbeck, G., Kellermann, K., Pothmann, R. & Schauseil-Zipf, U. (1992): Stellenwert der Valproattherapie bei Kindern mit West-Syndrom. In: *Valproinsäure*, eds. G. Krämer & M. Laub, pp. 149–154. Berlin, Heidelberg, New York: Springer-Verlag.

Kurokowa, T., Goya, N., Fukuyama, Y., Susuki, M., Seki T. & Ohtahara S. (1980): West syndrome and Lennox–Gastaut syndrome: a survey of natural history. *Pediatrics* **65,** 81–88.

Kuriyama, M., Konishi, Y., Fujii, Y., Yasujima, M., Sudo, M., Konishi, K., Nakamura, K. & Ichise, T. (1992): Treatment of infantile spasms with long-term low dose ACTH. *No-To-Hattatsu* **24,** 469–474.

Lacy. J.R. & Penry, J.K. (1976): *Infantile spasms.* New York: Raven Press.

Lagenstein, I., Willig, R.P. & Iffland, P. (1978): Behandlung frühkindlicher Anfälle mit ACTH und Dexmethason unter standardisierten Bedingungen. I. Klinische Ergebnisse Monatsschr. Kinderheilk 126, 492–499.

Lerman, P. & Kivity, S. (1982): The efficacy of corticotropin in primary infantile spasms. *J. Pediatr.* **101,** 294–296.

Livingston, J.H., Beaumont, D., Arzimanoglou, A. & Aicardi, J. (1989): Vigabatrin in the treatment of epilepsy in children. *Br. J. Clin. Pharmacol.* **27** (suppl. 1), 109–112.

Lombroso, C.T. (1983): A prospective study in infantile spasms: clinical and therapeutic correlations. *Epilepsia* **24,** 135–158.

Low, N.L. (1958): Infantile spasms with mental retardation. II. Treatment with cortisone and adrenocorticotropine. *Pediatrics* **22,** 1165–1169.

Luni, E., Dulac, O., Pajot, N. & Beaumont, D. (1989): Vigabitrin in the treatment of childhood epilepsies: a single-blind placebo-controlled study. *Epilepsia* **30.** 430–437.

Matsumoto, A., Watanabe, K., Negoro, T., Sugiura, M., Iwase, K., Hara, K. & Miyazaki, S. (1981): Long-term prognosis after infantile spasms: statistical study of prognostic factors in 200 cases. *Dev. Med. Child Neurol.* **23,** 51–65.

Mizutani, I. (1969): Clinical investigations of infantile spasms: long-term follow-up study, especially on the development of intelligence. *Dev. Med. Child Neurol.* **11,** 811–812.

Nolte, R. (1992): West-Syndrom. *Monatsschr. Kinderheilkd.* **140,** 446–450.

Nolte, R., Christen, H.J. & Doerrer, J. (1988): Preliminary report of a multi-center study on the West syndrome. *Brain Dev.* **10,** 236–242.

Nolte, R., Schöntag, K. & Scheffner, D. (1990): Standardisierte ACTH-Therapie bei Säuglingen mit West-Syndrom. Ergebnisse einer prospektiven, multizentrischen Studie. In: *Epilepsie 89,* ed. P. Wolf, pp. 409–414. Einhorn-Presse Verlag.

O'Donohoe, N. (1976): A 15-year follow-up of 100 children with infantile spasms. *Ir. J. Med. Sci.* 145–138.

Ohtahara, S., Yamatogi, Y., Ohtsuka, Y., Oka, E. & Ishida, T. (1980): Prognosis of West syndrome with special reference to Lennox syndrome: a developmental study. In: *Advances in epileptology: the Xth epilepsy international symposium*, eds. J. Wada & J.K. Penry, pp. 149–154. New York: Raven Press.

Ohtsuka, Y., Matsuda, M., Ogina, T., Kobayashi, K. & Ohtahara, S. (1987): Treatment of the West syndrome with high-dose pyridoxal phosphate. *Brain Dev.* **9,** 418–421.

Pavone, L., Incorpora, G., La Roas, M., Livolti, S. & Mollica, F. (1981): Treatment of infantile spasms with sodium dipropylacetic acid. *Dev. Med. Child Neurol.* **23,** 454–461.

Pietz, J., Benninger, C., Schäfer, H., Mittermaier, G., Sontheimer, D. & Rating, D. (1991): Hochdosierte Vitamin-B6-Behandlung bei BNS-Anfallsleiden. In: *Aktuelle Neuropädiatrie 1990*, ed. J. Lütschg, pp. 238–241. Berlin: Springer-Verlag.

Pinsard, N. (1980): Evolution à long terme du syndrome de West (à propos de 100 cas). *Gaslini* **12** (suppl. 1), 24–25.

Pollack, M.A., Zion, T.E. & Kellaway, P. (1979): Long-term prognosis of patients with infantile spasms following ACTH therapy. *Epilepsia* **20,** 255–260.

Prats, J.M., Garaizar, C., Rua, M.J., Garcia-Nieto, M.L. & Madoz, P. (1991): Infantile spasms treated with high doses of sodium valproate: initial response and follow-up. *Dev. Med. Child Neurol.* **33,** 617–625.

Riikonen, R. (1982): A long-term follow-up study of 214 children with the syndrome of infantile spasms. *Neuropediatrics* **13,** 14–23.

Riikonen, R. & Amnell, G. (1981): Psychiatric disorders in children with earlier infantile spasms. *Dev. Med. Child. Neurol..* **23,** 747–760.

Riikonen, R. & Donner, M. (1980): ACTH therapy in infantile spasms: side-effects. *Arch. Dis. Child* **55,** 664–672.

Seki, Y., Kawahara, Y. & Hirose, M. (1976): The long-term prognosis of infantile spasms followed in school age. *Folia Psychiatr. Neurol. Japan.* **30,** 297–306.

Siemes, H., Spohr, H.-L., Michael, T. & Nau, H. (1988): Therapy of infantile spasms: results of a prospective study. *Epilepsia* **29,** 553–560.

Siemes, H., Spohr, H.-L. & Michael, T (1993): Langzeitergebnisse der primären Valproattherapie von BNS-Krämpfen. In: *Epilepsie 92*, ed. H. Stefan, pp. 256–266. Berlin: Deutsche Sektion der Internationalen Liga geger Epilepsie.

Siemes, H., Brandl, U. & Spohr, H.-L. (1994): Vigabatrin in infantile spasms. In: *Vigabatrin*, eds. G. Krämer & D. Schmidt (in press). Berlin, Heidelberg, New York: Springer Verlag.

Singer, W.D., Rabe, E.F. & Haller, J. S. (1980): The effect of ACTH therapy upon infantile spasms. *J. Pediatr.* **96,** 485–489.

Snead, O.C., Benton, J.W. & Myers, G.J. (1983): ACTH and prednisone in childhood seizure disorders. *Neurology* **33,** 966–970.

Snyder, C.H. (1967): Infantile spasms: favorable response to steroid therapy. *JAMA* **201,** 198–200.

Sorel, L. & Dusaucy-Bauloye, A. (1958): A propos de 21 cas d'hypsarrhythmia de Gibbs: son traitement spectaculaire par l'ACTH. *Acta Neurol. Psychiatr. Belg.* **58,** 130–141.

Taft, T. & Cohen, H. (1971): Hypsarrhythmia and infantile autism: a clinical report. *J. Autism Dev. Disord.* **1,** 327–336.

Trojaborg, W. & Plum, P. (1960): Treatment of 'hypsarrhythmia' with ACTH. *Acta Pediatr. Scand.* **49,** 572–582.

Vasella, F., Pavlicova, E., Schneider, H.J., Rudin, H.J. & Karbowski, K. (1973): Treatment of infantile spasms and Lennox–Gastaut syndrome with clonazepam (Rivotril). *Epilepsia* **14,** 165–175.

Völzke, E., Doose, H. & Stephan, E. (1967): The treatment of infantile spasms and hypsarrhythmia with Mogadon. *Epilepsia* **8,** 64–70.

West, W.J. (1841): On a peculiar form of infantile convulsions. *Lancet* **1,** 724–725.

Willoughby, J.A., Thursten, D.L. & Holowach, J. (1966): Infantile myoclonic seizures: an evaluation of ACTH and corticosteroid therapy. *J. Pediatr.* **69,** 1136–1138.

Section VII

Psychogenesis and psychotherapy

Hysterical or 'pseudoepileptic' seizures are a big issue again since their similarity to focal seizures of frontal origin has been perceived. In this section, the present state of their diagnosis and management is described. As we are preparing to ask the intriguing question why frontal lobe epileptic and hysterical seizures are so similar, some other observations seem to cast doubt on the sharp line which is often assumed to separate the psychogenesis from the somatogenesis of seizures.

The well-known fact that epileptic seizures may be psychodynamically induced, i.e. psychogenic, is juxtaposed with its counterpart, observations of hysterical seizures provoked by an epileptic aura. To an aura, a variety of responses are possible which are to a greater or lesser extent subject to conscious control.

One of them, taking countermeasures to interrupt the ongoing aura, can be developed into a therapeutic strategy. Intriguingly, although at the onset of this treatment auras are still allowed to occur, this may eventually lead to complete abatement of seizures. The mechanism behind such a development remains to be explained.

At the end of a book where so much is said about secondary epileptogenesis and epilepsy as a disease process, the section closes with an antitethical hypothesis about possible mechanisms of negative feedback to the seizure generator which may exert a curative effect beyond the control of individual seizures.

Epileptic Seizures and Syndromes, Edited by Peter Wolf
© 1994 John Libbey & Company Ltd., pp. 633–642

Chapter 62

Diagnosis of pseudoepileptic seizures

Américo C. Sakamoto*, Hans Holthausen† and Soheyl Noachtar‡

**Department of Neurology, Ribeirão Preto Medical School, University of São Paulo, Brazil Campus Universitario, Ribeirão Preto-SP 14049–900, Brazil; †Epilepsie-Zentrum Bethel, Klinik Mara I, Maraweg 21, 33617 Bielefeld, Germany; ‡Ludwig – Maximilians, Universität München, Klinikum Grosshadern, Neurologische Poliklinik, 8090 München 70, Germany*

Introduction

Pseudoepileptic seizures (PESs) are *paroxysmal events* or *seizures* of definitely non-epileptic origin. An extensive list of terms have been employed to characterize these events but most authors refer to them as *psychogenic seizures* or simply *pseudoseizures*. Both terminologies are, however, incorrect or at least incomplete. Although the term psychogenic seizure has the obvious advantage of putting emphasis on its imputed pathogenic mechanism, it is indisputable that genuine epileptic seizures (ESs) can also be provoked by, or generated under, psychogenic stimuli and therefore be, in this sense, truly psychogenic seizures as well. On the other hand, the terminology pseudoseizure sounds equally unsatisfactory because these non-epileptic events are nevertheless still seizures, while the term pseudoseizure seems to imply a 'false seizure' rather than a 'falsely epileptic seizure'. In daily clinical practice, neurologists and psychiatrists need to have a clear terminology that precisely describes those events that are still seizures but of unquestionable non-epileptic origin. We personally prefer to use *pseudoepileptic seizure*, instead of other longer names like psychogenic pseudoepileptic seizures, non-epileptic psychogenic seizures, non-epileptic attack disorders, etc.

Like many other topics in medicine, the diagnosis of PES has over the years been greatly affected by the impact of the advent of new (diagnostic) technologies and of the recognition or better delineation of new clinical syndromes. We are here referring to the introduction of video-electroencephalographic monitoring techniques (video-EEG) into the diagnostic armamentarium, and the identification or better knowledge and understanding of previously unsuspected peculiar types of frontal lobe epileptic seizures (FLESs), whose phenomenology very closely resembles PESs.

In this chapter, then, we will mainly concentrate on discussing the contribution and consequences of these two factors, video-EEG and 'new' frontal lobe syndromes, to the diagnosis of PES. It is our understanding that classical criteria that many of us probably learned in our medical school days as of invaluable importance for this specific diagnosis (side-to-side head movements, for example) ought to be reconsidered in the light of 'new' information gathered from exhaustive video-EEG documentation of different sorts of paroxysmal events and especially the better understanding of frontal lobe epileptic manifestations. Lastly, we will also review apparently controversial data on serum prolactin measurements, which, in many instances and circumstances, seem to be of potential assistance in differentiating true ES from PES.

Clinical phenomenology (or video-EEG data)

> 'The characteristic of the convulsions which are called "hysterical", "hysteroid", "hystero-epileptic", or "hysteria major", is, as stated in the introductory chapter, that the spasmodic movements are of a more or less coordinated character. The grouping of muscular contractions is, in the main, such as may be produced by the will. Hence the spasm has a somewhat purposive aspect. Rigid fixation of the trunk and limbs alternates with wild movements, in which the limbs are thrown about; the arms strike out, the legs kick, the head is dashed from side to side' (Gowers, 1881).

This classical description of a typical PES was extracted from Gowers's chapter on 'Hysteroid or coordinated convulsions – hystero-epilepsy' (Gowers, 1881). In our days, however, many of us would probably agree that similar description could well be used to characterize subtypes of FLES. In other words, there is an imperative need for clear-cut (if possible) criteria for the differential diagnosis of the two conditions. In addition, Gowers elaborated one of the very first tables comparing diagnostic characters of epileptic *vs.* hysterical fits. During many decades his 'distinctive characters' were followed as guidelines and considered valid diagnostic criteria for the identification of PES. Video-EEG techniques further explored and refined the clinical semiology of these attacks, as can be appreciated in the initial video-EEG data.

Initial video-EEG data

In the early 1980s many reports focusing on video-EEG recordings of PES were published (Desai *et al.*, 1982; Guberman, 1982; Gulick *et al.*, 1982; King *et al.*, 1982; Luther *et al.*, 1982), dedicated either to the description of their main characteristics or to the comparative analysis of the clinical features of PESs *vs.* true ESs.

Guberman (1982), for example, reinforced the classical concept that motor manifestations of PES are non-stereotypic, asymmetrical, asynchronous and possibly modifiable by the examiner. He also emphasized that this type of spells could be induced by suggestion and that the return to a normal level of consciousness was usually abrupt.

Desai *et al.* (1982), in comparing clinical features of intractable complex partial seizures (CPSs) and seizures of unknown type discussed in detail the clinical phenomenology of a subgroup of six patients thought to have PESs and their diagnostic criteria. Motor behaviour was again the main issue, especially the absence of an atonic phase, irregularity of clonic jerks, body rolling and rocking, leg kicking and side-to-side head jerking. In addition, they suggested in their case no. 3 that response to verbal commands, recall of spoken words and preservation of consciousness during an attack with clear bilateral motor involvement would exclude the diagnosis of an ES. In their case no. 5 they suggested in addition that prolonged unresponsiveness and abduction of the arms followed by abrupt return to consciousness would also exclude ES. However, an important limitation of their study was that one of their major criteria for diagnosing PES was the deviation from characteristics of already known ES types, which, by itself, could have prevented them from recognizing any possibly unusual ES as a genuine ES. They also properly concluded that 'no single criterion is sufficient for an unequivocal diagnosis of psychogenic seizures', and, as a matter of fact, none of those above-mentioned features are nowadays considered as excluding the diagnosis of epilepsy. Also, importantly, they had already recognized that 'most epileptic seizures are relatively stereotyped, although some are quite bizarre and unusual'.

Gates *et al.* (1985) similarly compared 'convulsive' PES and generalized tonic–clonic seizures

(GTCSs) and claimed that they has identified 'useful bedside criteria for distinguishing a pseudo-seizure from a tonic–clonic seizure', namely, the quality of upper and lower extremity movements (whether in phase or out of phase), the time and nature of vocalization (at the start or middle of the seizure), pelvic thrust (forward or retropelvic), whole-body rigidity, eye manifestations and quality of head movements (especially side-to-side movements or unilateral turn). However, they pointed out that 'pelvic thrust (classically considered typical for PES) and rigidity were not useful as single variables'. Interestingly, they also demonstrated that a combination of variables (through multivariate discriminant analysis) significantly improved their classification schema.

All these clinical criteria were, however, not fundamentally different from the ones already established around the turn of the century, probably because most of the studies were still relying exclusively on classically well-known (pre-established) patterns of epileptic seizures for the diagnosis of ESs, or on the exclusion capacity of normal ictal and postictal EEGs. Therefore, the concept of 'hysterical-like' FLESs was not established yet. Consequently, most of these initial video-EEG studies are currently of little or no value for the clinical differentiation between PES and FLES.

Frontal lobe epilepsy

In dealing with the diagnosis of PES, it is necessary to review the clinical semiology of those FLESs whose phenomenology closely resembles pseudoepileptic attacks. For a more comprehensive and detailed description of FLES phenomenology, the readers are referred to the papers by Hajek and Wieser (1988) and Delgado-Escueta *et al.* (1991). Differential diagnosis between FLES and PES was really never a major issue until the landmark papers by Williamson *et al.* (1985) and Williamson and Spencer (1986) appeared. These authors take the credit of popularizing the notion that ESs can be bizarre and manifest as 'hysterical-like' episodes. According to them, these FLESs are characteristically brief, of sudden onset and offset, with little or no postictal confusion, stereotyped, with prominent motor automatisms (usually complex and of a sexual nature), and frequently associated with vocalization of variable complexity and preceded by non-specific warnings.

Although full documentation of such cases of FLESs through invasive techniques and postoperative seizure-free state is scarce in the literature, it is nevertheless widely accepted that ESs originating from mesial frontal cortex and orbital frontal cortex can produce 'hysterical-like' clinical phenomenology mimicking PESs.

Waterman *et al.* (1987), for example, reported on 12 such cases associated with ictal discharges in the mesial frontal lobes. Morris *et al.* (1988) reported on 11 patients with supplementary motor area (SMA) epileptic seizures, three of them exhaustively investigated through invasive subdural electrodes. These seizures usually began abruptly and often consisted of tonic posturing of one or more extremities, sometimes followed by rhythmic or clonic movements. Vocalization, grunting and twisting of the body also occurred frequently. Consciousness usually remained intact. Electrical cortical stimulation reproduced tonic posturing in two of these patients and vocalization in another one. They further stressed that 'SMA seizures are an important exception to the rule that consciousness is invariably impaired in patients with seizures in whom all four extremities are involved. Several of our patients were thought to have pseudoseizures because they broke the rule.' Fusco *et al.* (1990) also reported on eight similar cases, calling attention to their main behavioural manifestations: motor activity and vocalization. Motor behaviour was again usually complex and consisted of bilateral, asynchronous or rhythmic movements of limb and trunk, pelvic and whole-body movements, thrashing and kicking of legs, bicycling actions, pelvic torsion, violent rocking of trunk, kneeling, standing up and walking. Vocalization was also characteristic and consisted of grunting, shouting, screaming, moaning, howling, whistling sounds, talking gibberish, animal noises, etc. They, like other authors, also observed the predominance of the episodes during sleep. Many of these commplex motor manifestations were already demonstrated to be produced by electrical stimulation of SMA and anterior cingulate cortex in humans (Penfield & Jasper, 1954; Tailarach *et al.*, 1973; Van Buren & Fedio, 1976; Bancaud *et al.*, 1977). Based on all these data it is our understanding that the literature already contains good clinical and experimental evidence that frontal lobes, especially mesial frontal and orbital frontal cortex, can produce 'hysterical-like' ESs.

Pseudoepileptic seizure *vs.* frontal lobe epileptic seizure

Because mesial and orbitofrontal lobe seizures can mimic 'convulsive' PES, it becomes increasingly crucial to compare clinical features of both conditions under the same circumstances of observation, and ideally examined by the same group of observers. Very few papers have specifically addressed this question from this perspective (Kanner *et al.*, 1990; Wilkus *et al.*, 1990; Saygi *et al.*, 1992), including more recent articles on PES (Meierkord *et al.*, 1991; Leis *et al.*, 1992).

Kanner *et al.* (1990) specifically attempted to compare clinical phenomenology of SMA seizures (63 episodes in 12 patients) and PES (111 episodes in 44 patients) evaluated under similar conditions. By analysing a checklist of 45 descriptive categories and 950 qualifying options they found 'SMA seizures to be shorter in duration (five times shorter), stereotypic, tend to occur during sleep, and often present with a tonic contraction of upper extremities in abduction' and 'conversely, PES to be longer, non-stereotypic, and occur in awake state'. Tonic posturing occurred in both groups but tonic contraction of upper extremities in abduction was specific for SMA seizures, especially when occurring as an initial phenomenon. Oposthotonus was also observed in both groups but involved only the neck in SMA seizures and neck and trunk in PESs. Thrashing activity was also found to be slightly different, being shorter and stereotypic (within each patient) for the SMA group and longer and more elaborate in the PES group. They cautiously concluded that 'clinical phenomena may be useful in distinguishing PESs from SMA seizures, although the final diagnosis must be documented by neurophysiologic means'.

Wilkus *et al.* (1990) made a similar comparison between episodes recorded from two patients with CPSs of proved frontal lobe origin and two patients with PESs. Interestingly, they looked at not only the overall appearance of the episodes, but rather the exact sequence and time course of each clinical manifestation. Although the number of patients was too small to produce definitive conclusions, they found that true ESs were quite stereotypic while PESs, despite an overall stereotypic appearance, were more varied when detailed analysis of each individual feature of the seizures was broken down in terms of specific sequence and duration. It is our opinion that their observation warrants further investigation in larger groups of patients, provided multiple episodes from each patient are recorded and meticulous verification of stereotype or intraindividual consistency is observed.

Saygi *et al.* (1992) more recently also compared 63 FLESs in 11 patients and 29 PESs in 12 patients. They found no statistically significant difference between the two groups with respect to history of psychiatric disorder, ictal pelvic thrusting, kicking, pedalling, rocking of body, side-to-side head movements or rapid postictal recovery. Variables which favoured FLES were: nocturnal occurrence, short ictal duration, younger age at onset, stereotyped patterns of movements and magnetic resonance image (MRI) and EEG abnormalities. At the end, they concluded that 'no single criterion or even the whole clinical picture is sufficient to differentiate the most confusing group of partial epileptic seizures from pseudoepileptic seizures'.

Although controversial, the use of suggestion or induction techniques (Cohen & Suter, 1982) under video-EEG monitoring can sometimes be of great help in comparing clinical features of ES and PES, provided the recorded events are identical to the patients' habitual seizures. Of additional and decisive help are those instances when 'provoked' events can be stopped or clearly modified in their course by the examiner.

Prolactin data

Since the pioneer publication by Öhman *et al.* (1976), different groups of investigators have tried to correlate serum prolactin measurements in humans with the occurrence of various forms of epileptic and non-epileptic seizures (Trimble, 1978; Collins *et al.*, 1983; Wyllie *et al.*, 1984; Laxer *et al.*, 1985;

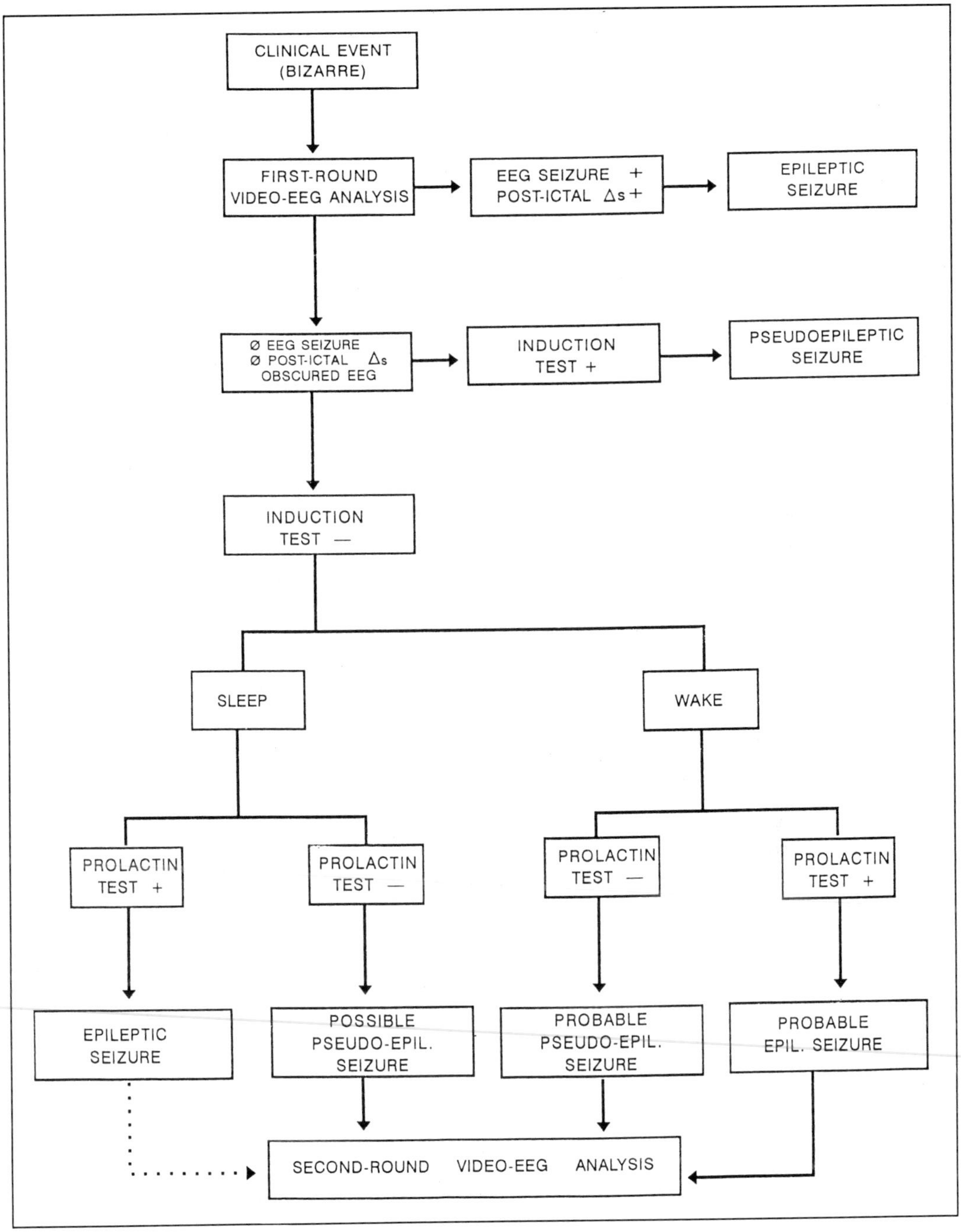

Fig. 1. Proposed algorithm for the differential diagnosis between pseudoepileptic seizures and true epileptic seizures .

Pritchard *et al.*, 1985; Sperling *et al.*, 1986; Rao *et al.*, 1989; Wroe *et al.*, 1989; Meierkord *et al.*, 1992). Although direct comparison of these studies is difficult because of marked methodological variability, especially heterogeneous patient selection, variable baseline and timing of prolactin measurements and diverse criteria for considering normal or abnormal prolactin level changes, it is nevertheless widely accepted that prolactin levels do increase after ESs and do not significantly increase after PESs. This conclusion is further supported by studies employing direct electrical stimulation of human limbic structures which showed parallel increase of prolactin levels, thus suggesting that stimulation (excitation) of limbic neurones increases prolactin release.

Electrical stimulation investigations in temporal lobe epileptic patients with depth electrodes implanted in to the amygdala and hippocampus have clearly demonstrated an increase in prolactin levels after effective stimulations or after seizures, while ineffective stimuli producing only brief after-discharges of less than 10 s duration had no effect on prolactin secretion (Gallagher *et al.*, 1987). Previously, Parro *et al.* (1980) obtained similar results by stimulating the amygdala in a similar group of epileptic patients with implanted depth electrodes. Sperling & Wilson (1986) conducted a more detailed study of electrical stimulation, involving 11 patients, with depth electrodes stereotaxically implanted into the basolateral amygdala, anterior, mid- and posterior hippocampus and hippocampal gyrus, in addition to extra electrodes eventually implanted into the SMA or the orbitofrontal or anterior cingulate cortex. They performed a total of 39 stimulations, mostly of the amygdala (22 stimulations) and anterior hippocampus (10 stimulations), but also of the mid-hippocampus (two stimulations), orbitofrontal cortex (two stimulations), cingulate gyrus (two stimulations) and SMA (one stimulation). Similarly, they observed that only two stimulations causing high-frequency regional limbic after-discharges lasting 20 and 60 s, respectively, were able to produce elevations on prolactin levels. All other stimuli had absolutely no effect, thus suggesting that only intense and extensive discharges involving limbic structures are effective in this respect, probably due to their secondary subcortical spread.

Many other clinical studies have also looked for correlations between prolactin levels and video-EEG-documented events. Wyllie *et al.* (1984) observed a threefold increase in prolactin levels after 80 per cent, 43 per cent and 10 per cent of GTCSs, CPSs and simple partial seizures (SPSs), respectively, in a group of 17 patients and 65 seizures. Additionally, they found that, despite no intergroup differences in the proportion of patients with abnormal prolactin levels, the subgroup of five patients presenting only GTCSs had mean levels 5.5 times greater than baseline, while the subgroup of four patients presenting solely CPSs had mean levels only 3.1 times greater than baseline. Based on these data they suggested the existence of a positive correlation between the degree of prolactin increase and the extent of the epileptic activity. Because prolactin levels were not changed after some ESs they also pointed out that normal prolactin values can not be used to definitively exclude the possibility of ESs.

Laxer *et al.* (1985) in another similar study, involving 70 patients and 85 seizures recorded through non-invasive and invasive video-EEG techniques, found that prolactin levels were significantly increased after any primarily or secondarily GTCSs, after any temporal lobe CPSs other than just aura or behavioural arrest, and not significantly increased after SPSs. In their study they also included a subgroup of patients with PESs which showed no significant increase in prolactin levels. In addition, they performed discriminant function analysis and demonstrated that PESs were correctly classified in 94.4 per cent and ESs in 65.5 per cent of the seizures. Contrary to the findings of Wyllie *et al.* (1984), they observed that progression into secondarily GTCS did not substantially affect prolactin levels in the temporal lobe epilepsy group, thus suggesting that extension/intensity of the epileptic activity plays an important but limited role in prolactin release.

Pritchard *et al.* (1985) similarly compared a group of six patients with ESs to another group of six patients with PESs and found mean postictal prolactin levels significantly higher for the epileptic group at 15, 30, 45 and 60 min postictally.

In another highly selected group of 16 epileptic patients with multicontact depth electrodes consistently and bilaterally implanted into the basolateral amygdala, anterior, mid- and posterior hippocampal pes and hippocampal gyrus, plus eventual additional depth electrodes implanted into the SMA or orbitofrontal or anterior cingulate cortex, Sperling *et al.* (1986) also looked for correlations between SPSs, CPSs, electrographic seizure patterns and postictal prolactin levels. In a total of 38 CPS in 15 patients they observed a minimum twofold postictal increase over baseline in all seizures. The ictal electrographic pattern started unilaterally in the mesial temporal region in 34 seizures then spread to the contralateral side in all instances. In the other four seizures, the ictal pattern was recorded simultaneously in both mesial temporal regions. There was no correlation between prolactin levels and seizure duration or type of ictal behaviour.

In the sample of 40 SPSs (auras), postictal prolactin levels were significantly elevated in only eight of those 10 seizures which were associated with unilateral high-frequency regional ictal electrographic discharges. In none of 20 auras associated with variable and low-frequency regional ictal discharges, focal discharges or a combination of low-frequency regional and focal discharges was there any postictal prolactin elevation. Neither was any increase observed in the other 10 auras associated with no limbic ictal EEG changes. Based on these findings, Sperling *et al.,* (1986) suggested that in the case of auras the intensity or 'high frequency' of the limbic discharges was a necessary condition for the prolactin elevation, while for the CPSs prolactin was invariably elevated.

In another study involving 33 patients, Wroe *et al.* (1989) found that prolactin levels above 1000 mU/l were highly suggestive of ESs and that the false negative rate was only 9 per cent for GTCSs but 38 per cent for CPSs.

More recently Meierkord *et al.* (1992) reported on prolactin levels in 10 patients with temporal lobe epileptic seizures (TLESs) and 11 patients with FLESs. Prolactin levels were found to be elevated after six out of eight CPSs of temporal lobe origin (75 per cent) and in only one out of eight CPSs of frontal lobe origin (12.5 per cent). Similar results had earlier been reported by Hammers (1990). This elevation was not related to the duration of seizures, gender, unilateral or bilateral ictal EEG features or the presence or absence of EEG spiking. Their data confirm that prolactin measurements are valuable for the diagnosis of CPSs of temporal lobe origin and suggest that they are of little help for the differential diagnosis between FLESs and PESs.

Overall one can assume that there is already a fairly good amount of data supporting an important role for prolactin measurements in the diagnosis of ESs and PESs. Strikingly, however, prolactin levels seem to remain unchanged after repetitive epileptic seizures (Jackel *et al.*, 1987) or even after status epilepticus (Tomson *et al.*, 1989). Possible explanations are depletion of stored prolactin by recent seizure activity (Jackel *et al.*, 1987) or activation of the dopaminergic system during prolonged or repeated epileptic seizures, which inhibits secretion of prolactin from the hypophysis (Tomson *et al.*, 1989). One should therefore be cautious, and not exclude the diagnosis of status epilepticus based on normal prolactin levels.

Concluding remarks

Neurologists and epileptologists are frequently solicited to establish the differential diagnosis between ES and PES. In most instances experienced clinicians can accomplish that without any major difficulty. However, in other circumstances, this can be an almost impossible task which defies even the most experienced epileptologists. Practical consequences of misdiagnosis in this field are obviously dramatic. A frontal lobe epilepsy patient could thus be misdiagnosed as having pseudoepileptic attacks and be denied a chance for appropriate treatment (including surgery) and an eventually seizure-free state. Probably he/she would receive unnecessary psychiatric treatment or psychotherapy from which no relief could be expected.

Many variables, such as sex, circumstances of occurrence (asleep or awake), precipitating factors, psychological or psychiatric profile, past history of sexual abuse, etc., can be of help but are definitely of no decisive influence in this differential diagnosis. On the other hand, the clinical phenomenology of both conditions is unfortunately too complex and variable to permit a safe diagnosis on clinical grounds alone. Classical signs, such as uncoordinated limb movements, side-to-side head movements, sphincter relaxation, pupil signs, avoidance response, type and timing of vocalization, etc., are equally not decisive. Although no single test can unequivocally differentiate both conditions in all cases, video-EEG and prolactin measurements seem to be the most helpful tests and therefore should be routinely performed.

Despite the limitless possibilities of different types of PESs, in clinical practice the major problem is really narrowed down to the differentiation between 'hysterical-like' FLESs (especially mesiofrontal and orbitofrontal seizures) and 'convulsive' PESs. For these cases we think that the utilization of a diagnostic algorithm, as proposed in Fig. 1, would probably be helpful. In this proposal every 'bizarre' clinical event should then be submitted to a first-round video-EEG analysis, looking in first place specifically for an unequivocal EEG seizure pattern or unquestionable postictal EEG changes. ESs are rarely devoid of any ictal or postictal EEG changes, including FLESs (Morris *et al.*, 1988).

In a second step, those cases with no EEG changes or obscured (by artefacts) ictal EEGs should be submitted to an induction test (under video-EEG monitoring). If habitual seizures are induced and the provoked events are clearly modifiable by the examiner (interrupted or modified in their course), the test is considered positive and diagnostic of PESs. Although ESs are reportedly also provokable and inhabitable by external and internal stimuli (Brown & Fenwick, 1989; Fenwick & Brown, 1989), it is nevertheless highly unlikely that they would also be modifiable under suggestion or devoid of any ictal EEG changes.

Patients with negative or doubtful induction tests should then be further investigated. They should all have serial prolactin measurements. A positive prolactin test (threefold increase, for example) strongly suggests an epileptic seizure, while a negative test definitely does not exclude this possibility. However, it does unquestionably make the possibility of PESs more likely.

A careful look into the circumstances of spontaneous occurrence of the seizures is sometimes helpful, especially their relationship to the sleep–wake cycle. Seizures that clearly occur out of sleep are more likely to be of epileptic origin. On the other hand, seizures that show in this respect a clear peri-ictal EEG–behavioural dissociation, for example alpha rhythm while apparently sleeping (Thacker *et al.*, 1993), are most probably PESs. This is also true for patients showing posterior alpha rhythm while apparently unresponsive. In practice, an always difficult situation is when the patient wakes up some minutes before presenting the seizure. There is always the possibility of an ES preceded by an aura (which wakes up the patient and usually produces no EEG seizure pattern) or, conversely, a PES which occurs in a patient who woke up minutes before the seizure for some other reason. In summary, seizures that unequivocally occur out of sleep and show a clear prolactin test (positive test) are certainly of epileptic origin. Seizures that occur while the patient is awake and similarly show a clear prolactin test are most probably ESs. Conversely, seizures that occur in wake or apparently sleeping patients and are associated with a negative prolactin test are most likely to be 'probable' or 'possible' pseudoepileptic events. All these doubtful cases should then be submitted to a second-round detailed video-EEG analysis, looking in multiple seizure recordings specifically for interevents and intra-individual stereotypy and consistency, in other words, exact sequence and duration of each component or fragment of the clinical event. Although this type of analysis has not been systematically tested in larger series, we think it is an attractive and promising approach and certainly warrants further systematic investigation. It is also our impression that many apparently chaotic or 'bizarre' seizures are surprisingly stereotypic when submitted to this type of detailed and second-by-second or 'frame-by-frame' video analysis.

References

Bancaud, J., Talairach, J., Geier, S., Bonis, A., Trottier, S. & Manrique, M. (1977): Manifestations comportamentales incuites par la stimulation électrique du gyrus cingulaire anterieur chez l'homme. *Rev. Neurol. (Paris)* **132,** 705–724.

Brown, S.W. & Fenwick, P.B.C. (1989): Evoked and psychogenic epileptic seizures: inhibition. *Acta Neurol. Scand.* **80,** 541–547.

Cohen, R.J. & Suter, C. (1982): Hysterical seizures: suggestion as a provocative EEG test. *Ann. Neurol.* **11,** 391–395.

Collins, W.C.J., Lanigan, O. & Callaghan, N. (1983): Plasma concentrations following epileptic and pseudoseizures. *J. Neurol. Neurosurg. Psychiatry* **46,** 505–508.

Delgado-Escueta, A.V., Swartz, B.E., Walsh, G.O., Chauvel, P., Bancaud, J. & Broglin, D. (1991): Frontal lobe seizures and epilepsies in neurobehavioral disorders. In: *Advances in neurology,* Vol. 55, eds. D. Smith, D. Treiman & M. Trimble, pp. 317–340. New York: Raven Press.

Desai, B.T., Porter, R.J. & Penry, J.K. (1982): Psychogenic seizures – a study of 42 attacks in six patients with intensive monitoring. *Arch. Neurol.* **39,** 202–209.

Fenwick, P.B.C. & Brown, S.W. (1989): Evoked and psychogenic epileptic seizures. I. Precipitation. *Acta Neurol. Scand.* **80,** 535–540.

Fusco, L., Iani, C., Faedda, M.T., Manfredi, M., Vigevano, F., Ambrosetto, G., Ciarmatori, C. & Tassinari, C.A. (1990): Mesial frontal lobe epilepsy: a clinical entity not sufficiently described. *J. Epilepsy* **3,** 123–135.

Gallagher, B.B., Flanigin, H.F., King, D.W. & Littleton, W.H. (1987): The effect of electrical stimulation of medial temporal lobe structures in epileptic patients upon ACTH, prolactin, and growth hormone. *Neurology* **37,** 299–303.

Gates, J.R., Ramani, V., Whalen, S. & Loewenson, R. (1985): Ictal characteristics of pseudoseizures. *Arch. Neurol.* **42,** 1183–1187.

Gowers, W.R. (1881): Epilepsy and other chronic convulsive diseases: their causes, symptoms, and treatment. London: J. & A. Churchill.

Guberman, A. (1982): Psychogenic pseudoseizures in non-epileptic patients. *Can. J. Psychiatry* **27** (5), 401–404.

Gulick, T.A., Spinks, I.P. & Wing, D.W. (1982): Pseudoseizures: ictal phenomena. *Neurology* **32,** 24–30.

Hajek, M. & Wieser, H.G. (1988): Extratemporal, mainly frontal, epilepsies: surgical results. *J. Epilepsy* **1,** 103–119.

Hammers, R. (1990): Prolaktinnegative Komplex-fokale Anfälle: Hinweis auf frontalen Ursprung? In: *Epilepsie 89,* ed. P. Wolf, pp. 52–58. , Reinbek: Einhorn-Press.

Jackel, R.A., Malkowicz, D., Trivedi, R., Sussman, N.M., Eskin, B.A. & Harner, R.N. (1987): Reduction of prolactin response with repetitive seizures. *Epilepsia* **28 (5),** 588.

Kanner, A.M., Morris, H.H., Lüders, H., Dinner, D.S., Wyllie, E., Medendorp, S.V. & Rowan, A.J. (1990): Supplementary motor seizures mimicking pseudoseizures: some clinical differences. *Neurology* **40,** 1404–1407.

King, D.W., Gallagher, B.B., Murvin, A.J., Smith, D.B., Marcus, D.J., Hartlage, L.C. & Ward, L.C. (1982): Pseudoseizures: diagnostic evaluation. *Neurology* **32,** 18–23.

Laxer, K.D., Mullooly, J.P. & Howell, B. (1985): Prolactin changes after seizures classified by EEG monitoring. *Neurology* **35,** 31–35.

Leis, A.A., Ross, M.A. & Summers, A.K. (1992): Psychogenic seizures: ictal characteristics and diagnostic pitfalls. *Neurology* **42,** 95–99.

Luther, J.S., McNamara, J.O., Carwile, S., Miller, P. & Hope, V. (1982): Pseudoepileptic seizures: methods and video analysis to aid diagnosis. *Ann. Neurol.* **12,** 458–462.

Meierkord, H., Will, B., Fish, D. & Shorvon, S. (1991): The clinical features and prognosis of pseudoseizures diagnosed using video-EEG telemetry. *Neurology* **41,** 1643–1646.

Meierkord, H., Shorvon, S., Lightman, S. & Trimble, M. (1992): Comparison of the effects of frontal and temporal lobe partial seizures on prolactin levels. *Arch. Neurol.* **49,** 225–230.

Morris, H.H., Dinner, D.S., Lüders, H., Wyllie, E. & Kramer, R. (1988): Supplementary motor seizures: clinical and electroencephalographic findings. *Neurology* **38,** 1075–1082.

Öhman, R., Walinger, J., Balldin, J., Wallin, L. & Abrahamsson, L. (1976): Prolactin response to electroconvulsive therapy. *Lancet* **ii,** 936–937.

Parro, A., Velasco, M., Cervantes, C., Muñoz, H., Cerbón, M.A. & Velasco, F. (1980): Plasma prolactin increase following electric stimulation of the amygdala in humans. *Neuroendocrinology* **31,** 60–65.

Penfield, W. & Jasper, H. (1954): *Epilepsy and the functional anatomy of the human brain.* Boston: Little, Brown.

Pritchard, P.B., Wannamaker, B.B., Sagel, J. & Daniel, C.M. (1985): Serum prolactin levels in evaluation of pseudoepileptic seizures. *Ann. Neurol.* **18,** 87–89.

Rao, M.R., Stefan, H. & Bauer, J. (1989): Epileptic but not psychogenic seizures are accompanied by simultaneous elevation of serum pituitary hormones and cortisol levels. *Neuroendocrinology* **49,** 33–39.

Saygi, S., Katz, A., Marks, D.A. & Spencer, S.S. (1992): Frontal lobe partial seizures and psychogenic seizures: comparison of clinical and ictal characteristics. *Neurology* **42,** 1274–1277.

Sperling, M.R. & Wilson, C.L. (1986): The effect of limbic and extralimbic electrical stimulations upon prolactin secretion in humans. *Brain Res.* **371,** 293–297.

Sperling, M.R., Pritchard, P.B., Engel, J., Jr, Daniel, C. & Sagel, J. (1986): Prolactin in partial epilepsy: an indicator of limbic seizures. *Ann. Neurol.* **20,** 716–722.

Talairach, J., Bancaud, J., Geier, S., Bordas-Ferrer, M., Bonis, A., Szikla, G. & Rusu, M. (1973): The cingulate gyrus and human behaviour. *Electroencephalogr. Clin. Neurophysiol.* **34,** 45–52.

Thacker, K., Devinsky, O., Perrine, K., Alper, K. & Luciano, D. (1993): Nonepileptic seizures during apparent sleep. *Ann. Neurol.* **33,** 414–418.

Tomson, T., Lindbom, U., Nilsson, B.Y., Svanborg, E. & Anderson, D.E.H. (1989): Serum prolactin during status epilepticus. *J. Neurol. Neurosurg. Psychiatry* **52,** 1435–1437.

Trimble, M.R. (1978): Serum prolactin in epilepsy and hysteria. *Br. Med. J.* **2,** 1682.

Van Buren, J.M. & Fedio, P. (1976): Functional representation on the medial aspect of the frontal lobes in man. *J. Neurosurg.* **44,** 275–289.

Waterman, K., Purves, S.J., Kosaka, B., Strauss, E. & Wada, J.A. (1987): An epileptic syndrome caused by medial frontal lobe seizure foci. *Neurology* **37,** 577–582.

Wilkus, R.J., Thompson, P.M. & Vossler, D.G. (1990): Bizarre ictal automatisms: frontal lobe epileptic or psychogenic seizures? *J. Epilepsy* **3,** 207–213.

Williamson, P.D. & Spencer, S.S. (1986): Clinical and EEG features of complex partial seizures of extratemporal origin. *Epilepsia* **27** (suppl. 2), 46–63.

Williamson, P.D., Spencer, D.D., Spencer, S.S., Novelly, R.A. & Mattson, R.H. (1985): Complex partial seizures of frontal lobe origin. *Ann. Neurol.* **18,** 497–504.

Wroe, S.J., Henley, R., John, R. & Richens, A. (1989): The clinical value of serum prolactin measurement in the differential diagnosis of complex parhal seizures. *Epilepsy Res.* **3,** 248–252.

Wyllie, E., Lüders, H., MacMillan, J.P. & Gupta, M. (1984): Serum prolactin levels after epileptic seizures. *Neurology* **34,** 1601–1604.

Epileptic Seizures and Syndromes, Edited by Peter Wolf
© 1994 John Libbey & Company Ltd., pp. 643–650

Chapter 63

Management of psychogenic and pseudoepileptic seizures

Tim Betts

Seizure Clinic, Neuropsychiatry Service and Epilepsy Liaison Service, Department of Psychiatry, University of Birmingham, Queen Elizabeth Psychiatric Hospital, Edgbaston, Birmingham B15 2QZ, UK

'Most people with non-epileptic seizures are the victims of misdiagnosis rather than the perpetrators of it.'

Introduction

Semantic differences in terminology between the United Kingdom, Europe and the United States of America make it necessary for me to define my terms.

The term psychogenic seizure in the United Kingdom means an epileptic seizure which is precipitated by some emotional or mood state (Fenwick, 1991) but does not imply that such a seizure is non-epileptic. In parts of the continent of Europe and in the United States, however, the term appears to be synonymous with that of a non-epileptic seizure (so-called pseudoepileptic seizure).

I consider that the appropriate term for a seizure that is not an epileptic one, whether it is convulsive or otherwise, is 'non-epileptic seizure' (NES), and that a person who has NES should be described as suffering from a 'non-epileptic attack disorder' (NEAD) (Betts, 1990). NEAD has attracted a great deal of attention recently: it is recognized that the condition is common, is often mistaken for epilepsy, and is of some economic importance since NEAD may continue for many years unless recognized and treated. Between 10–20 per cent of patients referred to specialist centres for epilepsy for assessment of chronic epilepsy may be expected to be suffering from NEAD (Ramani, 1986), although it is my clinical impression that this proportion is starting to fall, possibly because the pool of such patients in the area which my service covers has been partially drained and has not been replaced. NES are, however, still likely to be confused with epilepsy at the time of initial presentation (Sander *et al.*, 1990).

The topic of NES has been the subject of several recent reviews (Mulder, 1990; Savard & Andermann, 1990; Betts, 1990, 1993; Betts & Boden, 1991) and also the subject of two recent publications (Gram *et al.*, 1993; Rowan & Gates, 1993), these two books representing an European and an American view respectively. Most of the published literature concerns itself with the recognition of non-epileptic seizures: discussions about management often seem to stop at that point. There is certainly no consensus view on management (Mulder, 1990) and very few follow-up studies have been published looking at the natural history of these conditions or their prognosis following treatment (Betts & Boden, 1992a).

Review of the literature suggests that different centres are almost certainly seeing different types of NES with differing aetiology, and that the proportion of patients with NES that also have associated psychiatric symptoms also varies widely: there is little consensus therefore on the classification of NES or on management.

What follows, therefore, must, of necessity, be a personal view based on some 25 years of recognizing and managing NEAD. My experience may well be different from that of others, and I accept that we are as yet some way from a consensus about both recognition and management of these conditions.

I certainly believe that many doctors have fallen into the error of placing epilepsy upon a kind of pedestal (Betts, 1993) and have developed a belief in the 'sanctity' of epilepsy so that, when faced with a patient whose seizures have been labelled as epileptic for some time but which, on fuller examination, turn out to be non-epileptic, we tend to take a dismissive view of the patient (the commonly used term 'pseudoseizure' is certainly extremely pejorative). The patient is blamed for a mistake in diagnosis which is usually the physician's.

We are over-eager to make a diagnosis of epilepsy because by doing so we 'medicalize' otherwise disturbing and puzzling paroxysmal behaviour: having 'medicalized' this behaviour we can then treat it with drugs and no longer have to understand the meaning of the seizures or the psychopathalogy of the person who has the seizures. The patient is often grateful to receive a medical explanation for his or her behaviour (as is his or her family), and both are often rather puzzled and angry when the medical excuse is withdrawn from them. The answer to this lies in being able to make the correct diagnosis of epilepsy or non-epilepsy in the first place, but, as studies of first seizures have shown (Sander *et al.*, 1990), this may be difficult and their true nature may not be revealed for some considerable time, which makes life difficult for the patient, family and doctor and may pressurize the doctor into making an over-hasty decision about the nature of the patient's attacks. Rectifying such a mistake later can be difficult. I have suggested elsewhere (Betts, 1993) that it may be better to consider epilepsy as a variety of 'seizure disorders' rather than making it a primary diagnosis.

General management

There are five general factors in the management of NES which are important but which are often neglected.

The first is that there is a wide differential diagnosis to NES: they are not all the same, although much of the literature implies that they are. In managing an NES, one has to try to determine what kind one is dealing with.

Secondly, although a firm diagnosis of epilepsy can be made using modern diagnostic techniques it is not always possible to make a firm diagnosis of non-epilepsy: there is often a slight haze of doubt surrounding the diagnosis. As our knowledge of the wilder shores of epilepsy extends (principally in the recognition of the sometimes puzzling and strange behaviour that occurs during frontal lobe and other extratemporal seizures), we may have to change the diagnosis of non-epilepsy back to epilepsy. Clinicians managing NES have to live with this uncertainty and have to avoid undue dogmatism. It is often better to say to the patient 'none of our tests have confirmed your attacks are epileptic and it may be better for a while, therefore, to treat them as though they are not and see how we get along with that', rather than making some *ex cathedra* statement about the nature of the patient's seizures which has to be rather embarrassingly revised in the light of future evidence.

The third general factor about NES is that most, if not all of them, are of a psychological nature. Some people with NES will therefore also be suffering from recognizable psychiatric syndromes. It is important not to make the mistake of assuming that any patient with seizures who has recognizable psychiatric pathology is therefore suffering from NES. A commonly made mistake is that, in patients who have seizures and who have also suffered some kind of sexual abuse in the past, it is assumed that they have non-epileptic seizures. This is not so (Greig & Betts, 1992). Although in many patients both the psychological symptoms and non-epileptic attacks are part of a post-traumatic stress disorder, often relating to previous sexual abuse, actual epileptic seizures may also be precipitated by sexual abuse. The correct management is to manage the post-traumatic stress disorder as a whole rather than concentrating on either the seizures or the psychological symptoms (Betts & Boden, 1992b; Cartmill & Betts, 1992).

The fourth general factor is that many people with NES also have epilepsy. Different authors produce different figures for the prevalence of epilepsy in patients who also have NES (figures vary between 10 and 90 per cent – Betts, 1993), but because a patient has been shown to have NES it should not be assumed that all his or her seizures are therefore epileptic.

The fifth general point is not to make the diagnosis hurriedly but to review and consider the evidence carefully and to bear in mind that the diagnosis may have to be changed in the light of further evidence. The specific management of NES can be considered under the following headings.

Recognition

Recognition of the non-epileptic nature of a patient's seizures may sometimes be easy and depend purely on a description given by the patient or a witness or the physician's own observations. Panic attacks and faints, for instance, should be recognizable from the history given, although, if the history-taking is incompetent or there are specific features to the panic attack or to the faint which are not normally seen but which can occur (e.g. the prolonged unconsciousness that can occur if somebody faints in an upright position, or incontinence which sometimes accompanies a faint), the decision may be more difficult. Mostly the diagnosis of NES will be made after a period of investigation, using video monitoring and specialist electroencephalographic (EEG) investigation. It should be remembered that some seizures will not be confirmed as epileptic, however, unless invasive EEG monitoring is done, so that at some point in the investigatory cycle the physician has to balance the risks of further investigation against the benefits of an accurate knowledge of the nature of the patient's seizures. At some point, therefore, the physician will stop, either because of the lack of facilities to take investigation further or because it is felt that the risks of further investigation are not justified.

At this point, it may be possible for the physician to say that it is certain that the attacks are non-epileptic or it is certain that the attacks are epileptic (bearing in mind that it is rarely possible to be certain of non-epilepsy although it is possible to be certain of epilepsy). More probably, however, the physician will arrive at the conclusion that on the present basis of evidence the most likely diagnosis (which may of course be changed in the future if further evidence comes to light) is that the attacks are probably epileptic and should therefore be be treated as such or that they are probably non-epileptic. Sometimes, in my experience, it is impossible to know what the patient's seizures are and under those circumstances, if a reasonably full trial of anticonvulsant medication has been tried and has failed (and the patient is not suitable for further investigation for possible epilepsy surgery), then a behavioural approach should be tried. By and large, the behavioural approach for the treatment of epilepsy (Fenwick 1991; Betts 1993) is remarkably close to the behavioural treatment for NES. One is treating the seizure, whether it is epileptic or not, as an unwanted piece of behaviour which the patient can learn to extinguish by various behavioural or cognitive means. As indicated at the beginning of this chapter, I take the view that psychogenic seizures are epileptic seizures which are emotionally precipitated. If they are considered in this light, the management of such seizures is the same as the management of NES; there are such few differences that the accounts of the management of psychogenic seizures and of NES can run in parallel.

I think this inability to distinguish between the form of treatment for two different sorts of seizures is sometimes helpful in patient management because it is possible with patients with puzzling seizures to be able to say, 'It does not really matter whether your seizures are epileptic or not since the treatment is the same. Let's just get on and see if we can help you to stop them.'

Confrontation

Once a working diagnosis has been reached, the time has come to confront the patient with the new diagnosis. This is often mishandled, although Mulder (1990) has shown that a well-timed and executed confrontation may be all that is needed to help the patient's seizures stop and this is also my experience. It is also my experience, unfortunately, to see many patients in whom the confrontation has been mishandled so that an angry, humiliated and rejected patient is discharged from a clinic or a hospital having been told (or having been given the implication) that the seizures are imaginary or are 'put on' in some way. The patient is often then left to fend for himself or herself or is suddenly transferred to psychiatric care without an informed and proper explanation ever having been given.

If confrontation is to succeed, then, the patient must be taken into the physician's confidence early on in the investigation process so that the patient understands that the physician is trying to establish exactly what the patient's seizures are and is aware of the dangers of making a diagnosis of epilepsy when no such condition exists. The alternative diagnosis of NES should be painted in a positive light. 'If this turns out not to be epilepsy, that is good news because at least we will know what we are dealing with and there are things that we can do to help you stop your seizures.' The patient should not be made to feel that non-epilepsy is somehow discreditable or that he is faking (very few people in my experience deliberately simulate epileptic seizures; most people with NES are the victims of misdiagnosis rather than perpetrators of it).

Time should be set aside to confront the patient properly. His/her history should be reviewed, the results of the various diagnostic investigations discussed and then the conclusion drawn (hopefully with the patient agreeing) that it is best at this stage to assume the seizures are non-epileptic in nature. The physician will often be in a situation when he/she cannot be completely certain that seizures are non-epileptic and should get across in a positive way the fact that, although at the present time it is to be assumed that the seizures are non-epileptic, the diagnosis can be re-examined at a later date in the light of fresh evidence or if better investigatory facilities become available. The physician is sometimes faced with a different situation when he/she is saying to the patient 'although none of the tests we have done suggest that your seizures have an epileptic basis to them, their clinical appearance still makes me feel that it is right to continue treating then as though they are epileptic'.

Sufficient time should also be given to allow patients to ventilate their feelings about the change in diagnosis and to give an assurance that the patient will continue to be supported and that the change in diagnosis is a positive event and not a negative one.

For this reason, if the physician feels unable to continue to look after the patient, transfer of care to another physician should not be hurried and should not be seen as a rejection.

Interviews may need to be held with the patient's family and in a very similar manner the change in diagnosis explained and ventilated. It is important that the patient continues to be supported by his/her family and it is therefore important to get across both to the patient and to the family that, although the seizures are not epileptic, they are nevertheless real, that attempts will be made to find an explanation for them and that the patient continues to be worthy of medical care and support. Families must be steered away from thinking that the patient has lost face or that they have been cheated or that, without help, the patient can pull him/herself together and stop the seizures.

An aid to the confrontational process is showing the patient his or her own seizures on video (if video analysis of the patient's seizure behaviour has been done) or similar seizures from other patients can be used. People with epilepsy should also see their own (or similar) seizures (Betts, 1993).

This form of confrontation may need to be done several times and careful note must be made of the patient's emotional reaction to seeing his or her seizures (as this may eventually form part of the therapeutic process), but the confrontation is also used to talk through the seizure in such a way that the patient understands why it is considered not to be epileptic. This may also be done with the patient's family if necessary. It should be clear from the above that the confrontational process may take several interviews and may need to be carried out in the patient's home. Significant others in the patient's life and community care workers may also need to be informed of the nature of the patient's seizures. It is particularly important that the patient's general practitioner understands the nature of the seizures and how the diagnostic decision was arrived at, since he or she may need to support the patient in the community for some considerable time (Betts & Duffy, 1993).

Further investigation

As indicated earlier, it is important to try to establish not just that the patient has NES but what kind of NES he/she has. A full classification is presented in Betts (1993) but basically NES fall into four types.

A small proportion of non-epilepsy is actually some other kind of organic disorder masquerading as epilepsy; the management of these conditions will not be considered further here, although it should be remembered that a patient in this category may have quite severe emotional problems whilst adjusting to the new diagnosis.

A second group of patients (roughly a third of those with NES) have some kind of recognized psychiatric disorder (such as panic disorder or vasovagal attacks – obviously sometimes occurring in the setting of other psychiatric disorders) which has been misdiagnosed as epilepsy. Thirdly, some patients, again often with co-existing psychiatric or personality disorder, may be deliberately or unconsciously simulating epilepsy, although in my experience this is uncommon.

The remaining patients have what might be termed a *primary* NEAD, the commonest types being (1) sudden displays of aggression, rage or frustration ('tantrums'), which often become medicalized and usually occur in the setting of an immature personality or learning disability, (2) 'swoons', which are cutting-off behaviour in which the patient suddenly withdraws from contact from either his/her environment or from intrusive and unpleasant thoughts, and (3) so-called 'abreactive seizures', in which there is characteristic back-arching, pelvic thrusting and gasping and which seem, as with the swoon, to occur particularly in women who have suffered sexual abuse. These last two seizures, in particular, often occur in the setting of a chronic post-traumatic stress disorder related to previous abuse (Betts & Boden, 1992b; Cartmill & Betts, 1992). Although particularly likely to occur in women, they can be seen in men, and I have, for instance, one male patient with the swoon type of attack occurring in the setting of a post-traumatic stress disorder related to combat experience.

Behaviour reminiscent of tantrums, swoons and abreactive attacks can also be caused by epileptic discharge, particularly in the frontal lobes: often people with epilepsy also have significant psychopathology, including a past history of sexual abuse or post-traumatic stress disorder (Greig & Betts, 1992).

In addition to determining the type of non-epileptic attack the patient has, attempts must be made to try to understand its aetiology. This requires a full psychiatric history and examination, plus a search for precipitating events in the past which may have initially caused the seizures to occur. This may require special psychiatric techniques, such as repeatedly confronting the patient with the image of his/her seizure on videotape whilst trying to explore what is going on in the patient's mind in terms of both cognitive and behavioural cues before the seizure starts: this occasionally involves the use of abreactive techniques, sometimes chemical or, in my experience, more usually hypnotic. This exploratory work takes time and during it the patient's seizure frequency may temporarily increase. This has to be accepted as the price to be paid for understanding the patient. During the time of exploration a great deal of support may need to be given to the patient, significant others and the family: community workers will need to understand that this investigatory phase is important.

Even if it is clear that the seizures are not the result of some previous life trauma, it is necessary to explore the cognitive and behavioural cues that tell a patient that a seizure is coming on, because many NES can only be controlled if the behavioural and cognitive factors which are reinforcing and keeping the seizures going can be understood.

I have mentioned before the importance of keeping up morale in the patient, helping him/her not to lose face, making sure that he/she does not feel rejected and spending time abreacting and listening to the anger and other feelings that may occur at having the diagnosis changed. Some patients, partly because of reinforcement from physicians, have an emotional investment in the diagnosis of epilepsy (which equals medical respectability) and it may take some time for this entrenched view to be changed.

If patients are being treated for psychogenic seizures, it may also take some time for them to accept that emotional, behavioural or cognitive events may trigger off a seizure (and may take even longer for families to realize this), although in my experience people with epilepsy are much more accepting nowadays of psychological explanations for the precipitation of seizures than they were a few years ago. In such patients, detailed behavioural and cognitive analysis of events preceding seizures will be necessary before a treatment programme can be worked out, and exploration of emotional and environmental events occurring at the time of the first seizure may be invaluable. I have no doubt that some people with recurrent epilepsy started their seizures at a time of stress because they were carrying a tendency towards epilepsy in their brain (either because of genetic or structural predisposition), and the epilepsy started when it did because of concomitant stressful events. If these events are not explored, the emotional significance of the patient's seizures may not be understood and behavioural cognitive or emotional treatment of the patient's epilepsy will therefore be of no avail.

Specific treatments

The general ambience of management has already been described in terms of a non-rejecting attitude and trying to understand the thoughts and feelings of the patient at the time that seizures first started and before seizures now occur. Woven into this treatment package are specific treatments, their use depending to some extent on what the physician eventually feels determines the patient's non-epileptic attacks. These may be subsumed under behavioural, cognitive psychotherapeutic and counselling methods.

The principal behavioural treatment for NES (which can also be used in emotionally precipitated epileptic seizures) is operant conditioning. The use of operant conditioning is to prevent the reinforcement of seizure behaviour (either by ignoring seizures or by 'punishing' them). This can be an effective treatment for NES providing the full co-operation of other professionals, the patient's family and significant others in the patient's life can be recruited into the treatment process so that if the patient does have a seizure all parties know that they must completely ignore it. This is difficult enough to arrange in a hospital ward and much more difficult to arrange in the community (although see Betts and Duffy (1993) for an example of how this can be achieved). If one ignores seizure behaviour, the frequency of seizures will often initially rise to a crescendo and then fall rapidly, particularly if, at the same time, non-seizure behaviour is 'rewarded' (in other words, when the patient is not having a seizure he/she is engaged in pleasurable and rewarding activities). This can be a very successful treatment paradigm but, as already indicated, can be very difficult to achieve in certain settings.

In those NES which are precipitated by anxiety, behavioural techniques aimed at reducing anxiety may be very appropriate. These include breathing control techniques (hyperventilation can trigger off non-epileptic attacks as well as epileptic ones), cue-controlled arousal manipulation (Fenwick, 1991; Betts, 1994) and autohypnotic techniques (Betts, 1994). These techniques can be very successful but need full co-operation from the patient to achieve and also need practice. They can also be used in treating emotionally precipitated epileptic attacks (Fenwick, 1991; Betts, 1994).

Cognitive techniques involve helping the patient to recognize specific cognitive triggers to seizures. This may be a recurring negative thought, or a recurring memory of a previous trauma that precipitates a seizure. Behavioural and cognitive analysis is initially needed to understand what the trigger is and then the patient can apply either a behavioural method or a cognitive method (by interposing a positive thought against a negative one) to stop the progression of the seizure. Often a combination of behavioural and cognitive methods is necessary and again a cognitive analysis is needed before the technique can be used, and the patient needs to understand the method and to practise it if it is going to work.

In patients with post-traumatic stress disorder, counselling and psychotherapy may be needed. The events of the trauma need to be relived and associated emotions related to the experience discharged, and the patient needs to come to terms with the event. It is my experience that post-traumatic stress disorder is quite common in patients with certain types of NEAD and the attack disorder will not resolve unless the post-traumatic stress disorder is also managed. Patients with post-traumatic stress disorder related to sexual abuse have certain particular characteristics because so often the abuse occurred in childhood and the post-traumatic syndrome has been carried forward into adult life (Cartmill & Betts, 1992): for these patients counselling and psychotherapy may need to be intensive and prolonged but is often successful (Betts & Boden, 1992b).

For many patients the cause of their NES still exists in their environment and may still reinforce the seizure behaviour. In my experience (Betts & Boden, 1992a), although it is often possible to manage non-epileptic attacks in hospital and to almost completely suppress them in that setting, they will often return when the patient goes home because the patient is returning to an environment or the family setting which has caused the problem in the first place. Under these circumstances, family therapy (involving the whole family and preventing the scapegoating of the patient) is obviously very necessary but lack of community resources may prevent this important part of the patient's therapy.

Treatment of psychogenic seizures

As has been indicated, the basic principles of the behavioural, cognitive or emotional management of epileptic seizures induced by stress or by specific thoughts or emotions are very similar to the above programme. It requires close co-operation between patient and physician to recognize specific emotional events or feelings that may precipitate seizures (and therefore necessitates the keeping of a careful diary not just of seizures but of feelings and thoughts that have occurred before the seizure, and of specific situations in which the seizures seem to occur), and then the institution of a behavioural or cognitive programme aimed at recognizing the likelihood of a seizure occurring before it starts and using the appropriate first aid. Most of these methods probably relate to manipulating arousal as most seizures are probably arousal-mediated (Fenwick, 1991). This entails helping the patient to develop a technique which rapidly reduces arousal (relaxation) or which rapidly increases arousal (alerting). In my experience, cue control arousal manipulation seems to work best (Betts, 1993), as does reinforcing those control skills that the patient already has. Most of these techniques require the patient to have some warning of the seizure taking place, but this is not necessarily so and even patients with generalised tonic–clonic seizures can occasionally use these techniques if there is a reliable emotional precipitant. For a further description of these techniques with some case examples, see Betts (1993, 1994).

Conclusion

The psychological management of epileptic seizures and NES is very similar. It requires careful explanation and confrontation, building a trusting relationship with the patient, exploring the behavioural and cognitive cues that occur before a seizure takes place, exploring the underlying meaning of the seizure for the patient and exploring any events that were occurring in the patient's life at the time the seizures started. Then a series of behavioural and cognitive techniques can be applied, designed to help the patient recognize when a seizure is coming on and developing his/her skills in stopping it. Operant conditioning, particularly reinforcing seizure-free activity, is often necessary for both types of seizure, as are family support and therapy. Fostering a good relationship between the physician, the patient and his/her family family is essential. Under certain circumstances, when the nature of a patient's seizure is uncertain, behavioural and cognitive treatment may be a particularly good option to take.

For readers unfamiliar with the techniques described above, there is a videotape *(Same difference – non-epileptic seizures, pseudoseizures)*, VT number 1051, available from the Television and Film Unit, University of Birmingham, B15 2TT, which illustrates their use.

References

Betts, T. (1990): Pseudoseizures: seizures that are not epilepsy. *Lancet* **336,** 163–164.

Betts, T. (1993): Neuropsychiatry. In: *A textbook of epilepsy*, eds. A. Richens, J. Laidlaw & D. Chadwick, pp. 423–449. Edinburgh: Churchill Livingstone.

Betts, T. (1994): Lamotrigine in the context of non-pharmacological therapies for epilepsy. *Rev. Contemp. Pharmacother.* **5,** 141–146.

Betts, T. & Boden, S. (1991): Pseudoseizures (non-epileptic attack disorder). In: *Women and epilepsy*, ed. M. Trimble, pp. 234–258. Chichester: Wiley.

Betts, T. & Boden, S. (1992a): Diagnosis, management and prognosis of a group of 128 patients with non-epileptic attack disorder. Part 1. *Seizure* **1,** 19–26.

Betts, T. & Boden, S. (1992b): Diagnosis, management and prognosis of a group of 128 patients with non-epileptic attack disorder. Part II. Previous childhood sexual abuse in the aetiology of these disorders. *Seizure* **1,** 27–32.

Betts, T. & Duffy, N. (1993): Treatment of non-epileptic attack disorder (pseudoseizures) in the community. In: *Pseudo-epileptic seizures*, eds. L. Gram, S. Johannesson, P. Osterman and M. Sillanpää, pp. 109–121. Petersfield, UK: Wrightson Biomedical Publishing.

Cartmill, A. & Betts, T. (1992): Seizure behaviour in a patient with post-traumatic stress disorder following rape: notes on the aetiology of 'pseudoseizures'. *Seizure* **1,** 33–36.

Fenwick, P. (1991): Evocation and inhibition of seizures: behavioural treatment. In: *Advances in neurology*, Vol. 55, eds. D. Smith, D. Treiman & M. Trimble, pp. 163–183. New York: Raven Press.

Gram, L, Johannessen, S., Osterman, P. & Sillanpää, M. (eds.) (1993): *Pseudoepileptic seizures.* Petersfield, UK: Wrightson Biomedical Publishing.

Greig, E. & Betts, T. (1992): Epileptic seizures induced by sexual abuse: pathogenic and pathoplastic factors. *Seizure* **1,** 269–274.

Mulder, O. (1990): Management of pseudoepileptic seizures. In: *Comprehensive epileptology*, eds. M. Dam & L. Gram, pp. 495–504. New York: Raven Press.

Ramani, V. (1986): Intensive monitoring of psychogenic seizures, aggression and dyscontrol syndromes. In: *Advances in neurology*, Vol. 46, ed. R. Gumnit, pp. 203–207. New York: Raven Press.

Rowan, J. & Gates, J. (eds.) (1993): *Non-epileptic seizures.* Boston: Butterworth-Heinemann.

Sander, J., Hart, Y., Johnson, A. & Shorvon, S. (1990): National general practice study of epilepsy: newly diagnosed epileptic seizures in a general population. *Lancet* **336,** 1257–1271.

Savard, G. & Andermann, F. (1990): Convulsive pseudoseizures: a review of current concepts. *Behav. Neurol.* **3,** 133–141.

Epileptic Seizures and Syndromes, Edited by Peter Wolf
© 1994 John Libbey & Company Ltd., pp. 651–656

Chapter 64

Epileptogenic-hysterical (dissociative) seizures

Martin Schöndienst

Epilepsie-Zentrum Bethel, Klinik Mara I, Maraweg 21, 33617 Bielefeld, Germany

Introduction

In 1881, John Hughlings Jackson remarked in his paper on dissolution in postepileptic conditions: 'I beg the reader never to lose sight of the fact that our particular task is narrowed to the condition of patients when their paroxysms are over, when the discharges causing them have ceased. Sometimes patients act more or less elaborately in this post-paroxysmal stage. There is, for an example, epileptic mania (post-epileptic, I think). A consideration of causes of epilepsy on this aspect is very important, not only as illustrating dissolution, but in other ways. Unless we have studied many kinds of actions after epileptic seizures of different degrees of severity, and especially actions after the slightest, we shall overlook the epileptic nature of some of our patients' cases altogether; for example, we may mistake epilepsy for hysteria' (Jackson, 1958, p. 11).

Jackson's statement not only recalls his basic idea, which is almost forgotten, that ictal and postictal symptoms can essentially be understood as disintegration or dissolution processes. It also expresses a very keen awareness of the absolute differences between hysteria and epilepsy.

The gradual and increasingly successful identification of apparently hysterical phenomena as epileptic has played an important role in the history of epileptology. For example, even Friedman still placed pyknoepilepsy in the no man's land between hysteria and epilepsy, and conceived it as a benign disease whose non-epileptic character was indubitably confirmed by the fact that absences were situation-dependent. When in 1939 Jung detected 3/s spike waves in pyknoepilepsy, the epileptic nature of this disease 'as in petit mal seizures of true epilepsy' was ensured.

The latest important step toward what could be called an 'epileptification' of apparently hysterical phenomena was the recognition of seemingly hysterical fits as 'hypermotor' epileptic seizures with frontal involvement.

However, one group of patients have not profited from this increase in our knowledge. Their fits are characterized by a combination of both epileptic and hysterical (dissociative, see below) phenomena. Such transitional phenomena are difficult to grasp and give rise to problems of terminology as well as classification. Interestingly, in the same year (1881) that Jackson postulated the above-mentioned strict differentiation between epileptic and hysterical phenomena, Gowers (1902) introduced the term 'postepileptic hysteria'. He pointed out that the epileptic components that are found tend to be mild, and he cautioned against assuming an independent hysterical syndrome in epileptics exhibiting 'hysteroid convulsions' immediately following epileptic fits. These concise considerations were reintroduced by Rabe (1970), although he himself used the term '*Hysteroepilepsie*' to encompass such heterogeneous phenomena as combinations of hysterical and epileptic fits in patients with epileptic personality disorder, hysterical fits in so-called wakening epilepsy and even epileptogenic hysterical fits.

This chapter reports on a group of patients whose fits have an epileptic onset that is followed directly by a hysterical course.

We find a diagnosis of 'epileptogenic hysterical fits' sufficiently established when, after a definite epileptic onset, not only clinical symptoms (hesitant onset, undulating course, variability in the course of the fit, etc.) give clear indications of a pseudoepileptic event, but also the patients' electroencephalography (EEG) indicates a normal waking pattern during the period when they are not responsive.

This chapter refers to six patients in whom a direct transition from an epileptic to a pseudoepileptic fit could be assumed on the basis of these criteria. These case reports are used to discuss the following issues:

1. Is it appropriate to label certain seizures as epileptogenic-hysterical (dissociative)?
2. Is such a label more informative than the usual statement that expressive gestures are simply (post) ictal confusion, embellishment, or – in German – *Ausgestaltung?*
3. Is this an academic or theoretical problem or does it have therapeutic implications?

Illustrative case reports

Case 1. This patient, who presents a compulsive-schizoid personality, is a 27-year-old female librarian who has had a focal epilepsy of unknown aetiology since the age of 10. Her magnetic resonance tomography (MRT) shows slight volume reduction of the right temporal lobe and her interictal EEG reveals sharp waves in 99 per cent over the right and 1 per cent over the left temporal lobe. Her auras are accompanied by a non-lateralized seizure pattern, while her psychomotors seizures show alternating left and right temporal discharges. After her epileptic aura ('It's like a pressure in my stomach, a real fear that rises up as far as my memory'), she complains about a 'flowing in my body'. Then, she becomes non-responsive to communication, while the EEG is simultaneously showing normal waking activity. During this period, she wriggles her pelvis for several minutes. Afterwards, she first throws her legs up in the air one after the other, and then repeatedly flings up her body and her legs and lets them fall back on the bed.

The first consultation with this patient produced a characteristic problem: she had been told that she should come to me because of her psychogenic attacks. However, she knew little about the different forms of attack, and had no idea how to differentiate them. I also lacked this information, so that I almost felt that the double nature of these attacks was a phenomenon that did not permit description. So the first consultation ended in a rather helpless way. But there was a surprising change in the second. The patient had a similar seizure to the one described above, and I told her that it had seemed to me as if I had seen two seizures in one. Then she told me that the second one was meant to reduce her anxiety after the first; she had had a similar one, for example, 4 days earlier. For me, the most important aspect was that this patient's recognition of her seizure represented a perception with only immediate postictal access, that is, a state-dependent perception. Likewise, the recall for earlier, similar seizures also seemed to function like a state-dependent memory.

Case 2 is a 22-year-old woman with focal epilepsy of unknown aetiology since she was a neonate. She exhibits a right frontal sharp-wave focus and secondary bilateral synchrony. The MRT shows only minimal left ventricle dilatation. She has frequent 'gelastic fits' and long-lasting auras with fugue reactions that observers continuously perceived to be hysterical.

We observed long-lasting auras during which the patient switched between phases in which she complained about insufferable sensations of constrictions in her body and other phases during which she was unresponsive to tests despite a normal EEG.

She describes her own perception of the seizures in a curious way:

> When the fit doesn't really take off, it's like, I don't know, for hours everything is so strange and confused in my head, and I've a continuous urge to laugh. Then I have to run off somewhere, very quickly, so that, at times, I really fly down the stairs, mostly to the graveyard over there. Then sometimes I have to cry my heart out among the dead. And when the fit takes off, like an electric shock, it's wonderful. Then perhaps I'll see something I saw that day before my eyes, for example, the way a sparrow flew off. I'll see that over and over again, and then a hardness flows through my body as if I were a stone. It sounds crazy, but at the time, I feel like a wandering tree that springs from branch to branch.

Her frequent, protracted, agitated auras had shifted this patient's symptoms toward a hysterical personality and covered over and masked her actually extremely vulnerable, sensitive mental structure.

In this case, psychotherapy initially consisted in giving the patient time, a great deal of time, for the stumbling verbalization of the contents of the aura. These are perceived as foreign to the ego, dangerous and, above all, embarrassing. Toward the end of treatment, she once said, 'Now I know that I am not mad, but that it's the fits, so the auras don't give me this anxiety any more.'

This patient continues to have epileptic seizures but no more epileptogenic-hysterical ones, so that she was able to complete a vocational training. Previously, she had to receive in-patient psychiatric treatment most of the time.

Case 3 is a 19-year-old girl with an epilepsy with generalized and focal elements resulting from a hypotrophic premature birth. Her seizures take the form of myoclonic absences, tonic falls, and complex–focal seizures. Furthermore, she has a previous history of chronic sexual abuse from her own brother.

Her nurse gives a careful description of the seizures:

> The patient has a very pale face, and suddenly says that she is feeling strange. She smacks her lips, twitching in the corner of her mouth, glassy stare, now the eyelids begin to twitch slightly, she turns her head from side to side, has single twitches in her left arm and leg. When testing tonus, she first lets her leg be moved easily, suddenly it goes completely stiff. We take her to her bed. As soon as she is lying down, she panics completely, throws herself around, kicks in all directions, falls out of bed. This phase lasts for about 2–3 min. When she is lying on the floor she calms down.

Study group

We found epileptogenic-hysterical seizures in a total of six patients.

Table 1 presents some clinical aspects of this group. Five of the six patients were female. All epilepsies involved focal elements. Three of the patients had pure focal epilepsies. Multifocality was present in all cases. No preference for the right or left hemisphere could be observed. Isolated hysterical seizure phenomena occurred in only two patients. In the remaining four patients, they occurred exclusively in a temporal relationship to an epileptic seizure onset.

An interictal hysterical personality, currently labelled histrionic personality in Diagnostic and Statistical Manual of Mental Disorders (third edition, revised), was not present in any of the cases. Anxious, sensitive and depressive features were predominant.

Table 1. Six patients with 'epileptogenic-hysterical attacks': clinical aspects

	Age	Sex	Type of epilepsy	EEG discharges	Auras with anxiety	Isoloated hysterical attacks	Personality traits	Chronic sexual abuse
K.S.	27	Female	Focal, unknown aetiology	Right and left temporal	+	–	Schizoid-compulsive	?
H.H.	44	Female	Focal, unknown aetiology	Left and right temporo-parietal	+	–	Anxious-depressive	+
C.S.	22	Female	Focal, unknown aetiology	Right and left temporal	+	–	Sensitive	–
W.B.	19	Male	Generalized and focal components	Generalized and right frontal	+	–	Anxious-paranoic	– (but chronic violent abuse)
B.B.	21	Female	Generalized and focal components	Generalized and left temporal	+	+	Schizoid-depressive	+
B.M.	19	Female	Generalized and focal components	Generalized and right temporopsrietal	+	+	Anxious-dependent	+

All patients had auras with anxiety as a major symptom.

In three cases, chronic sexual abuse could be ascertained. A further case, the only boy in the group, was a victim of continuous family violence during childhood. No data are available on this aspect in the remaining two patients.

Table 2 presents the outcome of treatment for both epileptic and hysterical seizure symptoms.

Table 2. Outcome of six patients with 'epileptogenic-hysterical attacks'

	Pharmacotherapy of seizures	Psychotherapy received?	Results concerning the hysterical components of the attacks
K.S.	Still testing pharmacoresistance	–	
	Pharmacoresistant		
H.H.	Pharmacoresistant	+	Complete remission
C.S.	Seizure-free (VPA < 50 µg/ml,	+	Complete remission
W.B.	ethosux. < 30 mg/ml)	+	Considerable improvement
	Seizure-free (CBZ < 7.8 µg/ml,		
B.B.	ethosux. < 99 µg/ml	+	Complete remission
	Reduction of seizure frequency >		
B.M.	75% (PB < 39 µg/ml)	+	Considerable improvement

Of the three patients with epilepsy containing both generalized and focal elements, two have become seizure-free while one continues to have epileptic seizures. Of the three patients with pure focal epilepsy, two have been proved resistant to all first-choice drugs (carbamazepine, phenytoin and phenobarbital) in monotherapy with dosage up to subtoxic levels. In the remaining patient, effective drug therapy is still being sought. This last patient has only just begun psychotherapy. The other patients received psychotherapy for a minimum of several months. When necessary, attempts were made to modify unfavourable life conditions.

For the five patients who have already received psychotherapy, three of whom continue to have epileptic seizures, the treatment was highly successful, with full remission of hysterical components in their seizures in three patients.

Compared with other treatment outcomes in patients with pseudoseizures, which generally show a success rate of only between 50 and 60 per cent (see, e.g. Betts & Boden, 1992), psychotherapy in patients with epileptogenic-hysterical seizures seems, thus, to be surprisingly successful.

A note on psychotherapeutic techniques

Compared with epileptological procedures, one of the first differences consists in the type of exploration. One tries to clarify an epilepsy through specific questions, listening to the patient and observation. The results of such questioning are notably disappointing in persons with hysterical disorders. Part of the nature of these disorders is that both biographical and emotional contexts are dissociated. There are good reasons for this, although one cannot track them down with questions. The focus of attention must be shifted away from the disease to the person. This changes meanings. Events that are normally viewed as disruptions to exploration now gain psychodynamic significance. For example, a patient's circumlocutions reveal the way she/he talks round a topic that, in itself, must remain unmentioned. Or a patient's devaluation of others indicates a projection of self-contempt. Or the patient's idealization of another physician reveals his or her 'splitting' tendencies. Just like, of course, the willingness to receive flattery as a physician indicates one's own susceptibility to seduction.

However, particularly among abuse patients who have suffered early traumatization, it is essential to accept anger and anxiety in the client–therapist relationship. The treatment of hysterical patients with early trauma requires the therapist to be particularly open and involved in the relationship. If this is not understood, the result is the frequent alternation between distancing oneself and the particularly inappropriate willingness to become too much personally involved. When treatment does not produce any noticeable improvement, this also makes the therapist feel like a failure. One could almost say that the hysterical way of being ill always hurts the therapist in a way that is otherwise scarcely found in medicine.

Of central importance in the treatment of patients with epileptogenic-hysterical seizures seems to be, furthermore, to respect the intensive fears of disintegration in these patients. This fear of becoming mad arising from aura or seizure experiences is often so great that it is sometimes kept secret for years – particularly for this reason. It then requires a long and ego-strengthening process of building up a relationship until these fears can in any way be discussed without threat and finally alleviated.

Discussion

The concept of hysteria has been completely replaced by dissociation in current psychiatric classification. This has inverted, as it were, a trend that translated dissociative processes completely into hysterical ones at the beginning of this century and conceived them as defence reactions to conflictual sexual experiences. In fact, the accumulation of prior abuse in our patients was surprising. None the less, it is in line with the findings of Betts and Boden (1992), who reported a history of abuse in 54 per cent of patients with non-epileptic attack disorders in their important large-scale study.

The second decisive aetiological element in hysterical disturbances, the organic aspect, which Freud himself had also emphasized, fell victim, as it were, to a narrow reception of his theory. For, in *Brüchstuck einer Hysterie-Analyse* (1905) (Freud, 1972, p. 200), he wrote:

'As far as I can see, each hysterical symptom requires the contribution of both sides. It cannot arise without a certain somatic compliance, which is achieved by a normal or a diseased process . . . The mental processes in all neuroses are, to a broad extent, the same ones; only then do we have to consider the somatic compliance, which provides the mental processes with an escape route into the physical. When this cannot be achieved immediately, the complete state does not turn into a hysterical condition, but a mental symptom in the form of a compulsion, a phobia, or the like.'

During Freud's time, there were even more precise ideas on the form of this somatic compliance than we have today. As Freud stated in *Über Hysterie* (1893) (Freud, 1987, p. 195):

'Namely, one very frequently finds that the content and cause of hysterical phenomena are events ... that have gained great significance because they occurred in particularly important times when a disposition was enhanced through disease . . . Such "hypnoid states" are of short duration and, as it were, out of touch with the rest of the individual's mental life . . . Through our long experience with this, it would seem probable that every form of hysteria . . . involves a rudiment of the so-called double conscience and that the inclination toward this dissociation and thus toward the occurrence of abnormal states of consciousness, which we wish to label hypnoid, is the underlying phenomenon of hysteria.'

It is interesting to see that the early analytical concept of hysteria had also considered those characteristics that are conspicuous in our patients with epileptogenic-hysterical seizures: in particular, episodic states of double conscience, state-dependent awareness and memory, as well as traumatizing events.

Therefore, it could be considered that the dissociative concept provides a better description of the psychological process than concepts such as pseudoseizure, psychogenic attack or hysterical attack. Above all, it corresponds to modern psychiatric terminology. Therefore, it might actually have been better to have written about epileptogenic dissociative attacks.

Conclusions

The analyses can be summarized as follows:

1. Ictal or postictal hysterical embellishment should not be assigned merely to declining epileptic discharges or to a hysterically disposed personality.
2. Far more, it seems to point to severe psychological problems in the patients. These problems frequently consist in a conjunction of anxiety-arousing seizure experiences and early abuse.
3. Psychotherapy is necessary and apparently even more successful than in patients with isolated hysterical attacks
4. In our cases, psychotherapy was effective even when epileptic seizures continued.

Acknowledgement

Translated from German to English by Jonathan Harrow, Bielefeld University, including the quotations from Freud.

References

Betts, T. & Boden, S. (1992): Diagnosis, management and prognosis of a group of 128 patients with non-epileptic attack disorder, Part I. *Seizure* **1,** 19–26.

Freud, S. (1972): *Bruchstücke einer Hysterie-Analyse.* In: *Gesammelte Werke, Werke aus den Jahren 1904–1905,* Vol. 5, ed. S. Freud, pp. 162–286. London. Frankfurt: Imago Publishing.

Freud, S. (1987): Über den psychischen Mechanismus hysterischer Phänomene (Vortrag, 1893). In: *Gesammelte Werke, Nachtragsband, Texte aus den Jahren 1885 bis 1938,* ed. von A. Richards, pp. 181–195. Frankfurt: Fischer Verlag.

Friedmann, M. (1906): Über die gehäuften Kleinen nicht-epileptischen Absencen oder Kurzen narkoleptischen Anfälle. *Deutsche Zeitschr. f. Nervenheilk.* **30,** 462–492.

Jung, R. (1939): Über vegetative Reaktionen und Hemmungswirkungen von Sinnesreizen im Kleinen epileptischen Anfalle. *Nervenarzt* **12,** 169–185.

Gowers, W.R. (1902): *Epilepsie* II. Auflage, deutsche autorisierte Ausgabe von Dr M. Weiss, Leipzig, Wien. Franz Deuticke.

Jackson, J.H. (1958): *Selected writings,* Vol. 2, *Evolution and dissolution of the nervous system,* ed. J. Taylor. London: Staples Press.

Rabe, F. (1970): Die Kombination hysterischer und epileptischer Anfälle. In: *Das Problem der 'Hysteroepilepsie' in neuer Sicht,* Neurologie – Neurology Series, No. 5. eds. H.J. Bauer, H. Gänshirt & P. Vogel.Schriftenreihe Berlin, Heidelberg, New York: Springer-Verlag.

Epileptic Seizures and Syndromes, Edited by Peter Wolf
© 1994 John Libbey & Company Ltd., pp. 657–665

Chapter 65

Psychogenic epileptic seizures and behavioural treatment of epilepsy

Peter Fenwick

Institute of Psychiatry, Maudsley Hospital, Denmark Hill, London SE5 8AZ

Summary

Little attention has been given to the part played in seizure genesis by ongoing brain activity in either precipitating or inhibiting seizures. Although in the focal epilepsies the presence of pacemaker cells – damaged neurones which fire in the epileptic mode continuously – has been demonstrated both in animal models and in human epilepsy, seizures arise only spasmodically. Behaviour can be thought of as changes in the excitation and inhibition of populations of neurones. It is thus likely that these excitatory and inhibitory waves will either increase or decrease the likelihood of seizures arising. The conditioning of the neurones to fire volleys in a biofeedback paradigm in the conditioning of seizures in a classical Pavlovian sense and the occurrence of seizures in response to behavioural changes have also been shown in animal models of epilepsy and in humans. It has been demonstrated that many children can spontaneously both inhibit and generate their own seizures. Many adults too use behavioural strategies either to inhibit seizures or to stop them spreading. In some patients the voluntary generation of seizures may come to form a response to stress or to difficult life situations. Thus any complete epilepsy programme must take into account the patient, his/her behaviour and the relationship between seizures and behaviour.

Introduction

For many years it has been standard practice to teach each new generation of medical students that epilepsy is a medical condition and that seizures arise as a result of abnormal brain discharges, usually caused by a damaged area of brain tissue. Although it is becoming recognized that this model of seizure genesis is too simple, the close relationship between ongoing cerebral activity and the capacity of those cells involved in that activity to be diverted into a seizure process is not always recognized.

Lockard's model of seizure genesis

Lockard *et al.* (1980a) used aluminium hydroxide paste to produce focal epileptogenic lesions in the cortex of monkeys, and the area was implanted with microelectrodes. Lockhard defined two populations of epileptogenic cells in the damaged area. Group 1 cells were pacemaker cells – partially damaged neurones at the centre of the focus. These cells fired *continuously* in an abnormal, bursting mode and their activity was not modified to any significant extent by surrounding brain activity.

Group 2 cells were partially damaged neurones surrounding the focus. These cells could fire in both the bursting, epileptic mode and in a normal mode, and their activity could be modified by surrounding brain activity. Lockard suggested that in the genesis of a seizure, the continuously discharging group 1 cells recruited group 2 cells; abnormal discharges spread within the group 2 cells to produce a focal seizure. Secondarily generalized seizures occurred when normal neurones were recruited into the seizure discharge.

This model suggests that ongoing brain activity can alter the likelihood of a seizure either between group 1 and group 2 neurones, or between group 2 and normal brain cells. The activity of the neurones surrounding the focus determines the likelihood of a seizure occurring and spreading. Behaviour, which can be described in terms of excitation and inhibition of populations of neurones, must therefore be crucial in the genesis of seizure activity.

Spike-and-wave seizures

Avoli and Gloor (1982) proposed a cat penicillin model of spike-and-wave seizures. They showed that spike-and-wave generation is predominantly cortical and that the thalamus plays only a secondary role. These seizures can be modified by reticular formation stimulation, so the spike-wave generator is probably reticulocortical. If this is the case in humans (and there is indirect evidence that this may be so (Fenwick, 1981)), changes in reticular activity (which is altered by behaviour) could be expected to lead either to an increase or decrease of seizure discharges, and so to have a direct effect on seizure frequency.

Spike activity

Lockard *et al.* (1980a) have suggested that spike activity is caused by the synchronization of populations of group 1 neurones and that changes in spike frequency are related to seizure frequency. They have also shown that numbers of spikes occurring at any one time can be modified by, amongst other things, psychosocial processes. Spike firing in epileptic monkeys has been shown to increase significantly during and after their exposure to a more dominant monkey.

Evoked seizures

Evoked seizures are said to occur in about 5 per cent of people with epilepsy (Symonds, 1959), though in hospital populations the rate may be nearer 25 per cent (Fenwick, 1981). In susceptible individuals, any form of appropriate (usually rhythmic) peripheral stimulation may evoke a seizure (Newmark & Penry, 1979). Photosensitive epilepsy is one such example (Wilkins *et al.*, 1981a; Binnie *et al.*, 1985). Reading, eating, stimulation of the skin, movement, sounds and smells can all trigger seizures (Merlis, 1974; Fenwick, 1981). It could be predicted from Lockard's model that altering the level of activity within a damaged area of the cortex would allow group 1 neurones to recruit group 2 neurones and so trigger a seizure. This also carries the implication that alteration in the level of excitation in the area of an epileptic focus can prevent seizure activity from arising and spreading.

Psychogenic epileptic seizures

Psychogenic epileptic seizures are those generated by an action of mind. Fenwick (1981) has classified such seizures as either *primary* – those produced when the patient deliberately attempts to induce a seizure by an act of will – or *secondary* – those which occur when the subject is thinking, but not trying to induce a seizure. Secondary psychogenic epileptic seizures, caused by ongoing activity of mind, have also been called the 'thinking epilepsies'. Excitation of the seizure focus may occur during mental activity such as multiplication or addition (reviews in Merlis, 1974; Fenwick, 1981; see also Inoue *et al.*, Chapter 11). Wilkins *et al.* (1981b) have documented a case of a patient, in whom they were able to demonstrate a parietal lobe lesion, who, whenever doing mathematical calculations, would have an absence attack.

Primary

Psychogenic epileptic seizures are common in all types of epilepsy, whether or not they have a focal onset. Such seizures may be produced either by activating specific brain areas, in the case of focal seizures, or by using attention to alter arousal levels, in the case of generalized seizures. Many patients learn that by a willed action (usually the manipulation of attention) they can alter neuronal activity in brain areas surrounding the epileptogenic focus and produce a seizure.

1. A man aged 36 suffered from partial complex seizures commencing in his left temporal lobe, and accompanied by an epigastric aura and a feeling of sadness. He had discovered in adolescence that sad thoughts could trigger a secondary generalized seizure.
2. A 19-year-old youth with absence attacks would induce a shower of seizures when his mother was cross with him. He admitted doing this by suddenly swinging his attention to the periphery of his visual attentional field, producing a split in his concentration.
3. A 22-year-old man had tonic–clonic seizures which commenced with loss of consciousness and no focal features. He discovered that he could generate grand mal seizures by lying down and deliberately holding his mind empty. He would then awake in a confused postictal state, a sensation that he quite enjoyed.

A survey of 76 patients attending the epilepsy clinic at the Maudsley Hospital indicated that 25 per cent could generate their own seizures at will or knew what they had to do to bring a seizure on. There is a fine line between deliberate induction of seizures and allowing oneself the luxury of a mental state that you know is likely to induce a seizure. Over 50 per cent said that they had seizures when they were tense, depressed or tired, and over 30 per cent had them when they were angry, excited or bored.

Seizure inhibition

Seizure inhibition, like seizure generation, consists of both primary and secondary components. Primary seizure inhibition is the direct inhibition of seizures by an act of will: secondary seizure inhibition is the unintentional stopping of seizures by thoughts or actions which interfere with the generation of the seizure.

The use of external stimulation to inhibit seizure occurrence (primary inhibition) is well documented. (Efron, 1956; Forster *et al.*, 1969; de Weerdt & van Rijn, 1975; Forster, 1977a). Most patients have some mental strategy which helps inhibit their seizures. The Maudsley Hospital Epilepsy Clinic Survey showed that 36.4 per cent of 76 patients claimed that they could sometimes stop their seizures, 33.8 per cent could reduce the frequency of seizures, and 27.3 per could stop their seizures spreading. Although only 3.9 per cent said their mechanism invariably succeeded, the removal of specific precipitants can be very valuable.

1. A 42-year-old woman had her first grand mal seizure at the age of 16. Since the age of 6 or 7, she had had feelings of *déjà vu*, sometimes associated with feelings of guilt. She described her behavioural strategy, which in part consisted of helping her deal with her guilt, as the most powerful anticonvulsant she had ever been given.

When seizures arise from a different area of cortex, different inhibitory strategies will be needed.

2. A 28-year-old man had suffered for 2 years from focal motor seizures consisting of brief rhythmical leg jerking with little impairment of consciousness. He found that unsteadiness, produced either by poor balance when walking down an incline or by a sudden change in visual cues when he entered a large room, tended to precipitate an attack. When he was taught to improve his balance by keeping his gaze fixed in these situations, his seizure frequency was reduced.

Efron (1956) described a conditioned inhibition of seizures in a patient with temporal lobe epilepsy who experienced a stereotyped aura, with secondary genralization. The patient found she could abort a seizure by smelling an unpleasant odour, presumably by altering the excitability of cells surrounding the focus, thus preventing the spread of the seizure discharge. She was then conditioned to a bracelet presented at the same time as the smell. It was fortuitously discovered that seizure abortion also occurred if the patient merely thought about the bracelet. Her seizure frequency declined and she considered herself cured.

Indirect primary inhibition

Indirect primary inhibition of seizures occurs when the patient carries out a set of actions, either physical or mental, which stop the seizure occurring or generalizing, but which act in a non-specific way. The main mechanism of action is a change in alertness and therefore in reticular formation activity (Mostofsky & Balaschak, 1977). For example, focal seizures may be aborted if the person says 'no' to him/herself, or attends to something different at the onset of the aura. One patient found he could sometimes stop seizures generalizing by hitting his arm, though it is debatable whether this functioned by non-specific arousal or because local stimulation of the arm changed motor excitability. Prince (1966) and Tassinari (1969) have described the modification of focal cortical epileptogenic discharges by afferent impulses.

Deliberate alerting in boring situations has been know to produce a reduction in petit mal seizures, and is reviewed below (Jung, 1962; Ounsted *et al.*, 1966).

Secondary inhibition

Secondary inhibition occurs when thoughts or actions happen incidentally to reduce seizure frequency without the patient's conscious will. Maintaining interest or alertness often has this effect. S. Brown (pers. comm.) noted that children in a special school had fewer seizures in an interesting art class than in classes where their interest was less successfully held. Many patients report having fewer seizures when they are on holiday, or when their interest is held, for example while watching a film or at the theatre. Others find that they are more likely to remain seizure-free if they adopt a low-key lifestyle, without too much excitement or excess novelty. In the Maudsley Hospital questionnaire study referred to above, patients reported that excitement (40.8 per cent), anger (45.3 per cent) and tension and anxiety (58.4 per cent) increased the likelihood of a seizure.

It is postulated that all these effects are mediated through an alteration in the excitability of group 2 neurones, leading directly to seizure inhibition. Excitability of group 2 neurones is also modified by changes in reticular formation activity (Lockard, 1980a, b), which can result from interest or boredom, and so this too can alter the likelihood of seizure discharges.

Behaviour during focal seizures

Patients who have focal seizures, particularly if these are followed by complex automatisms, show a wide range of behaviour. The form an automatism takes is at least partly determined by the patient's thought content and surroundings. Forster and Liske (1963) cite the case of an organist who had a seizure while playing a hymn. He stopped during the aura and played a few bars of jazz before recommencing the hymn. Because the seizure discharges activate structures which are already involved in ongoing behaviour, behaviour in the later stages of an automatism may seem to be appropriate. Thus, patients who have partial complex seizures on the pavement seldom walk into the road.

Consciousness is impaired during an automatism, and most automatisms are brief (Knox, 1968; Theodore *et al.*, 1983). Memory is always impaired because for an automatism to arise there must have been a bilateral spread of the seizure discharge into both periamygdaloid–hippocampal structures (Jasper, 1964).

Psychological methods for treatment of epilepsy

Standard methods of behaviour modification could be expected to alter seizure activity because of the close relationship between seizure activity and the ongoing patterns of excitation and inhibition in the neuronal pools which surrounding the epileptogenic focus. Mostofsky (1981) and Mostofsky and Balaschak (1977) have reviewed this subject, and have defined three areas: reward management, self-control and psychophysiological treatments. However, in any conditioning programme there is likely to be more than one therapeutic factor leading to change. Any success brought about by the programme, for example, will improve the patient's self-image and enhance self-esteem. Consequent drug reduction will improve his/her alertness, well-being and chances of employment.

Reward management

Reward mangement includes overt reward (Flannery & Cautela, 1973; Zlutnick *et al.*, 1975; Balaschak, 1976; Iwata & Lorentszen, 1976); covert reward (Cautela, 1971; Daniels, 1975); denial of reward (Gardner, 1967; Daniels, 1975); punishment programmes (Bandler, 1957; Zlutnick, 1972; Adams *et al.*, 1973; Zlutnick *et al.*, 1975; Iwata & Lorentszon, 1976) and relief avoidance (Dorcas & Schaffer, 1945; Stevens, 1962; Ounstead *et al.*, 1966).

Self-control strategies

Self-control procedures enable the patient to gain control of his/her seizure activity by cognitive processes.

Self-control

As already described, most patients with epilepsy employ some cognitive strategies to inhibit seizure activity, both by avoiding situations likely to cause seizures and by trying to abort seizures once they have begun (Fenwick, 1988; Brown & Fenwick, 1989; Fenwick & Brown, 1989).

Relaxation and desensitization

Relaxation training usually involves teaching the patient to use progressive relaxation (Wolpe, 1969) if a seizure seems imminent. An extension of this method is relaxation and covert desensitization, in which the patient, while relaxed, imagines the occurrence of a seizure and the resultant anxiety. The consequent desensitization to the idea of a seizure occurring is believed to result in a reduction in seizure frequency (Parrino, 1971; Standage, 1972; Mostofsky, 1975; Cabral & Scott, 1976; Ince, 1976; Muthen, 1978; Brown & Fenwick, 1989). Flooding, a method which exposes the patient to seizure-provoking situations, has been used by Pinto (1972).

Psychotherapy

Both individual psychotherapy and group psychotherapy have been used and probably work at many different levels. Better life adjustment leads to greater relaxation and a sense of fulfilment, both powerful anticonvulsants, together with, in some patients, the reduction of covert seizure induction. Group psychotherapy may modify the patient's relationships with his/her peers and suggest alternative ways of dealing with problems and seizures and new cognitive strategies of seizure control (Gottschalk, 1953; Williams *et al.*, 1978).

Significant seizure reduction has been reported in five patients who have been shown videotapes of their seizures during treatment sessions (Feldman & Paul, 1976). Probably several psychological mechanics could have been involved (Mostofsky & Balaschak, 1977).

Psychophysiological

The induction of epileptic seizures in a classical Pavlovian conditioning paradigm has been demonstrated in cats and in humans. The classical methods of habituation and extinction have been applied to the control of epilepsy by Forster (1972). The aim is to extinguish the abnormal cortical discharges by stimulus exposure until habituation occurs. This has been tried in the visual, auditory and sensory modalities, with some success (Forster & Campos, 1964; Forster *et al.*, 1964; Booker *et al.*, 1965; Forster, 1977b). However, the conditioning of seizures is a fragile process and can be obliterated by one grand mal seizure.

Biofeedback

Anticonvulsant rhythms

Sterman (1973) suggested that biofeedback training to increase the 12–16 Hz sensorimotor rhythm had powerful anticonvulsant properties. Other authors (Finlay *et al.*, 1975; Siefert & Lubar, 1975; Lubar & Bhaler, 1976; Lubar, 1977) have used biofeedback with varying degrees of success. Some authors attributed any reduction in seizure frequency to non-specific factors rather than to enhancement in sensorimotor rhythm training (Finlay, 1977; Kuhlman & Allison, 1977; Sterman, 1977) and current opinion reflects this view. A study by Quy *et al.* (1979) finally laid the subject to rest (review in Fenwick, 1981).

Non-specific biofeedback

Other studies have used different rhythms in a conditioning programme, for example the alpha rhythm (Cabral & Scott, 1976). Whyler *et al.* (1976) increased fast low-voltage activity and suppressed slow-wave activity surrounding the epileptic focus, all with some success. Kaplan (1975) and Kuhlman and Allison (1977) successfully used augmentation of µactivity. Lockard *et al.* (1977) extended biofeedback techniques to their alumina-gel monkey model of epilepsy and found some change in seizure frequency, although this was not consistently beneficial. Again, any reduction in seizure activity was more likely to be non-specific rather than due to the direct alteration of cerebral rhythms. For a review see Fenwick (1981).

Conclusion

Epileptic seizures should not be thought of as arising randomly. The patient should be helped to see the way in which his/her seizures are intimately related to what he/she is feeling, doing or thinking. If a patient has focal epilepsy, a detailed clinical history should be taken to establish the position of the focus; this in turn will determine the relationship between the individual and his/her epilepsy and those aspects of his/her psychic life and behaviour which may either trigger or inhibit seizure activity. A complete treatment of epilepsy involves not just the giving of drugs, but also teaching the patient about brain function and the way his/her feelings, thinking and behaviour can all be used in the control of the seizures.

References

Adams, K.M., Klinge, V., Keiser T.W. (1973): The extinction of a self-injurious behaviour in an epileptic child. *Behav. Res. Ther.* **11,** 351–356.

Avoli, M. & Gloor, P. (1982): Role of the thalamus in generalised penicillin epilepsy: observations on decorticate cats. *Exp. Neurol.* **77** (2), 386–402.

Bandler, B., Kaufman, I., Dykens, J., Schleifer, M. & Shapiro, L. (1957): Seizures and the menstrual cycle. *Am. J. Psych.* **113,** 704–798.

Binnie, C., Findlay, J. & Wilkins, A. (1985): Mechanisms of epileptogenesis in photosensitive epilepsy implied by the effects of moving patterns. *Electroencephalogr. Clin. Neurophysiol.* **61,** 1–6.

Booker, H.E., Forster, F.M. & Klove, H. (1965): Extinction factors in startle (acoustico-motor) seizures. *Neurology* **15,** 1095–1103.

Brown, S. & Fenwick, P. (1989): Seizure inhibition. *Acta Scand. Neurol.* **80,** 541–545.

Cabral, R.J. & Scott, D.F. (1976): Effects of two desensitization techniques, biofeedback and relaxation, on intractable epilepsy: follow-up study. *J. Neurol. Neurosurg. Psychiatry* **39,** 504–507.

Cautela, J.R. (1971): Covert extinction. *Behav. Ther.* **2,** 192–200.

Daniels, L.K. (1975): The treatment of grand mal epilepsy by covert and operant conditioning techniques: a case study. *Psychosomatic* **16,** 65–67.

de Weerdt, C.J. & van Rijn, A.J. (1975): Conditioning therapy in reading epilepsy. *Electroencephalogr. Clin. Neurophysiol.* **39,** 417–420.

Dorcas, R.M. & Schaffer, G.W. (1945): Textbook of abnormal psychology, 3rd edn. Baltimore, MD: Williams and Williams.

Efron, R. (1956): The effect of olfactory stimuli in arresting uncinate fits. *Brain* **79,** 267–281.

Feldman, R.G. & Paul, N.L. (1976): Identity of emotional triggers in epilepsy. *J. Nerv. Mental Dis.* **162,** 345–353.

Fenwick, P. (1981): Precipitation and inhibition of seizures. In: *Epilepsy and psychiatry*, eds. E. Reynolds & M. Trimble, pp. 306–321. London: Churchill Livingstone.

Fenwick, P. (1988): The significance of a seizure. In: *Bridge between neurology and psychiatry*, eds. M.R. Trimble & E.H. Reynolds, pp. 247–262. London: Churchill Livingstone.

Fenwick, P. & Brown, S. (1989): Evoked and psychogenic epileptic seizures. 1. Precipitation. *Acta Scand. Neurol.* **80,** 525–540.

Finlay, W.W. (1977): Operant conditioning of the EEG in two patients with epilepsy: methodological and clinical considerations. *Pavlovian J. Biol. Sci.* **12,** 93–111.

Finlay, W.W., Smith, H.A. & Etherton, M.D. (1975): Reduction of seizures and normalisation of the EEG in a severe epileptic following sensorimotor biofeedback training: preliminary study. *Biol. Psychol.* **2,** 189–203.

Flannery, R.B., Jr & Cautela, J.R. (1973): Seizures: controlling the uncontrollable. *J. Rehab.* **39,** 34–36.

Forster, F.M. (1977a): Epilepsy evoked by higher cognitive functions: decision-making epilepsy. In: *Reflex epilepsy, behaviour therapy and conditioned reflexes*, pp. 124–134. Springfield: Charles C. Thomas.

Forster, F.M. (1977b): Reflex epilepsy. In: *Behaviour therapy and conditioned reflexes, (Minneapolis)* pp. 242–255, 318. Springfield: Charles C. Thomas.

Forster, F.M. (1972): Classification and conditioning treatment of the reflex epilepsies. *Int. J. Neurol.* **9,** 73–86.

Forster, F.M. & Campos, G.B. (1964): Conditioning foactors in stroboscopic-induced seizures. *Epilepsia* **5,** 156–165.

Forster, F.M. & Liske, E. (1963): Role of environmental clues in temporal lobe epilepsy. *Neurology* **13,** 301–305.

Forster, F.M., Ptacek, L.J., Peterson, W.G., Chun, R.W.M., Bengzon, A.R.A. & Campos, G.B. (1964): Stroboscopic-induced seizure discharges: modification by extinction techniques. *Arch. Neurol.* **11,** 603–608.

Forster, F.M., Paulsen, W. & Baughman, F. (1969): Clinical therapeutic conditioning in reading epilepsy. *Neurology* **19,** 71–77.

Gardner, J.E. (1967): Behaviour therapy treatment approach to a psychogenic seizure case. *J. Consult. Psychol.* **31,** 209–212.

Gottschalk, L.A. (1953): Effects of intensive psychotherapy on epileptic children. *Arch. Neurol. Psychiatr.* **70,** 361–384.

Ince, L.P. (1976): The use of relaxation training and a conditioned stimulus in the elimination of epileptic seizures in a child: a case study. *J. Behav. Ther. Exp. Pschiatry* **7,** 39–42.

Iwata, B.A. & Lorentzson, A.M. (1976): Operant control of seizure-like behaviour in an institutionalised retarded adult. *Behav. Ther.* **7,** 247–251.

Jasper, H. (1964): Some physiological mechanisms involved in epileptic automatism. *Epilepsia* **5,** 1–20.

Jung, R. (1962): Blocking of petit mal attacks by sensory arousal and inhibiton of attacks by an active change in attention during the epileptic aura. *Epilepsia* **3,** 435.

Kaplan, B.J. (1975): Biofeedback in epilepsy: equivocal relationship of reinforced EEG frequency to seizure reduction. *Epilepsia* **16,** 477–485.

Knox, S. (1968): Epileptic automatisms and violence. *Med. Sci. Law* **8,** 96–104.

Kuhlman, W.M. & Allison, T. (1977): EEG feedback training in the treatment of epilepsy: some questions and answers. *Pavlovian J. Biol. Sci.* **12,** 112–122.

Lockard, J.S. (1980a): A primate model of clinical epilepsy: mechanisms of action through quantification of therapeutic effects. In: *Epilepsy: a window to brain mechanisms,* eds. J.S. Lockard & A.A. Ward, pp. 11–50. New York: Raven Press.

Lockard, J.S. (1980b): Social primate model of epilepsy. In: *Epilepsy: a window to brain mechanisms,* eds. J.S. Lockard & A.A. Ward, pp. 165–190. New York: Raven Press.

Lockard, J.S., Whyler, A.R., Finch, C.A. & Hulbert, K.E. (1977): EEG operant conditioning in a monkey model. 1. Seizure data. *Epilepsia* **18** (4), 471–479.

Lubar, J.F. (1977): Electroencephalographic methodology and the management of epilepsy. *Pavlovian J. Biol. Sci.* **12,** 147–185.

Lubar, J.F. & Bhaler, J.F. (1976): Behavioural management of epileptic seizures following EEG biofeedback training of the senori-motor rhythm. *Biofeedback Self Regulation* **1,** 77–104.

Merlis, J.K. (1974): Reflex epilepsy. In: *Handbook of neurology,* Vol. 15, *The epilepsies,* ed. J.K. Merlis, pp. 440–456. Amsterdam: Elsevier.

Mostofsky, D.I. (1975): Teaching the nervous system. New York Univ. *Educ. Quart.* Spring, 8–13.

Mostofsky, D.I. (1981): Recurrent paroxysmal disorders of the central nervous system. In: *Handbook of clinical behaviour therapy,* eds. S. Turner, K. Calhoun & H. Adams, pp. 454–460. Chichester: John Wiley and Sons.

Mostofsky, D.I. & Balaschak, B.A. (1977): A psychobiological control of seizures. *Psychol. Bull.* **84,** 723–750.

Muthen, J. (1978): Psychological treatment of epileptic seizures. Thesis, Institute of Applied Psychology, Uppsala University, Sweden.

Newmark, M.E. & Penry, A.K. (1979): *Photosensitivity and epilepsy: a review.* New York: Raven Press.

Ounstead, C., Lee, D. & Hut, S.J. (1966): Electroencephalographic and clincal changes in an epileptic child during repeated photic stimulation. *Electroencephalogr. Clin. Neurophysiol.* **21,** 388–391.

Parrino, J.J. (1971): Reduction of seizures by desensitization. *J. Behav. Ther. Exp. Psychiatr.* **2,** 215–218.

Pinto, R. (1972): A case of movement epilepsy with agarophobia, treated successfully by flooding. *Br. J. Psychiatr.* **121,** 287–288.

Prince, D.A. (1966): Modification of focal cortical epileptogenic discharges by afferent impulses. *Epilepsia* **7,** 181–201.

Quy, R.J., Hut, S.J. & Foresst, S. (1979): Sensorimotor rhythm feedback training in epilepsy. *Biol. Psychol.* **9,** 129–149.

Siefert, A.R. & Lubar, J.F. (1975): Reduction of epileptic seizures through EEG biofeedback training. *Biol. Psychol.* **3,** 156–184.

Standage, K.F. (1972): Treatment of epilepsy by reciprocal inhibition of anxiety. *Guys Hosp. Rep.* **121,** 217.

Sterman, M.B. (1973): Neurophysiological and clinical studies of sensori-motor EEG biofeedback training: some effects of epilepsy. In: *Biofeedback: behaviour medicine,* ed. L. Birk, pp. 507–526. Boston: Grune and Stratton.

Sterman, M.B. (1977): Effects of sensorimotor EEG feedback training on sleep and clinical manifestation of epilepsy. In: *Biofeedback and behaviour,* eds. J. Beatty & H. Legewie, pp. 167–200. New York: Plenum Press.

Stevens, J.R. (1962): Endogenous conditioning to abnormal cerebral electrical transience in man. *Science* **137,** 974–976.

Symonds, C. (1959): Excitation and inhibition in epilepsy. *Brain* **82** (2), 133–146.

Tassinari, C.A. (1968): Suppression of focal spikes by somato-sensory stimuli. *Electroencephalogr. Clin. Neurophysiol.* **25,** 574.

Theodore, W., Porter, R. & Penry, K. (1983): Complex partial seizures: clinical characteristics and differential diagnosis. *Neurology* **33,** 1115–1121.

Whyler, A.R., Lockard, J.S., Ward, A.A. & Finch, C.A. (1976): Condition EEG desynchronisation and seizure occurrence in patients. *Electroencephalogr. Clin. Neurophysiol.* **41,** 501–512.

Wilkins, A.J., Binnie, C.D. & Darby, C.E. (1981a): Interhemispheric differences in photosensivtive epilepsy 1: pattern sensitivity thresholds. *Electroencephalogr. Clin. Neurophysiol.* **52,** 461–468.

Wilkins, A.J., Zifkin, B., Anderman, F. & McGovern, E. (1981b): Seizures induced by thinking. *Ann. Neurol.* **11,** 608–612.

Williams, D.T., Spiegel, H. & Mostofsky, D.I. (1978): Neurogenic and hysterical seizures in children and adolescents: differential diagnostic and therapeutic considerations. *Am. J. Psychiatr.* **135**, 82–86.

Wolpe, J. (1969): *The practice of behaviour therapy.* Elmsford, New York: Pergamon Press.

Zlutnick, S.I. (1972): The control of seizures by the modification of pre-seizure behaviour: the punishment of behavioural chain components (Doctoral dissertation, Utah State College). *Dissertation Abstracts International* **33,** 6B (Univ. Microfilms No. 72–31, 182).

Zlutnick, S.I., Mayville, W.J. & Moffat, S. (1975): Behavioural control of seizure disorders: the interruption of chained behaviour. In: *Behaviour therapy and health care: principles and applications*, eds. R.C. Katz & S.I. Zlutnick. Elmsford, New York: Pergamon Press.

Epileptic Seizures and Syndromes, Edited by Peter Wolf
© 1994 John Libbey & Comany Ltd., pp. 667–673

Chapter 66

Aura interruption: how does it become curative?

Peter Wolf

Epilepsie-Zentrum Bethel, Klinik für Anfallskranke, Mara I, Maraweg 21, 33617 Bielefeld, Germany

Summary

This chapter describes the history and methods of epilepsy therapy through counteracting the seizure spread after aura onset. Possible neurophysiological explanations include depolarization of neurones liable to be recruited by the seizure discharge and deliberate learned positive shift of the cortical DC potential, which is known to undergo a negative shift at seizure onset. Like all other therapies, this should also aim at complete seizure control in view of a possible cure. A tentative five-step development of therapeutic action is suggested which is derived from exemplary case reports where seizures remitted completely.

Introduction

In the previous chapter, a review was given of various psychological and behavioural treatments which are believed or have been demonstrated to be helpful in the management of epilepsy. It was shown that these procedures can reduce the frequency or severity of seizures, or both, and that an improvement of the patients' self-esteem may be a welcome additional benefit.

As in pharmacological and surgical epilepsy therapy, however, it must not be forgotten that complete control of seizures is the most important prerequisite for a substantial improvement of life quality, that it opens the only hope for a definite cure from the disease and that this, therefore, has to be the primary aim of all our therapeutic efforts. This standard must also be applied to the evaluation of behavioural therapy. The present chapter therefore looks into the power of one of these approaches, aura interruption, to obtain this goal.

Historical background and underlying theories

Of all therapies of epilepsy which are in use today, the arrest of seizures in development by the application of countermeasures has by far the longest tradition. Probably discovered by patients, it was mentioned as an established procedure by Hellenistic physicians, such as Aretaeus the Cappadocian and Galen, in the first and second centuries. It was well-known that seizures beginning distally in a limb and spreading from there to the brain could be interrupted by manipulations such as the application of ligatures. This may have contributed to the concept of 'sympathetic' epilepsy originating in the periphery, from where a 'pneumatic substance' spread through the body and to the brain like poison from the bite of a scorpion (Temkin, 1945), and the ligature was thought to arrest the spread of this substance.

This therapeutic approach remained in use throughout the history of medicine. Tissot (1770) mentions numerous examples. He still regarded the effectiveness of such procedures as a support of the concept of sympathetic epilepsy. One of the discoveries that seriously shattered this concept was the finding of Odier (1811, quoted from Gowers, 1881) that the ligature arrested 'a fit which is due to a cerebral tumour as effectually and more frequently than one due to any other cause'.

It thus became obvious that different explanations had to be found. Under the influence of Brown-Séquard's experiments, where, following a lesion of the spinal cord, external stimuli produced convulsions, Jackson (1870) suggested that a similar relation existed between a peripheral sensation 'preceding' the seizure and the 'internal discharge', the beginning of which was reflected in the 'outward spasm'. Such a relation, however, could only explain the action of a ligature applied between a first aura sensation and the onset of spasm, but not after its onset.

It was Gowers (1881) who conceived a totally new theory. According to him, 'the arrest must be effected, not in the limb convulsed, but in the centre in which the discharge is occurring, of which the local convulsion is the outward manifestation. The strong peripheral impression on the limb above the part convulsed probably raises the resistance in the nerve-cells of the corresponding parts of the brain and thus arrests the spread of the discharge. The effect of the ligature must first be exerted on the sensory centre, and through this on the motor centre. The two are connected intimately, and their mutual interaction must be constant, so that the condition of the motor centre is no doubt readily influenced through the sensory centre. Hence, a fit may be arrested by the ligature, whether it begins by a sensation or by a motion, i.e. whether the sensory or motor centre leads in the discharge. Additional observation is necessary to determine whether the ligature is more effective in one class of fits than in the other' (Gowers, 1881).

The knowledge and discussion of these phenomena were common among the British neurologists of the late nineteenth century. Case 2 of Horsley (see Chapter 1), the first patient operated for epilepsy without evidence of a lesion, transferred by Jackson solely on anatomical considerations based on the seizure semiology, could arrest his Jacksonian seizures, which began with flexor twitching of the thumb, by stretching the thumb or applying a ligature. For Horsley, this suggested 'the possibility of the so-called muscular sense being represented in the excito-motor area' (Horsley, 1886).

Little has to be added to the neurophysiological hypothesis of Gowers. His 'resistance in the nerve-cells' would today be viewed in terms of massive depolarization of the neurones involved due to which they are not recruitable for the spreading epileptic discharge (Speckmann, 1986).

Methods of seizure interruption

A ligature and passive stretching of a muscle in spasm are simple countermeasures which have often been reported. In other instances, much more intricate procedures are applied, such as in a patient in the care of first Brown-Séquard and then Jackson, who described it in great detail (1931, I, 6f); in this case, the help of a second person was necessary.

Gowers (1881) reported a variety of countermeasures (Table 1), of which the first three were often successful in seizures commencing in a limb. The last three were occasionally effective in 'attacks which begin by a general or bilateral aura, or by the epigastric sensation', and which can rarely be arrested. He points out, however, that nitrite of amyl, which had been given in view of vasal dilatation, was most successful in cases with a deliberate olfactory aura, and wonders if it could act through the olfactory nerve.

It is with Efron's report (1956, 1957) of the interruption of an aura by an olfactory stimulus applied before the appearance of a habitual olfactory hallucination that the most recent period of this therapeutic approach began. To use an olfactory stimulus had been his patient's own idea, and today we frequently follow the patients' own suggestions and experiences to develop an individually tailored strategy. About 62 per cent of patients with auras have their own experiences (Paulson, 1963; Reker, 1988), perhaps even more (Richard & Reiter, 1990). Most of these, however, suggest no specific relation to the probable region of seizure onset but belong to the realm of non-specific exercises of relaxation, concentration or both.

Table 1. Arrest of fits (according to Gowers)

Ligature proximal to convulsion
Forcible prevention of spasm
Other cutaneous stimulations (pinch, prick, rub)
Muscular exertion (e.g. quickly walking around the room)
Strong olfactory impression (ammonia, nitrite of amyl)
Strong gustatory sensation (chewing a piece of ginger; swallowing a handful of common salt)

With patients who have no experiences of their own and where the seizure semiology suggests no specific route, it has been useful to teach them self-regulation of the cortical slow direct current (DC) potential by means of biofeedback (Rockstroh *et al.*, 1993). At the onset of an epileptic seizure there is a negative DC shift, as was demonstrated by Caspers and Speckmann (1969) in experimental epilepsies. Figure 1 demonstrates that, in patients, this DC shift may occur not at aura onset but when the first overt seizure signs begin. This can explain why the method may still be efficient after the onset of the aura. The patients are trained to deliberately produce a positive DC shift as a response to an aura. The reported experiences of successful patients suggest that, perhaps, this method works in a way similar to relaxation procedures.

Case 1

A 33-year-old woman with a family history of epilepsy had had complex focal seizures with a typical epigastric aura since age 10, soon followed by sleep grand mal. The seizures were resistant to valproic acid (VPA), carbamazipine (CBZ) and diphenylhydantoin (DPH). With phenobarbital (PB) there was some reduction in seizure frequency with a relative increase of isolated auras.

The patient has learned very well how to influence her DC potential, and applies it highly successfully. Since more than 1 year ago, she has had one complete focal seizure, which took her by surprise at awakening, and the frequency of isolated auras is steadily decreasing.

To obtain a positive DC shift, she visualizes a vividly imagined scene from her childhood, with the prominent figure of an old woman, a person like one from a fairy-tale who used to be very kind to her when she brought her the mail and newspaper. This image induces an unparalleled feeling of warmth and well-being, she says.

Effectiveness of the procedure

To be effective, the countermeasures must often be applied in a specific way and at a specific time. The first clear account of this was given by Gowers (1881). He described in detail how a ligature could be easily practised, and pointed out that, if the commencing fit had got beyond the part to which the ligature was applied the attack was not arrested. Then too, it was important to apply the ligature regularly because it had been observed that, when it was omitted even only once, resulting in a general convulsion, the method lost its effect for ever.

In the patient of Efron (1956) it took some time to find the most effective olfactory stimulus, and its application had to be timed precisely. This is probably important for many patients. One of the questions concerning seizure interruption is why patients who have experienced the effectiveness of a countermeasure are not successful enough to arrest all seizures. One answer to this is that an unknown number of patients probably are as successful and are included in the large number of epileptics not in treatment (Zielinski, 1974). One of them was seen by the present author when he had

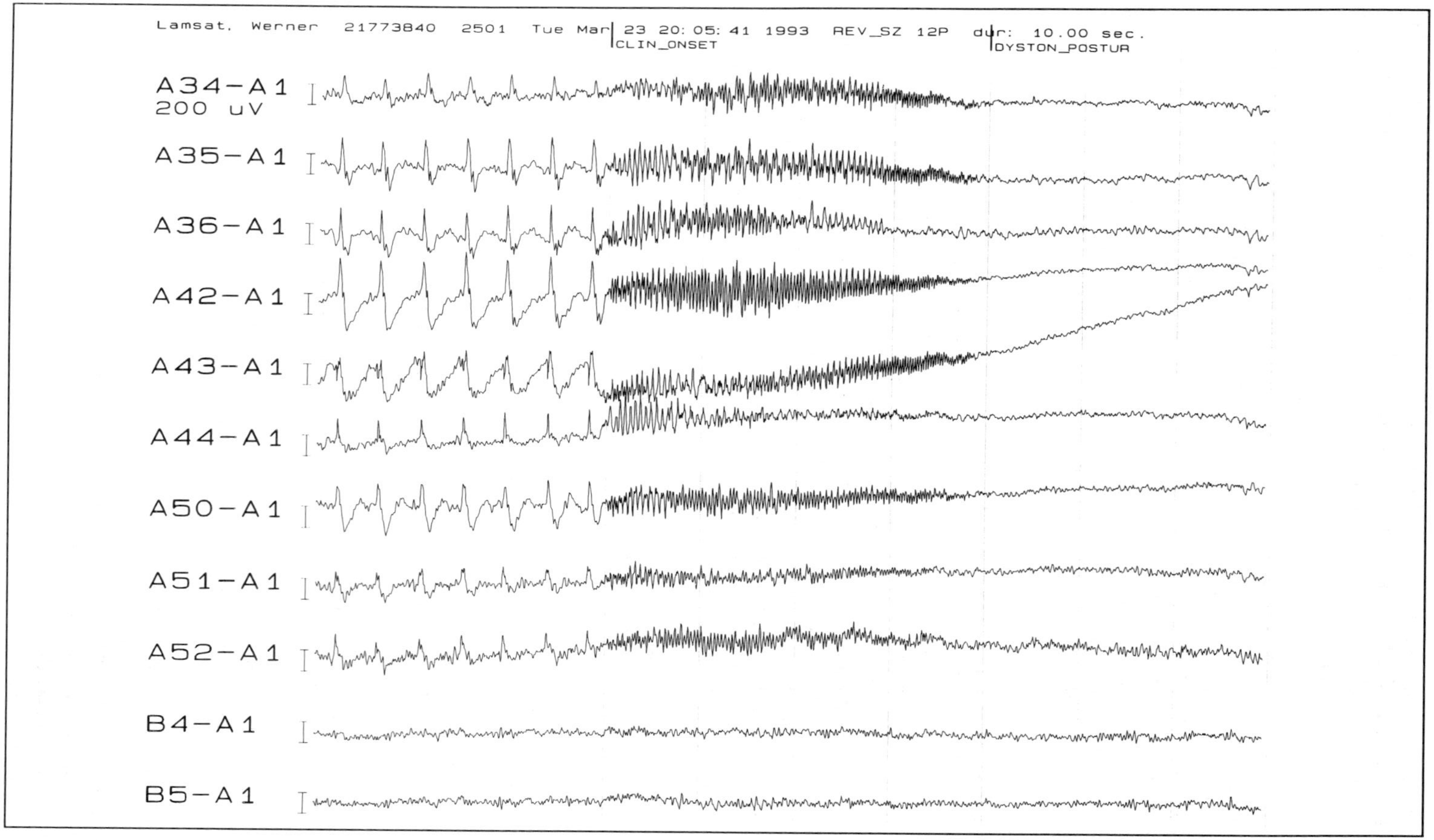

Fig. 1. Cortical DC registration from a subdural plate in a patient with focal tonic seizures of the left hand and arm, preceded by a somatosensory aura in the left hand. To the left, a typical aura has just set in, and the electrocorticogram shows rhythmic spike- and-wave discharge. The negative DC shift, however, does not occur before the onset of the motor seizure signs, accompanied by a tonic epileptiform pattern.The patient eventually became seizure-free after removal of a small area in the postcentral convolution exactly at electrode position A43, which produced a sensory deficit in the left hand. Numbers refer to electrode contacts on two plates (A and B). Unipolar montage with left ear reference. (Courtesy of Dr Hans Lüders.)

his first generalized tonic–clonic seizure (GTCS) after many years because just once he had failed to apply his own successful method of counteracting an aura, which consisted of a combination of physical relaxation and mental concentration. He had long since given up medication and seeing a doctor about his condition (Wolf, 1992).

The patients whom we see, and who are only sometimes successful, either find that they have seizures of variable 'strength', of which they only can arrest the weaker ones, or seem never to have applied countermeasures other than randomly. Improvement of antiepileptic drug regimen may attenuate the seizures and render them more accessible to countermeasures. Counselling and training programmes to teach these patients a systematic use of seizure arrest may be sufficient for a better therapeutic effect. In other cases, however, neurotic attitudes about the seizures may be an obstacle to the compliance with the procedure. Compliance is no less necessary in this line of treatment than in pharmacotherapy. A good example of the necessity to sometimes have seizure arrest embedded in a more comprehensive psychotherapy was given by Bühring and Welteke (1990).

Case 2

This 27-year-old patient had drug-resistant simple focal, complex focal and secondarily generalized seizures. High-level DPH reduced the seizure frequency but did not completely control even the secondary GTCS. During the focal seizures, he often showed aggressive behaviour. Attempts at interrupting the seizures at aura onset by hitting his left palm with his right fist were partially successful but resulted in an interictal state of high irritability and aggression. During a phase of psychotherapy he learned to accept and constructively deal with his aggressive impulses, and now found his own method of seizure interruption, which consisted in focusing on the epigastric sensation and trying to calm it down by touching his abdomen with his flat palms, breathing quietly and remembering a calming autosuggestive formula. With some training, this method became completely successful. The pivotal factor, however, was clearly the change in attitude towards the seizures and towards the possibility of their self-control.

Cure of epilepsy by seizure arrest

The ultimate therapeutic aim in epileptology is complete and persistent seizure control without further therapy. There is no therapeutic route which guarantees such an outcome. Thus, whereas many patients are indeed cured by the surgical removal of an epileptic focus, many others only remain free of seizures on the condition of further drug treatment. On the other hand, if complete seizure control has been reached by pharmacotherapy, it is often possible to diminish the dose of drugs, and finally discontinue them without a relapse. It is not known how cure is effected in these cases, as there is general agreement that the present antiepileptic drugs have no direct curative effect but just prevent seizures from happening. Treatment by seizure arrest, even if it is perfectly effective, is no real parallel to this because, here, minimal seizures are still allowed to occur: the auras or local seizures to which these patients respond. There is therefore some scepticism concerning a curative effect of such therapy, even of an indirect effect as with pharmacotherapy.

Thus, Jackson considered that successful ligatures perhaps only 'put off a fit' (1931, I, 16), although in one of his patients the development to a GTCS or focal seizures starting in the foot was consistently interrupted by the application of a complex arresting procedure (1931, I, 6f).

Gowers (1881) had more optimistic experiences. 'The repeated arrest of fits by the ligature may produce a permanent effect. I have a patient whose fits always commence in the hand by a sensation which passes up the arm, and could be arrested by the ligature applied just above the elbow. After employing the ligature in this manner for some months, he found that the fits, commencing in the same way, stopped of their own accord at the spot at which they had been repeatedly arrested by the ligature. They never stopped thus before the patient commenced the use of the ligature, which appeared to have produced a permanent increase of resistance at a certain part of the unstable nerve tissue.' He speculated that 'the permanent arrest of fits must be ascribed to a corresponding change in the 'functional nutrition' of the centre, but it is difficult to know what exactly he meant by this. He quotes attempts at obtaining a permanent effect by an extended peripheral irritation through the application of blisters but does not sound very much in favour of such a procedure. His own alternative trials, especially by daily faradization of the limb and by circular sinapisms (mustard plasters), were without success.

Efron (1957) in the second report on his patient gave the first detailed and highly interesting account of her eventual cure. The process was gradual. At first, an olfactory stimulus was found which was able to interrupt the patient's aura. Then, a routine was established to always apply the stimulus at the right moment. Next, as it was bothering to always sniff a perfume bottle, the stimulus was transferred by operant conditioning to a bracelet at which the patient glanced, and which would evoke the interruptive smell. The next step was that the smell was, if necessary, evoked by merely thinking of the bracelet. During this development, the auras had become constantly slighter but more frequent. At the same time, it became less and less necessary for the patient to deliberately evoke the arresting stimulus, and, in the next phase, the first indication of an aura would immediately and involuntarily be followed by the imagined smell. After that, the auras disappeared but the patient would still occasionally experience the smell, until that too stopped. It seems that the interruptive stimulus had become a conditioned response which was evoked by slighter and slighter and at last subexperiential stimuli. The more and more efficient and rapid inhibition must have had a negative feedback action on the discharging focus, the exact neurophysiological nature of which remains to be defined.

Such a development must obviously depend on a set of favourable circumstances, some of which can be defined while others remain obscure. It cannot be expected that such a development easily becomes routine. But it should be studied further in order to find out if and how it can be facilitated.

Case 3

We observed a similar but more rapid development in a boy aged 15 who had for 1½ years suffered from GTCS beginning with paraesthesias of the left half of the body, with onset in the hand, followed by a tonic convulsion of the left arm. During this aura, he tried in vain to suppress it by abrupt, massive movements. All physical and ancillary findings were normal. The seizures were resistant to phenytoin and VPA. At the highest tolerated concentration of CBZ (11.0 μg/ml) the GTCS stopped, but he went on having isolated auras with paraesthesias of the left arm and a tonic contraction of the hand, about three to four times per month. If these lasted longer than 10–12 s, he became afraid of having a convulsive seizure but found that he was now able to arrest the fit by clenching the fist or grasping a cool object with his left hand.

He was counselled to systematize this procedure and clench his fist always and immediately when he experienced an aura. In addition, he was told to exercise the procedure several times every day by imagining the aura and clenching his fist. For about half a year, he did not follow the advice and went on having simple focal seizures as above. He complied, however, with the repetition of the instruction, which resulted in a dramatic fall of seizure frequency over a period of 6 months, after which the seizures completely disappeared. He reported that he did not apply the method of arrest consciously any longer but found that he frequently caught himself having clenched his left fist without paying attention to it. He has now been seizure-free for 3 years, with a reduced dose of CBZ (serum level now 5.4 μg/ml), which will be stepwise further withdrawn. He was as unaware as the patient of Efron (1957) of what had happened in the ultimate phase of seizure abolishment.

These exemplary observations seem to suggest that epilepsy may be cured as a consequence of behavioural treatment with seizure arrest in response to aura. Such a development seems to depend on a sequence of successful therapeutic steps (Table 2). First, a countermeasure must be found which effectively arrests the seizures of the individual patient. Second, the patient must learn to apply the countermeasure systematically, with proper timing. Third, along with the patient's exercising the procedure, a stage needs to be reached where all seizures are arrested. Whereas all these steps require the patient's active co-operation, in a next stage the response becomes established firmly enough to be involuntarily evoked by the aura, in a reflex-like manner. Then, in an ultimate stage, the constant, increasingly rapid and increasingly effective inhibition of all seizure spread seems to be fed back to and to influence the seizure-generating mechanism itself.

Table 2. Aura interruption: how does it become curative?

1. Detection of an effective countermeasure
2. Systematic well-timed application of countermeasure
3. Successful arrest of all seizures
4. Conditioned reflex interruption
5. 'Unlearning' of seizures by negative feedback

Of such a negative feedback which would help the brain to 'unlearn' the production of seizures, only vague indications may be seen with antiepileptic pharmacotherapy (Wolf *et al.*, 1987). It could be the counterpart of the positive feedback which has been postulated in the early development of epilepsy, where, according to Gowers, seizures beget seizures (Reynolds, 1988). To understand the negative feedback and its role in the cure of epilepsy would be of the highest importance.

References

Bühring, M. & Welteke, H. (1990): Entwicklung eines systematischen Anfallsunterbrechungstrainings, dargestellt anhand einer exemplarischen Fallstudie. In: *Epilepsie 89*, ed. P .Wolf, pp. 216–220, Reinbek: Einhorn-Presse.

Caspers, H. & Speckmann, E.-J. (1969): DC potential shifts in paroxysmal states. In: *Basic mechanisms of the epilepsies*, eds. H.H. Jasper, A.A. Ward & A. Pope, pp. 375–388. London: Churchill.

Efron, R. (1956): The effect of olfactory stimulus in arresting uncinate fits. *Brain* **79,** 267–281.

Efron, R. (1957): The conditioned inhibition of uncinate fits. *Brain* **80,** 251–262.

Gowers, W.R. (1881): *Epilepsy and other chronic convulsive diseases.* London: Wood.

Horsley, V. (1886): Brain surgery. *Br. Med. J.* **2,** 670–674.

Jackson, J.H. (1931): *Selected writings.* London: Hodder & Stoughton.

Paulson, G.W. (1963): Inhibition of seizures. *Dis. Nerv. Syst.* **24,** 657–664.

Reker, M. (1988): Befragung von Anfallspatienten über ihre Erfahrungen mit der Unterdrückung Aura-eingeleiteter Anfälle. In: *Medizinisches und Theologisches zur Epilepsie. Bethel-Beiträge*, Vol. 38 pp.106–112. Bielefeld: Bethel-Verlag.

Reynolds, E.H. (1988): A single seizure: likely to return. *Br. Med. J.* **297,** 1422–1423.

Richard, A. & Reiter, J. (1990): *Epilepsy: a new approach.* New York: Prentice Hall Press.

Rockstroh, B., Elbert, Th., Birbaumer, N., Wolf, P., Düchting-Röth, A., Reker, M., Daum, J., Lutzenberger, W. & Dichgans, J. (1993): Cortical self-regulation in patients with epilepsies. *Epilepsy Res.* **14,** 63–72.

Speckmann, E.-J. (1986): *Experimentelle Epilepsieforschung.* Darmstadt: Wissenschaftliche Buchgesellschaft.

Temkin, O. (1945): *The falling sickness.* Baltimore: Johns Hopkins Press.

Tissot, S.A. (1770): *Traité de l'épilepsie.* Lausanne: Chapuis.

Wolf, P. (1992): Behavioral therapy of epileptic seizures. *Bol. Epileps.* **1,** 72–75.

Wolf, P., Röder-Wanner, U.U. & Noachtar, S. (1987): Response of polygraphic sleep to phenytoin treatment for epilepsy: a longitudinal study of immediate, short- and long-term effects. *Acta Neurol. Scand.* **76,** 157–167.

Zielinski, J.J. (1974): Epileptics not in treatment. *Epilepsia* **15,** 203–211.

Index

E

F

G

H

I